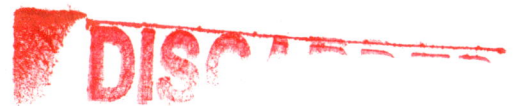

Handbook of
Health and
Rehabilitation
Psychology

Plenum Series in Rehabilitation and Health

SERIES EDITORS

Michael Feuerstein
*Uniformed Services University of the Health Sciences (USUHS)
Bethesda, Maryland*

and

Anthony J. Goreczny
*Highland Drive Veterans Affairs Medical Center
and University of Pittsburgh School of Medicine
Pittsburgh, Pennsylvania*

HANDBOOK OF HEALTH AND REHABILITATION PSYCHOLOGY
Edited by Anthony J. Goreczny

A Continuation Order Plan is available for this series. A continuation order will bring delivery of each new volume immediately upon publication. Volumes are billed only upon actual shipment. For further information please contact the publisher.

Handbook of Health and Rehabilitation Psychology

Edited by

Anthony J. Goreczny
*Highland Drive Veterans Affairs Medical Center
and University of Pittsburgh School of Medicine
Pittsburgh, Pennsylvania*

Plenum Press • New York and London

Library of Congress Cataloging-in-Publication Data

Handbook of health and rehabilitation psychology / edited by Anthony
J. Goreczny.
      p.   cm. -- (Plenum series in rehabilitation and health)
    Includes bibliographical references and index.
    ISBN 0-306-44970-6
    1. Clinical health psychology. 2. Medical rehabilitation-
  -Psychological aspects.   I. Goreczny, Anthony J. II. Series.
    R726.7.H36 1995
    616'.001'9--dc20   95-40862
                                                                CIP

ISBN 0-306-44970-6

© 1995 Plenum Press, New York
A Division of Plenum Publishing Corporation
233 Spring Street, New York, N. Y. 10013

All rights reserved

10 9 8 7 6 5 4 3 2 1

No part of this book may be reproduced, stored in a retrieval system, or transmitted in any form or by any means, electronic, mechanical, photocopying, microfilming, recording, or otherwise, without written permission from the Publisher

Printed in the United States of America

To my parents

Contributors

Daniel N. Allen, Department of Psychology, Highland Drive Veterans Affairs Medical Center, Pittsburgh, Pennsylvania 15206

Edna Alleyne, Community Health Program, Jackson State University, Jackson, Mississippi 39217

Bruce G. Bender, National Jewish Center for Immunology and Respiratory Medicine, Denver, Colorado 80206

Blaine L. Block, St. Elizabeth Regional Cancer Center, Dayton, Ohio 45408

Phillip J. Brantley, Department of Family Medicine, Louisiana State University Medical Center, Baton Rouge, Louisiana 70805

Ted L. Brasfield, Community Health Program, Jackson State University, Jackson, Mississippi 39217

Thomas G. Burish, Department of Psychology, Vanderbilt University, Nashville, Tennessee 37240

Eleanor B. Callon, Department of Family Medicine, Louisiana State University Medical Center, Baton Rouge, Louisiana 70805

Mark J. Chambers, The Sleep Clinic of Nevada, 1012 East Sahara, Las Vegas, Nevada 89104

Matthew M. Clark, Department of Psychiatry and Human Behavior, The Miriam Hospital, and Brown University School of Medicine, Providence, Rhode Island 02906

Cheza W. Collier, Addictive Behaviors Research Center, Department of Psychology, University of Washington, Seattle, Washington 98195

Thomas L. Creer, Department of Psychology, Ohio University, Athens, Ohio 45701

Margaret DeBon, The Universities Prevention Center, Department of Psychology, University of Memphis, Memphis, Tennessee 38152

Patricia M. Dubbert, Department of Psychology, Veterans Affairs Medical Center, and University of Mississippi School of Medicine, Jackson, Mississippi 39216

Terence E. Fitzgerald, Occupational Health Institute, Blue Ridge Rehabilitation Medicine, Asheville, North Carolina 28801

Robert R. Freedman, Department of Psychiatry and Behavioral Medicine, Wayne State University School of Medicine, and C. S. Mott Center, 275 East Hancock, Detroit, Michigan 48201

Douglas J. French, Department of Psychology, Ohio University, Athens, Ohio 45701

V. Diane Garrett, Behavioral Science Consultants, 5420 Corporate Boulevard, Suite 205, Baton Rouge, Louisiana 70808

James C. Gilchrist, St. Elizabeth Rehabilitation Center, St. Elizabeth Medical Center, Dayton, Ohio 45408

Virginia L. Goetsch, Department of Behavioral Medicine and Psychiatry, West Virginia University Health Sciences Center, Morgantown, West Virginia 26505

Michael G. Goldstein, Department of Psychiatry and Human Behavior, The Miriam Hospital, and Brown University School of Medicine, Providence, Rhode Island 02906

Anthony J. Goreczny, Highland Drive Veterans Affairs Medical Center and University of Pittsburgh School of Medicine, Pittsburgh, Pennsylvania 15206

Allen W. Heinemann, Department of Physical Medicine and Rehabilitation, Northwestern University Medical School, and Rehabilitation Institute of Chicago, Chicago, Illinois 60657

Polly B. Hitchcock, Department of Psychology, Louisiana State University, Baton Rouge, Louisiana 70803

Kenneth A. Holroyd, Department of Psychology, Ohio University, Athens, Ohio 45701

Warren T. Jackson, Department of Psychology, Louisiana State University, Baton Rouge, Louisiana 70803

Mary Casey Jacob, Departments of Psychiatry (Psychology), and Obstetrics and Gynecology, University of Connecticut Health Center, Farmington, Connecticut 06030

Kennis Jefferson, Community Health Program, Jackson State University, Jackson, Mississippi 39217

Robert D. Kerns, Psychology Service, West Haven Veterans Administration Medical Center, and Departments of Psychiatry, Neurology, and Psychology, Yale University, West Haven, Connecticut 06516

Robert C. Klesges, The Universities Prevention Center, Department of Psychology, University of Memphis, Memphis, Tennessee 38152

Linda R. Kostyak, Western Psychiatric Institute and Clinic, University of Pittsburgh Medical Center, Pittsburgh, Pennsylvania 15213

Wade Lancaster, Health Sciences Center, University of Virginia, Charlottesville, Virginia 22903

Kevin T. Larkin, Department of Psychology, West Virginia University, Morgantown, West Virginia 26506-6040

G. Alan Marlatt, Addictive Behaviors Research Center, Department of Psychology, University of Washington, Seattle, Washington 98195

Paul D. Nussbaum, Aging Research and Education Center, Lutheran Affiliated Services, 500 Wittenberg Way, Mars, Pennsylvania 16046

Colleen M. O'Halloran, Highland Drive Veterans Affairs Medical Center, Pittsburgh, Pennsylvania 15206

Donald B. Penzien, Department of Psychiatry, University of Mississippi Medical Center, Jackson, Mississippi 39216

Thomas G. Pickering, Cardiovascular Center, The New York Hospital–Cornell University Medical College, New York, New York 10021

Jeanetta C. Rains, Department of Psychiatry, University of Mississippi Medical Center, Jackson, Mississippi 39216

Shannon B. Sebastian, Department of Psychology, Louisiana State University, Baton Rouge, Louisiana 70803

Elizabeth M. Semenchuk, Department of Psychology, West Virginia University, Morgantown, West Virginia 26506-6040

Timothy W. Smith, Department of Psychology, University of Utah, Salt Lake City, Utah 84112

Nomita Sonty, Department of Psychology, National Rehabilitation Hospital, Washington, DC 20010

Barbara A. Stetson, Department of Psychology, Illinois Institute of Technology, Chicago, Illinois 60616

Janet S. St. Lawrence, Community Health Program, Jackson State University, Jackson, Mississippi 39217

Bradley T. Thomason, Department of Family and Preventive Medicine, Emory University School of Medicine, Atlanta, Georgia 30308

Denise M. Tope, Behavioral Medicine Institute, 5401 Kingston Pike, Suite 540, Knoxville, Tennessee 37919

Dennis C. Turk, Pain Evaluation and Treatment Institute, University of Pittsburgh School of Medicine, Pittsburgh, Pennsylvania 15213

Paula J. Varnado, Department of Psychology, Louisiana State University, Baton Rouge, Louisiana 70803

Steve Webne, Mental Health Association, 2401 21st Avenue South, Nashville, Tennessee 37212

Gerhard Werner, Highland Drive Veterans Affairs Medical Center and University of Pittsburgh School of Medicine, Pittsburgh, Pennsylvania 15206

Deborah J. Wiebe, Department of Psychology, University of Utah, Salt Lake City, Utah 84112

Donald A. Williamson, Department of Psychology, Louisiana State University, Baton Rouge, Louisiana 70803

Preface

Despite medical technological advances, the major killers with which we must currently contend have remained essentially the same for the past few decades. Stroke, cancer, and heart disease together account for the vast majority of deaths in the United States. In addition, due to improved medical care, many Americans who would previously have died now survive these disorders, necessitating that they receive appropriate rehabilitation efforts. One result of our own medical advances is that we must now accept the high costs associated with providing quality care to individuals who develop one of these problems, and we must avail ourselves to assist families of afflicted individuals.

Despite the relative stability of causes of death and disability, the health-care field is currently experiencing tremendous pressures, both from professionals within the field, who desire more and better technology than is currently available, and from the public and other payers of health care (e.g., insurance companies), who seek an end to increasing health-care costs. These pressures, along with an increased emphasis on providing evidence of cost-effectiveness and quality assurance, are substantially changing the way that health-care professionals perform their jobs.

There are also other areas of change that currently confront health-care professionals and will continue to do so in the future. First, the American population is getting older. In future years, the percentage of Americans who are 65 and older, and especially those who are 75 and older, will sharply rise. Because older adults tend to utilize health-care services more than people in other age groups, the burden on the health-care system will substantially increase. Second, the HIV virus presents an unprecedented challenge to Americans and to populations around the world. Not only is it a deadly virus for which we have no cure, but our behavior (e.g., IV drug use, unsafe sex practices) must change in order to slow the spread of the virus until we have found a cure. In addition, the cost of treating individuals afflicted with AIDS is enormous and will continue to increase, further taxing our medical-care system.

All of the changes described previously will require that health-care professionals learn new ways to continue to provide quality health care. First, with increased competition, health-care professionals must learn how to better market their services. Second, we must learn to utilize better technological advances to make our practices more efficient than they currently are and to assist us in our research efforts, thereby improving both the theoretical and clinical meaningfulness of our research.

One of the purposes of this handbook is to address the concerns we have listed. The next to last section of the book, Emerging Topics, contains chapters relevant to HIV, aging, computers, and marketing. Although these chapters contain information relevant to the current health-care climate, the information contained in these chapters will also help stimulate our thinking about future needs related to the logistics of health care.

Another primary purpose of the book is to update practitioners and researchers in the fields of rehabilitation psychology and health psychology. There have been some substantial changes and new information that will impact both our clinical treatments and our research initiatives. The first four sections of this handbook contain chapters about specific disorders or other important topics of relevance.

The intended audience for this volume is both researchers and clinicians. One expectation is that this handbook will offer clinicians suggestions for ways to improve their practices. Another intended effect is to stimulate research ideas and initiatives. Because the chapters in this handbook address both practical issues and theoretical ones, we can fulfill both purposes. In addition, students new to the fields of health psychology and rehabilitation psychology will find that the chapters provide excellent overviews of the topics.

A book of this magnitude does not come to fruition without the assistance of many individuals. It is to them that I extend my sincere gratitude and appreciation. First, I graciously thank Michel Hersen, who provided me with the inspiration to undertake this venture and whose guidance and assistance were invaluable. Next, the authors of the chapters provided excellent works, and their expertise is evident in their writing. The technical assistance provided by Eliot Werner and his staff at Plenum was second to none. I applaud the excellent support and professional manner in which Eliot and his staff handled all aspects of this handbook's preparation. Finally, I offer thanks to my wife, Kathleen, for her understanding during the many hours of preparation required for this text, and I appreciate the countless number of fun-filled diversions my two young children, Anthony and Danielle, provided us.

Contents

I. PSYCHOPHYSIOLOGICAL DISORDERS

1. Recent Developments in the Psychological Assessment and Management of Recurrent Headache Disorders 3

   Kenneth A. Holroyd and Douglas J. French

2. Recent Trends in Asthma Research 31

   Thomas L. Creer and Bruce G. Bender

3. Temporomandibular Disorders 55

   Dennis C. Turk, Donald B. Penzien, and Jeanetta C. Rains

4. Gastrointestinal Disorders 79

   V. Diane Garrett

5. Insomnia 99

   Mark J. Chambers

6. Raynaud's Disease and Phenomenon 117

   Robert R. Freedman

II. HEALTH PROMOTION

7. Smoking and Smoking Cessation: Current Conceptualizations and Directions for Future Research 135

   Margaret DeBon and Robert C. Klesges

8. Obesity: A Health Psychology Perspective 157

   Matthew M. Clark and Michael G. Goldstein

9. Anorexia and Bulimia Nervosa 175

   Donald A. Williamson, Shannon B. Sebastian, and Paula J. Varnado

10. Assessment and Modification of Coronary-Prone Behavior: A Transactional View of the Person in Social Context 197

    Timothy W. Smith

11. Hypertension 219

    Thomas G. Pickering

12. Cardiovascular Disorders 239

    Kevin T. Larkin and Elizabeth M. Semenchuk

13. Exercise and Physical Activity 255

    Patricia M. Dubbert and Barbara A. Stetson

14. Stress and Stress Management 275

    Phillip J. Brantley and Bradley T. Thomason

15. Preparation for Surgery 291

    Steve Webne

16. **Relapse Prevention** 307

   Cheza W. Collier and G. Alan Marlatt

III. REHABILITATION

17. **Toward an Integrative Diathesis–Stress Model of Chronic Pain** 325

    Robert D. Kerns and Mary Casey Jacob

18. **Spinal Cord Injury** 341

    Allen W. Heinemann

19. **Assessment and Conservative Treatment of Occupational Musculoskeletal Disability** 361

    Terence E. Fitzgerald and Nomita Sonty

20. **Assessment and Treatment of Multiple Sclerosis** 389

    Daniel N. Allen and Anthony J. Goreczny

21. **Traumatic Brain Injury** 431

    Eleanor B. Callon and Warren T. Jackson

22. **Cancer Rehabilitation: Concepts and Interventions** 457

    James C. Gilchrist and Blaine L. Block

IV. PSYCHOLOGICAL ASPECTS OF VARIOUS DISEASE STATES

23. **Recent Advances in Psychosocial and Behavioral Oncology** 481

    Denise M. Tope and Thomas G. Burish

24. **Psychological Aspects of Chronic-Maintenance Hemodialysis Patients** 497

   Phillip J. Brantley and Polly B. Hitchcock

25. **Diabetes Mellitus: Considerations of the Influence of Stress** 513

   Virginia L. Goetsch and Deborah J. Wiebe

26. **Systemic Lupus Erythematosus** 535

   Linda R. Kostyak

V. EMERGING TOPICS

27. **Theoretical Models Applied to AIDS Prevention** 555

   Janet S. St. Lawrence, Ted L. Brasfield, Kennis Jefferson, and Edna Alleyne

28. **Aging: Issues in Health and Neuropsychological Functioning** 583

   Paul D. Nussbaum

29. **Computer Applications in Behavioral Medicine** 605

   Gerhard Werner

30. **The Marketing of Professional Health-Care Services** 637

   Wade Lancaster

VI. EPILOGUE

31. **The Future of Psychology in Health Care** 663

   Anthony J. Goreczny and Colleen M. O'Halloran

Index 677

I
PSYCHOPHYSIOLOGICAL DISORDERS

1

Recent Developments in the Psychological Assessment and Management of Recurrent Headache Disorders

Kenneth A. Holroyd and Douglas J. French

Most people occasionally experience but are seldom disabled by headaches. However, epidemiological studies reveal that more than 8 million females and 2 million males are disabled with some frequency by migraine headaches alone (Stewart, Lipton, Celentano, & Reed, 1992). The number of new cases of disabling headaches each year has been estimated at more than 2 million, almost 1% of the population (Goldstein & Chen, 1982). It is thus not surprising that headache is one of the most frequent complaints presented in outpatient medical settings (DeLozier & Gagnon, 1975; Leviton, 1978). Because the vast majority of patients (probably over 95%) who seek medical assistance have headaches that do not result from any identifiable structural abnormality or disease state, a large industry has arisen to develop, produce, and market headache remedies.

Interest in the use of behavioral interventions in the management of recurrent headache disorders was stimulated two decades ago, when promising results were reported with biofeedback training (e.g., Birk, 1974; Budzynski, Stoyva, Adler, & Mullaney, 1973). In the subsequent two decades, both the benefits and limitations of behavioral interventions in the management of recurrent headache disorders have become better understood. Accepted notions about the role that psychological and

---

Kenneth A. Holroyd and Douglas J. French • Department of Psychology, Ohio University, Athens, Ohio 45701.
Handbook of Health and Rehabilitation Psychology, edited by Anthony J. Goreczny. Plenum Press, New York, 1995.

biological factors play in the development and amelioration of recurrent headache problems have also changed. In this chapter, topics likely to be of interest to clinicians and researchers alike are reviewed with the goal of highlighting developments that have occurred in the last decade.

DIAGNOSIS/CLASSIFICATION

The limitations of the classification system that has guided clinical diagnosis for the last 30 years became increasingly evident in the 1980s. Formulated in 1962 at the National Institutes of Health, this Ad Hoc Committee system provides prototypic descriptions of recurrent headache syndromes (Ad Hoc Committee on the Classification of Headache, 1962). This system was based on the muscle contraction model of tension headache and vascular model of migraine that were dominant at that time. A major practical limitation of the Ad Hoc Committee system has been that criteria for differential diagnosis were not made explicit, but rather left to clinical judgment.

Currently, the Headache Classification Committee of the International Headache Society (IHS, 1988) is completing an update of this classification system. Published in a provisional form (with final revisions anticipated in 1997), this classification system is hierarchical in nature, with 12 major diagnostic categories and 145 subcategories (see Table 1.1 for outline). It specifies criteria for each diagnostic category. Diagnostic categories, such as mixed tension and migraine headache, that were judged too ambiguous to be operationally defined were deleted. The updated system also adds diagnostic categories that have come into use since the earlier system was published (e.g., headache associated with substances or their withdrawal). Because the IHS system holds out the promise of improved diagnostic reliability, it is likely to be widely adopted by researchers, and, in fact, the provisional system has already been adopted in studies evaluating new treatments.

In spite of the improved clarity of the IHS system, its validity remains unknown. Usable operational criteria for each diagnostic category were developed only by severely restricting the number of criteria used in differential diagnosis. For example, diagnostic criteria for migraine without aura (formerly common migraine) and tension-type headaches (formerly muscle contraction or tension headache) are presented in Table 1.2. The experienced diagnostician has traditionally considered not only these diagnostic criteria, but also other diagnostic criteria (e.g., association with menstrual cycle, alcohol and other dietary triggers, family history, previous response to drug therapies) when making this differential diagnosis. Evidence that this restricted set of criteria is sufficiently specific to migraine and tension-type headache to function as criteria for differential diagnosis is currently not available. In fact, it is not universally agreed that these two syndromes are best conceptualized categorically rather than dimensionally (Bakal, 1982; Olesen, 1991; Raskin, 1988).

A definitive classification system for recurrent headache disorders probably awaits advances in our understanding of the pathophysiology of these disorders. Publication of the IHS system, however, has stimulated renewed interest in problems of diagnosis (e.g., Rasmussen, Jensen, & Olsen, 1992). The publication of operationally defined diagnostic criteria has also stimulated the development of computer software to assist in diagnosis (Penzien et al., 1991). In this decade, we will probably see the further development of computer diagnostic aids, including easy-to-use desktop expert systems capable of modeling the complex diagnostic and treatment decisions of experienced clinicians. In spite of the limitations of the IHS classification system, it is stimulating research that will likely improve current diagnostic procedures and ultimately advance our understanding of headache disorders.

Table 1.1. Headache Classifications of the International Headache Society's Headache Classification Committee

Migraine and tension-type headache:

1. Migraine
    1.1. Migraine without aura
    1.2. Migraine with aura
        1.2.1. Migraine with typical aura
        1.2.2. Migraine with prolonged aura
        1.2.3. Familial hemiplegic migraine
        1.2.4. Basilar migraine
        1.2.5. Migraine aura without headache
        1.2.6. Migraine with acute onset aura
    1.3. Opthalmoplegic migraine
    1.4. Retinal migraine
    1.5. Childhood periodic syndromes that may be precursor to or associated with migraine
        1.5.1. Benign paroxysmal vertigo of childhood
        1.5.2. Alternating hemiplegia of childhood
    1.6. Complications of migraine
        1.6.1. Status migrainosus
        1.6.2. Migrainous infarction
    1.7. Migrainous disorder not fulfilling above criteria
2. Tension-type headache
    2.1. Episodic tension-type headache
        2.1.1. Episodic tension-type headache associated with disorder of pericranial muscles
        2.1.2. Episodic tension-type headache unassociated with disorder of pericranial muscles
    2.2. Chronic tension-type headache
        2.2.1. Chronic tension-type headache associated with disorder of pericranial muscles
        2.2.2. Chronic tension-type headache unassociated with disorder of pericranial muscles
    2.3. Headache of the tension-type not fulfilling above criteria

Additional classifications:

3. Cluster headache and chronic paroxysmal hemicrania
4. Miscellaneous headaches unassociated with structural lesion
5. Headache associated with head trauma
6. Headache associated with vascular disorders
7. Headache associated with nonvascular intracranial disorders
8. Headache associated with substances or their withdrawal
9. Headache associated with noncephalic infection
10. Headache associated with metabolic disorder
11. Headache or facial pain associated with disorder of the cranium, neck, eyes, ears, sinuses, teeth, mouth, or other facial or cranial structures
12. Cranial neuralgias, nerve trunk pain, and deafferentiation pain

Source: Headache Classification Committee of the International Headache Society (1988).

Table 1.2. Diagnostic Criteria for Tension-Type Headache and Migraine without Aura

I. Tension-type headache

   Diagnostic criteria:

   A. At least 10 previous headache episodes fulfilling criteria B–D listed below.
   B. Headache lasting from 30 minutes to 7 days.
   C. At least two of the following pain characteristics:
      1. Pressing/tightening (nonpulsating) quality
      2. Mild or moderate intensity (may inhibit, but does not prohibit activities)
      3. Bilateral location
      4. No aggravation by walking stairs or similar routine physical activity
   D. Both of the following:
      1. No nausea or vomiting (anorexia may occur)
      2. Photophobia and phonophobia are absent, or one but not the other is present

II. Migraine without aura

   Diagnostic criteria:

   A. At least five attacks fulfilling B–D listed below.
   B. Headache attacks lasting 4–72 hours (untreated or unsuccessfully treated)
   C. Headache has at least two of the following characteristics:
      1. Unilateral location
      2. Pulsating quality
      3. Moderate or severe intensity (inhibits or prohibits daily activities)
      4. Aggravation by walking stairs or similar routine physical activity
   D. During headache at least one of the following:
      1. Nausea and/or vomiting
      2. Photophobia and phonophobia

Source: Headache Classification Committee of the International Headache Society (1988).

PATHOPHYSIOLOGY

In the last decade, the role of central mechanisms in the pathophysiology of recurrent headache disorders has received increasing attention. Models of tension and migraine headaches formulated by H. G. Wolff in the 1940s emphasized peripheral muscular or vascular responses and remained unchallenged for 40 years. However, in the 1980s, the muscle contraction model of tension headache was challenged by the failure to detect postulated abnormalities of muscle activity (see reviews by Andrasik, Blanchard, Arena, Saunders, & Barron, 1982; Haynes, Cuevas, & Gannon, 1982), and the vascular model of migraine was challenged by the failure to find postulated changes in cerebral blood flow (Olesen, Larsen, & Lauritzen, 1981). At the same time, attention was being drawn to the possible role of central mechanisms in recurrent headache disorders, including disturbed central modulation of afferent nociceptive inputs and spreading depression—a gradual, spreading depolarization of cerebral neurons (Olesen, 1991). It thus began to appear plausible that a defect in brain stem pain-modulating systems or abnormalities of cerebral neuronal function, rather than abnormalities of peripheral muscular or vascular activity, might play a prominent etiological role in recurrent headache disorders (Olesen & Edvinsson, 1988; Raskin, 1988).

Recently, several efforts have been made to integrate these hypotheses in a multifactorial model that gives equal weight to peripheral and central influences (Moskowitz, 1990; Olesen, 1991). For example, Olesen (1991) argued that recurrent tension headaches can result from defective central pain modulation, peripheral muscle abnormalities, or a combination of central and peripheral factors. Similarly, migraines are postulated to result either from significant changes in vascular activity or from smaller vascular changes that only produce pain when afferent inputs from vascular sources are magnified at a central level.

Technical advances in the next decade are likely to permit a more definitive evaluation of both central and peripheral factors in the pathophysiology of recurrent headache disorders. Recent studies have identified pericranial muscle abnormalities in recurrent tension headache sufferers, suggesting that the failure to detect abnormalities in previous studies may have resulted from the use of recording methods that are insensitive to the muscle abnormalities of interest (e.g., Langemark & Olesen, 1987; Schoenen, Jamart, Gerard, Lenarduzzi, & Delwaide, 1987). Advances in the measurement of cerebral blood flow have also allowed investigators to identify regional cerebral blood-flow changes associated with the focal neurological symptoms, or aura, that precede the onset of headache in some migraine sufferers (Olesen, 1991). Subsequent improvements in measurement techniques will likely allow investigators to resolve controversies about the role of vascular and neuronal phenomena in migraine headaches.

It will be necessary to develop methods of assessing central pain-modulation deficits or to manipulate these deficits with highly selective pharmacological agents if we are to examine the role central pain modulation plays in recurrent headache disorders. The most promising development for psychophysiologists in this regard is the successful measurement of deficits in centrally mediated pericranial muscle reflexes in tension headache sufferers (Schoenen et al., 1987). It appears likely that a variety of drugs that selectively influence specific 5HT1 (serotonin) receptor sites in the brain will also become available in the 1990s. Thus, we will likely see important advances in our understanding of the pathophysiology of recurrent headache disorders in the next decade.

PSYCHOLOGICAL ASSESSMENT

Two decades ago, psychological assessment focused almost exclusively on the identification of psychopathology in the recurrent headache sufferer. Although epidemiological research *has* confirmed an association between recurrent headache disorders and depression and anxiety disorders (e.g., Merikangas, Angst, & Isler, 1990), only a small proportion of recurrent headache sufferers seen in general practice settings exhibit signs of psychological disturbance (Andrasik et al., 1982). Moreover, for many of these patients, the psychological problems are probably a consequence of living with recurrent headaches rather than a factor precipitating headache problems, as was earlier assumed. In the last decade, the focus of psychological assessment has broadened beyond the identification of psychopathology (Penzien, Rains, & Holroyd, 1993).

Examples of this more recent work include efforts to assess (1) the impact of headaches on the individual's life (disability/quality of life), (2) beliefs that might influence adaptation to recurrent headache problems (headache locus of control/self-efficacy), and (3) stresses and coping activities that might influence recurrent headache problems (stress/coping). Recent work in each of these areas is reviewed later.

Disability/Quality of Life

If the benefits and side effects of different therapies are to be compared, methods of assessing the impact of recurrent headache problems on daily functioning and quality of life need to be developed. When data from migraine sufferers were compared to other data from the Medical Outcomes Study (Stewart et al., 1989), migraine headaches were found to have a greater impact on role functioning (i.e., activities as a worker or homemaker), social activities, and mental health than the five other chronic diseases that were examined (arthritis, diabetes, myocardial infarction, gastrointestinal disorders, and hypertension; Osterhaus & Townsend, 1991). Unfortunately, little information is available about the ability of widely used drug or nondrug therapies to ameliorate the social and psychological problems associated with migraines, because treatment studies have focused narrowly on the impact of treatments on pain.

One problem is that available instruments have not been designed to assess disability or changes in quality of life that only occur episodically (i.e., during headache episodes). Existing instruments thus may underestimate the impact of recurrent headaches on an individual's life. In an attempt to remedy this problem, the Recurrent Illness Impairment Profile (Wittrock, Penzien, Moseley, & Johnson, 1991) assesses functioning in social, behavioral, cognitive, and recreational arenas, both during headaches of different severity and when the individual is headache-free. The availability of such measures will likely encourage investigators to more broadly evaluate the impact of drug and nondrug therapies on quality of life.

Expectancies

Locus of control and perceived self-efficacy beliefs may play a role in determining how an individual adapts to recurrent headache problems, and changes in these beliefs induced by behavior therapies may mediate the improvements observed with treatment. At least this is the hypothesis that has guided the recent development of expectancy measures used with recurrent headache sufferers. These measures appear to be showing greater promise than more general measures that assess expectancies about an individual's overall health (Wallston, 1992). *Locus of control* refers to the belief that headache episodes and headache relief are either within the individual's control (e.g., triggered by diet or self-imposed work pressures) or are outside the individual's control, influenced by either chance or fate (e.g., hormonal fluctuations, inherited vulnerability) or by the actions of health professionals (rather than by the individual's actions). Initial findings suggest that even when severity of headache problems is statistically controlled, locus-of-control beliefs predict medication consumption, psychological consequences of headache episodes (e.g., depression), and preference for self-regulatory or drug therapies (Martin, Holroyd, & Penzien, 1990). Self-regulatory treatments, but not prophylactic drug therapies, appear to change locus-of-control beliefs toward a more internal direction (Holroyd, Nash, Pingel, Cordingley, & Jerome, 1991; Penzien et al., 1989), and changes in locus-of-control beliefs may play a role in mediating improvements in headache activity produced by biofeedback training (Holroyd et al., 1984).

There is some ambiguity about what is meant by self-efficacy, because perceived self-efficacy might refer to confidence in one's ability to prevent headaches, manage headaches, or tolerate headaches. Social learning theory postulates that relevant self-efficacy expectations would influence emotional responses to headache episodes as well as efforts to cope with headache problems, thus influencing the individual's adaptation to recurrent headaches (Bandura, 1986). A recent study provides initial support for this hypothesis with the finding that self-efficacy (with respect to preventing headaches) accounted for significant variance in psychological distress and coping beyond that explained by locus-of-control beliefs, even when severity of headache problems was controlled statistically (Martin, Holroyd, & Rokiki, 1992). Other findings raise the possibility that changes in self-efficacy and locus-of-control beliefs during biofeedback training play a role in mediating improvements in headache activity observed with behavior therapies (Holroyd et al., 1984).

Stress and Coping

In spite of the fact that stress has been acknowledged as a precipitant of headaches for at least 40 years, investigators have only recently begun to examine this relationship. Recurrent headache sufferers report a greater number of daily life stressors than controls (e.g., Holm, Holroyd, Hursey, & Penzien, 1984), but most studies have been unable to shed much light on the details of this relationship. Using time series analysis, however, Moseley and colleagues (Moseley et al., 1991) revealed that daily life stressors tend to precede migraine episodes by a few days but tend to occur concurrently with tension headache episodes. This may explain why tension headache sufferers are more likely to identify a relationship between stress and headache episodes than are migraine sufferers.

Recurrent headache sufferers also are more likely than matched headache-free controls to report use of potentially ineffective strategies for coping with stress and strategies that are unlikely to resolve problems effectively, such as problem avoidance, wishful thinking, and social withdrawal (Ehde & Holm, 1992; Holm et al., 1984). For example, Ehde and Holm found that 70% to 80% of recurrent migraine and tension headache sufferers could be identified solely by the ways they appraise and cope with daily-life stress. It is unclear at this point whether avoidant coping precedes headache problems or is an adaptation to recurrent headaches. In either case, avoidant coping could help maintain headache problems and thus be an appropriate target for self-management therapy.

The focus on the psychological aspects of headache rather than on the mental health of the headache sufferer is likely to continue in the 1990s. Quality-of-life and expectancy measures are likely to be increasingly employed in clinical trials of new therapies. Measures of daily-life stress and coping also deserve continued attention, but existing data probably do not justify their use in the routine assessment of the recurrent headache sufferer.

NONPHARMACOLOGICAL TREATMENT

The most widely used nonpharmacological therapies for tension headache include relaxation training and electromyograph (EMG) biofeedback training, while for migraine headache, relaxation training and thermal ("handwarming") biofeedback training are the nonpharmacological treatments of choice. The effectiveness of these therapies was reasonably well established a decade ago. Preliminary support for the use of cognitive therapy in the management of tension headache and cephalic vasomotor biofeedback training in the management of migraine was also available. In the last 10 years, information about the short- and long-term effectiveness of these therapies has continued to cumulate. Thus, conclusions that were tentative a decade ago can be drawn with considerably more confidence today. In the last decade, three other developments stand out:

1. The development of more cost-effective methods of delivering nonpharmacological therapies
2. The improved identification of patients who fail to respond to standard nonpharmacological treatments
3. An emerging interest in the integration of pharmacological and nonpharmacological therapies.

Each of these developments will be addressed. However, we will first provide a current review of evidence supporting the effectiveness of the primary nonpharmacological treatments.

Relaxation/Biofeedback Therapies

Over 100 studies have evaluated the most widely used relaxation and biofeedback therapies. Drawing on recent meta-analyses of this literature, Table 1.3 presents the average improvements reported across studies with each treatment (Holroyd & Penzien, 1986; Penzien, Holroyd, Hursey, Holm, & Wittchen, 1985). Only data from studies that used daily headache recordings are included in the averages reported in Table 1.3, because studies that use other outcome measures (e.g., clinician's improvement ratings, patient's global reports of headache activity) may overestimtae improvement (Blanchard, Andrasik, Neff, Jurish, & O'Keefe, 1981; Holroyd & Penzien, 1990).

For recurrent tension headaches, it can be seen that relaxation training, EMG biofeedback training, and the combination of these two interventions each yield about a 50% reduction in tension headache activity. In contrast, untreated patients who simply record their headaches show virtually no improvement. Reductions in tension headache activity reported with relaxation and EMG biofeedback therapies are also more than twice as large as those reported with the most commonly used pseudotherapy control procedure (noncontingent or "false" biofeedback).

For recurrent migraines, it can be seen that improvements reported with relaxation training and with biofeedback training are substantially larger than those observed in untreated patients. However, results reported with the combination of relaxation training and thermal biofeedback training (55% reduction in migraine activity) are significantly larger than results reported with either relaxation or biofeedback training alone (36% reduction averaged across the remaining three treat-

Table 1.3. Average Improvement by Type of Treatment and Type of Headache

Type of treatment	Average % improvement	Treatment groups (*n*)	Improvement range (%)
Tension-type headache			
Combined EMG biofeedback and relaxation training	57	9	29 to 88
EMG biofeedback training	46	26	13 to 87
Relaxation training	45	15	17 to 94
Noncontingent biofeeedback training control	15	6	−14 to 40
Headache monitoring control	−4	10	−28 to 12
Migraine			
Combined relaxation training and thermal biofeedback	56	35	11 to 93
Relaxation training	37	38	5 to 81
Thermal biofeedback training	35	14	−8 to 80
Cephalic vasomotor biofeedback training	34	11	2 to 82
Headache monitoring control	3	15	−30 to 33

Source: Holroyd and Penzien (1986); Penzien et al. (1985).

ments). Meta-analysis of available studies thus suggests that the combination of relaxation training and thermal biofeedback training may be the nonpharmacological treatment of choice for recurrent migraines.

In contrast, the handful of studies that have directly compared the effectiveness of relaxation/thermal biofeedback training to either relaxation training alone or biofeedback training alone have not provided consistent support for the superiority of relaxation/thermal biofeedback training (e.g., Blanchard & Andrasik, 1987; Gauthier, Bois, Allaire, & Drolet, 1981; Sargent, Solbach, Coiyne, Spohn, & Fergerson, 1986). Differences in treatment protocols and in patient populations across studies may have mitigated against finding differences in treatment effectiveness in some studies. For example, some studies appear to have included a significant number of patients who were unlikely to benefit dramatically with the use of nonpharmacological treatment alone (e.g., patients experiencing headaches complicated by analgesic overuse), thereby reducing the likelihood that differences in the effectiveness of various nonpharmacological treatments would be detected. Other studies appear to have included too few patients to possess adequate statistical power. In any case, the hypothesis that combined relaxation/thermal biofeedback training is more effective than either relaxation training or biofeedback training alone must be considered tentative.

Cognitive-Behavior Therapy

Support for the use of cognitive-behavior therapy in the management of recurrent tension headaches continued to grow in the last decade. However, the value of cognitive-behavior therapy remains unproven in the management of recurrent migraines. The markedly different treatment protocols used in studies evaluating cognitive-behavior therapy and the small number of patients treated in some of these studies continue to limit the conclusions that can be drawn from this literature.

The rationale for cognitive-behavior therapy derives from the observation that the way individuals cope with stress can precipitate, exacerbate, and maintain headache episodes or influence headache-related disability. Cognitive-behavior therapy is thus used to teach recurrent headache sufferers to (1) identify stressful circumstances that precipitate or aggravate headaches and employ more effective coping strategies for managing these stressors; (2) more effectively cope with headaches when they do occur; and (3) manage the psychological consequences (e.g., depression and disability) of headaches (Holroyd & Andrasik, 1982).

Tension-Type Headache

Studies that have compared the effectiveness of cognitive therapy with relaxation or EMG biofeedback training indicate that cognitive therapy alone can effectively reduce tension headache activity (Holroyd & Andrasik, 1978; Holroyd, Andrasik, & Westbrook, 1977; Murphy, Lehrer, & Jurish, 1990). In practice, of course, cognitive therapy is likely to be introduced subsequent to or combined with relaxation therapy. It is thus significant that results from two of the three available studies suggest that cognitive therapy adds to the effectiveness of relaxation therapy (Appelbaum et al., 1990; Blanchard et al., 1990b; Tobin, Holroyd, Baker, Reynolds, & Holm, 1988). Cognitive-behavior therapy also has yielded more positive results than amitriptyline HCL, the most widely used preventive medication (Holroyd et al., 1991).

Cognitive-behavioral interventions have been hypothesized to be of greatest value when chronic daily stress, depression, or adjustment problems aggravate tension-type headaches or interfere with the application of self-regulation skills acquired during biofeedback or relaxation training (Holroyd & Andrasik, 1982). Some initial support for this hypothesis was reported by Tobin and colleagues (Tobin et al., 1988), who found high levels of daily-life stress, as assessed by the Hassles Scale (DeLongis, Coyne, Dakof, Folkman, & Lazarus, 1982), limited patients' response to relaxation training but did not interfere with combined relaxation/cognitive-behavior therapy.

Results from small-scale studies now suggest that cognitive-behavior therapy may be the preferred treatment for many recurrent tension-type headache sufferers. Larger scale studies are thus needed that evaluate brief cognitive-behavior therapy both by itself and in combination with preventive medication in medical settings where most recurrent headache disorders are treated.

Migraine

In contrast to the positive results obtained with cognitive-behavior therapy in the management of recurrent tension headaches, the value of cognitive-behavior therapy remains uncertain in managing recurrent migraines. Although cognitive-behavior therapy appears to yield improvements in migraine activity (e.g., Sorbi, Tellegen, & DuLong, 1989), evidence that cognitive therapy can enhance the effectiveness of combined relaxation/thermal biofeedback therapy is lacking (Blanchard et al., 1990a, 1990c; Lake, Rainey, & Pfapsdorf, 1979). Cognitive-behavior therapy procedures may require further modification to be of value in the management of recurrent migraine. However, the possibility that cognitive-behavior therapy adds little to the effectiveness of standard relaxation/thermal biofeedback therapies must also be entertained.

Maintenance of Treatment Gains

In the last decade, information indicating that improvements achieved with nonpharmacologic treatments are often well maintained continued to accumulate slowly. It is now well established that improvements achieved with behavioral treatments tend to be maintained, at least for the 3- to 9-month follow-up periods that have most frequently been evaluated. In fact, improvements in tension headache activity were slightly larger at follow-up (54% reduction in headache activity) than at immediate posttreatment evaluation (45% reduction) in 22 patient samples treated with relaxation training and/or EMG biofeedback training (Holroyd & Penzien, 1986). Similarly, improvements in migraine activity were slightly larger at follow-up (41% reduction) than immediately following treatment (36% reduction) in 43 patient samples treated with relaxation or biofeedback therapies (Penzien et al., 1985). The maintenance of improvements following cognitive-behavior therapy has been less frequently evaluated, but existing studies report good maintenance (e.g., Blanchard et al., 1990b; Holroyd & Andrasik, 1978; Holroyd et al., 1977; Richardson & McGrath, 1989; Sorbi et al., 1989; Tobin et al., 1988).

Positive, but less definitive, statements can be made about the *long-term* maintenance of improvements achieved with behavioral treatments. In five of six studies that employed daily headache recordings, reductions in tension headache activity of 50% or greater were still observed 1–3 years following relaxation, EMG biofeedback, or cognitive therapy (Andrasik, Blanchard, Neff, & Rodichok, 1984; Andrasik & Holroyd, 1983; Blanchard et al., 1988; Blanchard, Appelbaum, Guarnieri, Morrill, & Dentinger, 1987a; Holroyd & Andrasik, 1983). On the other hand, one study reported poor maintenance 1 year following combined relaxation/EMG biofeedback training (Reinking & Hutchings, 1981). In nine studies that employed daily headache recordings, reductions in migraine activity of at least 45% were still observed 1–3 years following relaxation training, biofeedback training, or cognitive-behavior therapy (Andrasik et al., 1984; Blanchard, Guarnieri, Andrasik, Neff & Rodichok, 1987b; Blanchard et al., 1988; Holroyd et al., 1989c; Friedman & Taub, 1985; Gauthier & Carrier, 1991; Knapp, 1982; Medina, Diamond, & Franklin, 1976; Silver, Blanchard, Williamson, Theobold, & Brown, 1979; Sorbi et al., 1989). In three studies, reductions in migraine activity of this magnitude were still observed 5–7 years following treatment (Blanchard et al., 1987a; Gauthier & Carrier, 1991; Lisspers & Ost, 1990).

The problem in interpreting long-term follow-up data is that 20% to 60% of patients typically are lost to follow-up, and other patients may have initiated medical treatment during the follow-up period. However, even when these methodological problems have been addressed, long-term follow-up results have been quite positive (e.g., Gauthier & Carrier, 1991; Holroyd, Holm, & Penzien, 1989; Sorbi et al., 1989). It thus appears that improvements achieved with behavioral treatments are frequently well maintained.

Neither monthly booster sessions nor brief monthly contacts appear to enhance the maintenance of improvements, possibly because, as noted previously, relatively good maintenance has been reported without such interventions (Andrasik et al., 1984; Blanchard et al., 1988). In a 5-year retrospective follow-up of over 400 patients, maintenance appeared to be best in younger patients (less than 30 years of age), females, and in patients who had not exhibited excessive medication use prior to treatment (Diamond, Medina, Diamond-Falk, & DeVeno, 1979). These results suggest that variables associated with initial treatment response may also be associated with maintenance. In the only other study that has examined individual differences in maintenance (Sorbi et al., 1998), high levels of posttreatment life stress (assessed with the Life Events Inventory) were associated with poor maintenance following relaxation training ($r = -.69$), whereas low "self-motivation" (measurement not described) was associated with poor maintenance following cognitive-behavior therapy ($r = .71$). Unfortunately, initial treatment response was not controlled in either study, so initial treatment response and maintenance may have been confounded in these studies. Additional information is clearly needed about factors predictive of long-term maintenance.

Alternate Formats for Treatment Delivery

In the 1980s, investigators began to explore ways to reduce the cost and increase the availability of behavioral treatments. Two promising avenues are limited-contact and small-group treatment administration.

Limited-Contact Treatment

In a limited-contact, or "home-based" treatment format, self-regulation skills are introduced in periodic clinic sessions, but written materials and auidotapes are used to teach patients at home most of what is typically taught in clinic sessions (Blanchard & Andrasik, 1985; Lascelles, McGrath, Sullivan, & Wesk, 1991; Nash & Holroyd, 1992). As a result, only 3–4 (monthly) clinic sessions may be required to complete limited-contact behavioral treatment. This is in contrast to the 10–20 (often weekly) clinic sessions required for completely therapist-administered, or "clinic-based" treatment. Of course, if therapist contact could be completely eliminated, treatment cost could be further reduced and treatments made even more widely available. However, to date, self-administered treatments have been plagued by poor compliance and poor treatment results (Kohlenberg, 1984; Larsson, Melin, & Döberl, 1990). It appears that some therapist contact is necessary to address problems inevitably encountered in learning and using self-regulation skills.

With tension-type headache, positive results have been reported with limited-contact (e.g., 3 therapist sessions and 2 phone contacts) relaxation therapy and cognitive-behavior therapy (Chesney & Shelton, 1976; Holroyd et al., 1991; Tobin et al., 1988). However, two reports that directly compared therapist-administered (e.g., 16 sessions of therapist instruction) and limited-contact relaxation training reported marginal results with the limited-contact treatment format (Larsson & Melin, 1988; Teders, Blanchard, Andrasik, Jurish, Neff, & Arena, 1984). Teders and associates, for example, reported only a 23% reduction in headache activity (and no significant reduction in medication use) with limited-contact relaxation training (3 clinic sessions and 2 phone contacts). These latter findings suggest that more work may be needed to determine the most effective way to administer relaxation training in a limited-contact treatment format and to identify patients who are likely to benefit from limited-contact treatment.

Limited-contact treatments have yielded positive results more consistently with migraine than with tension-type headache. Studies that compared the effectiveness of limited-contact and therapist-administered thermal biofeedback/relaxation training have found these two treatment administration procedures equally effective in reducing migraine activity (Blanchard & Andrasik, 1985; Gauthier, Paillé, & Roberge, 1990; Jurish, Blanchard, Andrasik, Teders, Neff, & Arena, 1983). For example, Gauthier et al. (1990) found that thermal biofeedback was as effectively administered in a limited-contact format (3 therapist sessions and 2 phone contacts) as a therapist-administered format (14 therapist sessions).

Limited-contact treatment can be more easily integrated into routine medical practice than therapist-administered treatment and therefore can be made more available and affordable than therapist-administered treatment. The limited available research suggests that limited-contact treatment is a viable alternative for many recurrent headache sufferers and that both limited-contact treatment and therapist-administered treatment produce improvements that appear to be equally well maintained (Blanchard et al., 1988; Gauthier et al., 1990). Nonetheless, a significant proportion of patients will continue to require therapist-administered treatment. Individuals who excessively use analgesic medication, are clinically depressed, or suffer from particularly refractory headache problems may be particularly likely to require a therapist-centered treatment. Other patients simply do not persist in efforts to learn or apply self-regulation skills without regular contact with a health professional. Additional information is therefore needed about the optimal design of limited-contact treatment formats and about patient characteristics that predict a successful response to limited-contact treatment.

Small-Group Treatment

Administration of behavioral treatment in groups is a widely recognized method of reducing the cost of treatment. One study found that thermal biofeedback training can be as effectively administered to migraine sufferers in small groups as individually (Gauthier, J. Coté, G. Coté, & Drolet, in press). Relaxation and cognitive-behavior therapies have also proven effective in reducing recurrent tension headaches when administered in small groups (e.g., Chesney & Shelton, 1976; Holroyd & Andrasik, 1978). However, to the best of our knowledge, no study has directly compared the effectiveness of relaxation training or cognitive-behavior therapy when administered in individual versus small-group formats.

Where patient flow is adequate and cost issues are of concern, it may be feasible to reduce the cost of treatment and to make good use of health professionals' time by administering treatment in small groups rather than individually. However, this requires that health professionals are not only able to administer behavioral treatments, but that they also are adept at handling problems that arise in group treatment (Rose, 1990).

Special Populations

Behavioral treatments were evaluated initially in adult headache sufferers ranging in age from 18 to 55. The management of recurrent headache problems in children and older adults has only recently been subjected to controlled study.

Pediatric Populations

Pediatric migraine occurs in about 3% of adolescents and 1% of young children (e.g., Bille, 1962; Sillanpaa, 1983), and most of what is known about the management of pediatric headaches in general is the result of studies conducted on children with migraines. Tension-type headache has only rarely been studied in pediatric populations, either because few young children suffer from severe tension-type headaches (McDonald, 1986) or because parents are less likely to seek treatment for children suffering from tension-type headache than from migraine (Labbé & Williamson, 1984).

Migraine. Combined relaxation/thermal biofeedback training appears to be as effective, or possibly more effective, with children as with adults (Blanchard & Andrasik, 1985; Labbé & Williamson, 1984; Mehegan, Masek, Harrison, Russo, & Leviton, 1984). Blanchard & Andrasik, for example, reported an 82% reduction in migraine activity with relaxation/thermal biofeedback training and a 45% reduction in migraine activity with relaxation training alone in a sample of children 8 to 16 years of age. Positive results with this type of treatment and a reluctance to use drug therapies in young children raise the possibility that relaxation/thermal biofeedback training might be the treatment of choice for pediatric migraine.

Improvements reported with relaxation training alone tend to be less impressive than improvements reported with combined relaxation/thermal biofeedback training. In the largest controlled evaluation of relaxation training to date, 99 children and adolescents (aged 9 to 17), received either relaxation therapy or a one-session treatment that focused on managing migraine triggers. The one-session treatment consisted of reviewing headache diary recordings and offering strategies for coping with migraine triggers (McGrath et al., 1988). Improvements observed with relaxation training tended to be larger in magnitude (55% reduction in migraine activity) than those achieved with the one-session treatment (34% reduction), but these improvements were not significantly different.

Especially valuable for the pediatric headache sufferer would be an effective limited-contact treatment, because it would allow many young headache sufferers who do not now receive treatment to receive help in the school setting. Fortunately, limited-contact treatment appears feasible with children, at least when there is a supportive family environment. An early pilot study (Burke & Andrasik, 1989) compared the effectiveness of therapist-administered (10 clinic sessions) with child-administered and parent-administered thermal biofeedback training (each requiring only 3 clinic sessions) in 9 migraine sufferers 10 to 14 years of age. Two of 3 patients receiving the therapist-administered and child-administered treatments, and all 3 patients receiving the parent-administered treatment achieved greater than 50% reduction in migraine activity. In a larger study, therapist-administered (8 clinic sessions) and patient-administered (1 clinic contact plus weekly phone contacts)' treatment packages combining relaxation training and cognitive-behavior therapy yielded equivalent results (48% and 50% reduction in migraine activity, respectively) in 87 adolescents, 11 to 18 years of age (McGrath, Humphreys, Keene, Goodman, Lascelles, Cunningham, & Firestone, 1992). In this study, both treatments produced better results than were observed with a brief treatment that focused only on modifying migraine triggers (6% reduction). Larger scale evaluations of limited-contact relaxation/thermal biofeedback training and treatment packages such as the one developed by McGrath and colleagues appear warranted. Of particular interest would be treatments administered in school versus clinic settings.

Tension-Type Headache. The limited available data suggest that behavioral treatments can be effective in controlling pediatric tension-type headache. Werder & Sargent (1984) reported that nine adolescents (mean age of 15) treated with combined relaxation and biofeedback therapies reduced tension headache hours by 39% at the end of 2 months of treatment and by 95% at 1-year follow-up. In a reanalysis of data from three controlled studies, Larsson and Melin (1988) further concluded that therapist-administered relaxation training produced larger improvements (63% reduction in headache activity) in adolescents (aged 16 to 18) than did group discussion or information-only treatments. More information is clearly needed regarding the prevalence of tension-type headaches in children as well as the effectiveness of behavioral treatments for children with tension-type headaches.

Geriatric Population

Epidemiological data suggest that the incidence of recurrent headache disorders may peak between 25 to 45 years of age and then decline significantly (Rasmussen, Jensen, Schroll, & Olesen, 1991; Stewart et al., 1992). However, older headache sufferers are likely to have other medical disorders that can aggravate headache problems or complicate treatment (Hale, May, Marks, Moore, & Stewart, 1987), and they may be more likely than their younger counterparts to receive a tension-type headache diagnosis as opposed to a migraine diagnosis (Solomon, Kunkel, & Frame, 1990).

Early research suggested that older tension-type headache sufferers were unresponsive to relaxation training or EMG biofeedback training (Blanchard & Andrasik, 1985; Holyroyd & Penzien, 1986). For example, in one retrospective analysis, patients over 55 years of age rarely benefited from either relaxation or EMG biofeedback therapies (Blanchard & Andrasik, 1985). However, more recent findings suggest that older patients may do quite well with behavior therapies when treatment administration is altered. More detailed explanations of treatment procedures, frequent reviews of the material covered, and additional time to practice elementary skills before introduction of more advanced skills may help the older patient benefit from self-regulatory treatments (Arena, Hightower, & Chong, 1988; Kabela, Blanchard, Appelbaum, & Nicholson, 1989).

Older adult headache sufferers remain understudied. There have been no controlled evaluations of behavior therapies involving an adequate number of older patients to permit an estimate of the effectiveness of these therapies. Controlled evaluations of behavior therapies appear warranted because drug therapy is often complicated in the older patient and may be limited by the large number of side effects.

Treatment Nonresponders

In the last decade, there was an increase in research aimed at the identification of factors associated with a poor response to existing therapies. One third to one half of patients fail to show a clinically significant improvement with behavioral treatment. The lack of consistent outcomes reported across studies using the same behavioral treatment also appears to result, in large part, from the greater inclusion of nonresponsive patients in some study samples than in others (Holroyd & Penzien, 1986). The development of effective treatments for patients unresponsive to traditional behavioral therapies is likely to be a priority in the next decade. Three factors associated with poor treatment response include excessive medication use, a continuous headache pattern, and concurrent psychiatric disorder.

Excessive Medication Use

Excessive analgesic or abortive medication use can both aggravate headache problems and limit the benefits obtained from drug and nondrug therapies (e.g., Kudrow, 1982; Mathew, Kurman, & Perez, 1989; Michultka, Blanchard, Appelbaum, Jaccard, & Dentinger, 1989; Rapoport, 1988). In a retrospective review of patient records, for example, "high medication users" (defined by a score of 40 or higher on an adaptation of the summary medication index developed by Coyne, Sargent, Segerson, & Obourn, 1976), were significantly less likely than low medication users (with scores of 10 or less) to benefit from psychological treatments, such as relaxation or biofeedback training (Michultka et al., 1989). Only 29% of high-medication users showed a 50% or greater reduction in headache activity, while 55% of low-medication users showed this level of improvement.

Unfortunately, it is not currently possible to specify precisely at what level of use analgesic or ergotamine drugs begin to aggravate headache problems. Scholz, Diener and Geiselhart (1988) examined medication use in 39 patients whose daily headaches appeared to be aggravated by their medication use, and concluded that daily use of 3–4 mg. of either ergotamine or dihydroergotamine or 1000 mg. of either acetaminophen or salicylic acid was very likely to aggravate, rather than ameliorate headaches. Both the Second International Workshop on Drug-Related Headache (Diener & Wilkinson, 1988) and the Classification Committee of the International Headache Society (1988) formulated diagnostic criteria specifically for headaches that are complicated by chronic use of analgesic or abortive medications (see Table 1.4). It can be seen that the two sets of diagnostic criteria differ. For example, in one, the quantity of medication consumed serves as the criterion for diagnosis, and in the other, the number of days on which medication is consumed serves as the diagnostic criterion. An additional problem for the clinician is that the diagnosis of headaches aggravated by chronic medication use cannot be made with confidence on the initial visit, because this diagnosis requires that withdrawal from the offending medication result in an improvement in headache problems.

If a patient's headaches are complicated by excessive medication use, withdrawal from the offending medications is likely to be essential to effective treatment. Two clinical series (Baumgartner, Wesseley, Bingol, Maly, & Holzner, 1989; Diener et al., 1989) provide preliminary support for the inclusion of supervised withdrawal from analgesic and abortive medications in treatment programs, at least for patients who consume very high levels of these medications (an average 35 to 40 doses per week). Diener et al. concluded from retrospective patient ratings obtained at long-term follow-up ($\bar{X} = 35$ months) that 69% of patients showed a 50% reduction in headache activity, a 50% reduction in medication use, or both. Baumgartner et al. similarly judged 61% of patients to have significantly reduced both medication use and headache activity at follow-up ($\bar{X} = 17$ months). Neither study included compar-

Table 1.4. Diagnostic Criteria for Headaches Aggravated by Chronic Medication Use

IHS criteria[a]	2nd International Workshop criteria[b]
Headache characteristics	
1. More than 14 headache days/month 2. Headache is diffuse, pulsating, and distinguished from migraine by absent attack pattern and/or absent associated symptoms—for ergotamine-induced headache	1. More than 20 headache days/month 2. Daily headache duration exceeds 10 hours
Relationship to medication use	

1. Ergotamine
  a. Onset is preceded by daily ergotamine intake (oral ≥ 2mg, rectal ≥ 1mg)
2. Analgesics
  a. At least 50 g/month of aspirin or equivalent
  b. At least 100 tablets/month of analgesics combined with barbiturates or other nonnarcotic compounds
  c. Narcotic analgesic use
3. Headache disappears within 1 month after withdrawal of substance
	1. Intake of analgesics or abortive medication on more than 20 days per month
	
	2. Regular intake of analgesics and/or ergotamine in combination with barbiturates, codeine, caffeine, antihistamines, or tranquilizers
	
	3. Increase in the severity and frequency of headaches after discontinuation of drug intake

[a]Headache Classification Committee of the International Headache Society (1988).
[b]Diener and Wilkinson (1988).

ison or control groups; therefore, these findings must be interpreted cautiously. Nonetheless, the patients represented in these studies are often unresponsive to treatment, so the improvement figures reported in these studies are encouraging.

Continuous Headaches

Patients with almost continuous headaches appear to be less responsive to relaxation or biofeedback therapies than patients who experience well-defined episodes of headache activity (Bakal, Demjen, & Kagonov, 1981; Blanchard, Appelbaum, Radnitz, Jaccard, & Dentinger, 1989; Holroyd et al., 1988; Jacob, Turner, Szekely, & Edelman, 1983). For example, Blanchard et al. found that patients who recorded almost continuous (one or fewer headache-free days during a 4-week baseline), at times intensely painful headaches, were less likely to benefit from relaxation or EMG biofeedback than were patients with episodic headaches (two or more headache-free days per week). While 13% of the patients with continuous headaches showed at least a 50% reduction in headache activity, more than 50% of the patients with episodic headaches evidenced a 50% reduction in headache activity. Only about 10% of the near-continuous headache sufferers in this study met criteria for excessive medication use; therefore, continuous headaches in most of these patients could not be assumed to be a product of medication overuse.

Investigators do not agree about how near-continuous headaches (also termed chronic daily headache or benign, almost daily headache) need to be conceptualized. It is unclear whether this headache pattern represents a new disorder or group of disorders or is a severe expression of a combination of disorders already included in the existing classification system. In some settings, the largest portion of patients with near-continuous headaches reports a history of at least occasional migraines, leading some authors to suggest that migraines transformed or evolved into a new disorder (Mathew, Reuveni, & Perez, 1987). Others contend that these patients are more accurately conceptualized as suffering from both migraines and tension-type headaches or, when medication use contributes to the occurrence of almost daily headaches, from analgesic-complicated headaches. The second largest group of patients with near-continuous headaches report no history of migraine, and there is relative agreement that many of these patients suffer from chronic, tension-type headaches. A problem with existing studies of near-continuous headaches is that criteria for identifying near-continuous headaches vary across studies, ranging from a requirement of 15 or more headache-days a month to a requirement that headache occur daily.

Standardized criteria for identifying near-continuous headaches need to be developed and used across studies so that results from specialized headache treatment centers and from primary-care facilities can be compared. More information is also needed about risk factors that predict the development of near-continuous headaches in patients whose headaches begin with episodic migraine or tension-type headaches. Finally, controlled studies that evaluate methods of improving the effectiveness of behavioral treatments with patients who have near-continuous headaches are needed. It would be helpful, for example, to know what proportion of these patients can be helped by extended relaxation training or EMG biofeedback training, cognitive-behavior therapy, or the combination of prophylactic medication and behavioral treatment.

Concurrent Psychiatric Disorder

Patients with elevated scores on psychological tests that assess depression or psychiatric disturbance have done poorly with behavioral treatment in some studies (e.g., Blanchard et al., 1985; Jacob et al., 1983) but not in others (Ford, Strobel, Strong, & Szarek, 1983). At this point, it is not clear if abnormal psychological test scores are strongly associated with excessive medication use or near-continuous headaches. One series of studies in a general population of recurrent headache patients suggests this is not the case. Patients with near-continuous headaches showed only small elevations in Beck Depression Inventory scores and Minnesota Multiphasic Personality Inventory (MMPI) scores (Blanchard et al., 1989), whereas patients who were identified as using medication excessively did not differ significantly from controls on these measures (Michultka et al., 1989). In contrast, a study conducted at a specialized headache treatment center (Mathew et al., 1989) reported that patients with near-continuous headaches, particularly patients who remained unresponsive to treatment, exhibited a high incidence of both elevated MMPI profiles (100% of unresponsive patients) and excessive analgesic use. These patients also tended to report a history of parental alcoholism and sexual or physical abuse, and one third exhibited an abnormal response to the Dexamethasone Suppression Test. Assessment of the relationships between abnormal psychological test scores and both excessive analgesic use and near-continuous headaches is essential, as is an elucidation of relationship between psychopathology and treatment outcome.

Compliance with treatment regimens can be a significant problem with patients who also are handicapped by a psychiatric disorder. Clinical impressions suggest that brief psychotherapy focusing on the management of acute psychiatric symptoms can facilitate the management of recurrent headache problems in these patients, but no confirming research data are available. Other ideas for adapting existing treatment techniques for use with this population need to be articulated, and these modified treatments need evaluation.

INTEGRATING DRUG AND NONDRUG THERAPIES

Surprisingly little attention has been devoted to evaluating treatment strategies that integrate drug and nondrug treatments. As a result, only tentative statements can be made about the relative effectiveness of widely used drug and nondrug therapies and about the benefits and costs of combining these two therapeutic modalities. Obstacles that have limited research in this area were identified by Holroyd (1993) and include (1) the limited number of investigators who are knowledgeable about both drug and nondrug therapies; (2) cultures that evolve in clinical settings that inhibit experimentation with multimodal treatment strategies; and (3) the tendency of both professional journals and associations to deemphasize interprofessional communication that might stimulate interest in combined treatment strategies.

Comparative and Combined Effects

Migraine

Probably the best estimate of the comparative effectiveness of pharmacological and nonpharmacological treatments in the management of adult migraines can be obtained by comparing the outcomes achieved with the most intensively evaluated and widely used treatments within each category. Accordingly, improvement scores from a recent meta-analysis integrating results from 25 clinical trials of propranolol and 35 clinical trials of relaxation/thermal biofeedback training (over 2,400 migraine sufferers) are presented in Table 1.5. Improvements reported with both propranolol and relaxation/thermal biofeedback training are significantly larger than

Table 1.5. Average Percentage Improvement in Migraine Headache for Treatment and Control Groups Using Daily Headache Records as Outcome Measures

	Treatment conditions			
	Relaxation/biofeedback	Propranolol	Placebo	Untreated
Average patient improvement[a] (%)	43.3	43.7	14.3	2.1
Range of scores (%)	11 to 87	26 to 65	−23 to 32	−30 to 33

[a]Average improvement in headache activity weighted by sample size.
Source: Holroyd and Penzien (1990).

improvements reported with placebo or observed in untreated migraineurs. However, these two therapies do not differ in effectiveness, each yielding about 43% reduction in migraine activity. Available clinical trials thus provide substantial support for the effectiveness of both propranolol and relaxation/thermal biofeedback training, but no empirical support that these two treatment modalities differ in effectiveness.

In spite of the fact that pharmacological and nonpharmacological therapies are frequently administered conjointly in specialized headache treatment centers, only three studies have examined the effectiveness of such combined treatments. Two of these studies found the combination of propranolol and relaxation/thermal biofeedback training to be highly effective, yielding more than 70% average reduction in migraine activity, significantly better than was observed with relaxation/biofeedback training alone (Holroyd et al., in press; Mathew, 1981). Data from one study further raise the possibility that combined treatment might allow as many as two thirds of patients to effectively control migraines with only a low propranolol dose (60 mg/day) and enable some patients to subsequently discontinue propranolol after a few months of drug therapy without suffering a relapse of migraine problems (Holroyd, 1993). In the third study to evaluate combined treatment, and the only study to examine the long-term effects of a combined therapy, amitriptyline initially enhanced the effectiveness of biofeedback training. However, beginning at month 8 and continuing through the 24-month observation period, results achieved with biofeedback training alone were superior to results obtained with the combination of amitriptyline and biofeedback training (Reich & Gottesman, 1993). It is not clear why poorer results were observed with the combined treatment than with biofeedback alone. However, several investigators caution that patients who receive combined pharmacological/nonpharmacological treatment might attribute their improvement to drug therapy and cease or reduce use of self-regulation skills, thereby reducing the effectiveness of the combined treatment (Hollon & DeRubeis, 1981). In any case, these latter findings highlight the need for information about long-term treatment effects of combined treatments.

Pediatric Migraine. Pharmacological and nonpharmacological therapies for pediatric migraine have been compared in only one study. In this study (Olness, MacDonald, & Uden, 1987), classic migraine sufferers aged 6 to 12 years combined receiving relaxation and self-hypnosis training (5 treatment sessions), evidenced significantly better treatment outcome than those patients receiving propranolol (3 mg/kg/day). In fact, whereas combined relaxation/self-hypnosis produced better results than placebo, results achieved with propranolol and placebo did not differ from one another.

Other studies also suggest that nonpharmacological treatments deserve greater attention in the management of pediatric migraine. Results reported in clinical trials of propranolol appear to be poorrer in children than in adults. Two (Forsythe, Gillies, & McCarran, 1984; Olness et al., 1987) of three (Ludvigsson, 1974) available double-blind trials of propranolol found that propranolol and placebo did not differ in effectiveness for children, whereas propranolol has consistently been found superior to placebo for adults (Table 1.5). As noted, combined relaxation and thermal biofeedback and other combination therapies yield improvements with pediatric migraine that often equal or exceed improvements reported with adult migraine (Guarnieri & Blanchard, 1990; Labbé & Williamson, 1984; McGrath et al., 1992; Richter et al., 1986; Werder & Sargent, 1984). These findings, and the difficulties inherent with drug therapies in pediatric populations (Andrasik, Blake, & McCarran, 1986), argue for more intensive study of behavioral interventions in pediatric populations.

Tension-Type Headache

Limited information is available concerning the relative effectiveness of the most widely used drug and nondrug therapies for recurrent tension headaches. The most informative of the three available studies compared stress management training (administered in a limited-therapist-contact treatment format) and amitriptyline (individualized dose of 25–75 mg/day; Holroyd et al., 1991). Both stress management training and amitriptyline yielded significant improvements in tension headache activity (56% and 27% reduction in headache activity, respectively). However, stress management yielded better results than amitriptyline on several variables, including headache index, somatic complaints, side effects, and perceptions of control of headache activity.

The two remaining studies with tension-type headache are limited by their reliance on muscle relaxants that are not considered by most investigators to be the preferred agents for managing recurrent tension-type headaches. In the first of these studies (Paiva et al., 1982), significant improvements were observed with both 12 sessions of EMG biofeedback and with diazepam (dose unspecified). An important note is that although patients relapsed when diazepam was discontinued, they did not relapse when biofeedback was ended. In the second study (Larsson et al., 1990), chlormezanone (400 mg/day) failed to enhance the effectiveness of self-administered relaxation training. However, both relaxation training and the combined relaxation/chlormezanone therapies yielded poor results (14% and 9% reduction in headache activity, respectively).

Additional research is needed to elucidate the benefits and limits of promising combined pharmacological/nonpharmacological therapies for migraine and to evaluate similar combined therapies with tension-type headache. In addition, more information is needed about the differing treatment-effect profiles of pharmacological and nonpharmacological treatments. Initial findings suggest behavioral treatments may produce improvement more slowly than pharmacological treatments (Holroyd et al., 1988, 1992; Reich & Gottesman, 1993), yield fewer side effects than pharmacological treatments (but require more time and effort to complete), and produce positive psychological effects not observed with pharmacological treatment (Holroyd et al., 1991).

Medication Adherence

Poor adherence limits the effectiveness of drug therapy for many recurrent headache sufferers. Packard and O'Connell (1986) concluded, on the basis of 100 patient interviews, that over 50% of headache sufferers fail to properly adhere to drug treatment regimens. Fitzpatrick, Hopkins, and Harvard-Watts (1983) similarly found that 1 year after initiating drug therapy, only 24% of patients reported they had used heachache medications as instructed. These observations suggest that psychological interventions might be of value in facilitating patients' effective use of prescribed medications.

The one study that has focused on improving adherence focused on problems encountered in using ergotamine (Holroyd et al., 1989b). Ergotamine presents special problems, because the effective use of this medication requires rather complex self-management skills: accurate identification of migraine onset, a method of keeping medication readily available, correct timing of medication intake, and the control of intake to prevent overuse. In the Holroyd et al. study, patients received either a brief adherence intervention or standard ergotamine therapy. The adherence intervention consisted of a meeting with an allied health professional following the neurologist's prescription of ergotamine, three telephone calls to identify and remedy problems with ergotamine use, and a workbook to help identify and correct adherence problems. Patients who received the adherence intervention attempted to abort 70% of migraine attacks and showed clinically significant reductions in migraine activity (40%). In contrast, patients who received standard ergotamine therapy attempted to abort only about 40% of their migraine attacks and showed smaller reduction in migraine activity (26%). These results suggest that interventions to facilitate the chronic headache sufferer's effective use of prescribed medications deserve more attention than they have received to date. For many patients, brief interventions that successfully improve adherence with existing medical regiments could yield greater benefits than will new pharmacological agents.

CONCLUSION

The value of behavioral interventions in the management of migraine and tension-type headaches now can be considered reasonably well established. In the last decade, evidence that standard relaxation and biofeedback therapies are effective and produce lasting reductions in headache activity has continued to cumulate. At present, however, these therapies remain unavailable in most family medicine or general neurology settings, although they are almost universally available at more specialized headache treatment centers. In the next decade, greater attention will therefore need to be paid to the integration of established behavioral therapies into general medical practice where they can offered to patients who have not yet developed more intractable or complicated headache problems. The relatively recent development of limited-contact treatment formats will likely facilitate this integration. Little attention, however, has yet been devoted to the training of nurses or other health professionals to administer these interventions in general practice milieus; thus, at this point, it is uncertain how easily these treatments can be exported to new settings.

Although the value of behavior therapy in the management of recurrent headache disorders has been established, our understanding of headache disorders and their management remains rudimentary. Efforts to further enhance the effectiveness of behavioral interventions might profit by identifying subgroups of patients that are nonresponsive to behavioral interventions. For some of these nonresponsive patients, such as the patient who relies excessively on analgesic or abortive medications, behavioral interventions might play a preventative as well as therapeutic role in their care. Research also is needed to identify effective strategies for integrating behavioral and pharmacological treatments. Little more is known today about the comparative effectiveness and combined effects of pharmacological and nonpharmacological treatments than was known a decade ago, and this has limited the acceptance of behavioral therapies by the medical profession. More information also is needed about the therapeutic mechanisms underlying the improvements produced by behavioral treatments. Progress in understanding therapeutic mechanisms has the potential not only to enhance our understanding of behavioral treatments, but also may stimulate the development of more effective treatments. Finally, basic research is needed that will shed light on the ways psychological and biological variables interact in producing severe problem headaches. In the last decade, our ability to manage recurrent, disabling headaches has improved noticeably. In the next decade, we hope that further practical advances in headache management will be accompanied by similar advances in our understanding of the nature of headache disorders and their treatment.

REFERENCES

Ad Hoc Committee on the Classification of Headache. (1962). Classification of headache. *Journal of American Medical Association, 179,* 717–718.

Andrasik, F., Blake, D. D., & McCarran, M. S. (1986). A biobehavioral analysis of pediatric headache. In N. A. Krosnegor, J. D. Arastch, & M. F. Cataldo (Eds.), *Child health behavior: A behavioral pediatrics perspective* (pp. 394–434). New York: Wiley.

Andrasik, F., Blanchard, E. B., Arena, J. G., Saunders, N. L., & Barron, K. D. (1982). Psychophysiology of recurrent headache: Methodological issues and new empirical findings. *Behavior Therapy, 13,* 407–429.

Andrasik, F., Blanchard, E. B., Neff, D. F., & Rodichok, L. D. (1984). Biofeedback and relaxation training for chronic headache: A controlled comparison of booster treatments and regular contacts for long-term maintenance. *Journal of Consulting and Clinical Psychology, 52,* 609–615.

Andrasik, F., & Holroyd, K. A. (1983). Specific and nonspecific effects in the biofeedback treatment of tension headache: 3-year follow-up. *Journal of Consulting and Clinical Psychology, 51,* 634–636.

Appelbaum, K. A., Blanchard, E. B., Nicholson, N. L., Radnitz, C., Kirsch, C., Michultka, D., Attanasio, V., Andrasik, F,. & Dentinger, M. P. (1990). Controlled evaluation of the addition of cognitive strategies to a home-based relaxation protocol for tension headache. *Behavior Therapy, 21,* 293–303.

Arena, J. G., Hightower, N. E., & Chong, G. C. (1988). Relaxation therapy for tension headache in the elderly: A prospective study. *Psychology and Aging, 1,* 96–98.

Bakal, D. A. (1982). *The psychobiology of chronic headache.* New York: Springer.

Bakal, D. A., Demjen, S., & Kaganov, J. A. (1981). Cognitive behavioral treatment of chronic headache. *Headache, 21,* 81–86.

Bandura, A. (1986). *Social foundations of thought and action: A social cognitive theory.* Englewood Cliffs, NJ: Prentice-Hall.

Baumgartner, C., Wesseley, P., Bingol, C., Maly, J., & Holzner, F. (1989). Long-term prognosis of analgesic withdrawal in patients with drug-induced headaches. *Headache, 29,* 510–514.

Bille, B. (1962). Migraine in school children. *Acta Paediatrica Scandinavica, 51,* 1–151.

Birk, L. (Ed.). (1974). *Biofeedback: Behavioral medicine.* New York: International Universities Press.

Blanchard, E. B., & Andrasik, F. (1985). *Management of chronic headache: A psychological approach.* Elmsford, NY: Pergamon Press.

Blanchard, E. B., & Andrasik, F. (1987). Biofeedback treatment of vascular headache. In J. P. Hatch, J. D. Rugh, & J. G. FIsher (Eds.), *Biofeedback studies in clinical efficacy* (pp. 1–79). New York: Plenum Press.

Blanchard, E. B., Andrasik, F., Evans, D. D., Neff, D. F., Appelbaum, K. A., & Rodichok, L. D. (1985). Behavioral treatment of 250 chronic headache patients: A clinical replication series. *Behavior Therapy, 16,* 308–327.

Blanchard, E. B., Andrasik, F., Neff, D. F., Jurish, S. E., & O'Keefe, D. M. (1981). Social validation of the headache diary. *Behavior Therapy, 12,* 711–715.

Blanchard, E. B., Appelbaum, K. A., Guarnieri, P., Morrill, B., & Dentinger, M. P. (1987a). Five-year prospective follow-up on the treatment of chronic headache with biofeedback and/or relaxation. *Headache, 27,* 580–583.

Blanchard, E. B., Appelbaum, K. A., Guarnieri, P., Neff, D. F., Andrasik, F., Jaccard, J., & Barron, K. D. (1988). Two studies of the long-term follow-up of minimal-threapist contact treatments of vascular and tension headache. *Journal of Consulting and Clinical Psychology, 56,* 427–432.

Blanchard, E. B., Appelbaum, K. A., Radnitz, C. L., Jaccard, J., & Dentinger, M. P. (1989). The refractory headache patient—I. Chronic, daily, high-intensity headache. *Behaviour Research and Therapy, 27,* 403–410.

Blanchard, E. B., Appelbaum, K. A., Radnitz, C. L., Michultka, D., Morrill, B., Kirsch, C., Hillhouse, J., Evans, D. D., Guarnieri, P., Attanasio, V., Andrasik, F., Jaccard, J., & Dentinger, M. P. (1990b). A placebo-controlled evaluation of abbreviated progressive muscle relaxation and relaxation combined with cognitive therapy in the treatment of tension headache. *Journal of Consulting and Clinical Psychology, 58,* 210–215.

Blanchard, E. B., Appelbaum, K. A., Radnitz, C. L., Morrill, B., Michultka, D., Kirsch, C., Guarnieri, P., Hillhouse, J., Evans, D. D., Jaccard, J., & Barron, K. D. (1990c). A controlled evaluation of thermal biofeedback and thermal biofeedback combined with cognitive therapy in the treatment of vascular headache. *Journal of Consulting and Clinical Psychology, 58,* 216–224.

Blanchard, E. B., Appelbaum, K. A., Nicholson, N. L., Radnitz, C. L., Morrill, B., Michultka, D., Kirsch, C,. Hillhouse, J., & Dentinger, M. P. (1990a). A controlled evaluation of the addition of cognitive therapy to a home-based biofeedback and relaxation treatment of vascular headache. *Headache, 30,* 371–376.

Blanchard, E. B., Guarnieri, P., Andrasik, F., Neff, D. F., & Rodichok, L. D. (1987b). Two-, three-, and four-year follow-up on the self-regulatory treatment of chronic headache. *Journal of Consulting and Clinical Psychology, 55,* 257–259.

Budzynski, T. H., Stoyva, J. M., Adler, C. S., & Mullaney, D. J. (1973). EMG Biofeedback and tension headache: A controlled outcome study. *Psychosomatic Medicine, 6,* 509–514.

Burke, E. J., & Andrasik, F. (1989). Home- vs. clinic-based biofeedback treatment for pediatric migraine: Results of treatment through one-year follow-up. *Headache, 29,* 434–440.

Chesney, M. A., & Shelton, J. L. (1976). A comparison of muscle relaxation and electromyogram biofeedback treatments for muscle contraction headache. *Journal of Behavior Therapy and Experimental Psychiatry, 7,* 221–225.

Coyne, L., Sargent, J., Segerson, J., & Obourn, R. (1976). Relative potency scale for analgesic drugs: Use of psychophysical procedures with clinical judgments. *Headache, 16,* 70–71.

DeLongis, A., Coyne, J. C., Dakof, G., Folkman, S., & Lazarus, R. S. (1982). Relationship of daily hassles, uplifts, and major life events to health status. *Health Psychology, 1,* 119–136.

DeLozier, J. E., & Gagnon, R. O. (1975). *National Ambulatory Medical Care Survey: 1973 summary.* Washington, DC: U.S. Government Printing Office.

Diamond, S., Medina, J., Diamond-Falk, J., & DeVeno, T. (1979). The value of biofeedback in the treatment of chronic headache: A five-year restrospective study. *Headache, 19,* 90–96.

Diener, H. C., Dichgans, J., Scholz, E., Geiselhart, S., Gerber, W. D., & Bille, A. (1989). Analgesic-induced chronic headache: Long-term results of withdrawal therapy. *Journal of Neurology, 236,* 9–14.

Diener, H. C., & Wilkinson, M. (Eds.). (1988). *Drug-induced headache.* New York: Springer-Verlag.

Ehde, D. M., & Holm, J. E. (1992). Stress and headache: Comparisons of migraine, tension and headache-free subjects. *Headache Quarterly, Current Treatment and Research, 3,* 54–60.

Fitzpatrick, R. M., Hopkins, A. P., & Harvard-Watts, O. (1983). Social dimensions of healing: A longitudinal study of outcomes of medical management of headaches. *Social Science Medicine, 17,* 501–510.

Ford, M. R., Strobel, C. F., Strong, P., & Szarek, B. L. (1983). Quieting response training: Predictors of long-term outcome. *Biofeedback and Self-Regulation, 8,* 393–408.

Forsythe, W., Gillies, D., & McCarran, M. (1984). Propranolol in the treatment of childhood migraine. *Developmental Medicine and Child Neurology, 19,* 90–96.

Friedman, H., & Taub, H. A. (1985). Extended follow-up study of the effects of brief psychological procedures in migraine therapy. *American Journal of Clinical Hypnosis, 28,* 27–33.

Gauthier, J., Bois, R., Allaire, D., & Drolet, M. (1981). Evaluation of skin temperature biofeedback training at two different sites for migraine. *Journal of Behavioral Medicine, 4,* 407–419.

Gauthier, J. G., & Carrier, S. (1991). Long-term effects of biofeedback on migraine headache: A prospective follow-up study. *Headache, 31*(9), 605–612.

Gauthier, J., Coté, G., Coté, A., & Drolet, M. (in press). Group versus individual thermal biofeedback in the treatment of migraine: A comparative outcome study. *Headache.*

Gauthier, J., Paillé, S., & Roberge, C. (1990). Minimal therapist contact and clinic-based biofeedback in the treatment of migraine. *Canadian Psychology, 31,* 411.

Goldstein, M., & Chen, T. C. (1982). Epidemiology of disabling headache. In M. Critchley, A. R. Friedman, S. Goring, & F. Sicuter (Eds.), *Advances in neurology* (pp. 30–42). New York: Raven Press.

Guarnieri, P., & Blanchard, E. B. (1990). Evaluation of home-based thermal biofeedback treatment of pediatric migraine headache. *Biofeedback and Self-Regulation, 15,* 179–184.

Hale, W. E., May, F. E., Marks, R. G., Moore, M. P., & Stewart, R. B. (1987). Headache in the elderly: An evaluation of risk factors. *Headache, 27,* 272–276.

Haynes, S. N., Cuevas, J., & Gannon, L. R. (1982). The psychophysiological etiology of muscle-contraction headache. *Headache, 22,* 122–132.

Headache Classification Committee of the International Headache Society. (1988). Classification and diagnostic criteria for headache disorders, cranial neuralgias, and facial pain. *Cephalalgia, 8*(Suppl. 7), 13–92.

Hollon, S. D., & DeRubeis, J. (1981). Placebo–psychotherapy combinations: Inappropriate representations of psychotherapy in drug–psychotherapy comparative trials. *Psychology Bulletin, 90,* 467–477.

Holm, J. E., Holroyd, K. A., Hursey, K. G., & Penzien, D. G. (1984). *Tension headache versus headache-free subjects: An evaluation of stressful events, cognitive appraisal, and coping strategies.* Philadelphia, PA: Society of Behavioral Medicine.

Holroyd, K. A. (1993). Integrating pharmacologic and non-pharmacologic treatments. In C. D. Tolison & R. S. Kunkel (Eds.), *Headache diagnosis and interdisciplinary treatment* (pp. 309–320). New York: Urban & Schwartzenberg.

Holroyd, K. A., & Andrasik, F. (1978). Coping and the self-control of chronic tension headache. *Journal of Consulting and Clinical Psychology, 5,* 1036–1045.

Holroyd, K. A., & Andrasik, F. (1982). A cognitive–behavioral approach to recurrent tension and migraine headache. In P. E. Kendall (Ed.), *Advances in cognitive–behavioral research and therapy* (pp. 275–320). New York: Academic Press.

Holroyd, K. A., & Andrasik, F. (1983). Do the effects of cognitive therapy endure? A two-year follow-up of tension headache sufferers treated with cognitive therapy or biofeedback. *Cognitive Therapy and Research, 6,* 325–334.

Holroyd, K. A., Andrasik, F., & Westbrook, T. (1977). Cognitive control of tension headache. *Cognitive Therapy and Research, 1,* 121–133.

Holroyd, K. A., Cordingley, G. E., Pingel, J. D., Jerome, A., Theofanous, A. G., Jackson, D. K., & Leard, L. (1989b). Enhancing the effectiveness of abortive therapy: A controlled evaluation of self-management training. *Headache, 29,* 148–153.

Holroyd, K. A., France, J. L., Cordingley, G. E., Rokiki, L., Kvaal, S., Lipchik, G. L., & McCool, H. R. (in press). Enhancing the effectiveness of relaxation-thermal biofeedback training with propranolol hydrochloride. *Journal of Consulting and Clinical Psychology.*

Holroyd, K. A., Holm, J. E., Hursey, K. G., Penzien, D. B., Cordingley, G. E., Theofanous, A. G., Richardson, S. C., & Tobin, D. L. (1988). Home-based behavioral treatment versus abortive pharmacological treatment. *Journal of Consulting and Clinical Psychology, 56,* 218–223.

Holroyd, K. A., Holm, J. E., & Penzien, D. B. (1989a). Long-term maintenance of improvements achieved with (abortive) pharmacological and nonpharmacological treatments for migraine: Preliminary findings. *Biofeedback and Self-Regulation, 14,* 301–308.

Holroyd, K. A., Holm, J. F., Penzien, D. B., Cordingley, G. E., Hursey, K. G., Martin, N. J., & Theofanous, A. (1989c). Long-term maintenance of improvements achieved with (abortive) pharmacological and nonpharmacological treatments for migraine: Preliminary findings. *Biofeedback and Self-Regulation, 14,* 301–308.

Holroyd, K. A., Nash, J. M., Pingel, J. D., Cordingley, G. E., & Jerome, A. (1991). A comparison of pharmacological (amitriptyline HCL) and nonpharmacological (cognitive–behavioral) therapies for chronic tension headaches. *Journal of Consulting and Clinical Psychology, 59,* 387–393.

Holroyd, K. A., & Penzien, D. B. (1986). Client variables in the behavioral treatment of recurrent tension headache: A meta-analytic review. *Journal of Behavioral Medicine, 9,* 515-536.

Holroyd, K. A., & Penzien, D. B. (1990). pharmacological vs. nonpharmacological prophylaxis of recurrent migraine headache: A meta-analytic review of clinical trails. *Pain, 42,* 1–13.

Holroyd, K. A., Penzien, D. B., Hursey, K. G., Tobin, D. L., Rogers, L., Holm, J. E., Marcille, P. J., Hall, J. R., & Chlia, A. G. (1984). Change mechanisms in EMG biofeedback training: Cognitive changes underlying improvements in tension headache. *Journal of Consulting and Clinical Psychology, 52,* 1039–1053.

Jacob, R. G., Turner, S. N., Szekely, B. C., & Edelman, B. H. (1983). Predicting outcome of relaxation therapy in headaches: The role of "depression." *Behavior Therapy, 14,* 457–465.

Jurish, S. E., Blanchard, E. B., Andrasik, F., Teders, S. J., Neff, D. F., & Arena, J. G. (1983). Home- versus clinic-based treatment of vascular headache. *Journal of Consulting and Clinical Psychology, 51,* 743–751.

Kabela, E., Blanchard, E. B., Appelbaum, K. A., & Nicholson, N. L. (1989). Self-regulatory treatment of headache in the elderly. *Biofeedback and Self-Regulation, 14,* 219–228.

Knapp, T. W. (1982). Treating migraine by training in temporal artery vaso-constriction and/or cognitive behavioral coping: A 1-year follow-up. *Journal of Psychosomatic Research, 26,* 551–557.

Kohlenberg, R. J. (1984, August). *Self-help treatment of migraine headache: An outcome study.* Paper presented at the American Psychological Association Convention, Washington, DC.

Kudrow, L. (1982). Paradoxical effects of frequent analgesic use. In M. Critchley, A. P. Friedman, S. Gorini, & F. Sicuteri (Eds.), *Advances in neurology: Headache: Physiopathological and clinical concepts* (pp. 335–341). New York: Raven Press.

Labbé, A. E., & Williamson, D. A. (1984). Treatment of childhood migraine using autogenic feedback training. *Journal of Consulting and Clinical Psychology, 52,* 968–976.

Lake, A., Rainey, J., & Papsdorf, J. D. (1979). Biofeedback and rational emotive therapy in the management of migraine headache. *Journal of Applied Behavioral Analysis, 12,* 127–140.

Langemark, M., & Olesen, J. (1987). Pericranial tenderness in tension headache: A blind, controlled study. *Cephalalgia, 7,* 249–255.

Larsson, B., & Melin, L. (1988). The psychological treatment of recurrent headache in adolescents— Short-term outcome and its prediction. *Headache, 28,* 187–195.

Larsson, B., Melin, L., & Döberl, A. (1990). Recurrent tension headache in adolescents treated with self-help relaxation training and muscle relaxant drug. *Headache, 30,* 665–671.

Lascelles, M. A., McGrath, P. J., Sullivan, M.J.L., & Wesk, A. (1991). Self-administered treatments for adolescents with headache: Description, applications and limitations. *Headache Quarterly—Current Treatment and Research, 2,* 196–200.

Leviton, A. (1978). Epidemiology of headache. In B. S. Schoenberg (Ed.), *Advances in neurology* (Vol. 19, pp. 341–352). New York: Raven Press.

Lisspers, J., & Ost, L. G. (1990). Long-term follow-up with migraine treatment: Do the effects remain up to six years? *Behaviour Research and Therapy, 28,* 313–322.

Ludvigsson, J. (1974). Propranolol used in prophylaxis of migraine in children. *Acta Neurologica Scandinavica, 50,* 109–115.

Martin, N., Holroyd, K., & Penzien, D. (1990). The headache-specific locus-of-control scale: Adaptation to recurrent headaches. *Headache, 30,* 729–734.

Martin, N., Holroyd, K., & Rokiki, L. (1993). The Headache Self-Efficacy Scale. *Headache, 33,* 244–248.

Mathew, N. T. (1981). Prophylaxis of migraine and mixed headache: A randomized controlled study. *Headache, 21,* 105–109.

Mathew, N. T., Kurman, R., & Perez, F. (1989). Intractable chronic daily headache: A persistant neurobeavioral disorder. *Cephalalgia, 9*(Suppl. 1a), 180–181.

Mathew, N. T., Reuveni, V., & Perez, F. (1987). Transformed or evolutive headache. *Headache, 27,* 102–106.

McDonald, J. T. (1986). Childhood migraine: Differential diagnosis and treatment. *Postgraduate Medicine, 80,* 301–306.

McGrath, P. J,. Humphreys, P., Goodman, J. T., Keene, D., Firestone, P., Jacob, P., & Cunningham, S. J. (1988). Relaxation prophylaxis for childhood migraine: A randomized placebo-controlled trial. *Developmental medicine and Child Neurology, 30,* 626–631.

McGrath, P. J,. Humphreys, P,. Keene, D., Goodman, J. T., Lascelles, M. A., Cunningham, S. J., & Firestone, P. (1992). The efficacy and efficiency of a self-administered treatment for adolescent migraine. *Pain, 49,* 321–324.

Medina, J. L., Diamond, S., & Franklin, M. A. (1976). Biofeedback therapy for migraine. *Headache, 16,* 115–118.

Mehegan, J. E., masek, B. J., Harrison, R. H., Russo, D. C., & Leviton, A. (1984). *Behavioral treatment of pediatric headache.* Unpublished manuscript, Boston Children's Hospital, Boston, MA.

Merikangas, K. R., Angst, J,. & Isler, H. (1990). Migraine and psychopathology. *Archives of General Psychiatry, 47,* 894–852.

Michultka, D. M., Blanchard, E. B., Appelbaum, K. A., Jaccard, J., & Dentinger, M. P. (1989). The refractory headache patient: 2 high medication consumption (analgesic rebound) headache. *Behaviour Research and Therapy, 27,* 411–420.

Moseley, T. H., Penzien, D. B., Johnson, C. A., Brantley, P. J., Wittrock, D. A., Andrew, M. E., & Payne, T. J. (1991). Time series analysis of stress and headache. *Cephalgia, 11,* 306–307.

Moskowitz, M. A. (1990). Basic mechanisms of headache. *Neurology Clinics, 8,* 801–815.

Murphy, A. I., Lehrer, P. M., & Jurish, S. (1990). Cognitive coping skills training and relaxation training as treatments for tension headaches. *Behavior Therapy, 21,* 89–98.

Nash, J., & Holroyd, K. (1992). Home-based behavioral treatment for recurrent headache: A cost-effective alternative. *American Pain Society Bulletin, 2,* 1–6.

Olesen, J. (1991). Clinical and pathophysiological observations in migraine and tension-type headache explained by integration of vascular, supraspinal and myofacial inputs. *Pain, 46,* 125–132.

Olesen, J., & Edvinsson, L. (Eds.). (1988). *Basic mechanisms of headache.* Amsterdam: Elsevier.

Olesen, J., Larsen, B., & Lauritzen, M. (1981). Focal hyperemia followed by spreading oligemia and impaired activation of rCBF in classic migraine. *Annals of Neurology, 9,* 344–352.

Olness, K., MacDonald, J. T., Uden, D. L. (1987). Comparison of self-hypnosis and propranolol in the treatment of juvenile migraine. *Pediatrics, 79,* 593–597.

Osterhaus, J. T., & Townsend, R. J. (1991). The quality of life of migraineurs: A cross sectional profile. *Cephalalgia, 11*(Suppl. 1), 103–104.

Packard, R. C., & O'Connell, P. (1986). Medication compliance among headache patients. *Headache, 26,* 416–419.

Paiva, T., Nunes, J. S., Moreira, A., Santos, J., Teixeira, J., & Barbosa, A. (1982). Effects of frontalis EMG biofeedback and diazepam in the treatment of tension headache. *Headache, 22,* 216–220.

Penzien, D. B., Andrew, M. E., Knowlton, G. E., McAnulty, R. D., Rains, J. C., Johnson, C. A., Hursey, K. G,. & Jacks, S. D. (1991). Computer-aided system for headache diagnosis with the IHS headache diagnostic criteria: Development and validation. *Cephalgia, 11*(Suppl. 11), 325–326.

Penzien, D. B., Holroyd, K. A., Hursey, K. G., Holm, J. E., & Wittchen, H. U. (1985). *Behavioral treatment of recurrent migraine: A meta-analysis of over five-dozen group outcome studies.* Paper presented at the meeting of the Association for Advancement of Behavior Therapy, November, Houston, TX.

Penzien, D. B., Johnson, C. A., Carpenter, D. E., Prather, R. C., Beckham, J. C., Porzelius, J. Campos, P. E., Perkins, T. S., Krug, L., Pbert, L., Payne, T. J., & Holroyd, K. (1989). *Home-based behavioral treatment vs. propranolol for recurrent migraine: Preliminary findings.* Paper presented at the meeting of the Society for Behavioral Medicine, March, San Francisco, CA.

Penzien, D. D., Rains, J. C., & Holroyd, K. (1993). Psychological assessment of the recurrent headache sufferer. In C. D. Tollison & R. S. Kunkel (Eds.), *Headache: Diagnostic and interdisciplinary treatment* (pp. 39–50). Baltimore, MD: Urban & Schwartzenberg.

Rapoport, A. M. (1988). Analgesic rebound headache. *Headache, 28,* 662–665.

Raskin, N. H. (1988). *Headache.* New York: Churchill Livingstone.

Rasmussen, B. K., Jensen, R., & Olesen, J. (1991). A population-based analysis of the diagnostic criteria at the International Headache Society. *Cephalgia, 11,* 129–134.

Rasmussen, R., Jensen, M., Schroll, & Olesen, J. (1991). Epidemiology of headache in a general population—A prevalence study. *Journal of Clinical Epidemiology, 44,* 1147–1157.

Reich, B. A., & Gottesman, M. (1993). Biofeedback and psychotherapy in the treatment of muscle contraction/tension-type headache. In C. D. Tolison & R. S. Kunkel (Eds.), *Headache diagnosis and interdisciplinary treatment* (pp. 167–180). New York: Urban & Schwartzenberg.

Reinking, R. H., & Hutchings, D. (1981). Follow-up to "Tension headaches: What form of therapy is most effective?" *Biofeedback and Self-Regulation, 6,* 57–62.

Richardson, G. M., & McGrath, P. J. (1989). Cognitive–behavioral therapy for migraine headaches: A minimal-therapist-contact approach versus a clinic-based approach. *Headache, 29,* 352–357.

Richter, I. L., McGrath, P. J., Humphreys, P. J., Goodman, J. T., Firestone, P., & Keene, D. (1986). Cognitive and relaxation treatment of pediatric migraine. *Pain, 25,* 195–203.

Rose, S. D. (1990). *Working with adults in groups.* San Francisco: Jossey-Bass.

Sargent, J., Solbach, P., Coyne, L., Spohn, H., & Fegerson, J. (1986). Results of a controlled, experimental, outcome study of non-drug treatments with a control of migraine headaches. *Journal of Behavioral Medicine, 9,* 291–323.

Schoenen, J., Jamart, B., Gerard, P., Lenarduzzi, P., & Delwaide, P. (1987). Exteroceptive suppression of temporalis muscle activity in chronic headache. *Neurology, 37,* 1834–1836.

Scholz, E., Diener, H. C. & Geiselhart, S. (1988). Drug-induced headache—Does a critical dosage exist? In H. C. Diener & M. Wilkinson (Eds.), *Drug-induced headache* (pp. 29–43). New York: Springer-Verlag.

Sillanpaa, M. (1983). Prevalence of headache in puberty. *Headache, 23,* 10–14.

Silver, B. V., Blanchard, E. B., Williamson, D. A., Theobald, P. E., & Brown, D. A. (1979). Temperature biofeedback and relaxation training in the treatment of migraine headaches: One-year follow-up. *Biofeedback and Self-Regulation, 4,* 359–366.

Solomon, G. D., Kunkel, R. S., & Frame, J. (1990). Demographics of headache in elderly patients. *Headache, 30,* 273–276.

Sorbi, M., Tellegen, B., & DuLong, A. (1989). Long-term effects of training and relaxation and stress-coping in patients with migraine: A three-year follow-up. *Headache, 29,* 111–121.

Stewart, A., Greenfield, S., Hays, R., Wells, K., Rogers, W. H., Berry, S., McGlynn, E. A., & Ware, J. E. (1989). Functional status and well-being of patients with chronic conditions. *Journal of the American Medical Association, 262,* 907–913.

Stewart, W. F., Lipton, R. B., Celentano, D. D., & Reed, J. L. (1992). Prevalence of migraine headache in the United States: Relationship to age, income, race and other sociodemographic factors. *Journal of the American Medical association, 267,* 64–69.

Teders, S. J., Blanchard, E. B., Andrasik, F., Jurish, S. E., Neff, D. F., & Arena, J. G. (1984). Relaxation training for tension headache: Comparative efficacy and cost-effectiveness of a minimal therapist contact versus a therapist delivered procedure. *Behavior Therapy, 15,* 59–70.

Tobin, D. L., Holroyd, K. A., Baker, A., Reynolds, R.V.C., & Holm, J. E. (1988). Development and clinical trial of a minimal contact, cognitive–behavioral treatment for tension headache. *Cognitive Therapy and Research, 12*(4), 325–339.

Wallston, K. A. (1992). Hocus-pocus: The focus isn't strictly on locus: Rotter's social learning theory modified for health. *Cognitive Therapy and Research, 16*(2), 183–199.

Werder, D. S., & Sargent, J. D. (1984). A study of childhood headache using biofeedback as treatment alternative. *Headache, 24,* 122–126.

Wittrock, D. A., Penzien, D. B., Moseley, J. H., & Johnson, C. A. (1991). The recurrent illness impairment profile: Preliminary results using the headache version. *Headache Quarterly, Current Treatment and Research 2,* 138–139.

2

Recent Trends in Asthma Research

Thomas L. Creer and Bruce G. Bender

INTRODUCTION

If there is one word that peppers any discussion of asthma, it is *complex*. The term repeatedly reappears throughout recent discussions of the disorder, whether it occurs in proposing how to define the condition or in describing the pathophysiology of the condition. Furthermore, it is a rare conversation among scientists who investigate asthma, especially those who have studied the disorder for a period of time, that does not end with participants shaking their heads and muttering something about how complex asthma seems to have become. Readers will come to appreciate this complexity during the following brief discussion of three topics: definition of asthma, characteristics of the disorder, and model of pathophysiology.

DEFINITION OF ASTHMA

Researchers have made several attempts to define asthma. Committees composed of experts in the field have met on several occasions in an attempt to arrive at a consensual agreement on a definition of the condition. All attempts have failed. Busse and Reed (1988) noted reasons for this failure. They pointed out that clinicians treating patients need a different definition than either epidemiologists concerned with populations or immunologists investigating pathogenesis of the disor-

---

Thomas L. Creer • Department of Psychology, Ohio University, Athens, Ohio 45701. **Bruce G. Bender** • National Jewish Center for Immunology and Respiratory Medicine, Denver, Colorado 80206. *Handbook of Health and Rehabilitation Psychology,* edited by Anthony J. Goreczny. Plenum Press, New York, 1995.

der. The frames of reference are so diverse and the types of information required so different, it is not surprising that agreement is impossible. The difficulty in defining asthma further increases because of "the complexity and heterogeneity of the genetic, environmental, psychosocial, physiologic, and molecular biologic factors in its pathogenesis, course, and manifestations" (p. 969). Attempts to define asthma in terms of its cause have also failed because the cause of the disorder is unknown.

In an attempt to reach agreement, experts have proposed several operational definitions for asthma. These definitions may include a listing of criteria, such as the proposed definitions of the Allergy Foundation of America or the American Thoracic Society (Busse & Reed, 1988; Reed & Townley, 1983), or a simple statement, such as that by Canny and Levison (1990). There are problems with both approaches; with multiple criteria, arriving at an operational definition that totally excludes other respiratory disorders has been unachievable. For example, differences between chronic bronchitis and asthma can be subtle and obscure (Bernstein, 1983). This has meant that one fourth of adults with chronic bronchitis will meet most established criteria for asthma as well. Levison (1991) cautioned that misdiagnosis of asthma is common in children because clinicians often confuse asthma with chronic bronchitis and bronchiolitis. For this reason, Canny and Levison (1990) offered a general definition of asthma: "We propose that any child, regardless of age, with recurrent (three or more) episodes of wheezing and/or dyspnea should be considered as having asthma until proven otherwise" (p. 406). Definitions with multiple criteria are necessary for research purposes; they may, however, provide little value to clinicians who concentrate on treatment of patients. Simple statement definitions, such as the one Canny and Levision proposed are too general for scientific purposes but are invaluable to clinicians. These definitions only reflect operational descriptions of asthma. Arriving at an operational definition of an asthma attack, required for assessment of the condition, involves a totally separate process that entails obtaining agreement among medical personnel, behavioral scientists, and patients (Creer, 1992).

CHARACTERISTICS OF ASTHMA

Despite difficulties in defining asthma, most experts agree on the intermittent, variable, and reversible nature of the disorder. There is, however, considerable heterogeneity, both among patients and within individual patients, regarding these characteristics.

Intermittency of Attacks

The frequency of attacks varies from patient to patient and, for a given individual, from time to time. One patient may suffer a burst of attacks during a period of a few days and then go several months, even years, between attacks. Another patient may have perennial asthma and experience attacks most days throughout the year. Frequency of attacks experienced by patients is a function of several variables, including number and diversity of stimuli that trigger their asthma, degree of hyperreactivity of their airways, degree of control established over their disorder, and patient variables, such as medication compliance and symptom discrimination.

Variability of Attacks

Variability of asthma refers both to severity of a patient's asthma and to intensity of discrete attacks. Use of the term in this framework is somewhat confusing because it is not always clear whether the label refers to the general condition of patients or to specific attacks they experience. Creer, Reynolds, and Kotses (1991) pointed out that asthma severity presents two major concerns to medical and behavioral scientists. First, there is no standard way of classifying either a given attack or the overall asthma of a patient as mild, moderate, or severe. Although authors use such classification terms throughout the literature on asthma, there are no common criteria for their use. Second, lack of operational definitions regarding severity, both of asthma and separate attacks, complicates the matter of assessing the condition over time. Finally, Renne and Creer (1985) warn that patients acquire different expectations because of the severity of their asthma. If their attacks are mild, they anticipate all future episodes will be mild. They therefore do not prepare to cope with more severe attacks. On the other hand, a single severe attack can color expectations of patients regarding future attacks. Creer (1979) noted that, in most cases, patients who panic during their attacks acquired that behavioral pattern because of a single severe attack when they or those around them became very frightened.

Reversibility of Attacks

McFadden (1980) referred to reversibility as the *sine qua non* of asthma; it distinguishes asthma from other types of respiratory disorders, particularly emphysema, in which reversibility does not occur. As with the other characteristics of asthma, however, the reversibility characteristic presents additional enigmas. First, reversibility is a relative condition. Although the majority of asthma patients show complete reversibility of airway obstruction, others do not attain total reversibility of their asthma, even with intensive therapy (Loren et al., 1978). Second, the spontaneous remission of some attacks makes it virtually impossible to prove with certainty a cause-effect relationship between changes in a patient's asthma and a given treatment for the disorder (Creer, 1982).

PATHOPHYSIOLOGY OF ASTHMA

Difficulties defining asthma and characteristics of the disorder reveal something about the intricacies of asthma. A brief description of current knowledge and thought concerning the pathogenesis of asthma results in a broader perspective of the perplexing nature of asthma. It is important that behavioral scientists understand current trends if they are to make a contribution to unraveling the mystery of asthma. Figure 2.1 presents a model of asthma. Description of the aspects of this model follow.

Stimuli

Reed and Townley (1983) listed irritants, exercise and cold air, respiratory infections, allergens, aspirin and related substances, and situations and emotional

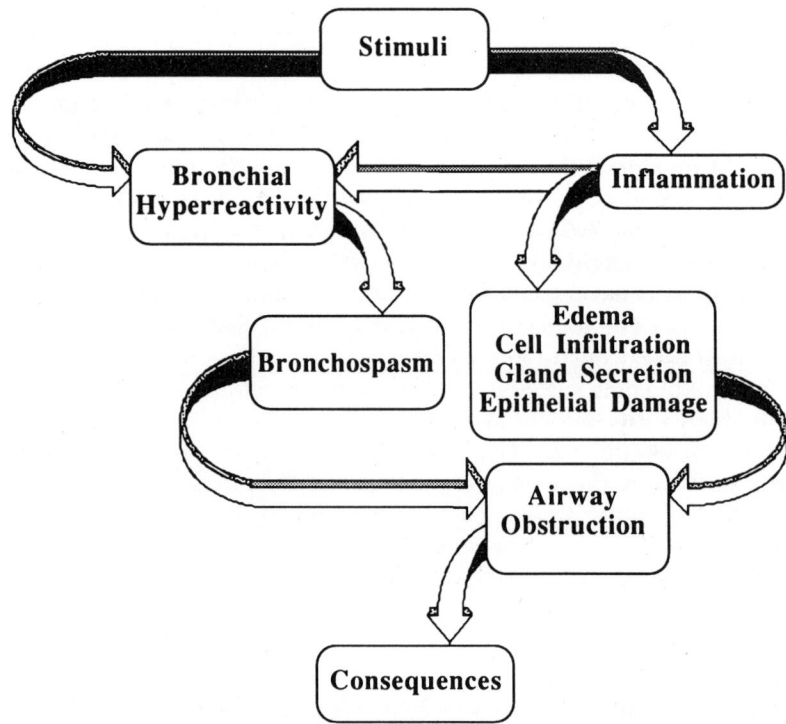

Figure 2.1. Model of asthma.

responses as potential stimuli involved in pathogenesis of asthma. The initial three categories of stimuli affect everyone with asthma; the last three categories affect only some patients and vary substantially among individuals. The exact stimulus or stimuli that provoke a given attack vary both across and within patients. Thus, it is frivolous to say with certainty that a stimulus or set of stimuli "caused" asthma; the best that one can accomplish is to identify stimuli correlated with a specific attack (Creer & Kotses, 1990). Finally, to tighten the Gordian knot regarding causes of asthma, Reed and Townley noted that "some episodes of asthma do not have a recognizable stimulus" (p. 813).

Linkage of Stimuli to Responses

Reed and Townley (1983) discussed several factors that link stimuli to the physiological responses that comprise asthma. There exist two prominent physiological events: inflammation and bronchial hyperreactivity. In recent years, researchers have given increased attention to the concept that airway inflammation underlies asthma. As Madison (1991) explained, "Inflammation of the airways, whether it be stimulated by immunologic or nonimmunologic mechanisms, may be the critical event that promotes the development of asthma in general" (p. 175). Ellis (1988) regarded increased bronchial reactivity or hyperresponsiveness as "a fundamental and intrinsic characteristic of all individuals with asthma, both children and adults" (p. 1039). This means that asthma patients are more responsive than normal patients to a wide diversity of stimuli. Precisely how inflammation occurs in the airways and how it relates to bronchial hyperresponsiveness is unknown (Madison, 1991). There are a number of cells and mediators that may play a role in this relationship; discussion of these mediators is beyond the purview of this chapter, however.

Figure 2.1 provides a working model of asthma that is of value to both medical and behavioral scientists. To the former, it illustrates current research and thought concerning asthma; the model depicts the prototype that will guide medical scientists in developing effective approaches to the management of asthma. To achieve this goal, they will focus on stimuli, airway obstruction, and factors linking stimuli to airway obstruction. The focus of behavioral scientists will remain both on stimuli correlated with airway obstruction and consequences of asthma. Before describing selected topics regarding stimuli and consequences related to asthma, however, we will briefly discuss psychological and behavioral assessment.

ASSESSMENT

Depending on the aims of the investigator, clinicians and researchers can utilize several approaches to assess adults with asthma. One example includes the Revised Asthma Problem Checklist (Creer et al., 1989), a 76-item paper-and-pencil instrument used to elicit information related to asthma from adults and children, as well as members of their families. It is helpful in identifying potential problems that might be amenable to behavioral or medical intervention. The instrument has solid validity and reliability (Creer, 1992; Creer et al., 1989). In addition, the instrument provides a 5-point rating scale for each item; this permits use of the instrument as an outcome measure. The Asthma Self-Efficacy Scale (Tobin, Wigal, Winder, Holroyd, & Creer, 1987) is a valid and reliable 80-item paper-and-pencil instrument designed to measure patients' self-efficacy concerning their ability to control asthma. It, too, is useful both as a screening instrument and an outcome measure. Finally, investigators have used commercially available instruments, such as the Minnesota Multiphasic Personality Inventory (MMPI). One example of such use is a research project that assessed whether patients who have a near-fatal attack differ from control patients who do not have such experiences (Boulet, Deschesnes, Turcotte, & Gignac, 1991).

More than has been the case with adults, investigators have directed a considerable amount of research in the last two decades toward elucidating the psychological implications of childhood asthma. These studies have included psychological characteristics of asthmatic children and their families, effects of asthma upon psychological development, and mediating effects of children's psychological variables upon adaptation to illness and treatment. Investigators in the field have utilized a variety of dependent measures for psychological and behavioral assessment of childhood asthma. For many investigators, a well-developed instrument used with a variety of pediatric populations can be the best choice for a valid and reliable assessment of psychological functioning in asthmatic children. Creer (1991b) identified a list of published psychological instruments that can be useful to investigators evaluating personality (e.g., Personality Inventory for Children, California Psychological Inventory, Child Anxiety Scale, Children's Depression Inventory, Piers–Harris Children's Self-Concept Scale), intelligence (e.g., Kaufman Assessment Battery for Children, Porteus Mazes, Wechsler Intelligence Scale for Children–Revised), general achievement (e.g., Wide-Range Achievement Test–Revised, Woodcock Johnson Psycho-Educational Battery), and neuropsychologic functioning (e.g., Halstead–Reitan Neuropsychological Test Battery for Children, Luria–Nebraska Neuropsychological Battery).

Some questions in pediatric asthma require information that general-purpose psychological instruments cannot provide. Specifically, concerns about medication compliance, medication side effects, effects of anoxia on the brain, family dysfunction, quality of life, and asthma self-management have required utilization of less widely published experimental measures, and, in some cases, necessitated development of asthma-specific measures. In the following sections, we describe aspects of several of these topics, including compliance, medication side-effects, and quality of life.

STIMULI

A wealth of studies have attempted to identify and, at times, change behaviors that correlate either with the onset of asthma or factors that trigger the disorder. Review of such studies could address several topics including smoking, illicit drug use, and suggestion. However, we selected four topics for discussion: medication compliance, avoidance and escape from triggers of asthma, risk-factor analysis, and emotional responses.

Medication Compliance

In the past decade, almost all research conducted on medication compliance or adherence and asthma has utilized children as subjects. Discussions of relative benefits of various medications used to treat childhood asthma frequently fail to consider patient adherence. Noncompliance is not simply a matter of inconvenience affecting a small number of patients. Patient compliance in the use of prescribed medications to control chronic illness is, on average, 50% (Eraker, Kirscht, & Becker, 1984). Noncompliance of medication used to control chronic illness is particularly problematic when benefits of medication use are not immediately apparent after dosing and when patients do not believe that medication intervention will effectively change the course of their illness (Conrad, 1985). Frequency of dosing is also a factor; adherence generally decreases when patients must take medications two or three times per day (Cramer, Mattson, Prevey, Scheyer, & Ouellette, 1989). Given the high rate of noncompliance, conclusions about drug effectiveness from clinical trials may be erroneous (Sbarbaro & Steiner, 1991). Investigators from one study noted that adherence among asthmatic patients was so variable that valid conclusions about drug effectiveness were available for only 10 of 34 patients (29%) in their study (Mawhinney et al., 1991).

The inaccuracy in methods of assessing compliance complicates attempts to understand the relationship between medications, compliance, and control of asthma. Pill counts and diary cards, frequent compliance measures used in research, are often inaccurate. One investigation demonstrated a 36% discrepancy between pill counts and physiological measures of antacid consumption in ulcer patients (Roth,

Carson, & Hsi, 1970). Another technique, similar to pill counts, involves weighing canisters of aerosolized medications to determine whether amount of medication used by patients is consistent with physicians' prescriptions, one recent study found 13.7% of participants discharged several bursts of aerosol into the air on their way to a scheduled appointment to give an artificial appearance of compliance (Rand et al., 1992). A second measure of patient compliance, the drug diary, may be equally deceptive. In a study of 19 asthmatic patients treated with aerosolized medications, patients failed to record their medication usage in their drug diaries and over-reported appropriate usage by more than 50% (Mawhinney et al., 1991). Unfortunately, because pill counts, canister weighing, and diary cards generally underestimate overall patient adherence in use of medication, conclusions drawn from studies using them may be invalid.

Inaccurate self-reporting of compliance in clinical investigations indicates a need for more objective measures of patient compliance in such studies. One such approach is to directly measure presence of a specific drug in the bloodstream. Investigators can easily measure theophylline directly through blood serum assays (Ellis, 1988). This is not the case for all asthma medications, however. In some cases, pharmacists can add a riboflavin tracer to medications to assess compliance (Creer, 1991a). This approach is objective, direct, and quantifiable. However, several factors complicate measurement of theophylline or riboflavin in the blood. These complicating factors include variable rates of absorption, metabolism, and elimination; interactions between the measured drug and other substances; and timing of measurement. Blood assay techniques also have other limitations; parents may become reluctant to have blood drawn from their children, and parents may give the appearance of adherence by increasing their children's medication consumption immediately before an appointment.

Recent studies have employed electronic technology to significantly advance objective evaluation of patient compliance in the use of both pill and aerosolized medications for treating asthma. Several such investigations have utilized a nebulizer chronolog, a portable device that houses a standard nebulizer canister and records date and time of each use of aerosolized medication (Mawhinney et al., 1991; Spector et al., 1986; Tashkin et al., 1991). Other studies have utilized advanced methodologies (e.g., microprocessors) for recording date and time of medication removal from pill containers (Cramer et al., 1989; Eisen, Miller, & Woodward, 1990). The use of microprocessors to record medication use moves significantly beyond previous compliance methodology by providing the capacity not only to determine how much medication patients have consumed, but also patterns of medication usage. For example, one recent study (Rand et al., 1992) followed 115 patients with respiratory obstructions. Intriguingly, canister weight change classified 83% of the patients as having satisfactory or better adherence, and 73% of the patients reported appropriate daily use of their inhalers on their diary cards. Information recorded by their nebulizer chronologs, however, indicated that only 15% of the individuals used the inhaler appropriately.

The assessment of compliance may also extend to aspects of asthma self-management other than medication utilization. For example, clinicians frequently ask patients to take various steps to monitor their asthma symptoms at home and to alter activities, take medications, or contact their physician, depending upon results of this self-monitoring. Peak flow meters allow children or adult asthmatics to measure pulmonary efficiency at home (Wright & McKerrow, 1959). However, recent evidence indicates that although use of objective measures of air flow obstruction can lead to improvement in patient conditions (Bauman et al., 1989), many patients are noncompliant in following directions for use of peak flow meters in home management (Clark, Evans, & Mellins, 1992). Microprocessor-based technology to monitor home peak flow measurement, similar to devices used to evaluate medication compliance, may soon be available.

Avoidance or Escape from Asthma Triggers

Patients can learn to avoid stimuli known to trigger their asthma. By doing so, they may be able to prevent unnecessary attacks or, in the case of ongoing episodes, to escape from the stimuli that may have precipitated their asthma. A number of studies have demonstrated that children with asthma can learn to avoid stimuli that precipitate their asthma, such as allergens or irritants (e.g., Baum & Creer, 1986; Creer et al., 1988). In the study by Baum and Creer, for example, 24% of a sample of children with asthma indicated that they attempted to avoid or escape from stimuli correlated with their asthma as the initial step in their management of attacks. Following training, the percentage jumped to 73%, thus demonstrating that a brief educational intervention was effective in teaching patients to avoid or escape from known precipitants of their attacks. Creer, Renne, and Christian (1976) summarized findings showing that, when allowed to participate in physical activities, children with asthma learned to gauge their participation to avoid exercise-induced asthma. Plaut (1988) presented several illustrations of children who learned to avoid exercise-induced asthma by taking preventative steps, such as premedicating themselves, as prescribed by their physicians, before participating in events that could precipitate attacks. Specific instructions on how to avoid triggers of their asthma are a major component in both self-management programs (Creer et al., 1988) and self-help manuals for the disorder (Plaut, 1988). Recently, Creer (1991c) suggested that, in some cases, patients with asthma could avoid asthma attacks by preparing for the likelihood that they might experience asthmatic episodes. The author suggested two strategies to assist in such preparation. First, asthmatic patients need to monitor their respiratory responses during peak periods when they might experience asthma; this would be the case especially with patients who experience seasonal asthma. The use of peak flow meters, with values recorded twice daily in an asthma diary, would serve this purpose. Second, patients and their families would benefit by taking the following steps as they approach a season or event when attacks are most likely to occur: (1) prepare to avoid and escape known precipitants; (2) review treatment protocols with their physicians and be certain that necessary medications are available; and (3) rehearse asthma management steps.

Risk-Factor Analysis

Risk-factor analysis is based on the premise that the only certainty about asthma is the probable nature of the condition. Characteristics of asthma, such as intermittency of attacks, severity, and degree of reversibilty, represent probabilistic variables. The combinations and permutations of these variables set limits that one can achieve in controlling asthma. Table 2.1 summarizes research that investigators undertook to

Table 2.1. Risk-Factor Analysis of Precipitating Stimuli for Asthma

Stimuli	Probability equation	References
PEFR	$P_t(A) = F(P_{t-k}, B_{t-k})$	Taplin & Creer, 1978 Harm et al., 1985 Kotses et al., 1991 Pinzone et al., 1991
Medication compliance	$P_t(A) = F(B_{t-k})$	Creer, 1979 Kotses et al., 1991 Pinzone et al., 1991

Environmental factors
  Mold
  Ragweed
  Temperature change
  Dust
	$P_t(A) = F(E_{t-k})$	Stout et al., 1991
		Kotses et al., 1991

Emotional factors Anxiety	$P_t(A) = F(Em_{t-k})$	Kotses et al., 1991
Exercise	$P_t(A) = F(P_{t-k}, B_{t-k})$	Kotses et al., 1991 Pinzone et al., 1991

Note. $P_t(A)$ = Probability of asthma at a given moment; F = Function; P = Physiological; B = Behavior; E = Environment; Em = Emotion; $t-k$ = Past history.

determine the probability that known precipitants of patients' attacks or respiratory responses can predict likelihood of patients' future attacks. Researchers based initial studies in attack prediction on patients' responses, namely their peak flow values. Peak-flow values, also called peak expiratory flow rates (PEFR) and obtained with a peak flow meter, provide a measure of *pulmonary physiology,* defined as the fastest air flow rate sustained by a patient for at least 10 milliseconds during forced exhalation (Wright & McKerrow, 1959). Taplin and Creer (1978) reported the initial demonstration of use of peak flow values to predict asthma. They entered peak flow values into a conditional probability equation to predict occurrence of asthma with two children. The investigators individually determined for each child, the baserate, or prior probability of likelihood of an attack, and a critical peak flow value that most enhanced predictability of asthma. The investigators then calculated two conditional probabilities for each subject: (1) the probability of asthma occurring in a 12-hour period following a flow rate less than or equal to the critical value, and (2) the probability of asthma occurring in a 12-hour period following a flow rate greater than the critical value. Using this procedure, Taplin and Creer (1978) obtained approximately a 300% increase over the base rate in predicting asthma in their subjects. Harm, Kotses, and Creer (1985) extended the procedure with 25 asthmatic children and found the average improvement in predictability probability was approximately 500%.

Recent studies have investigated the possibility that variables other than PEFR can predict attacks. Pinzone, Carlson, Kotses, and Creer (1991) examined medication compliance and exercise data to predict asthma attacks in 10 patients. They found that exercise predicted probability of attacks in 2 of 5 subjects with exercise-induced asthma; however, they found that medication compliance was not predictive of asthma attacks even though Creer (1979) earlier found that missing a medication dose predicted 100% of the attacks one child experienced. Pinzone and her colleagues reported that peak flow values predicted attacks in 9 of their 10 subjects; furthermore, exercise and time of day further enhanced prediction of attacks. Stout, Kotses, Carlson, and Creer (1991) examined the degree to which asthma attacks correlated with seven environmental variables determined for each of 17 adults with asthma. Using stepwise regression procedures, the investigators found that cladosporium mold, ragweed pollen, and temperature change were significant predictors of attacks. Stout and co-workers concluded that knowledge of the probability of occurrence of known risk or predictor factors, unique to each individual, could predict likelihood that an individual would experience asthma within a present time frame.

Research on risk prediction has three implications (Creer, 1991c; Creer, Kotses, & Wigal, 1992). First, physicians can use information gathered in these studies not only to refine their predictions of future attacks of individual patients, but also to tailor strategies to allow patients to prevent some attacks. Second, with the experimental basis of attack prediction firmly established, treatment team members can help develop simple tactics to permit patients to predict, on the basis of changes they detect through self-monitoring, the probability of experiencing an asthma attack within a set period of time. When patients keep accurate information on environmental, physiological, and behavioral stimuli unique to them, they can determine through simple arithmetic the likelihood of whether they will experience asthma in a coming period of time. Finally Kotses et al. (1991) employed risk factor data to develop individualized self-management programs for 8 patients with asthma. Baseline data revealed which stimuli correlated with patients' attacks; team members then entered this information into an equation to determine the probability that the identified stimuli would produce asthma in individual patients within a predetermined period of time. Subsequently, investigators randomly assigned subjects to either an experimental or control group. Experimental patients received a brief intervention program aimed at preventing attacks. Although this project involved only a small number of patients, results showed a 22% decrease in number of attacks in the experimental group. A refinement of this procedure led to even more impressive findings with 30 asthmatic patients (H. Kotses, personal communication, May 1, 1992).

Emotional Reactions

The role of emotions in asthma has mystified both patients and scientists for centuries. There is little doubt that emotional reactions can influence asthma, although most individuals generally believe that emotions affect an ongoing attack rather than serve as a stimulus for an asthmatic episode. The real problem, and the reason that emotions and asthma are such a conundrum, is that there is no satisfactory way to assess emotions. There are four reasons for the dilemma (Creer & Kotses,. 1990). First, it is impossible to standardize the stimuli that could induce emotions or the emotional reactions that could trigger an attack. These stimuli are ideosyncratic to each patient. Second, it would be difficult to quantitatively assess the emotional response that occurs with presentation of a given stimulus. This will vary from patient to patient and as a function of the context within which presentation of the stimulus occurs. Third, it is often difficult to determine, in the real world, whether an emotional reaction is the cause or consequence of asthma. Finally, the nature of the relationship between emotions and asthma is a complex physiological enigma. Plausible pathways through which emotional events could precipitate attacks include hyperventilation, hypocapnia, vagal bronchoconstriction, changes in adrenal or cortical function, and endocrine activity (Reed & Townley, 1983). Scientists may never elucidate the exact pathways by which emotions exert an effect on asthma. As R. Cherniack and L. Cherniack (1983) pointed out, it is impossible to provide a complete description of the neural mechanisms involved in human respiration because scientists cannot ethically conduct experiments required to obtain the pertinent information.

CONSEQUENCES

A large number of consequences of asthma are of interest to behavioral scientists. These include (1) behavioral deficits, including lack of symptom discrimination, nonassertiveness, and depression; (2) behavioral excesses, particularly anger, anxiety, panic, and hospital overuse; and (3) cognitive deficits, such as ignorance of asthma and its treatment, overreliance on memory, self-efficacy beliefs, and lack of decision-making skills (Creer & Kotses, 1990; Creer et al., 1992). We elected to discuss two topics because they are both representative and current regarding the potential contribution psychologists and other behavioral scientists can make to the management of asthma. These are the psychological side effects of asthma medications and quality of life.

Psychological Side Effects of Asthma Medications

Physicians can treat asthma with a variety of medications that may relieve bronchospasm, protect the airways from irritant stimuli, prevent pulmonary hyperresponsivity, and decrease inflammation. Although drugs can provide powerful beneficial changes in pulmonary and inflammatory responses, some drugs also have substantial undesirable physiological and psychological side effects. Two medications, theophylline and systemic corticosteroids, have been the subject of particular concern and investigation because of purported psychological side effects. The discussion that follows is a review of attempts to evaluate psychological side effects accompanying these two medications and assessment questions raised by this body of research.

Theophylline

Researchers have been concerned in recent years about possible theophylline-induced changes in children's mood, behavior, and ability to learn (American Asthma Report, 1989; Rachelefsky et al., 1986). Crucial to the question of psychological side effects of theophylline and other asthma medications is the issue of subjectivity. When a group of parents of asthmatic children answered questions about medication side effects, half of the respondents complained that their children experienced restlessness and/or hyperactivity when they took theophylline (American Asthma Report, 1989). A variety of unblinded case reports and case-review studies have also suggested that theophylline use with asthmatic patients may result in depression

(Murphy, Dillon, & Fitzgerald, 1980), stammering (McCarthy, 1981), psychosis (Wasser, Bronheim, & Richardson, 1981), impaired motor skills (Springer, Goldenberg, Ben Dov, & Godfrey, 1985), and weakened impulse control (Firestone & Martin, 1979). However, blinded, controlled studies present a different picture of theophylline side effects. These studies have reported side effects that include decreased classroom adaptation (Furukawa et al., 1984; Rachelefsky et al., 1986), impaired visual–spatial planning (Springer et al., 1985), diminished motor steadiness (Joad, Ahrens, Lindgren, & Weinberger, 1986), and impaired memory and concentration (Furukawa et al., 1988).

In most cases, treatment-related differences were small and there was little consistency across studies. Most intriguing has been the inability of parents to identify theophylline-related changes in their children's behavior when blinded to theophylline versus placebo treatments. Two double-blind, randomized, placebo-controlled crossover studies found no theophylline-related changes on comprehensive batteries of psychological tests (Rappaport et al., 1989; Schlieper, Alcock, Beaudry, Feldman, & Leikin, 1991). In another study, parents reported their belief that theophylline caused undesirable changes in their children's behavior but were unable to blindly discriminate placebo-versus theophylline-phase behavior using a standardized questionnaire (Bender & Milgrom, 1992). Results from these studies, when contrasted with results from the survey of parents in the American Asthma Report (1989), suggest that parents' blinded, objective observations of their children do not support the parents' beliefs that theophylline causes significant behavior change in their asthmatic children.

Corticosteroids

Psychological side effects of corticosteroids have been the subject of even greater controversy than side effects due to theophylline. The adult literature, comprising primarily case reports and case-review studies, indicates that 3% of hospitalized adult patients treated with prednisone experience psychosis. Furthermore, a dose–response relationship appears to be present; patients who receive more than 40 mg per day of prednisone have a significantly greater risk for development of serious psychiatric symptoms than those on lower dosages (Boston Collaborative Drug Surveillance Program, 1972; Ling, Perry, & Tsuang, 1981).

Although few controlled studies of steroid side effects in adults exist, there are several controlled studies of side effects in pediatric populations. Findings from these studies indicate virtually no episodes of significant psychiatric reactions to steroids. However, subtle mood (Bender, Lerner, & Kollasch, 1988; Bender, Lerner, & Poland, 1991; Harris, Carel, Rosenberg, Joshi, & Leventhal, 1986) and memory changes in children do occur, appear dose-related (Bender et al., 1988), and are more likely to occur in children who have a history of emotional dysfunction or come from dysfunctional families (Bender et al., 1991). Although steroid side effects reported among children appear quite different from those reported among adults, it is difficult to determine whether these reflect actual age-mediated differences or different methodologies of these two bodies of literature. As seen in the theophylline side-effects studies, unblinded reports of medication-related psychological problems are subjective and may reflect considerable distortion.

Implications for Further Assessment of Medication Side Effects

We can identify several important conclusions from the often confusing literature addressing theophylline and corticosteroid psychological side effects. Research studies cannot overemphasize the importance of blinded studies. Whether patients tend to develop strong belief systems about their illness and its treatment (Becker et al., 1979), find cause-and-effect relationships between medications and psychological problems that have no objective support, or undergo evaluation for side effects in the course of a research program or for clinical purposes, blinded, placebo controlled procedures are the only means of eliminating subjectivity.

When conducting a blinded evaluation of medication side effects with asthmatic children, it is essential to include parents' observations of their children's behavior wherever possible. Parents have opportunity to observe a wide sampling of behavior outside the laboratory. Also, although parents are often reluctant to relinquish their beliefs that behavior problems seen in their children are attributable to asthma medications, they may be more willing to accept findings that contradict these beliefs if the findings consist, in part, of their own blinded observations. Teachers' observations can also be quite helpful in assessing potential medication side effects, because teachers observe children in settings requiring impulse control, concentration, and learning, behaviors purportedly compromised by some medications. One study found that ratings of teachers, but not parents, could discriminate behavior of children taking theophylline from that of children taking a placebo (Rachelefsky et al., 1986).

The areas of behavior and psychological functioning purportedly affected by theophylline or corticosteroids overlap considerably. Comprehensive evaluation of potential side effects must include a battery of tests measuring each potentially affected area, including attention, impulsivity and physical activity level, memory and learning, visual–motor skills, and self-reported mood. Studies by Rappaport et al. (1989) and Bender and colleagues (1988, 1991, 1992) are representative of this comprehensive battery approach to testing medication side effects; in each case, the investigators chose instruments meeting three criteria: (1) the tests measured behaviors purportedly affected by the medication; (2) administration of the tests could occur on repeated occasions without large practice effects; and (3) most of the tests were relatively time efficient, allowing administration of the entire battery on repeated occasions without placing exhaustive demands on patients. Bender et al. (1988) noted that children's responses to many tests change from the first to the second testing occasion as children become familiar with the test, and these authors recommended administration of baseline practice trials of those tests utilized for repeated evaluation of side effects in order to eliminate this initiation effect.

Quality of Life

Of increasing interest in evaluating patients with asthma, as well as other chronic illnesses, is assessment of *quality of life*. This term has particular appeal in outcome studies, because it suggests the possibility of assessing patients' overall adaptations. In studies evaluating relative effectiveness of various asthma treatment regimens, quality-of-life measures may provide a means of comparison that moves beyond measures of pulmonary function and specific symptoms to provide a broader picture of how individual patients perceive the impact of the illness on their lives.

Although quality-of-life assessment is a burgeoning area of research, numerous problems continue to plague the area. The greatest problem in quality-of-life assessment is definition. The quality-of-life concept is complex and may involve many potential components, including illness symptoms, impact on work, income, social life, sexual activity, physical activity, and subjective mood states (e.g., happiness, well-being, frustration). As the combinations of questions from these areas vary between instruments, the instruments differ in what they measure and, not surprisingly, in their outcomes (Williams & Wood-Dauphinee, 1989). Because quality-of-life measures vary considerably, they are not interchangeable. Two similar studies of treatment outcome using different quality-of-life instruments may draw different conclusions about treatment effectiveness and impact of illness on the lives of individual patients.

Lohr (1989) suggested that all quality-of-life instruments fall somewhere on a measurement continuum depending on whether they utilize restrictive or global concepts. Instruments that fall on the restrictive end of the continuum attempt to evaluate impact of illness on specific areas of functioning (e.g., physical activity), whereas those at the global end attempt to capture a broader and more subjective picture of life adaptation. The global approach has distinct advantages and disadvantages; it appears to move closer to the goal of quality-of-life research (i.e., evaluating broad impact of illness on the individual patient's life) but carries the disadvantages described in the previous paragraph. The restrictive approach, focusing upon one area of a patient's life, lends itself more easily to operational definition; the measurement objective is clearer and more specific, and the researchers are therefore more confident they know what it is they are measuring.

Two quality-of-life instruments recently developed for use specifically in asthma populations demonstrate the heterogeneity of such instruments. The Living with Asthma Questionnaire is a 68-item instrument that includes self-evaluation of both mood (e.g., feeling worried) and somatic (e.g., breathing obstruction) symptoms (Hyland, Finnis, & Irvine, 1991). The authors identified 11 factor-analyzed domains that include social-leisure activities, sports, sleep, holidays, work and other activities, colds, mobility, effects on others, medication usage, doctors, and dysphoric states and attitudes. The Asthma Quality-of-Life Questionnaire, a shorter instrument containing 32 items, also purports to measure quality of life in asthmatic adults (Juniper et al., 1992). In this case, the factor-analyzed subscales include asthma symptoms, responses to environmental stimuli, need to avoid stimuli, limitation of activities, and emotional dysfunction. No information is yet available, beyond examination of specific item content, regarding comparability of these two instruments. It is not clear that either instrument measures a well-defined, global quality-of-life construct, and it is impossible to judge relative outcomes of two different studies of asthma treatment effectiveness if each study uses a different instrument. Other instruments that investigators have used to evaluate quality of life in asthma patients, including the Asthma Symptom Checklist (Kinsman, Luparello, O'Banion, & Spector, 1973) and the Attitudes to Asthma Scale (Sibbald, 1989), are subject to similar criticisms regarding variability and provide little understanding of the underlying concepts or theoretical framework upon which researchers based development of the instruments.

At this point, we must conclude that scientific research has not yet achieved successful measurement of a singular quality-of-life construct. Interestingly, most recently developed quality-of-life instruments generate several subscales purportedly measuring a variety of adaptation dimensions and shy away from a single, overall quality-of-life score. The result is that most of these instruments attempt to do in a single questionnaire what other studies accomplish with the battery approach, but they do it less well. The battery approach, reflecting the more traditional approach to assessment of psychological adaptation in any chronically ill population, involves selection of a series of separate measures of illness symptoms, emotional functioning, social adjustment, and physical activity level. For example, Downey, Erhardt, Gruen, Bell, and Morishima (1989) described the psychological adaptation of Turner's syndrome women after utilizing a battery of self-administered questionnaires and clinician-produced ratings that separately assessed social effectiveness, social support, sexual experiences, psychiatric symptomatology, and overall psychological functioning. The advantages of the battery approach are evident. Researchers and clinicians can utilize well-developed instruments designed to measure one area of psychological functioning and subjected to numerous studies of theoretical and measurement properties with considerably greater confidence than a single instrument that attempts to measure all areas. It may appear both time- and cost-effective to use a single quality-of-life questionnaire, perhaps fulfilling an investigator's dream for an almost effortless, but comprehensive, evaluation of treatment outcome. However, until considerably more development of quality-of-life measurements has occurred, researchers need to use such instruments in outcome studies with great caution; outcome research would be most beneficial if it used these instruments without other outcome measures to allow for comparison and validation of the quality-of-life instruments.

SELF-MANAGEMENT

Self-management of asthma consists of performance of self-initiated competencies by patients to permit them to become partners with medical and behavioral personnel in the control of asthma. We achieve this aim only after patients have learned to integrate current medical and behavioral knowledge and expertise into their own framework of information, abilities, skills, and expectations regarding management of asthma. Self-management techniques have found a fertile home in the treatment of asthma; clinical researchers have developed and tested at least two dozen educational and self-management programs for childhood asthma alone (Wigal, Creer, Kotses, & Lewis, 1990). Although there were methodological shortcomings in many of these first-generation programs, overall, they demonstrated that self-management skills and competencies permit patients to become partners with health-care personnel in the control of asthma (Creer, Wigal, Kotses, & Lewis, 1990).

Figure 2.2 depicts a recently proposed second-generation model for self-management of asthma (Creer et al., 1992). We present the model for two reasons. First, it permits us to synthesize the topics we have discussed into a common conceptual structure. The model reflects progress made by behavioral and medical scientists in synthesizing their scholarship and abilities to develop strategies for controlling asthma. Second, the model allows us to suggest future directions that

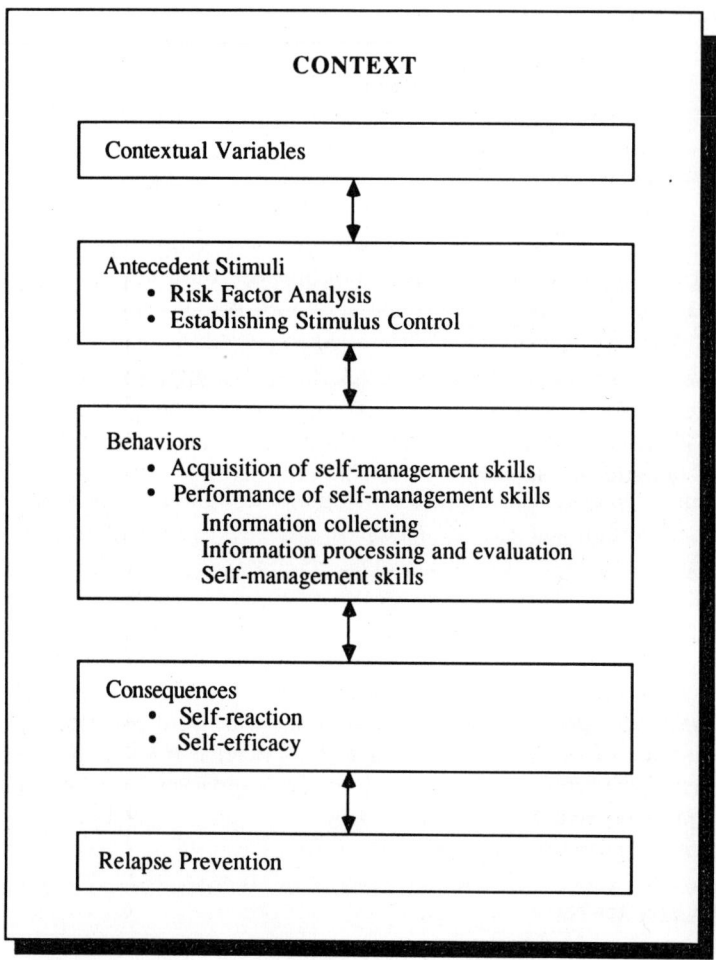

Figure 2.2. Schema of second-generation model of asthma self-management.

clinicians and researchers must take to reduce the impact of many of the stimulus variables and consequences we presented. We confess that the present integration of behavioral and medical knowledge, as summarized in Figure 2.2, will generate more questions than answers.

Context

Context consists of the setting where a particular event or set of events occur. The importance of context with respect to asthma and asthma attacks has received recognition for many years (Creer & Christian, 1976); indeed, many behavioral scientists now propose that researchers consider context within any behavioral study (e.g., Sulzer-Azaroff & Mayer, 1991). Context frames all events depicted in Figure 2.2. With asthma, context forms a complex matrix that entails numerous self-management skills, such as preventing attacks by taking prescribed maintenance medications, avoiding known triggers of asthma, reacting to abort attacks, and developing positive expectations regarding the ability to make a contribution to controlling one's asthma. Context consists of contingency relationships among four events: contextual variables, antecedent stimuli, behavior, and consequences. The significance of the components becomes apparent in discussing each component.

Contextual Variables

There are three types of contextual variables:

Setting Events. Setting events refer to complex antecedent stimuli, events, and stimulus–response interactions (Sulzer-Azaroff & Mayer, 1991). For example, many physicians advise patients to take prescribed medications in order to prevent attacks. Whether they follow this advice constitutes medication compliance. Many patients make efforts to comply; others are likely to be more nonadherent than adherent to medication instruction. Although we know prevalence rates of compliance, there is need for systematic investigation of variables that comprise adherent behavior. At the same time, most patients know what stimuli trigger their asthma. To many patients, these stimuli are discriminative stimuli associated with attacks; some patients, in fact, develop personal ways of assessing the probability that occurrence of a stimulus or stimuli could precipitate an attack. We need to know more about how stimuli become discriminative stimuli to patients as well as the type of expectations patients acquire about known triggers of their asthma.

Establishing Operations. Establishing operations are stimuli or events that either alter rates of responses previously associated with reinforcers or change effectiveness of reinforcers. Medication compliance again provides an apt illustration. If patients perceive that medications prevent, halt, or lessen severity of attacks, drugs become reinforcers; patients are therefore likely to be compliant. If patients expect that medications will not manage their asthma or if they perceive that drugs have adverse side effects, medications are not reinforcing; in these cases, patients are apt to be nonadherent. Another type of establishing operation relevant to use of medications is the sunk cost effect (Arkes, 1991). This implies that patients will continue using medications even when they perceive the medications are not achieving desired effects; such overuse of medications is particularly a problem with inhaled medications. Although we know the behavior occurs, there again has been no systematic investigation of this decision-making error.

Establishing Stimuli. Establishing stimuli (S_E) are stimuli paired with an establishing operation; the response or stimulus change they evoke becomes conditioned stimuli for that operation. An S_E cues or prompts occurrence of the establishing operation (Sulzer-Azaroff & Mayer, 1991). An example of an S_E is a nebulizer that dispenses asthma medications. When patients experience asthma, they seek out their nebulizer because the device has become a conditioned stimulus for relieving episodes. When the nebulizer is not immediately present, however, patients may desperately seek it because they recognize no change is apt to occur in their asthma without medication. This circumstance is also an establishing stimulus. If a patient does not quickly find and use the nebulizer, an asthma attack is not only likely to intensify, but the patient is apt to develop inappropriate behavioral patterns, such as panic, that interfere with control of future attacks.

Antecedent Stimuli

Contingencies are relationships between responses and stimuli that precede or accompany responses (i.e., antecedents) and events that follow those responses (i.e., consequences). Our interest has focused on antecedent stimuli and consequences.

Risk-Factor Analysis. We discussed the significance of risk-factor analysis in predicting probability of asthma attacks in patients. Greater knowledge and application of risk-factor analysis will permit physicians to tailor more effective treatment programs for individual patients.

Establishing Stimulus Control. This term refers to changing antecedent events in order to alter occurrence of a response. This could entail that patients both narrow and reduce the impact some antecedent stimuli have in triggering attacks and establish other antecedent stimuli to increase control of asthma. Clinicians can take two approaches (Creer et al., 1992). First, we can teach patients to modify old antecedents by changing their perceptions of antecedent stimuli to their attacks, teaching them to avoid or escape from their precipitants, narrowing stimulus control, and initiating behavioral changes. Second, we can teach patients to arrange antecedents by such steps as environmental programming, initiating positive self-instruction while eliminating negative self-statements, generating patients' precommitment to help control their asthma, and establishing stimulus generalization. The latter is particularly important in self-management if we expect to achieve the goal of teaching patients to manage their asthma across settings.

Behavior

Self-management involves both acquisition of self-management skills and subsequent performance of those skills. The process of acquisition and performance requires separate assessment. Acquisition involves gaining knowledge of asthma, its management, and the role patients can take in helping to control the disorder. Teaching patients about asthma and its management was the backbone of the two-dozen programs developed for childhood asthma (Wigal et al., 1990). Performance is the subsequent translation by patients from knowledge of what they have learned will help manage asthma to initiating specified behaviors. Performance involves several steps, including information collection, information processing and evaluation, and implementation of specific self-management skills.

Information Collection. Patients must collect valid and reliable data about themselves and their asthma. Earlier, we noted that patients do not always provide accurate information about themselves; there are frequent discrepancies between what patients report and what mechanical measures indicate regarding use of asthma medications. Despite this caveat, we must emphasize that data collected by patients yield both the best and worst information gathered about their asthma. For this reason, instruction in information gathering must be at the core of any patient-education effort.

Information Processing and Evaluation. Information processing and evaluation are also crucial functions in self-management; patients must make pertinent judgments and decisions about their asthma based on information they have collected about the condition. We know decision-making strategies that are common to Gold Standard Physicians and Gold Standard Patients (Creer, 1990). Research is lacking in determining how health-care providers and patients can apply more refined strategies and heuristics of decision making, such as those in other aspects of medicine (Arkes, 1991), to change some of the stimuli and response factors we have described throughout this chapter.

Self-Management Skills. Performance of self-management skills rests on the foundation of self-instruction or self-statements by patients to themselves. Self-instruction includes prompting, directing, and maintenance of performance of self-management competencies. Self-instruction is important in two respects: controlling attacks and promoting coping strategies. To an increasing degree, establishing control over attacks entails patients performing, in a stepwise manner, strategies their physicians suggest for the management of asthma. Coping strategies involve performance of proven self-management tactics and techniques. It is our hope that second-generation asthma self-management programs incorporate more of the techniques that researchers have developed in the past decade for self-regulation of a variety of problems (Creer et al., 1992). These would include greater emphasis of relaxation skills; systematic desensitization, including self-desensitization by adolescents and adults; skill rehearsal; modeling, sometimes with guided participation; linking or unlinking chains of behavior; self-reinforcement, particularly coupled with self-instruction; rehearsal; and application of Premack's Principle (e.g., teaching patients to guide their behavior by making occurrence of a less probable response contingent upon performance of a more probable response) (Premack, 1959).

Consequences

What occurs when patients perform self-management skills to help manage their asthma requires more systematic investigation. Patients must learn to review and evaluate their performance in an objective and accurate manner. We cite the example of medication compliance as a topic with a prime need for such attention. The attention patients direct toward evaluating their performance is called *self-reaction* (Bandura, 1986). Based on evaluation of their performance, patients can establish realistic expectations about their performance as well as evaluate whether they require more training and expertise. *Self-efficacy* is the belief that one can adequately perform specific skills in a given situation (Bandura, 1977). Accurate methods of assessing self-efficacy are increasingly evaluated in studies of asthma self-management (e.g., Tobin et al., 1987); it is imperative that research programs assess self-efficacy to a greater degree in future programs.

Relapse Prevention

Marlatt (1982) suggested a relapse prevention model as a paradigm for understanding patient relapse. In current context, *relapse* refers to violation of self-imposed rules or sets of rules that patients have learned to use in managing their asthma. When developing asthma intervention programs, clinicians could incorporate instruction in specific self-management techniques, such as the following:

1. Taking any prescribed prophylactic medication
2. Avoiding of high-risk situations
3. Escaping from high-risk situations
4. Mastering performance of self-management skills
5. Rehearsing asthma self-management competencies between attacks
6. Avoiding factors that weaken self-management performance (e.g., reliance upon memory)
7. Taking remedial steps when necessary
8. Developing new coping strategies as appropriate.

We anticipate that not only will investigators research the potential role of relapse prevention in control of asthma, but also that it will become a key component of all second-generation asthma self-management programs (Creer et al., 1992).

REFERENCES

Anonymous. (1989). *The American Asthma Report.* New York: Research and Forecasts, Inc.

Arkes, H. (1991). Costs and benefits of judgment errors: Implications for debiasing. *Psychological Bulletin, 110,* 486–498.

Bandura, A. (1977). Self-efficacy: Toward a unifying theory of behavioral change. *Psychological Review, 84,* 191–215.

Bandura, A. (1986). *Social foundations of thought and action: A social cognitive theory.* Englewood Cliffs, NJ: Prentice-Hall.

Baum, D., & Creer, T. L. (1986). Medication compliance in children with asthma. *Journal of Asthma, 23,* 49–59.

Bauman, A. E., Craig, A. R., Dunsmore, J., Browne, G., Allen, D. H., & Vandenberg, R. (1989). Removing barriers to effective self-management of asthma. *Patient Education and Counseling, 14,* 217–226.

Becker, M. H., Maiman, L. A., Kirscht, J. D., Haefner, D. L., Drachman, R. H., & Taylor, D. W. (1979). Patient perceptions and compliance: Recent studies of the health belief model. In R. B. Hayes, D. W. Taylor, & D. L. Sackett (Eds.), *Compliance in health care* (pp. 79–109). Baltimore, MD: Johns Hopkins University.

Bender, B. G., Lerner, J. A., & Kollasch, E. (1988). Mood and memory changes in asthmatic children receiving corticosteroids. *American Academy of Childhood and Adolescent Psychiatry, 27,* 720–725.

Bender, B. G., Lerner, J. A., & Poland, J. E. (1991). Association between corticosteroids and psychologic change in hospitalized asthmatic children. *Annals of Allergy, 66,* 414–419.

Bender, B., & Milgrom, H. (1992). Theophylline-induced behavior change in children: An objective evaluation of parents' perceptions. *Journal of the American Medical Association, 267,* 2621–2624.

Bernstein, I. L. (1983). Asthma in adults: Diagnosis and treatment. In E. Middleton, Jr., C. E. Reed, & E. F. Ellis (Eds.), *Allergy: Principles and practice* (pp. 901–934). St. Louis, MO: Mosby.

Boston Collaborative Drug Juvenile Program. (1972). Acute adverse reactions in relation to dosage. *Clinical Pharmacology, 13,* 694–698.

Boulet, L.-P., Deschesnes, F., Turcotte, H., & Gignac, F. (1991). Near-fatal asthma: Clinical and physiologic features, perception of bronchoconstriction, and psychologic profile. *Journal of Allergy and Clinical Immunology, 88,* 838–846.

Busse, W. W., & Reed, C. E. (1988). Asthma: Definitions and pathogenesis. In E. Middleton, Jr., C. E. Reed, E. F. Ellis, N. F. Adkinson, Jr., & J. W. Yunginer (Eds.), *Allergy: Principles and practice* (pp. 969–998). St. Louis, MO: Mosby.

Canny, G. J., & Levison, H. (1990). Childhood asthma: A rational approach to treatment. *Annals of Allergy, 64,* 406-416.

Cherniack, R. M., & Cherniack, L. (1983). *Respiration in health and disease* (3rd ed.). Philadelphia: Saunders.

Clark, N. M., Evans, D., & Mellins, R. B. (1992). Patient use of peak flow monitoring. *Annual Review of Respiratory Disease, 144,* 722–725.

Conrad, P. (1985). The meaning of medications: Another look at compliance. *Social Science and Medicine, 20,* 29–37.
Cramer, J. A., Mattson, R. H., Prevey, M. L., Scheyer, R. D., & Ouellette, V. L. (1989). How often is medication taken as prescribed? *Journal of the American Medical Association, 261,* 3273–3277.
Creer, T. L. (1979). *Asthma therapy: A behavioral health-care system for respiratory disorders.* New York: Springer.
Creer, T. L. (1982). Asthma. *Journal of Consulting and Clinical Psychology, 50*(6), 912–921.
Creer, T. L. (1990). Strategies for judgment and decision making in the management of childhood asthma. *Pediatric Asthma and Allergy Immunology, 4,* 253–264.
Creer, T. L. (1991a). Medication compliance and asthma. *Journal of Respiratory Diseases, 12,* 543–548.
Creer, T. L. (1991b). Psychologic and behavioral assessment of childhood asthma. Part I: Psychologic instruments. *Pediatric Asthma, Allergy, and Immunology, 5,* 317–328.
Creer, T. L. (1991c). The application of behavioral procedures to childhood asthma: Current and future perspectives. *Patient Education and Counseling, 17,* 9–22.
Creer, T. L. (1992). Psychological and behavioral assessment of childhood asthma: Part II. Behavioral approaches. *Pediatric Asthma, Allergy, and Immunology, 6,* 21–34.
Creer, T. L., Backial, M., Burns, K. L., Leung, P., Marion, R. J., Miklich, D. R., Morrill, C., Taplin, P. S., & Ullman, S. (1988). Living with Asthma: Part I. Genesis and development of a self-management program for childhood asthma. *Journal of Asthma, 25,* 335–362.
Creer, T. L., & Christian, W. P. (1976). *Chronically-ill and handicapped children: Their management and rehabilitation.* Champaign, IL: Research Press.
Creer, T. L., & Kotses, H. (1990). An extension of the Reed and Townley cocneption of the pathogenesis of asthma: The role of behavioral and psychological stimuli and responses. *Pediatric Asthma, Allergy, and Immunology, 2,* 169–184.
Creer, T. L., Kotses, H., & Wigal, J. K. (1992). A second-generation model of asthma self-management. *Pediatric Asthma, Allergy, and Immunology, 6,* 143–165.
Creer, T. L., Renne, C. M., & Christian, W. P. (1976). Behavioral contributions to rehabilitation and childhood asthma. *Rehabilitation Literature, 37,* 226–232, 247.
Creer, T. L., Reynolds, R.V.C., & Kotses, H. (1991). *A handbook for asthma self-management: A leader's guide to living with asthma.* Athens, OH: Ohio University Press.
Creer, T. L., Wigal, J. K., Kotses, H., & Lewis, P. D. (1990). A critique of 19 self-management programs for childhood asthma: Part II. Comments regarding the scientific merit of the programs. *Pediatric Asthma, Allergy, and Immunology, 4,* 41–55.
Creer, T. L., Wigal, J. K., Tobin, D. L., Kotses, H., Snyder, S. E., & Winder, J. A. (1989). The Revised Asthma Problem Behavior Checklist. *Journal of Asthma, 26,* 17–29.
Downey, J., Ehrhardt, A. A., Gruen, R., Bell, J. J., & Morishima, A. (1989). Psychopathology and social functioning in women with Turner syndrome. *Journal of Nervous and Mental Disease, 177,* 191–201.
Eisen, S. A., Miller, D. K., & Woodward, R. S. (1990). The effect of prescribed daily dose frequency on patient medication compliance. *Archives of Internal Medicine, 150,* 1881–1884.
Ellis, E. F. (1988). Asthma in infnacy and childhood. In J. E. Middleton, Jr., C. E. Reed, E. F. Ellis, J.N.F. Adkinson, & J. W. Yunginer (Eds.), *Allergy: Principles and practice* (pp. 969–998). St. Louis, MO: Mosby.
Eraker, S. A., Kirscht, J. P., & Becker, M. H. (1984). Understanding and improving patient compliance. *Annals of Internal Medicine, 100,* 258–268.
Firestone, P., & Martin, J. (1979). An analysis of the hyperactive syndrome: A comparison of hyperactive, behavior problem, asthmatic, and normal children. *Journal of Abnormal Child Psychology, 7,* 261–273.
Furukawa, C. T., DuHamel, T. R., Weimer, L., Shapiro, G. G., Pierson, W. E., & Bierman, C. W. (1988). Cognitive and behavioral findings in children taking theophylline. *Journal of Allergy and Clinical Immunology, 81,* 83–88.
Furukawa, C. T., Shapiro, G. G., DuHamel, T., Weiner, L., Pierson, W. E., & Bierman, C. W. (1984). Learning and behavior problems associated with theophylline therapy. *Lancet, 1,* 621.
Harm, D. L., Kotses, H., & Creer, T. L. (1985). Improving the ability of peak expiratory flow rates to predict asthma. *Journal of Allergy and Clinical Immunology, 76*(5), 688–694.
Harris, J. C., Carel, C. A., Rosenberg, L. A., Joshi, P., & Leventhal, B. G. (1986). Intermittent high dose corticosteroid treatment in childhood cancer. *Journal of the American Academy of Child Psychiatry, 25,* 120–124.

Hyland, M. E., Finnis, S., & Irvine, S. H. (1991). A scale for assessing quality of life in adult asthma sufferers. *Journal of Psychosomatic Research, 35,* 99–110.

Joad, J., Ahrens, R. C., Lindgren, S. D., & Weinberger, M. M. (1986). Extrapulmonary effects of maintenance therapy with theophylline and inhaled albuterol in patients with chronic asthma. *Journal of Allergy and Clinical Immunology, 78*(6), 1147–1153.

Juniper, E. G., Guyatt, G. H., Epstein, R. S., Ferrie, P. J., Jaeschke, R., & Hiller, T. K. (1992). Evaluation of impairment of health related quality of life in asthma: Development of a questionnaire for use in clinical trials. *Thorax, 47,* 76–83.

Kinsman, R. A., Luparello, T., O'Banion, K., & Spector, S. (1973). Multidimensional analysis of the subjective symptomatology of asthma. *Psychosomatic Medicine, 35,* 250–267.

Kotses, H., Stout, C., Wigal, J. K., Carlson, B., Creer, T. L., & Lewis, P. (1991). Individualized asthma self-management: A beginning. *Journal of Asthma 28,* 287–289.

Levison, H. (1991). Canadian consensus on the treatment of asthma in children. *Canadian Medical Association Journal, 145,* 1440–1445.

Ling, M.H.M., Perry, P. J., & Tsuang, M. T. (1981). Side effects of corticosteroid therapy. *Archives of General Psychiatry, 38,* 471–477.

Lohr, K. N. (1989). Conceptual background and issues in quality of life. In F. Mosteller & J. Falotico-Taylor (Eds.), *Quality of life and technology assessment* (pp. 1–6). Washington, DC: National Academy Press.

Loren, M. L., Leung, P. K., Cooley, R. L., Chai, H., Bell, T. D., & Buck, V. M. (1978). Irreversibility of obstructive changes in severe asthma in children. *Chest, 74,* 126–129.

Madison, J. M. (1991). Chronic asthma in the adult: Pathogenesis and pharmacotherapy. *Seminars in Respiratory Medicine, 12,* 175–184.

Marlatt, G. A. (1982). Relapse prevention: A self-control program for the treatment of addictive behaviors. In R. B. Stuart (Ed.), *Adherence, compliance and generalization in behavioral medicine.* New York: Brunner/Mazel.

Mawhinney, H., Spector, S. L., Kinsman, R. A., Siegel, S. C., Rachalefsky, G. S., Katz, R. M., & Rohr, A. S. (1991). Compliance in clinical trials of two nonbronchodilator antiasthma medications. *Annals of Allergy, 66,* 294–299.

McCarthy, M. M. (1981). Speech effects of theophylline. *Pediatrics, 68,* 749.

McFadden Jr., E. R. (1980). Asthma: Pathophysiology. *Seminars in Respiratory Medicine, 1,* 297–303.

Murphy, M. B., Dillon, A., & Fitzgerald, M. X. (1980). Theophylline and depression. *British Medical Journal, 281,* 1322.

Pinzone, H. A., Carlson, B. W., Kotses, H., & Creer, T. L. (1991). Prediction of asthma episodes in children using peak expiratory flow rates, medication compliance, and exercise. *Annals of Allergy, 67,* 461–647.

Plaut, T. F. (1988). *Children with asthma: A manual for parents* (2nd ed.). Amherst, MA: Pedipress.

Premack, D. (1959). Toward empirical behavioral laws: Positive reinforcement. *Psychological Review, 66,* 219–233.

Rachelefsky, G., Wo, J., Adelson, J., Spector, S., Katz, R., Siegel, S., & Rohr, A. (1986). Behavior abnormalities and poor school performance due to oral theophylline usage. *Journal of Allergy and Clinical Immunology, 77,* 145.

Rand, C. S., Wise, R. A., Nides, M., Simmons, M. S., Bleecker, E. R., Kusek, J. W., Li, V. C., & Tashkin, D. P. (1992). Metered-dose inhaler adherence in a clinical trial. *American Review of Respiratory Disease, 146,* 1559–1564.

Rappaport, L., Coffman, H., Guare, R., Fenton, T., DeGraw, C., & Twarog, F. (1989). Effects of theophylline on behavior and learning in children with asthma. *American Journal of Diseases of Children, 143,* 368–372.

Reed, C. F., & Townley, R. G. (1983). Asthma: Classification and pathogenesis. In E. Middleton Jr., C. E. Reed, & E. F. Ellis (Eds.), *Allergy: Principles and practice* (pp. 811–831). St. Louis, MO: Mosby.

Renne, C. M., & Creer, T. L. (1985). Asthmatic children and their families. In M. L. Walraich & D. K. Routh (Eds.), *Advances in developmental and behavioral pediatrics* (pp. 41-81). Greenwich, CN: JAI Press.

Roth, H. P., Carson, H. S., & Hsi, B. P. (1970). Measuring intake of a prescribed medication: A bottle count and tracer technique compared. *Clinical Pharmacology and Therapeutics, 11,* 228–237.

Sbarbaro, J. A., & Steiner, J. F. (1991). Noncompliance with medications: Vintage wine in new (pill) bottles. *Annals of Allergy, 66,* 273–275.

Schlieper, A., Alcock, D., Beaudry, P., Feldman, W., & Leikin, L. (1991). Effect of therapeutic plasma concentrations of theophylline on behavior, cognitive processing, and affect in children with asthma. *Journal of Pediatrics, 118,* 449–455.

Sibbald, B. (1989). Patient self-care in acute asthma. *Thorax, 44,* 97–101.

Spector, S. L., Lewis, C. E., Feldman, C. H., Haynes, R. B., Hindi-Alexander, M., Kinsman, R. A., Menendez, R. A., & Sbarbaro, J. A. (1986). Workshop 6: Compliance factors. *Journal of Allergy and Clinical Immunology, 78,* 529–533.

Springer, C., Goldenberg, B., Ben Dov, I., & Godfrey, S. (1985). Clinical, physiologic, and psychologic comparison of treatment by cromolyn or theophylline in childhood asthma. *Journal of Allergy and Clinical Immunology, 76,* 64–69.

Stout, C., Kotses, H., Carlson, B. W., & Creer, T. L. (1991). Predicting asthma in individual patients. *Journal of Asthma, 28,* 41–47.

Sulzer-Azaroff, B., & Mayer, G. R. (1991). *Behavior analysis for lasting change.* Ft. Worth, TX: Holt, Rinehart & Winston.

Taplin, P. S., & Creer, T. L. (1978). A procdure for using peak expiratory flow-rate data to increase the predictability of asthma episodes. *The Journal of Asthma Research, 16*(1), 15–19.

Tashkin, D., Rand, C., Nides, M., Simmons, M., Wise, R., Coulson, A. H., Li, V., & Gong, H. (1991). A nebulizer chronolog to monitor compliance with inhaler use. *The American Journal of Medicine, 91*(Suppl. 44), 33–36.

Tobin, D. L., Wigal, J. K., Winder, J. A., Holroyd, K. A., & Creer, T. L. (1987). A self-efficacy scale for asthma. *Annals of Allergy, 59*(10), 273–277.

Wasser, W. G., Bronheim, H. E., & Richardson, B. K. (1981). Theophylline madness. *Annals of Internal Medicine, 95,* 191.

Wigal, J. K., Creer, T. L., Kotses, H., & Lewis, P. D. (1990). A critique of 19 self-management programs for childhood asthma: Part I. The development and evaluation of the programs. *Pediatric Asthma, Allergy, and Immunology, 4,* 17–39.

Williams, J. I., & Wood-Dauphinee, S. (1989). Assessing quality of life: Measures and utility. In F. Mosteller & J. Falotico-Taylor (Eds.), *Quality of life and technology assessment* (pp. 65–115). Washington, DC: National Academy Press.

Wright, B. M., & McKerrow, C. B. (1959). Maximum forced expiratory flow rate as a measure of ventilatory capacity: With a description of a new portable instrument for measuring it. *British Medical Journal, 2,* 1041–1047.

3

Temporomandibular Disorders

Dennis C. Turk, Donald B. Penzien, and Jeanetta C. Rains

NATURE OF TEMPOROMANDIBULAR DISORDERS

Temporomandibular disorders (TMDs) represent a range of clinical problems with a set of common features that involve masticatory musculature and/or the temporomandibular joint. The most common initial symptom is pain, usually localized in the muscles of mastication, the preauricular area (in front of the ear), the temporomandibular joint (TMJ), or all three areas. Chewing or other jaw functions usually aggravate the pain. Other common symptoms include jaw ache, earache, headache, and facial pain. In addition to complaints of pain, patients with TMDs frequently evidence a limited range of, or deviant mandibular movement on opening and joint sounds (e.g., clicking, popping, grating, or crepitus). Dentists frequently observe the presence of excessive wear on the teeth of TMD patients. This excessive wear may result from bruxing (i.e., grinding and repeated clenching of the teeth). Bruxing causes excessive levels of muscle tension and when prolonged, may result in structural changes in the temporomandibular joint. TMDs commonly fall into four major categories depending on the presumed site of pathophysiology:

1. Myofascial pain dysfunction (MPD) disorders of the muscles of mastication
2. Internal derangement (ID) of the contents of the joint space, implying anatomical disturbance of the disc—condyle relationship and consequent changes in the mechanics of the joint—pathologic placement
3. Degenerative joint disorders (DJD) and other changes of the condyle and other bony components of the joint
4. Fractures, infections, and tumors of the joint.

Dennis C. Turk • Pain Evaluation and Treatment Institute, University of Pittsburgh School of Medicine, Pittsburgh, Pennsylvania 15213.   **Donald B. Penzien and Jeanetta C. Rains** • Department of Psychiatry, University of Mississippi Medical Center, Jackson, Mississippi 39216.
Handbook of Health and Rehabilitation Psychology, edited by Anthony J. Goreczny. Plenum Press, New York, 1995.

Basic Anatomy and Physiology

To understand the classes of TMDs enumerated previously, it is helpful to have a basic understanding of the anatomy and physiology that may relate to various symptoms. When the mouth opens and shuts, the U-shaped mandible (lower jaw) moves. At the ends of the mandible are joints that connect with the temporal bones of the head; thus, the name of the joint is the temporomandibular joint (TMJ). As the jaw opens, the condyles (knob-like ends of the jaw bones) first rotate within the hollows of articular fossa (located just in front of the ear) and then slide forward along the lower edges of the temporal bones. To assist this movement, a separate piece of cartilage (articular disk) rests on the top of each condyle. The disk moves with the condyle as it rotates and slides, conforming to the varying space between the bones. The chewing muscles control the joint motions. The teeth determine the relationship of the jaws when the mouth is closed and subsequently affect the motions of the joint.

TMJs may develop a variety of disorders that affect the joints themselves (degeneration of the condyles or inflammation of the lubricating fluid that lines the capsules containing the TMJs or the tissue that connects the disk to the temporal bone behind it), the muscles and connective tissues (myofascial pain), and other tissues surrounding the joints (displacement of the articular disk). These may occur separately or together, and they reinforce each other. The affected structure or structures hypothetically cause the range of symptoms that TMD sufferers report.

In this chapter we review the prevalence of TMDs and examine some of the diagnostic problems and the most prevalent etiological models. We also examine the contributions of psychological factors in TMDs. We review the efficacy of the diverse range of therapeutic interventions that practitioners use to treat TMDs and consider the mechanisms for the efficacy of common treatments. We also provide guidelines for the treatment of TMD sufferers.

Epidemiology of TMD

Studies have shown a relatively high prevalence of the common TMD signs and symptoms with estimates ranging from 28–81% of the general population. Schiffman, Fricton, Haley, and Shapiro (1990) found that in a nonclinical sample of nursing students, 69% had a clinically determinable TMD. In a population-based epidemiological study, Von Korff, Dworkin, LeResche, and Kruger (1987) reported a 12% prevalence rate of TMD-related pain among adults. Despite the high prevalence rates of TMD pain, Schiffman et al. (1990) noted that only 6% of their sample of nursing students had symptoms severe enough to warrant treatment, and Von Korff et al. (1987) observed that only 23% of those with TMD-related pain actually sought treatment. Thus, it is important not to equate the identification of symptoms in a population with the need or desire for treatment. It appears that most patients with clinically detectable signs function adequately without significant symptoms and do not need treatment. Despite the high prevalence of TMD signs and symptoms it has been suggested that only about 5% of these individuals are in need of treatment (e.g., Schiffman et al., 1990).

Although there is no reason to suspect that the prevalence of TMD has increased in recent years, the number of persons seeking treatment for TMD has risen dramatically. It may be that dentists are more frequently recommending that patients be treated (Al-Hasson, Ismail, & Ash, 1986) and the increased volume of patients seeking treatment may, in a circular fashion, encourage a greater number of practitioners to provide treatment. Conversely, the greater availability of treatment may lead to still greater treatment seeking.

Researchers have not yet sufficiently defined predisposing factors to accurately identify patients at risk for developing TMDs, nor can we identify patients who are likely to experience greater symptom severity. In addition, research has not clarified what factors are etiological or contributory in nature. Some factors will be risk factors only; others may be causal in nature, whereas other factors may result from or be purely coincidental to the problem. Thus, factors may represent predisposing, initiating, or perpetuating factors and have different roles in the progression of TMDs (McNeill, Mohl, Rugh, & Tanaka, 1990).

Unfortunately, we have limited knowledge regarding the history or the natural course of TMDs. The signs and symptoms of TMDs may represent transient and self-limiting problems, and they may thus resolve without serious long-term effects (Greene & Laskin, 1983); however, a portion of patients with TMDs develop a chronic pain syndrome (Dworkin & Burgess, 1987; National Institutes of Health Consensus Development Conference, 1986). Data are not yet available to develop clear-cut guidelines to establish who warrants treatment.

Epidemiological studies suggest that signs and symptoms of TMDs are equally distributed between males and females. It is primarily females in the 25–44 year old age group, however, who seek treatment, and the ratio of females to males in clinics approaches 7:1 (Rugh & Solberg, 1985).

Diagnostic Problems

Although clinicians have written about TMD for over six decades, there is a lack of consensus regarding what constitutes a clinically significant TMD syndrome. Attempts to differentiate TMD patients from nonpatients by simply counting the number of signs and symptoms have not been rewarding. One can distinguish clinical cases from controls most readily by report of pain, pain in response to palpations, restricted vertical range of motion of the mandible, and clicking joint sounds. The latter, however, are not present in the majority of persons seeking treatment for TMD-related pain (Dworkin et al., 1990a). Moreover, these symptoms are quite common in asymptomatic subjects (Kircos, Ortendahl, Mar, & Arakawa, 1987). Researchers have also seriously questioned the importance of bruxing, a behavior they previously characterized as a central feature of TMD (Marbach, Raphael, Dohrenwend, & Lennon, 1990). Bruxing, a high-frequency behavior, is common among asymptomatic patients (Moss, Ruff, & Sturgis, 1984). Similarly, even though there appears to be strong support for the presence of osteoarthrosis in a larger portion of TMD patients, a comparable percentage of symptom-free patients (e.g., nontemporomandibular joint dysfunction symptoms) also show radiographic evidence of osteoarthrosis in the TMJ (Ericson & Lundberg, 1968).

Further compounding the diagnostic dilemma is that signs and symptoms of different categories of TMD overlap considerably, and more than one clinical problem can be present in the same patient at the same time (Dworkin, LeResche, & DeRouen, 1988). Thus, the relevance of joint sounds, pain on palpation of masticatory muscles, bruxing, and radiographic evidence of degenerative changes for TMD is unclear even though the most prominent etiological models, which we describe later, emphasize the presence of these signs and symptoms.

Psychometric Problems

A number of the previously noted diagnostic problems directly relate to the available systems for assessing oral dysfunction/structural abnormalities (OD/SA). Shortcomings of the diagnostic assessment procedure include reliance upon patients' subjective reports and use of unstandardized examination and diagnostic procedures that involve clinician interpretation based on uncalibrated methods. In addition, some clinicians incorrectly assume that the hypothesized diagnostic criteria are consistently present.

Dworkin et al. (1988) noted that there exists a lack of data available on the reliability of many OD/SA indices practitioners use to derive classification systems. They examined the reliability of TMD examination methods and found that even with standardized examination protocols, the reliability of assessment of occlusal status, pain on palpation, and certain clinical findings is poor prior to specific calibration training (Dworkin et al., 1990b). Dworkin et al. (1988) also demonstrated the relatively low test–retest reliability of typical diagnostic criteria.

The validity of many assessment procedures also remains undetermined, Van der Weele and Dibbets (1987) presented data that seriously challenge the validity of one of the most commonly used TMD indices, which Helkimo (1974) proposed. There even exists little agreement regarding the diagnostic approach that is best for classification. LeResche, Dworkin, Sommers, and Truelove (1991) contrasted two common TMD classification schemes and found great variability in the prevalence rates and little concordance in the assignment of classification between the two schemes (kappa .02, only slightly better than chance). This presents a major problem because differing diagnostic criteria can contribute to lack of comparability across studies.

The lack of reliability and validity within the realm of clinical practice results in patients being offered widely divergent diagnostic explanations, prognostic judgments, and therapeutic regimens depending on who conducts the assessment. The heterogeneity of clinical procedures among practitioners for evaluating and treating TMD patients reflects the deficiencies in reliable scientific data concerning the relative cost, effectiveness, and safety of alternative strategies for managing TMDs.

In 1969, Laskin wrote,

> There are two aspects of successful management of any disease process: one is the establishment of an accurate diagnosis; the other is an understanding of its etiology so that a rational treatment plan can be formulated. Unfortunately, in the management of many problems involving the temporomandibular joint, we have not been highly successful in either of these areas. (p. 152)

Despite a large volume of research, Laskin's comment is equally relevant today—over 25 years later. Even with the duly noted limitations, it remains important to consider the two primary etiological models that have guided research and treatment of TMD.

ETIOLOGICAL MODELS OF TMD

Since the 1930s with the identification of TMDs as a problem, researchers have proposed two competing etiological models. A number of factors are used to classify subgroups of TMD patients. A common approach is to view TMDs as consisting of two independent subgroups depending on presumed etiology: myogenic (muscle) or arthralgic (joint). The myogenic group is characterized by muscular hyperarousal due to stress and muscular abnormalities resulting from parafunctional habits (e.g., bruxing; Laskin, 1979). The arthralgic category consists of subdivisions of specific structural abnormalities (Moss, Garrett, & Chiodo, 1982). The approaches for classifying patients with orofacial pain are deductive, and researchers have based them on *a priori* notions of causality. Each of the two models provide theoretical support for different treatments.

Structural Disharmony or Biomechanical Model

The structural disharmony or biomechanical model maintains that certain dental–occlusal abnormalities of the somatognathic system lead to abnormal jaw muscle and joint function with eventual pain. Structural disharmonies include malocclusion, craniomandibular malalignment, and condylar displacement but do not include degenerative joint disease or anatomical derangements of the intracapsular TMJ structures due to trauma. This model suggests that TMDs result primarily from structural disharmonies and that psychological distress, when detected, is a consequence of the discomfort and frustrations that result from the disorder (Clark & Adler, 1985). Treatment includes physical correction of occlusal problems and consists of a variety of techniques to reposition the jaw in central occlusion position.

Research on the Structural Model

The etiological role of malocclusion (how the teeth and jaw function in relation to each other) and position of the jaw, the basis for the structural disharmony model, has been challenged. For example, several studies have reported no association between occlusion and TMDs (for a review see Clark and Adler, 1985). Studies of asymptomatic subjects have shown great variation in condyle–fossa relationship and even between left and right TMJs within the same person (D. Blaschke & T. Blaschke, 1981). One research study also demonstrated that the prevalence of internal derangements of the condyle in the fossa (anterior and posterior deviation of more than 1 mm) was the same for symptomatic and asymptomatic patients (Bean & Thomas, 1987). Bean and Thomas concluded that, contrary to the suggestion of the structural model, condylar position in the fossa is of questionable significance with regard to the etiology of TMDs.

Psychophysiological or Myofascial Pain–Dysfunction Model

The psychophysiological, myofascial pain–dysfunction (MPD) model proposes that, except for obvious degenerative arthritic conditions and problems resulting from external trauma, TMDs occur primarily because of psychological stress rather than occlusal abnormalities. Laskin (1969) hypothesized that when an individual is confronted with aversive stimulation that is very intense or recurrent and the individual lacks adequate coping skills, a stereotypic response pattern may develop in a unfavorably disposed body system. The combination of centrally induced increases in muscle tension and the presence of parafunctional habits such as bruxing result in muscle fatigue and spasm that produce the pain and dysfunction. It has been suggested that excessive stress can result in masticatory muscle hyperactivity that may manifest as various forms of parafunctional habits, such as bruxing. These high-force activities may lead to muscle and joint pain, limited range of motion, and joint sounds (Haber, Moss, Kuczmierczk, & Garrett, 1983). Similar symptoms, however, can occasionally also result from muscular overcontraction or trauma.

According to Laskin (1969), although MPD syndrome starts as a functional disorder, it can ultimately lead to organic changes in the TMJ and masticatory muscles and even cause possible alterations in the dentition. In MPD, this unfavorable disposition may result from overutilization of masticatory muscles (e.g., bruxism) or a structural problem (e.g., internal derangement of the TMJ). As the response continues, the sympathetic nervous system becomes dysregulated and the sustained hyperactivity of these muscles may lead to local ischemia and reflex muscle spasm. With sustained muscular hyperactivity, pain develops as a consequence of local ischemic hypoxia and pain-eliciting irritants from hypoxic cells (e.g., lactic acid). These irritants may cause nociceptive receptors to become increasingly sensitized. The resulting muscle pain then may act as a new stressor and thus perpetuate a vicious pain–tension–pain cycle. Secondary organic changes may become self-perpetuating because they result in altered oral patterns with attendant reinforcement of the initial spasm and pain.

In short, MPD results from the interaction of potentially stressful environmental events, anxiety, inadequate coping abilities, and a predisposing organic or psychological condition that elicits muscle tension, which when it persists, produces the TMD symptoms. Laskin (1969) reported that because "Initiating factors for the MPD syndrome are generally emotional, rather than physical, (and) treatment must be directed toward this aspect of the problem . . ." (p. 148).

Research on the MPD Model

Experimentally, psychophysiological models of TMD predict that when patients with masticatory pain experience stressful stimuli, they will exhibit elevated and prolonged reactions, relative to health controls, in the muscles of mastication. Additionally, from a symptom-specificity perspective, muscular hyperreactivity to stress will occur primarily in masticatory muscles. Furthermore, muscular reactions to stress and the magnitude of these muscular reactions will more closely relate to psychological variables (e.g., depression and anxiety) than physical variables (e.g., degree of TMJ abnormality).

Investigators have performed a great deal of research to evaluate the adequacy of the psychophysiological, MPD model. Several studies (Dahlstrom, Carlsson, Gale, & Jansson, 1985; Kapel, Glaros, & McGlynn, 1989; Katz et al., 1989; Mercuri, Olson, & Laskin, 1979; Moss & Adams, 1984; Rugh & Montgomery, 1987; Thomas, Tiber, & Schireson, 1973; Yemm, 1969) have examined the role of muscular activity in the facial muscles and TMD. Overall, the studies have yielded mixed results. Several investigators (Kapel et al., 1989; Mercuri et al., 1979; Rugh & Montgomery, 1987; Thomas et al., 1973) have reported baseline EMG differences in masticatory muscles between TMD patients and healthy controls, whereas others (Moss & Adams, 1984; Yemm, 1969) have not found significant baseline differences between patients and controls. Reynolds (1988) examined five different studies and concluded that a mean of 34% (range 3% to 100%!) of TMD patients displayed resting elevated baseline levels of masseter and/or temporalis muscular arousal.

Similarly, the evidence is equivocal regarding whether TMD patients, in comparison to control subjects, show significantly greater EMG increases when they experience psychologically stressful stimuli. Several studies have controlled baseline differences, and some of these studies have demonstrated no significant EMG increases in response to psychological stressors (Kapel et al., 1989; Moss & Adams, 1984), whereas other studies have reported that TMD patients display significantly higher EMG levels during stressful stimuli relative to the EMG level of control subjects (Dahlstrom et al., 1985; Katz et al., 1979; Mercuri et al., 1979; Thomas et al., 1973).

The association between levels of muscle tension and clinical symptoms is unclear. For example, studies using biofeedback for TMD have not demonstrated a co-occurrence of pain reduction and reduction in masseter EMG activity (Funch & Gale, 1984). Close inspection of two noteworthy studies (Dohrmann & Laskin, 1978; Stenn, Mothersill, & Brooke, 1979) suggests that their patients' improvement following EMG biofeedback training and stress management training did not result from lowered day-to-day masseter muscle activity. Researchers have reported similar results with EMG biofeedback treatment for chronic headaches and back pain. A long list of methodological flaws, however, prevents one from making firm conclusions (see Flor & Turk, 1989 for an extended review).

Turk and his colleagues have conducted a series of studies in an attempt to correct the methodological problems that have confounded research on the importance of stress induced muscular arousal in TMD patients. In one of these investigations (Turk & Rudy, 1986), subjects were exposed to three experimental tasks that were counterbalanced across subjects to minimize potential carryover effects between tasks: (1) a standardized neutral image that placed subjects in their living room with the television on; (2) an experimenter-guided personally relevant stressful image of a recent stressful epxerience that the subject discussed previously during the psychological intake interview; and (3) a general stress task, mental arithmetic, during which time subjects counted backward silently by 7's from 543. During each task the investigators obtained simultaneous EMG recordings bilaterally from masseter and temporalis muscles as well as from several non-pain-specific muscle sites (e.g., forearm). Each task followed a baseline phase and preceded a return-to-baseline phase. Subjects also rated their current stress, muscle tensions, and pain levels following each task.

In the Turk and Rudy (1986) study, TMD patients' baseline levels of muscle arousal did not differ from healthy controls or non-TMD-pain patients. During the stress tasks, the TMD patients exhibited high levels of masseter and temporalis muscular activity and a delayed return to baseline levels. In contrast, the healthy controls and non-TMD-pain patients displayed no significant elevations in the masseter or temporalis muscle tension levels during the stress tasks. Recently, Flor, Birbaumer, Schulte, and Roos (1991), using virtually the same methodology and procedure, replicated these results, suggesting that although TMD patients do not have higher resting muscle tension levels than normals, TMD patients do exhibit site-specific muscular arousal to stressful stimuli.

Another study (Rudy, Turk, & Flor, 1988) utilized 40 patients with either normal ($n = 20$) or abnormal (e.g., displaced discs; $n = 20$) TMJ computed axial tomography (CT) results. Analysis of masseter and temporalis EMGs indicated no baseline EMG differences between the TMD patients and 10 healthy controls and no differential responding to the neutral image. TMD patients, however, did display significant site-specific EMG elevations in response to the two stress tasks relative to the controls. Patients' EMG increases were significantly higher for personally relevant stress tasks than for the mental arithmetic. Interestingly, abnormalities of the TMJ based on CTs did not relate to muscular hyperarousal during baseline or stress tasks. Furthermore, during the stress tasks, significant EMG changes for non-site-specific muscles did not occur. Thus, although it is common to differentiate TMD patients based on joint abnormalities, these data demonstrate that muscle arousal to stress can occur regardless of the presence or absence of structural abnormalities.

It is also interesting that Rudy et al. (1988) found significantly different posttask pain ratings between patients even though their levels of stress and muscle tension were equivalent. The normal CT group reported significantly higher posttask pain levels for both stress conditions. These results indicate that even though EMG increases during the psychological stress tasks were quite small, a subset of TMD patients (those with normal CTs) perceived these masticatory muscle tension increases as painful.

Thus, although there is some research to support the psychophysiological, MPD model, the psychophysiological results are mixed. Moreover, parafunctional activities such as bruxing, that hypothetically play an important role in MPD do not appear to significantly relate to perceived pain intensity (Harkins, Bush, Price, & Hamer, 1991; Marbach et al., 1990).

In summary, there exists a paucity of research on the validity of either structural or psychophysiological models. Consequently, there is little basis for differentiating between the structural-model dysfunction syndrome and MPD-syndrome patients in terms of etiology. As we note later, there is little evidence to support the differential efficacy of treatments based on either of these two prevalent models. Thus, currently, decisions regarding treatment are empirical, depending upon the preferences of the practitioner.

ROLE OF PSYCHOLOGICAL FACTORS IN TMD

Researchers have implicated psychological factors in several aspects of TMDs. Psychological factors may explain why some patients seem to experience more distress with symptoms and why only a small percentage of patients with symptoms actually seek treatment. From the psychophysiological, MPD model, stress-related muscle hyperactivity and oral habits may serve as etiological factors. Moreover, psychological variables, such as depression and secondary gain, may help explain why some patients do not respond to conventional therapy. As appears to characterize the entire literature of TMD, however, research evaluating the role of psychological characteristics in TMD is both controversial and contradictory (Greene, Olson, & Laskin, 1982).

Emotional Distress in the General Category of TMD

Many individuals associate the presence of psychological disturbances (e.g., depression, anxiety) with orofacial pain syndromes (Dworkin, Truelove, Bonica, & Sola, 1990c). Some individuals have suggested that differences among TMD patients most likely relate to specific psychological traits, psychopathological features, or maladaptive behavior patterns (e.g., Butterworth & Deardorff, 1987; Lipton & Marbach, 1984).

Examination of research that specifically attempts to identify significant psychological variables among TMD patients has proven equivocal (Moss et al., 1982; Rugh & Solberg, 1976). For example, Oakley et al. (1989) reported that 28% of 107 patients with TMD showed signs of depression (Beck Depression Inventory scores over 9; $M = 8.71$, $SD = 8.40$) and 24% evidenced "high anxiety" (Spielberger State–Trait Anxiety Inventory [Spielberger, Gorsuch, & Lushene, 1970], trait anxiety greater than the 83rd percentile). In a retrospective study, Gallagher, Marbach, Raphael, Dohrenwend, and Cloitre (1991) reported that 41% of female TMD patients suffered from major depression. Keefe and Dolan (1986) compared groups of MPD and back pain patients and reported that both groups had high mean scores for anxiety, depression, obsessive–compulsiveness, and somatization, and there were no differences between these two groups, despite the fact that back pain patients evidence more disability as a result of their condition.

Many others, however, have found little difference in psychological distress between TMD patients and other patients with identified organic pathology or even healthy controls. Rugh and Solberg (1976) reviewed 15 studies that investigated the personality characteristics of TMD patients, and Speculand and Goss (1985) reviewed 10 additional studies examining psychological factors in TMD. These reviews concluded that there was no clear TMD "personality profile" and that although elevated levels of anxiety and depression were common among TMD patients, such problems were not consistently found. Based on the diversity of findings and the lack of consistent results, the authors concluded that there is little evidence that TMDs correlate with any specific personality traits. In contrast to Keefe and Dolan (1986), Merskey et al. (1987) and Egan and Betrus (1986) suggested that TMD patients may actually have *lower* rates of psychological disorder than other chronic pain populations.

Similar inconsistency is apparent when comparing TMD patients with healthy controls. Beaton, Egan, Nakagawa-Kogan, and Morrison (1991) reported that, on average, TMD patients complain of *more* psychological symptoms than healthy controls, whereas Schnurr, Brooke, and Rollman (1990) reported that orofacial pain patients *do not differ* from healthy controls with regard to personality, coping, skills, or attitudes toward health. Moreover, TMD patients are no different from other pain patients on diverse psychological measures.

Subgroups of TMD Patients Based on Psychological Factors

Several investigators have attempted to identify subgroups of TMDs based on psychological characteristics of patients or psychopathology using the MMPI and Symptom Checklist-90 Revised (SCL-90R; Butterworth & Deardorff, 1987; Lipton & Marbach, 1984). For example, Butterworth and Deardorff identified three subgroups of TMD patients when performing cluster analysis on SCL-90R scores. One group demonstrated no clinical elevations (39%), a second group (44%) demonstrated elevations of the SCL-90R somatization, depression, and anxiety scales, and a third group (26%) demonstrated significant elevations on many scales, indicating significant emotional problems. It is important to note that Butterworth and Deardorff's Groups 2 and 3 reported more severe pain that Group 1. Thus, the three subgroups of patients appear to represent a continuum of psychological distress that relates to increasing severity of pain and interference with life (see Rudy, Kerns, & Turk, 1988) rather than discrete categories based on types of psychopathology.

Despite the use of psychological measures with TMD patients, psychologists have not yet demonstrated the validity of using such measures to differentiate patients, nor have investigators published replications of subgroups based on these measures (Turk, 1990). Controlled studies of TMD patients have shown few case-control differences on traditional psychological measures (Marbach, Lennon, & Dohrenwend, 1988; Salter, Brooke, Merskey, Fichter, & Kapasianyk, 1983). Furthermore, the literature currently available does not permit clarification of whether differences that are present are consequences or antecedents of the chronic illness experience.

Review of the chronic pain literature reveals that a number of psychological or behavioral factors, in addition to physical and psychological pathology, play a role in reports of pain and disability that accompany chronic pain. Specifically, research suggests that patients' perceptions of pain, the impact of pain on their lives, and perceived control of pain, as well as responses of significant others to pain behaviors and level of activity, all contribute to the patients' disability. Increasingly, health-care professionals view TMDs as multifactorial problems with structural (occlusion), functional (clenching and grinding teeth), external trauma, arthritic deterioration, and psychological factors (e.g., anxiety, tension) as interrelated causes (Solberg, 1986). Thus, investigators need to undertake classification of TMD *patients* rather than merely undertaking classification of disease according to presumed physical and psychological etiology.

Recently proposed classification systems have suggested the use of comprehensive, multiaxial diagnostic approaches for pain patients in general (Turk & Rudy, 1987, 1988) and TMD patients in particular (Rudy, Turk, Zaki, & Curtin, 1989). This approach involves systematic consideration of several parameters of illness simultaneously and requires establishment of an appropriate scale for each parameter or axis.

Turk and Rudy (1987, 1988) have proposed a classification system for chronic pain that emphasizes the empirical integration of physical, psychosocial, and behavioral data in assessing chronic pain. These investigators have labeled this approach the Multiaxial Assessment of Pain (MAP). Their primary hypothesis maintained that certain modal patterns in psychological assessment data recur in chronic pain patients and that these patterns represent homogeneous subgroups of chronic pain patients that are, at least to some extent, independent of medical diagnosis.

In order to assess the psychosocial and behavioral factors, Turk and Rudy (1988) used the West Haven–Yale Multidimensional Pain Inventory (MPI; Kerns, Turk, & Rudy, 1985). The MPI consists of a set of empirically derived scales that assesses chronic pain patients' appraisals of pain severity and impact, mood state, response from significant others, and interference with activities.

In the first study (Turk & Rudy, 1987), these researchers performed a hierarchical cluster analysis on the MPI scales in order to group heterogeneous samples of chronic pain patients according to similarities between their profile patterns. On the basis of this analysis, the investigators identified four distinct patient profiles. Bayesian posterior probabilities then classified a second sample of patients, and these statistical procedures assigned over 90% of the sample, to one of the four groups that the cluster analysis identified in the first sample. The descriptive labels identifying the four group profiles are (1) "Disabled" (DI; 29% of the sample), (2) "Dysfunctional" (DYS; 28%), (3) "Interpersonally Distressed" (ID; 21%), and (4) "Adaptive Copers" (AC; 19%).

The DI and DYS groups differed from the other subgroups by high levels of pain severity, life interference, and affective distress, and low ratings of life control and general activity. The DI and DYS groups differed from each other primarily on the basis of physical pathology, with the DI groups revealing higher levels of physical pathology. The ID group was characterized by low levels of perceived social support, and the AC group displayed low levels of interference and affective distress along with high levels of perceived life control and general activity.

Turk and Rudy (1987) noted that the four groups did not differ significantly from each other on gender, age, or pain chronicity. The groups did differ on physical pathology, with the DI and DYS groups demonstrating significantly more physical pathology than the AC and ID groups. However, even when controlling for physical pathology by using it as a covariate, the groups remained significantly distinct.

In another study (Turk & Rudy, 1988), subgroups of chronic pain patients also emerged through cluster analyses; in this study, however, the investigators did not include physical pathology in the cluster analysis. The analyses identified three groups that were virtually identical to those in the previous study, with the exception that the DYS group combined a larger proportion of patients (43%) than the earlier study. With physical pathology excluded from the analysis, the DI and DYS groups collapsed into a single group. In a similar study examining TMD patients, Rudy et al. (1988) identified three subgroups of patients that were analogous to the DYS, ID, and AC groups in the Turk and Rudy (1988) study.

Turk and Rudy (1990) examined the robustness of the MAP taxonomy by concurrently studying several different pain syndromes, specifically, chronic low back pain (BP), head pain (HP), and TMD patients. As expected, the mean scores on each of the MPI scales were significantly different for each of the three diagnostic samples. However, when controlling statistically for mean differences, the scale intercorrelations between the diagnostic groups were equivalent.

When controlling for group mean scores, the statistical procedures classified a higher percentage of BP patients (62% of the sample) than TMD and HP patients (46% and 44%, respectively) into the DYS group and a smaller percentage of BP patients relative to TMD and HP patients as AC (20%, 32%, and 31%, respectively). There were no between-group differences in the percentage of patients classified as ID (18%, 22%, and 25%, respectively). All three diagnostic groups, however, appeared in each of the MAP clusters. Thus, it is possible that TMD, HP, and BP patients classified within the same subgroup may be more similar to each other than patients with the same diagnoses who fall into different subgroups.

Rudy et al. (1989) contrasted the three subgroups of TMD patients (i.e., DYS, ID, AC) and concluded that the between-cluster differences were independent of age, pain chronicity, common TMD symptoms (e.g., joint sounds, intercisal opening, pain on palpation of the muscles of mastication), and computed axial tomography information. These results call into question the validity of relying predominantly upon physical factors for establishing TMD diagnoses and question the utility of basing treatment decisions exclusively on physical factors. Rather, these findings emphasize the importance of psychosocial and behavioral factors in treatment decision making.

The identification of three subgroups of TMD patients based on psychosocial and behavioral factors has important implications for treatment. These results suggest that clinicians might optimize treatment outcomes for TMD patients by tailoring interventions to match the psychological characteristics of the patients rather than relying predominantly upon psychopathological or physical factors *per se* when formulating treatment plans.

Association of Psychological Distress and Subcategories of TMD

As discussed by Eversole, Stone, Matheson, and Kaplan (1985), research on psychological factors and TMD has unfortunately proceeded as if TMD patients are homogeneous with respect to physical pathology—the "illusion of homogeneity." They predicted that level of psychological distress would vary by physical subcategory of TMD (e.g., myofascial pain dysfunction, internal derangements, degenerative joint disease). In addressing this isue, Eversole et al. examined the MMPI profiles of MPD, TMJ internal derangements, and atypical facial pain patients. They found that both the MPD and the atypical pain groups showed significant elevations for the first three scales of the MMPI beyond the internal derangement group. A number of subsequent studies have reported results consistent with the view expressed by Eversole et al. For example, Bush, Whitehill, and Martelli (1989), Harness and Peltier (1992), Keefe and Dolan (1986), Lundeen, Sturdevant, and George (1987), and McCreary, Clark, Merril, Flack, and Oakley (1991) reported that (1) differences in levels of psychological distress were evident between categories of TMD patients, and (2) MPD patients perceived higher levels of anxiety than TMJ patients.

Once again, however, the research is inconsistent. Marbach and Lund (1981) compared three subgroups of facial pain patients based upon physical pathology: MPD, arthritis of the temporomandibular joints, and trigeminal neuralgia. They found no differences between the groups, and none of the groups reported "high" levels of depression. LeResche et al. (1991) compared the psychological profiles of groups of patients with either MPD, internal derangement, or degenerative joint disease and found physical pathology unrelated to levels of stress, anxiety, depression, or somatic concerns. However, using a more stringent set of diagnostic criteria, they found that MPD patients evidenced higher levels of anxiety, depression, and somatization than the internal derangement and degenerative joint disease groups.

Some of the inconsistencies in the literature undoubtedly are the result of the use of assessment instruments for which no norms exist for TMD populations. Furthermore, such instruments often include somatic items that may reflect prolonged pain and medication use rather than psychopathology or response of patients to the apparent inability of clinicians to ameliorate pain or definitely identify the cause of pain.

We must be cautious in interpreting studies of psychological symptoms in TMD patients because investigators performing the studies usually failed to control for severity of pain. When McCreary et al. (1991) did control for pain severity, the differences between the TMJ and MPD groups on anxiety and depression disappeared, and the groups only differed significantly on somatic concerns. Similarly, when Marbach and Lund (1981) compared patients with MPD, degenerative joint disease, and trigeminal neuralgia with controls, they found no differences among the groups on measures of emotional distress. Rather, they did find that patients with severe pain were more anxious and depressed than patients with minor pain.

In general, studies suggest that the level of psychopathology is no greater in MPD patients than in controls, but MPD patients appear to respond with greater facial muscle arousal to stressful stimuli. The pattern of scores on pain and distress measures in MPD patients is consistent with a psychophysiological model of disorder. In several studies, the MPD group reported significantly higher levels of psychological distress. However, MPD patients' elevated anxiety and depression may not relate solely to their pain levels. MPD patients are often preoccupied with worries about physical functioning and fearful about something going wrong with their bodies. Furthermore, they often avoid dealing with distressing aspects of their lives. Such suppression of emotional difficulties might contribute to excessive muscle tension and may facilitate dysfunctional oral habits such as clenching and bruxing.

Even though researchers have identified subgroups of TMD patients based on structural and psychological variables, at the present time nearly all patients who present with the classical signs of TMDs tend to receive similar treatments and the treatments they receive depend upon the preferences and prejudices of the clinicians from whom they seek treatment. To date, there is little conclusive evidence that (1) there are subgroups of TMD patients based on behavioral patterns or psychopathology, and (2) TMD patients who differ on the identification of radiographic signs of joint abnormalities differ on any psychosocial, psychopathological, or behavioral variables.

Rugh (1982) summarized by saying,

> There is convincing evidence that psychological factors play a significant role in the etiology and maintenance of masticatory pain and dysfunction. These effects are mediated through (a) muscle hyperactivity, (b) altered perception and tolerance of pain, (c) secondary gains, (d) depression, (e) personality characteristics, (f) anxiety, and (g) parafunctional habits. However, masticatory pain and dysfunction cannot be understood by a study of only psychological factors. (p. 90)

ASSESSMENT OF TMD PATIENTS

A thorough assessment of chronic TMD patients routinely includes careful behavioral and psychosocial evalaution (Rugh, 1982). It is usually helpful if the oral history includes questions to evaluate behavioral, social, emotional, and cognitive factors that may initiate, sustain, or result from the patient's condition. A number of psychological and behavioral factors to recognize during screening and comprehensive evaluations could necessitate further evaluation by a mental health professional (see Table 3.1).

Table 3.1. Indications for Psychological Assessment of TMD Patients

Psychological assessment of TMD patients is indicated when:
- There is clinically significant anxiety or depression.
- There is evidence of drug abuse.
- There have been repeated failures with conventional therapies.
- There is evidence of secondary gain.
- Major life events have produced TMD symptoms.
- Pain duration is greater than 6 months.
- There is a history of stress-related disorders.
- There is inconsistency in response to drugs.
- There are inconsistent, inappropriate, and vague reports of pain.
- There appears to be an exaggeration or overdramatization of symptoms (pain behaviors).
- Symptoms vary with life events.

TREATMENT EFFICACY

Traditionally, most TMD treatment varied according to the clinician's favorite theory (e.g., occlusal disharmonies, psychophysiology). As we discuss later, the available evidence (Greene & Laskin, 1983) suggests that almost any treatment can be effective for a substantial proportion of TMD patients (70–80% success rate) and these results seem to endure (94% maintenance), at least in the short term. However, this suggestion that 20% to 30% of patients fail to benefit from treatment and some studies have reported significant relapse over time (Zaki, Turk, & Rudy, 1992).

Biofeedback and Relaxation Training

Because of the emphasis of the psychophysiological model on stress and muscular activity in TMD, clinicians often use EMG biofeedback in conjunction with relaxation therapy in the treatment of TMD (e.g., Carlsson, Gale, & Ohman, 1975; Dohrman & Laskin, 1978; Pierce & Gale, 1988). Unfortunately, however, some studies have not supported the efficacy of EMG biofeedback training (e.g., Moss, Wedding, & Sanders, 1983; Peck & Kraft, 1977). For example, Moss and associates reported that relaxation training was more important than biofeedback, which added little to relaxation training.

Furthermore, research suggests that although biofeedback may benefit some patients, other patients may need additional psychological interventions. For example, Gessel (1975) treated patients with EMG biofeedback training and recommendations for home practice of progressive muscle relaxation training. In this study, 65% of patients reported satisfactory reduction in symptoms. The 35% who reported unsuccessful treatment also reported higher levels of depression and marked impairment in activities of daily living. Such data suggest that an additional intervention for depression might be necessary as a supplement or alternative to biofeedback. This study emphasized that TMD patients are not a homogeneous group; different patients may require specific treatments directed toward their individual problems.

Several investigators (e.g., Crockett, Foreman, Alden, & Blasberg, 1986; Funch & Gale, 1984) have noted that although a number of behavioral techniques effectively treat TMD patients, there is little evidence for the superiority of relaxation training, biofeedback training, or cognitive–behavioral therapy. The only advantage of biofeedback over these other approaches is that biofeedback appears to help patients learn more quickly (Gale, 1986).

Researchers need to be circumspect when interpreting the results of the biofeedback and stress management studies. In most of these studies, the follow-up periods have been short. This is problematic in that there is some evidence suggesting that the beneficial effects of EMG biofeedback training are not long lasting, with EMG levels often returning to pretreatment levels on termination of treatment (Mohl, Ohrbach, Crow, & Gross, 1990).

Interocclusal Appliances

Splint therapy using a wide range of interoral appliances is the preferred mode of intervention for those who adhere to the structural, occlusal disharmonies model.

A number of investigators have evaluated the efficacy of various splints, and a few studies have directly compared splints with biofeedback training and relaxation training. Some studies have reported that splints were more efficacious than relaxation training and biofeedback training (e.g., Okeson, Kemper, Moody, & Haley, 1983). However, in the study by Okeson et al., the relaxation treatment comprised giving patients a 20-minute tape of a relaxation procedure with instructions to practice once a day. Thus, patients did not receive an optimally administered form of relaxation treatment. In addition, Hijzen, Slangen, and Van Houweligen (1986) found EMG biofeedback training to be more effective than splints.

Crockett et al. (1986) reported no difference between EMG biofeedback training, relaxation training, transcutaneous electrical nerve stimulation, and a splint and physiotherapy exercise program. All treatments produced reductions in EMGs during resting and task (physical and psychological stress) conditions. Similarly, Dahlstrom and Carlsson (1982, 1984) found no difference in the efficacy of splints and EMG biofeedback training.

Finally, Zaki et al. (1992) noted that splints appeared more effective than stress management training and EMG biofeedback training at posttreatment; however, by 6-month follow-up, the patients treated with splints demonstrated significant relapse on depression and a trend toward relapse on pain. The patients treated with stress management and biofeedback treatment maintained their initial results and showed additional improvements surpassing the splint therapy at the follow-up.

Predictors of Outcome

One problem with the previously reported results is that they focus on group effects. It is probable that different patients respond optimally to different treatments. For example, Gale and Funch (1984) and Zaki et al. (1992) reported that the best predictors of treatment outcome for TMD were psychosocial factors, not clinical and demographic factors. Funch and Gale (1984) noted that patients who evidenced the most successful outcomes (both short- and long-term) were more motivated (as per clinician ratings of compliance and cooperation), were less depressed, and reported higher levels of internal locus of control than other patients.

Results from some studies have shown that younger patients with symptoms of TMD are more likely to benefit from relaxation training than older patients with longer histories of TMDs (Funch & Gale, 1984; Gessel & Alderman, 1971). Conversely, Funch and Gale reported that those who were successful with EMG biofeedback training were older, more likely to be married, and had symptoms for a longer period than those who were less successful with biofeedback. In addition, patients who reported bruxing behavior were more likely to succeed with relaxation therapy and less likely to succeed with EMG biofeedback training. Turk and Rudy (1986) observed that TMD patients classified in the DYS group, relative to the ID and AC groups, exhibited the highest levels of hypermuscular arousal in response to stress. These results suggest that dysfunctional patients might benefit more than ID and AC patients from combined stress management and EMG biofeedback training.

Results such as these just cited emphasize the importance of not treating TMD patients as homogeneous. Rather, clinicians need to individualize treatments to match patients' characteristics. Interestingly, the variables that appear to relate to treatment efficacy are psychological rather than physiological parameters.

Treatment Nonresponders

It is important to reiterate that 20–30% of TMD patients are nonresponsive to conservative treatment. Schwartz, Greene, and Laskin (1979) suggested that nonresponsive patients with MPD syndrome are more psychologically disturbed than patients who do respond to treatment. The researchers found that nonresponders evidenced higher scores on the depression and psychopathic deviant scales of the MMPI. Gessel (1975) noted that more depressed patients did not fare as well with biofeedback as those who were less depressed and suggested that the more depressed patients might need additional interventions to supplement treatment. We have found similar results in the first author's laboratory (Zaki et al., 1992), and studies are currently under way to determine whether specific interventions to treat depression can enhance the effects of splints and stress management and biofeedback. Olson and Malow (1987) found that nonresponders to conventional TMD therapies (i.e., splints) did well with a combined EMG biofeedback training and cognitive–behavioral therapy program, and patients receiving this combined treatment program fared better than patients receiving EMG biofeedback training alone. The addition of psychotherapy may enhance the effects of biofeedback because it focuses on patients' problems in living that may lead to stress and muscle tension, whereas biofeedback alone simply teaches patients to relax.

It appears that TMD patients who have more complex problems (e.g., high levels of depression, interpersonal problems) may require more comprehensive approaches than they obtain from any one modality. Thus, it might serve us well to rephrase "Which treatment is effective?" to "Which treatment is most effective for patients with what particular characteristics?"

Mechanisms of Change

The fact that splint therapy is successful cannot serve as proof that a malocclusion exists and the structural theory is correct. One clinical report evaluated the effectiveness of maxillary occlusal splints on two groups of patients with TMJ dysfunction and found equal effectiveness (80% successful for both groups) whether or not the subjects showed any evidence of occlusal interference (cited in Clark, 1987). Similarly, studies demonstrating the efficacy of behavioral methods do not provide adequate support for the importance of muscular arousal. Researchers have not definitively demonstrated the hypothesized association between elevated muscular arousal and TMD symptoms, and many patients maintain benefits following treatment even though they do not demonstrate alterations in muscular activity (Burdette & Gale, 1988; Dahlstrom, Carlsson, Gale, & Jansson, 1984; Dalen, Ellerben, Espelid, & Gronningsaeter, 1986; Hijzen et al., 1986).

The results of a study by Burdette and Gale (1988) are instructive. The investigators examined the effects of EMG biofeedback training on patients with TMD. Their results did not support a direct association between change in the level of tonic EMG activity or muscle tension and the relief of pain. The treatment-failure group achieved as dramatic a decrease in resting EMG activity during therapy as did the treatment-success group, without experiencing the same degree of symptom relief. Thus, lowering tonic, resting EMG activity alone does not appear sufficient to ensure successful therapy for TMD patients.

Research conducted by Laskin and his colleagues has demonstrated that a wide range of conservative treatment approaches can effectively reduce symptoms of TMD (e.g., anxiolytic medication, oral appliances, relaxation training, transcutaneous electrical nerve stimulation, and psychological counseling). However, they have also reported similar results with the use of outright placebo treatments (i.e., nonactive drug; Greene & Laskin, 1971, 1972a), a nonoccluding biteplate (Greene & Laskin, 1972b), nonfunctional biofeedback (Dohrmann & Laskin, 1978), and mock equilibration (Goodman, Green, & Laskin, 1976). Goodman et al. noted that mock equilibration involving an elaborate rationale, the construction of dental casts on the first visit, and grinding on the nonoccluding surfaces on the teeth by a slow-speed handpiece on two subsequent visits, produced total or nearly total remission of the pain symptoms in 64% of the patients. The use of a placebo splint—an acrylic maxillary appliance worn supposedly to separate the malocculuding teeth and rest the muscle but therapeutically does not improve occlusion or muscle tension produced similar levels of improvement (Greene & Laskin, 1972a). Laskin and Greene (1972b) also showed that 52% of patients reported pain reduction from a placebo drug given with an elaborate rationale.

The fact that patients apparently can successfully manage TMD symptoms through such diverse interventions suggests that something other than structural change is responsible for the treatment effects. Moreover, the efficacy of such a diversity of interventions suggests that no specific single treatment is necessary for a successful treatment outcome. It is plausible that there exist nonspecific factors common to all treatments for TMD, namely attention, a credible rationale, placebo effects, reduction of anxiety and tension, and cognitive awareness of the oral cavity and patients' maladaptive behaviors. It is also possible that some of the noted effects are due to the general tendency for this type of disorder to improve over time.

Regression to the mean is also a likely factor in the reported success with these diverse intervention. People tend to seek treatment when symptoms are at their worst and this, coupled with the natural history of the disorder likely leads to significant symptom improvement over time. For example, Salter, Brooke, and Merskey (1986) reported that untreated patients fared as well as patients receiving combinations of physical therapy modalities (e.g., ultrasound and occlusal splints) at 3-month follow-up. In this study, the distribution of outcomes did not vary as a function of whether the patients reported receiving any treatment. Therefore, various interventions may overestimate rates of successful treatment.

RECOMMENDATIONS FOR TREATMENT OF TMD PATIENTS

The major goals of management of TMD include reduction of pain, restoration of normal jaw function, reduction of need for future health care, reduction in use of analgesic medication, and restoration of normal lifestyle functioning. We can best achieve these goals by designing programs to treat the physical disorder and reduce the contributing psychological factors. The treatment must address not only the objective symptoms but also the psychosocial factors in the patient's life that motivated him or her to seek treatment.

Optimal treatment will likely involve careful patient education about jaw habits, jaw posture, and the relationship between stress, muscle activity, and painful symptoms in order to assist the patient in observing, reducing, and avoiding injurious activity. TMDs are generally benign conditions (Greene & Laskin, 1988). It is important to reassure the patient that he or she does not have cancer or a progressive, debilitating disease. Such assurance can help relieve anxiety about the persistence or grave nature of the symptoms.

In many instances, to relieve painful symptoms, the patient must combine the more physical or somatic techniques, such as interocclusal appliances and physical modalities, with educational–behavioral techniques, such as exercises, relaxation training, stress management training, and avoidance of harmful activity. The failure to combine appropriate techniques is a major reason patients sometimes fail to achieve long-lasting pain relief. Purely physical and somatic treatment often yields transient relief at best.

Stress management training is an important component as it can achieve the following:

1. Teach patients about physiological symptoms and sources of stress as well as stressful habit patterns (e.g., bruxism)
2. Provide practical skills for habit change and relaxation technique
3. Underscore the importance of cognition and perception as these processes relate to stress (maladaptive or negative thought patterns)
4. Emphasize the concepts of voluntary self-regulation and self-responsibility.

In addition to identifying the symptoms of stress, it is equally important to help patients become aware of the sources of stress.

CONCLUDING COMMENTS

As discussed in the initial section of this chapter, a major problem in the TMD literature that may account for many of the inconsistent results is the lack of agreement regarding criteria for different diagnostic subgroups of TMD. The fact that dentists have only recently paid attention to the reliability of examination ratings (e.g., pain upon muscle palpation) they use to diagnose TMD compounds the problems within the literature. In the face of unreliable diagnostic judgments and large variability in treatment methods among clinicians, "doctor shopping" may seem entirely rational to patients suffering from TMD.

Given the current state of knowledge of TMD, clinicians have little empirical basis for making treatment decisions. The most prudent course at present is, at least initially, to use the least intrusive and most conservative treatments. Furthermore, it is advisable to use a combined treatment approach that incorporates occlusal splints, education about jaw functioning, and EMG biofeedback and stress management training. In summary, the challenge to clinicians treating TMD patients is to sort out the complex physical and psychiatric differential diagnoses and develop tailored treatment approaches that fit the idiosyncracies of each patient.

Investigators need to focus future research on treating recalcitrant TMD patients, identifying the characteristics of those patients who fail to benefit from the usual modalities, and matching treatments to patients' characteristics. To date, investigators have not consistently identified nonresponders prior to the initiation of treatment (cf. Millstein-Prentkly & Olson, 1979). Some of the cited evidence provides preliminary leads, and the use of measures such as the MPI and the identification of subgroups appears to offer a promising approach (Turk, 1990).

ACKNOWLEDGMENT

Support for completion of this chapter was provided in part by grant DE07514 from the National Institute of Dental Research.

REFERENCES

Al-Hasson, H. K., Ismail, A. I., & Ash, M. M., Jr. (1986). Concerns of patients seeking treatment for TMJ dysfunction. *Journal of Prosthetic Dentistry, 56,* 217–221.
Bean, L. R., & Thomas, C. A. (1987). Significance of condylar positions in patients with temporomandibular disorders. *Journal of the American Dental Association, 114,* 76–77.
Beaton, R. D., Egan, K. J., Nakagawa-Kogan, H., & Morrison, K. N. (1991). Self-reported symptoms of stress with temporomandibular disorders: Comparisons to healthy men and women. *Journal of Prosthetic Dentistry, 65,* 289–293.
Blaschke, D., & Blaschke, T. (1981). A method of determining temporomandibular joint bony relationships. *Journal of Dental Research, 60,* 35–43.
Burdette, B. H., & Gale, E. N. (1988). The effects of treatment on masticatory muscle activity and mandibular posture in myofascial pain–dysfunction patients. *Journal of Dental Research, 67,* 1126–1130.
Bush, F. M., Whitehill, J. M., & Martelli, M. F. (1989). Pain assessment in temporomandibular disorders. *Journal of Craniomandibular Practice, 7,* 137–143.
Butterworth, J. C., & Deardorff, W. W. (1987). Psychometric profiles of craniomandibular pain patients: Identifying specific subgroups. *Journal of Craniomandibular Practice, 5,* 225–232.
Carlsson, S. G., Gale, E. N., & Ohman, A. (1975). Treatment of temporomandibular joint syndrome with biofeedback training. *Journal of the American Dental Association, 91,* 602–605.
Clark, G. T., & Adler, R. (1985). A critical evaluation of occlusal therapy: Occlusal adjustment procedures. *Journal of the American Dental Association, 110,* 743–750.
Crockett, D. J., Foreman, M. E., Alden, L., & Blasberg, B. (1986). A comparison of treatment modes in the management of myofascial pain dysfunction syndrome. *Biofeedback and Self-Regulation, 11,* 279–291.
Dahlstom, L., & Carlsson, S. G. (1982). Comparison of effects of electromyographic biofeedback and occlusal splint therapy on mandibular function. *Scandinavian Journal of Dental Research, 90,* 151–156.
Dahlstom, L., & Carlsson, S. G. (1984). Treatment of mandibular dysfunction: The clinical usefulness of biofeedback in relation to splint therapy. *Journal of Oral Rehabilitation, 11,* 277–284.
Dahlstrom, L., Carlsson, S. G., Gale, E. N., & Jansson, T. G. (1984). Clinical and electromyographic effects of biofeedback training in mandibular dysfunction. *Biofeedback and Self-Regulation, 9,* 451–463.
Dahlstrom, L., Carlsson, S. G., Gale, E. N., & Jansson, T. G. (1985). Stress-induced muscular activity in mandibular dysfunction: Effects of biofeedback training. *Journal of Behavioral Medicine, 8,* 191–200.
Dalen, K., Ellerben, B., Espelid, J., & Gronningsaeter, A. (1986). EMG feedback in the treatment of myofascial pain dysfunction syndrome. *Acta Odontologica Scandinavica, 44,* 279–288.
Dohrmann, R. J., & Laskin, D. M. (1978). An evaluation of electomyographic biofeedback in the treatment of myofascial pain–dysfunction. *Journal of the American Dental Association, 96,* 656–662.
Dworkin, S. F., & Burgess, J. A. (1987). Orofacial pain of psychogenic origin: Current concepts and classification. *Journal of the American Dental Association, 115,* 565–571.
Dworkin, S. F., Huggins, K. H., LeResche, L. R., Von Korff, M., Howard, J., Truelove, E. L., & Sommers, E. (1990a). Epidemiology of signs and symptoms in temporomandibular disorders: Clinical signs in cases and controls. *Journal of the American Dental Association, 120,* 273–281.
Dworkin, S. F., LeResche, L. R., & DeRouen, T. (1988). Reliability of clinical measurement in temporomandibular disorders. *Clinical Journal of Pain, 4,* 89–100.

Dworkin, S. F., LeResche, L., DeRouen, T., Von Korff, M., Truelove, E. L., Sommers, E., & Huggins, K. H. (1990b). Assessing clinical signs of temporomandibular disorders: Reliability of clinical examiners. *Journal of Prosthetic Dentistry, 63,* 574–579.

Dworkin, S. F., Truelove, E. L., Bonica, J. J., & Sola, A. (1990c). Facial and head pain caused by myofascial and temporo-mandibular disorder. In J. J. Bonica (Ed.), *The management of pain* (pp. 727–725). Philadelphia: Lea & Febiger.

Egan, K. J., & Betrus, P. (1986). Psychological functioning in five pain syndromes: Tension headache, backache, migraine, temporomandibular and gastrointestinal pain syndromes. *Clinical Journal of Pain, 2,* 233–238.

Ericson, S., & Lundberg, M. (1968). Structural changes in the finger, wrist, and temporomandibular joint: A comparative study. *Acta Ondontologica Scandinavica, 26,* 111–119.

Eversole, L. R., Stone, C. E., Matheson, D., & Kaplan, H. (1985). Psychometric profiles and facial pain. *Oral Surgery, Oral Medicine, and Oral Pathology, 60,* 269–274.

Flor, H., Birbaumer, N., Schulte, W., & Roos, R. (1991). Stress-related electromyographic responses in patients with chronic temporomandibular pain. *Pain, 46,* 145–152.

Flor, H., & Turk, D. C. (1989). Psychophysiology of chronic pain patients: Do chronic pain patients exhibit symptom-specific psychophysiological responses? *Psychological Bulletin, 105,* 215–259.

Funch, D. P., & Gale, E. N. (1984). Biofeedback and relaxation therapy for chronic temporomandibular joint pain: Predicting successful outcomes. *Journal of Consulting and Clinical Psychology, 52,* 928–935.

Gale, E. N. (1986). Behavioral approaches to temporomandibular disorders. *Annals of Behavioral Medicine, 8,* 11–17.

Gale, E. N., & Funch, D. P. (1984). Factors associated with successful outcome from behavioral therapy for chronic temporomandibular (TMJ) pain. *Journal of Psychosomatic Research, 28,* 441–448.

Gallagher, R. M., Marbach, J. J., Raphael, K. G., Dohrenwend, B. P., & Cloitre, M. (1991). Is major depression comorbid with temporomandibular pain and dysfunction syndrome? A pilot study. *Clinical Journal of Pain, 7,* 219–225.

Gessel, A. H. (1975). Electromyographic biofeedback and tricyclic antidepressants in myofascial pain–dysfunction syndrome: Psychological predictors of outcome. *Journal of the American Dental Association, 91,* 1048–1052.

Gessel, A. H., & Alderman, M. M. (1971). Management of myofascial pain–dysfunction syndrome of the temporomandibular joint by tension control training. *Psychosomatics, 12,* 302–309.

Goodman, P., Greene, C. S., & Laskin, D. M. (1976). Response of patients with myofascial pain–dysfunction syndrome to mock equilibration. *Journal of the American Dental Association, 92,* 755–758.

Greene, C. S., & Laskin, D. M. (1971). Meprobamate therapy for the myofascial pain dysfunction syndrome: A double-blind evaluation. *Journal of the American Dental Association, 82,* 587–590.

Greene, C. S., & Laskin, D. M. (1972a). Splint therapy for the myofascial pain–dysfunction (MPD) syndrome: A comparative study. *Journal of the American Dental Association, 84,* 624–628.

Greene, C. S., & Laskin, D. M. (1972b). Therapeutic effects of diazepam fascial pain–dysfunction (MPD) patients. Program and abstracts of papers, International Association of Dental Research, Abstract Nos. 193, 50.

Greene, C. S., & Laskin, D. M. (1983). Long-term evaluation of treatment for myofascial pain–dysfunction syndrome: A comparative analysis. *Journal of the American Dental Association, 107,* 235–238.

Greene, C. S., & Laskin, D. M. (1988). Long-term status of TMJ clicking in patients with myofascial pain and dysfunction. *Journal of the American Dental Association, 117,* 461–465.

Greene, C. S., Olson, R. E., & Laskin, D. M. (1982). Psychological factors in the etiology, progression, and treatment of MPD syndrome. *Journal of the American Dental Association, 105,* 443–448.

Haber, J. D., Moss, R. A., Kuczmierczk, A. R., & Garrett, J. C. (1983). Assessment and treatment of stress in myofascial pain–dysfunction syndrome: A model for analysis. *Journal of Oral Rehabilitation, 10,* 187–196.

Harkins, S. W., Bush, F. M., Price, D. D., & Hamer, R. M. (1991). Symptom report in orofacial pain patients: Relation to chronic pain, experimental pain, illness behavior, and personality. *Clinical Journal of Pain, 7,* 102–113.

Harness, D. M., & Peltier, B. (1992). Comparison of MMPI scores with self-report of sleep disturbance and bruxism in the facial pain population. *Journal of Craniomandibular Practice, 10,* 70–74.

Helkimo, M. (1974). Studies of function and dysfunction of the masticatory system: II. Index of anamnestic and clinical dysfunction and occlusal state. *Swedish Dental Journal, 67,* 101–121.

Hijzen, T. H., Slangen, J. L., & Van Houweligen, H. C. (1986). Subjective, clinical and EMG aspects of biofeedback and splint treatment. *Journal of Oral Rehabilitation, 13*, 529–539.

Kapel, L., Glaros, A. G., & McGlynn, F. D. (1989). Psychophysiological responses to stress in patients with myofascial pain–dysfunction syndrome. *Journal of Behavioral Medicine, 12*, 297–406.

Katz, J. O., Rugh, J. P., Hatch, J. P., Langlais, R. P., Terezhalmy, G. T., & Borcherding, S. H. (1989). Effect of experimental stress on masseter and temporalis muscle activity in human subjects with temporomandibular disorders. *Archives of Oral Biology, 34*, 393–398.

Keefe, F. J., & Dolan, E. (1986). Pain behavior and pain coping strategies in low back pain and myofascial pain dysfunction syndrome patients. *Pain, 24*, 49–56.

Kerns, R. J., Turk, D. C., & Rudy, T. E. (1985). The West Haven–Yale Multidimensional Pain Inventory (WHYMPI). *Pain, 23*, 245–256.

Kircos, L. T., Ortendahl, D. A., Mark, A. S., & Arakawa, M. (1987). Magnetic resonance imaging of the TMJ disk in asymptomatic volunteers. *Journal of Oral and Maxillofacial Surgery, 45*, 852–854.

Laskin, D. M. (1969). Etiology of the pain–dysfunction syndrome. *Journal of the American Dental Association, 79*, 147–153.

Laskin, D. M. (1979). Myofascial pain–dysfunction: Etiology. In B. G. Sarnat & D. M. Laskin (Eds.), *The temporomandibular joint: A biological basis for clinical practice* (pp. 289–299). Springfield, IL: Charles C. Thomas.

LeResche, L., Dworkin, S. F., Sommers, E. E., & Truelove, E. L. (1991). An epidemiologic evaluation of two diagnostic classification schemes for temporomandibular disorders. *Journal of Prosthetic Dentistry, 65*, 131–137.

Lipton, J. A., & Marbach, J. J. (1984). Predictors of treatment outcome in patients with myofascial pain–dysfunction syndrome and organic temporomandibular joint disorders. *Journal of Prosthetic Dentistry, 51*, 387–393.

Lundeen, T. F., Sturdevant, J. R., & George, J. M. (1987). Stress as a factor in muscle and temporomandibular joint pain. *Journal of Oral Rehabilitation, 14*, 447–455.

Marbach, J. J., Lennon, M. C., & Dohrenwend, B. P. (1988). Candidate risk factors for temporomandibular pain and dysfunction syndrome: Psychosocial, health behavior, physical illness, and injury. *Pain, 34*, 139–147.

Marbach, J. J., & Lund, P. (1981). Depression, anhedonia and anxiety in temporomandibular joint and other facial pain syndromes. *Pain, 11*, 73–84.

Marbach, J. J., Raphael, K. G., Dohrenwend, B. P., & Lennon, M. C. (1990). The validity of tooth grinding measures: Etiology of pain dysfunction syndrome revisited. *Journal of the American Dental Association, 120*, 327–333.

McCreary, C. P., Clark, G. T., Merril, R., Flack, V., & Oakley, M. E. (1991). Psychological distress and diagnostic subgroups of temporomandibular disorder patients. *Pain, 44*, 29–34.

McNeill, C., Mohl, N. D., Rugh, J. D., & Tanaka, T. T. (1990). Temporomandibular disorders: Diagnosis, management, education, and research. *Journal of the American Dental Association, 120*, 253–263.

Mercuri, L. G., Olson, R. E., & Laskin, D. M. (1979). The specificity of response to experimental stress in patients with myofascial pain and dysfunction syndrome. *Journal of Dental Research, 58*, 1866–1871.

Merskey, H., Lau, C. L., Russell, E. S., Brooke, R. I., James, M., Lappano, S., Neilsen, J., & Tilsworth, R. H. (1987). Screening for psychiatric morbidity. The pattern of psychological illness and premorbid characteristics in four chronic pain populations. *Pain, 30*, 141–157.

Millstein-Prentkly, S., & Olson, R. E. (1979). Predictability of treatment outcome in patients with myofascial pain–dysfunction (MPD) syndrome. *Journal of Dental Research, 58*, 1341-1346.

Mohl, N. D., Ohrbach, R. K., Crow, H. C., & Gross, A. J. (1990). Devices for the diagnosis and treatment of temporomandibular disorders. Part III: Thermography, ultrasound, electrical stimulation, and electromyographic biofeedback. *Journal of Prosthetic Dentistry, 63*, 472–477.

Moss, R. A., & Adams, H. E. (1984). Physiological reactions to stress in subjects with and without myofascial pain dysfunction symptoms. *Journal of Oral Rehabilitation, 11*, 219–232.

Moss, R. A., Garrett, J., & Chiodo, J. F. (1982). Temporomandibular joint dysfunction and myofascial pain dysfunction: Parameters, etiology and treatment. *Psychological Bulletin, 92*, 331–346.

Moss, R. A., Ruff, M. H., & Sturgis, E. T. (1984). Oral behavioral patterns in facial pain, headache, and non-headache populations. *Behavior Research and Therapy, 22*, 683–687.

Moss, R. A., Wedding, D., & Sanders, S. H. (1983). The comparative efficacy of relaxation training and masseter EMG feedback in the treatment of TMJ dysfunction. *Journal of Oral Rehabilitation, 10,* 9–17.

National Institutes of Health Consensus Development Conference. (1986). *The integrated approach to the management of pain.* NIH Consensus Development Statement, vol. 3, no. 3. Washington, DC: U.S. Government Printing Office.

Oakley, M. E., Clark, G. T., McCreary, C. P., Solberg, W. K., Flack, V. F., & Pullinger, A. G. (1989). Dentists' ability to detect psychological problems in patients with temporomandibular disorders and chronic pain. *Journal of the American Dental Association, 118,* 727–730.

Okeson, J. P., Kemper, J. T., Moody, P. M., & Haley, J. V. (1983). Evaluation of occlusal splint therapy and relaxation procedures in patients with temporomandibular disorders. *Journal of the American Dental Association, 107,* 420–424.

Olson, R. E., & Malow, R. M. (1987). Effects of biofeedback and psychotherapy on patients with myofascial pain dysfunction who are nonresponsive to conventional treatments. *Rehabilitation Psychology, 32,* 195–204.

Peck, C. L., & Kraft, G. (1977). Electromyographic biofeedback for pain related to muscle tension. *Archives of Surgery, 112,* 889–193.

Pierce, C. J., & Gale, E. N. (1988). A comparison of different treatments for nocturnal bruxism. *Journal of Dental Research, 67,* 597–601.

Reynolds, M. D. (1988). Is the concept of temporomandibualr joint pain–dysfunction syndrome valid? *Journal of Craniomandibular Practice, 6,* 299–307.

Rudy, T. E. (1990). Psychophysiological assessment in chronic orofacial pain. *Anesthesia Progress, 37,* 82–87.

Rudy, T. E., Kerns, R. D., & Turk, D. C. (1988). Chronic pain and depression: Toward a cognitive–behavioral mediation model. *Pain, 25,* 129–140.

Rudy, T. E., Turk, D. C., & Flor, H. (1988, May). *Stress and chronic TMJ pain: A psychophysiological analysis.* Paper presented at the joint meeting of the Canadian and American Pain Societies, Toronto, Canada.

Rudy, T. E., Turk, D. C., Zaki, H. S., & Curtin, H. D. (1989). An empirical taxometric alternative to traditional classification of temporomandibular disorders. *Pain, 36,* 311–320.

Rugh, J. D. (1982). Psychological factors in the etiology of masticatory pain and dysfunction. In D. Laskin (Ed.), *The President's Conference on the examination, diagnosis, and management of temporomandibular disorders* (pp. 85–94). Chicago: American Dental Association.

Rugh, J. D., & Montgomery, G. T. (1987). Physiological reactions of patients with TM disorders vs. symptom-free controls on a physical stress task. *Journal of Craniomandibular Disorders and Facial Oral Pain, 1,* 243–250.

Rugh, J. D., & Solberg, W. K. (1976). Psychological implications in temporomandibular pain and dysfunction. *Oral Science Review, 1,* 3–15.

Rugh, J. D., & Solberg, W. K. (1985). Oral health status in the United States: Temporomandibular disorders. *Journal of Dental Education, 49,* 398–405.

Salter, M. W., Brooke, R. I., & Merskey, H. (1986). Temporomandibular dysfunction syndrome: The relationship of clinical and psychological data to outcome. *Journal of Behavioral Medicine, 9,* 97–109.

Salter, M., Brooke, R. I., Merskey, H., Fichter, G. F., & Kapasianyk, D. H. (1983). Is the temporomandibular pain and dysfunction syndrome a disorder of the mind? *Pain, 17,* 151–166.

Schiffman, E., Fricton, J. R., Haley, D., & Shapiro, B. L. (1990). The prevalence and treatment needs of subjects with temporomandibular disorders. *Journal of the American Dental Association, 120,* 295–303.

Schnurr, R. F., Brooke, R. I., & Rollman, G. B. (1990). Psychosocial correlates of temporomandibular joint pain and dysfunction. *Pain, 42,* 153–165.

Schwartz, R. A., Greene, C. S., & Laskin, D. M. (1979). Personality characteristics of patients with myofascial pain–dysfunction (MPD) syndrome. *Journal of Dental Research, 58,* 1435–1439.

Solberg, W. K. (1986). Temporomandibular disorders: Background and the clinical problem. *British Dental Journal, 160,* 157–161.

Speculand, B., & Goss, A. M. (1985). A review of psychological factors in temporomandibular joint dysfunction pain. *International Journal of Oral Surgery, 14,* 131–137.

Spielberger, C., Gorsuch, R., & Lushene, N. (1970). *Manual for the State-Trait Anxiety Inventory.* Palo Alto, CA: Consulting Psychologist's Press.

Stenn, P. G., Mothersill, K. J., & Brooke, R. I. (1979). Biofeedback and cognitive behavioral treatment of myofascial pain dysfunction. *Behavior Therapy, 10,* 29–36.

Thomas, L. J., Tiber, N., & Schireson, S. (1973). The effects of anxiety and frustration on muscular tensions related to the temporomandibular joint syndrome. *Oral Surgery, 36,* 763–768.

Turk, D. C. (1990). Customizing treatment for chronic pain patients: Who, what, and why. *Clinical Journal of Pain, 6,* 255–270.

Turk, D. C., & Rudy, T. E. (1986, March). *Stress, chronic pain, and muscular reactivity.* Paper presented at the 7th Annual Meeting of the Society of Behavioral Medicine, San Francisco, CA.

Turk, D. C., & Rudy, T. E. (1987). Toward a comprehensive assessment of chronic pain patients: A multiaxial approach. *Behaviour Research and Therapy, 24,* 237–249.

Turk, D. C., & Rudy, T. E. (1988). Toward and empirically derived taxonomy of chronic pain patients: Integration of psychological assessment. *Journal of Consulting and Clinical Psychology, 56,* 233–238.

Turk, D. C., & Rudy, T. E. (1990). Robustness of an empirically derived taxonomy of chronic pain patients. *Pain, 43,* 27–36.

Van der Weele, T., & Dibbets, J.M.H. (1987). Helkimo's index: A scale or just a set of symptoms? *Journal of Oral Rehabilitation, 14,* 229–237.

Von Korff, M., Dworkin, S. F., LeResche, L., & Kruger, A. (1987). Epidemiology of temporomandibular disorders: TMD pain compared to other pain sites. *Pain, Suppl. 4,* S123.

Yemm, R. (1969). Temporomandibular disorders and masseter muscle response to stress. *British Dental Journal, 127,* 508–510.

Zaki, H. S., Turk, D. C., & Rudy, T. E. (1992). A comparison of splint and biofeedback treatments for TMJ pain. *Journal of Dental Research, 71,* 259. [Abstract]

4

Gastrointestinal Disorders

V. Diane Garrett

Disorders of the gastrointestinal (GI) tract constitute a major health problem in the United States. A report from the National Foundation for Ileitis and Colitis (1986) suggested that more than 34 million Americans have diseases of the GI tract. GI diseases account for approximately 15% of all admissions to general hospitals and 200 thousand absences from work per day. As many as 60% of all consultations to physicians result from GI complaints. Moreover, GI disorders are a major cause of death in the United States, resulting in approximately 200 thousand deaths yearly. Estimated economic costs (both medical costs and losses from reduced work productivity) are greater than $50 billion annually.

Investigators have, for many years, hypothesized that the GI tract is a primary site of behavioral responses to environmental stimuli (Wolf & Welsh, 1972). Early analytic theory emphasized the importance of feeding and toilet training in childhood as a major factor in the development of adult personality (C. Tollison & J. Tollison, 1984). Investigators have suggested that social learning and operant and classical conditioning are possible mechanisms that contribute to the expression of psychophysiological disorders, including digestive diseases (Whitehead, Fedoravicius, Blackwell, & Wooley, 1979). As a result, researchers commonly conceptualized several of the gastrointestinal disorders as subject to the impact of environmental events.

Nonetheless, psychologists in behavioral medicine have made surprisingly few attempts to reliably delineate the psychological problems associated with these disorders or to develop sound behavioral interventions for individuals with GI complaints. Increasing interest in the field of behavioral medicine and the expanding

---

V. Diane Garrett • Behavioral Science Consultants, 5420 Corporate Boulevard, Suite 205, Baton Rouge, Louisiana 70808.
Handbook of Health and Rehabilitation Psychology, edited by Anthony J. Goreczny. Plenum Press, New York, 1995.

role of psychologists in health-care facilities suggest research involving assessment and treatment of digestive diseases affords numerous opportunities to psychologists.

This chapter provides a discussion of four GI disorders—irritable bowel syndrome, Crohn's disease, peptic ulcer disease, and esophageal motility disorders—and a brief description of each disorder, its clinical presentation, a review of the psychological factors associated with the disorder, and an examination of treatment methods employed with each disorder.

IRRITABLE BOWEL SYNDROME

Definition and Description

Irritable bowel syndrome (IBS) is a non-life-threatening disorder characterized by disturbed intestinal motility accompanied by either diarrhea *or* constipation and pain that has no known organic basis (Schuster, 1989). Associated symptoms include complaints of bloating, excessive flatulance, dyspepsia, and a sense of incomplete evacuation, urgency, or fecal incontinence (Mitchell & Drossman, 1987). The disorder is generally episodic with alternating periods of remission and exacerbation.

Hypotheses concerning the etiology of IBS include abnormalities of colon motility, abnormal myoelectrical wave activity, and endocrine abnormalities (see Thompson, 1984, and Whitehead and Schuster, 1985, for reviews). However, no general agreement exists concerning the underlying pathophysiological mechanisms of the disorder (Whitehead & Schuster, 1985). Clinicians can make a diagnosis of IBS only after organic bowel disease is ruled out.

Currently, medical treatment involves symptomatic treatment with bulking agents, anxiolytics, antidepressants, smooth muscle relaxants, or anticholinergic drugs (Bennett & Wilkinson, 1985; Latimer, 1983; Whitehead & Schuster, 1985). However, traditional medical treatment has limited success (Mitchell & Drossman, 1987).

IBS is the most common nonorganic diagnosis made by gastroenterologists (Mitchell & Drossman, 1987) and affects 8% (Whitehead, Winget, Fedoravicius, Wooley, & Blackwell, 1982) to 17% (Drossman, Sandler, McKee, & Lovitz, 1982) of American adults yearly. Individuals with IBS are typically female (Fielding, 1977), and the onset of the disorder generally occurs during young adulthood (Latimer, 1983).

Role of Psychological Factors

Experts frequently associate IBS with psychological symptoms, and as many as 70% to 80% of individuals with IBS exhibit elevated scores on psychological tests (Whitehead & Crowell, 1991). Moreover, one group of researchers reported the presence of overt psychiatric disorders in this population to be as high as 100% (Latimer et al., 1981), leading some investigators to describe IBS as the somatic expression of a psychiatric disorder (see Walker, Roy-Byrne, and Katon, 1990, for a review). In addition, as many as 50% of patients report symptom exacerbation in response to environmental stress (Whitehead & Crowell, 1991). This relationship indicates psychological factors play a role in the disorder.

Several investigators have reported IBS patients obtain elevations on scales assessing somatization, interpersonal sensitivity, depression, hostility, and anxiety (e.g., Whitehead, Bosmajian, Zonderman, Costa, & Schuster, 1988; Wise, Cooper, & Ahmed, 1982). Typical MMPI profiles for this population have elevations on Scales 1 (hypochondriasis), 2 (depression), and 3 (hysteria; West, 1970), and researchers employing the Eysenck Personality Inventory have reported high levels of neuroticism (e.g., Latimer et al., 1981).

However, in an excellent review, Whitehead and Crowell (1991) concluded that based on psychological testing results, no consistent pattern of psychological complaints exists in IBS. The typical MMPI profile of IBS patients, for example, also is common in many other patient groups (e.g., patients with chronic pain). Moreover, whether the psychological complaints precede the IBS symptoms, or conversely, the IBS symptoms precede the psychological distress, remains unresolved in the literature.

Standardized interviews have generally failed to identify specific psychiatric diagnoses among individuals with IBS. In their review, however, Whitehead and Crowell (1991) reported higher rates of depression and somatization among those with IBS relative to a community sample, whereas the prevalence of generalized anxiety disorder was not different between the groups.

Recently, several researchers have indicated a self-selection bias may contribute to the reportedly high rates of psychological complaints among patients with IBS. That is, those individuals who seek medical treatment for their IBS complaints may differ psychologically from nonpatients with IBS symptoms. Two separate studies found individuals who present for treatment of IBS complaints do report more psychological distress than IBS sufferers in the community who do not present as patients for treatment (Drossman et al., 1988; Whitehead et al., 1988). In addition, the level of psychological distress reported by IBS clinic patients was no different from clinic patients with lactose malabsorption, a genetic GI disorder with symptoms similar to IBS (Whitehead et al., 1988). This finding suggests IBS patients do not differ psychologically from individuals with organic GI disorders. Other recent studies have also failed to find significant psychopathology in IBS patients (Talley et al., 1990).

The psychological symptoms experienced by individuals with IBS may influence whether they seek medical attention but might not relate to IBS *per se*. Thus, a self-selection bias might have contaminated previous psychological investigations, resulting in an overestimate of psychological problems in this population.

Regardless of the degree of psychopathology present, 50% to 85% of IBS patients report stress leads to exacerbation of symptoms (Whitehead & Schuster, 1985). Stress related to employment and family or relationship problems may contribute significantly to symptom intensity (Chaudhary & Truelove, 1962; Hill & Blendis, 1967). Several authors report stress related to loss in early childhood (e.g., parental death, divorce, separation) may etiologically relate to IBS (Hill & Blendis, 1967; Hislop, 1971). Investigators have also reported individuals with IBS evidence higher stress levels than both non-GI-disordered individuals and individuals with inflammatory bowel disease (Fava & Pavan, 1976/1977; Mendeloff, Monk, Siegel, & Lillienfeld, 1970).

Scientists have proposed several mechanisms to explain the stress–IBS relation. Calloway, Fonagy, Pounder, and Morgan (1983) suggested air swallowing, associated with anxiety (in response to stress), may result in altered bowel activity (i.e., increased flatulence, bowel distension, and colon motility). Others (Whitehead & Schuster, 1985) suggested IBS patients are biologically predisposed to respond with colon hyperreactivity. Exposure to environmental stressors may then interact with a biological predisposition, resulting in IBS symptoms. Maintenance of symptoms in the absence of stressors could subsequently result from classical conditioning effects.

Individuals with ISB frequently display a pattern of learned illness behavior. Liss, Alpers, and Woodruff (1973) reported 28% of their sample carried a diagnosis of hysteria (i.e., DSM-III-R Somatization Disorder), suggesting a learned component to the somatic complaints. Whitehead et al. (1982) also found a high incidence of learned illness behavior in IBS subjects. Persons with IBS were significantly more likely to report a variety of somatic complaints, including skin rashes, peptic ulcers, high blood pressure, headaches, and other pain than were individuals with peptic ulcers. IBS patients also expressed more concerns about acute illnesses and reported an early history of positive reinforcement for illness behaviors. In addition, acute problems hospitalized IBS patients at twice the rate of peptic ulcer patients. Mendeloff et al. (1970) and Sandler, Drossman, Nathan, and McKee (1984) reported results similar to Whitehead et al. (1982).

Treatment

Researchers have investigated psychological treatment of IBS more thoroughly than any other GI disorder (see Blanchard, Schwarz, & Radnitz, 1987, for an excellent review). Research indicates multicomponent behavioral interventions involving education about bowel function, progressive muscle relaxation, and self-instructional training are as effective as medical treatments in alleviating the GI symptoms associated with IBS. Moreover, these treatments have the additional benefit of reducing anxiety levels (Bennett & Wilkinson, 1985). Others have reported similar results (Wise et al., 1982).

Some studies have investigated the efficacy of biofeedback on IBS symptoms. Furman (1973) reported training in bidirectional biofeedback of bowel sounds was successful in 5 patients with IBS. Although later attempts to replicate this study failed, patients treated unsuccessfully with bowel-sound biofeedback evidenced symptomatic improvement when subsequently treated with EMG biofeedback and progressive muscle relaxation (Weinstock, 1976). EMG biofeedback alone may reduce the number of abnormal stools in IBS patients and, when used with stress management training, may significantly decrease psychological distress associated with IBS (Giles, 1978).

Although the studies previously discussed suggest psychological interventions may improve the distress and GI symptoms accompanying IBS, the lack of control groups in these studies makes conclusions regarding the effectiveness of treatment difficult. Moreover, one study reported the placebo response rate in individuals with IBS to be as high as 72% (Whitehead & Schuster, 1985), suggesting the need for controlled group-outcome studies.

Blanchard and his colleagues have conducted the majority of controlled group-outcome studies that involve IBS patients. Using a multicomponent treatment program that consisted of progressive muscle relaxation, thermal biofeedback, patient education, and training in cognitive coping strategies, Neff and Blanchard (1987) treated 10 IBS patients for 12 individual sessions while 9 additional patients served as a symptom-monitoring control group (i.e., patients monitored GI symptoms daily for 12 weeks). Following treatment, 6 of the 10 treated patients exhibited clinical improvement (i.e., a 50% reduction in presenting GI symptoms), whereas only one subject in the control condition evidenced the 50% reduction criterion. The investigators later treated subjects in the control group with the treatment package previously administered to the experimental group. Control subjects subsequently exposed to the treatment package exhibited rates of improvement similar to those of the experimental group.

Follow-up studies using the Neff and Blanchard (1987) treatment package indicate maintenance of treatment benefits from 1 to 4 years (Blanchard, Schwarz, & Neff, 1988; Schwarz, Blanchard, & Neff, 1986; Schwarz, Taylor, Scharff, & Blanchard, 1990). In addition, Blanchard and Schwarz (1987) adapted the treatment package to a group format and obtained positive results similar to those they obtained with the individually administered treatment.

To address the high rate of placebo response in individuals with IBS, Blanchard and colleagues (1992) recently investigated the relative effectiveness of their multicomponent treatment package and an attention–placebo control (pseudomeditation and EEG alpha-suppression biofeedback). They also included a symptom-monitoring control group. Individuals in both the attention–placebo and experimental groups exhibited reductions in GI symptoms and in anxiety and depression scores at posttreatment. However, the results of this study revealed no benefits of the multicomponent treatment package over the attention–placebo control group.

Blanchard et al. (1992) reported two possible explanations for these results. The lack of difference between groups may have been secondary to a placebo response by those subjects in the attention–placebo group. Alternately, subjects in the attention–placebo condition may have transformed that condition into an active treatment. Anecdotal reports by subjects as well as psychophysiological data suggest this may have been the case. Unfortunately, the investigators did not include a formal test of treatment conditions.

These studies suggest behavioral interventions may positively influence subjective ratings of psychological distress and GI symptoms in patients with IBS. Furthermore, the work by Blanchard and his colleagues (1992) indicates that patients with IBS can maintain improvements resulting from behavioral interventions. However, researchers need to employ "dismantling" designs to determine the active treatment components. In addition, investigators need to develop methodology to detect subject transformation of placebo conditions.

CROHN'S DISEASE

Definition and Description

Crohn's disease (CD) is a chronic, life-threatening disease resulting in edema and inflammation that progresses to ulceration of the intestinal mucosa and necrotic breakdown of the entire thickness of the bowel (Binder & Katz, 1977). Although scientists have postulated bacterial, hereditary, psychosomatic, metabolic, and allergenic causes of CD, the etiology of the disorder remains unknown (Cohn, Lederman, & Shore, 1970). Symptomatically, CD patients present with abdominal pain, diarrhea, fever, vomiting associated with weight loss, chronic GI bleeding, anemia, and protein and/or vitamin deficiencies. Periods of remission and exacerbation characterize the clinical course of the illness.

Clinicians employ medical treatments in an attempt to reduce inflammation of the submucosa using steroid treatment, adrenocorticotrophic hormone (ACTH), or azathioprine (an immunosuppressive agent). Treatment may also require surgical intervention to eliminate complications of the disease (Latimer, 1978).

CD affects nearly 2 million Americans. The incidence of CD is approximately 6 per 100 thousand of the population with a prevalence rate of 75 per 100 thousand (Gerbert, 1980). However, evidence suggests these figures may underestimate the problem (Korelitz, 1982; Winship et al., 1979) and indicate the incidence may be increasing. Age at onset of the disorder peaks between the second and fourth decade with equal prevalence in males and females (Mekhjian, Switz, Melnyk, Rankin, & Brooks, 1979).

Role of Psychological Factors

Clinicians have debated the role of psychological factors in CD since the disease was first described in 1932 (Crohn, Ginzburg, & Oppenheimer, 1932). Investigators have proposed that psychological factors have a role in the etiology of the disease and in the exacerbation of symptoms. Although interest in psychological variables as etiological factors has waned, considerable discussion continues concerning the role of psychopathology in the ongoing disease process. Most of this research has focused on the presence of psychopathology in individuals with CD or the role of stress on symptom expression. A brief review of these two areas of research follows. The interested reader may also wish to consult an excellent review by Schwarz and Blanchard (1990).

Several studies based on retrospective chart review (R. Schwartz & I. Schwartz, 1982; Whybrow, Kane, & Lipton, 1968) and psychiatric interviews (Crocket, 1952; Goldberg, 1970) have suggested higher than expected rates of psychopathology (particularly anxiety and depression) in patients with CD. Objective measures have also indicated the presence of psychopathology in CD patients. For example, Sheffield and Carney (1976) administered the Eysenck Personality Inventory and the Manifest Anxiety Scale to patients with CD, chronic nonpsychosomatic medical diseases, psychosomatic disorders, and neurotic diagnoses. CD patients were less neurotic than patients diagnosed as psychoneurotic, and there were no differences between CD patients and the psychosomatic group in terms of anxiety or neuroticism. However, CD patients were more anxious and neurotic than the chronic nonpsychosomatically ill group, suggesting individuals with CD are more similar to patients with psychosomatic disorders than to other medically ill groups.

In the initial phase of a two-phase study, McKegney, Gordon, and Levine (1970) found that 58% of CD patients required psychiatric consultation, 20% required psychotherapy, and 53% had psychiatric diagnoses. In Phase 2 of the study, the investigators interviewed 19 CD patients and administered to these patients the Cornell Medical Index (CMI). Of this group of patients, 53% required psychiatric consultation, 10% required psychotherapy, and 47% had psychiatric diagnoses.

Analysis of the CMI data indicated that the investigators rated 32% of the CD group as moderately to severely disturbed. These authors also reported a strong positive correlation between severity of emotional disturbance and severity of the disease process.

Helzer, Chammas, Norland, Stillings, and Alpers (1984) also investigated the association between psychological factors and CD. In this study the clinicians classified significantly more CD patients than chronically ill control subjects as depressed. Furthermore, 52% of the CD group had a diagnosable psychiatric disorder (compared to 30% of the control group). However, Helzer et al. (1984) reported no interaction between CD symptoms and psychiatric disorder. Although those CD patients with diagnosed psychiatric disorders did tend to have more severe diseases, the relation was not significant.

The studies in the preceding literature review suggest a significant degree of psychological involvement in CD. Based on their review of the literature, Schwarz and Blanchard (1990) concluded that while depression, anxiety, and neurosis appear to occur frequently in this population, no consistent pattern of psychopathology is apparent. Several additional points remain unclear:

1. Whether psychiatric involvement in CD is higher than in other chronic illness groups
2. Whether the psychological problems that patients with CD experience predate the onset of the disease
3. How psychological factors interact with the disease process.

Although some data suggest the incidence of psychiatric involvement in CD is somewhat higher than in other chronic illness groups (Helzer et al., 1984; Sheffield & Carney, 1976), the issue is far from resolved (Schwarz & Blanchard, 1990). The degree of psychopathology found in CD may simply be a function of having a chronic illness, and may have little or no relation to CD *per se*. Without carefully controlled studies to address this issue, researchers can shed little light on the question of psychological involvement in CD.

A second area of research interest has been the influence of stress (i.e., environmental events) on CD. Although some researchers have published reports that stressful life events relate to the *onset* of the disorder (e.g., Parfitt, 1967; Sperling, 1960), most studies suggest that stress influences the course of the disease by leading to an *exacerbation* of the primary symptoms of the disorder (Cohn et al., 1970; Crocket, 1952; Ford, Glober, Castelnuovo-Tedesco, 1969; McKegney et al., 1970; Whybrow et al., 1968). A review of these early studies suggests as many as 64% to 92% of individuals with CD experience exacerbation of symptoms in response to stress. Only one study (Crocket, 1952) found a lower (19%) association between stress and symptom expression.

These early studies suggest that individuals with CD are particularly susceptible to the effects of environmental events. However, we must cautiously evaluate the conclusions drawn from this body of literature because it relies exclusively on the individuals' verbal recall of stressful events or a retrospective chart review to determine the degree of stress–symptom involvement (Garrett, Brantley, Jones, & McKnight, 1991). In addition, the early studies included no standardized means of assessing stressful events.

More recently, several studies have employed improved methodology to investigate the stress–disorder relation in CD. However, in contrast to the earlier studies, the results of recent work are inconclusive. Using a standardized measure of major life events (i.e., the Paykel Life Events Questionnaire), Helzer et al. (1984) found no relation between disease severity at the time of interview and major life events occurring during the 6 months prior to assessment. Although the researchers used a standardized means of assessing stress, the Helzer et al. study was, unfortunately, retrospective.

To address the potential error introduced by retrospective recall of events, several studies have employed prospective designs. Like Helzer et al. (1984), North, Alpers, Helzer, Spitznagel, and Clouse (1991) found no association between major stressful events and exacerbation of CD in a two-year study. Conversely, Duffy et al. (1991) reported that exposure to major stressful events relates to CD symptoms and significantly increases risk of disease exacerbation. However, health-related concerns comprised the majority of the stress measure, and stress accounted for only 7% of the variation in disease activity.

Several investigators (e.g., DeLongis, Coyne, Dakof, Folkman, & Lazarus, 1982) suggested that minor stressful events or "hassles" account for a greater percentage of variance in prediction of physical symptoms than major stressful events. To examine the relation between daily minor stress and CD symptoms, Garrett et al. (1991) had patients monitor stress and symptoms daily for 28 days. Although the between-subject analyses indicated a significant positive relation between daily minor stress and symptoms, only 3 of 10 subjects evidenced significant individual within-subject correlations. Similarly, Greene, Blanchard, and Suls (1989) had patients monitor CD symptoms and minor stress for 7 consecutive days each month for a 6-month period. The monitoring revealed a positive association between symptoms and minor stress for 6 of 9 subjects.

In summary, although early studies suggest a strong stress–disorder relationship, methodological problems confound the results and subsequent conclusions. Recent research regarding the influence of stress on CD is mixed and more difficult to interpret. However, in conjunction with the results of prospective investigations examining major stressful events (i.e., Duffy et al., 1991; North et al., 1991), the studies examining the role of minor stress (i.e., Garrett et al., 1991; Greene et al., 1989) suggest stress influences only a subset of patients with CD. In order to further understand the stress–symptom relation in this disease, researchers must conduct additional investigations.

Treatment

Scientists have conducted relatively little research on the effectiveness of psychological interventions with CD patients. Given the prevalence of psychopathology and the potential role of stress in the disease, this lack of research represents a significant gap in the literature.

In the earliest available treatment study, supportive psychotherapy and psychoanalytically oriented group therapy provided improvements in anxiety, mood, and depression in patients with CD (Freyberger, Kunsebeck, Lempa, Wellmann, & Avenarius, 1985), but a medically treated control group did not evidence these changes. However, the investigators did not provide any data regarding changes in CD symptoms following treatment.

Using a control group outcome study, Milne, Joachim, and Niedhardt (1986) treated 80 patients with ulcerative colitis (UC) or CD using six sessions of stress management training, including communication skills, planning skills, and autogenics. The investigators followed these patients at 4-month intervals for 1 year. Results indicated reduced scores on measures of disease activity and illness-related stress for the treated group, but the untreated control group evidenced no changes. However, the investigators did not match subjects for pretreatment symptom severity; therefore, it is unclear if changes in symptom scores represent treatment effects or regression to the mean (Schwarz & Blanchard, 1990).

Finally, Schwarz and Blanchard (1991) treated patients with inflammatory bowel disease (i.e., both UC and CD patients; IBD) using their multicomponent treatment program, originally developed for use with IBS patients (see section on IBS treatment; Neff & Blanchard, 1987). Following an 8-week treatment program, treated patients exhibited improvement of five or eight symptoms with abdominal pain showing a statistically significant reduction. However, the symptom-monitoring control group improved on all 8 symptoms (four statistically significant reductions). Moreover, when control subjects subsequently participated in the treatment program, patients evidenced *increased* problems on symptoms!

The symptom-monitoring control group produced greater symptomatic change than the treatment group, suggesting that relative to symptom monitoring, psychological treatment of IBD may be harmful. However, Schwarz and Blanchard (1991) also reported that pretreatment psychological distress was higher for CD than UC patients and that the investigators did not equate the two groups in the study for disease type. Consequently, CD patients comprised 70% of the treatment group whereas only 30% of the symptom-monitoring group had CD. The surprising results of this study may, therefore, be the result of differences in response to treatment between the two types of patients with inflammatory bowel disease. Finally, a noteworthy finding is that all patients, regardless of response to treatment, rated themselves as better able to cope with the demands of the disease following treatment.

Clearly the issue of psychological interventions with CD is far from resolved. Although patients may report subjective improvement, current psychological treatments have relatively little influence on the primary GI symptoms of CD. Future research needs to determine if differences between UC and CD patients exist and if the detrimental effect reported by Schwarz and Blanchard (1991) is a consistent finding.

PEPTIC ULCER DISEASE

Definition and Description

Peptic ulcer disease (PUD) refers to ulcerating lesions in the stomach (gastric ulcers; GU) or duodenum (duodenal ulcers; DU). Ulcer lesions result when a breakdown in mucosal defensive factors expose the mucosa to the aggressive action of gastric acid and pepsin (Dajani, 1986). Duodenal ulcers are approximately four times more common than gastric ulcers (Kurata & Haile, 1984) and are more reactive to stress (Whitehead & Schuster, 1985). The remainder of this chapter, therefore, is about DU.

The classic symptoms of DU involve epigastric pain beginning 1–3 hours after eating. Food or antacids may relieve the pain associated with DU (Whitehead & Schuster, 1985); however, some DU patients may be asymptomatic (Soll, 1989); complications of DU include persistent nausea and vomiting, hemorrhage, or perforation.

Most current etiological theories of PUD focus on a multiple-causation–interaction model. Researchers have proposed genetic influences interact with environmental or lifestyle factors (e.g., smoking, stress, presence or bacteria), leading to increased acid secretion and compromised mucosal integrity. The interaction of psychosocial, behavioral, physiological, and genetic variables results in development of an ulcer (Walker, Luther, Samloff, & Feldman, 1988). Endoscopy and radiographic examination assist in the accurate diagnosis of DU (Soll, 1989).

Medical treatment of DU focuses on relief of symptoms, healing of the ulcer, and preventing recurrence or complications (Soll, 1989). Current treatment of choice for DU is oral administration of H_2-receptor antagonists (e.g., cimetidine or ranitidine; Scharschmidt, 1987), and this treatment produces significant healing in 71% of DU patients (Winship, 1978). Other medical treatments include antacids and psychotropic medication (e.g., anxiolytics and antidepressants; Haggerty & Drossman, 1985).

PUD is a relatively common disorder affecting approximately 4 million Americans per year (Whitehead & Schuster, 1985). Clinicians diagnose 200 thousand new cases of DU each year, and an estimated 10% of the adult population will develop PUD during their lifetime. DU is 1.5 to 3 times more likely in males than females (Sol, 1989).

Role of Psychological Factors

Alexander, French, and Pollack (1968) suggested that individuals with PUD experience internal conflict secondary to unresolved dependency needs (see Schindler & Ramchandani, 1991 for a review). Theorists hypothesize that the externalized response to this internal conflict involves an aggressive, confident approach, culminating in the stereotype of individuals who have PUD as hard-driving business persons (Whitehead & Schuster, 1985).

Empirical data, however, has not supported this stereotype. Moreover, Whitehead and Schuster (1985) reported that individuals with PUD are likely the opposite of the hard-driving business person. Passivity, conformity, shyness, and introversion are more characteristic of individuals with PUD (see Whitehead and Schuster, 1985 for a review). A recent investigation also found no relationship between Type A coronary-prone behavior and PUD (Langeluddecke, Goulston, & Tennant, 1987), again suggesting the stereotype is incorrect.

Studies examining psychopathology among patients with PUD have found elevations on scales assessing hypochondriasis, depression, dependency, and social isolation in conjunction with low scores on ego strength (Feldman, Walker, Green, & Weingarden, 1986). Other researchers have reported high levels of anxiety in this population (e.g., Langeluddecke et al., 1987; Magni, DiMario, Rizzardo, Pulin, & Naccarato, 1986). However, aside from increased levels of depression, anxiety, and dependence, individuals with PUD do not exhibit a characteristic psychopathological profile (Whitehead & Schuster, 1985).

Researchers and clinicians alike have found that a major area of interest is the role of stress in ulcer formation. Some investigators have reported that the development of ulcers is more common during periods of intense stress (e.g., war) and among urban as opposed to rural populations (see Pflanz, 1971 for a review). Moreover, PUD is more common among individuals with high-stress jobs (Cobb & Rose, 1973; Richard & Fell, 1975).

Research also indicates stressful events have a greater role in DU than in gastric ulcer. Patients with DU report a significantly greater number of stressful events occurring in the 6 months preceding the onset of their illness than GU patients (Sapira & Cross, 1982). Conversely, Feldman et al. (1986) found no greater frequency of stressful life events for PUD patients compared to controls, but subjective ratings of the impact of the events were significantly more negative for PUD patients. Thus, it is possible that individuals with PUD do not experience a greater number of stressful life events than others but that the impact of those events is greater.

In summary, research indicates patients with PUD are likely shy, passive individuals who are somewhat more anxious and depressed than nonpatients. Moreover, the role of stressful life events and their impact on PUD suggests this group is particularly vulnerable to the effects of stress; however, scientists have not yet delineated the means by which stress has its effects on this population.

Treatment

Since the introduction of cimetidine and ranitidine in the medical management of DU, researchers have conducted relatively few studies involving psychological treatment of DU. The high success rates of these drugs, in combination with high rates of spontaneous healing in DU (Scheurer et al., 1977), have decreased researchers' interest in developing behavioral interventions. Based on their review of the literature, Whitehead and Schuster (1985) suggested this disinterest is premature. Recurrence of DU throughout the lifetime of the patient is common. Although traditional medical treatment has beneficial short-term effects, behavioral interventions offer strategies for coping with stress that an exclusively biomedical approach does not provide. Teaching DU patients to deal more effectively with environmental stressors may alter the natural course of the disorder and decrease its rate of recurrence.

Chappell, Stephano, Rogerson, and Pike (1936) conducted the earliest available controlled study of behavioral intervention with PUD patients. The investigators treated 32 patients who had either GU or DU with a treatment package that included education concerning the relationship between GI functioning and emotions, distraction techniques, contingency management (i.e., extinction of social reinforcement for pain complaints and illness behavior), use of positive self-statements, and positive expectancy of improvement. Ninety-four percent of the patients were asymptomatic after treatment compared to 10% of individuals in a control group. The investigators conducted a 3-year follow-up of 28 treated patients and found that 10 of the 28 had experienced no ulcer-related symptoms since treatment, and 26 of the 28 patients rated themselves as improved. Patients in the control group did not maintain the treatment gains.

Beaty (1976) reported successful treatment of DU patients using EMG biofeedback, daily relaxation practice, and *in vivo* exposure to idiosyncratically defined stressors. Six-month follow-up indicated patients were free of pain and medication usage. Aleo and Nicassio (1978) used a similar treatment approach for 12 weeks with 4 DU patients. They reported ulcer healing and elimination of pain in 3 of the 4 patients. The fourth subject exhibited a reduction in ulcer size and pain intensity. Based on research indicating the causal role of excess gastric acid secretion in DU, some investigators have evaluated using biofeedback of pH levels (Welgan, 1974). However, this treatment is time-consuming and impractical for most practitioners.

More recently, Brooks and Richardson (1980) provided 11 male DU patients with anxiety-management training and assertiveness training, while 11 other patients served as an attention–placebo control group. Sixty days posttreatment, the treated group reported less severe ulcer symptoms, fewer days of pain, and a reduction in antacid medication usage. Treated patients were also less anxious and more assertive at posttreatment assessment. However, examination of X-ray studies showed no difference between the groups at follow-up, suggesting no physiological changes accompanied treatment. Nonetheless, these researchers found a decrease in ulcer recurrence in the behaviorally treated patients at a 3½-year follow-up assessment. The authors concluded that relatively brief behavioral treatment had beneficial effects on the natural course of the disease by decreasing recurrence of the ulcers. Berbalk, Kollenbaum, and Volkel (1984) also obtained positive results using stress inoculation training as the active treatment program.

In summary, a review of the available literature suggests psychological interventions positively influence DU by decreasing recurrence of the disease. Researchers need to develop treatment protocols to compare traditional medical treatment, psychological interventions, and combined medical and psychological treatments of DU so that they can identify an optimal course of patient management for this pervasive disorder.

ESOPHAGEAL MOTILITY DISORDERS

Definition and Description

Esophageal motility disorders (EMDs) result from abnormalities in activity of smooth or striated muscles in the esophagus or secondary to systemic disease (Nelson & Castell, 1988). The four primary EMDs include: achalasia, diffuse esophageal spasm, nutcracker esophagus, and hypertensive lower esophageal sphincter (for a description of these disorders, refer to Nelson and Castell, 1988 and Richter and Castell, 1988). Etiology of achalasia involves degeneration of the neurons controlling esophageal motility and vagal stimulation. However, the etiology of the remaining EMDs is less well understood (Clouse, 1991). Clinicians utilize esophageal manometric recordings to diagnose these disorders. The disorders are most common in adulthood, and patients are often 40–50 years of age when their physicians make the diagnosis (Clouse, 1989).

Although each EMD varies somewhat in its clinical presentation, the primary symptoms of all EMDs are chest pain and dysphagia to both liquids and solids (Nelson & Castell, 1988). As many as 80% of patients with the disorder typically report substernal chest pain as the primary symptom (Clouse, 1989). Patients use a variety of words to describe the pain, ranging from dull to colicky. However, pain may mimic angina pectoris, because it often radiates into the neck and arms (Richter & Castell, 1988). Approximately 50% of patients with noncardiac chest pain may have an EMD (Richter & Castell, 1988; Young, Richter, Bradley, & Anderson, 1987).

Current medical treatment for EMDs typically involves reassuring patients that the cause of their chest pain is noncardiac in nature. Other medical interventions may involve oral administration of nitrates, anticholinergics, psychotropics (e.g., sedatives and antidepressants), or calcium-channel blocking agents. Severe cases may require more intensive treatment, such as esophageal dilatation or surgery.

Role of Psychological Factors

Researchers have investigated the role of psychological factors less extensively in EMDs than in other GI disorders. Nonetheless, several studies suggest esophageal motility is subject to the influence of environmental events. Esophageal contractions occur in the presence of startling noises, and stressful interviews can induce abnormal contractions in normal subjects (Schuster, 1983). One study also reported that dichotic listening tasks and the cold pressor test result in increased amplitude of esophageal contractions (Ayres, Robertson, Naylor, & Smith, 1989). Moreover, Anderson, Dalton, Bradley, and Richter (1989) found that cognitive stress led to a significantly greater increase in esophageal contraction amplitude in patients with nutcracker esophagus than in healthy controls or chest-pain patients without manometric abnormalities.

Psychiatric diagnoses also occur frequently in this population. Clouse and Lustman (1983) found that 84% of patients with abnormal esophageal manometric recordings met criteria for diagnosis of a psychiatric disorder according to DSM-III criteria, whereas only 31% of patients with normal manometric patterns met diagnostic criteria. Most commonly reported diagnoses were depression, anxiety (generalized anxiety disorder and panic disorder), and somatization disorders (Clouse & Lustman, 1983). Katon et al. (1988) also reported high rates of psychiatric diagnoses (79%) in this population, with depression and anxiety disorders most common. Colgan et al. (1988) reported similar results.

Psychological test results also support the association of abnormal esophageal motility and psychological factors. Richter, Obrecht, Bradley, Young, and Anderson (1986), using the Millon Behavioral Health Inventory, compared 20 patients with nutcracker esophagus and 20 patients with IBS to control groups consisting of 20 patients with structural esophageal abnormalities, and two groups of 20 healthy volunteers. Patients with EMD and IBS differed significantly from the three control groups on scales assessing somatic anxiety and gastrointestinal susceptibility.

Treatment

The studies in the previous section suggest psychological variables are a factor in EMD. Yet, researchers have performed few studies that investigate the influence of psychological interventions with these disorders. To date, only case studies involving behavioral treatment of EMDs are present in the literature.

In the earliest reported study, Jacobson (1927) described the successful treatment of three patients with DES using progressive muscle relaxation. Later, Latimer (1981) used both relaxation and biofeedback in a female patient with DES. Relaxation training reduced esophageal spasm from an initial 10 hours per week to 1 hour per week, but the patient continued to complain of dysphagia. Biofeedback of peristaltic contractions did not reduce the patient's complaints of dysphagia, but Latimer noted that spasm of the lower esophageal sphincter remitted when the patient swallowed twice in rapid succession. The patient was instructed to continue this "double-swallow" technique, and she subsequently experienced a further reduction of symptoms to approximately 6 minutes per week. Interestingly, abnormal manometric patterns continued despite the presence of subjective clinical improvement.

More recently, Shabsin, Katz, and Schuster (1988) treated a 27-year-old female patient with a 12-year history of vigorous achalasia using a behavioral pain-management program. Prior to treatment, the patient reported four to five episodes of chest pain per week. Initial treatment involved six 1-hour sessions of relaxation training, including progressive muscle relaxation, autogenic techniques, and frontalis EMG and finger temperature biofeedback. Following the relaxation training, the patient received 10 sessions of behavioral modification with the goal of increasing activity levels and decreasing pain behaviors. The patient also received cognitive restructuring techniques to decrease the subjective experience of pain. Follow-up at 12 weeks and 1-year posttreatment indicated the patient was asymptomatic. However, like the Latimer (1981) study, manometric patterns did not change in this patient.

The results of these investigations with two of the primary EMDs suggest behavioral techniques can successfully decrease subjective distress associated with DES and achalasia. As noted, improvements occur in the absence of manometric changes, suggesting that psychological factors play an important role in maintaining the symptoms of some patients with EMD. Researchers need to conduct additional studies to determine if subjective improvement in the absence of physiological change is a consistent finding with EMD patients or representative of only a subset of individuals with EMDs. In addition, researchers need to perform investigations using placebo treatment and no-treatment control groups before any firm statements about the effectiveness of behavioral treatment with EMDs are made.

CONCLUSIONS

Psychological factors appear to have an important, if still poorly understood, role in GI disorders. Although researchers and clinicians who work with GI disorders report that anxiety, depression, and neurosis are common in these populations, the nature of the relation between existing psychopathology and the disorders remains elusive. Moreover, recent work by Drossman et al. (1988) and Whitehead et al. (1988) suggests previous reports of psychopathology rates in IBS are overestimates secondary to selection bias. Whether this hypothesis holds true for other GI disorders remains untested.

A consistent finding in the literature is the role of environmental stress in these disorders. Stress appears to have an important role in IBS, DU, and perhaps CD. Although further research regarding the role of stress in CD is essential, the direction of recent work (Garrett et al., 1991; Greene et al., 1989) is promising. Effective treatment of EMD using relaxation also suggests an influence of stress in these disorders. Investigators in the area need to conduct additional research using prospective controlled designs.

The psychological treatment literature for GI disorders also appears promising.

Symptoms associated with IBS, the most thoroughly researched GI disorder, respond to behavioral treatment strategies and are maintained over time (e.g., Blanchard et al., 1992). Furthermore, behavioral interventions with DU may provide a useful adjunctive therapy to medical management. Available evidence suggests psychological treatment with DU patients may reduce the recurrence of the disorder (Brooks & Richardson, 1980) and consequently improve the quality of life of these patients. In addition, although treatment of EMDs is in its infancy, the available case studies suggest these disorders warrant further attention from psychologists in behavioral medicine. Finally, investigators have only recently begun to study the psychological treatment of CD, and it remains an area for fruitful research.

REFERENCES

Aleo, S., & Nicassio, P. (1978). Auto-regulation of duodenal ulcer: A preliminary report of four cases. *Proceedings of the 9th Annual Meeting of the Biofeedback Society of America* (pp. 278–281). Denver, CO: Biofeedback Society of America.

Alexander, F., French, T. M., & Pollack, G. (1968). *Psychosomatic specificity: Experimental study and results.* Chicago: University of Chicago Press.

Anderson, K. O., Dalton, C. B., Bradley, L. A., & Richter, J. E. (1989). Stress induces alteration of esophageal pressures in healthy volunteers and non-cardiac chest pain patients. *Digestive Diseases and Sciences, 34,* 83–91.

Ayres, R. C., Robertson, D. A., Naylor, K., & Smith, C. L. (1989). Stress and oesophageal motility in normal subjects and patients with irritable bowel syndrome. *Gut, 30,* 1540–1543.

Beaty, E. T. (1976). Feedback-assisted relaxation training as a treatment for peptic ulcers. *Biofeedback and Self-Regulation, 1,* 323–324 (Abstract).

Bennett, P., & Wilkinson, S. (1985). A comparison of psychological and medical treatment of the irritable bowel syndrome. *British Journal of Clinical Psychology, 24,* 215–216.

Berbalk, H., Kollenbaum, V.-E., & Volkel, H. (1984). Biochemical effects of "stress-innoculation": An important and neglected method of therapeutic control demonstrated on a group of ulcer patients. *Zeitschrift fur Klinische Psychologie. Forschung und Praxis, 13,* 276–7287 (From *Psychological Abstracts,* 1985, 72, Abstract No. 18035).

Binder, S. C., & Katz, B. (1977). Regional enteritis: A review of the literature. *The Ohio State Medical Journal, 73,* 661–666.

Blanchard, E. B., & Schwarz, S. P. (1987). Adaptation of a multicomponent treatment for irritable bowel syndrome to a small-group format. *Biofeedback and Self-Regulation, 12,* 63–73.

Blanchard, E. B., Schwarz, S. P., & Neff, D. F. (1988). Two-year follow-up of behavioral treatment of irritable bowel syndrome. *Behavior Therapy, 19,* 67–73.

Blanchard, E. B., Schwarz, S. P., & Radnitz, C. R. (1987). Psychological assessment and treatment of irritable bowel syndrome. *Behavior Modification, 11,* 348–372.

Blanchard, E. B., Schwarz, S. P., Suls, J. M., Gerardi, M. A., Scharff, L., Greene, B., Taylor, A. E., Berreman, C., & Malamood, H. S. (1992). Two controlled evaluations of multicomponent psychological treatment of irritable bowel syndrome. *Behavior Research and Therapy, 30,* 175–189.

Brooks, G. R., & Richardson, F. C. (1980). Emotional skills training: A treatment program for duodenal ulcer. *Behavior Therapy, 11,* 198–207.

Calloway, S. P., Fonagy, P., Pounder, R. E., & Morgan, M. J. (1983). Behavioural techniques in the management of aerophagia in patients with hiatus hernia. *Journal of Psychosomatic Research, 27,* 499–502.

Chappell, M. N., Stefano, J. J., Rogerson, J. S., & Pike, F. H. (1936). The value of group psychological procedures in the treatment of peptic ulcer. *American Journal of Digestive Diseases and Nutrition, 3,* 813–817.

Chaudhary, N. A., & Truelove, S. C. (1962). The irritable colon syndrome: A study of the clinical features, predisposing causes, and prognosis in 130 cases. *Quarterly Journal of Medicine, 31,* 307–323.

Clouse, R. E. (1989). Motor disorders. In M. H. Sleisenger, & J. S. Fordtran (Eds.), *Gastrointestinal disease: Pathophysiology, diagnosis, management* (pp. 559–593). Philadelphia: Saunders.

Clouse, R. E. (1991). Psychiatric disorders in patients with esophageal disease. *Medical Clinics of North America, 75,* 1081–1096.

Clouse, R. E., & Lustman, P. J. (1983). Psychiatric illness and contraction abnormalities of the esophagus. *New England Journal of Medicine, 309,* 1337–1342.

Cobb, S., & Rose, R. M. (1973). Hypertension, peptic ulcer, and diabetes in air traffic controllers. *Journal of the American Medical Association, 224,* 489–492.

Cohn, E. M., Lederman, I. I., & Shore, E. (1970). Regional enteritis and its relation to emotional disorders. *American Journal of Gastroenterology, 54,* 378–387.

Colgan, S. M., Schofield, P. M., Whorwell, P. J., Bennett, D. H., Brooks, N. H., & Jones, P. E. (1988). Angina-like chest pain: A joint medical and psychiatric investigation. *Postgraduate Medicine, 64,* 734–746.

Crocket, R. W. (1952). Psychiatric findings in Crohn's disease. *Lancet, 1,* 946–949.

Crohn, B. B., Ginzburg, L., & Oppenheimer, G. D. (1932). Regional ileitis. *Journal of the American Medical Association, 99,* 1323.

Dajani, E. Z. (1986). Is peptic ulcer a prostaglandin deficiency disease? *Human Pathology, 17,* 106–107.

DeLongis, A., Coyne, J. C., Dakof, G., Folkman, S., & Lazarus, R. S. (1982). Relationship of daily hassles, uplifts, and major life events to health status. *Health Psychology, 1,* 119–136.

Drossman, D. A., McKee, D. C., Sandler, R. S., Mitchell, M., Cramer, E. M., Lowman, B. C., & Burger, A. L. (1988). Psychosocial factors in the irritable bowel syndrome. *Gastroenterology, 95,* 701–708.

Drossman, D. A., Sandler, R., McKee, D. C., & Lovitz, A. J. (1982). Bowel patterns among subjects not seeking health care. *Gastroenterology, 83,* 529–534.

Duffy, L. C., Zielezny, M. A., Marshall, J. R., Byers, T. E., Weiser, M. M., Phillips, J. F., Calkins, B. M., Ogra, P. L., & Graham, S. (1991). Relevance of major stress events as an indicator of disease activity prevalence in inflammatory bowel disease. *Behavioral Medicine, 17,* 101–110.

Eysenck, H. J., & Eysenck, S.B.G. (1968). *Eysenck Personality Inventory.* San Diego: Educational and Industrial Testing Service.

Fava, G. A., & Pavan, L. (1976/1977). Large bowel disorders: Illness configuration and life events. *Psychotherapy and Psychosomatics, 27,* 93–99.

Feldman, M., Walker, P., Green, J. L., & Weingarden, K. (1986). Life events stress and psychosocial factors in men with peptic ulcer disease: A multidimensional case-controlled study. *Gastroenterology, 91,* 1370–1379.

Fielding, J. F. (1977). The irritable bowel syndrome. *Clinical Gastroenterology, 6,* 607–622.

Ford, C. V., Glober, G. A., & Castelnuovo-Tedesco, P. (1969). A psychiatric study of patients with regional enteritis. *Journal of the American Medical Association, 208,* 311–315.

Freyberger, H., Kunsebeck, H.-W., Lempa, W., Wellman, W., & Avenarius, H.-J. (1985). Psychotherapeutic interventions in alexithymic patients with special regard to ulcerative colitis and Crohn patients. *Psychotherapy and Psychosomatics, 44,* 72–81.

Furman, S. (1973). Intestinal biofeedback in functional diarrhea: A preliminary report. *Journal of Behavior Therapy and Experimental Psychiatry, 4,* 317–321.

Garrett, V. D., Brantley, P. J., Jones, G. N., & McKnight, G. T. (1991). The relation between daily stress and Crohn's disease. *Journal of Behavioral Medicine, 14,* 87–96.

Gerbert, B. G. (1980). Psychological aspects of Crohn's disease. *Journal of Behavioral Medicine, 3,* 41–58.

Giles, S. L. (1978). Separate and combined effects of biofeedback training and brief individual psychotherapy in the treatment of gastrointestinal disorders. *Dissertations Abstracts International, Part B,* 2495.

Goldberg, D. (1970). A psychiatric study of patients with diseases of the small intestine. *Gut, 11,* 459–465.

Greene, B., Blanchard, E. B., & Suls, J. (1989). *Long-term monitoring of psychosocial stress and inflammatory bowel disease symptoms in patients with inflammatory bowel disease.* Poster presented at the 23rd Annual Meeting of the Association for Advancement of Behavior Therapy, Washington, DC.

Haggerty, J. J., & Drossman, D. A. (1985). Use of psychotropic drugs in patients with peptic ulcer. *Psychosomatics, 26,* 277–284.

Helzer, J. E., Chammas, S., Norland, C. C., Stillings, W. A., & Alpers, D. H. (1984). A study of the association between Crohn's disease and psychiatric illness. *Gastroenterology, 86,* 324–330.

Hill, O. W., & Blendis, L. (1967). Physical and psychological evaluation of "non-organic" abdominal pain. *Gut, 12,* 221–229.

Hislop, I. G. (1971). Psychological significance of the irritable colon syndrome. *Gut, 12,* 452–457.

Jacobson, E. (1927). Spastic esophagus and mucous colitis: Etiology and treatment by progressive relaxation. *Archives of Internal Medicine, 39,* 433–445.

Katon, W., Hall, M. L., Russo, J., Cormier, L., Hollifield, M., Vitaliano, P. P., & Beitman, B. D. (1988). Relationship of psychiatric illness to coronary arterioigraphic results. *American Journal of Medicine, 84,* 1–9.

Korelitz, B. I. (1982). Epidemiological and psychosocial aspects of inflammatory bowel disease with observations on children, families, and pregnancy. *American Journal of Gastroenterology, 77,* 929–933.

Kurata, J. H., & Haile, B. M. (1984). Epidemiology of peptic ulcer disease. *Clinical Gastroenterology, 13,* 289.

Langeluddecke, P., Goulston, K., & Tennant, C. (1987). Type A behavior and other psychological factors in peptic ulcer disease. *Journal of Psychosomatic Research, 31,* 335–340.

Latimer, P. R. (1983). *Functional gastrointestinal disorders: A behavioral medicine approach.* New York: Springer.

Latimer, P. R. (1978). Crohn's disease: A review of the psychological and social outcome. *Psychological Medicine, 8,* 649–656.

Latimer, P. R. (1981). Biofeedback and self-regulation in the treatment of diffuse esophageal spasm: A single-case study. *Biofeedback and Self-Regulation, 6,* 181–189.

Latimer, P. R., Sarna, D., Campbell, D., Latimer, M., Waterfall, W., & Daniel, E. E. (1981). Colonic motor and myoelectrical activity: A comparative study of normal subjects, psychoneurotic patients, and patients with irritable bowel syndrome. *Gastroenterology, 80,* 893–901.

Liss, J. L., Alpers, D., & Woodruff, R. A., Jr. (1973). The irritable colon syndrome and psychiatric illness. *Diseases of the Nervous System, 34,* 151–157.

Magni, G., DiMario, F., Rizzardo, R., Pulin, S., & Naccarato, R. (1986). Personality profiles of patients with duodenal ulcer. *American Journal of Psychiatry, 143,* 1297–1300.

McKegney, F. P., Gordon, R. O., & Levine, S. M. (1970). A psychosomatic comparison of patients with ulcerative colitis and Crohn's disease. *Psychosomatic Medicine, 32,* 153–165.

Mekhjian, H. S., Switz, D. M., Melnyk, C. S., Rankin, G. B., & Brooks, R. K. (1979). Clinical features and natural history of Crohn's disease. *Gastroenterology, 77,* 898–906.

Mendeloff, A. I., Monk, M., Siegel, C. I., & Lilienfeld, A. (1970). Illness experience and life stresses in patients with irritable colon and with ulcerative colitis: An epidemiologic study of ulcerative colitis and regional enteritis in Baltimore, 1960–1964. *New England Journal of Medicine, 282,* 14–17.

Milne, B., Joachim, G., & Niedhardt, J. (1986). A stress management programme for inflammatory bowel disease patients. *Journal of Advanced Nursing, 11,* 561–567.

Mitchell, C. M., & Drossman, D. A. (1987). The irritable bowel syndrome: Understanding and treating a biopsychosocial illness disorder. *Annals of Behavioral Medicine, 9,* 13–18.

National Foundation for Ileitis and Colitis. (June/July 1986). *News from National.* New York: Author.

Neff, B. F., & Blanchard, E. B. (1987). A multi-component treatment for irritable bowel syndrome. *Behavior Therapy, 18,* 70–83.

Nelson, J. B., & Castell, D. O. (1988). Esophageal motility disorders. *Disease-A-Month, 34,* 301–389.

North, C. S., Alpers, D. H., Helzer, J. E., Spitznagel, E. L., & Clouse, R. E. (1991). Do life events or depression exacerbate inflammatory bowel disease? *Annals of Internal Medicine, 114,* 381–386.

Parfitt, H. L. (1967). Psychiatric aspects of regional enteritis. *Canadian Medical Association Journal, 97,* 807.

Pflanz, M. (1971). Epidemiological and sociocultural factors in the etiology of duodenal ulcer. *Advances in Psychosomatic Medicine, 6,* 121–151.

Richard, W. C., & Fell, R. D. (1975). Health factors in police job stress. In W. H. Kroes & J. J. Hurrell (Eds.), *Job stress and the police officer: Identifying stress reduction techniques* (pp. 76–187, HEW Publication No. NIOSH). Washington, DC: U.S. Government Printing Office.

Richter, J. E., & Castell, D. O. (1988). Esophageal disease as a cause of noncardiac chest pain. In G. H. Stollerman, W. J. Harrington, J. T. LaMont, J. J. Leonard, & M. D. Siperstein (Eds.), *Advances in internal medicine* (pp. 311–335). Chicago: Year Book Medical Publishers.

Richter, J. E., Obrecht, W. F., Bradley, L. A., Young, & Anderson. (1986). Psychological comparison of patients with nutcracker esophagus and irritable bowel syndrome. *Digestive Diseases and Sciences, 31,* 131–138.

Sandler, R. S., Drossman, D. A., Nathan, H. P., & McKee, D. C. (1984). Symptoms complaints and health care seeking behavior in subjects with bowel dysfunction. *Gastroenterology, 87,* 314–318.

Sapira, J. D., & Cross, M. R. (1982). Pre-hospitalization life change in gastric ulcer (GU) versus duodenal ulcer (DU). *Psychosomatic Medicine, 44,* 121 (Abstract).

Scharschmidt, B. F. (1987). Peptic ulcer disease: Pathophysiology and current medical management. *Western Journal of Medicine, 146,* 724–733.

Scheurer, U., Witzel, L., Halter, F., Keller, H.-M., Huber, R., & Galeazzi, R. (1977). Gastric and duodenal ulcer healing under placebo treatment. *Gastroenterology, 72,* 838–841.

Schindler, B. A., & Ramchandani, D. (1991). Psychologic factors associated with peptic ulcer disease. *Medical Clinics of North America, 75,* 865–876.

Schuster, M. M. (1983). Esophageal spasm and psychiatric disorder. *New England Journal of Medicine, 309,* 1382–1383.

Schuster, M. M. (1989). Irritable bowel syndrome. In M. H. Sleisenger & J. S. Fordtran (Eds.), *Gastrointestinal disease: Pathophysiology, diagnosis, management* (pp. 1402–1418). Philadelphia: Saunders.

Schwartz, R. A., & Schwartz, I. K. (1982). Psychiatric disorders associated with Crohn's disease. *International Journal of Psychiatry in Medicine, 12,* 67–73.

Schwarz, S. P., & Blanchard, E. B. (1990). Inflammatory bowel disease: A review of the psychological assessment and treatment literature. *Annals of Behavioral Medicine, 12,* 95–105.

Schwarz, S. P., & Blanchard, E. B. (1991). Evaluation of a psychological treatment for inflammatory bowel disease. *Behavior Research and Therapy, 29,* 167–177.

Schwarz, S. P., Blanchard, E. B., & Neff, D. F. (1986). Behavioral treatment of irritable bowel syndrome: A 1-year follow-up study. *Biofeedback and Self-Regulation, 11,* 189–198.

Schwarz, S. P., Taylor, A. E., Scharff, L., & Blanchard, E. B. (1990). Behaviorally treated irritable bowel syndrome patients: A four-year follow-up. *Behavior Research and Therapy, 28,* 331–335.

Shabsin, H. S., Katz, P. O., & Schuster, M. M. (1988). Behavioral treatment of intractable chest pain in a patient with vigorous achalasia. *American Journal of Gastroenterology, 83,* 970–973.

Sheffield, B. F., & Carney, M.W.P. (1976). Crohn's disease: A psychosomatic illness? *British Journal of Psychiatry, 128,* 446–450.

Soll, A. H. (1989). Duodenal ulcer and drug therapy. In M. H. Sleisenger, & J. S. Fortran (Eds.), *Gastrointestinal disease: Pathophysiology, diagnosis, management* (pp. 814–879). Philadelphia: Saunders.

Sperling, M. (1960). The psycho-analytic treatment of a case of chronic regional ileitis. *International Journal of Psychoanalysis, 41,* 612.

Talley, N. J., Phillips, S. F., Bruce, B., Twomey, C. K., Zinsmeister, A. R., & Melton, L. J., III. (1990). Relation among personality and symptoms in nonulcer dyspepsia and the irritable bowel syndrome. *Gastroenterology, 99,* 327–333.

Thompson, W. G. (1984). The irritable bowel. *Gut, 25,* 305–320.

Tollison, C. D., & Tollison, J. W. (1984). Psychological aspects of selected medical disorders. In H. E. Adams & P. B. Sutker (Eds.), *Comprehensive handbook of psychopathology* (pp. 917–938). New York: Plenum Press.

Walker, E. A., Roy-Byrne, P. P., & Katon, W. J. (1990). Irritable bowel syndrome and psychiatric illness. *American Journal of Psychiatry, 147,* 565–570.

Walker, P., Luther, J., Samloff, I. M., & Feldman, M. (1988). Life events stress and psychosocial factors in men with peptic ulcer disease: II. Relationships with serum pepsinogen concentration and behavioral risk factors. *Gastroenterology, 94,* 323–340.

Weinstock, S. A. (1976). The re-establishment of intestinal control in functional colitis. *Biofeedback and Self-Regulation, 1,* 324.

Welgan, P. R. (1974). Learned control of gastric acid secretions in ulcer patients. *Psychosomatic Medicine, 36,* 411–419.

West, K. L. (1970). MMPI correlates of ulcerative colitis. *Journal of Clinical Psychology, 26,* 214–229.

Whitehead, W. E., Bosmajian, L., Zonderman, A. B., Costa, P. T., Jr., & Schuster, M. M. (1988). Symptoms of psychologic distress associated with irritable bowel syndrome: Comparison of community and medical clinic samples. *Gastroenterology, 95,* 709–714.

Whitehead, W. E., & Crowell, M. D. (1991). Psychologic considerations in the irritable bowel syndrome. *Gastroenterology Clinics of North America, 20,* 249–267.

Whitehead, W. E., Fedoravicius, A. S., Blackwell, B., & Wooley, S. (1979). A behavioral conceptualization of psychosomatic illness: Psychosomatic symptoms as learned responses. In J. R. McNamara (Ed.), *Behavioral approaches to medicine: Application and analysis* (pp. 65–99). New York: Plenum Press.

Whitehead, W. E., & Schuster, W. (1985). *Gastrointestinal disorders: Behavioral and physiological basis for treatment.* Orlando, FL: Academic Press.

Whitehead, W. E., Winget, C., Fedoravicius, A. S., Wooley, S., & Blackwell, B. (1982). Learned illness behavior in patients with irritable bowel syndrome and peptic ulcer. *Digestive Diseases and Sciences, 27,* 202–208.

Whybrow, P. C., Kane, F. J., Jr., & Lipton, M. A. (1968). Regional ileitis and psychiatric disorder. *Psychosomatic Medicine, 30,* 209–221.

Winship, D. H. (1978). Cimetidine in the treatment of duodenal ulcer: Review and commentary. *Gastroenterology, 74,* 402–406.

Winship, D. H., Summers, R. W., Singleton, J. W., Best, W. R., Becktel, J. M., Lenk, L. F., & Kern, F., Jr. (1979). National Cooperative Crohn's Disease Study: Study design and conduct of the study. *Gastroenterology, 77,* 829–834.

Wise, T. M., Cooper, J. N., & Ahmed, S. (1982). The efficacy of group therapy for patients with irritable bowel syndrome. *Psychosomatics, 23,* 465–469.

Wolf, S., & Welsh, J. D. (1972). The gastrointestinal tract as a response system. In N. S. Greenfield & R. A. Sternbach (Eds.), *Handbook of Psychophysiology* (pp. 419–456). New York: Holt, Rinehart & Winston.

Young, L. D., Richter, J. E., Bradley, L. A., & Anderson, K. O. (1987). Disorders of the upper gastrointestinal system: An overview. *Annals of Behavioral Medicine, 9,* 7–12.

5

Insomnia

Mark J. Chambers

DEFINITION AND EPIDEMIOLOGY

Insomnia is a clinical problem that has proved difficult to define. Generally considered to be a complaint or symptom rather than a disorder, insomnia can result from one or more of a multitude of causes. The current nosology of the American Sleep Disorder Association (ASDA) includes over 40 diagnostic classifications that could potentially relate to insomnia complaints; however, the term *insomnia* actually identifies only a handful of these diagnoses (American Sleep Disorders Association, 1990).

Most experts have agreed that any definition of insomnia must include a subjective complaint of difficulty with sleep initiation and/or maintenance. What constitutes "difficulty," however, has been less clear. Morin and Kwentus (1988) proposed very specific standards, such as a sleep-onset latency of greater than 30 minutes, wake time during the night of more than 30 minutes, or a total sleep time of less than 6.5 hours. Borkovec (1982), on the other hand, argued that because of the extreme variability in amount of sleep different individuals need, an objective definition of insomnia is inappropriate. He instead recommended defining insomnia as "a subjective complaint of disturbed sleep or disrupted daily functioning due to poor sleep . . . regardless of objective sleep parameters" (p. 880). Coates and Thoresen (1981) agreed that complaints of disturbed sleep need not relate to objective evidence; however, their definition of insomnia emphasizes presence of "a *complaint* of daytime fatigue *attributed* to poor sleep" (p. 241).

Because ASDA nosology does not regard insomnia as a single entity, a precise definition of insomnia has continued to be elusive. The more common insomnia diagnoses, such as *psychophysiological insomnia* and *idiopathic insomnia*, do not

---

Mark J. Chambers • The Sleep Clinic of Nevada, 1012 East Sahara, Las Vegas, Nevada 89104.
Handbook of Health and Rehabilitation Psychology, edited by Anthony J. Goreczny. Plenum Press, New York, 1995.

require objective verification of a sleep complaint, nor do they specify required values for nocturnal sleep parameters, such as sleep onset latency or total sleep time. On the other hand, the diagnosis of *short sleeper* (an individual who requires significantly less sleep than the population mean) is contingent on total sleep time being less than 75% of the age-related norm. (It is interesting to note that a complaint of insomnia does not preclude this diagnosis.) Also, *sleep state misperception,* a complaint of insomnia not confirmed by objective testing, requires a "normal sleep pattern," defined as a sleep latency of less than 15 or 20 minutes and a total sleep time greater than 6.5 hours.

Official nosology, therefore, would not recognize individuals complaining of insomnia but exhibiting so-called normal sleep patterns as insomniacs (even though the classification system acknowledges that some individuals require considerably more sleep than others). Conversely, individuals demonstrating substantially less sleep than the norm could be either insomniacs or short sleepers; the diagnostic criteria do not necessarily distinguish between the two. For the purposes of this chapter, therefore, the term *insomnia* refers to a subjective complaint of reduced sleep time or poor sleep quality *and* an associated complaint of subsequent daytime consequences (e.g., fatigue, sleepiness, impaired functioning). This chapter will examine, in detail, relationships between this subjective complaint and objective indexes of nocturnal sleep and daytime functioning.

This chapter will not discuss sleep disturbances directly associated with specific medical (e.g., sleep apnea, chronic pain) or psychiatric (e.g., major depression, schizophrenia) disorders, nor will it address circadian rhythm disorders or insomnia resulting from external factors, such as drug or alcohol use or inadequate sleeping environments. Instead, it will focus attention on those variants of insomnia with no clear etiology, sometimes referred to as *primary insomnia.*

Unfortunately, lack of consensus regarding an operational definition of insomnia has confounded attempts to obtain estimates of the prevalence of insomnia. As a result, studies employing broad, far-reaching definitions of insomnia have yielded higher prevalence rates than studies taking more conservative approaches. Some reports have estimated the prevalence of insomnia at over 30% (Bixler, A. Kales, Soldatos, J. Kales, & Healey, 1979; Mellinger, Balter, & Uhlenhuth, 1985; Welstein, Dement, Redington, Guilleminault, & Mitler, 1983), based on responses to somewhat vague questions regarding nocturnal sleep patterns (e.g., "Do you have a hard time falling asleep?"). In contrast, Ford and Kamerow (1989) obtained a prevalence rate of only 10.2% by specifying that sleep disturbances must have lasted for a minimum of 2 weeks.

Liljenberg, Almqvist, Hetta, Roos, and Ågren (1988), using even more restrictive criteria (e.g., subjective sleep deficits of at least 1 hour), estimated the prevalence of chronic insomnia to be less than 5%. In light of this latter finding, it is important to note that although 30.7% of the Welstein et al. (1983) subjects had "insomnia-like sleep problems," only 4.3% answered "yes" to the question, "Would you say you have insomnia?" Ford and Kamerow (1989) also noted that of those individuals labeled as insomniacs by some studies, only a small proportion had actually pursued treatment for sleep-related complaints, which suggests that most did not regard their sleep patterns as a serious problem.

Although researchers have disagreed on the prevalence of insomnia, there has been somewhat better agreement on other characteristics of the insomniac population. Research has consistently found that insomnia complaints, including both difficulty falling asleep and problems with nocturnal awakenings, are more prevalent among women than men (Bixler et al., 1979; Ford & Kamerow, 1989; Liljenberg et al., 1988; Mellinger et al., 1985; Welstein et al., 1983). Also, elderly individuals appear more prone to report sleep problems than younger individuals (Bixler et al., 1979; Ford & Kamerow, 1989; Mellinger et al., 1985); difficulties with sleep maintenance are particularly prominent among older people (Bixler et al., 1979; Welstein et al., 1983). There is also some evidence that complaints of disturbed sleep are more common among lower socioeconomic status (SES) individuals (Bixler et al., 1979; Ford & Kamerow, 1989) and those with less education (Bixler et al., 1979), relative to higher SES individuals and those with more education, respectively. Approximately 6% of the population reports having spoken to a physician about trouble sleeping in a given year, and about half of that group acknowledges receipt of a prescription for sleeping pills (Institute of Medicine, 1979; Welstein et al., 1983).

THEORETICAL FORMULATIONS OF PRIMARY INSOMNIA

In recent years, investigators have advanced several competing theories concerning the etiology of chronic insomnia. Some authorities have speculated that physiological hyperarousal is responsible for insomniacs' complaints of disturbed sleep. Others have argued that cognitive activation at bedtime results in extended wakefulness. Several authors have assumed that disturbed nocturnal sleep is the result of emotional conflict and personality dysfunction. Much of the currently available evidence, however, suggests that complaints of primary insomnia may not be due to true sleep deficits. Instead, the daytime fatigue reported by insomniacs may be a reaction to stress and anxiety associated with subjective impressions that sleep is inadequate, even though the physiological need for sleep is being met. We now examine each of these theoretical views in detail.

Physiological Hyperarousal

The view that insomnia may be a manifestation of physiological hyperarousal owes much to a study by Monroe (1967). Monroe's data demonstrated elevations in rectal temperature, phasic vasoconstrictions, body movements, and basal skin resistance among poor sleepers, relative to good sleepers. However, Monroe classified subjects on the basis of responses to a questionnaire about sleep habits; none of the so-called poor sleepers actually considered themselves insomniacs. Also, as Borkovec (1982) noted, a circadian rhythm phase shift could have been responsible for both the elevated nocturnal physiological activity and reports of disturbed sleep. Borkovec's argument received support from data showing that although insomniacs may have higher levels of presleep physiological activation than controls, these differences diminish with the approach of sleep onset (Freedman & Sattler, 1982).

Results of other studies have not been consistent with the hyperarousal hypothesis. Adam, Tomeny, and Oswald (1986) failed to find significant differences between poor and good sleepers in nocturnal body temperature, pulse rate, muscle metabolism, urinary cortisol, or adrenaline excretion. Johns, Gay, Masterton, and Bruce (1971) also found no significant differences in rectal temperature but reported their poor sleepers had elevated adrenocortical activity. Other studies have been unable to obtain significant correlations between frontalis EMG and sleep latency (Good, 1975; Haynes, Follingstad, & McGowan, 1974).

Clinicians have utilized behavioral insomnia treatments such as progressive relaxation and biofeedback based on the assumption that lowered physiological arousal will lead to better sleep. Although some studies have indicated that these techniques can be effective, there is little evidence that they work by reducing arousal. Most treatment-outcome research has failed to reveal significant correlations between improvement in nocturnal sleep and changes in physiological parameters such as heart rate, respiration rate, or EMG (Borkovec & Fowles, 1973; Borkovec, Grayson, O'Brien, & Weerts, 1979; Coursey, Frankel, Gaardner, & Mott, 1980; Hauri, 1981; Haynes et al., 1974; Lick & Heffler, 1977). In addition, some studies have shown that false feedback is as effective as true biofeedback in treating insomnia complaints (Nicassio, Boylan, & McCabe, 1982; VanderPlate & Eno, 1983).

Researchers have often cited the hyperarousal hypothesis to explain a somewhat anomalous characteristic of primary insomnia: the lack of significant daytime sleepiness. Although subjective reports of daytime fatigue among insomniacs are routine, objective recordings using the Multiple Sleep Latency Test (MSLT) have not found that insomniacs are sleepier during the day than normal controls (Seidel et al., 1984; Seidel & Dement, 1982; Stepanski, Zorick, Roehrs, Young, & Roth, 1988; Sugerman, Stern, & Walsh, 1985). This finding is especially surprising in light of the fact that research has consistently found increased sleepiness among normal sleepers following even modest reductions in nocturnal sleep time (Carskadon & Dement, 1981, 1982). Some authors, therefore, have proposed that the chronic hyperarousal hypothesized to disturb the sleep of insomniacs at night may also keep them awake during the day (Seidel & Dement, 1982; Stepanski et al., 1988). A study by Stepanski, Zorick, Peters, and Roth (1990) tested this postulate of the hyperarousal hypothesis by comparing MSLT scores of insomniacs and normals following one night of total sleep deprivation. The hypothesis implicitly predicts that insomniacs will not become as sleepy as normal sleepers under such conditions because the hypothesized hyperarousal of insomniacs would supposedly counteract the effects of sleep deprivation. This was not the case, however; the insomniacs demonstrated an increase in sleepiness comparable to that of the good sleepers.

Some critics have argued that the MSLT may not be an appropriate test of sleepiness for insomniacs, pointing out that anxiety about falling asleep may keep them awake despite their physiological sleepiness. However, studies employing boring tasks or no-demand instructions have also failed to yield significant evidence of daytime sleepiness (Hauri & Wisbey, 1990; Schneider-Helmert, 1987). Thus, the bulk of the evidence appears to support the conclusions of Coates and Thoresen (1981), Lichstein and Fischer (1985), and Turner (1986) that the hyperarousal hypothesis has not proven to be a useful theoretical framework for understanding the etiology of insomnia.

Cognitive Activation

It is not uncommon for insomnia patients to report difficulties "turning off" their thoughts at bedtime. Such anecdotal reports have undoubtedly provided the impetus for research examining the extent to which cognitive intrusions may cause and maintain insomnia. Lichstein and Rosenthal (1980), for example, found that insomniacs are considerably more likely to attribute their sleeping difficulties to cognitive rather than somatic arousal, but these authors failed to acknowledge that patients' subjective impressions regarding the causes of their insomnia may not be reliable. Nicassio, Mendlowitz, Fussell, and Petras (1985) reported a strong relationship between sleep latency and questionnaire items related to cognitive arousal, but conclusions regarding causation would be premature, especially given that the sleep latencies in this study derived from subjective reports.

Other studies have suggested that quality, rather than quantity, of mental activity may be what distinguishes insomniacs from normals. Insomniacs, relative to good sleepers, tend to have more negative, obsessive thoughts (Kuisk, Bertelson, & Walsh, 1989; Shealy, 1979; Van Egeren, Haynes, Franzen, & Hamilton, 1983), thoughts that may include concerns about being able to sleep (Borkovec, 1982). Still, these studies do not establish a causal relationship between cognitive activity and disturbed sleep. In contrast, Freedman and Sattler (1982) found no differences in presleep cognitive activity between insomniacs and controls. These authors suggested that excessive nocturnal rumination may simply be an epiphenomenon of sleeplessness rather than a true cause. In other words, alert insomniacs may be more susceptible to obsessive thinking while lying awake in bed than are drowsy good sleepers who are closer to sleep onset.

Experimental efforts to establish a relationship between cognitive activation and disturbed sleep have yielded equivocal results. In one study, students assigned the task of giving a speech on a specific topic had more difficulty falling asleep for a daytime nap than controls not given such an assignment, presumably because of the anxiety and cognitive efforts prompted by the task (Gross & Borkovec, 1982). However, students given the same task but not supplied the topic fell asleep with much less difficulty. Thus, the longer sleep latencies among the group given the topic may not necessarily have represented an inability to sleep. Instead, students who knew the topic beforehand may have intentionally stayed awake in order to prepare for the speech. In a similar experimental paradigm, Haynes, Adams, and Franzen (1981) attempted to induce disturbed sleep through neutral cognitions (mental arithmetic) and concluded that the results were not consistent with a cognitive-activation model of insomnia.

Other work in this area has focused on relationships between cognitive activity and subjective components of insomnia complaints, prompted by research findings that insomniacs tend to overestimate sleep latency and underestimate total sleep time (Carskadon et al., 1976; Coates et al., 1983; Frankel, Coursey, Buchbinder, & Snyder, 1976; Hauri & Fisher, 1986). Borkovec (1982) proposed that excessive, uncontrollable mental activity may cause insomniacs to overestimate the passage of time, resulting in an exaggeration of sleep latency and nocturnal wake time. This hypothesis received support from data in a study conducted by Borkovec and Hennings (1978); the authors demonstrated that insomniacs do not perform as well on a time estimation task as tense individuals with no complaints of insomnia. These same authors also showed that progressive relaxation training improves time estimation accuracy of insomniacs, suggesting that the primary mechanism of relaxation training as a treatment for insomnia may be a function of its effect on patients' subjective impressions regarding amount of time spent awake in bed at night while attempting to sleep.

Emotional and Personality Dysfunction

The sleep disorders literature is replete with data indicating poorer mental health and greater personality problems among insomniacs than among good sleepers, even in the absence of specific psychiatric diagnoses. Depressed mood and anxiety are common among insomniacs (Adam et al., 1986; Ford & Kamerow, 1989; Hauri & Fisher, 1986; Kales et al., 1984; Mellinger et al., 1985; Morin & Gramling, 1989; Vollrath, Wicki, & Angst, 1989; Zammit, 1988). Also, insomnia patients consistently yield a greater number of pathological scale elevations on the MMPI (Levin, Bertelson, & Lacks, 1984; Schneider-Helmert, 1987; Shealy, Lowe, & Ritzler, 1980). Many investigators have viewed the psychological characteristics common to insomnia patients as having a causal relationship to reported sleep disturbances. Berlin (1985), for example, suggested that insomnia results from an inability of patients to "discharge emotional arousal during the day" (p. 69). Similarly, Healey et al. (1981) proposed that insomnia relates to "unresolved and internalized psychological conflicts" (p. 447).

It is important to note, however, that relationships between psychological characteristics and insomnia have only been correlational; this does not necessarily imply causation. Also, the magnitude of emotional disturbance (e.g., MMPI scale scores) among insomniacs does not correlate significantly with nocturnal sleep parameters such as sleep latency or total sleep time (Carskadon et al., 1976; Shealy et al., 1980). Perhaps the most relevant data on this issue come from a study by Stepanski et al. (1989), who compared nocturnal sleep and personality features of two groups: complaining insomnia patients presenting for treatment, and individuals with insomnia-like sleep patterns, specifically recruited for the study. Stepanski and his colleagues found that although the groups had similar nocturnal sleep, the patient group demonstrated significantly greater evidence of psychopathology and personality disturbance than did the subjects who had not actively sought treatment.

The results of the Stepanski et al. (1989) study reveal that insomnia patients represent a self-selected group (by virtue of the fact that they choose to seek treatment) and therefore may not be representative of the insomniac population as a whole. Thus, the psychological distress so often seen in insomnia patients may not actually cause disturbed sleep but may simply be a factor that motivates them to get help. The Stepanski group considered this possibility in its conclusions, stating that in pursuing treatment, insomnia patients may actually be "seeking relief from their psychological symptoms, which they perceive to be related to their poor sleep" (p. 426). This position is consistent with the results of other studies that found no significant differences on the MMPI between controls and experimentally recruited insomniacs (Adam et al., 1986; Seidel et al., 1984).

Are Insomniacs Sleep Deprived?

The definition proposed earlier in this chapter characterized insomnia as a subjective complaint of inadequate nocturnal sleep accompanied by reports of daytime fatigue or other forms of compromised functioning. However, as discussed previously, insomniacs' subjective estimates regarding their sleep are often erroneous relative to data provided by objective recordings; on average, the actual difference in total sleep time between self-described insomniacs and noncomplaining sleepers is only about 35 minutes (Chambers & Keller, 1993). Moreover, several studies have failed to detect significant daytime sleepiness among insomniacs (Seidel & Dement, 1982; Seidel et al., 1984; Stepanski et al., 1988; Sugerman et al., 1985) despite the fact that restricted nocturnal sleep in otherwise normal sleepers consistently results in increased daytime sleepiness (Carskadon & Dement, 1981, 1982). These and other findings have begun to call into question the assumption that insomniacs' complaints are the result of insufficient sleep at night.

Authors such as Adam et al. (1986) and Coates and Thoresen (1981) have observed that objective differences in sleep time between insomniacs and normals do not seem consistent with the magnitude of most insomnia patients' daytime complaints. Insomniacs typically report that the consequences of their poor sleep include symptoms such as fatigue, forgetfulness, poor coordination, difficulty concentrating, and low productivity (Hauri & Fisher, 1986; Kales et al., 1984; Zammit, 1988). Objective testing, however, has failed to reveal consistent performance deficits in daytime functioning among insomniacs, relative to controls (Adam et al., 1986; Mendelson, Garnett, Gillin, & Weingartner, 1984; Mendelson et al., 1984; Schneider-Helmert, 1987; Seidel et al., 1984; Sugerman et al., 1985). In fact, when both insomniacs and controls rate their respective levels of functioning at a specific moment in time (as opposed to broad, global, retrospective assessments), differences in subjective symptomatology between the two groups disappear (Mendelson, James, Garnett, Sack, & Rosenthal, 1986).

Several investigators have found that insomniacs tend to complain of numerous somatic symptoms in addition to those attributed to the insomnia itself (Adam et al., 1986; Hauri & Fisher, 1986; Kales et al., 1984; Piccione, Tallarigo, Zorick, Wittig, & Roth, 1981; Zammit, 1988). Piccione et al. (1981) interpreted these findings to mean that insomniacs are "emotionally overresponsive and likely to complain of a variety of somatic complaints in the absence of serious medical illness" (p. 263). Given that insomniacs obtain roughly the same amount of nocturnal sleep as normals and show no objective evidence of daytime sleepiness or impaired functioning, their subjective daytime complaints of fatigue appear consistent with Piccione et al.'s assessment. Thus, it is reasonable to conclude, particularly in light of the personality problems and emotional distress typically found among insomnia patients, that the fatigue and daytime functioning deficits of which insomniacs complain may be somatized symptoms that have no true physiological basis.

Some experts (Chambers & Keller, 1993; Lichstein, 1988; Lichstein & Fischer, 1985; Lichstein & Rosenthal, 1980) have posited that many insomnia patients may simply be naturally short sleepers who require less sleep than the population norm. In the absence of daytime sleepiness, patients who sleep 5 or 6 hours per night may not need more sleep, even though they complain of insomnia and daytime dysfunction. Lichstein (1988) has termed these individuals *insomnoids*, and he has speculated that anxiety resulting from the belief that their sleep is somehow abnormal may be a major component of their daytime distress. He has also noted that in their attempts to obtain the 8 hours of sleep they believe they must have, insomnoids may spend hours of frustrating, anxious wakefulness in bed each night. The stress associated with this behavior, according to Lichstein, may be responsible for much of the fatigue and other difficulties experienced by insomniacs the following day. Recent research data (Chambers & Kim, 1993) support this hypothesis.

CLINICAL MANAGEMENT OF PRIMARY INSOMNIA

The multifaceted nature of insomnia renders it particularly difficult to manage in clinical settings. Clinicians can best achieve successful resolution of insomnia complaints through careful and thorough assessment of the complaints and their possible causes followed by a tailored treatment approach that addresses the specific needs and circumstances of individual patients.

Evaluating an Insomnia Complaint

Medical Examination

Almost any medical problem or physical symptom has the potential to disturb sleep (Coates & Thoresen, 1981). For this reason, medical examinations are an indispensable first step in the investigation of insomnia complaints. Exams need to include a review of medications being used to treat other medical conditions because many medications have sleep-related side effects. Drugs with stimulant properties, including over-the-counter pain relievers containing caffeine, may disturb nocturnal sleep, especially if used at night. Medications with short half-lives, taken at bedtime, may lose their effectiveness before the end of the sleep period, and the subsequent rebound can result in a middle-of-the-night arousal. Some daytime medications may also contribute to complaints of insomnia, particularly if sedation or drowsiness results. Patients using such medications may mistakenly attribute their poor alertness during the day to inadequate sleep, even when nocturnal sleep remains essentially undisturbed.

Ironically, chronic use of prescription sleeping medications may be the most common and significant medical factor in the maintenance of persistent insomnia complaints. Despite patients' insistence to the contrary, sedative–hypnotics produce only slight increases in the amount of nocturnal sleep, and these effects diminish with time (Gillin & Mendelson, 1981). Development of tolerance may lead to use of higher and higher doses, but even with such increases, the quality and quantity of sleep may be worse than before patients initiated use of the drug. When habitual users attempt to stop taking their sleeping pills, however, the increased sleep disturbance associated with withdrawal effects leads them to conclude that they cannot sleep without pharmacological assistance. Failing to realize that withdrawal is only temporary, they typically resume medicating their sleep problems before they have had an opportunity to get an accurate view of their sleep without drugs.

Medical examinations also provide an opportunity to rule out presence of a primary organic sleep disorder (although it is imperative that psychologists not automatically assume that examining physicians have done this). *Sleep apnea*, a disorder characterized by frequent interruptions in respiration throughout the night, can result in significant sleep fragmentation leading unsuspecting patients to report insomnia problems (Fredrickson & Krueger, 1994). Symptoms suggesting presence of sleep apnea include loud and disruptive snoring, morning headaches, a sore throat or dry mouth upon awakening, and observations by the patient's sleeping partner of pauses in breathing during sleep.

Restless legs syndrome and *periodic limb movement disorder,* two conditions that often occur in tandem, are also common organic causes of chronic insomnia (Fredrickson & Krueger, 1994). In the first, patients describe restless, crawling, or itching sensations in their legs that appear when they lie down to sleep at night. These feelings, which may also be present in the daytime during periods of extended inactivity, usually subside somewhat with movement of the legs. Periodic limb movements, on the other hand, occur only during sleep. In most cases, the patient's bed partner observes rhythmic twitching of the legs (or less commonly, the arms) at intervals of 20–30 seconds. In the absence of a bed partner, patients may identify the presence of periodic limb movements by extreme disturbance of the bed covers in the morning or problems with leg cramping upon awakening. Repeated, unexplained arousals during the night or excessive daytime sleepiness may also indicate a physiological sleep dysfunction. If a clinician suspects the presence of an organic sleep disorder, it is prudent to refer those patients to a sleep disorders center for an overnight evaluation.

Sleep History

The initial focus of the sleep-history interview must be the nature of the sleep problem itself. Is the problem with falling asleep, staying asleep, or both? How often does the problem occur and under what circumstances? When did the problem first appear? Did any other unusual or significant events coincide with the onset of the problem? To date, what treatments has the patient attempted to alleviate the problem? What are the daytime consequences of the sleep problem? Does the patient have any irrational fears, erroneous beliefs, or distorted perceptions regarding sleep or the insomnia problem?

Clinicians must also always assess practices and habits related to sleep hygiene, such as daytime napping and use of caffeine, alcohol, and nicotine. In addition, patients' sleep schedules frequently provide valuable clues regarding the nature and causes of insomnia complaints. A patient who regularly spends 10 hours in bed each night, for example, would be almost certain to have difficulty initiating sleep or have extended wake time during the night. An individual who habitually sleeps late on weekends may have a delayed sleep phase, making it more difficult to fall asleep at a reasonable hour during the week. Nocturnal behaviors may also be relevant. What does the patient do in the middle of the night when unable to sleep? Individuals with a habit of lying in bed worrying or solving problems may be exacerbating their sleeping difficulties by associating the bed with sleep-incompatible activities. (See Lacks [1987] for more detail on the sleep history interview.)

Finally, interviewers must give some attention to patients' emotional functioning and psychiatric status, although it is possible to overemphasize this component of an insomnia complaint. Presence of emotional distress or a psychiatric diagnosis does not automatically account for a patient's report of disturbed nocturnal sleep. In cases involving severe psychiatric disturbance, such as a major depressive disorder or a psychotic condition, the treatment team should consider psychiatric intervention, including pharmacotherapy. For other diagnoses, such as anxiety or personality disorders, psychotherapy may be the treatment indicated, but clinicians must not assume that psychotherapy alone, in the absence of behavior therapy specifically for the sleep problem will result in satisfactory resolution of an insomnia complaint (Spielman & Glovinsky, 1991).

Sleep Logs

Patients' global, retrospective reports regarding their sleep patterns can be unreliable. For this reason, daily sleep logs for a period of 1–2 weeks usually help clarify the nature and severity of the insomnia (Lacks & Morin, 1992). At a minimum, logs need to include information about bedtimes and awakening times, sleep latency, total sleep time, number and length of awakenings during the night, and ratings concerning the quality of sleep and level of restedness the following day. When applicable, patients may also need to note daytime events, such as caffeine and alcohol intake, drug use, naps, or scheduling of meals or exercise. Finally, patients must carefully document use of sleeping pills and other medications that may affect sleep.

In addition to their role in assessment and diagnosis, sleep logs can be a valuable component of the treatment process. Records kept during the evaluation phase can provide baseline sleep data against which patient and clinician can compare subsequent therapeutic gains. Regular monitoring may also prompt a patient to realize that the problem is not as severe as imagined, thereby resulting in a reduction of anxiety about sleep. Clinicians must not assume, however, that sleep logs provide an entirely accurate measure of patients' nocturnal sleep patterns because insomniacs tend to overestimate sleep latency and underestimate total sleep time (Carskadon et al., 1976; Coates et al., 1983; Frankel et al., 1976; Hauri & Fisher, 1986). Clinicians need to view particularly extreme reports (e.g., no sleep at all for a week or more) with skepticism (McCall & Edinger, 1992). Still, sleep logs do correlate significantly with objective measures of sleep latency and total sleep time (Lacks, 1988). Moreover, accurate measurement of nocturnal sleep may not always be as important as patients' subjective impressions of their problems, especially given that objectively normal sleep sometimes accompanies complaints of insomnia.

Treatment of Primary Insomnia

In recent years, clinical researchers have introduced numerous behavioral therapies for treatment of chronic insomnia, only a few of which the following sections review. Although many of these approaches have statistically significant effects on subjective complaints of insomniacs (Murtagh & Greenwood, 1995), some researchers have questioned the clinical significance of objective changes in sleep latency and total sleep time that have resulted from these techniques (Coates & Thoresen, 1981; Morin & Kwentus, 1988). Also, there is evidence that behavioral insomnia therapies may rely strongly on placebo effects and patient expectations (Chambers & Keller, 1993; Lichstein & Fischer, 1985). On the other hand, treatment-outcome studies have given insufficient attention to the daytime complaints that inevitably accompany reports of insomnia; some evidence indicates that behavioral treatment approaches may have direct effects on this aspect of the problem while having little effect on nocturnal sleep parameters.

In constructing treatment programs for insomnia complaints, patients' individual needs and circumstances must dictate the choice of therapeutic techniques. It is important to keep in mind that the ultimate goal of therapy is to improve the quality of patients' waking lives, not necessarily to increase total sleep time or reduce sleep latency. As discussed previously, many insomniacs may actually be meeting their physiological need for sleep, and undue emphasis in therapy on increasing total sleep time may only increase these patients' sleep-related anxiety, anxiety that may have been a major factor in the decision to seek treatment. In such cases, cognitive intervention may be an important supplement to other behavioral techniques.

Stimulus Control

Stimulus control is perhaps the most widely used and researched of the behavioral techniques currently available for treating insomnia. Developed by Bootzin (1972), this approach assumes that insomnia may result from a conditioned response of wakefulness and arousal associated with stimuli of the bed and bedroom. According to stimulus control theory, certain behaviors and responses can become conditioned as a result of repeated pairings with particular stimuli. In the case of insomnia, this theory hypothesizes that an insomniac's practice of lying awake in bed night after night results in the bed becoming associated with alertness rather than sleepiness. Stimulus control therapy attempts to counteract this conditioning by ensuring that stimuli of the bed become paired only with sleep.

In stimulus control treatment, patients receive instructions to go to bed only when sleepy and to use the bed for no activities other than sleep (sexual activity is the sole exception). If unable to sleep, patients are to remain in bed no longer than about 10 minutes, after which time they are to get up and engage in relaxing activities in another room until they are ready to sleep. This treatment also includes instructions to maintain regular morning awakening times and avoid napping during the day. Research has consistently found that this approach is equal or superior in effectiveness to most other behavioral approaches in reducing sleep latency (Bootzin, 1984; Espie, Lindsay, Brooks, Hood, & Turvey, 1989; Lacks, Bertelson, Gans, & Kunkel, 1983; Lacks & Powlishta, 1989; Morin & Azrin, 1987; Turner & Ascher, 1982). This approach has also been successful in the treatment of sleep maintenance problems (Lacks, Bertelson, Sugerman, & Kunkel, 1983; Schoicket, Bertelson, & Lacks, 1988).

There has been some question, however, as to whether the efficacy of stimulus control is actually due to classical conditioning processes. Espie et al. (1989), for example, noted that because many treatment-outcome studies rely on sleep latency as the dependent variable, the stimulus control instruction to get into bed only when sleepy may be a "virtual guarantee" of reduced sleep onset latency. Also, Haynes, Adams, West, Kamens, and Safranek (1982) found no relationship between sleep-incompatible behaviors (e.g., reading in bed) and sleep onset latency. In discussing these results, the authors speculated that instructions to engage in some other activity when unable to sleep may actually work by modifying insomniacs' "attributions of control of sleep-processes, level of concern about sleep difficulties, or other competing cognitive events associated with sleep-onset periods" (p. 338). This hypothesis received support from the finding that countercontrol therapy (i.e., instructions to engage in a nonarousing activity in bed when unable to sleep) is as effective as stimulus control therapy in treating chronic insomnia (Zwart & Lisman, 1979).

Sleep Restriction

Postulating that excessive time in bed (TIB) may be a factor that perpetuates chronic insomnia, Spielman, Saskin, and Thorpy (1987) developed and tested a treatment approach that systematically restricts TIB. In sleep restriction therapy, patients monitor their baseline sleep patterns via sleep logs for 2 weeks. From these records, the therapist calculates an average total sleep time (TST), which is then prescribed as the nightly TIB (e.g., if initial TIB is 6 hours, the bedtime is set for 6 hours prior to the required wake-up time). During treatment, patients calculate daily sleep efficiency (TST/TIB). If the mean sleep efficiency for a 5-day period exceeds .90, patients increase TIB by 15 minutes. However, if mean sleep efficiency drops below .85, patients reduce TIB to the mean TST of the previous 5 days.

The 35 patients treated with sleep restriction therapy in the seminal Spielman et al. (1987) study demonstrated significant decreases in sleep latency and wake time during the night along with an increase in mean sleep efficiency from .67 to .87. Other studies (Edinger, Hoelscher, Marsh, Ionescou-Pioggia, & Lipper, 1990; Morin, Kowatch, & Wade, 1989; Rubinstein et al., 1990; Schmidt-Nowara, Beck, & Jessop, 1991) have reported similar findings. However, changes in TST have generally been small or nonsignificant. Spielman et al. (1987), for example, reported a mean increase in TST of only 23 minutes. Hoelscher and Edinger (1988), treating a small sample of older adults, yielded no significant TST changes, as measured by both subjective estimates and objective measures. At least two studies (Morin et al., 1989; Rubinstein et al., 1990) have obtained increases in subjective estimates of TST while recording *decreases* of 20 to 30 minutes in actual TST. Still, patients treated with sleep restriction generally report better quality sleep and less fatigue during the day, relative to baseline (Edinger et al., 1990; Morin et al., 1989; Schmidt-Nowara et al., 1991; Spielman et al., 1987).

Research on sleep restriction therapy clearly illustrates that treatment-related changes in insomnia patients' daytime symptomatology do not necessarily depend on increased TST. This supports the hypothesis that actual amount of nocturnal sleep obtained by insomniacs is not the primary factor responsible for daytime complaints. Instead, as Chambers (1992) and Lichstein and Fischer (1985) have proposed, stress induced by insomniacs' anxious efforts to sleep at night may result in fatigue the following day that patients then interpret to be a consequence of inadequate sleep. Techniques such as stimulus control and sleep restriction, thus, may help relieve this stress by reducing the number of frustrating wakeful hours spent each night in bed.

Relaxation Training and Biofeedback

As discussed previously in this chapter, assumptions regarding the possible relationship between physiological tension and nocturnal sleep disturbance have led to the use of treatment strategies designed to reduce this tension. Several studies have demonstrated that relaxation training results in significant subjective improvement in sleep latency or total sleep time, relative to baseline or no-treatment controls (Bootzin, 1984; Borkovec & Hennings, 1978; Borkovec & Weerts, 1976; Borkovec et al., 1979; Carr-Kaffashan & Woolfolk, 1979; Espie et al., 1989; Friedman, Bliwise, Yesavage, & Salom, 1991; Lick & Heffler, 1977; Shealy, 1979; Woolfolk & McNulty, 1983). A few studies have also verified objective improvements in sleep as a result of treatment (Borkovec & Weerts, 1976; Borkovec et al., 1979; Coursey et al., 1980; Freedman & Papsdorf, 1976). Actual changes in sleep latency, however, have been a modest 10–25 minutes.

Some studies have compared the efficacy of relaxation training to that of other behavioral treatments for insomnia. With respect to changes in nocturnal sleep, research has found that relaxation training is inferior to both stimulus control (Bootzin, 1984; Espie et al., 1989; Lacks et al., 1983) and sleep restriction (Friedman et al., 1991). Espie et al. (1989), however, reported significant improvements for relaxation training, but not stimulus control, in subject ratings of restedness and enjoyment of sleep. There has been some question as to whether the tension-release component of relaxation training is essential in the treatment of insomnia. Borkovec et al. (1979) found tension-release relaxation training superior to identical training without tension-release in the reduction of sleep latency. Woolfolk and McNulty (1983), on the other hand, failed to find a significant impact for the presence of tension-release in the relaxation treatment of sleep initiation problems.

Biofeedback has also demonstrated some promise as a treatment for insomnia, but, as with relaxation training, objective improvements have not been substantial (Coursey et al., 1980; Freedman & Papsdorf, 1976; Hauri, 1981; Hauri, Percy, Hellekson, Hartmann, & Russ, 1982). A few studies have compared the efficacy of biofeedback with that of relaxation training (Coursey et al., 1980; Freedman & Papsdorf, 1976; Nicassio et al., 1982), but neither approach emerged as clearly superior. With regard to the type of biofeedback that is most effective, neither Hauri (1981) nor Nicassio et al. (1982) found frontalis EMG biofeedback superior to control in reducing sleep latency. Hauri (1981) also examined theta EEG and sensorimotor (SMR) feedback and reported them to be similarly ineffective in significantly reducing sleep latency. After additional analysis, however, Hauri found that theta feedback could be useful if limited to "tense" insomniacs, whereas SMR feedback appeared efficacious only for subjects already sufficiently relaxed prior to treatment. Hauri et al. (1982) subsequently replicated this finding.

Cognitive Restructuring

Patients' cognitions are often of considerable importance in the presentation of an insomnia complaint, regardless of whether an actual sleep disturbance exists. For this reason, many authors have maintained that cognitive interventions can be valuable, and perhaps even primary, components of insomnia treatment programs (e.g., Chambers, 1992; Lichstein & Fischer, 1985; Morin & Kwentus, 1988). Even if insomnia is due to an identifiable organic disorder, the anxiety and fear often associated with a chronic sleep problem, if left unaddressed, may prevent successful resolution of the insomnia.

Patients' expectations and beliefs can have a significant role in the ultimate outcome of treatment. Therapists must therefore encourage patients to set reasonable goals for therapy, both in terms of the ultimate outcome and the speed at which they obtain their goals. As previously discussed, many reports of insomnia may result from a lower than average need for sleep. Patients who are not sleepy during the day, even if they complain of fatigue or other problems with daytime functioning, may actually be obtaining all the sleep they require. For such patients, it is often the anxiety and frustration experienced while attempting to sleep, rather than a lack of sleep, that is responsible for the daytime tiredness. Thus, cognitive interventions that prompt patients to view their sleep patterns as a lessened *need* to sleep, rather than an *inability* to sleep, may help reduce this anxiety. When clinicians advise insomnia patients to give up trying to sleep and accept their sleep as normal, they report less sleep-related anxiety at night and better sleep efficiency (Fogle & Dyal, 1983).

Improving insomnia patients' perspective of their daytime functioning can also relieve the performance anxiety they may experience. These patients may tend to selectively recall mistakes and other performance problems following a poor night of sleep. Therapists can therefore encourage patients to note instances of satisfactory performance on such days an remind them that they may forget mistakes made following good sleep or attribute these mistakes to other causes. Clinicians must also be aware that insomniacs often alter their usual daytime routines following a night of insomnia, claiming that they feel too tired to go to work or socialize with friends. Clinicians must urge such patients to perform all of their normal activities during the day, regardless of how much or how little sleep they obtained the previous night. Patients who follow this advice generally react with surprise when they discover how little their "sleep problem" has impaired their functioning. As a result, their fears regarding insomnia and its consequences diminish.

CONCLUSION

Sleep is a universal human experience. Perhaps because of this, misconceptions and erroneous assumptions may be more common about sleep than for other psychological and medical phenomena. These misconceptions can have serious consequences, particularly when they exacerbate patients' anxieties about insomnia. For this reason, treating clinicians must be able to supply insomnia patients with sensible, accurate information and advice about sleep. Insomnia does not cause serious physical or mental illness, nor is it likely to be an early symptom of a terminal disease. Ironically, it may be that worry about sleep and the concomitant stress pose the most serious threat to the health of chronic insomniacs. In many cases, therapists can successfully address chronic insomnia complaints through appropriate cognitive and behavioral interventions. Success does not necessarily translate into increases in sleep time, however; instead, the goal of therapy is to improve patient satisfaction with waking functioning.

REFERENCES

Adam, K., Tomeny, M., & Oswald, I. (1986). Physiological and psychological differences between good and poor sleepers. *Journal of Psychiatric Research, 20,* 301–316.

American Sleep Disorders Association. (1990). *ICSD—International classification of sleep disorders: Diagnostic and coding manual.* Rochester, MN: Author.

Berlin, R. M. (1985). Psychotherapeutic treatment of chronic insomnia. *American Journal of Psychotherapy, 39,* 68–74.

Bixler, E. O., Kales, A., Soldatos, C. R., Kales, J. D., & Healey, S. (1979). Prevalence of sleep disorders in the Los Angeles metropolitan area. *American Journal of Psychiatry, 136,* 1257–1262.

Bootzin, R. R. (1972). A stimulus control treatment for insomnia. *Proceedings of the 80th Annual Convention of the American Psychological Association, 7,* 395–396.

Bootzin, R. R. (1984). Evaluation of stimulus control instructions, progressive relaxation, and sleep hygiene as treatments for insomnia. In W. P. Koella, E. Rüther, & H. Schulz (Eds.), *Sleep '84: Proceedings of the 7th European Congress on Sleep Research* (pp. 142–144). Stuttgart: Verlag.

Borkovec, T. D. (1982). Insomnia. *Journal of Consulting and Clinical Psychology, 50,* 880–895.

Borkovec, T. D., & Fowles, D. C. (1973). Controlled investigation of the effects of progressive and hypnotic relaxation on insomnia. *Journal of Abnormal Psychology, 82,* 153–158.

Borkovec, T. D., Grayson, J. B., O'Brien, G. T., & Weerts, T. C. (1979). Relaxation treatment of pseudoinsomnia and idiopathic insomnia: An electroencephalographic evaluation. *Journal of Applied Behavior Analysis, 12,* 37–54.

Borkovec, T. D., & Hennings, B. L. (1978). The role of physiological attention-focusing in the relaxation treatment of sleep disturbance, general tension, and specific stress reaction. *Behaviour Research and Therapy, 16,* 7–19.

Borkovec, T. D., & Weerts, T. C. (1976). Effects of progressive relaxation on sleep disturbance: An electroencephalographic evaluation. *Psychosomatic Medicine, 38,* 173–180.

Carr-Kaffashan, L., & Woolfolk, R. L. (1979). Active and placebo effects in treatment of moderate and severe insomnia. *Journal of Consulting and Clinical Psychology, 47,* 1072–1080.

Carskadon, M. A., & Dement, W. C. (1981). Cumulative effects of sleep restriction on daytime sleepiness. *Psychophysiology, 18,* 107–113.

Carskadon, M. A., & Dement, W. C. (1982). Nocturnal determinants of daytime sleepiness. *Sleep, 5,* S73–S81.

Carskadon, M. A., Dement, W. C., Mitler, M. M., Guilleminault, C., Zarcone, V. P., & Spiegel, R. (1976). Self-reports versus sleep laboratory findings in 122 drug-free subjects with complaints of chronic insomnia. *American Journal of Psychiatry, 133,* 1382–1388.

Chambers, M. J. (1992). Therapeutic issues in the behavioral treatment of insomnia. *Professional Psychology: Research and Practice, 23,* 131–138.

Chambers, M. J., & Keller, B. (1993). Alert insomniacs: Are they really sleep deprived? *Clinical Psychology Review, 13,* 649–666.

Chambers, M. J., & Kim, J. Y. (1993). The role of state-trait anxiety in insomnia and daytime restedness. *Behavioral Medicine, 19,* 42–46.

Coates, T. J., & Thoresen, C. E. (1981). Treating sleep disorders: Few answers, some suggestions, and many questions. In S. M. Turner, K. S. Calhoun, & H. E. Adams (Eds.), *Handbook of clinical behavior therapy* (pp. 240–289). New York: Wiley.

Coates, T. J., Killen, J. D., Silverman, S., George, J., Marchini, E., Hamilton, S., & Thoresen, C. E. (1983). Cognitive activity, sleep disturbance, and stage specific differences between recorded and reported sleep. *Psychophysiology, 20,* 243–250.

Coursey, R. D., Frankel, B. L., Gaarder, K. R., & Mott, D. E. (1980). A comparison of relaxation techniques with electrosleep therapy for chronic, sleep-onset insomnia: A sleep-EEG study. *Biofeedback and Self-Regulation, 5,* 57–73.

Edinger, J. D., Hoelscher, T. J., Marsh, G. R., Ionescou-Pioggia, M., & Lipper, S. (1990). Treating sleep maintenance problems in older adults. *Sleep Research, 19,* 218.

Espie, C. A., Lindsay, W. R., Brooks, D. N., Hood, E. M., & Turvey, T. (1989). A controlled comparative investigation of psychological treatments for chronic sleep-onset insomnia. *Behaviour Research and Therapy, 27,* 79–88.

Fogle, D. O., & Dyal, J. A. (1983). Paradoxical giving up and the reduction of sleep performance anxiety in chronic insomniacs. *Psychotherapy: Theory, Research, and Practice, 20,* 21–30.

Ford, D. E., & Kamerow, D. B. (1989). Epidemiologic study of sleep disturbances and psychiatric disorders: An opportunity for prevention? *Journal of the American Medical Association, 262,* 1479–1484.

Frankel, B. L., Coursey, R. D., Buchbinder, R., & Snyder, F. (1976). Recorded and reported sleep in chronic primary insomnia. *Archives of General Psychiatry, 33,* 615–623.

Fredrickson, P. A., & Krueger, B. R. (1994). Insomnia associated with specific polysomnographic findings. In M. H. Kryger, T. Roth, & W. C. Dement (Eds.), *Principles and practice of sleep medicine* (2nd ed., pp. 523–534). Philadelphia: W. B. Saunders.

Freedman, R., & Papsdorf, J. D. (1976). Biofeedback and progressive relaxation treatment of sleep-onset insomnia: A controlled, all-night investigation. *Biofeedback and Self-Regulation, 1,* 253–271.

Freedman, R. R., & Sattler, H. L. (1982). Physiological and psychological factors in sleep-onset insomnia. *Journal of Abnormal Psychology, 91,* 380–389.

Friedman, L., Bliwise, D. L., Yesavage, J. A., & Salom, S. R. (1991). A preliminary study comparing sleep restriction and relaxation treatments for insomnia in older adults. *Journal of Gerontology, 46,* P1–P8.

Gillin, J. C., & Mendelson, W. B. (1981). Sleeping pills: For whom? When? How Long? In G. C. Palmer (Ed.), *Neuropharmacology of central nervous system and behavioral disorders* (pp. 285–316). New York: Academic Press.

Good, R. (1975). Frontalis muscle tension and sleep latency. *Psychophysiology, 12,* 465–467.

Gross, R. T., & Borkovec, T. D. (1982). Effects of a cognitive intrusion manipulation on the sleep-onset latency of good sleepers. *Behavior Therapy, 13,* 112–116.

Hauri, P. (1981). Treating psychophysiologic insomnia with biofeedback. *Archives of General Psychiatry, 38,* 752–758.

Hauri, P., & Fisher, J. (1986). Persistent psychophysiologic (learned) insomnia. *Sleep, 9,* 38–53.

Hauri, P. J., Percy, L., Hellekson, C., Hartmann, E., & Russ, D. (1982). The treatment of psychophysiologic insomnia with biofeedback: A replication study. *Biofeedback and Self-Regulation, 7,* 223–235.

Hauri, P., & Wisbey, J. (1990). The MSLT in insomnia. *Sleep Research, 19,* 234.

Haynes, S. N., Adams, A., & Franzen, M. (1981). The effects of presleep stress on sleep-onset insomnia. *Journal of Abnormal Psychology, 90,* 601–606.

Haynes, S. N., Adams, A. E., West, S., Kamens, L., & Safranek, R. (1982). The stimulus control paradigm in sleep-onset insomnia: A multimethod assessment. *Journal of Psychosomatic Research, 26,* 333–339.

Haynes, S. N., Follingstad, D. R., & McGowan, W. T. (1974). Insomnia: Sleep patterns and anxiety level. *Journal of Psychosomatic Research, 18,* 69–74.

Healey, E. S., Kales, A., Monroe, L. J., Bixler, E. O., Chamberlin, K., & Soldatos, C. R. (1981). Onset of insomnia: Role of life-stress events. *Psychosomatic Medicine, 43,* 439–451.

Hoelscher, T. J., & Edinger, J. D. (1988). Treatment of sleep-maintenance insomnia in older adults: Sleep period reduction, sleep education, and modified stimulus control. *Psychology and Aging, 3,* 258–263.

Institute of Medicine. (1979). *Sleeping pills, insomnia, and medical practice.* Washington, DC: National Academy of Sciences.

Johns, M. W., Gay, T.J.A., Masterton, J. P., & Bruce, D. W. (1971). Relationship between sleep habits, adrenocortical activity and personality. *Psychosomatic Medicine, 33,* 499–508.

Kales, J. D., Kales, A., Bixler, E. O., Soldatos, C. R., Cadieux, R. J., Kashurba, G. J., & Vela-Bueno, A. (1984). Biopsychobehavioral correlates of insomnia: V. Clinical characteristics and behavioral correlates. *American Journal of Psychiatry, 141,* 1371–1376.

Kuisk, L. A., Bertelson, A. D., & Walsh, J. K. (1989). Presleep cognitive hyperarousal and affect as factors in objective and subjective insomnia. *Perceptual and Motor Skills, 69,* 1219–1225.

Lacks, P. (1987). *Behavioral treatment for persistent insomnia.* Elmsford, NY: Pergamon Press.

Lacks, P. (1988). Daily sleep diary. In M. Hersen & A. S. Bellack (Eds.), *Dictionary of behavioral assessment techniques* (pp. 162–164). Elmsford, NY: Pergamon Press.

Lacks, P., Bertelson, A. D., Gans, L., & Kunkel, J. (1983). The effectiveness of three behavioral treatments for different degrees of sleep onset insomnia. *Behavior Therapy, 14,* 593–605.

Lacks, P., Bertelson, A. D., Sugerman, J., & Kunkel, J. (1983). The treatment of sleep-maintenance insomnia with stimulus–control techniques. *Behaviour Research and Therapy, 21,* 291–295.

Lacks, P., & Morin, C. M. (1992). Recent advances in the assessment and treatment of insomnia. *Journal of Consulting and Clinical Psychology, 60,* 586–594.

Lacks, P., & Powlishta, K. (1989). Improvement following behavioral treatment for insomnia: Clinical significance, long-term maintenance, and predictors of outcome. *Behavior Therapy, 20,* 117–134.

Levin, D., Bertelson, A. D., & Lacks, P. (1984). MMPI differences among mild and severe insomniacs and good sleepers. *Journal of Personality Assessment, 48,* 126–129.

Lichstein, K. L. (1988). Sleep compression treatment of an insomnoid. *Behavior Therapy, 19,* 625–632.

Lichstein, K. L., & Fischer, S. M. (1985). Insomnia. In M. Hersen & A. S. Bellack (Eds.), *Handbook of clinical behavior therapy with adults* (pp. 319–352). New York: Plenum Press.

Lichstein, K. L., & Rosenthal, T. L. (1980). Insomniacs' perceptions of cognitive versus somatic determinants of sleep disturbance. *Journal of Abnormal Psychology, 89,* 105–107.

Lick, J. R., & Heffler, D. (1977). Relaxation training and attention placebo in the treatment of severe insomnia. *Journal of Consulting and Clinical Psychology, 45,* 153–161.

Liljenberg, B., Almqvist, M., Hetta, J., Roos, B.-E., & Ågren, H. (1988). The prevalence of insomnia: The importance of operationally defined criteria. *Annals of Clinical Research, 20,* 393–398.

McCall, W. V., & Edinger, J. D. (1992). Subjective total insomnia: An example of sleep state misperception. *Sleep, 15,* 71–73.

Mellinger, G. D., Balter, M. B., & Uhlenhuth, E. H. (1985). Insomnia and its treatment: Prevalence and correlates. *Archives of General Psychiatry, 42,* 225–232.

Mendelson, W. B., Garnett, D., Gillin, J. C., & Weingartner, H. (1984). The experience of insomnia and daytime and nighttime functioning. *Psychiatry Research, 12,* 235–250.

Mendelson, W. B., Garnett, D., & Linnoila, M. (1984). Do insomniacs have impaired daytime functioning? *Biological Psychiatry, 19,* 1261–1264.

Mendelson, W. B., James, S. P., Garnett, D., Sack, D. A., & Rosenthal, N. E. (1986). A psychophysiological study of insomnia. *Psychiatry Research, 19,* 267–284.

Monroe, L. J. (1967). Psychological and physiological differences between good and poor sleepers. *Journal of Abnormal Psychology, 72,* 255–264.

Morin, C. M., & Azrin, N. H. (1987). Stimulus control and imagery training in treating sleep-maintenance insomnia. *Journal of Consulting and Clinical Psychology, 55,* 260–262.

Morin, C. M., & Gramling, S. E. (1989). Sleep patterns and aging: Comparison of older adults with and without insomnia complaints. *Sleep and Aging, 4,* 290–294.

Morin, C. M., Kowatch, R. A., & Wade, J. B. (1989). Behavioral management of sleep disturbances secondary to chronic pain. *Journal of Behavior Therapy and Experimental Psychiatry, 20,* 295–302.

Morin, C. M., & Kwentus, J. A. (1988). Behavioral and pharmacological treatments for insomnia. *Annals of Behavioral Medicine, 10,* 91–100.

Murtagh, D.R.R., & Greenwood, J. M. (1995). Identifying effective psychological treatments for insomnia: A meta-analysis. *Journal of Consulting and Clinical Psychology, 63,* 79–89.

Nicassio, P. M., Boylan, M. B., & McCabe, T. G. (1982). Progressive relaxation, EMG biofeedback and biofeedback placebo in the treatment of sleep-onset insomnia. *British Journal of Medical Psychology, 55,* 159–166.

Nicassio, P. M., Mendlowitz, D. R., Fussell, J. J., & Petras, L. (1985). The phenomenology of the pre-sleep state: The development of the pre-sleep arousal scale. *Behaviour Research and Therapy, 23,* 263–271.

Piccione, P., Tallarigo, R., Zorick, F., Wittig, R., & Roth, T. (1981). Personality differences between insomniac and non-insomniac psychiatry outpatients. *Journal of Clinical Psychiatry, 42,* 261–263.

Rubinstein, M. L., Rothenberg, S. A., Maheswaran, S., Tsai, J. S., Zozula, R., & Spielman, A. J. (1990). Modified sleep restriction therapy in middle-aged and elderly chronic insomniacs. *Sleep Research, 19,* 276.

Schmidt-Nowara, W. W., Beck, A. A., & Jessop, C. A. (1991). An experimental evaluation of sleep restriction to treat chronic insomnia and reduce hypnotic use. *Sleep Research, 20,* 323.

Schneider-Helmert, D. (1987). Twenty-four-hour sleep–wake function and personality patterns in chronic insomniacs and healthy controls. *Sleep, 10,* 452–462.

Schoicket, S. L., Bertelson, A. D., & Lacks, P. (1988). Is sleep hygiene a sufficient treatment of sleep-maintenance insomnia? *Behavior Therapy, 19,* 183–190.

Seidel, W. F., Ball, S., Cohen, S., Patterson, N., Yost, D., & Dement, W. C. (1984). Daytime alertness in relation to mood, performance, and nocturnal sleep in chronic insomniacs and noncomplaining sleepers. *Sleep, 7,* 230–238.

Seidel, W. F., & Dement, W. C. (1982). Sleepiness in insomnia: Evaluation and treatment. *Sleep, 5* (Suppl. 2), S182–S190.

Shealy, R. C. (1979). The effectiveness of various treatment techniques on different degrees and durations of sleep-onset insomnia. *Behaviour Research and Therapy, 17,* 541–546.

Shealy, R. C., Lowe, J. D., & Ritzler, B. A. (1980). Sleep onset insomnia: Personality characteristics and treatment outcomes. *Journal of Consulting and Clinical Psychology, 48,* 659–661.

Spielman, A. J., & Glovinsky, P. B. (1991). The varied nature of insomnia. In P. J. Hauri (Ed.), *Case studies in insomnia* (pp. 1–15). New York: Plenum Press.

Spielman, A. J., Saskin, P., & Thorpy, M. J. (1987). Treatment of chronic insomnia by restriction of time in bed. *Sleep, 10,* 45–56.

Stepanski, E., Koshorek, G., Zorick, F., Glinn, M., Roehrs, T., & Roth, T. (1989). Characteristics of individuals who do or do not seek treatment for chronic insomnia. *Psychosomatics, 30,* 421–427.

Stepanski, E., Zorick, F., Peters, M., & Roth, T. (1990). Effects of sleep deprivation on alertness in chronic insomnia. *Sleep Research, 19,* 297.

Stepanski, E., Zorick, F., Roehrs, T., Young, D., & Roth, T. (1988). Daytime alertness in patients with chronic insomnia compared with asymptomatic control subjects. *Sleep, 11,* 54–60.

Sugerman, J. L., Stern, J. A., & Walsh, J. K. (1985). Daytime alertness in subjective and objective insomnia: Some preliminary findings. *Biological Psychiatry, 20,* 741–750.

Turner, R. M. (1986). Behavioral self-control procedures for disorders of initiating and maintaining sleep (DIMS). *Clinical Psychology Review, 6,* 27–38.

Turner, R. M., & Ascher, L. M. (1982). Therapist factor in the treatment of insomnia. *Behaviour Research and Therapy, 20,* 33–40.

VanderPlate, C., & Eno, E. N. (1983). Electromyograph biofeedback and sleep onset insomnia: Comparison of treatment and placebo. *Behavioral Engineering, 8,* 146–153.

Van Egeren, L., Haynes, S. N., Franzen, M., & Hamilton, J. (1983). Presleep cognitions and attributions in sleep-onset insomnia. *Journal of Behavioral Medicine, 6,* 217–232.

Vollrath, M., Wicki, W., & Angst, J. (1989). The Zurich study. VIII. Insomnia: Association with depression, anxiety, somatic syndromes, and course of insomnia. *European Archives of Psychiatry and Neurological Sciences, 239,* 113–124.

Welstein, L., Dement, W. C., Redington, D., Guilleminault, C., & Mitler, M. M. (1983). Insomnia in the San Francisco Bay Area: A telephone survey. In C. Guilleminault & E. Lugaresi (Eds.), *Sleep/wake disorders: Natural history, epidemiology, and long-term evolution* (pp. 73–85). New York: Raven Press.

Woolfolk, R. L., & McNulty, T. F. (1983). Relaxation treatment for insomnia: A component analysis. *Journal of Consulting and Clinical Psychology, 51,* 495–503.

Zammit, G. K. (1988). Subjective ratings of the characteristics and sequelae of good and poor sleep in normals. *Journal of Clinical Psychology, 44,* 123–130.

Zwart, C. A., & Lisman, S. A. (1979). An analysis of stimulus control treatment of sleep-onset insomnia. *Journal of Consulting and Clinical Psychology, 47,* 113–118.

6

Raynaud's Disease and Phenomenon

Robert R. Freedman

INTRODUCTION

The primary symptom of Raynaud's phenomenon is episodic digital vasospasms provoked by exposure to cold and/or emotional stress (Freedman & Ianni, 1983a). Attacks generally last for several minutes and consist of blanching followed by cyanosis and rubor. The disorder is four times more common in women than in men and has an estimated prevalence of 4.3% in the United States (Weinrich, Marieg, Keil, McGregor, & Diat, 1990). The term *Raynaud's disease* denotes the primary form of the disorder in which symptoms are not the result of an identifiable disease process, such as scleroderma or other collagen vascular diseases. When the symptoms occur secondarily to another disease, we use the term *Raynaud's phenomenon*.

PHYSIOLOGICAL CONTROL OF FINGER BLOOD FLOW

We can best understood the pathophysiology of Raynaud's disease in context of physiological mechanisms controlling finger blood flow. Digital vasculature is almost entirely cutaneous and plays a fundamental role in regulation of body temperature. The palmar surfaces and tips of fingers are rich in arteriovenous anastomoses (or shunts) that function in parallel with capillary beds. These shunts have capacities that enable them to rapidly vary their lumen sizes and rates of blood flow in response to changes in external temperature. They accomplish this mainly through

---

Robert R. Freedman • Department of Psychiatry and Behavioral Medicine, Wayne State University School of Medicine, and C. S. Mott Center, 275 East Hancock, Detroit, Michigan 48201.
Handbook of Health and Rehabilitation Psychology, edited by Anthony J. Goreczny. Plenum Press, New York, 1995.

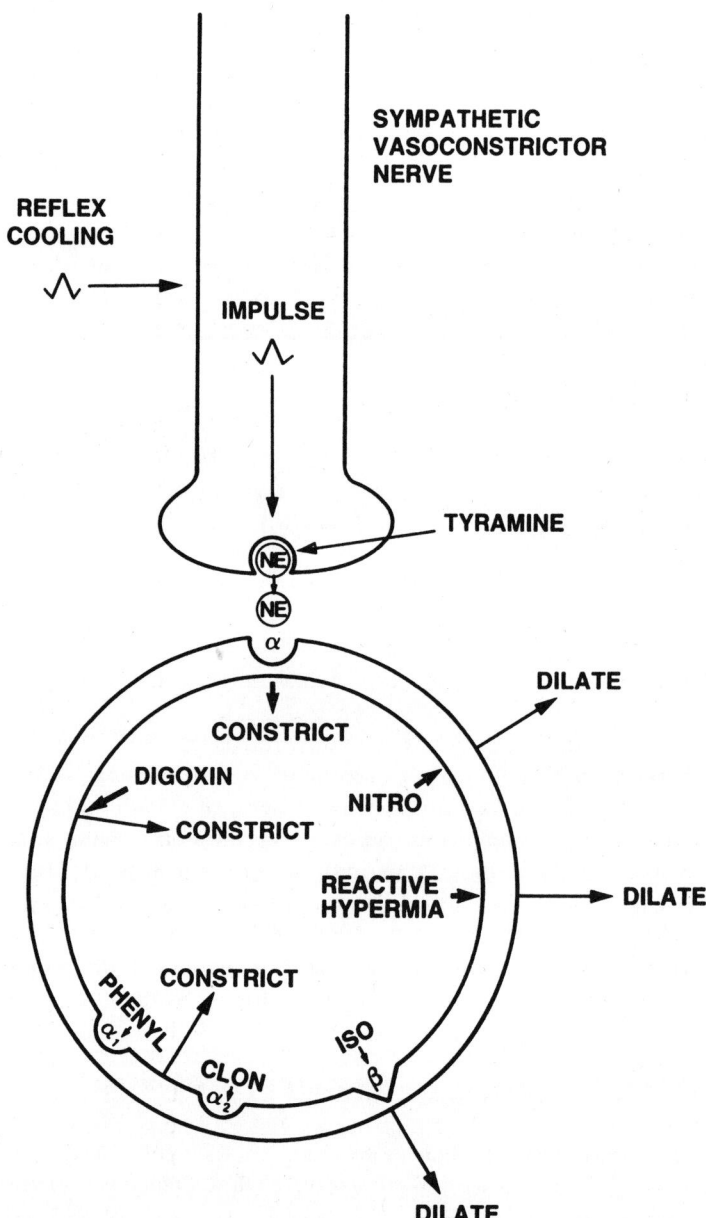

Figure 6.1. Control of digital blood flow. Reflexive cooling causes digital vasoconstriction through liberation of norepinephrine (NE) from sympathetic nerve endings, which indirect heating can reduce. Injection of tyramine causes vasoconstriction by displacing NE from nerves. Interaction of circulating NE or synthetic agonists, such as phenylephrine (PHENYL) or clonidine (CLON), with α-1- and α-2-adrenergic receptors can also cause vasoconstriction. Synthetic β-adrenergic agonists, such as isoproterenol (ISO), cause vasodilation through interaction with β-receptors. Reactive hyperemia produces vasodilation through accumulation of unknown compounds during ischemia (Freedman, 1989).

sympathetic adrenergic vasoconstrictor nerves (Figure 6.1). Body cooling causes reflex finger vasoconstriction through increased neural activity and, conversely, body heating produces vasodilation through withdrawal of this activity. Sympathetic nervous system (SNS) activity also affects finger capillary blood flow, but to a lesser extent than arteriovenous shunt flow (Coffman, 1972). There are no known vasodilating nerves in human fingers, although such nerves do exist in the skin of forearms (Shepherd, 1963).

Interactions of circulating vasoactive substances with α- and β-adrenergic receptors produce vasoconstriction and vasodilation, respectively, and thereby control finger blood flow. Circulating catecholamines, released from the adrenal medulla and other nerve endings "upstream," act at α-adrenergic receptors to produce vasoconstriction. These α receptors are probably closer to the lumen than those that respond to norepinephrine released from sympathetic nerve endings. α and β receptors consist of subtypes based on their relative sensitivities to different agonists. Researchers have discovered a β-adrenergic vasodilating mechanism in finger by injecting isoproterenol, a synthetic β-adrenergic agonist, in the brachial artery and then blocking this effect with propranolol, a β-adrenergic antagonist (Cohen & Coffman, 1981). However, researchers have not yet found an endogenous ligand that acts at these β receptors.

Sensitivities of vascular adrenergic receptors change according to temperature and represent one means of local control of blood flow (Freedman, Sabharwal, Moten, & Migály, 1992). Other local influences include changes in blood gases and metabolism, myogenic tone, and the axon reflex (Vanhoutte, 1980).

PATHOPHYSIOLOGY

Although scientists do not know the etiology of Raynaud's disease, researchers in the field have advanced two main theories to explain it. Raynaud (1888) felt that increased SNS activity caused an exaggerated vasoconstrictive response to cold, while Lewis (1929) thought that a "local fault" caused small peripheral blood vessels to be hypersensitive to local cooling. Investigations of plasma catecholamine levels in Raynaud's disease patients have generally not supported Raynaud's theory. Studies of plasma epinephrine and norepinephrine in Raynaud's disease patients have found levels that were higher (Peacock, 1959), lower (Surwit & Allen, 1983), or not different (Kontos & Wasserman, 1969) from those of nonaffected individuals! Additionally, microelectrode studies of skin nerve sympathetic activity found no differences between patients with primary Raynaud's disease and control subjects during cold pressor tests or other sympathetic stimuli (Fagius & Blumberg, 1985).

Research conducted in our laboratory has supported the theory of Lewis. We found no differences between patients with primary Raynaud's disease and control subjects in their responses to a variety of sympathetic stimuli, such as reflex cooling, indirect heating, or intra-arterial infusions of tyramine, a compound that causes indirect release of norepinephrine from sympathetic nerve endings (Freedman, Sabharwal, Desai, Wenig, & Mayes, 1989a). In the same investigation, we demonstrated that patients had significantly greater digital vasoconstrictive responses to intra-arterial phenylephrine (an α_1-adrenergic agonist) and clonidine (an α_2-adrenergic agonist) than did normal control subjects. These results suggest that patients with primary Raynaud's disease have increased peripheral vascular α_1- and α_2-adrenergic receptor sensitivity and/or density compared with nonaffected individuals. Several studies of platelet α_2-adrenergic receptors also found increased receptor density in Raynaud's disease patients relative to controls (Edwards, Phinney, Taylor, Keenan, & Porter, 1987; Graafsma et al., 1991; Keenan & Porter, 1983).

In a subsequent study, we produced vasospastic attacks in 9 of 11 patients with primary Raynaud's disease and in 8 of 10 patients with scleroderma (Freedman, Mayes, & Sabharwal, 1989b). The vasospastic attacks, photographed using an automatic camera, received scores by three independent raters. Local injection of lidocaine anesthetized two fingers on one hand, and plethysmography demonstrated effectiveness of the nerve blocks. Frequency of vasospastic attacks in nerve-blocked fingers was not significantly different than in corresponding intact fingers on the contralateral hand. These findings clearly demonstrate that vasospastic attacks of Raynaud's disease and phenomenon can occur without involvement of efferent digital nerves and argue against the etiologic role of sympathetic hyperactivity.

In vitro studies (Flavahan, Lindblad, Verebeuren, Shepherd, & Vanhoutte, 1985; Flavahan & Vanhoutte, 1986; Harker et al., 1990) have shown that cooling modulates contractile responses mediated by α-adrenergic receptors, depending on species and blood vessels involved. We therefore examined effects of cooling on α_1 and α_2 adrenergic responses in Raynaud's disease patients using brachial artery infusions of

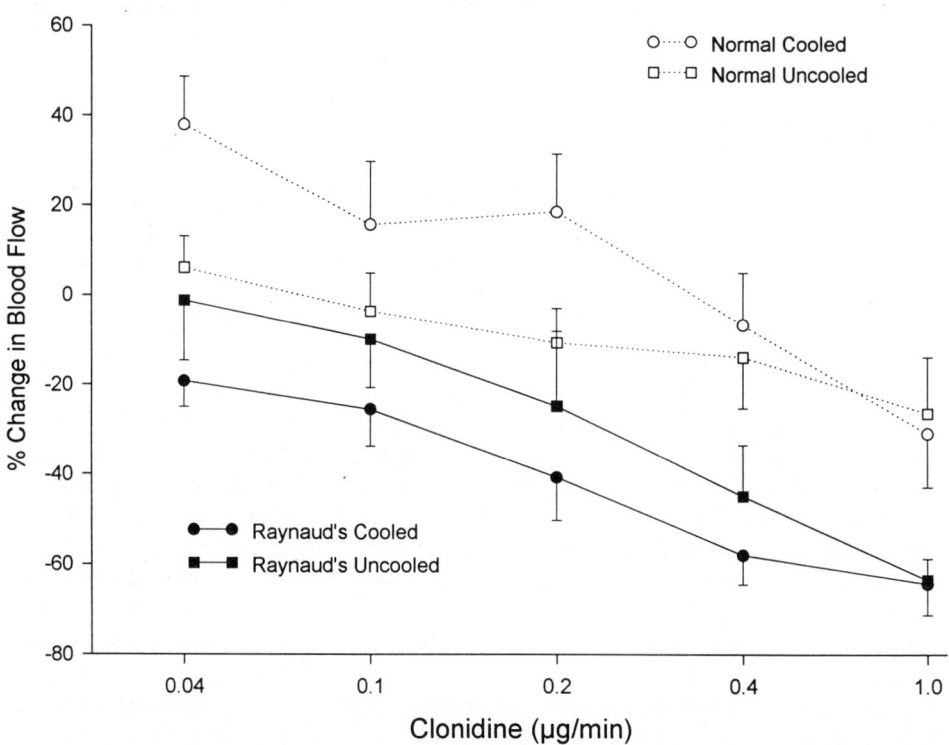

Figure 6.2. Finger blood flow responses to intra-arterial clonidine in cooled and intact fingers in 17 Raynaud's disease patients and 12 normal volunteers (means ± SEM).

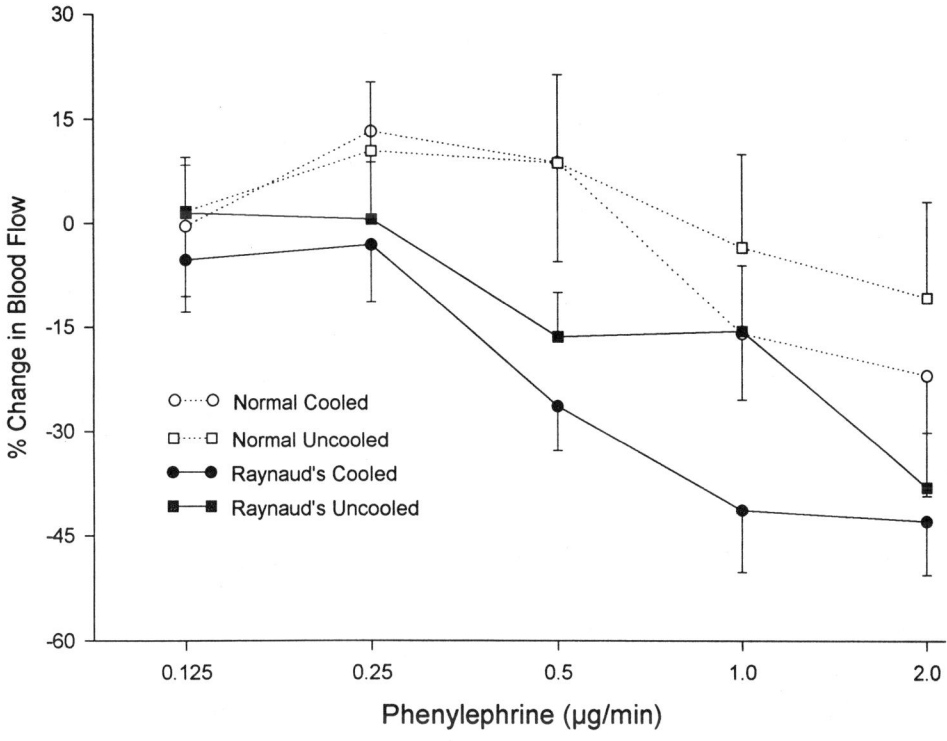

Figure 6.3. Finger blood flow responses to intra-arterial phenylephrine in cooled and intact fingers in 17 Raynaud's disease patients and 12 normal volunteers (means ± SEM).

α_1 and α_2 adrenergic agonists (Freedman, Moten, Migárly, & Mayes, 1992). We studied 17 primary Raynaud's disease patients and 12 female normal volunteers by administering clonidine HCl and phenylephrine HCl through a brachial artery catheter. Venous occlusion plethysmography measured blood flow in cooled and uncooled fingers. Cooling potentiated α_2 adrenergic vasoconstriction in patients ($p < .05$) but depressed this response in controls ($p < .01$); see Figure 6.2. Cooling did not significantly affect vasoconstrictive responses to phenylephrine, but vasoconstrictive responses were significantly greater in both cooled and uncooled fingers of patients than in corresponding fingers of controls ($p < .05$); see Figure 6.3. These results suggest that cold-induced sensitization of peripheral vascular α_2-adrenergic receptors constitutes the "local fault" by which cooling triggers vasospastic attacks of Raynaud's disease. Normal catecholamine elevations acting upon hypersensitive vascular α_1- and α_2-adrenergic receptors explain the phenomenon of attacks induced by emotional distress.

In summary, the most recent evidence strongly suggests that peripheral vascular α_2 adrenoceptors that are hypersensitive to cold locally trigger vasospastic attacks of Raynaud's disease. Moreover, because vascular α_1- and α_2-adrenoceptors are hypersensitive in Raynaud's disease patients in the basal state, normal catecholamine elevations produced by emotional stress or by reflex cooling can also trigger vasospastic attacks.

FAMILIAL AGGREGATION OF IDIOPATHIC RAYNAUD'S DISEASE

Research has demonstrated that α-adrenoceptor function is under considerable genetic control in humans (Propping & Friedl, 1983). As a first step toward identifying a genetic component in idiopathic Raynaud's disease, we sought to determine if this syndrome showed significant familial aggregation. Thirty consecutive patients (26 women, 4 men), classified as having idiopathic Raynaud's disease, served as probands in this investigation. All met the Allen and Brown (1932) criteria for primary Raynaud's, had negative antinuclear tests, and evidenced nail fold capillaries with no evidence of connective tissue disease. We then constructed pedigrees for all probands. First-degree relatives of probands and nonconsanguineous relatives completed questionnaires to determine presence of Raynaud's symptoms and absence of secondary disorders. When possible, relatives underwent medical examinations. The probands had 217 first-degree relatives of whom 46 (17 men, 29 women) received a diagnosis of Raynaud's disease. This represents a prevalence of 21.2% (30.8% if including probands). There were 237 nonconsanguineous relatives who served as controls. Of these, 5 (3 men, 2 women) received diagnoses of Raynaud's disease (2.1%). A chi-square test showed that prevalence of Raynaud's disease was significantly ($p < .0001$) higher among probands' relatives than among nonconsanguineous controls. This finding demonstrates significant familial aggregation of primary Raynaud's disease. Because consanguineous and nonconsanguineous relatives presumably shared similar environments, this aggregation is most likely due to genetic factors.

MEDICAL TREATMENTS FOR RAYNAUD'S DISEASE

Pharmacological treatments for Raynaud's disease have received review elsewhere (Coffman, 1991). Briefly, nifedipine is presently the drug of first choice for patients with primary Raynaud's disease. Nifedipine is a calcium show-channel blocker that reduces influx of calcium into cells, thereby decreasing vasoconstriction. Research has demonstrated that nifedipine decreases frequency, duration, and intensity of vasospastic attacks in about two thirds of primary and secondary Raynaud's patients treated.

Because serotonergic vasoconstriction is also present in human fingers, physicians have used ketanserin, a serotonergic S_2 antagonist, to treat primary and secondary Raynaud's patients. However, a very large double-blind study of primary and secondary Raynaud's patients produced disappointing results (Coffman et al., 1989). Reduction in attack frequency with ketanserin was only 34%, compared with a placebo rate of 18%, and there were no changes in severity or duration of vasospastic attacks. Moreover, there were no changes in finger blood measurements during cold or warm conditions.

Some patients have undergone surgical sympathectomies as a means of abolishing reflex sympathetic activity, but vascular tone generally recovers within a period of a few weeks (Robertson & Smithwick, 1951). Our recent finding that vasospastic attacks can occur in primary and secondary Raynaud's patients despite digital nerve blockade raises serious questions regarding the physiological rationale for sympathectomy.

EFFECTS OF TEMPERATURE BIOFEEDBACK IN NORMAL INDIVIDUALS

Toward the end of developing nonpharmacological treatments for Raynaud's and other disorders, many investigators began to study effects of temperature biofeedback in normal volunteers. The first studies combined effects of various procedures, such as monetary rewards and suggestions of thermal imagery. Taub and Emurian (1976) described an uncontrolled investigation in which they trained subjects to increase and decrease hand temperature using feedback. The authors claimed that subjects usually learned desired responses within four sessions and that average temperature change was approximately 1.2°C.

Two subsequent controlled studies (Surwit, Shapiro, & Feld, 1976) failed to demonstrate significant finger temperature increases using biofeedback and monetary rewards. Although subjects were able to produce significant temperature declines averaging 2.0°C, they were not able to demonstrate significant temperature increases. Increasing the number of training sessions failed to improve performance. The authors hypothesized that a ceiling effect might have accounted for failure to produce significant vasodilation, so they performed a subsequent study in a cooler environment. However, this manipulation failed to improve performance.

Keefe and colleagues have demonstrated significant temperature elevations using finger temperature feedback and other procedures in a series of controlled studies. In the first investigation (Keefe, 1975), subjects received 12 brief training sessions of temperature feedback to either raise or lower their finger temperature relative to that of their forehead. Subjects demonstrated significant finger temperature elevations and declines, averaging +1.0°C and −0.8°C, respectively. Keefe (1978) then studied six groups of 10 subjects each, who were randomly assigned to receive combinations of temperature feedback, thermal suggestions, and response-specific instructions. Subjects given either feedback and response-specific instructions, feedback and thermal suggestions, or no feedback and thermal suggestions were able to produce significant elevations (+0.8–1.1°C) in finger temperature and maintain their responses during follow-up sessions 1 and 2 weeks later. In the final study (Keefe & Gardner, 1979), subjects given brief temperature feedback training sessions again demonstrated significant within-session temperature elevations, but increasing the number of sessions to 20 did not increase magnitude of finger temperature responses.

For effects of finger temperature feedback to be clinically useful, they obviously must be reproducible without use of instruments and outside laboratories. Stoffer, Jensen, and Nesset (1979) trained normal subjects to increase finger temperature using true feedback, false feedback, or no feedback. During a posttraining test of voluntary control without feedback, only the contingent group demonstrated significant finger temperature elevations (+0.4°C). We (Freedman & Ianni, 1983b) then conducted a series of studies to determine if subjects could sustain temperature elevations outside the laboratory and to examine the role of relaxation in temperature biofeedback. In the first experiment, subjects received six 56-minute sessions of finger temperature feedback, frontalis EMG feedback, tape-recorded autogenic training, or simple instructions to increase finger temperature. We tested ability to increase finger temperature without feedback before and after training and outside the laboratory with ambulatory monitoring equipment. Temperature feedback subjects showed significant vasodilation during the first 12 minutes of the first training session only. Other groups showed no vasodilation whatsoever. Subjects as a whole showed significant within-session decreases in frontalis EMG level, respiration rate, and heart rate. During posttraining laboratory voluntary control tests, only the temperature feedback group produced significant finger temperature elevations, but subjects in this group could not sustain this effect when retested outside the laboratory. We concluded that the temperature feedback response was not sufficiently robust to generalize outside the laboratory.

We considered the possibility that excessively lengthy sessions could have impeded effects of training. Kluger and Tursky (1982) also found that feedback-induced vasodilation occurred early in training sessions and then declined. We therefore performed a second study in which we shortened training sessions to 32 minutes each. Subjects then received either 6 or 10 training sessions in finger temperature feedback or instructions to increase finger temperature. In this study, temperature feedback subjects significantly increased finger temperatures during all training sessions ($+0.42°C$), whereas those who received instructions only demonstrated no such effects. Increasing the number of training sessions from 6 to 10 had no effect. Subjects in the instructions-only group demonstrated significant heart rate and muscle tension decreases during training, whereas temperature feedback subjects did not. In this study, temperature feedback subjects showed significant vasodilation during posttraining laboratory voluntary control tests ($+0.56°C$) as well as outside the laboratory with ambulatory monitoring ($+2.4°C$), effects not shown by the instructions-only group. Thus, decreasing the session length resulted in a more robust laboratory training effect and also enhanced generalization of feedback-induced vasodilation to a setting outside the laboratory.

In contrast to finger temperature feedback, researchers have conducted much less work on relaxation methods to produce finger-temperature increases in nonpatient populations. Blizard, Cowings, and Miller (1975) did not find significant vasodilation during six sessions of autogenic training. Boudewyns (1976) did find significant finger-temperature elevations during brief tape recorded relaxation instructions.

Thus, nonpatient populations can achieve significant peripheral vasodilation using finger temperature feedback training, although there is less evidence that relaxation procedures can produce this effect. Subjects trained in finger temperature feedback can retain this response over time and reproduce it without feedback as well as outside laboratories. Interestingly, feedback-induced vasodilation appears early in training and does not seem to increase over extended training sessions. Indeed, studies utilizing brief training periods (Freedman & Ianni, 1983b; Keefe, 1978; Keefe & Gardner, 1979; Kluger & Tursky, 1982; Stoffer et al., 1979) find training effects superior to those of investigations utilizing longer training periods (Freedman & Ianni, 1983b; Surwit, 1977; Surwit, Shapiro, & Feld, 1976).

Physiological relaxation, as indicated by declines in heart rate, respiration rate, muscle tension, or skin conductance level, does not seem to be necessary for feedback-induced vasodilation. Work discussed later in this chapter shows than an active β-adrenergic vasodilating mechanism is involved in feedback-induced vasodilation and does not operate through the efferent sympathetic nervous pathway.

BEHAVIORAL TREATMENT OF RAYNAUD'S DISEASE

Despite evidence that peripheral vascular α-adrenergic responsiveness is high among patients with Raynaud's disease, it has not yet been possible to design pharmacological agents that specifically target digital blood vessels. Thus, side effects, such as hypotension, headaches, and flushing, have limited the usefulness of some drugs. In contrast, behavioral treatments for Raynaud's disease have been very promising and appear to have no adverse effects.

Behavioral treatments for Raynaud's disease have endeavored to increase finger temperature and/or blood flow and ameliorate symptoms through relaxation procedures, such as autogenic training (Surwit, Pilon, & Fenton, 1978), or through finger temperature biofeedback (Freedman & Ianni, 1983b; Freedman, Sabharwal, Ianni, Desai, Wenig, & Mayes, 1988). In the first controlled study (Surwit, Pilon, & Fenton, 1978), the investigators randomly assigned patients to receive either autogenic training (self-suggestion of warm imagery) alone or in combination with temperature feedback. In addition, for a 1-month period, half the subjects served as a waiting-list control group for the other half; after 1 month, control subjects then received treatment. Subjects as a whole showed improvement on a cold stress test and reported decreased attack frequencies (10%–32%), but there were no group differences on these measures. A subsequent study (Keefe, Surwit, & Pilon, 1980) comparing progressive relaxation, autogenic training, or a combination of both also found no differences between treatment groups.

Because prior investigations utilized various combinations of behavioral procedures, we conducted a study (Freedman, Ianni, & Wenig, 1983) in which we compared effects of temperature feedback alone with those of autogenic training or frontalis EMG feedback. We also studied a fourth procedure in which subjects received temperature feedback during mild cold stress to the finger. We hypothesized that this procedure would enhance generalization of the feedback response to the natural environment, where patients must produce the response under cold conditions. Patients who received temperature feedback alone or under cold stress showed significant elevations in finger temperature and significant declines in reported symptom frequency the following winter (66.8% and 92.5%, respectively). Those who received EMG feedback or autogenic training showed neither significant vasodilation nor symptomatic improvement, but did demonstrate declines in muscle tension, heart rate, and reported stress levels. Patients in the temperature feedback groups did not show declines in the latter three measures, but did maintain symptomatic improvement at 2- and 3-year follow-up periods (Freedman, Ianni, & Wenig, 1985). Thus, effects of finger temperature biofeedback are physiologically different from those of autogenic training, frontalis EMG feedback, or simple instructions to increase finger temperature. Temperature feedback produces digital vasodilation without bradycardia or decreased muscle tension, whereas the other techniques produced bradycardia and lower EMG levels but did not increase finger temperature. Research has uncovered a β-adrenergic mechanism that may explain increased digital blood flow in absence of decreased generalized physiological arousal (Cohen & Coffman, 1981). We therefore tested involvement of this mechanism during temperature feedback in Raynaud's disease patients and nonpatient controls by local β-blockade of vasodilation with intra-arterial infusions of propranolol (Freedman et al., 1988). We first randomly assigned 18 patients with idiopathic Raynaud's disease and 16 control subjects to receive 10 sessions of temperature feedback or autogenic training. Following training, in a separate session, we placed a catheter in the right brachial artery using local anesthetic and connected the catheter to two infusion pumps, one containing 0.9% saline solution and the other containing propranolol. The experimenter remotely controlled the pumps, housed in a sound-proofed box, from a polygraph in a separate room. Venous occlusion plethysmography assessed finger blood flow in both hands. After baseline recordings, the experimenter activated temperature-feedback signals or the autogenic tape. After 6 minutes, the experimenter switched the infusion from saline to propranolol (0.5 mg/min.) for 2 minutes, then saline for 4 minutes, propranolol (same dose) for 2 minutes, and saline for 4 minutes. These changes occurred without the subjects' knowledge. Significant bilateral vasodilation occurred in temperature feedback subjects, and propranolol significantly reduced vasodilation in infused, but not control hands. Magnitudes of these effects were not significantly different in Raynaud's disease and control subjects. There were no significant blood flow changes at all in patients or control subjects who received autogenic training. There were no significant heart rate or blood pressure changes in the temperature feedback group; the autogenic group showed a significant decline in heart rate during autogenic instructions. Thus, feedback-induced vasodilation involves a β-adrenergic mechanism. Raynaud's patients who received temperature feedback showed significant increases in finger temperature and capillary blood flow and significant declines in attack frequency (mean = 81%), which subjects maintained at 1- and 2-year follow-ups.

The only known efferent vasomotor nerves in human fingers are adrenergic (Figure 6.1); neurogenic vasoconstriction results from interaction of released norepinephrine with postjunctional α-adrenergic receptors. Our finding of a β-adrenergic mechanism in temperature biofeedback thus raised the question of whether neural mechanisms mediate feedback-induced vasodilation. Because it is possible to block digital nerves by local injection of an anesthetic, a method was available to test this hypothesis. Because digital nerve blockade raises finger blood flow to near ceiling levels, we reduced it to midrange by infusing norepinephrine (NE; 0.25 μg/min) in the right brachial artery. To control for all manipulations, we measured blood flow in three fingers; right, nerve-blocked + NE; right, no block + NE; left, no block, no NE. We then repeated the propranolol infusion of the previous study (Figure 6.4). In two separate studies of normal subjects ($N = 8, N = 9$) and a subsequent study with Raynaud's disease patients ($N = 10$), we found that neither nerve-blockade nor norepinephrine attenuated vasodilation produced by temperature feedback, but propranolol did reduce vasodilation. Thus, digital nerves do not appear to mediate the β-adrenergic vasodilating mechanism of temperature feedback.

To further examine possible changes in SNS activity during temperature feed-

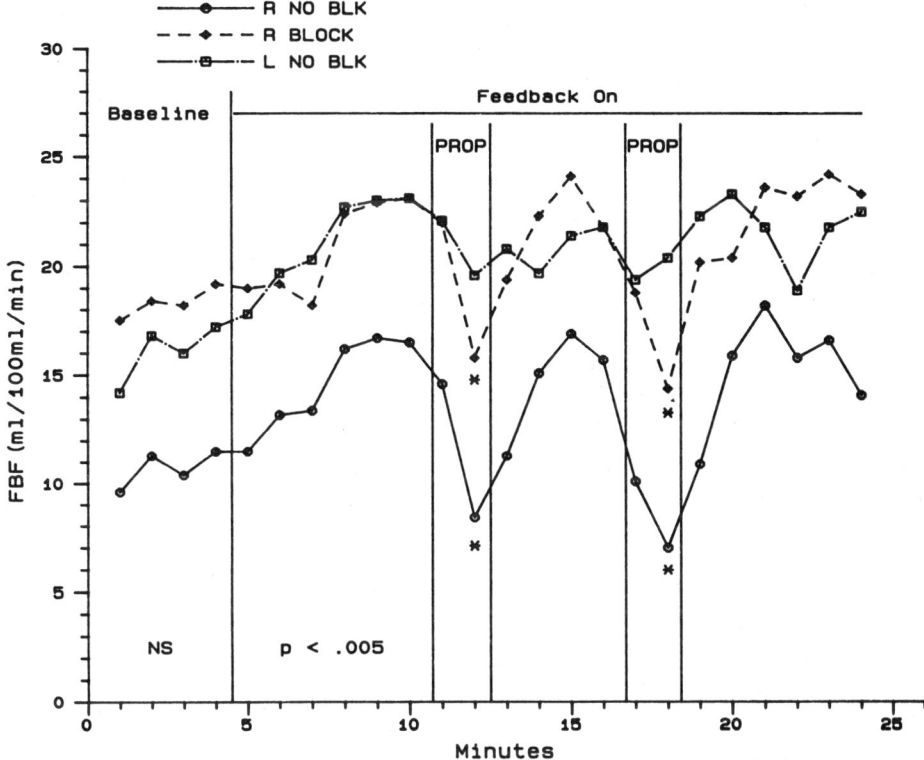

Figure 6.4. Blood flow (FBF) in three fingers during last 4 minutes of baseline period and subsequent temperature feedback period. Nerves in right second finger (R block) received anesthetic. During baseline period, FBF did not significantly change (NS). When feedback began, FBF in all three fingers increased significantly ($p < .005$). Propranolol (PROP) infused in right brachial artery (.5 mg for 2 min.) caused significant ($p < .01$) reduction in FBF in infused hand (*) but not left hand (Freedman, Sabharwal, Ianni, Desai, Wenig, & Mayes, 1988).

back and autogenic training, we recently measured plasma levels of epinephrine (E) and NE during these procedures (Freedman, Keegan, Migály, Galloway, & Mayes, 1991). An IV needle was inserted into a vein on the back of the hand and connected via nonthrombogenic tubing to a Cormed blood withdrawal pump located in an adjacent room so that subjects could not observe collection of blood. We subsequently analyzed plasma levels of E and NE by the HPLC-EC method. Thirty-one randomly assigned patients with idiopathic Raynaud's disease received eight 32-minute sessions of either finger temperature feedback ($N = 16$) or autogenic training ($N = 15$) over 28 days. Sessions 1 and 8 involved continuous blood draws. During training, feedback patients evidenced significant temperature and blood flow elevations ($p < .001$) but autogenic patients did not show such changes. There were no significant effects for NE and E for either group.

This investigation provides no evidence that SNS activation, as reflected by measures of plasma catecholamines, is lower during behavioral treatments for primary Raynaud's disease. These results are consistent with previous findings that catecholamine levels are not consistently high in Raynaud's patients (Kontos & Wasserman, 1969; Surwit & Allen, 1983), vasospastic attacks can occur during sympathetic nerve blockade (Freedman, Mayes, & Sabharwal, 1989a), and sensitization of peripheral vascular α-adrenergic receptors is involved (Freedman et al., 1989b). Furthermore, our findings are consistent with recent evidence that a nonneural, β-adrenergic mechanism mediates, at least in part, feedback-induced vasodilation (Freedman et al., 1988). Future research needs to attempt identification of the ligand responsible for this vasodilation and its precise mechanism of action.

SECONDARY RAYNAUD'S PHENOMENON

Behavioral and medical treatments for Raynaud's phenomenon have been less successful than those for the primary form of the disorder. In case studies (Freedman, Lynn, Ianni, & Hale, 1981), we showed that scleroderma patients treated with finger temperature feedback were able to increase digital temperature and show some symptomatic improvement. However, a subsequent controlled investigation produced disappointing results (Freedman, Ianni, & Wenig, 1984). Twenty-four randomly assigned patients meeting the American Rheumatism Association (now the American College of Rheumatology) classification criteria for systemic sclerosis (Freedman, Ianni, & Wenig, 1983) received 10 sessions of training in finger temperature feedback, EMG feedback, or autogenic training using the procedures of our previous study. Subjects receiving finger temperature feedback showed significant increases in finger temperature during training and during a posttraining voluntary control test, whereas those receiving EMG feedback or autogenic training did not. Following treatment, however, no group showed significant reductions in frequency of reported vasospastic attacks. There were no group differences in data obtained during ambulatory monitoring or laboratory cold stress tests. Reasons for failure of temperature feedback to reduce symptoms in scleroderma patients are not apparent. However, it is likely that underlying pathophysiology of secondary Raynaud's phenomenon is different from that of the primary disease.

Scientists have performed fewer pharmacological studies on secondary than on primary Raynaud's patients. Several small-scale studies (Belch et al., 1983) reported positive results of prostaglandin I2 and E1 infusions on secondary Raynaud's patients. However, it was necessary to administer compounds by intravenous infusion. Most studies of nifedipine on Raynaud's disease also included secondary patients. Although results were generally positive, it was not always possible to distinguish between primary and secondary patients in some published reports.

CONCLUSIONS

Research on pathophysiology of Raynaud's disease now shows that vasospastic attacks do not result from SNS hyperactivity, but probably from hypersensitivity of peripheral vascular α_2-adrenergic receptors to cooling. Additionally, peripheral vascular α_1-adrenoceptors are hypersensitive in Raynaud's disease patients in the basal state. Thus, normal catecholamine elevations produced by emotional stress or by reflex cooling can also trigger vasospastic attacks. We recently found significant familial aggregation of Raynaud's disease, suggesting a genetic basis for this disorder. Pathophysiology of secondary Raynaud's phenomenon remains poorly understood.

The most efficacious treatment for primary Raynaud's disease now appears to be temperature biofeedback without addition of other treatments. Several controlled group-outcome studies have shown that primary Raynaud's patients given temperature biofeedback alone achieved reported symptom frequency reductions ranging from 67% to 92%, which patients maintained at 2- and 3-year follow-ups. Addition of other procedures, such as autogenic training or progressive relaxation, to temperature biofeedback produced less satisfactory results, as did the use of progressive relaxation and autogenic training alone. These results are superior to those of most pharmacological studies and do not have concomitant difficulties of side effects. Our finding that attacks can occur even during digital nerve blockade seriously challenges the use of sympatholytic drugs and surgical sympathectomies.

During investigations on mechanisms of temperature biofeedback, we showed that feedback-induced vasodilation does not result from reductions in SNS activation. Early studies in our laboratory did not find expected reductions in heart rate, skin conductance level, or reported arousal in Raynaud's patients or normal subjects given temperature feedback. We subsequently demonstrated that sympathetic nerves do not mediate feedback-induced vasodilation, but, rather, a β-adrenergic mechanism appears responsible for vasodilation. Consistent with these findings, we most recently found that plasma levels of norepinephrine and epinephrine do not significantly change during temperature feedback or autogenic training in Raynaud's disease patients.

Research on etiology and treatment of Raynaud's phenomenon has been less successful than work on the primary form of the disorder. Due to difficulty performing invasive procedures in patients with secondary Raynaud's phenomenon, researchers have little knowledge regarding pathophysiology of vasospastic attacks in such patients. However, histological studies have shown luminal narrowing due to intimal proliferation of connective tissue, thickening of basement membranes, and fibrosis of adventitia in these patients (Rodnan, 1979). *In vivo* observation of skin capillaries reveals consistent abnormalities in secondary patients (Maricq et al., 1980) and very low levels of finger capillary blood flow (Coffman & Cohen, 1971). In light of these findings, it may be difficult to achieve consistent vasodilation in secondary Raynaud's patients, although clinical researchers must conduct further research on this problem.

In conclusion, knowledge of pathophysiology of Raynaud's disease has advanced considerably in the last decade. Numerous studies have shown temperature biofeedback is an efficacious treatment for this disorder and delineated some aspects of its mechanism. Nonetheless, investigators must conduct further research in this area and on the less understood problems of Raynaud's phenomenon.

ACKNOWLEDGMENT

Research conducted by the author was supported by grants HL-23828 and HL-30604 from the NIH.

REFERENCES

Allen, E., & Brown, G. (1932). A critical review of minimal requisites for diagnosis. *American Journal of Medical Science, 183,* 187–195.

Belch, J.J.F., Newman, P., Drury, J. K., McKenzie, F., Capell, H., Leiberman, P., Forbes, C. D., & Prentice, C.R.M. (1983). Intermittent epoprostenol (prostacyclin) infusion in patients with Raynaud's syndrome. *Lancet,* 313–315.

Blizard, D. A., Cowings, P., & Miller, N. E. (1975). Visceral responses to opposite types of autogenic-training imagery. *Biological Psychology, 3,* 49–55.

Boudewyns, P. (1976). A comparison of the effects of stress vs. relaxation instruction on the finger temperature response. *Behavior Therapy, 7,* 54–67.

Coffman, J. D. (1972). Total and nutritional blood flow in the finger. *Clinical Science, 42,* 243–250.

Coffman, J. D. (1979). Vasodilator drugs in peripheral vascular disease. *New England Journal of Medicine, 300,* 713–717.

Coffman, J. D. (1991). Raynaud's phenomenon. *Hypertension, 17,* 593–602.

Coffman, J. D., Clement, D. L., Creager, M. A., Dormady, J. A., Janssens, M.M.-L., McKedry, R.J.R., Murray, G. D., & Nielsen, S. L. (1989). International study of ketanserin in Raynaud's phenomenon. *American Journal of Medicine, 87,* 264–268.

Coffman, J. D., & Cohen, A. S. (1971). Total and capillary fingertip blood flow in Raynaud's phenomenon. *New England Journal of Medicine, 285,* 259–263.

Cohen, R., & Coffman, J. (1981). Beta-adrenergic vasodilator mechanism in the finger. *Circulation Research, 49,* 1196–1201.

Edwards, J. M., Phinney, E. S., Taylor, L. M., Keenan, E. J., & Porter, J. M. (1987). α_2-adrenoceptor levels in obstructive and spastic Raynaud's syndrome. *Vascular Surgery, 5,* 38–45.

Fagius, J., & Blumberg, H. (1985). Sympathetic outflow to the hand in patients with Raynaud's phenomenon. *Cardiovascular Research, 19,* 249–253.

Flavahan, N. A., Lindblad, L. E., Verebeuren, T. J., Shepherd, J. T., & Vanhoutte, P. M. (1985). Cooling and α_1- and α_2-adrenergic responses in cutaneous veins: Role of receptor reserve. *American Journal of Physiology, 249,* H950–H955. (*Heart Circ Physiol, 18*)

Flavahan, N. A., & Vanhoutte, P. M. (1986). Effect of cooling on alpha$_1$- and alpha$_2$-adrenergic responses in canine saphenous and femoral veins. *Journal of Pharmacology and Experimental Therapeutics, 239,* 139–147.

Freedman, R. R. (1989). Raynaud's disease. In G. Turpin (Ed.), *Handbook of clinical psychophysiology* (pp. 469–494). London: Wiley.

Freedman, R. R., & Ianni, P. (1983a). Role of cold and emotional stress in Raynaud's disease and scleroderma. *British Medical Journal, 287,* 1499–1502.

Freedman, R. R., & Ianni, P. (1983b). Self-control of digital temperature: Physiological factors and transfer effects. *Psychophysiology, 20,* 682–688.

Freedman, R. R., Ianni, P., & Wenig, P. (1983). Behavioral treatment of Raynaud's disease. *Journal of Consulting and Clinical Psychology, 151,* 539–549.

Freedman, R. R., Ianni, P., & Wenig, P. (1984). Behavioral treatment of Raynaud's phenomenon in scleroderma. *Journal of Behavioral Medicine, 7,* 343–353.

Freedman, R. R., Ianni, P., & Wenig, P. (1985). Behavioral treatment of Raynaud's disease: Long-term follow-up. *Journal of Consulting and Clinical Psychology, 53,* 136.

Freedman, R. R., Keegan, D., Migály, P., Galloway, M. P., & Mayes, M. (1991). Plasma catecholamines during behavioral treatments for Raynaud's disease. *Psychosomatic Medicine, 53,* 433–439.

Freedman, R. R., Lynn, S., Ianni, P., & Hale, P. (1981). Biofeedback treatment of Raynaud's disease and phenomenon. *Biofeedback and Self-Regulation, 6,* 355–365.

Freedman, R. R., Mayes, M. D., & Sabharwal, S. C. (1989a). Induction of vasospastic attacks despite digital nerve block in Raynaud's disease and phenomenon. *Circulation, 80,* 859–862.

Freedman, R. R., Mayes, M., & Sabharwal, S. (1989b). Digital nerve blockade in Raynaud's disease. *Circulation, 80,* 1923–1924.

Freedman, R. R., Moten, M., Migály, P., & Mayes, M. (1993). Cold-induced potentiation of α_2-adrenergic vasoconstriction in idiopathic Raynaud's disease. *Arthritis and Rheumatism, 36,* 685–689.

Freedman, R. R., Sabharwal, S. C., Desai, N., Wenig, P., & Mayes, M. (1989a). Increased α-adrenergic responsiveness in idiopathic Raynaud's disease. *Arthritis and Rheumatism, 32,* 61–65.

Freedman, R. R., Sabharwal, S. C., Ianni, P., Desai, N., Wenig, P., & Mayes, M. (1988). Nonneural beta-adrenergic vasodilating mechanism in temperature biofeedback. *Psychosomatic Medicine, 50,* 394–401.

Freedman, R. R., Sabharwal, S. C., Moten, M., & Migály, P. (1992). Local temperature modulates α_1- and α_2-adrenergic vasoconstriction in man. *American Journal of Physiology: Heart and Circulatory Physiology, 263,* H1197–H1200.

Graafsma, S. J., Wollersheim, H., Droste, H. T., ten Dam, M.A.G.J., van Tits, L.J.H., Reyenga, J., de Miranda, J.F.R., & Thien, T. (1991). Adrenoceptors on blood cells from patients with primary Raynaud's phenomenon. *Clinical Science, 80,* 325–331.

Harker, C.T.P., Ousley, E. J., Harris, J., Edwards, M., Taylor, L. M., & Porter, J. M. (1990). The effects of cooling on human saphenous vein reactivity to adrenergic agonists. *Journal of Vascular Surgery, 12,* 45–49.

Keefe, F. (1975). Conditioning changes in differential skin temperature. *Perceptual and Motor Skills, 40,* 283–288.

Keefe, F. (1978). Biofeedback vs. instructional control of skin temperature. *Journal of Behavioral Medicine, 1,* 323–335.

Keefe, F., & Gardner, E. (1979). Learned control of skin temperature: Effects of short and long-term biofeedback training. *Behavior Therapy, 10,* 202–210.

Keefe, F., Surwit, R., & Pilon, R. (1980). Biofeedback, autogenic training, and progressive relaxation in the treatment of Raynaud's disease: A comparative study. *Journal of Applied Behavior Analysis, 13,* 3–11.

Keenan, E. J., & Porter, J. M. (1983). α_2-adrenergic receptors in platelets from patients with Raynaud's syndrome. *Surgery, 94,* 204–209.

Kluger, M., & Tursky, B. (1982). A strategy for improving finger temperature biofeedback training. *Psychophysiology, 19,* 329 (Abstract).

Kontos, H. A., & Wasserman, A. J. (1969). Effect of reserpine in Raynaud's phenomenon. *Circulation, 39,* 259–266.

Lewis, T. (1929). Experiments relating to the peripheral mechanism involved in spasmodic arrest of circulation in the fingers, a variety of Raynaud's disease. *Heart, 15,* 7–101.

Maricq, H., LeRoy, E., D'Angelo, W., Medsger, T., Rodnan, G., Sharp, G., & Wolfe, J. (1980). Diagnostic potential of *in vivo* capillary microscopy in scleroderma and related disorders. *Arthritis and Rheumatism, 23,* 183–189.

Peacock, J. H. (1959). Peripheral venous blood concentration of epinephrine and norepinephrine in primary Raynaud's disease. *Circulation Research, 7,* 821–827.

Propping, P., & Friedl, W. (1983). Genetic control of adrenergic receptors on human platelets: A twin study. *Human Genetics, 64,* 105–109.

Raynaud, M. (1888). *New research on the nature and treatment of local asphyxia of the extremities* (T. Barlow, Trans.). London: New Syndenham Society.

Robertson, C., & Smithwick, R. (1951). The recurrence of vasoconstrictor activity after limb sympathectomy in Raynaud's disease and allied vasomotor states. *New England Journal of Medicine, 245,* 317–320.

Rodnan, G. (1979). Progressive systemic sclerosis (scleroderma). In D. McCarty (Ed.), *Arthritis and allied conditions* (pp. 762–810). Philadelphia: Lea & Febinger.

Shepherd, J. T. (1963). *Physiology of the circulation in human limbs in health and disease.* Philadelphia, Saunders.

Stoffer, G. R., Jensen, J.A.S., & Nesset, B. L. (1979). Effects of contingent versus yoked temperature feedback on voluntary temperature control and cold stress tolerance. *Biofeedback and Self-Regulation, 4,* 51–61.

Surwit, R. (1977). Simple versus complex feedback displays in the training of digital temperature. *Journal of Consulting and Clinical Psychology, 45,* 146–147.

Surwit, R. S., & Allen, L. M. (1983). Neuroendocrine response to cold in Raynaud's syndrome. *Life Science, 32,* 995–1000.

Surwit, R., Pilon, R., & Fenton, C. (1978). Behavioral treatment of Raynaud's disease. *Journal of Behavioral Medicine, 1,* 323–335.

Surwit, R. S., Shapiro, D., & Feld, J. L. (1976). Digital temperature autoregulation and associated cardiovascular changes. *Psychophysiology, 13,* 242–248.

Taub, E., & Emurian, C. S. (1976). Feedback-aided self-regulation of skin temperature with a single feedback locus. *Biofeedback and Self-Regulation, 1,* 147–168.

Vanhoutte, P. M. (1980). Physical factors of regulation. In D. Bohr, A. Somylo, & H. Sparks (Eds.), *Handbook of physiology* (Vol. 2). Baltimore: American Physiological Society.

Weinrich, M. C., Maricq, H. R., Keil, J. E., McGregor, A. R., & Diat, F. (1990). Prevalence of Raynaud's phenomenon in the adult population of South Carolina. *Journal of Clinical Epidemiology, 43,* 1343–1349.

II
HEALTH PROMOTION

7

Smoking and Smoking Cessation
Current Conceptualizations and Directions for Future Research

Margaret DeBon and Robert C. Klesges

Cigarette smoking is the number one preventable cause of death in the United States. Smoking is a major contributor to risk of heart disease, malignant neoplasms, and stroke, the three leading causes of death in the United States (U.S. Department of Health and Human Services, 1987). Recent estimates indicate that smoking accounts for at least 400 thousand premature deaths each year and causally relates to 170 thousand deaths from cardiovascular disease, 130 thousand deaths from cancer, and 50 thousand deaths from chronic obstructive pulmonary disease (U.S. Department of Health and Human Services, 1988; U.S. Department of Health, Education, and Welfare, 1979). Of most recent concern is the effect of passive smoking, which may account for up to 53 thousand nonsmoker deaths per year (U.S. Department of Health and Human Services, 1986).

Despite these figures and knowledge of health consequences of cigarette smoking, at least 53 million Americans continue to smoke and approximately 1 million (3 thousand teenagers a day) start smoking annually (Pierce, Fiore, Novotny, Hatziandrea, & Davis, 1989; U.S. Department of Health and Human Services, 1990). Given current trends in smoking and their impact at both the individual and national level, the focus of this review is fourfold. First, we present a discussion of the reasons why people continue to smoke. Next, we discuss the most widely used pharmacological and behavioral treatments for smoking cessation along with strengths and weak

---

Margaret DeBon and Robert C. Klesges • The Universities Prevention Center, Department of Psychology, University of Memphis, Memphis, Tennessee 38152.
Handbook of Health and Rehabilitation Psychology, edited by Anthony J. Goreczny. Plenum Press, New York, 1995.

nesses of each approach. Third, we discuss the latest strategies for relapse prevention. Finally, we address smoking and related issues in one group at high risk for smoking, namely women.

THEORETICAL MODELS OF CONTINUED SMOKING

People continue to smoke for a variety of individual (e.g., reinforcers of smoking) and social reasons (Shiffman & Jarvick, 1987; U.S. Department of Health and Human Services, 1988). Media also reinforce decisions to smoke, despite the ban of cigarette advertisements on television in the United States (Davis, 1987; Flay, 1987; Tye, Warner, & Glantz, 1987). Moreover, people continue to smoke because there are both powerful behavioral and biological factors associated with smoking as well as strong negative consequences to smoking cessation (Klesges, Benowitz, & Meyers, 1991; Lichtenstein & Brown, 1980; U.S. Department of Health and Human Services, 1988).

BEHAVIORAL MODELS OF CONTINUED SMOKING

The primary behavioral reason for sustained smoking is that smoking is possible under a wide variety of circumstances and settings (Lichtenstein & Brown, 1980). As such, smokers learn to associate smoking with many daily activities (e.g., drinking, driving, talking on the telephone, work breaks, and socializing). Another behavioral factor associated with continued smoking is that advantages of continued smoking are immediate and adverse consequences of smoking are remote and probabilistic. The consequences of smoking cessation are acute and usually quite negative (Klesges et al., 1991). A third behavioral component to continued smoking is sheer strength of the smoking habit due to practice effects (U.S. Department of Health and Human Services, 1990). If the average smoker smokes one pack of cigarettes a day, they are lighting up and smoking approximately 7,300 times a year (Klesges et al., 1991). Finally, weight control is another reason for continued smoking. As we discuss in more detail later, weight control is a major factor in continuation of smoking as well as a possible factor in smoking relapse (Klesges et al., 1991).

BIOLOGICAL MODELS OF CONTINUED SMOKING

The most compelling biological factor in sustained cigarette smoking is that nicotine is a highly addictive drug. It enhances release of neurotransmitters that produce behavioral arousal and activate the sympathetic nervous system (Klesges et al., 1991; U.S. Department of Health and Human Services, 1988). Other biological factors associated with continued smoking are the reported increases in concentration and problem-solving abilities, improvement in selective attention and reaction time, and mood-lifting effect of nicotine (U.S. Department of Health and Human Services, 1988). In addition, smokers develop a substantial tolerance to arousal effects of continued smoking (Benowitz, Porchet, & Jacob, 1989) and experience withdrawal symptoms when they discontinue nicotine use. Furthermore, smokers tend to maintain idiosyncratic blood levels of nicotine from day to day that provide optimal personal comfort (Benowitz, 1988), and they tend to compensate for reduced number of cigarettes and increased elimination of nicotine (Benowitz & Jacob, 1985; Benowitz, Jacob, Kozlowski, & Yu, 1986) by either increasing number of cigarettes smoked or by altering smoking topography (e.g., inhaling deeper, increased puff duration). Taken together, there is no other substance that has the combination of addictive and repetitive/reinforcement qualities of nicotine.

SOCIAL MODELS OF CONTINUED SMOKING

Although society's tolerance for smoking is becoming progressively more negative (e.g., social and legal restrictions regarding places available for smoking are more common), there are still socially reinforcing aspects of smoking. Smoking relapse, for example, does not have the negative social consequences of alcoholism relapse. More important, most exposure to smoking-specific cues center around social activities; hence, smokers tend to associate with smokers, and former smokers tend to relapse around other smokers.

In discussing factors associated with sustained smoking, however, one must not overlook the power that the media have in proliferation of cigarette smoking. Cigarette manufacturers spend up to $3 billion per year in advertising and promotional activities (Federal Trade Commission, 1989). Cigarette advertisers have the highest national expenditures in outdoor media, second highest in magazines, and third in newspapers (Davis, 1987). Moreover, several advertising campaigns have apparently targeted women and minorities as well as blue-collar workers. Cigarette manufacturers have increased their emphasis in magazines reaching blue-collar workers (e.g., *Popular Mechanics*) and decreased advertisements in "upscale" magazines, such as *U.S. News and World Report.* The "upscale" magazines saw advertising decreases from 23% in 1984 to 17% in 1985, whereas blue-collar magazines demonstrated a 2.3% increase from 1984 to 1985. In a recent study by Isbell and Klesges (1992), the researchers found that tobacco companies have drastically increased the number of advertisements in magazines that have largely black and female readerships. In contrast, advertisements in magazines read primarily by white males have generally decreased. The results of both these studies indicate that cigarette advertisements, at least in magazines, are targeting people who may be at high risk for smoking.

It is not only the number of advertisements alone that indicate cigarette companies are targeting specific populations; content of these advertisements is also an important issue. For example, a 1987 article in *Advertising Age* discussed a Phillip Morris Company campaign test-marketed in Switzerland. The campaign promoted the cigarette, "Star," as a "fashion accessory, much like a piece of jewelry or a scarf." In fact, plans are to change the packaging several times a year to coincide with seasonal changes in women's clothing.

Perhaps the most disturbing aspect of tobacco advertising is the exposure to, or targeting of, children and adolescents. Companies have targeted these groups via several subtle, and not-so-subtle, ways. For example, candy cigarettes promote cigarette brands indirectly to children and teach them at an early age to model behaviors of adult smokers. Cigarette companies clearly direct advertising logos and symbols at children and youth, placing such logos and symbols on children's toys, video arcade games, and candy products. In one recent study, researchers found that children between ages 3 to 5 recognized the Disney Channel logo significantly more than Old Joe the Camel (the logo for Camel cigarettes). However, by age 6, children recognize Old Joe as well as Mickey Mouse (Fischer, Schwartz, Richards, Gildstein, & Rojas, 1991). In addition, 30.4% of the 3-year-olds and 91.3% of the 6-year-olds correctly identified Old Joe as a cigarette logo. These findings are particularly disturbing when the expected percentage for random guessing was only 8.3%. Furthermore, in a study by DiFranza and colleagues (1991), the authors found that cartoon advertisements using Old Joe the Camel were far more successful at marketing this brand of cigarette to children than to adults. For example, children were more likely than adults in the study to recognize Old Joe and successfully identify the advertised product.

SMOKING CESSATION STRATEGIES

It is with knowledge of both behavioral and physiological factors that promote smoking that clinicians were able to develop current treatment strategies for smoking cessation. The majority of smoking interventions are either pharmacological, behavioral, or combined behavioral/pharmacological strategies.

Pharmacological Approaches

In the past 20 years, smoking cessation interventions have turned more toward pharmacological approaches combined with behavioral counseling. There are a number of pharmacological agents available (e.g., phenylpropanolamine (PPA), mecamylamine, clonidine, fluoxetine, tryptophan, and d-fenfluramine). Two experimental drugs that have received recent interest are clonidine and PPA. The use of clonidine in smoking cessation reportedly reduced tobacco withdrawal symptoms, including intensity of nicotine cravings (Glassman, Jackson, Walsh, Rouse, & Rosefeld, 1984; Ornish, Zisook, & McAdams, 1988). However, in other studies, results have been variable. Although some investigators have demonstrated this nonreceptor antagonist is more effective than an oral placebo (Glassman et al., 1988), others have found little or no benefit in trials using oral or transdermal clonidine (Davison et al., 1988; Franks, Harp, & Bell, 1989).

PPA, an over-the-counter drug commonly found in most cold and sinus medicines and diet aids, has, in gum form, effectively reduced postcessation weight gain in women relative to placebo gum and no-gum controls (R. Klesges, L. Klesges, Meyers, Klem, & Isbell, 1990). In addition, abstinence rates were significantly greater in the PPA group in comparison to the other conditions. In a follow-up study (Klesges et al., 1992), the investigators found that PPA reduces postcessation weight gain in both men and women relative to no-gum controls; they also found a significant dose–response relationship for withdrawal symptoms among female participants.

By far, however, the most widely used pharmacological agent for treatment of smoking cessation is some type of replacement nicotine. Nicotine replacement therapy in the form of 2 mg prolacrilex gum and transdermal patches are currently the only two products approved by the Food and Drug Administration for treatment of smoking cessation. Meta-analysis have demonstrated that nicotine gum is effective for smoking cessation (Hughes, 1991; Kottke, Battista, DeFriese, & Brekke, 1988; Lam, Sze, Sacks, & Chalmers, 1987) and for reducing withdrawal symptoms, particularly with heavy smokers. In smoking cessation clinics, success rates at 6 months were 27% for nicotine gum and 18% for placebo gum. Tonnesen and colleagues (1988) found 4 mg nicotine gum was more effective than 2 mg gum in heavy smokers, and the rate of effectiveness for 4 mg gum with heavy smokers was comparable to the rate of effectiveness obtained with 2 mg gum in smokers with medium or low levels of dependency. However, nicotine gum is not without it's disadvantages. These disadvantages include the following:

1. The instructions for chewing the gum are very particular, and there is the potential problem of misuse and inadequate instruction leading to several troublesome side effects (Lichtenstein & Glasgow, 1992).
2. Caffeine, a commonly used substance, affects pH balance of the mouth, and this can subsequently alter absorption of nicotine (Armitage & Turner, 1970).
3. There are some restrictions on who may use the gum (e.g., there are recommendations against its use for sufferers of temporomendibular joint disease, denture wearers, and pregnant or nursing women; *Physicians' Desk Reference*, 1990).
4. There is a dose-dependent relationship; therefore, users must be willing to chew the gum frequently enough to reach therapeutic nicotine levels in the bloodstream (Lichtenstein & Glasgow, 1992). However, this is less likely to be a problem with introduction of 4 mg gum in this country.
5. Nicotine gum, if not chewed properly, may produce side effects, including hiccups, gastrointestinal upset, nausea, and mouth sores (*Physicians' Desk Reference*, 1990, pp. 1127–1130).

Another form of nicotine replacement therapy are nicotine patches. Unfortunately, there are only a few studies evaluating the effectiveness of nicotine patches (Buchkremer, Bents, Horstman, Opitz, & Tolle, 1989; Daughton et al., 1991; Hurt, Lauger, Offord, Kottke, & Dale, 1990; J. Rose, Jarvick, & K. Rose, 1984; Tonnesen, Norregaard, Simonsen, & Sawe, 1991; Transdermal Nicotine Study Group, 1991). However, what is known is that transdermal patches demonstrate significant differences between active and placebo patches in quit rates and withdrawal symptoms (Daughton et al., 1991; Hurt et al., 1990; Rose et al., 1984; Tonnesen et al., 1991; Transdermal Nicotine Study Group, 1991). In addition, Daughton and colleagues (1991) demonstrated that nicotine patches, used in conjunction with low-intervention therapy, significantly enhance cessation rates relative to placebo patches.

Unfortunately, patches are not as effective as nicotine gum in reducing postcessation withdrawal symptoms, such as weight gain (Daughton et al., 1991; Hughes, 1991; Kottke et al., 1988; Lam et al., 1987; Tonnesen et al., 1991). At the current time, the mechanism by which use of the gum reduces postcessation weight gain is not clear. Some possibilities are that chewing gum decreases intake of specific foods, alters eating habits, or perhaps the fact that absorption sites are different plays a role. Another disadvantage of patches is that they may cause skin irritation and do not allow for self-dosing. Currently, there is debate about 16-hour patches versus 24-hour patches. One benefit to 24-hour patches is that they suppress morning nicotine cravings; 16-hour patches do not do this. However, continuous administration over a 24-hour period might induce tolerance, and overdosing can affect quality of sleep (Benowitz, 1991). Recently, one double-blind study compared 16-hour and 24-hour nicotine patches (Daughton et al., 1991). The study revealed no significant differences in quit rates between groups at 4 weeks and 6 months. Quit rates for 24-hour patch wearers were 30% and 22%, respectively, and 35% and 31%, respectively for the group wearing 16-hour patches.

Given the efficacy and popularity of both of these approaches (i.e., nicotine patches and gum), clinicians need more information regarding these treatment strategies and whom they are most likely to benefit. To date, no study has directly compared efficacy of patches versus nicotine gum. Table 7.1 presents hypothesized and theorized advantages and disadvantages of patches versus nicotine gum.

As in Table 7.1, nicotine patches may provide better compliance rates than nicotine gum. However, the gum provides ability for self-dosing, greater withdrawal-symptom reduction, less postcessation weight gain, and the gum may have higher efficacy rates (Daughton et al., 1991; Hall, Tunstall, Ginsberg, Benowitz, & Jones, 1987; Hughes, 1991; Hurt et al., 1990; Tonnesen et al., 1991; Transdermal Nicotine Study Group, 1991). However, the observation that patches are more widely accepted and easier to use may minimize any differences in efficacy. Nicotine gum is considerably less expensive than patches and comparable in monthly budgeting to what a one pack/day smoker would spend on cigarettes. As with all drugs, one must not minimize issues regarding side effects, and, as previously noted, both of these nicotine delivery systems have potentially serious side effects. In addition, certain medical conditions contraindicate use of one or both systems. It is important to note

Table 7.1. Advantages and Disadvantages of the Nicotine Patch versus Nicotine Gum

Characteristic	Nicotine patch	Nicotine gum
Compliance	Thought to be better	Thought to be worse
Acceptance	Thought to be better	Thought to be worse
Variability of dose	Excellent	Poor
Symptom reduction	Good	Excellent
Self-dosing	Poor	Excellent
Efficacy		
Initial	35–61%	56–64%
6 month	22–26%	23–35%
12 month	17–29%	25–38%
Cost (1 month)	$120	$80
Reduction of postcessation weight gain	Poor	Good
Side effects	Yes	Yes
Use in:		
TMJ	Yes	No
Pregnancy	No	No
Cardiovascular disease	No	No
Chronic dermatologic disorders	No	Yes
Hypertension	No	No

that in the case of pregnancy, however, nicotine replacement therapy is likely to be a lesser risk to the fetus than cigarette smoking in two ways: (1) neither mother nor fetus will experience exposure to the high levels of carbon monoxide produced by cigarette smoking, and (2) the delivery system in nicotine replacement is slower than in smoking; thus, nicotine replacement will not produce as high a level of nicotine concentration in the brain, or as intense physiological effects as would smoking (Benowitz, 1991).

Behavioral Strategies

There is a vast literature on behavioral treatment strategies for smoking cessation. For example, Schwartz (1987), when reviewing only those studies from 1978 to 1985, cited a total of 883 references for smoking cessation. Discussing all the strategies in behavioral stop-smoking programs is beyond the scope of this review, and excellent reviews of the literature exist (see Schwartz). However, we have observed some common ingredients and conclusions regarding the literature. First, most contemporary stop-smoking programs are multicomponent by nature. Although intensity varies from program to program, content generally does not. Most of these programs include all or some of the following components: self-monitoring, contingency contracting, stimulus control, social support, relaxation or stress management, and relapse prevention. Clinicians have adopted the multicomponent approach because research has demonstrated that multicomponent smoking cessation programs are more effective than programs broken down into their parts or single strategy treatments (Lando, 1982; Schwartz, 1987). Long-term abstinence can reach as high as 50% in multicomponent programs (U.S. Department of Health and Human Services, 1988). That is,

> We seem to have finally learned the lesson that minor differences (in treatments) will not lead to major differences (in outcomes). . . . Studies have consistently failed to identify that one elusive "magic bullet" intervention component. (Lichtenstein & Glasgow, 1992)

A second observation about stop-smoking programs is that literature reviews of smoking treatments indicate the area consists of treatments in which "everything works and nothing works." That is, most, if not all, approaches to smoking cessation are successful in getting a substantial number of people to quit initially (U.S. Department of Health and Human Services, 1989, 1990). However, all programs have a significant amount of relapse (Glasgow & Lichtenstein, 1987; Lichtenstein, 1982; Pechacek, 1979, Schwartz, 1987). Hunt, Barnett, and Branch (1971) reported that approximately 65% of all quitters relapse within 3 months of quitting, another 10% relapse 3- to 6-months postcessation, and about 3% relapse 6- to 12-months postcessation. Moreover, even 1 year after prolonged abstinence, relapse occurs in about one third of quitters (U.S. Department of Health and Human Services, 1990).

Another conclusion regarding stop-smoking programs is the increased popularity of combined behavioral and pharmacological treatments. Hughes (1991) evaluated efficacy of nicotine gum use in conjunction with psychological therapy relative to therapy alone. Results indicated that the combined approach significantly increased quit rates relative to the therapy-only group. Hughes hypothesized that the combination of the therapy component designed to improve relapse prevention skills with the decrease in withdrawal symptoms from the gum produces more positive effects.

These conclusions lead us to ask, "What new technologies are available for helping people behaviorally to stop smoking." As pointed out by Shiffman (1992), the answer is "Very little." In the late 1960s and 1970s, we saw a wide proliferation of effective stop-smoking techniques, such as stimulus control strategies, controlled smoking, and aversive strategies. However, since then, very few new strategies have evolved. Two exceptions to this general trend are relapse prevention and targeting of individuals at high risk. These are both significant advances in the stop-smoking literature and merit further discussion.

The term *relapse prevention* has become a fixture in behavioral science since publication of Marlatt and Gordon's *Relapse Prevention: Maintenance Strategies in the Treatment of Addictive Behaviors* (1985). Relapse prevention consists of non-pharmacological approaches concerned with maintenance of abstinence rather than just initial attainment of cessation (U.S. Department of Health and Human Services, 1988). Unfortunately, at least in practice in smoking-cessation programs, it has not been successfully implemented. Research has indicated that relapse rates are as high as 75–80% for smokers who achieve cessation (Garvey, Heinhold, & Rosner, 1989; Hughes, Hymowitz, Ochene, Simon, & Vogt, 1981; U.S. Department of Health and Human Services, 1990). Relapse occurs in high-risk (tempting) situations (Niaura et al., 1988; O'Connell & Martin, 1987; Shiffman, 1984), when the quitter experiences severe withdrawal symptoms (Swan et al., 1988; U.S. Department of Health and Human Services, 1990), due to abstinence-violation effect (Curry, Marlatt, & Gordon, 1987; Marlatt & Gordon, 1985), or due to unacceptable postcessation weight gain (Hall, Ginsberg, & Jones, 1986; R. Klesges, Meyers, L. Klesges, & LaVasque, 1989).

One commonly used strategy to aid in prevention of relapse is social support. Social support involves enlistment of friends, co-workers, peers, family, or fellow quitters to provide support during the quit attempt and abstinence. Most studies have demonstrated that social support predicts continued abstinence (Prochaska & DiClemente, 1983, 1985) and that perceived level of social support relates to smoking cessation and maintenance (Coppotelli & Orleans, 1985; U.S. Department of Health and Human Services, 1990). However, in one review of five studies (Lichtenstein, Glasgow, & Abrams, 1986), the authors found a relationship between social support and smoking cessation but no significant differences between regular buddy groups and groups trained to be more facilitative.

Another new concept in smoking-cessation programs is targeting and tailoring programs to a select set of smokers. For targeting and tailoring components, we rely heavily on the works of Prochaska and DiClemente (1982, 1983, 1985; DiClemente et al., 1991). They recently demonstrated very strong support for the stages-of-change model of smoking cessation (Prochaska & DiClemente, 1991). They suggest that clinicians may need to tailor stop-smoking interventions to specific stages. For instance, smokers in the precomtemplation stage (i.e., when individuals are smoking and not considering a quit attempt) and contemplation stage (i.e., when smokers are seriously considering a quit attempt but are not currently ready to do so), may require less intense, but longer programs, in order to move them successfully into the action stage. On the other hand, action-stage smokers (i.e., those who are considering quitting in the next 30 days or those who have already quit) may benefit from more intense, shorter, action-oriented types of intervention.

Given that few new strategies exist to help patients stop smoking, we must meet this challenge by testing new and alternative smoking-cessation programs. For example, there is a need to tailor stop-smoking programs to meet the needs of specific groups that continue to maintain high prevalence rates of smokers (e.g., heavy smokers, minorities, women, and adolescent girls). For example, in the case of heavy smokers (>24 cigarettes/day), an intense stop-smoking program with a combined pharmacological–behavioral approach would probably be most beneficial. Targeting specific groups has proved successful in the past with white males. In 1965, 50.2% of American men were smokers; in 1987, that figure has declined to 31.7% (U.S. Department of Health and Human Services, 1989). The decrease in prevalence among males is likely due to both the decline in number of teenage males who start smoking and the increase in number of adult males who quit (U.S. Department of Health and Human Services, 1990).

To summarize, we have a significant amount of information regarding whites and males. In addition, the literature is full of information about moderate smokers. Currently, we need more information regarding other groups of smokers. Of particular concern is the alarming prevalence rates among U.S. minority groups. Black Americans have a higher rate of smoking (34.8%) than any other ethnic/racial group in the United States, and they evidence the highest rate of mortality and morbidity from cardiovascular disease and cancer (U.S. Department of Health and Human Services, 1988). Smoking prevalence among Native Americans, non-Hispanic whites, and Hispanic whites ranges from nearly 26% to 30% (U.S. Department of Health and Human Services, 1988). Moreover, it is not surprising that recent studies indicate that higher educated and more affluent smokers have higher quit rates than their less educated and affluent counterparts (U.S. Department of Health and Human Services, 1989). As such, future research needs to focus on smoking behaviors of the less educated and affluent groups and address issues unique to them, whether those issues be social, cultural, or biological.

Finally, researchers need to specifically design smoking-cessation programs toward women and adolescent girls. Overall, although smoking rates have decreased in the past few decades, smoking rates have decreased more slowly for women than men (U.S. Department of Health and Human Services, 1988). The slower rate of decline among females is due to an increase in smoking among adolescent girls (U.S. Department of Health and Human Services, 1990). In the next section, we discuss information and challenges specific to adolescent girls and adult, female smokers as well as possible solutions.

Women and Smoking

This final section addresses four key issues related to women and smoking. First, we discuss the importance of targeting cessation programs for females. Second, we provide information about what researchers in the field know regarding why adolescent girls start smoking. Third, we discuss why women continue to smoke and relapse, and last, we discuss issues related to helping women quit.

Targeting women in smoking-cessation programs is important for two reasons: (1) women are more likely to take up smoking than men, and (2) they may be less likely to quit (American Cancer Society, 1986; Blake et al., 1989; U.S. Department of Health and Human Services, 1990). In 1987, an estimated 26.5% of American women smoked cigarettes (U.S. Department of Health and Human Services, 1988). That figure is down from nearly 32% in 1965, a 17% drop in incidence rates. However, during the same period, American men displayed a 37% drop in smoking prevalence. We can expect, if current trends continue, that more women than men will be smoking in the United States by 1995 (American Cancer Society, 1990).

Current smoking rates among women have resulted in a dramatic rise in lung cancer deaths in U.S. women; in fact, lung cancer deaths now exceed the number of breast cancer deaths. An estimated 146 thousand women will die in 1992 from lung cancer (American Cancer Society, 1992). Since 1987, more women have died from lung cancer than breast cancer, a disease that had been the leading cause of cancer deaths among women for over 40 years (American Cancer Society, 1992). In addition, cigarette smoking will account for approximately 200 thousand deaths in women in 1992 (American Cancer Society, 1992). This figure does not include smoking related deaths from cardiovascular disease, chronic obstructive pulmonary disease, and stroke. Moreover, recent studies have raised the possibility that there are weak positive relationships between cigarette smoking and breast cancer (Hiatt & Fireman, 1986; London et al., 1989; U.S. Department of Health and Human Services, 1990) and between cigarette smoking and cervical cancer (Brock et al., 1988; Nischan, Ebeling, & Schindler, 1988; U.S. Department of Health and Human Services, 1990). Another cigarette smoking risk for women concerns use of oral contraceptives. Even though low doses are being used in current oral contraceptive preparations, women who smoke and use birth control pills are more likely to suffer stroke and are at high risk for cardiovascular disease (U.S. Department of Health and Human Services, 1990).

In addition to cardiovascular disease and cancer risks, women who smoke are endangering their reproductive health as well as that of their unborn children. Research has shown that nicotine inhibits estrogen synthesis, decreases fertility, and brings about early menopause (Barbieri, Gochberg, & Ryan, 1986; Barbieri, McShane, & Ryan, 1986; Baron, LaVecchia, & Levi, 1990; U.S. Department of Health and Human Services, 1980, 1990). Pregnant women who smoke are at higher risk for spontaneous abortion, fetal death, and children with low birthweight (Campbell & Gray, 1987; Daling et al., 1985; Kleinman, Pierre, Madans, Land, & Schramm, 1988; H. A. Pattinson, Taylor, & H. M. Pattinson, 1991). Women who stop smoking prior to or within the first 3 to 4 months of pregnancy reduce low birthweight risk to that of women who never smoked (Cooper, 1989, cited in U.S. Department of Health and Human Services, 1990; Kleinman & Madans, 1985; Rush & Cassano, 1983; U.S. Department of Health and Human Services, 1990). However, a reduction in frequency of smoking without complete abstinence has demonstrated little or no benefit for pregnant women with regard to birthweight of their children (Hebel, Fox, & Sexton, 1988; U.S. Department of Health and Human Services, 1990).

Why Do Girls Start Smoking?

Surveys conducted in 1985 by the National Institute on Drug Abuse (American Cancer Society, 1986) indicate that approximately 26% of the teenage population surveyed smoked. Some experts in this area have argued that this figure is an underestimation of nearly 5% because dropouts tend to have higher prevalence rates and the figures do not take into consideration smoking experimentation (Kandel, 1980; Pirie, Murray, & Luepher, 1988; U.S. Department of Health and Human Services, 1988). Others have argued that 80–90% of all children have experimented with cigarettes and that 20–40% of all adolescents become regular smokers (Baugh,

Hunter, Webber, & Berenson, 1982; Flay, d'Avernas, Best, Kersell, & Ryan, 1983; U.S. Department of Health and Human Services, 1988). Recently, smoking initiation rates among females have consistently exceeded initiation rates among males (U.S. Department of Health and Human Services, 1988). Perhaps most disturbing is that the average age of smoking onset in females has continuously declined in the last 50 years (U.S. Department of Health and Human Services, 1980). The Surgeon General's Report (1980) indicated that from 1968 to 1974, the age of smoking initiation dropped for adolescent girls from 15–16-years-old to 12–14-years-old. Compounding these statistics is the finding that early substance use is more likely to lead to continued and heavy use (Brunswick & Boyle, 1979; O'Rourke & Stone, 1971).

What, then, precipitates smoking onset in adolescents? We do know that smoking is a complex behavior, and adolescents start to smoke for many reasons. Researchers have identified several factors as predictors of adolescent smoking. These factors include the following:

1. Smoking status of parents and friends (Chassin, Presson, Montello, Sherman, & McGrew, 1986; Covington & Omelich, 1988)
2. Adolescent perception of other smokers (Chassin, Presson, Sherman, Corty, & Olshavsky, 1984; Collins et al., 1987; Sussman et al., 1988)
3. Low levels of social support and low performance expectations in school as well as other areas of life (D'Onofrio, Their, Schnur, Buchanan, & Omelich, 1982)
4. Rebellious or risk-taking behaviors (Chassin et al., 1986; Collins et al., 1987)
5. Value of smoking in altering appearance of one's characteristics (e.g., images of toughness, maturity, and independence; Bland, Dewley, & Day, 1975)
6. Physiological effects of smoking (Freidman, Lichtenstein, & Biglan, 1985; Leventhal, Brown, Shacham, & Engquist, 1979).

A study by Covey and Tam (1990) found that in addition to friends' smoking status, depressive mood and living in a single-family home were also predictive of adolescent smoking.

Very little is known about the unique determinants of smoking onset in girls. One recent study (Camp, Klesges, & Relyea, 1993) found that white adolescent females were more likely to report that smoking helped control body weight. This study reported that over 40% of the sample endorsed the belief that smoking can aid in weight and/or appetite suppression. Camp and colleagues (1993) found that 45.7% of participants who believed smoking can help control weight were white females; this percentage is significantly higher than that of black females (10%), black males (13.5%), and white males (29.9%). In addition, Camp et al. found that weight control beliefs correlated with regular versus experimental cigarette use even when the experimenters controlled for other determinants of smoking onset. This confirms findings of Charlton (1984, cited in Gritz, Klesges, & Meyers, 1989) that the heaviest regular smokers were most likely to agree that smoking controls weight.

Why Women Continue to Smoke and Relapse

There is an emerging literature on both behavioral and biological factors that maintain smoking and contribute to relapse in women. To date, there are five promising areas that may help us understand why women smoke. First, from a biological perspective, the constituents of cigarette smoking play a role in maintenance of smoking behavior. As stated previously, nicotine is an addictive substance that produces a variety of changes in the autonomic nervous system and therefore produces stimulation. In addition, data from some studies indicate that females metabolize nicotine slower than males (Benowitz & Jacob, 1984; Kozlowski, Fracher, & Lei, 1982). Slower nicotine metabolic rates would elevate nicotine serum levels for longer periods and perhaps produce greater metabolic effects of smoking in females (U.S. Department of Health and Human Services, 1990). This may be one possible explanation for the greater weight reducing properties of smoking witnessed in females than males (U.S. Department of Health and Human Services, 1988; Williamson et al., 1991).

Weight gain and fear of weight gain is a second reason for continued smoking in women. Studies have documented that smokers weigh less than nonsmokers, those who quit smoking gain weight, and those who start smoking lose weight (R. Klesges, Meyers, L. Klesges, & LaVasque, 1989; U.S. Department of Health and Human Services, 1988). On average, smokers weigh about 7 pounds less than nonsmokers (U.S. Department of Health and Human Services, 1988) and smoking cessation leads to an average weight gain of about 5 pounds (U.S. Department of Health and Human Services, 1990). However, some ex-smokers are at higher risk for large weight gain, namely whites, women, and heavy smokers (U.S. Department of Health and Human Services, 1990). Women, on average, gain 8 pounds postcessation, whereas men experience only a 6-pound gain (Williamson et al., 1991). Incredibly, one study reported that black women gain approximately 27 pounds postcessation (Cutter, R. Klesges, & L. Klesges, 1992).

Fear of weight gain is also a factor associated with smoking relapse and initiation as well as continued smoking (Camp et al., 1993; R. Klesges & L. Klesges, 1988; Weekley, Klesges, & Relyea, 1992). R. Klesges and L. Klesges (1988) found that at least one third of smokers report continued smoking for weight-related reasons, and women, in particular, are likely to initiate smoking to reduce weight (Camp et al., 1993; Charlton, 1984). Concern about body-weight issues is a strong predictor of smokers who do not have a history of cessation attempts (Klesges et al., 1988) and among smokers who do not intend to quit in the future (Weekley et al., 1992).

A third possible reason for continued smoking or smoking relapse in women is caffeine. Reports linking caffeine use and smoking are unequivocal (Cameron & Boehmer, 1982; Conway, Vickers, Ward, & Rahe, 1981; Siegelaub, & Seltzer, 1974; Wingerd & Sponzilli, 1977, cited in Istvan & Matavazzo, 1984; U.S. Department of Health and Human Services, 1988); in addition, caffeine consumption may also relate to smoking relapse (Brandon, Tiffany, Obremski, & Baker, 1990). As reported in U.S. Department of Health and Human Services (1990), smoking cessation leads to decreases in caffeine elimination (Benowitz, Hall, & Modin, 1989; Brown, Jacob, Wilson, & Benowitz, 1988); thus, increased caffeine levels may mimic nicotine withdrawal symptoms due to caffeine overdose (Sachs & Benowitz, 1990, cited in U.S. Department of Health and Human Services, 1990). Recent evidence suggests that smoking women may have higher caffeine intake levels than men (R. Klesges & L. Klesges, 1992). As such, they may be particularly prone to caffeine effects during cessation. In addition, it is important to note that oral contraceptives increase the half-life of caffeine up to 11 hours (Abernathy & Todd, 1985, cited in Somani & Gupta, 1988).

Work in the area of negative affect has also been of benefit in understanding why women smoke. Women, relative to men, smoke more for pleasure and to reduce negative affect (Frith, 1971; Ikard & Tomkins, 1973; Livson & Leino, 1988). Studies have also demonstrated that women use fewer active coping strategies in dealing with stress than men do (Billings & Moos, 1981; Folkman & Lazarus, 1980; Stone & Neal, 1984) and that "upset episodes," precipitated by negative affect, are more likely to result in relapse (Shiffman, 1986).

Last, in the past several years, research has investigated the menstrual cycle as an important variable in understanding women's smoking behavior. The menstrual cycle consists of several different phases marked by changes in the female sex hormones, estrogen and progesterone. These hormonal changes are responsible for onset of menses (i.e., menstrual phase), follicle development (i.e., follicular phase), rupture of the follicle and release of the ovum (i.e., ovulation), and finally, development of the corpus luteum (i.e., luteal phase). Currently, there is a small body of preliminary data that suggests smoking behavior and withdrawal symptomatology change in relationship to menstrual cycle. Steinberg and Cherek (1989) noted that smoking topography increased significantly during the menstrual phase relative to all other phases. Other studies have also demonstrated changes in cigarette consumption during the cycle (Mello, Mendelson, & Palmieri, 1987; O'Hara, Porter, & Anderson, 1989; Steinberg & Cherek, 1989), but some studies have found no differences in smoking behavior during the cycle (DeBon, R. Klesges, & L. Klesges, 1993; Pomerleau, Garcia, & Pomerleau, 1992). In a study of withdrawal symptoms, O'Hara et al. (1989) found that women who quit during the luteal phase showed significantly higher scores of withdrawal symptoms than those who quit in the first 15 days of their cycle. Furthermore, they found that luteal phase quitters reported significantly more withdrawal symptoms than male quitters. Pomerleau, Garcia, and Pomerleau (1992) reported results similar to O'Hara et al. (1989). Pomerleau and colleagues found that menstrual and withdrawal symptoms were more pronounced during the late luteal/abstinence condition than during early follicular and mid- to late follicular phases. In a cigarette smoking and alcohol study, Mello et al. (1987) found that three fourths of premenstrual women increased smoking, and reports of physical discomfort were higher in women who smoked less during this phase. In a recent study by DeBon et al. (1993) that evaluated symptoms in smoking and nonsmoking women over the menstrual cycle, the investigators found effects for both smoking status and cycle phase; women who smoked had higher mean symptom scores over all phases of the menstrual cycle than their nonsmoking counterparts. In addition, as expected, mean symptom scores were significantly higher during menses and the late luteal phase.

Helping Women Quit: What Works

We currently know very little about what helps women quit and maintain abstinence. Unfortunately, we know that women generally have lower success rates in achieving and maintaining smoking cessation than men (Gritz, 1978; Horowitz, Hindi-Alexander, & Wagner, 1985; Hurt, Offord, & Hepper, 1988). Further research is necessary to aid in tailoring and targeting smoking-cessation programs for women and girls. These programs need to address weight-control concerns, social support, cognitive coping skills, and relapse prevention as well as collect more data on smoking-behavior changes over the menstrual cycle.

Future menstrual cycle studies may provide clear information about optimal times for cessation attempts. Future research might include randomized studies comparing follicular and luteal quitting, the relationship between premenstrual syndrome and smoking, and possible interactions between smoking, alcohol consumption, and the menstrual cycle. One major problem in this area of study is design limitations and inconsistent definitions of cycle phases. These inconsistent definitions of phase may contribute to the variable results obtained to date.

Also warranting further consideration in the ovarian-cycle field is the potential three-way relationship between cycle phase, smoking behavior, and negative affect. As stated previously, women smoke and relapse in response to negative affect (Ikard & Tomkins, 1973; Livson & Leino, 1988; Shiffman, 1986), and negative affect increases prior to menses (Schecter, Bachman, Vaitukaitus, Phillips, & Saperstein, 1989). In addition to collecting more preliminary data on these three variables and how they interact, smoking cessation programs need to address these factors both individually and as a group.

Regarding negative affect and the menstrual cycle, smoking-cessation programs may enlist social support, cognitive coping-skills training, and stress- and anger-management components. Cessation programs with behavioral and pharmacological approaches alone may not be effective in helping women quit. Livson and Leino (1988) suggested that because women may view smoking as a stress modulator and a respite opportunity from the burdens of both their new and "traditional" roles, smoking-cessation programs need techniques that are responsive to these beliefs.

Recent research has indicated that social support is an effective strategy in smoking cessation with women but not men (Fisher et al., 1991). Fisher and associates, in comparing a social-support approach to smoking cessation with a self-knowledge/self-management approach, found that women in the social-support condition were more successful in abstaining than their female counterparts in the self-management condition. In addition, the investigators found no such difference for men; men in the study responded the same to both treatment strategies. Moreover, DiLorenzo, Powers, Cormier, Herbig, and Fisher (1990) found that social support as an aid to smoking cessation was more important for female quitters and relapsers than for their male counterparts. Although both male and female quitters report greater social support for quitting than relapsers, women quitters report considerably more social support than female relapsers; this difference is only marginally significant between male quitters and relapsers. These findings suggest that the more assistance and support women get, the more likely they are to be successful quitters.

In addition, it appears that women benefit more from programs that have a relapse prevention component rather than those stressing absolute abstinence. In a study by Curry, Marlatt, Gordon, and Baer (1988), comparing a relapse prevention approach to the typical absolute abstinence model, women were more successful in relapse-prevention programs than with the absolute abstinence approach. Twenty percent of long-term abstainers in the absolute abstinence condition were women, relative to 78% in the relapse prevention condition. They also found that even though participants in the relapse-prevention program lapsed sooner than their absolute abstinence counterparts, relapse-prevention program participants were more likely to quit again within the next year. In addition, analyses indicated that women were 4.5 times as likely to quit in a relapse-prevention approach than in the absolute abstinence program. For men, the opposite was true; the absolute abstinence approach was more likely (2.3 times) to help men quit than the relapse-prevention strategy.

Future cessation programs for women need to address the weight gain associated with cessation. Cessation programs may accomplish this by using pharmacological agents or by incorporating weight-control strategies into the cessation program. It is important to note, however, that recent smoking-cessation treatment studies (Hall, 1994; Pirie, 1994) including a weight-control component, found no effect on postcessation weight gain or cessation rates. Moreover, the weight-control program had either no effect or a negative effect on smoking-cessation rates. Perhaps the additional burden of a weight-control program may overload participants to the point that added intervention is detrimental to cessation (Gritz et al., 1994). In addition, both the menstrual cycle literature and the smoking-cessation literature demonstrate change in total food consumption and changes in types of foods consumed. Here, again, lies another complex interaction that warrants further study; that is, does food intake vary if cessation attempts occur at different phases of the cycle? Future studies need to evaluate pharmacological and behavioral approaches to dealing with these issues.

When discussing postcessation weight gain and women, the special needs of black women warrant additional attention. As stated previously, black women gain, on average, up to 27 pounds postcessation (Cutter et al., 1992). This fact, coupled with high rates of obesity among black women may contribute to, or exacerbate, health problems (e.g., diabetes, hypercholesterolemia). Black women have one of the highest incidence rates of obesity in the U.S. (National Heart, Lung, and Blood Institute, 1990). Relative to white women, black women are between 1.6 to 2.5 times more likely to be obese (Heckler, 1985; Kumanyika, 1987; Wadden et al., 1990). Considering health consequences associated with obesity, this area is in great need of further investigation.

Finally, in response to the challenge of helping adolescent girls to quit, perhaps the least is known in this area. As with women, studies investigating several factors, such as weight control, negative affect, and social support among adolescent girls, as well as more investigations into factors associated with smoking initiation are necessary in order to better understand this group and develop effective treatments. These studies also need to include white and nonwhite girls. A recent study by Headen, Bauman, Deane, and Koch (1991) found that there are racial differences in adolescent smoking onset. For example, they found that friends' smoking relates to smoking initiation among white adolescents but not among blacks. Additionally, whites initiated smoking at a younger age than blacks. Unfortunately, this study did not evaluate the role of weight and weight-related concerns. Perhaps, given that the age of initiation is decreasing for girls, prevention programs need to begin as early as age 10. However, program developers must be aware that recent research has shown that "programs not related to age-specific realities will be viewed as 'stupid' and 'useless' and ignored" (Ritenbaugh, 1992).

In summary, intervention has made much progress in the "war" on smoking, particularly with male smokers. However, the focus of future research needs to be on women, adolescent girls, minorities, heavy smokers, and blue-collar workers. In addition to strategies mentioned in this chapter, such as relapse prevention, pharmacological agents, and targeted and tailored programs, the media, legislature, and society as a whole need to aid in smoking cessation and, in particular, in prevention of smoking initiation among teens. Laws restricting public smoking, bans on cigarette advertising aimed at children and adolescents, and restricted access to cigarettes by youths are just some of the ways in which we can further curtail smoking.

REFERENCES

Abernathy, D. R., & Todd, E. L. (1985). Impairment of caffeine clearance by chronic use of low-dose estrogen-containing oral contraceptives. *European Journal of Clinical Pharmacology, 28,* 425–428.

American Cancer Society (1986). Women and smoking. *Healthline, 5,* 12–13.

American Cancer Society (1990). *Cancer facts and figures—1990.* 7–11.

American Cancer Society (1992). *Cancer facts and figures—1992.* 8–12.

Armitage, A. K., & Turner, D. M. (1970). Absorption of nicotine in cigarette and cigar smoke. *Nature, 226,* 1231–1232.

Barbieri, R. L., Gochberg, J., & Ryan, K. J. (1986). Nicotine, cotinine, and anabasine inhibit aromatase in human trophoblast *in vitro. Journal of Clinical Investigation, 77,* 727–1733.

Barbieri, R. L., McShane, P. M., & Ryan, K. J. (1986). Constituents of cigarette smoke inhibit human granulosa cell aromatase. *Fertility and Sterility, 46,* 232–236.

Baron, J. A., LaVecchia, C., & Levi, F. (1990). The anti-estrogenic effect of cigarette smoking in women. *American Journal of Obstetrics and Gynecology, 162,* 502–514.

Baugh, J. G., Hunter, S. M., Webber, L. S., & Berenson, G. S. (1982). Developmental trends of first cigarette smoking experience of children: The Bogalusa Heart Study. *American Journal of Public Health, 72,* 1161–1164.

Benowitz, N. L. (1988). Pharmacologic aspects of smoking and nicotine addiction. *New England Journal of Medicine, 319,* 1318–1330.

Benowitz, N. L. (1991). Nicotine replacement therapy during pregnancy. *Journal of the American Medical Association, 266,* 3174–3177.

Benowitz, N. L., Hall, S. M., & Modin, G. (1989). Persistent increase in caffeine concentrations in people who stop smoking. *British Medical Journal, 298,* 1075–1076.

Benowitz, N. L., & Jacob, P. III. (1984). Daily intake of nicotine during cigarette smoking. *Clinical Pharmacology and Therapeutics, 35,* 499–504.

Benowitz, N. L., & Jacob, P. III. (1985). Nicotine renal excretion rate influences nicotine intake during cigarette smoking. *Journal of Pharmacology and Experimental Therapeutics, 234,* 153–155.

Benowitz, N. L., Jacob, P. III., Kozlowski, L., & Yu, L. (1986). Influence of smoking fewer cigarettes on exposure to tar, nicotine, and carbon monoxide exposure. *New England Journal of Medicine, 314,* 1310–1313.

Benowitz, N. L., Porchet, H., & Jacob, P. III. (1989). Nicotine dependence and tolerance in man: Pharmacokinetic pharmacodynamic investigations. In A. Norberg, K. Fuxe, B. Holmstedt, & A. Sundell (Eds.), *Progress in Brain Research, 79,* 279–287. Amsterdam: Elsevier.

Billings, A. G., & Moos, R. H. (1981). The role of coping responses and social resources in attenuating the stress of life events. *Journal of Behavioral Medicine, 4,* 139–157.

Blake, S. M., Klepp, K. I., Pechacek, T. F., Folsom, A. R., Luepker, R. V., Jacobs, D. R., & Mittlemark, M. B. (1989). Differences in smoking cessation strategies between men and women. *Addictive Behaviors, 14,* 409–418.

Bland, J. M., Bewley, B. R., & Day, I. (1975). Primary schoolboys: Image of self and smoker. *British Journal of Preventive and Social Medicine, 29,* 262–266.

Brandon, T. H., Tiffany, S. T., Obremski, K. M., & Baker, T. B. (1990). Post-cessation cigarette use: The process of relapse. *Addictive Behaviors, 15,* 107–114.

Brandon, T. H., Zelman, D. C., & Baker, T. B. (1987). Effects of maintenance sessions on smoking relapse: Delaying the inevitable? *Journal of Consulting and Clinical Psychology, 55,* 780–782.

Brock, K. E., Berry, G., Mock, P. A., Maclennan, R., Truswell, A. S., & Brinton, L. A. (1988). Nutrients in diet and plasma and risk of *in situ* cervical cancer. *Journal of National Cancer Institute, 80,* 580–585.

Brown, C. R., Jacob, P. III, Wilson, M., & Benowitz, N. L. (1988). Changes in rate and pattern of caffeine metabolism after cigarette smoking. *Clinical Pharmacology and Therapeutics, 43,* 488–491.

Brunswick, A. F., & Boyle, J. M. (1979). Patterns of drug involvement: Developmental and secular influences on age at initiation. *Youth and Society, 11,* 139–162.

Buchkremer, G., Bents, H., Minneker, E., & Opitz, K. (1989). Combination of behavioral smoking cessation with transdermal nicotine substitution. *Addictive Behaviors, 14,* 229–238.

Cameron, P., & Boehmer, J. (1982). And coffee too. *International Journal of the Addictions, 17,* 569–574.

Camp, D. E., Klesges, R. C., & Relyea, G. (1993). The relationship between body weight concerns and adolescent smoking. *Health Psychology, 12,* 24–32.

Campbell, O. M., & Gray, R. H. (1987). Smoking and ectopic pregnancy: A multinational case-control study. In M. J. Rosenberg (Ed.), *Smoking and reproductive health* (pp. 70–75). Littleton, MA: PSG.

Charlton, A. (1984). Smoking and weight control in teenagers. *Public Health London, 98,* 277–281.

Chassin, L., Presson, C. C., Montello, D., Sherman, S. J., & McGrew, J. (1986). Changes in peer and parent influence during adolescence: Longitudinal versus cross-sectional perspectives nonsmoking initiation. *Developmental Psychology, 22,* 327–334.

Chassin, L., Presson, C. C., Sherman, S. J., Corty, E., & Olshavsky, R. W. (1984). Predicting the onset of cigarette smoking in adolescents: A longitudinal study. *Journal of Applied Social Psychology, 14,* 224–243.

Collins, L. M., Sussman, S., Rauch, J. M., Dent, C. W., Johnson, C. A., Hansen, W. B., & Flay, B. R. (1987). Psychosocial predictors of young adolescent smoking: A sixteen-month, three-wave longitudinal study. *Journal of Applied Social Psychology, 18,* 554–573.

Conway, T. L., Vickers, R. R., Ward, H. W., & Rahe, R. H. (1981). Occupational stress and variation in cigarette, coffee, and alcohol consumption. *Journal of Health and Social Behavior, 22,* 155–165.

Cooper, L. (1989). *An epidemiologic assessment of low birth weight and smoking behavior in a black urban population.* Unpublished doctoral dissertation, University of Maryland, Bethesda, MD.

Coppotelli, H. C., & Orleans, C. T. (1985). Partner support and other determinants of smoking cessation maintenance among women. *Journal of Consulting and Clinical Psychology, 54,* 342–346.

Covey, L. S., & Tam, D. (1990). Depressive mood, the single-parent home, and adolescent cigarette smoking. *American Journal of Public Health, 80,* 1330–1333.

Covington, M. V., & Omelich, C. L. (1988). I can resist anything but temptation: Adolescent expectations for smoking cigarettes. *Journal of Applied Social Psychology, 18,* 203–227.

Curry, S. J., Marlatt, G. A., & Gordon, J. R. (1987). Abstinence violation effect: Validation of an attributional construct with smoking cessation. *Journal of Consulting and Clinical Psychology, 55,* 145–149.

Curry, S. J., Marlatt, G. A., Gordon, J. R., & Baer, J. S. (1988). A comparison of alternative theoretical approaches to smoking cessation and relapse. *Health Psychology, 7,* 545–556.

Cutter, G., Klesges, R. C., & Klesges, L. M. (1992). *Race, gender, and its relationship to postcessation weight gain.* Manuscript submitted for editorial review.

Daling, J. R., Weiss, N. S., Voigt, L., Spandoni, L. R., Soderstrom, R., Moore, D. E., & Stadel, B. V. (1985). Tubal infertility in relation to prior induced abortion. *Fertility and Sterility, 43,* 389–394.

Daughton, D. M., Heatley, S. A., Prendergast, J. J., Causey, D., Knowles, M., Rolf, C. N., Cheney, R. A., Hatlelid, K., Thompson, A. B., & Rennard, S. I. (1991). Effect of transdermal nicotine delivery as an adjunct to low-intervention smoking cessation therapy. A randomized, placebo-controlled, double blind study. *Archives of Internal Medicine, 151,* 749–752.

Davis, R. M. (1987). Current trends in cigarette advertising and marketing. *New England Journal of Medicine, 316,* 725–732.

Davison, R., Kaplan, K., Fintel, D., Parker, M., Anderson, L., & Haring, O. (1988). The effect of clonidine on the cessation of cigarette smoking. *Clinical and Pharmacological Therapeutics, 44,* 265–267.

DeBon, M., Klesges, R. C., & Klesges, L. M. (1993). The effects of smoking status and the menstrual cycle on energy balance. *Proceedings of the 14th Annual Convention of the Society of Behavioral Medicine, 133* (Abstract).

DeBon, M., Klesges, R. C., & Klesges, L. M. (in press). Symptomatology across the menstrual cycle in smoking and nonsmoking women. *Addictive Behaviors.*

DiClemente, C. C., Prochaska, J. O., Fairhurst, S. K., Velicer, W. F., Velasquez, M. M., & Rossi, J. S. (1991). The process of smoking cessation: An analysis of precontemplation, contemplation, and preparation stages of change. *Journal of Consulting and Clinical Psychology, 59,* 295–304.

DiFranza, J. R., Richards, Jr., J. W., Paulman, P. M., Wolf-Gillespie, N., Fletcher, C., Jaffe, R. D., & Murry, D. (1991). RJR Nabisco's cartoon camel promotes camel cigarettes to children. *Journal of the American Medical Association, 266,* 3149–3153.

DiLorenzo, T. M., Powers, R. W., Cormier, J. F., Herbig, L. J., & Fisher, E. B. (1990). The role of social support and competence skills in smoking cessation among women. *1990 World Conference on Lung Health.*

D'Onofrio, C. N., Their, H. D., Schnur, A. E., Buchanan, D. R., & Omelich, C. L. (1982). The dynamics of adolescent smoking behavior. *World Smoking and Health, 7,* 18–24.

Federal Trade Commission. (1989). *1988 Federal Trade Commission Report to Congress.* Washington DC: Government Printing Office.

Fischer, P. M., Schwartz, M. P., Richards, J. W., Goldstein, A. O., & Rojas, T. H. (1991). Brand logo recognition by children aged 3 to 6 years. *Journal of the American Medical Association, 266,* 3145–3148.

Fisher, E. B., Rehberg, H. R., Beaupre, P. M., Hughes, C. R., Levitt-Gilmore, T., Davis, J. R., & DiLorenzo, T. M. (1991, November). Gender differences in response to social support in smoking cessation. *Association for Advancement of Behavior Therapy, 11.*

Flay, B. R. (1987). Mass media and smoking cessation: A critical review. *American Journal of Public Health, 77,* 153–158.

Flay, B. R., d'Avernas, J. R., Best, J. A., Kersell, M. W., & Ryan, K. B. (1983). Cigarette smoking: Why young people do it and ways of preventing it. In P. J. McGrath & P. Firestone (Eds.), *Pediatric and adolescent behavioral medicine: Issues in treatment* (pp. 76–92). New York: Springer.

Folkman, S., & Lazarus, R. S. (1980). An analysis of coping in a middle-aged community sample. *Journal of Health and Social Behavior, 21,* 219–239.

Franks, P., Harp, J., & Bell, B. (1989). Randomized, controlled trial of clonidine for smoking cessation in a primary care setting. *Journal of the American Medical Association, 262,* 3011–3013.

Freidman, L. S., Lichtenstein, E., & Biglan, A. (1985). Smoking onset among teens: An empirical analysis of initial situations. *Addictive Behaviors, 10,* 1–13.

Frith, C. D. (1971). Smoking behavior and its relation to the smokers immediate experience. *British Journal of Social and Clinical Psychology, 10,* 73–78.

Garvey, A. J., Heinhold, J. W., & Rosner, B. (1989). Self-help approaches to smoking cessation: A report from the normative aging study. *Addictive Behavior, 14,* 23–33.

Glasgow, R. E., & Lichtenstein, E. (1987). Long-term effects of behavioral smoking cessation interventions. *Behavior Therapy, 18,* 297–324.

Glassman, A. H., Jackson, W. K., Walsh, B. T., Rouse, S. P., & Rosenfeld, B. (1984). Cigarette craving, smoking withdrawal and clonidine. *Science, 226,* 864–866.

Glassman, A. H., Stetner, F., Walsh, B. T., Raizman, P. S., Fleiss, J. L., Cooper, T. B., & Covey, L. S. (1988). Heavy smokers, smoking cessation, and clonidine: Results of a double-blind, randomized trial. *Journal of the American Medical Association, 259,* 2863–2866.

Gritz, E. R. (1978). Women and smoking: A realistic appraisal. In J. L. Schwartz (Ed.), *International conference on smoking cessation.* New York: American Cancer Society.

Gritz, E. R., Klesges, R. C., & Meyers, A. W. (1989). The smoking and body weight relationship: Implications for intervention and postcessation weight control. *Annals of Behavioral Medicine, 11,* 144–153.

Gritz, E. R., St. Jeor, S., Bennett, G., Biener, L., Blair, S., Brunner, R. L., DeHorn, A., Foreyt, J., Haire-Joshu, D., Hall, S., Hill, D. R., Jensen, J., Kristeller, J., Marcus, B. H., Nides, M., Pirie, P., Solomon, L., Stillman, F., Ernst, J., & Zeigler-Mealer, C. D. (1994). Task Force III: Implications with respect to prevention and interventions. *Health Psychology, 12.*

Hall, S. M. (1994). Preventing weight gain after smoking cessation. *Health Psychology.*

Hall, S. M., Ginsberg, D., & Jones, R. T. (1986). Smoking cessation and weight gain. *Journal of Consulting and Clinical Psychology, 54,* 342–346.

Hall, S. M., Tunstall, G., Ginsberg, D., Benowitz, N., & Jones, R. T. (1987). Nicotine gum and behavioral treatment: A placebo controlled trial. *Journal of Consulting and Clinical Psychology, 55,* 603–605.

Headen, S. W., Bauman, K. E., Deane, G. D., & Koch, G. G. (1991). Are the correlates of smoking initiation different for Black and White adolescents? *American Journal of Public Health, 81,* 854–857.

Hebel, J. R., Fox, N. L., & Sexton, M. (1988). Dose-response of birth weight to various measures of maternal smoking during pregnancy. *Journal of Clinical Epidemiology, 41,* 483–489.

Heckler, M. M. (1985). *Report of the secretary's task force on Black and minority health.* Bethesda, MD: U.S. Department of Health and Human Services.

Hiatt, R. A., & Fireman, B. H. (1986). Smoking, menopause, and breast cancer. *Journal of National Cancer Institute, 78,* 833–838.

Horowitz, M. B., Hindi-Alexander, M., & Wagner, T. J. (1985). Psychosocial mediators of abstinence, relapse, and continued smoking: A one-year follow-up of a minimal intervention. *Addictive Behaviors, 10,* 29–39.

Hughes, G. H., Hymowitz, N., Ochene, J. K., Simon, N., & Vogt, T. M. (1981). The multiple risk factor. Intern trial (MRFIT) intervention on smoking. *Preventive Medicine, 10,* 476–500.

Hughes, J. R. (1991). Combined psychological and nicotine gum treatment for smoking: A critical review. *Journal of Substance Abuse, 3,* 337–350.

Hughes, J. R., Gust, S. W., Keenan, R., Fenwick, J. W., Skoog, K., & Higgins, S. T. (1991). Long-term use of nicotine vs. placebo gum. *Archives of Internal Medicine, 151,* 1993–1998.

Hunt, W. A., Barnett, L. W., & Branch, L. G. (1971). Relapse rates in addiction programs. *Journal of Clinical Psychology, 427,* 455–456.

Hurt, R. D., Lauger, G. G., Offord, K. P., Kottke, T. E., & Dale, L. C. (1990). Nicotine-replacement therapy with use of a transdermal nicotine patch-A randomized double-blind placebo-controlled trial. *Mayo Clinic Proceedings, 65,* 1529–1537.

Hurt, R. D., Offord, K. P., & Hepper, N.G.G. (1988). Long-term follow-up of persons attending community-based smoking-cessation program. *Mayo Clinic Proceedings, 63,* 681–690.

Ikard, F. F., & Tomkins, S. (1973). The experience of affect as a determinant of smoking behavior: A series of validity studies. *Journal of Abnormal Psychology, 81,* 172–181.

Isbell, T. R., & Klesges, R. C. (1992). Cigarette advertising and smoking rates in women and minorities *Proceedings of the 13th Annual Convention of the Society of Behavioral Medicine,* 104 (Abstract).

Istvan, J., & Matavazzo, J. D. (1984). Tobacco, alcohol, and caffeine use: A review of their interrelationships. *Psychological Bulletin, 95,* 301–326.

Kandel, D. B. (1980). Drug and drinking behavior among youth. *American Review of Sociology, 6,* 235–285.

Kleinman, J. C., & Madans, J. H. (1985). The effects of maternal smoking, physical stature, and educational attainment on the incidence of low birth weight. *American Journal of Epidemiology, 121,* 843–855.

Kleinman, J. C., Pierre, M. B., Jr., Madans, J. H., Land, G. H., & Schramm, W. F. (1988). The effects of maternal smoking on fetal and infant mortality. *American Journal of Epidemiology, 127,* 274–281.

Klesges, R. C., Benowitz, N. L., & Meyers, A. W. (1991). Behavioral and biobehavioral aspects of smoking and smoking cessation: The problem of post cessation weight gain. *Behavior Therapy, 22,* 179–199.

Klesges, R. C., & Klesges, L. M. (1988). Cigarette smoking as a dietary strategy in a university population. *International Journal of Eating Disorders, 7,* 413–419.

Klesges, R. C., Klesges, L. M., Isbell, T. R., Klem, M. L., DeBon, M., & Shuster, M. L. (1992). The effects of phenylpropanolamine on symptoms associated with smoking withdrawal *Proceedings of the 13th Annual Convention of the Society of Behavioral Medicine,* 103 (Abstract).

Klesges, R. C., Klesges, L. M., Meyers, A. W., Klem, M., & Isbell, T. (1990). The effects of phenylpropanolamine on dietary intake, physical activity, and body weight following smoking cessation. *Clinical Pharmacology and Therapeutics, 47,* 747–754.

Klesges, R. C., Meyers, A. W., Klesges, L. M., & La Vasque, M. E. (1989). Smoking, body weight, and their effects on smoking behavior: A comprehensive review of the literature. *Psychological Bulletin, 106,* 1–27.

Klesges, R. C., Ray, J., & Klesges, L. M. (1992). *The relationship between caffeine intake and cigarette smoking: An analysis of the Second National Health and Nutrition Examination Survey (NHANESII).* Manuscript submitted for editorial review.

Klesges, R. C., Somes, G. W., Pascale, R., Klesges, L. M., Murphy, M., Brown, K., & Williams, E. (1988). Knowledge and beliefs regarding the consequences of cigarette smoking and their relationships to smoking status in a biracial sample. *Health Psychology, 7,* 387–401.

Kottke, T. E., Battista, R. N., DeFriese, G. H., & Brekke, M. L., (1988). Attributes of successful smoking cessation interventions in medical practice: A meta-analysis of 39 controlled trials. *Journal of the American Medical Association, 259,* 2882–2889.

Kozlowski, L. T., Fracher, R. C., & Lei, H. (1982). Nicotine yields of cigarettes. Plasma nicotine levels in smokers and public health. *Preventive Medicine, 11,* 240–244.

Kumanyika, S. (1987). Obesity in Black women. *Epidemiologic Reviews, 9,* 31–50.

Lam, W., Sze, P. C., Sacks, H. S., & Chalmers, T. C. (1987). Meta-analysis of randomized controlled trials of nicotine chewing gum. *Lancet, 2,* 27–30.

Lando, H. A. (1982). A factorial analysis of preparation, aversion, and maintenance in the elimination of smoking. *Addictive Behaviors, 7,* 143–154.

Leventhal, H., Brown, D., Shacham, S., & Engquist, G. (1979). Effects of preparatory information about sensations, threats of pain, and attention on cold pressor distress. *Journal of Personality and Social Psychology, 37,* 688–714.

Lichtenstein, E. (1982). The smoking problem: A behavioral perspective. *Journal of Consulting and Clinical Psychology, 50,* 804–819.

Lichtenstein, E., & Brown, R. A. (1980). Smoking cessation methods: Review and recommendations. In W. R. Miller, (Ed.), *The addictive behaviors: Treatment of alcoholism, drug abuse, smoking, and obesity* (pp. 56–72). Oxford, England: Pergamon.

Lichtenstein, E., & Glasgow, R. E. (1992). Smoking cessation: What have we learned in the past decade? *Journal of Consulting and Clinical Psychology, 60,* 518–527.

Lichtenstein, E., Glasgow, R. E., & Abrams, D. B. (1986). Social support in smoking cessation: In search of effective interventions. *Behavior Therapy, 17,* 607–619.

Livson, N., & Leino, E. V. (1988). Cigarette smoking motives: Factorial structure and gender differences in a longitudinal study. *International Journal of Addictions, 23,* 535–544.

London, S. J., Golditz, G. A., Stampfer, M. J., Willett, W. C., Rosner, B. A., & Speizer, F. E. (1989). Prospective study of smoking and risk of breast cancer. *Journal of National Cancer Institute, 81,* 1625–1631.

Marlatt, G. A., & Gordon, J. R. (1985). *Relapse prevention: Maintenance strategies in the treatment of addictive behaviors.* New York: Guilford.

Mello, N. K., Mendelson, J. H., & Palmieri, S. L. (1987). Cigarette smoking by women: Interactions with alcohol use. *Psychopharmacology, 93,* 8–15.

National Heart, Lung, and Blood Institute. (1990, August). *Obesity and cardiovascular disease in minority populations.* NHLBI Consensus Workshop, Bethesda, MD.

Niaura, R. S., Rohsenow, D. J., Binkoff, J. A., Monti, P. M., Pedraza, M., & Abrams, D. B. (1988). Relevance of cue reactivity to understanding alcohol and smoking relapse. *Journal of Abnormal Psychology, 97,* 133–152.

Nischan, P., Ebeling, K., & Schindler, C. (1988). Smoking and invasive cervical cancer risk. *American Journal of Epidemiology, 128,* 74–77.

O'Connell, K. A., & Martin, E. J. (1987). Highly tempting situations associated with abstinence, temporary lapse, and relapse among participants in smoking cessation programs. *Journal of Consulting and Clinical Psychology, 55,* 367–371.

O'Hara, P., Portser, S. A., & Anderson, B. P. (1989). The influence of menstrual cycle changes on the tobacco withdrawal syndrome in women. *Addictive Behaviors, 14,* 595–600.

O'Rourke, T. W., & Stone, D. B. (1971). A prospective study of trends in youth smoking. *Journal of Drug Education, 1,* 49–61.

Ornish, S. A., Zisook, S., & McAdams, L. A. (1988). Effects of transdermal chlonidine treatment on withdrawal symptoms associated with smoking cessation. *Archives of Internal Medicine, 320,* 898–903.

Parry, J. (1987, October 12). Fashion smokes glow in Switzerland, *Advertising Age,* p. 68.

Pattinson, H. A., Taylor, P. J., & Pattinson, H. M. (1991). The effect of cigarette smoking on ovarian function and early pregnancy outcome. *Fertility and Sterility, 55,* 780–783.

Pechacek, T. F. (1979). Modification of smoking behavior. In *Smoking and health: A report of the U.S. Surgeon General.* (Department of Health, Education, and Welfare Publication No. PHS 79-50066). Washington, DC: U.S. Government Printing Office.

Physicians' Desk Reference. (1990). Oradell, NJ: Medical Economics Books.

Pierce, J. P., Fiore, M. C., Novotny, T. E., Hatziandreu, E. J., & Davis, R. M. (1989). Trends in cigarette smoking in the U.S. project to year 2000. *Journal of the American Medical Association, 261,* 61–65.

Pirie, P. L. (1994). Effects of nicotine gum on postcessation weight gain. *Health Psychology.*

Pirie, P. L., Murray, D. M., & Luepher, R. V. (1988). Smoking prevalence in a cohort of adolescents, including absentees, dropouts, and transfers. *American Journal of Public Health, 78,* 176–178.

Pomerleau, C. S., Garcia, A. W., & Pomerleau, O. F. (1992). The effects of menstrual cycle phase on nicotine intake and on biochemical and subjective measures in women smokers: A preliminary report. *Psychoneuroendocrinology, 17,* 627–636.

Pomerleau, C. S., Garcia, A. W., & Pomerleau, O. F. (1992). Effects of menstrual phase and nicotine abstinence on symptomatology in women smokers. *Proceedings of the 13th Annual Convention of the Society of Behavioral Medicine, 63,* (Abstract).

Prochaska, J. O., & DiClemente, C. C. (1982). Transtheoretical therapy: Toward a more integrative model of change. *Psychotherapy: Theory, Research, and Practice, 19,* 276–288.

Prochaska, J. O., & DiClemente, C. C. (1983). Stages and processes of self-change of smoking: Toward an integrative model of change. *Journal of Consulting and Clinical Psychology, 51,* 390–395.

Prochaska, J. O., & DiClemente, C. C. (1985). Common processes of self-change in smoking, weight control, and psychological distress. In S. Shiffman & T. A. Wills (Eds.), *Coping and substance use.* (pp. 367–386). Orlando, FL: Academic Press.

Rose, J. E., Jarvick, M. E., & Rose, K. D. (1984). Transdermal administration of nicotine. *Drug and Alcohol Dependency, 13,* 209–213.

Ritenbaugh, C. (1992). Smoking and weight control among adolescent females: Implications for prevention *Proceedings of the 13th Annual Convention of the Society of Behavioral Medicine, 63,* (Abstract).

Rush, D., & Cassano, P. (1983). Relationship of cigarette smoking and social class to birth weight and perinatal mortality among all births. *Journal of Epidemiology and Community Health, 37,* 249–255.

Sachs, D.P.L., & Benowitz, N. L. (1990). The nicotine withdrawal syndrome: Nicotine absence or caffeine excess? In L. S. Harris (Ed.), *Problems of drug dependency.* National Institute on Drug Addiction Research Monograph Series.

Schecter, D., Bachman, G. A., Vaitukaitus, J., Phillips, D., & Saperstein, D. (1989). Perimenstrual symptoms: Time course of symptom intensity in relation to endocrinologically defined segments of the menstrual cycle. *Psychomatic Medicine, 51,* 173–194.

Schwartz, J. L. (1987, April). *Review and Evaluation of Smoking Cessation Methods: U.S. and Canada 1978–1985.* U.S. Department of Health and Human Services, Public Health Service (National Institutes of Health Publication No. 87-2940). Washington, DC: U.S. Government Printing Office.

Shiffman, S. (1984). Coping with temptations to smoke. *Journal of Consulting and Clinical Psychology, 52,* 261–267.

Shiffman, S. (1986). A cluster-analytic classification of smoking relapse episodes. *Addictive Behaviors, 11,* 295–307.

Shiffman, S. (1992). Smoking: New directions in clinical research. *Proceedings of the 13th Annual Convention of the Society of Behavioral Medicine,* 29 (Abstract).

Shiffman, S., & Jarvick, M. E. (1987). Situational determinants of coping in smoking relapse crises. *Journal of Applied Social Psychology, 17,* 3–15.

Somani, S. M., & Gupta, P. (1988). Caffeine: A new look at an age-old drug. *International Journal of Clinical Pharmacology, Therapy, and Toxicology, 26,* 521–533.

Steinberg, J. L., & Cherek, D. R. (1989). Menstrual cycle and cigarette smoking behavior. *Addictive Behaviors, 14,* 173–179.

Stolerman, I. P., Goldfarb, T., Fink, R., & Jarvik, M. E. (1973). Influencing cigarette smoking with nicotine antagonists. *Psychopharmacologia, 28,* 247–259.

Stone, A. A., & Neal, J. M. (1984). New measure of daily coping: Development and preliminary results. *Journal of Personality and Social Psychology, 46,* 802–806.

Sussman, S., Dent, C. W., Mestel-Rauch, J., Johnson, C. A., Hansen, W. B., & Flay, B. R. (1988). Adolescent nonsmokers, triers, and regular smokers estimates of cigarette smoking prevalence: When do overestimates occur and by whom? *Journal of Applied Social Psychology, 18,* 537–551.

Swan, F., Denk, C., Parker, S., Carmelli, D., Furze, C., & Rosenman, R. (1988). Risk behaviors for late relapse in male and female ex-smokers. *Addictive Behaviors, 13,* 253–256.

Tonnesen, P., Fryd, V., Hansen, M., Helsted, J., Gunnersen, A. B., Forchammer, H., & Stockner, M. (1988). Effect if nicotine chewing gum in combination with group counseling on the cessation of smoking. *New England Journal of Medicine, 318,* 15–18.

Tonnesen, P., Norregaard, J., Simonsen, K., & Sawe, U. (1991). A double-blind trial of a 16-hour transdermal nicotine patch in smoking cessation. *New England Journal of Medicine, 325,* 311–315.

Transdermal Nicotine Study Group. (1991). Transdermal nicotine for smoking cessation: Six-month results from two multicenter controlled clinical trials. *Journal of the American Medical Association, 266,* 3133–3138.

Tye, J. B., Warner, K. E., & Glantz, S. A. (1987, Winter). Tobacco advertising and consumption: Evidence of a causal relationship. *Journal of Public Health Policy,* 492–507.

U.S. Department of Health, Education, and Welfare. (1979). *Health: United States.* U.S. Department of Health, Education, and Welfare, Public Health Service, Office of the Assistant Secretary for Health, Office on Smoking and Health. Washington, DC: U.S. Government Printing Office.

U.S. Department of Health and Human Services. (1986). *The health consequences of involuntary smok-*

ing: A report of the Surgeon General (DHHS Publication No. CDC 86-8397). Washington, DC: U.S. Government Printing Office.

U.S. Department of Health and Human Services. (1987). *Smoking, tobacco, and health* (DHHS Publication No. CDC 87-8397). Washington, DC: U.S. Government Printing Office.

U.S. Department of Health and Human Services. (1988). *The health consequences of smoking.* A report of the Surgeon General (DHHS Publication No. 88-8406). Washington, DC: U.S. Government Printing Office.

U.S. Department of Health and Human Services. (1989). *Reducing the health consequences of smoking.* A report of the Surgeon General (DHHS Publication No. CDC 89-8411). Washington, DC: U.S. Government Printing Office.

U.S. Department of Health and Human Services. (1990). *The health benefits of smoking cessation.* A report of the Surgeon General (DHHS Publication No. CDC 90-8416). Washington, DC: U.S. Government Printing Office.

U.S. Department of Health and Human Services. (1980). *The health consequences of smoking for women.* A report of the Surgeon General (DHHS Publication No. CDC 80-8397). Washington, DC: U.S. Government Printing Office.

Wadden, T. A., Stunkard, A. J., Rich, L., Rubin, C. J., Sweidel, G, & McKinney, S. (1990). Obesity in black adolescent girls: A controlled clinical trial of treatment by diet, behavior modification, and parental support. *Pediatrics, 85,* 345–352.

Weekley, C. K., Klesges, R. C., & Relyea, G. (1992). Smoking as a weight control strategy and its relationship to smoking status. *Addictive Behaviors, 17,* 259–271.

Williamson, D. F., Madans, J., Anda, R. F., Kleinman, J. C., Giovino, G. A., & Byers, T. (1991). Smoking cessation and severity of weight gain in a national cohort. *New England Journal of Medicine, 324,* 739–745.

Wingerd, J., & Sponzilli, E. E. (1977). Concentrations of serum protein fractions in white women: Effects of age, weight, smoking, tonsillectomy, and other factors. *Clinical Chemistry, 23,* 1310–1317.

8

Obesity
A Health Psychology Perspective

Matthew M. Clark and Michael G. Goldstein

INTRODUCTION

Obesity is a public health problem because of the medical complications associated with it, its prevalence, and recidivism following treatment (Brownell & Wadden, 1992). Presence of obesity correlates with hypertension, diabetes mellitus, certain forms of cancer, cardiovascular disease, sleep apnea, arthritis, gout, and gall bladder disease (Hubert, Feinleib, McNamara, & Castelli, 1983). Approximately 25% of the American population is obese, and obesity is rapidly becoming the most common form of nutritional imbalance in some Third World countries, such as Kenya (Atkinson, 1990). Treatment studies have yielded high attrition rates and poor long-term results (Hovell et al., 1988; Wadden, Stunkard, & Liebschutz, 1988). Obesity involves a complex interaction of physiological, genetic, psychological, sociocultural, and environmental factors. Recently, individual differences that may influence patient treatment-matching recommendations have received attention (Brownell & Wadden, 1992). This chapter reviews the literature and discusses guidelines for patient–treatment matching for obese adults.

DEFINITION OF OBESITY

Obesity is an excess of body fat. However, direct measurement of body fat is impractical for most clinicians (Kraemer, Berkowitz, & Hammer, 1990). The most widely indirect measurement used in America is the Metropolitan Life Insurance

---

Matthew M. Clark and Michael G. Goldstein • Department of Psychiatry and Human Behavior, The Miriam Hospital, and Brown University School of Medicine, Providence, Rhode Island 02906.
Handbook of Health and Rehabilitation Psychology, edited by Anthony J. Goreczny. Plenum Press, New York, 1995.

Company Height–Weight Tables (Andres, Elahi, Tobin, Muller, & Brant, 1985). These tables provide ranges of desirable weight by gender, height, and build. Use of these tables, however, limits international comparisons, and appropriateness of what is "desirable" is controversial (Kraemer et al., 1990). Body mass index (BMI), weight in kilograms divided by height in meters squared (kg/m^2), appears to be the best indirect measure available to clinicians because it is reliable, valid, and facilitates comparisons between studies. However, different scientists have used different BMI ranges in defining obesity (Sichieri, Everhart, & Hubbard, 1992). It appears that most scientists agree that a BMI > 30 denotes medically significant obesity (Blackburn & Kanders, 1987) and a BMI < 25 indicates a lean individual, but a consensus does not exist on classification of a BMI in the range 25–30 (Sichieri et al., 1992). This lack of consensus leads to confusion in interpreting research findings. Given high recidivism following weight loss and potential for health consequences subsequent to weight regain, careful assessment of individuals who are 5% to 20% overweight is necessary to accurately determine if these individuals are obese and if treatment is appropriate (Garner & Wooley, 1991). To further complicate this issue, recent research has indicated that relative to amount of body fat, distribution of body fat may have as much or more influence on health status. Upper-body obesity, or abdominal obesity, relates to cardiovascular disease, diabetes, and cholesterol more than does lower-body obesity, or gluteal–femoral obesity. These relationships are independent of BMI (Haffner, Mitchell, Stern, Hazuda, & Patterson, 1992; Seidell et al., 1992).

CAUSES OF OBESITY

Genetic Factors

Researchers have demonstrated that there is a strong genetic component to obesity (Brownell & Wadden, 1992). For example, identical twins are more similar than fraternal twins on BMI regardless of whether they grew up together or apart (Stunkard, Harris, Pedersen, & McClearn, 1990). Genetic factors appear to strongly influence both fat distribution (Bouchard et al., 1990) and metabolic rate (Ravussin et al., 1988). Stunkard et al. (1990), in reviewing the literature, concluded that genetic factors may account for as much as 70% of the variance in BMI.

Physiological Factors

Relationship between energy expenditure and energy intake ultimately determines gain or loss of body mass. The major determinants of 24-hour energy expenditure (24EE) are resting metabolic rate (RMR), thermic effect of food (TEF), and thermic effect of physical activity. RMR and TEF account for about 70% and 10%, respectively, of daily energy expenditure in sedentary individuals (Ravussin & Bogardus, 1992). Prospective studies have demonstrated that low RMR, controlled for body weight and composition, is a risk factor for subsequent weight gain and development of obesity. Although the main determinant of RMR is fat-free body mass, there are considerable differences in RMR between individuals that age, gender, or fat-free body mass cannot explain. Genetic factors may be important mediators of these differences. Research has also demonstrated that TEF is lower in obese individuals relative to normal-weight people, although it is unclear whether this represents a cause or consequence of obesity (Segal, Lacayanga, Dunaif, Gutin, & Pi-Sunyer, 1989).

Several interactive physiological systems, including the brain and its neurotransmitters, the gastrointestinal tract, the endocrine system, and adipose tissue together mediate regulation of body weight (Vasselli & Maggio, 1988). Vasselli and Maggio hypothesized that size and number of fat cells influence regulation of appetite and body weight. Their research has suggested that when fat cells diminish in size as a result of weight loss, feeding increases. Because most obese individuals have an increased number of fat cells, and because dieting cannot decrease total fat cell number, physiological mechanisms that seek to maintain lipid stores by preventing a reduction in fat cell size may inhibit efforts to achieve and maintain weight loss.

Several medical conditions can cause or contribute to obesity. these include endocrine disorders, such as hypothyroidism, Cushing's syndrome, hyperinsulinism, hypogonadism, growth hormone deficiency, hypothalamic syndromes, polycystic ovary syndrome, and pseudohypoparathyroidism (Bray, 1989). Obesity also relates to several rare genetic syndromes characterized by dysmorphic features, reproductive abnormalities, and varying degrees of mental retardation (Bray, 1989). Many medications appear related to weight gain, especially psychoactive medications (e.g., tricyclic antidepressants, phenothiazines, lithium), antihistamines, steroids, estrogens, and progesterone (Bray, 1989; Clark, Ruggiero, Pera, Goldstein, & Abrams, 1993).

Nicotine intake is another important physiological determinant of weight. Smokers weigh less than nonsmokers; nonsmokers who start smoking lose weight, and most smokers gain weight following smoking cessation (Klesges, Benowitz, & Meyers, 1991). Weight gain associated with smoking cessation results, in part, from the increase in metabolic rate associated with nicotine administration (Klesges et al., 1991). Nicotine's anorectic properties may also contribute to its effects on food intake.

Psychological Factors

General personality or psychological characteristics do not distinguish groups of obese individuals from groups of nonobese individuals (Moore & Rodin, 1986; Sallade, 1973; Wise & Gordon, 1977). However, psychological distress (Fitzgibbon & Kirschenbaum, 1991), psychiatric comorbidity (Agras, 1991), or binge eating (Marcus, Wing, & Hopkins, 1988) may influence weight status of a subgroup of obese individuals.

Binge Eating Disorder is rapid consumption of a large amount of food in a discrete period of time (DSM-IV; American Psychiatric Association, 1994) plus perceived loss of control during binge episodes. Frequently, binge eaters experience negative affect and make negative self-statements subsequent to a binge episode (Wilson, Nonas, & Rosenblum, 1993). Obese binge eaters report a greater sense of loss of control over eating, a greater fear of not being able to resist eating, a greater fear of gaining weight, more dissatisfaction with their weight, and more avoidance of seeing their bodies than nonbinging obese individuals. Furthermore, there is a higher prevalence of psychiatric comorbidity in obese binge eaters (Marcus et al., 1990) and greater psychological disturbance as measured by the MMPI (W. Dahlstrom, Welsch, & L. Dahlstrom, 1972) compared to nonbinging obese individuals.

Subsequently, obese binge eaters lose less weight (Keefe, Wychogrod, Weinberger, & Argas, 1984) and are more likely to drop out of the treatment (Marcus,

Wing, & Hopkins, 1988) compared to nonbinging obese individuals. Although estimates of binge eating in obese populations seeking treatment in hospital and university-based weight-management programs range from 20% to 55% (Telch, Agras, Rossiter, Wilfley, & Kenardy, 1990), prevalence of binge eating in a community sample of obese individuals may be as low as 2% (Spitzer et al., 1993). Further research is necessary to assess prevalence of binge eating in the general obese population and to clarify interrelationships of binge eating, psychopathology, psychological distress, and treatment outcome.

A subset of obese binge eaters purge, fast, overexercise, or use diuretics or laxatives to compensate for binge episodes, and these individuals, therefore, may meet criteria for bulimia nervosa. Stunkard (1986) estimated that up to 5% of obese individuals who seek treatment for weight management meet these criteria. Additionally, Stunkard found that up to 10% of obese individuals in treatment programs meet criteria for night-eating syndrome, characterized by morning anorexia, evening hyperphagia, and insomnia.

Courtois (1988) associated bulimia and compulsive overeating with a history of sexual abuse, and our clinical experience confirms this hypothesis. Obesity may have the psychologically positive effect of minimizing sexual contact (either verbal or physical) and enhancing feelings of safety or security. Subsequently, weight loss may cause psychological distress as individuals experience increased sexual attention from others, increased feelings of vulnerability, or increased numbers of flashbacks. However, these difficulties do not apply to all obese individuals who have histories of sexual abuse; therefore, further research is necessary to clarify which individuals may experience psychological distress subsequent to weight loss.

Physical Activity

Obese individuals are less physically active than lean individuals (Brownell & Wadden, 1992; Romieu et al., 1988). However, whether these findings are a cause or consequence of obesity is unclear. What is clear is that exercise increases energy expenditure, suppresses appetite, improves psychological and cardiovascular functions (Doyne et al., 1987; Paffenbarger, Hyde, Wing, & Steinmetz, 1984; Pavlou et al., 1989b), enhances weight loss, and improves maintenance results (Pavlou, Krey, & Steffee, 1989a).

Energy Intake

It is unclear whether obese individuals differ (i.e., eat more) from lean individuals in amount of calories they consume. Studies examining caloric intake of obese and nonobese individuals have failed to report differences in reported intake or differences in accuracy of their reporting of caloric intake (Klesges, Hanson, Eck, & Durff, 1988). Researchers have examined both total caloric intake and dietary fat intake. Because human bodies convert dietary fat to body fat more efficiently than our bodies convert carbohydrates to body fat (Dreon et al., 1988), increased fat intake may contribute to development of obesity. Dreon and colleagues reported that while total caloric intake did not relate to percent body fat, fat intake did positively correlate with percent body fat. In a separate sample of 141 females, total caloric intake did not correlate with relative weight, but a higher intake of fat did relate to relative weight (Romieu et al., 1988). Curb and Marcus (1991) reported that total caloric intake did not correlate to differences in BMI or subscapular skinfold thickness but that fat intake did positively correlate to BMI and skin folds. Therefore, although total caloric intake may not differ between obese and nonobese individuals, obese individuals may have higher fat intakes than nonobese individuals.

Summary

The preceding sections describe a myriad of factors that contribute to the etiology of obesity. Although genetic factors likely account for a large percentage of the variance in BMI, a complex web of psychological, behavioral, sociocultural, and physiological factors influence development and clinical course of obesity. Identifying and understanding similarities and differences among obese individuals is a challenge for both researchers and clinicians. The complex nature of obesity underscores the importance of multidimensional assessment and treatment and suggests that patient–treatment matching may be an integral component of clinical care.

TREATMENT

Goals of Treatment

Medical Goals

Although a consensus panel at the National Institutes of Health (1985) recommended weight reduction for individuals with body weights in excess of 20%, there is little evidence to suggest that weight loss results in decreases in mortality (National Institutes of Health Technology Assessment Conference Panel, 1992). However, incidence and severity of non-insulin-dependent diabetes mellitus and hypertension in overweight individuals do decrease in response to weight loss. Weight loss has positive effects on lipid levels, and, among very obese individuals, weight loss may result in improved functional status and decreased incidence and severity of sleep apnea.

Because weight loss is not without risk (National Institutes of Health Technology Assessment Conference panel, 1991), we believe it is best for clinicians to limit weight loss treatment to individuals who are more than 20% overweight (or with a BMI greater than 28) or who have current health problems that may decrease in response to weight loss. The goal of weight-loss programs must not be to attain individuals' "ideal weights" or even to achieve weights below the level of obesity. More modest goals, such as improving health or functional status and decreasing reliance on medications (e.g., antihypertensives, oral hypoglycemic agents), are more realistic and appropriate. To decrease risk of adverse effects, weight-loss programs must limit rate of weight loss and provide medical monitoring and supervision, especially when programs include caloric restriction or when individuals have conditions (e.g., diabetes, hypertension, cardiac disease, gallstones) that increase risks of weight loss.

Nutritional Goals

Diet has a significant influence on health (Surgeon General's Report on Nutrition and Health, 1988). In fact, 5 of the top 10 causes of death in the United States—

coronary heart disease (CHD), some types of cancer, stroke, diabetes mellitus, and atherosclerosis—relate to dietary intake. It is difficult to determine exact causal relationships, but a diet that is high in caloric, fat, cholesterol, and sodium intake and low in complex carbohydrates and fiber appears to contribute significantly to the diseases listed in the Surgeon General's Report on Nutrition and Health. As stated earlier, fat intake relates to degree of obesity, and, from 1910 to 1976, Americans increased their fat intake by 31% (Dreon et al., 1988).

Because increasing consumption of foods rich in complex carbohydrates and fiber and reducing consumption of total fat, saturated fat, and cholesterol may lead to improved health, one goal of treatment must be to improve nutritional intake. Furthermore, because high fat intake, rather than excessive caloric intake, characterizes obesity, weight management programs must include education about importance of nutrition and strategies for diet compositional changes (Miller, 1991).

Physical Activity Level

Increased physical activity improves individuals' health statuses, and exercise plays a crucial role in weight loss and weight maintenance. Paffenbarger and colleagues (1984, 1986) reported in an analysis of 16,936 Harvard alumni that exercise level inversely related to death from all causes, cardiovascular diseases (including CHD and stroke), and respiratory diseases. The benefit of exercise was independent of other lifestyles factors: obesity, smoking, or hypertension. Exercise also increases feelings of well being. Doyne and colleagues (1987) demonstrated effectiveness of an exercise program in the treatment of clinical depression. The authors randomly assigned 40 women to 8-week running (aerobic), weightlifting (nonaerobic), or wait-list control conditions. Both exercise conditions significantly reduced depression, as measured by the Beck Depression Inventory and the Hamilton Rating Scale for Depression. Clearly, increasing physical activity level has a positive impact upon physical and psychological health. Additionally, exercise has specific advantages for weight management. Exercise increases energy expenditure, improves metabolism, reduces body fat, reduces appetite, minimizes loss of lean tissue during weight loss, increases weight loss, and predicts success in weight-loss programs (Brownell, 1984; Pavlou et al., 1989b). Pavlou et al. (1989a) reported that individuals who exercised at least three times per week are successful in maintaining weight loss. Craighead and Blum (1989) reported that subjects who participated in a combined behavior therapy and supervised exercise program maintained significantly larger weight loss at a 1-year follow-up compared to a standard behavioral intervention that included exercise contracting. Finally, Wing and colleagues (1988) reported that participation in a supervised exercise program improved weight loss and weight maintenance (1-year follow-up) following a 10-week behavioral intervention.

Psychological and Behavioral Goals

Eating Habits

As stated earlier, some obese individuals experience episodes of binge eating. Because feelings of self-condemnation, guilt, and shame frequently follow binge episodes, reduction in frequency of binge episodes will likely be beneficial to those individuals who engage in binge eating. It may be that establishment of regular healthy eating habits will reduce frequency of binge episodes and lower the levels of dysphoria associated with binge eating (Telch et al., 1990).

Body Image

Research has consistently documented existence of negative attitudes toward fatness and discrimination toward obesity (Wright & Whitehead, 1987). The ideal body in our culture is both thin and physically fit (Brownell, 1991). Brownell stated that there are two widely held assumptions regarding body shape: (1) with the right combination of diet and exercise, every individual can reach their ideal; and (2) upon reaching this ideal, individuals will receive rewards. These beliefs can affect obese individuals in two ways: first, they may experience negative body image as a consequence of their obesity; and, second, they may set unreasonably thin goal weights for themselves. Not all obese individuals experience negative body image, but a subpopulation does report body image disturbance (Stunkard & Wadden, 1992). For some individuals, losing weight improves body image, whereas others may benefit from treatment specifically addressed at improving body image. Setting unrealistic goal weights may contribute to attrition, a sense of failure, low self-esteem, and even weight regain (Brownell, 1991; Brownell & Wadden, 1992). The challenge in this area is to assist individuals in challenging society's negative perception of obesity and to help individuals reduce potential consequences of negative body image. Brownell and Wadden (1992) recommended that clinicians assist patients in setting realistic goals, and the authors compiled questions clinicians can ask to assist in this area. They recommended that clinicians inquire about family history of obesity, the lowest weight an individual has maintained as an adult, clothing size, and feelings about appearance to assist clients in establishing a reasonable goal weight.

Psychological Status

In general, obese individuals do not differ from nonobese individuals on measures of psychopathology. However, our society does discriminate against obesity (Wadden & Stunkard, 1985), and some obese individuals report psychological distress secondary to their obesity. Some obese individuals experience distress for more general reasons (e.g., relationship issues, employment issues). Participation in a behavioral weight-management program usually results in decreased anxiety and depression. Marcus et al. (1988) reported that subjects experienced a reduction in psychological distress (as measured by the Beck Depression Inventory and the Symptom Checklist-90) following a 10-week behavioral weight-control program. However, we do not fully understand the psychological changes associated with weight loss, and further research is necessary to clarify how weight loss affects general psychological status.

Comprehensive Assessment

Given the complexity of obesity and importance of individual needs, treatment teams must complete comprehensive assessment to determine treatment goals and make decisions about the most appropriate interventions. We recommend that practitioners assess: (1) psychological factors, (2) physiological factors, (3) activity level, and (4) nutritional intake.

Psychological Evaluation

As described earlier in this chapter, psychological distress, psychiatric comorbidity, binge eating, purging, body image, history of sexual abuse, and goal weight may all impact treatment outcome. Therefore, clinicians must assess these areas. To accomplish this goal, we recommend that clinicians complete a standard psychosocial assessment with special attention focused on assessment of potential body image disturbance, binge eating, purging, night eating, or substance abuse. Upon assessment, questions about treatment expectations are appropriate. Some individuals may have unreasonable expectations, either in terms of goal weight or necessary (or lack thereof) lifestyle changes, or regarding other areas of their lives (e.g., personal relationships, self-esteem, mood, or professional goals) that they anticipate will change subsequent to weight loss. Exploration of any negative consequences of previous weight-loss experiences and potential changes in relationships is appropriate. Treatment is frequently in group settings; therefore, clinicians must ask individuals about previous group experiences and assess them regarding appropriateness for group treatment (i.e., personality disorders). Presence of psychiatric comorbidity is not necessarily a contraindication to weight loss, provided individuals are in adjunctive treatment for their comorbid psychiatric disorders and their current level of functioning does not prohibit adherence (i.e., actively psychotic individuals or individuals abusing alcohol). For individuals in treatment with other mental health professionals, signing written releases of information so that therapists can communicate with one another generally enhances assessment and facilitates coordination of care.

Medical Evaluation

All patients with obesity must have medical evaluations before participating in weight-management programs. It is best if physicians who have had special training in diagnosis and treatment of obesity and who are part of a comprehensive interdisciplinary treatment program perform the evaluations. At a minimum, physicians must screen patients to (1) determine if any of the physiological factors or medical conditions listed previously as potential causes of obesity are present, (2) identify illnesses or conditions that would require more intensive medical and behavioral monitoring during active weight loss (e.g., diabetes, hypertension, gallstones, sleep apnea, pulmonary disease), (3) identify contraindications to active weight loss (e.g., acute or unstable illness), (4) determine patients' capacities to participate in an exercise program, and (5) choose the most appropriate modalities for treatment. In addition, medical evaluations provide opportunities to assess other risk factors for disease (e.g., lipid assessment). Interested readers may refer to other sources (for more detailed descriptions of the medical evaluation of obesity (Bray, 1989; Clark et al., 1993).

Activity-Level Evaluation

Increasing physical-activity level will improve weight loss and enhance weight maintenance. Assessment of individuals' current levels of structured (i.e., an aerobic class) and lifestyle (i.e., walking up stairs instead of using an elevator) activity is appropriate. Exploration of readiness to exercise and self-efficacy about ability to exercise may also provide valuable information (Marcus, Selby, Niaura, & Rossi, 1992). Prior to initiating an exercise program, patients must receive medical clearance from their physicians.

Nutritional Evaluation

Prior to intervention, it is best if individuals record their food intake. This allows assessment of current caloric, fat, sodium, and fiber intake and establishes a baseline to which clinicians can compare future food records. We recommend that individuals record food eaten, amount, calories, time, setting, and mood.

Patient–Treatment Matching

Treatment teams can use results from comprehensive assessments to appropriately match patients to treatments. There are several models for making treatment decisions: classification systems, stepped-care approaches, patient–treatment matching, and an integrated three-step decision-making process (Brownell & Wadden, 1992). An approach that integrates patients' level of obesity and their psychological/psychiatric status (see Figure 8.1) may be most appropriate, however. In general, we recommend that

1. Patients who are 0–20% overweight focus on lifestyle changes (e.g., smoking cessation, increasing activity level, or nutritional improvements).
2. Patients who are 20–40% overweight follow balanced-deficit diets.
3. Patients who are 40–100% overweight consider hospital-based very-low-calorie diet programs.
4. Patients who are greater than 100% overweight consider either hospital-based VLCD programs or surgeries.

In general, because group treatment is cost-effective and efficacious, it is the treatment modality of choice, except where contraindicated due to psychiatric comorbidity or lifestyle factors.

Treatment Modalities

There are a range of commercial treatment programs, self-help groups (e.g., Overeaters Anonymous), commercial products (over-the-counter fasting products and diet pills), and unsupervised diets (either from books or magazines) available to consumers. Data on efficacy on these programs is minimal (Brownell & Wadden, 1992). This review focuses on modalities on which empirical results are available.

Behavioral Programs

A behavioral approach, behavior therapy, behavior modification, or the more recent cognitive–behavioral therapy usually serves as the foundation for all treatment. Treatment components include self-monitoring, stimulus control, eating more slowly, disruption of eating chains, cognitive restructuring, planning non-food-related activities, exercise instruction, nutritional education, problem solving, strategies for enhancing social support, and relapse prevention training (Brownell & Wadden, 1986; Foreyt, 1987).

Caloric Intervention

Balanced-Deficit Diet. Generally, individuals receive recommendations to consume low-fat, low-sodium, high-fiber diets with 50–55% of calories from carbohydrates, 30% or less from fat, and 15–20% from protein (Wadden, Van Itallie, & Blackburn, 1990). Generally, individuals consume 1,200–1,800 calories per day (Wing, Shoemaker, Marcus, McDermott, & Gooding, 1990). Individuals must view dietary changes as lifelong lifestyle changes, not as a "diet" that someone goes "on and off" (Kayman, Bruvold, & Stern, 1990). At present, most behavior therapy and balanced-deficit diet (BDD) programs last 16–20 weeks, and the average weight loss is 1–1.5 lbs. per week (Brownell & Wadden, 1986) with about 65% of this weight loss maintained for 1 year (Brownell & Wadden, 1992). However, at 3 to 5 years, individuals have generally returned to baseline weights.

Very-Low-Calorie Diets. Diets consisting of less than 800 calories per day are very-low-calorie diets (VLCDs; Wadden, Stunkard, & Brownell, 1983). The two most common types of VLCD are the liquid protein diet, on which individuals drink a supplemented product, or the protein-sparing modified fast, on which individuals consume lean meat, fish or fowl, and vitamins. Studies have reported similar weight losses from both types of VLCD (Wadden, Stunkard, Brownell, & Day, 1985). Generally, individuals lose 2–5 lbs. per week on a VLCD (Blackburn, Lynch, & Wong, 1986). When used in comprehensive behavioral programs, patients maintain 67% of weight loss at one year (Wadden & Stunkard, 1986) but only about 20% of weight loss at 3-year follow-up (Wadden et al., 1988).

Surgical Interventions

A multidisciplinary consensus panel convened by the National Institutes of Health recommended surgical interventions for obesity only for patients who are more than 100% overweight and previously failed at least one comprehensive nonsurgical treatment program (Consensus Development Conference Panel, 1991). This panel also recommended that only a multidisciplinary team with access to medical, surgical, psychiatric, and nutritional expertise select candidates for surgery. Patients selected for surgery must be willing to adhere to postoperative regimens, make lifelong changes in their eating behaviors, and undergo lifelong medical surveillance after surgery. Finally, the panel recommended that only surgeons with substantial experience in these procedures who work in settings with adequate support for all aspects of assessment and management perform these surgeries.

Vertical banded gastroplasty (VBG) and gastric bypass are the two procedures currently believed to produce the best results and fewest complications (Consensus Development Conference Panel, 1991; Kral, 1989). A recent study found that patients receiving gastric bypass had maintained a 50% loss of excess weight at 3-year follow-up (Hall et al., 1990). Research comparing surgery with nonsurgical treatment of severe obesity is lacking, however.

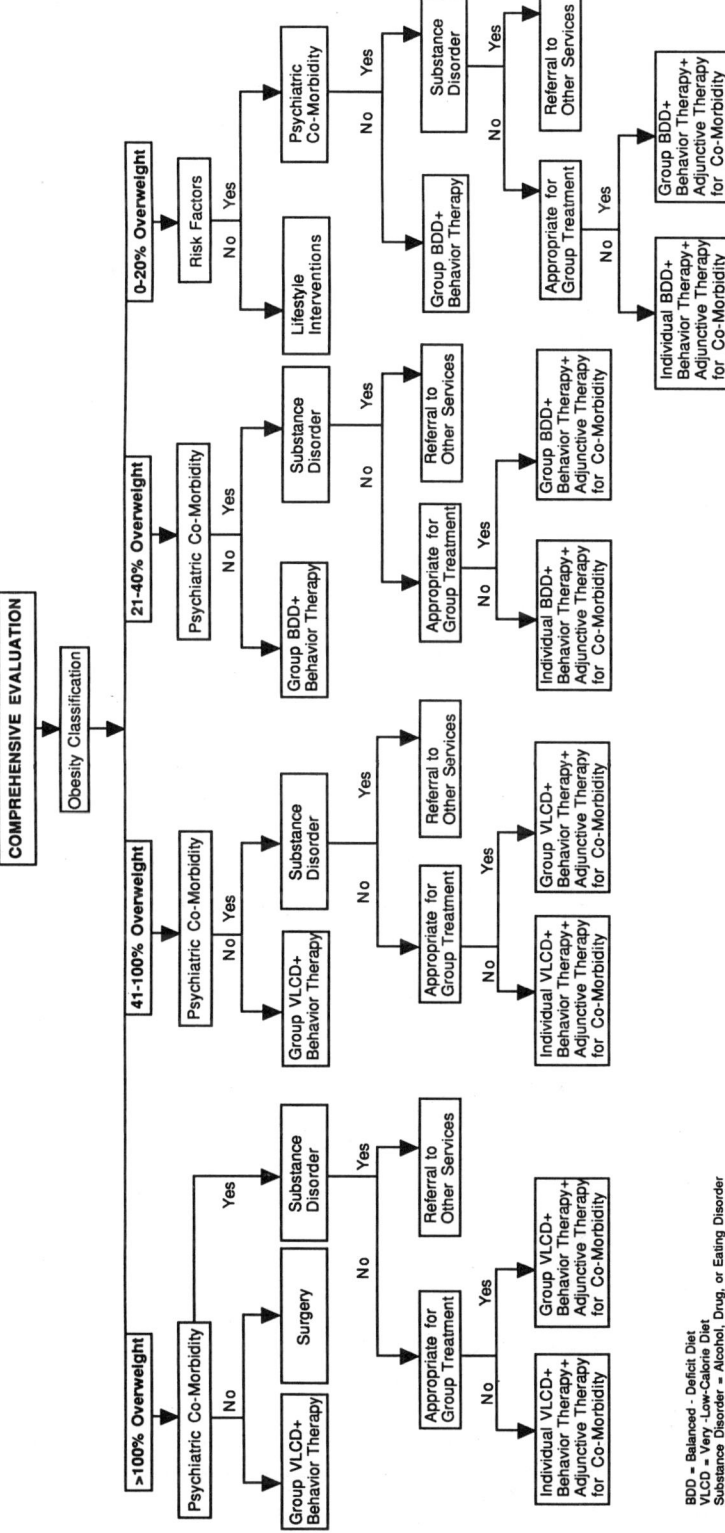

Figure 8.1. Patient–treatment matching in weight management. Adapted from Clark, Ruggiero, Pera, Goldstein, and Abrams (1993). Reprinted by permission.

Pharmacotherapy

The Food and Drug Administration (FDA) has labeled appetite-suppressing drugs as "short-term" adjunct to treatment of obesity (Bray, 1991). These drugs, which are central nervous system stimulants, produce an average weight loss of 0.6 lbs. per week more than placebo (Nauss-Karol & Sullivan, 1988). However, weight gain occurs after withdrawal of these agents, especially if patients receive pharmacological treatment without behavioral treatment (Craighead, Stunkard, & O'Brien, 1981). Moreover, they have potential to cause tolerance, withdrawal, and dependence. Some researchers have found that drugs affecting the neurotransmitter serotonin (e.g., fenfluramine, dexfenfluramine, and fluoxetine) are effective as adjuncts to obesity treatment with less abuse potential than central nervous system stimulants (Bray, 1992; Weintraub & Bray, 1989). However, weight gain also follows cessation of serotinergic agents (Bray, 1992).

There is considerable controversy as to whether weight loss clinics should use drugs chronically to treat obesity (Bray, 1991; Nauss-Karol & Sullivan, 1988). Weintraub and Bray (1989) argued that weight gain that follows cessation of appetite-suppressing drug therapy is an expected consequence of having a chronic "disease," such as obesity. They asserted that clinicians must not expect drug treatment to "cure" obesity, only to help control it. They drew parallels between use of these drugs to treat obesity and use of lipid-lowering agents to treat hypercholesterolemia. In both cases, cessation of drug therapy usually leads to reversal of treatment effects. However, these authors also noted that there are few clinical trials that demonstrate effectiveness and safety of the chronic use of these agents. Until such evidence is available, we do not recommend routine use of these agents. In all cases, treatment programs must link pharmacological therapy with behavioral and environmental interventions that address the multiple factors that produce and maintain obesity.

There are a number of other groups of medications currently under investigation for their potential benefit regarding treatment of obesity. Interested readers may refer to other sources for a discussion of potential usefulness of these agents (Bray, 1992; Nauss-Karol & Sullivan, 1988).

Weight Cycling

Research studies have indicated that weight cycling (weight loss followed by weight regain) increases abdominal obesity (Rodin, Radke-Sharpe, Rebuffe-Scrive, & Greenwood, 1990), lowers metabolic rate (Steen, Oppliger, & Brownell, 1988), and increases mortality for cardiovascular disease (Lissner et al., 1991). Other studies, however, have not found metabolic consequences (Melby, Schmidt, & Corrigan, 1990; Schotte, Cohen, & Singh, 1990) of weight cycling. Although studies have yielded conflicting results, weight-cycling may have a negative impact on physical and psychological health, and clinicians and patients must therefore be aware of potential consequences of weight cycling.

Maintenance

Recidivism among obese individuals attempting to lose weight and maintain those losses is high, as previously discussed, and we therefore recommend that

(1) treatment providers inform prospective patients of these high relapse rates, (2) treatments incorporate strategies for relapse prevention, and (3) patients participate in structured maintenance programs. However, which treatment strategies facilitate maintenance is unclear at this time. Weight loss is usually time-limited, while weight maintenance is lifelong. It may be that different skills are necessary for maintenance compared to the skills needed for weight loss. Only recently have investigators begun to examine which treatment components enhance maintenance. Wing and colleagues (1988) reported that participation in a 3-day-per-week supervised exercise program during a 10-week behavioral program improved weight maintenance at 1-year follow-up. Guare and colleagues (1989) reported that completing food records and changing eating habits assisted individuals in maintaining their weight loss. Wing, Marcus, Epstein, and Jawad (1991) demonstrated that obese women treated with their obese spouses and obese men treated alone demonstrated enhanced maintenance compared to obese women treated alone and obese men treated with their obese spouses. Perri and colleagues (1988) demonstrated effectiveness of a 1-year structured maintenance program that combined aerobic exercise, social support, therapist contact, weigh-ins, self-monitoring, and problem-solving skills. Further research is necessary to identify, in general, which treatment components facilitate maintenance and also to identify specific treatment components that facilitate maintenance for specific subgroups (e.g., male vs. female, bingers vs. nonbingers) of obese individuals.

SUMMARY

Obesity relates to increased morbidity and mortality. Genetics, physiology, nutrition, fat intake, physical activity level, culture, social support, eating habits, binge episodes, body image, psychological status, psychiatric comorbidity, substance usage, and medications all influence weight status. Recidivism following treatment is high. Perhaps greater attention to individual factors that influence weight loss or weight maintenance will improve treatment outcome. We recommend patients undergo comprehensive assessments to assist in matching of patients to treatment modalities. Practitioners need to assess potential benefits of weight loss versus potential benefits of other lifestyle changes (e.g., quitting smoking, improving self-esteem, or increasing physical activity level) and assess potential psychiatric comorbidity in making treatment recommendations. Once treatment teams make a decision to initiate weight loss, these teams may best serve patients by focusing on long-term lifestyle changes that consist of reducing dietary-fat intake, increasing physical activity level, establishing healthy eating habits, reducing frequency of binge episodes, improving body image, seeking adjunctive treatment for psychological/psychiatric issues when warranted, and making lifelong commitments to weight management.

Future research needs to examine (1) long-term strategies for increasing physical activity level in the obese population, (2) the role of binge eating in obesity, (3) exploration of different models of patient–treatment matching, (4) exploration of medications that may be beneficial, (5) strategies for improving maintenance, (6) the role of patient–treatment matching in maintenance, and (7) relationships between psychiatric comorbidity and treatment outcomes.

REFERENCES

Agras, W. S. (1991, March). *Overweight people are not all the same: How types and differences should guide interventions.* Paper presented at the Annual Convention of the Society of Behavioral Medicine, Washington, DC.

Andres, R., Elahi, D., Tobin, J. D., Muller, D. C., & Brant, L. (1985). Impact of age on weight goals. *Annals of Internal Medicine, 103,* 1030–1033.

Atkinson, R. (1990, November). *Cost-effectiveness of the treatment of obesity.* Paper presented at a Conference on Treatment of the Patient with Medically Significant Obesity, Atlanta, GA.

Blackburn, G. L., & Kanders, B. S. (1987). Medical evaluation and treatment of the obese patient with cardiovascular disease. *American Journal of Cardiology, 60,* 55G–58G.

Blackburn, G. L., Lynch, M. E., & Wong, S. L. (1986). The very-low-calorie diet: A weight-reduction technique. In K. D. Brownell & J. P. Foreyt (Eds.), *Handbook of eating disorders* (pp. 198–212). New York: Basic Books.

Bouchard, C., Tremblay, A., Despres, J.-P., Nadeau, A., Lupien, P. J., Theriault, G., Dussault, J., Moorjani, S., Pinault, S., & Fournier, G. (1990). The response to long-term overfeeding in identical twins. *New England Journal of Medicine, 322,* 1477–1482.

Bray, G. A. (1989). Classification and evaluation of the obesities. *Medical Clinics of North America, 73,* 161–183.

Bray, G. A. (1991). Barriers to the treatment of obesity. *Annals of Internal Medicine, 115,* 152–153.

Bray, G. A. (1992). Drug treatment of obesity. *American Journal of Clinical Nutrition, 55,* 538S–544S.

Brownell, K. D. (1984). Behavioral, psychological, and environmental predictors of obesity and success at weight reduction. *International Journal of Obesity, 8,* 543–550.

Brownell, K. D. (1991). Dieting and the search for the perfect body: Where physiology and culture collide. *Behavioral Assessment, 22,* 1–12.

Brownell, K. D., & Wadden, T. A. (1986). Behavior therapy for obesity: Modern approaches and better results. In K. D. Brownell & J. P. Foreyt (Eds.), *Handbook of eating disorders* (pp. 180–197). New York: Basic Books.

Brownell, K. D., & Wadden, T. A. (1991). The heterogeneity of obesity: Fitting treatments to individuals. *Behavior Therapy, 22,* 153–177.

Brownell, K. D., & Wadden, T. A. (1992). Etiology and treatment of obesity: Understanding a serious, prevalent, and refractory disorder. *Journal of Consulting and Clinical Psychology, 60,* 505–517.

Clark, M. M., Ruggiero, L., Pera, V., Goldstein, M. G., & Abrams, D. B. (1993). Assessment, classification and treatment of obesity: A behavioral medicine perspective. In A. Stoudemire & B. S. Fogel (Eds.), *Principles of medical psychiatry* (2nd ed., pp. 903–926). New York: Oxford University Press.

Consensus Development Conference Panel. (1991). Gastrointestinal surgery for severe obesity: Consensus Development Conference statement. *Annals of Internal Medicine, 115,* 956–961.

Courtois, C. (1988). *Healing the incest wound: Adult survivors in therapy.* New York: Norton.

Craighead, L. W., & Blum, M. D. (1989). Supervised exercise in behavioral treatment for moderate obesity. *Behavior Therapy, 20,* 49–59.

Craighead, L. M., Stunkard, A. J., & O'Brien, R. (1981). Behavior therapy and pharmacotherapy of obesity. *Archives of General Psychiatry, 38,* 763–768.

Curb, J. D., & Marcus, E. B. (1991). Body fat and obesity in Japanese Americans. *American Journal of Clinical Nutrition, 53,* 1552S–1555S.

Dahlstrom, W. G., Welch, G. S., & Dahlstrom, L. E. (1972). *An MMPI handbook: Vol. 1. Clinical interpretation* (2nd ed.). Minneapolis: University of Minnesota Press.

Doyne, E. J., Ossip-Klein, D. J., Bowman, E. D., Osborn, K. M., McDouglass-Wilson, I. B., & Neimeyer, R. A. (1987). Running versus weight lifting in the treatment of depression. *Journal of Consulting and Clinical Psychology, 5,* 748–754.

Dreon, D. M., Frey-Hewitt, B., Ellsworth, N., Williams, P. T., Terry, R. B., & Wood, P. D. (1988). Dietary fat: Carbohydrate ratio and obesity in middle-aged men. *American Journal of Clinical Nutrition, 47,* 995–1000.

Fitzgibbon, M. L., & Kirschenbaum, D. S. (1991). Distressed binge eaters as a distinct subgroup among obese individuals. *Addictive Behaviors, 16,* 441–451.

Foreyt, J. P. (1987). Issues in the assessment and treatment of obesity. *Journal of Consulting and Clinical Psychology, 55,* 677–684.

Garner, D. M., & Wooley, S. C. (1991). Confronting the failure of behavioral and dietary treatments for obesity. *Clinical Psychology Review, 11,* 729–780.

Guare, J. C., Wing, R. R., Marcus, M. D., Epstein, L. H., Burton, L. R., & Gooding, W. E. (1989). Analysis of changes in eating behavior and weight loss in type II diabetic patients. *Diabetes Care, 12,* 500–503.

Haffner, S. M., Mitchell, B. D., Stern, M. P., Hazuda, H. P., & Patterson, J. K. (1992). Public health significance of upper body adiposity for non-insulin-dependent diabetes mellitus in Mexican Americans. *International Journal of Obesity, 16,* 177–184.

Hall, J. C., Watts, J. M., O'Brien, P. E., Dunstan, R. E., Walsh, J. F., Slavotinek, A. H., Elmslie, R. G. (1990). Gastric surgery for morbid obesity: The Adelaide study. *Annals of Surgery, 211,* 419–427.

Hovell, M. F., Koch, A., Hofstetter, R., Sipan, C., Faucher, P., Dellinger, A., Borok, G., Forsythe, A., & Felitti, V. J. (1988). Long-term weight loss maintenance: Assessment of a behavioral and supplemented fasting regimen. *American Journal of Public Health, 78,* 663–666.

Hubert, H. B., Feinleib, M., McNamara, P. M., & Castelli, W. P. (1983). Obesity as an independent risk factor for cardiovascular disease: A 26-year follow-up of participants in the Framingham Heart Study. *Circulation, 67,* 968–977.

Kayman, S., Bruvold, W., & Stern, J. S. (1990). Maintenance and relapse after weight loss in women: Behavioral aspects. *American Journal of Clinical Nutrition, 52,* 800–807.

Keefe, P. H., Wychogrod, D., Weinberger, E., & Argas, W. S. (1984). Binge eating and outcome of behavioral treatment of obesity: A preliminary report. *Behaviour Research and Therapy, 22,* 319–321.

Klesges, R. C., Benowitz, N. L., & Meyers, A. W. (1991). Behavioral and biobehavioral aspects of smoking and smoking cessation: The problem of postcessation weight gain. *Behavior Therapy, 22,* 179–199.

Klesges, R. C., Hanson, C. L., Eck, L. H., & Durff, A. C. (1988). Accuracy of self-reports of food intake in obese and normal-weight individuals: Effects of parental obesity on reports of children's dietary intake. *American Journal of Clinical Nutrition, 48,* 1252–1256.

Kraemer, H. C., Berkowitz, R. I., & Hammer, L. D. (1990). Methodological difficulties in studies of obesity: I. Measurement issues. *Annals of Behavioral Medicine, 12,* 112–118.

Kral, J. G. (1989). Surgical treatment of obesity. *Medical Clinics of North America, 73,* 251–264.

Marcus, B. H., Selby, V. C., Niaura, R. S., & Rossi, J. S. (1992). Self-efficacy and the stages of exercise behavior change. *Research Quarterly for Exercise and Sport, 63,* 60–66.

Marcus, M. D., Wing, R. R., & Hopkins, J. (1988). Obese binge eaters: Affect, cognitions, and response to behavioral weight control. *Journal of Consulting and Clinical Psychology, 56,* 433–439.

Melby, C. L., Schmidt, W. D., & Corrigan, D. (1990). Resting metabolic rate in weight-cycling collegiate wrestlers compared with physically active noncycling control subjects. *American Journal of Clinical Nutrition, 52,* 409–414.

Miller, W. C. (1991). Diet composition, energy intake, and nutritional status in relation to obesity in men and women. *Medicine and Science in Sports and Exercise, 23,* 280–284.

Moore, R. S., & Roden, J. (1986). The influence of psychological variables in obesity. In K. D. Brownell & J. P. Foreyt (Eds.), *Handbook of eating disorders* (pp. 99–121). New York: Basic Books.

National Institutes of Health Consensus Development Panel on the Health Implications of Obesity. (1985). Health implications of obesity: National Institutes of Health Consensus Development Conference statement. *Annals of Internal Medicine, 103,* 1073–1077.

National Institutes of Health Technology Assessment Conference Panel. (1992). Methods for voluntary weight loss and control. *Annals of Internal Medicine, 116,* 942–949.

Nauss-Karol, C., & Sullivan, A. C. (1988). Pharmacological approaches to the treatment of obesity. In R. T. Frankle & M.-U. Yang (Eds.), *Obesity and weight control: The health professional's guide to understanding and treatment* (pp. 275–296). Rockville, MD: Aspen.

Paffenbarger, R. S., Hyde, R. T., Wing, A. L., & Hsieh, C.-C. (1986). Physical activity, all-cause mortality, and longevity of college alumni. *New England Journal of Medicine, 314,* 605–613.

Paffenbarger, R. S., Hyde, R. T., Wing, A. L., & Steinmetz, C. H. (1984). A natural history of athleticism and cardiovascular health. *Journal of the American Medical Association, 252,* 491–495.

Pavlou, K. N., Krey, S., & Steffee, W. P. (1989a). Exercise as an adjunct to weight loss and maintenance in moderately obese subjects. *American Journal of Clinical Nutrition, 49,* 1115–1123.

Pavlou, K. N., Whatley, J. E., Jannace, P. W., DiBartolomeo, J. J., Burrows, B. A., Duthie, E.A.M., & Lerman, R. H. (1989b). Physical activity as a supplement to a weight-loss dietary regimen. *American Journal of Clinical Nutrition, 49,* 1110–1114.

Perri, M. G., McAllister, D. A., Gange, J. J., Jordan, R. C., McAdoo, W. G., & Nezu, A. M. (1988). Effects of four maintenance programs on the long-term management of obesity. *Journal of Consulting and Clinical Psychology, 56,* 529–534.

Ravussin, E., & Bogardus, C. (1992). A brief overview of human energy metabolism and its relationship to essential obesity. *American Journal of Clinical Nutrition, 55,* 242S–245S.

Ravussin, E., Lillioja, S., Knowler, W. C., Christin, L., Freymond, D., Abbott, W.G.H., Boyce, V., Howard, B. V., & Bogardus, C. (1988). Reduced rate of energy expenditure as a risk factor for body-weight gain. *New England Journal of Medicine, 318,* 467–472.

Rodin, J., Radke-Sharpe, N., Rebuffe-Scrive, M., & Greenwood, M.R.C. (1990). Weight cycling and fat distribution. *International Journal of Obesity, 14,* 303–310.

Romieu, I., Willett, W. C., Stampfer, M. J., Colditz, G. A., Sampson, L., Rosner, B., Hennekens, C. H., & Speizer, F. E. (1988). Energy intake and other determinants of relative weight. *American Journal of Clinical Nutrition, 47,* 406–412.

Sallade, J. (1973). A comparison of the psychological adjustment of obese vs. nonobese children. *Journal of Psychosomatic Research, 7,* 89–96.

Schotte, D. E., Cohen, E., & Singh, S. P. (1990). Effects of weight cycling on metabolic control in male outpatients with non-insulin-dependent diabetes mellitus. *Health Psychology, 9,* 599–605.

Segal, K. R., Lacayanga, I., Dunaif, A., Gutin, B., & Pi-Sunyer, F. X. (1989). Impact of body fat mass and percent fat on metabolic rate and thermogenesis in men. *American Journal of Physiology, 256,* E573–E579.

Sichieri, R., Everhart, J. E., & Hubbard, V. S. (1992). Relative weight classifications in the assessment of underweight and overweight in the United States. *International Journal of Obesity, 16,* 303–312.

Spitzer, R. L., Yanouski, S., Wadden, T., Wing, R., Marcus, M. M., Stunkard, A., Devlin, M., Mitchell, J., Hasin, D., & Horne, R. L. (1993). Binge Eating Disorder: Its further validation in a multisite study. *International Journal of Eating Disorders, 13,* 137–153.

Steen, S. N., Oppliger, R. A., & Brownell, K. D. (1988). Metabolic effects of repeated weight loss and regain in adolescent wrestlers. *Journal of American Medical Association, 260,* 47–50.

Stunkard, A. J. (1986). Obesity. In R. Michels, A. M. Cooper, S. B. Guze, L. L. Juddy, G. L. Klerman, A. J. Solnit, & A. J. Stunkard (Eds.), *Psychiatry* (pp. 1–13). Philadelphia: Lippincott.

Stunkard, A. J., Harris, J. R., Pedersen, N. L., & McClearn, G. E. (1990). The body-mass index of twins who have been reared apart. *New England Journal of Medicine, 322,* 1483–1487.

Stunkard, A. J., & Wadden, T. A. (1992). Psychological aspects of severe obesity. *American Journal of Clinical Nutrition, 55,* 524S–532S.

Surgeon General's Report on Nutrition and Health: Summary and Recommendations. (1988). *Rhode Island Medical Journal, 71,* 391–401.

Telch, C. F., Agras, W. S., Rossiter, E. M., Wilfley, D., & Kenardy, J. (1990). Group cognitive–behavioral treatment for the non-purging bulimic: An initial evaluation. *Journal of Consulting and Clinical Psychology, 58,* 629–635.

Vasselli, J. R., & Maggio, C. A. (1988). Mechanisms of appetite and body-weight regulation. In R. T. Frankle & M.-U. Yang (Eds.), *Obesity and weight control: The health professional's guide to understanding and treatment* (pp. 17–34). Rockville, MD: Aspen.

Wadden, T. A., & Stunkard, A. J. (1985). Social and psychological consequences of obesity. *Annals of Internal Medicine, 103,* 1062–1067.

Wadden, T. A., Stunkard, A. J., & Brownell, K. D. (1983). Very low calorie diets: Their efficacy, safety, and future. *Annals of Internal Medicine, 99,* 675–684.

Wadden, T. A., Stunkard, A. J., Brownell, K. D., & Day, S. C. (1985). A comparison of two very-low-calorie diets: Protein-sparing-modified fast versus protein-formula-liquid diet. *American Journal of Clinical Nutrition, 41,* 533–539.

Wadden, T. A., Stunkard, A. J., & Liebschutz, J. (1988). Three-year follow-up of the treatment of obesity by very low calorie diet, behavior therapy, and their combination. *Journal of Consulting and Clinical Psychology, 56,* 925–928.

Wadden, T. A., Van Itallie, T. B., & Blackburn, G. L. (1990). Responsible and irresponsible use of very-low-calorie diets in the treatment of obesity. *Journal of the American Medical Association, 263,* 83–85.

Weintraub, M. T., & Bray, G. A. (1989). Drug treatment of obesity. *Medical Clinics of North America, 73,* 237–249.

Wilson, G. T., Nonas, C. A., & Rosenblum, G. (1993). Assessment of binge-eating in obese patients. *International Journal of Eating Disorders, 13,* 25–33.

Wing, R. R., Epstein, L. H., Paternostro-Bayles, M., Kriska, A., Nowalk, M. P., & Gooding, W. (1988). Exercise in a behavioral weight control programme for obese patients with type 2 (non-insulin-dependent) diabetes. *Diabetologia, 31,* 902–909.

Wing, R. R., Marcus, M. D., Epstein, L. H., Jawad, A. (1991). A "family-based" approach to the treatment of obese type II diabetic patients. *Journal of Consulting and Clinical Psychology, 59,* 156–162.

Wing, R. R., Shoemaker, M., Marcus, M. D., McDermott, M., & Gooding, W. (1990). Variables associated with weight loss and improvements in glycemic control in type II diabetic patients in behavioral weight control programs. *International Journal of Obesity, 14,* 495–503.

Wise, T. N., & Gordon, J. (1977). Sexual functioning in the hyperobese. *Obesity/Bariatric Medicine, 6,* 84–87.

Wright, E. J., & Whitehead, T. L. (1987). Perceptions of body size and obesity: A selected review of the literature. *Journal of Community Health, 12,* 117–129.

9

Anorexia and Bulimia Nervosa

Donald A. Williamson, Shannon B. Sebastian, and Paula J. Varnado

The eating disorders, anorexia and bulimia nervosa, have been the focus of extensive research throughout the last 15 years. This chapter discusses issues related to diagnosis, prevalence, etiology, assessment, and treatment. The emphasis is on recent research advances. A final section pertaining to future directions describes new areas of research that are emerging in the 1990s.

DIAGNOSIS AND COMORBIDITY

Sir William Gull first described anorexia nervosa as a recognized psychiatric syndrome in 1874. Throughout history, there have been reports of cases that resemble what the psychiatric community now characterizes as anorexia nervosa. The Greek physician Galen first described bulimia and termed the condition *bulimis*. Initially, clinicians regarded bulimia as a form of anorexia nervosa. In the 1960s and 1970s, bulimia received many labels, such as *bulimarexia, dysorexia,* and *dietary chaos syndrome*. In 1980, the third edition of the Diagnostic and Statistical Manual of Mental Disorders (DSM-III; American Psychiatric Association, 1980) recognized the disorder as a distinct syndrome termed *bulimia*. Thus, despite reports of anorexia and bulimia throughout the history of medicine, refinements in the operational definitions of these syndromes have occurred only since 1980. The following section reviews the changes in the defining characteristics of anorexia and bulimia nervosa that have occurred with the publication of the DSM-III and its revision DSM-III-R (American Psychiatric Association, 1987).

Donald A. Williamson, Shannon B. Sebastian, and Paula J. Varnado • Department of Psychology, Louisiana State University, Baton Rouge, Louisiana 70803.
Handbook of Health and Rehabilitation Psychology, edited by Anthony J. Goreczny. Plenum Press, New York, 1995.

DSM-III and DSM-III-R Changes

The central feature of anorexia nervosa is patients' intense fear of "fatness" that motivate extreme methods of weight loss despite often being very thin. The DSM-III-R defines *anorexia nervosa* as a disorder characterized by a refusal to maintain body weight over a minimal normal weight for age and height. An intense fear of gaining weight, body-image distortion, and amenorrhea are also requirements for a diagnosis of anorexia nervosa. The primary change in the diagnostic criteria from DSM-III to DSM-III-R was that DSM-III-R adopted less stringent weight-loss criteria (i.e., from "25% below original body weight" in DSM-III to "body weight 15% below that expected for age and height" in DSM-III-R). We recommend a criterion of 15% below normal body weight or a body mass index of less than 18 (Williamson, 1990) for this diagnostic requirement.

DSM-III first introduced the term *bulimia*. In DSM-III-R, the name of the syndrome changed to *bulimia nervosa* to reflect its relationship to anorexia nervosa. The essential feature of bulimia nervosa is recurrent episodes of binge eating that occur at least twice per week for 3 months. Following these binges, individuals utilize purgative methods (i.e., self-induced vomiting, laxative/diuretic abuse, strict dieting, and exercise) in order to prevent weight gain. Persistent concern with body size and weight must also be present for a diagnosis of bulimia nervosa (American Psychiatric Association, 1987). These DSM-III-R criteria are very different from those adopted in DSM-III. In DSM-III, extreme weight-control methods were not necessary for a diagnosis of bulimia. In order to ensure a level of clinical severity, the authors of DSM-III-R added the requirement that bingeing occur at least twice weekly for at least 3 months. DSM-III-R also includes the requirement of persistent overconcern with body shape and weight to emphasize the notion that preoccupation with body size as seen in anorexia nervosa is also present in bulimia nervosa. The authors of DSM-III-R eliminated the DSM-III requirements that self-deprecating thoughts follow a binge and awareness of an abnormal eating pattern and replaced these requirements with the necessary condition that individuals experience a feeling of "lack of control over eating behavior" during binges. One consequence of the changes in the DSM-III-R diagnostic criteria for anorexia and bulimia nervosa was the exclusion of many individuals with eating disorders to the category Eating Disorder Not Otherwise Specified. We discuss this issue later in the chapter.

Comorbidity

Depression, interpersonal sensitivity, various personality disorders, and anxiety are only a few of the additional problems that frequently accompany eating disorders (Williamson, 1990). Clinical studies have consistently found an association between eating disorders and depression (e.g., Hinz & Williamson, 1987). Williamson, Prather, Upton, Davis, Ruggiero, and Van Buren (1987) found that level of depression covaried with purging frequency.

Recent studies have found a high comorbidity of personality disorders with eating disorders. Piran, Lerner, Garfinkel, Kennedy, and Brouillete (1988) studied the presence of personality disorders in a sample of 38 bulimics and 30 anorexics. A personality disorder diagnosis was evident in 97.4% of bulimics; borderline (39.5%) and histrionic (13.5%) personality disorders were common. In the anorexic sample,

86.7% received a diagnosis of personality disorder; the most often diagnosed personality disorders were avoidant (33%) and dependent (10%) personality disorders.

Researchers have also linked anxiety to eating disorders. The most prominent anxiety is the fear of weight gain (Steere, Butler, & Cooper, 1990). Obsessive–compulsive habits are also prominent in anorexics and bulimics. Hudson, Pope, Yurgelun-Todd, Jonas, and Frankenburg (1987) found that 33% of their bulimic sample ($n = 51$) met diagnostic criteria for obsessive–compulsive disorder.

PREVALENCE OF ANOREXIA AND BULIMIA NERVOSA

Prevalence estimates of eating disorders have varied substantially due to secretiveness surrounding eating disorders and disagreements about defining characteristics of both anorexia and bulimia nervosa (Yates, 1989). Studies of prevalence have consistently reported that eating disorders are most prevalent in young females. Eating disorders are especially common among women who endure a substantial amount of scrutiny regarding physical fitness, such as athletes, ballerinas, and cheerleaders (Heatherton & Baumeister, 1991).

Earlier estimates regarding prevalence of bulimia utilized the DSM-III criteria that are less stringent than current DSM-III-R criteria. This resulted in an overestimate of the prevalence of bulimia nervosa as defined by DSM-III-R. Recent investigations have found the incidence of bulimia nervosa to be about 2–4% of young women and adolescents. For example, Rand and Kuldau (1992) estimated the incidence of bulimia nervosa, as defined by DSM-III-R criteria, by performing structured interviews of 2,115 adults in the general population. Among women aged 18 to 30 years, the incidence of bulimia nervosa was 4.1%.

Reports of anorexia nervosa have dramatically increased over the past two decades. From 1965 to 1985, prevalence estimates of anorexia nervosa nearly doubled (Jones, Fox, Babigian, & Hutton, 1980). Overall, estimates suggest that 1 out of every 100 females will develop anorexia nervosa during their lifetime. Males comprised 5% to 10% of all anorexia nervosa patients (Yates, 1989).

ETIOLOGY OF ANOREXIA AND BULIMIA NERVOSA

Psychodynamic Theories

In the 1950s, psychodynamic theories attributed eating disorders to fixation in the oral stage of development and rejection of femininity. Psychodynamic theories have conceptualized eating disorders as stemming from a need for control and interpersonal achievement. Restrictive dieting is theoretically an attempt to control one's body, especially during puberty when the body is changing rapidly (Bruch, 1985). These theories postulate that eating disorder patients fear food and weight gain due to a subconscious fear of losing control of bodily urges, such as hunger (Goodsitt, 1985).

Other psychodynamic theories propose that eating disorders stem from inadequate early mother–child interactions. Lerner (1983) suggested that food becomes a symbol for the distressed mother–child relationship, and bingeing and purging signify indecisiveness between loving and hating the mother.

Empirical evidence for psychodynamic theories of anorexia and bulimia nervosa is sparse. Strauss and Ryan (1987) investigated the proposition that anorexics and bulimics manifest poor autonomy and individuation. They found that, relative to controls, anorexics and bulimics do indeed experience more difficulty developing autonomy and individuation. However, Teusch (1988) found that bulimics are adequately autonomous. Overall, further research is necessary before theorists can make strong conclusions about the validity of psychodynamic theories of anorexia and bulimia nervosa.

Family Theories

Early family theories postulated that anorexia and bulimia nervosa were the result of destructive forces within the family. Recent family theories have observed that similar patterns of familial distress exist in families of children with eating disorders as well as in families of children with other psychological problems. Nevertheless, family theories describe families of anorexic and bulimic children as overprotective, enmeshed, rigid, and lacking in problem-solving skills. Poor communication skills and inadequate affective expression are also common family problems. Bulimic patients often report that they feel rejected, neglected, and blamed by their families (Humphrey, 1988). Relative to families of anorexic patients, families of bulimics are less cohesive, more conflictual, and more negative in daily interactions. Families of bulimics tend to have high expectations of success for their children, and such expectations result in anxiety and depression in the children (Yates, 1989).

Researchers have not yet firmly established the precise role played by family dysfunction in the etiology of eating disorders. For example, family problems may not be the cause, but rather the result of disordered eating habits. Head and Williamson (1990) found that a restrictive and conflictual family environment more strongly related to secondary psychopathology than the primary eating-disorder symptoms (e.g., bingeing, purging, body-image disturbances, etc.). Based upon existing scientific evidence, we must not assume that familial dysfunction is inevitable in families of eating-disordered patients. Nor can we conclude that family problems directly cause eating disorders.

Cognitive–Behavioral Theories

Brownell (1991) emphasized the role of emphasis on thinness as influential in the etiology of anorexia and bulimia nervosa. Physical fitness in our culture symbolizes success and acceptance. However, when physiological and genetic limitations prevent acquisition of the "ideal body," individuals develop alternative means of weight loss (e.g., vomiting, laxative abuse, or excessive exercise), and the onset of anorexia or bulimia nervosa is often the result.

In addition to the influence of sociocultural ideals, cognitive–behavioral theories maintain that anxiety about weight gain drives behaviors associated with anorexia and bulimia nervosa. Anxiety develops primarily due to distorted cognitions that stem from fear of negative evaluation, low self-esteem, attitudes toward weight, body-image distortion, and formation of rigid food rules. Prominent automatic thoughts include, "I feel fat" and "Thinness will make me happy."

Anorexics and bulimics engage in purgative behavior, excessive exercise, and dietary restriction in an attempt to control weight gain and, thus, alleviate anxiety. Anorexics attempt to avoid weight gain through restrictive eating; bulimics engage in periods of dietary restriction interrupted by bingeing and purging (Williamson, 1990).

In anorexia, dietary restraint, or starvation, results in suppressed appetite. Therefore, the anorexic is able to intake fewer calories and, at the same time, reduce anxiety about potential weight gain. In bulimia, following termination of dietary restraint, binge eating occurs due to energy deprivation, craving, and hunger. A cycle then develops in which fear of weight gain leads to purging and further dietary restraint; subsequently, hunger, emotional distress, or consumption of forbidden foods again "breaks" the period of dietary restraint, and the cycle continues.

Anxiety increases following bingeing due to fear of weight gain, and purging serves the function of reducing this anxiety. Therefore, purging occurs as an ultimate means of anxiety reduction. In bulimia, the consequences of purging include decreased nutrients in the body and lowered metabolic rate. Thus, not only does the probability of repeated bingeing increase, but when bingeing occurs, weight gain becomes more likely. Eventually a cyclical pattern of bingeing and purging develops that serves to regulate anxiety stemming from fear of fatness (Williamson, 1990).

According to most cognitive–behavioral theories of eating disorders, purgative habits and dieting get negatively reinforced by reduction of anxiety and worry about weight gain. In addition, normal hedonic effects of eating as well as reduction of negative affect theoretically maintain binge eating (Heatherton & Baumeister, 1991). Cognitive distortions about weight, body shape, and eating also presumably play a role in maintenance of anorexia and bulimia nervosa. There is ample empirical evidence in support of cognitive–behavioral models of eating disorders. Several studies of the cognitive–behavioral model of bulimia nervosa have documented that increased anxiety follows eating and decreased anxiety follows purging (see Williamson, Prather, Goreczny, Davis, & McKenzie, 1989c). Also, controlled investigations of bulimia nervosa (Dritschel, Williams, & Cooper, 1991) and anorexia nervosa (Garner & Bemis, 1982) have found evidence of distorted cognitions specific to food, eating, and body shape.

Body-Image Theories

Body-image theories are a variation of cognitive–behavioral models of anorexia and bulimia nervosa. Slade (1985) described body image as a disturbance in accuracy of perception of body image and body concept. Components of body image include distortion of body size and body-size dissatisfaction. Slade (1982) proposed that disturbances of body image are the primary motivation that determines the psychopathological behavior of anorexia and bulimia nervosa. He proposed that body image concerns function as a setting event (antecedent) and a negative reinforcer (consequence) for weight control. In Slade's model, aesthetic preference for thinness sets the occasion for dieting. Subsequent successful weight loss negatively reinforces dieting as a means to avoid fatness. Also, a patient's body image improves with weight loss, and this further reinforces restrictive eating patterns.

Rosen (1992) and Thompson (1992) have taken Slade's ideas further. Rosen suggested that eating abnormalities and weight control are essential features of eating disorders but are secondary to overconcern with shape and weight. He and Thompson have proposed that anorexia and bulimia nervosa are two manifestations of a general body-image disorder similar to body dysmorphic disorder. Thompson proposed three components to body-image disorder: affective, cognitive, and behavioral. He hypothesized that selective attention to information consistent with the belief that one has an unattractive body shape maintains body image distortions. Subsequently, negative automatic thoughts develop and contribute to low self-esteem, anxiety, and depression. Individuals dissatisfied with their body shapes may attempt to control anxiety associated with their bodies through avoidance behavior, such as not wearing revealing clothes, limiting socialization, or not allowing others to see or touch specific parts of their bodies (Rosen, 1992).

In a review of studies addressing the role of body-image disorder as a causal agent in anorexia and bulimia nervosa, Thompson (1992) found that body-image disorder had a direct effect on eating disturbance but not on global psychological functioning. Thompson concluded that the relationship between body-image disorder and eating disturbance is strong. He postulated that automatic comparison of one's body shape to an ideal shape or to the shape of others is a primary determinant of development of body-image disorder.

One prediction of body-image theory is that body image is overactive in eating disordered subjects. In a study contrasting bulimics and controls, McKenzie, Williamson, and Cubic (1993) tested this prediction. They found that following activation of weight fears, the body-image distortion of bulimics increased whereas control subjects remained unaffected. Patient ratings of ideal body size did not change in response to activation of weight fears. The authors proposed that perceived (actual) body size may be reactive to environmental variables, but ideal body size may be a stable characteristic.

Based upon current research findings, Rosen (1992) and Thompson (1992) proposed a DSM-IV category for body-image disorder. The rationale for the new category stems from current overlapping characteristics of Body Dysmorphic Disorder, Anorexia Nervosa, Bulimia Nervosa, Sexual Disorder Not Otherwise Specified, and Delusional Disorder (Somatic Type). In summary, in the past decade, empirical support for the significance of body image in the etiology and maintenance of anorexia and bulimia nervosa has flourished. Researchers, such as Rosen, have suggested that it may be more appropriate to think of anorexia and bulimia nervosa as body-image disorders. There is, however, considerable disagreement about the significance of body-image disturbances for the eating disorders (see Hsu & Sobkiewicz, 1989).

Biological Theories

Numerous physiological changes occur in anorexic and bulimic patients due to inadequate nutrition. For example, anorexic patients exhibit elevated levels of plasma cortisol, diminished rates of cortisol metabolism, and diminished responses to dexamethasone. Empirical investigations of physiological changes in anorexia and bulimia nervosa have resulted in four classes of biological theories: neurotransmitter, neuroendocrine, endorphin, and metabolic theories. A brief description of the biological correlates of anorexia and bulimia nervosa and empirical evidence in support of each theory follows.

Neurotransmitter Theories

Investigators have proposed that three different neurotransmitter systems may play a role in th etiology and maintenance of anorexia and bulimia nervosa. Neurotransmitters hypothetically involved include norepinephrine, serotonin, and endogenous opiates. Norepinephrine and serotonin theories rely on evidence that anorexics and bulimics, relative to non-eating-disordered individuals, have low levels of these two neurotransmitters (Fava, Copeland, Schweiger, & Herzog, 1989). In low-weight patients, norepinephrine and serotonin levels return to normal shortly after initial weight gain. Evidence reported by Yates (1989) found low levels of norepinephrine in anorexic women at long-term follow-up. Researchers have not yet offered acceptable explanations for this finding. Other neurotransmitter theories have proposed that insatiety during binge episode reflects deficiencies in serotonin. Evidence in support of this theory shows that bulimic patients exhibit a slower turnover rate of serotonin than do anorexic patients (Kaye, Ebert, & Gwirtsman, 1984).

Endogenous-opiate neurotransmitter theories propose that elevated opiates in the cerbrospinal fluid (CSF) of anorexic patients result in inhibition of catecholamines and luteinizing hormone (Garfinkel & Kaplan, 1985). When nondieting individuals receive beta endorphins, appetite increases. During periods of starvation, increased levels of opiates appear to decrease appetite. However, opiate antagonists have not been effective in reducing preoccupation with dieting, fear of weight gain, and resistance to treatment among eating-disordered patients (Yates, 1989).

Neuroendocrine Theories

Neuroendocrine theories of anorexia and bulimia nervosa consist of corticotropin releasing hormone (CRH) and peptide hormone theories. CRH theory attributes dietary restriction in anorexia nervosa to elevated concentrations of CRH in the CSF. Evidence reported by Fava et al. (1989) found CRH levels in the CSF of 7 anorexia nervosa patients were significantly higher than CRH levels of controls.

In bulimia nervosa, neuroendocrine theories explain that the absence of satiation in binge episodes results from insufficient secretion of the peptide hormone cholecystokinin, a hormone that reduces food intake in laboratory animals (Fava et al., 1989). A recent study by Geracioti and Liddle (1988) found that following ingestion of a liquid meal, cholecystokinin levels were significantly lower in a group of bulimic patients than in control subjects.

Endorphin Theories

Endorphin theories propose that purgative behavior in bulimic patients results in increased levels of plasma beta endorphin. Yates (1989) suggested that elevated levels of endorphins may result from vomiting, rapid caloric intake, or stress experienced by the stomach muscles. The release of endorphins creates the sensation of euphoria experienced by some bulimic patients after vomiting or excessive exercise. Some investigators have conceptualized bulimia nervosa as an addictive disorder. According to this conceptualization, the disorder perpetuates due to a recurring desire for the euphoria that results from endorphin release.

Metabolic Theories

Metabolic theories have examined the effects of weight change on cerebral glucose metabolism. Herholz and Emrich (1987) concluded that caudate metabolism is greater bilaterally when anorexics are at a low weight relative to measurements following weight gain. These authors suggested that a global increase in brain metabolism explains the clinical observation of hypervigilance in anorexic patients.

In summary, strong evidence exists in support of the role of neuroendocrine systems in eating. Although data from animal studies appear promising, further research on humans is necessary. Schlundt and Johnson (1990) suggested that future investigations of physiological mechanisms of anorexia and bulimia nervosa strive for a unified physiological conceptualization of the two disorders because it is unlikely that two separate feedback systems mediate anorexia and bulimia nervosa.

Genetic Theories

Family Studies

Clinical observation of family resemblance in body composition, body shape, and bone structure lends support to the hypothesis that eating disorders aggregate in families and that genetics may play a role. In an extensive review of research to date, Schlundt and Johnson (1990) concluded that anorexia nervosa is more common in families in which a female relative suffers from an eating disorder. However, researchers have not firmly established how the transmission of genetic characteristics occurs.

Twin Studies

Twin studies have investigated the genetic transmission of anorexia and bulimia. In anorexia nervosa, concordance rates for monozygotic pairs have ranged from 44% to 50% as compared to dizygotic pairs averaging 7% (Scott, 1986). Researchers have found lower concordance estimates for bulimia nervosa. Kendler, MacLean, Neale, Kessler, Heath, and Eaves (1991) found a bulimia concordance rate of 23% for monozygotic pairs and 9% for dizygotic pairs. Although these results appear promising, investigators have not yet conducted studies examining twins reared apart. Therefore, an environmental confound exists because it is possible that learning experiences of monozygotic twins were more similar than those of dizygotic twins.

Overall, empirical evidence from familial and genetic studies suggests that there may be genetic transmission of a determinant of anorexia and bulimia nervosa and that this determinant is more likely to affect females and identical twins. The precise transmitted characteristic is unclear, however. Genetic vulnerability may predispose individuals to personality type, psychiatric disturbance, body-image disturbance, or hypothalamic dysfunction.

ASSESSMENT OF ANOREXIA AND BULIMIA NERVOSA

There are many similarities between the types of eating disorders, and differential diagnosis can often be difficult. Psychometricians have developed several structured interviews, self-report symptom inventories, and body-image assessment techniques to aid in this process. Table 9.1 summarizes some of the most commonly used assessment instruments.

Table 9.1. Summary of Assessment Procedures for Eating Disorders

Name	Authors	Purpose	Description
A. Structured interviews			
CEDRI	Palmer, Christie, Cordle, Davis, & Kendrick (1987)	Assess core psychopathology of anorexia and bulimia nervosa.	35 questions; 4-point rating scale for symptoms
EDE	Cooper & Fairburn (1987)	Assess current eating disorder symptomatology. Good psychometrics.	62 questions; 7-point rating scale for symptoms
IDED	Williamson (1990)	Evaluate core psychopathology of anorexia nervosa, bulimia nervosa, and compulsive binge eating, for diagnosis using DSM-III-R criteria. Good psychometrics.	54 questions; 7-point rating scale for symptoms
B. Self-report measures			
BULIT	Smith & Thelen (1984)	Measure bulimic symptoms.	36 items; multiple choice
EAT	Garner & Garfinkel (1979)	Assess anorexic attitudes.	40 items; multiple choice
EDI	Garner & Olmstead (1984)	Measure the cognitive and behavioral components of anorexia and bulimia nervosa.	64 items; multiple choice
C. Body image measures			
BSQ	Cooper, Taylor, Cooper, & Fairburn (1987)	Assess frequency of thoughts or feelings about dissatisfaction with body shape.	34 items; self-report; 6-point frequency scale
BIATQ	Cash, Lewis, & Keeton (1987)	Measures positive and negative body-image cognitions.	52 items; 5-point rating scale
BSRQ	Butters & Cash (1987) Cash & Green (1986)	Assesses attitudes about appearance, health, and physical fitness.	140 items; 5-point rating scale
BIA	Williamson, Davis, Bennett, Goreczny, & Gleaves (1989)	Estimates of current body size, ideal body size, and discrepancy between the two.	9 silhouettes

Note: CEDRI = Clinical Eating Disorder Rating Instrument; EDE = Eating Disorder Examination; IDED = Interview for Diagnosis of Eating Disorders; BULIT = Bulimia Test; EAT = Eating Attitudes Test; EDI = Eating Disorder Inventory; BSQ = Body Shape Questionnaire; BIATQ = Body Image Automatic Thoughts Questionnaire; BSRQ = Body–Self Relations Scale; BIA = Body Image Assessment.

Structured Interviews

Only a few structured interviews are available to aid in diagnosis of eating disorders. Table 9.1 summarizes these instruments. Structured interviews allows for systematic gathering of information relevant for diagnosis, such as information about eating habits. Clinicians must also obtain relevant historical information, however.

Clinical Eating Disorder Rating Instrument

Palmer, Christie, Cordle, Davies, and Kendrick (1987) developed the Clinical Eating Disorder Rating Instrument (CEDRI) for the purpose of diagnosing anorexia and bulimia nervosa. In addition to eating behaviors and attitudes, the CEDRI assesses additional symptomatology, such as depression, anxiety, obsessions, and psychoses. The developers reported high interrater reliability, but they used a small sample size ($n = 11$) to develop the CEDRI.

Eating Disorder Examination

Cooper and Fairburn (1987) developed a structured interview that assesses patients' symptomatology over the past 4 weeks. They initially developed this semistructured interview to assess current bulimic symptomatology and to serve as a treatment-outcome measure. Research has shown that the EDE discriminates eating disorders from controls, and eating disorders from weight-preoccupied women. Five subscales exist, and psychometric research has shown adequate internal consistency.

Interview for Diagnosis of Eating Disorders

The Interview for Diagnosis of Eating Disorders (IDED) is a structured interview designed to gather information for diagnosis of anorexia and bulimia nervosa based on DSM-III-R criteria and to assess compulsive binge eating based on proposed diagnostic criteria (Williamson, 1990). The developer designed questions to assess symptoms as well as obtain a detailed history. Interviewers rate each DSM-III-R criterion on a 7-point rating scale. Williamson, Davis, Norris, and Van Buren (1990) reported that interrater reliability for symptoms (on 38 clinical subjects) was .85 or greater, and diagnostic agreement was 100% on those 38 subjects.

Self-Report Symptom Inventories

A variety of self-report inventories currently exist to assist in assessment of eating disorders. Table 9.1 summarizes characteristics of some of the commonly used measures. A complete review of these self-report inventories is beyond the scope of this chapter. Descriptions of some of the more widely used tests follow.

Bulimia Test

The Bulimia Test (BULIT; Smith & Thelen, 1984) measures symptoms of bulimia as specified by DSM-III (American Psychiatric Association, 1980). Test–retest reliability is good and concurrent validity is satisfactory. Factor analysis of the BULIT has revealed six factors: (1) vomiting; (2) bingeing; (3) negative feelings about bingeing; (4) menstrual problems; (5) preference for high-calorie, easily ingested food; and (6) weight fluctuations (Thelen, Mann, Pruit, & Smith, 1987). The BULIT recently underwent revision (BULIT-R) to accommodate to DSM-III-R criteria (Thelen, Farmer, Wonderlich, & Smith, 1991). Research has shown the BULIT-R is reliable and valid and correlates highly ($r = .99$) with the original test.

Eating Attitudes Test

The Eating Attitudes Test (EAT) assesses anorexic attitudes regarding eating (Garner & Garfinkel, 1979). The EAT contains three factors: (1) dieting, (2) bulimia and food preoccupation, and (3) oral control or restraint. It discriminates anorexics and bulimics from normals. Research has established reliability and concurrent validity of the EAT.

Eating Disorder Inventory

The Eating Disorder Inventory (EDI) measures cognitive and behavioral characteristics of anorexia and bulimia nervosa (Garner & Olmstead, 1984). The EDI contains eight subscales: (1) drive for thinness, (2) bulimia, (3) body dissatisfaction, (4) ineffectiveness, (5) perfectionism, (6) interpersonal distrust, (7) interoceptive awareness, and (8) maturity fears. The EDI yields a profile that clinicians can compare to anorexic or college-age female norms.

Body-Image Assessment

Many researchers consider the concept of body-image disturbance a core feature of anorexia and bulimia nervosa. DSM-III-R criteria for the eating disorders describe this construct as a disturbance in the way individuals experience their own body weight, size, or shape, or persistent overconcern with body shape and weight. Schlundt and Johnson (1990) concluded that, in general, women with anorexia and bulimia nervosa tend to view themselves as larger than they actually are, desire to be thinner, and feel dissatisfied with various body areas. Several assessment procedures designed to measure body-image disturbance currently exist. These include perceptual methods, questionnaires, and silhouettes.

Perceptual methods require subjects to make a judgment about the size of their body and reproduce that image. Clinicians can compute a Body Perception Index by dividing estimated size by actual size and multiplying by 100. This gives a ratio of over- or underestimation of the body or body parts. Various perceptual assessment methods exist, including (1) marking width of body parts on paper (Askevold, 1975); (2) manipulation of light beams (Ruff & Barrios, 1986); and (3) distorting lenses, mirrors, or video cameras (Touyz, Beumont, Collins, McCabe, & Jupp, 1984).

Many questionnaires are available that assess various aspects of body-image disturbance. These include the Body Shape Questionnaire (BSQ; P. Cooper, Taylor, Z. Cooper, & Fairburn, 1987), the Body Image Automatic Thoughts Questionnaire (BIATQ; Cash, Lewis, & Keeton, 1987), and the Body–Self Relations Questionnaire (BSRQ; Butters & Cash, 1987; Cash & Green, 1986). The BSQ assesses frequency of thoughts or feelings about dissatisfaction with body shape. The BIATQ measures positive and negative body-image cognitions. The BSRQ elevates attitudes about appearance, health, and physical fitness. Table 9.1 describes each of these questionnaires.

Williamson, Davis, Bennett, Goreczny, and Gleaves (1989a) developed a relatively simple measure called the Body Image Assessment (BIA). The BIA consists of nine silhouettes, on separate cards, depicting the female body. The cards range in size from very thin to very obese. Clinicians determine current body size (CBS) and ideal body size (IBS) estimates based on selection of body figures. The developers established normative data for women of differing heights and weights. This enables researchers to evaluate the extent to which the bulimics and anorexics select body silhouettes that deviate from normals. Recent research has shown that the discrepancy between CBS and IBS highly correlates with body-size dissatisfaction.

TREATMENT-OUTCOME RESEARCH

Researchers and clinicians who work with eating-disorder patients have developed several treatments for anorexia and bulimia nervosa. Controlled outcome studies that exist consist primarily of bulimic patients, however. It is very difficult to conduct controlled outcome studies for anorexia nervosa because the health risks associated with the disorder preclude the use of no-treatment or placebo control conditions. Most of the extant treatment-outcome studies have utilized cognitive–behavioral and pharmacological therapies. Table 9.2 summarizes these studies.

Psychological Therapy

Cognitive-behavior therapy (CBT) consists of cognitive therapy (CT) which focuses upon identification and alteration of irrational and dysfunctional attitudes, and behavioral components, such as stimulus control (SC) procedures and exposure with response prevention (ERP). Cognitive therapy for anorexia and bulimia nervosa attempts to modify irrational beliefs about food, weight, and body shape (Agras, Schneider, Arnow, Raeburn, & Telch, 1989; Fairburn, Kirk, O'Connor, & Cooper, 1986; Freeman, Barry, Dunkeld-Turnbull, & Henderson, 1988; Lee & Rush, 1986; Leitenberg, Rosen, Gross, Nudelman, & Vara, 1988; Wilson, Rossiter, Kleifield, & Lindholm, 1986; Wolf & Crowther, 1992; Yates & Sambrillo, 1984). Stimulus control procedures involve changing antecedent stimuli to the eating response (e.g., only eating at a certain time and place). Agras et al. (1989), Fairburn et al. (1988), Wolf and Crowther (1992), and Yates and Sambrillo (1984) have utilized SC as a component of CBT. Rosen and Leitenberg (1982) first described the use of ERP as a treatment for eating disorders. Since that time, other investigators have often included ERP as a behavioral component of treatment (Agras et al., 1989; Leitenberg et al., 1988; Wilson et al., 1986). This procedure involves prevention of the purging response that follows bingeing or eating forbidden foods. Although many of the reviewed studies utilized CBT and BT, the components of the treatments were somewhat different for each study. We discuss these differences in the review. Table 9.2 presents a summary of the controlled-outcome studies that have used cognitive–behavioral therapy.

Support for cognitive–behavioral interventions is extensive. In a review of behavioral treatments for bulimia nervosa, Rosen (1987) concluded that the average

Table 9.2. Summary of Controlled Treatment-Outcome Studies for Bulimia Nervosa

Name	Treatment(s)	Length/Follow-up	Results
A. Psychological therapy			
Lacey (1983)	BT (contracting) vs. control (dietary diary only).	10 weeks; 2 year f-u	Treatment program 93% success; 71% abstaining bingeing and purging at f-u.
Yates & Sambrillo (1984)	CT (CT, relaxation, and assertiveness) vs. CBT	6 weeks; 6 week f-u	No group differences.
Kirkley, Schneider, Agras, & Bachman (1985)	CB vs. nondirective.	16 weekly sessions	Both reduced bingeing and purging, but CBT significantly better and fewer dropouts; 38% abstained from bingeing and purging.
Lee & Rush (1986)	CBT vs. waiting-list control	6 weeks 2× weekly; 4 mo. f-u	Significant reductions in bingeing & purging; 26% abstinent.
Fairburn, Kirk, O'Connor, & Cooper (1986)	CGT vs. short-term psychotherapy.	19 sessions over 18 weeks; 12 mo. f-u	Both decreased purging; CBT better on general psychopathology and subjective state.
Wilson, Rossiter, Kleifield, & Lindholm (1986)	CT vs. CBT (CT + ERP)	16 weeks; 12 mo. f-u	CBT + ERP better at posttreatmennt and f-u; 71% of CBT + ERP reported no bingeing.
Wolchik, Weiss, & Katzman (1986)	Short-term group treatment focused on psychological problems rather than bingeing and purging.	7 weeks; 10 week f-u	Purging decreased; bingeing decreased; no improvement in waiting-list control.
Freeman, Barry, Turnbull, & Henderson (1988)	BT (graded tasks) vs. CBT vs. group (educational) vs. no treatment	15 weeks; 12 mo. f-u	All 3 treatments effective; appeared to be no advantage in adding cognitive elements; 77% stopped bingeing and purging.
Leitenberg, Rosen, Gross, Nudelman, & Vara (1988)	ERP (clinic) vs. ERP (multiple settings) vs. CBT without ERP vs. waiting-list control.	24 sessions over 14 weeks; 6 mo. f-u	All treatments effective with slight advantage for CBT + ERP for reduction of purging and bingeing on test meal.
Agras, Schneider, Arnow, Raeburn, & Telch (1989)	Waiting-list control vs. self-monitoring vs. CBT vs. CBT + ERP.	14 sessions over 12 weeks; 6 mo. f-u	All treatments effective with CBT most improvement; frequency of purging declined 77%; 56% abstinent from bingeing and purging; ERP had a deleterious effect.
Wolf & Crowther (1992)	CBT vs. BT (identifying the antecedents of bulimic behavior) vs. waiting-list control.	10 sessions 2× weekly; 3 mo. f-u	Both effective in decreasing bingeing and purging; BT maintained better at f-u; CBT evidenced additional changes.

(*continued*)

Table 9.2. (Continued)

Name	Treatment(s)	Length/Follow-up	Results
B. Pharmacotherapy			
Pope, Hudson, Jonas, & Yurgelun-Todd (1983)	Imipramine vs. placebo.	6 weeks; 1–8 mo. f-u	Imipramine 90% moderate to marked decrease in bingeing; 35% abstinent; further improvement at f-u with continued usage.
Walsh, Stewart, Gladis, & Glassman (1984)	Phenelzine vs. placebo.	8 weeks; 3–15 mo. f-u	56% of phenelzine subjects abstinent from bingeing; 60% of subjects followed relapsed after discontinuing the drug.
Hughes, Wells, Cunningham, & Ilstrup (1986)	Desipramine vs. placebo.	6 weeks; 1 mo. f-u	Desipramine decreased bingeing 91%; continued improvement with continued usage.
Agras, Dorian, Kirkley, Arnow, & Bachman (1987)	Imipramine vs. placebo.	16 weeks; no f-u	Imipramine decreased purging 72%.
Horne, Ferguson, Pope, Hudson, Lineberry, Ascher, & Cato (1988)	Bupropion vs. placebo.	8 weeks; no f-u	Bupropion decreased bingeing 67%; 30% abstinent from bingeing and purging.
Walsh, Gladis, Roose, Stewart, Stetner, & Glassman (1988)	Phenelzine vs. placebo.	10 weeks; no f-u	64% reduction in bingeing; not related to depression; 14/24 relapsed after discontinued.
Mitchell, Pyle, Eckert, Pomeroy, & Zimmerman (1990)	Imipramine vs. placebo vs. CBT + Imipramine or placebo.	12 weeks; f-u Pyle et al. (1990)	All active treatments decreased bingeing and purging; CBT superior and combination with medication only better in decreasing anxiety and depression.
Pyle, Mitchell, Eckert, Hatsukami, Pomeroy, & Zimmerman (1990)	CBT + Imipramine or placebo for maintenance.	16 weeks; no f-u	Initial treatment with CBT + Imipramine or placebo had lower relapse; attendance of support group or imipramine not associated with outcome.

Note: CBT = Cognitive–Behavioral Therapy; CT = Cognitive Therapy; BT = Behavior Therapy; ERP = Exposure with Response Prevention; f-u = follow-up.

reduction in vomiting at the end of treatment was 70%. In a 1- to 5-year follow-up study that examined effects of cognitive–behavioral therapy for anorexia nervosa, a majority (83%) of the subjects reported a "good" to "intermediate" outcome (Kennedy & Garfinkel, 1989). Fifty percent of subjects weighed above 85% of their recommended body weight and 54% had regular menses.

Williamson, Prather, Bennett, Davis, Watkins, and Grenier (1989b) conducted an uncontrolled evaluation of inpatient and outpatient CBT for bulimia nervosa. Both treatment conditions included ERP and CT. Inpatient follow-up was at 6 months, whereas outpatient follow-up was at 3 months. Both formats resulted in significant improvement. Whereas inpatients evidenced a rapid improvement, outpatients gradually improved. Follow-up results suggested that the two formats of CBT had relatively equivalent outcomes.

In two of the studies reviewed, there were no identified differences between CBT and non-CBT in the reduction of bingeing and purging (Fairburn et al., 1986; Freeman et al., 1988). Fairburn et al. concluded that CBT was superior, however, because of a reduction in general psychopathology associated with the CBT condition. Kirkley, Schneider, Agras, and Bachman (1985) compared CBT with a nondirective group. Whereas both therapies decreased bingeing and purging, the CBT group had fewer dropouts and decreased bulimic behaviors by a significantly larger amount than the nondirective group. (It is important to note that CBT was slightly different in each of these studies. We describe these differences in detail later.) Each of the non-CBT therapies focused on education and nutritional information. Wolchik, Weiss, and Katzman (1986) found that a psychoeducational approach that focused on information about bulimia, coping strategies, self-esteem, anger, cultural expectations of thinness, and body image was effective in decreasing bingeing and depression. Thus, research has consistently found CBT is superior to waiting-list controls (Agras et al., 1989; Lee & Rush, 1986; Leitenberg et al., 1988; Wolf & Crowther, 1992) and no-treatment controls (Freeman et al., 1988; Lacey, 1983).

In our review of the literature, we identified five studies that have examined whether addition of specific behavioral techniques (usually ERP) to CBT enhances effectiveness of treatment (Agras et al., 1989; Leitenburg et al., 1988; Wilson et al., 1986; Wolf & Crowther, 1992; Yates & Sambrillo, 1984). These studies have yielded inconsistent results. Yates and Sambrillo (1984) examined CBT, which included education, CT, assertion training, realistic perception of weight gain, and relaxation, versus CBT plus BT, which added stimulus-control techniques, response delay of bingeing, and response prevention of bingeing using incompatible behaviors. There were no differences between the two treatments. Wilson et al. (1986), on the other hand, found that CBT, which included ERP, was superior to CT at 1-year follow-up; 71% of the bulimics reported no bingeing posttreatment as opposed to 33% of those in the CT condition. Leitenberg et al. (1988) found similar results. These investigators compared four groups: (1) CBT and ERP in a single setting (clinic), (2) CBT and ERP in multiple settings (clinic, homes, and restaurants), (3) CBT with no ERP (self-monitoring, nutritional information, and CT), and (4) waiting-list control. All active treatment groups showed improvement; however, the CBT plus ERP groups had slightly better outcomes at follow-up on vomiting behavior and amount of food consumed at test meal. On the other hand, Agras et al. (1989) concluded that addition of ERP can have a deleterious effect on CBT (CT and SC). Wolf and Crowther (1992) also compared CBT (CT, problem solving, and stress management) versus a behavior therapy program that focused on identifying antecedents and consequences of bulimic behavior and used stimulus-control techniques. Although the clinical investigators encouraged use of ERP at home for the groups, therapy sessions did not involve ERP. When compared to a waiting-list control group, both therapy groups experienced decreases in bingeing, purging, and body dissatisfaction along with increases in feelings of general adequacy, security, and control. However, the CBT group additionally displayed less concern and preoccupation with dieting and greater confidence in identifying sensations of hunger and satiety at the end of treatment relative to pretreatment. Freeman et al. (1988) compared BT, which consisted of three meals per day, modification of eating behavior using graded tasks, and relaxation versus CBT, which included CT plus the behavioral component. CBT, BT, and a group condition that focused on support and education were superior to a waiting-list control with 71% of subjects no longer bingeing.

Investigators have also compared CBT to other psychotherapies. Kirkley et al. (1985) compared CBT and a nondirective group therapy that discussed nutritional information but included nonspecific instructions for behavior change. The CBT consisted of increasing eating regularity, delaying vomiting, increasing variety of foods eaten, stimulus-control techniques, altering the vomiting ritual, eating fear foods, and relaxation. Although both treatments decreased bingeing and purging, the CBT group demonstrated significantly less bingeing and purging and had fewer dropouts than the nondirective group. Thirty-eight percent of the CBT group and 11% of the nondirective group abstained from bingeing and purging at 3-month follow-up. Another study compared CBT (CT, stimulus control, and information) to a short-term focal therapy based on the central idea that eating problems constitute a maladaptive solution to "underlying difficulties." The focal therapy group also included an educational component (Fairburn et al., 1986). Both groups improved despite relatively brief therapy; however subjects in the CBT group improved to a greater degree than the focal therapy group, specifically in level of general psychopathology and subjective state.

Lacey (1983) compared CBT to a no-treatment control. CBT had the goal of increasing eating to three meals per day, decreasing bingeing and purging through contracting, and limiting the intake of carbohydrates. The group therapy was insight-oriented. The CBT condition was superior to the no-treatment control in decreasing bingeing and purging. Subjects maintained established gains through 2-year follow-up.

Overall, the majority of studies has shown that CBT is superior to waiting-list and no-treatment control. However, two studies with treatment phases for 15 and 18 weeks revealed no substantial advantage over other forms of psychotherapy in decreasing bingeing and purging. These non-CBT protocols each included an educational component about bulimia nervosa and eating habits. The addition of ERP has also produced conflicting results. It is unclear what specific components of treatment are responsible for successful outcome. There is a need for further process research to identify these components.

Pharmacological Therapy

Pharmacotherapy has shown a great deal of promise with bulimia nervosa, but not for anorexia nervosa. Fava et al. (1989) concluded that no drug, including antipsychotic and anticonvulsant medications, has consistently been effective for treatment of anorexia nervosa. Yates (1990), on the other hand, concluded that cyproheptadine, an appetite stimulant, shows the most promise as a medication for restricting anorexics because of its safety and minimal side effects. Halmi, Eckert, LaDu, and Cohen (1986) investigated the effects of cyproheptadine and amitriptyline on anorexia nervosa. The authors reported that cyproheptadine decreased the number of days required for anorexics to obtain required weight gain.

Walsh (1991) concluded that all medications with antidepressant properties significantly decrease frequency of bingeing and purging in both depressed and nondepressed bulimics. A variety of tricyclics and monoamine oxidase inhibitors (MAOIs) have been the subject of study. Table 9.2 summarizes the controlled-outcome studies of pharmacological therapy.

Four studies have examined the effects of imipramine on bulimia nervosa (Agras, Dorian, Kirkley, Arnow, & Bachman, 1987; Mitchell et al., 1990; Pope, Hudson, Jonas, & Yurgelun-Todd, 1983; Pyle et al., 1990). Treatment phases have ranged from 6 to 16 weeks, and imipramine has consistently resulted in decreased bingeing and purging. Mitchell et al. (1990) investigated the additive effects of imipramine or placebo to CBT. Both groups that included active CBT were superior to pharmacotherapy alone, although all of the active treatments decreased bingeing and purging. The researchers found no evidence that addition of pharmacotherapy enhanced effectiveness of CBT. In an extension of this study, Pyle et al. (1990) found that subjects who received initial treatment with CBT had the lowest relapse rate during maintenance. Attendance to support group or imipramine alone during follow-up did not associate with better outcome.

Two other antidepressants, desipramine and bupropion have also been effective for decreasing bingeing (Horn et al., 1988; Hughes, Wells, Cunningham, & Ilstrup, 1986). Two other studies concluded that phenelzine, a MAOI, is superior to placebo in decreasing binge frequency (Walsh et al., 1988; Walsh, Stewart, Roose, Gladis, & Glassman, 1984).

Overall, research has shown that antidepressants effectively decrease bingeing and purging. Craighead and Agras (1991) concluded that antidepressants appear to enhance dietary restraint, whereas CBT decreases dietary restraint. The authors stated that these modalities appear incompatible and suggested long-term pharmacological treatment as an alternative to CBT. Consistent with this recommendation, research has shown antidepressant treatment continues to produce improvement for as long as 8 months (Pope et al., 1983). Research has also shown antidepressants are effective regardless of whether subjects are depressed. However, we could find no pharmacological studies with long-term follow-up of at least 1 year after discontinuation of medication. One study that revealed the need for such follow-up (Walsh et al., 1984) found that 60% of their subjects relapsed after discontinuation of antidepressant medication. Thus, there is need for pharmacological studies with long-term follow-up that does not include active medication maintenance as well as long-term studies of maintaining bulimic subjects on antidepressant medications.

FUTURE DIRECTIONS

Proposed Changes in Diagnostic Criteria

As noted earlier, changes of diagnostic criteria in DSM-III-R had the effect of increasing the number of cases with diagnoses of eating disorder NOS. In our outpatient eating clinic, we use very stringent operational definitions for anorexia and bulimia nervosa. For example, we require purgative habits for a diagnosis of bulimia nervosa and a weight level 15% below normal or a BMI of less than 18 for a diagnosis of anorexia nervosa. As a consequence of using such stringent adherence to DSM-III-

R criteria, we diagnosed 46% (72 out of 155 consecutive referrals) of cases referred since 1987 as eating disorder NOS. Changes in diagnostic criteria for DSM-IV may partially remediate this problem (American Psychiatric Association, 1994). DSM-IV establishes two subtypes of anorexia: bulimic subtype and restricting subtype. Also, DSM-IV includes two subtypes for bulimia nervosa: purging type and nonpurging type, and new diagnostic category called binge eating disorder. The description of binge eating disorder includes the following symptoms/characteristics: (1) most cases are obese, (2) recurrent uncontrollable binge eating, (3) loss of control over eating, (4) distress about binge eating, and (5) a minimum of at least two binge-eating episodes over the past 6 months. Patients diagnosed with binge eating disorder must not meet the diagnostic criteria for bulimia nervosa and must not abuse diet pills in an attempt to avoid weight gain.

DSM-IV criteria also strengthen the descriptions of eating disorder NOS by providing two examples: subthreshold anorexia nervosa and subthreshold bulimia nervosa. These subthreshold eating disorders meet most, but not all, of the criteria for anorexia and bulimia nervosa (e.g., absence of amenorrhea for anorexia or binge eating that occurs less than twice per week for bulimia). In a recent test of these changes, Williamson, Gleaves, and Savin (1992) found supportive evidence for the new diagnostic subtypes. Cluster analyses classified eating disorder NOS subjects as binge eating disorder, nonpurging bulimia nervosa, and subthreshold anorexia nervosa. Of particular significance was the finding of a very homogeneous group of binge eaters that differentiated from nonpurging bulimia nervosa with 100% reliability.

Information-Processing Paradigm

Research concerning the psychopathology of eating disorders has consistently found fear of fatness is a central motivational factor for dieting, purging, and behaviors to check body size (Williamson, 1990). In recent years, several groups of researchers (e.g., Schlundt & Johnson, 1990; Vitousek & Hollon, 1990; Williamson, Barker, & Norris, 1993) have suggested that information-processing methodology might provide a paradigm for furthering research on the psychopathology of eating disorders. Other researchers have found this approach quite useful in the study of anxiety disorders and depression (Haaga, Dyck, & Ernst, 1991; McNally, 1990). This cognitive approach relies upon experimental methodologies for evaluating biases of memory, attention, and inferential thinking that reflect the concerns of an individual. In the case of anorexia and bulimia nervosa, one might predict that fear of fatness/overconcern with body size will associate with an attentional bias toward body-related and food-related stimuli. Several tests of this prediction using a modified Stroop color-naming task (Ben-Tovim, Walker, Fok, & Yap, 1989; Channon, Hemsley, & DeSilva, 1988), and a dichotic listening task (Schotte, McNally, & Turner, 1990) have yielded positive findings for this prediction. Also, Williamson, Gleaves, and Lawson (1991) reported a judgment bias in bulimia nervosa for reporting overeating at progressively larger caloric amounts.

The information-processing paradigm predicts that ambiguity about body-related or food-related stimuli may set the occasion for misinterpretation of such stimuli by eating-disorder subjects. Arkes (1991) described how such judgment/evaluative biases might arise. *Associative biases* are likely to occur with highly elaborated memories. Body concerns qualify as highly elaborated memories for eating-disorder patients. Activation of elaborated memories are likely to activate extraneous memories via association, thereby resulting in biased judgments about body size and amount of food consumed. *Psychophysical biases* occur when the person has a heightened sensitivity to certain stimuli (e.g., body-related cues) that result in distorted judgments about intensity of the stimulus. We believe that such cognitive processes may result in *automatic,* nonconscious reactions that have become known as body-image distortion; irrational cognitions related to body, food, and exercise; and body dysphoria. If this conclusion is correct, it would help explain why anorexics and bulimics behave as though their unreasonable ideas and behavior toward body size/appearance are perfectly reasonable and why they seem surprised that anyone might think differently.

Applications of the information-processing paradigm to the eating disorders have only begun. We recommend that researchers in the area of eating disorders develop very precise cognitive models (e.g., Williamson et al., 1993) so that empirical tests of the model can utilize very precise predictions.

REFERENCES

Agras, W. S., Dorian, B., Kirkley, B. G., Arnow, B., & Bachman, J. (1987). Imipramine in the treatment of bulimia: A double-blind controlled study. *International Journal of Eating Disorders, 6,* 29–38.

Agras, W. S., Schneider, J. A., Arnow, B., Raeburn, S. D., & Telch, C. F. (1989). Cognitive–behavioral and response-prevention treatments for bulimia nervosa. *Journal of Consulting and Clinical Psychology, 57,* 215–221.

American Psychiatric Association. (1980). *Diagnostic and statistical manual of mental disorders* (3rd ed.). Washington, DC: Author.

American Psychiatric Association. (1987). *Diagnostic and statistical manual of mental disorders* (3rd ed. rev.). Washington, DC: Author.

American Psychiatric Association. (1994). *Diagnostic and statistical manual of mental disorders* (4th ed.). Washington, DC: Author.

Arkes, H. R. (1991). Costs and benefits of judgement errors: Implications for debiasing. *Psychological Bulletin, 110,* 486–498.

Askevold, F. (1975). Measuring body image. *Psychotherapy and Psychosomatics, 26,* 71–77.

Ben-Tovim, D. I., Walker, M. K., Fok, D., & Yap, E. (1989). An adaptation of the Stroop test for measuring shape and food concerns in eating disorders: A quantitative measure of psychopathology? *International Journal of Eating Disorders, 8,* 686–687.

Brownell, K. D. (1991). Dieting and the search for the perfect body: Where physiology and culture collide. *Behavior Therapy, 22,* 1–12.

Bruch, H. (1985). Four decades of eating disorders. In D. M. Garner & P. E. Garfinkel (Eds.), *Handbook of psychotherapy for anorexia and bulimia* (pp. 7–18). New York: Guilford.

Butters, J. W., & Cash, T. F. (1987). Cognitive–behavioral treatment of women's body image dissatisfaction. *Journal of Consulting and Clinical Psychology, 55,* 889–897.

Cash, T. F., & Green, G. K. (1986). Body weight and body image among college women: Perception, cognition, and affect. *Journal of Personality Assessment, 50,* 290–301.

Cash, T. F., Lewis, R. J., & Keeton, P. (1987, March). *Development and validation of the Body-Image Automatic Thoughts Questionnaire: A measure of body related cognitions.* Paper presented at the meeting of the Southeastern Psychological Association. Atlanta, GA.

Channon, S., Hemsley, D., & DeSilva, P. (1988). Selective processing of food words in anorexia nervosa. *British Journal of Clinical Psychology, 27,* 259–260.

Cooper, Z., & Fairburn, C. G. (1987). The Eating Disorder Examination: A semi-structured interview of the assessment of the specific psychopathology of eating disorders. *International Journal of Eating Disorders, 6,* 1–8.

Craighead, L. W., & Agras, W. S. (1991). Mechanisms of action in cognitive–behavioral and pharmacological interventions for obesity and bulimia nervosa. *Journal of Consulting and Clinical Psychology, 59,* 115–125.

Dritschel, B. H., Williams, K., & Cooper, P. J. (1991). Cognitive distortions amongst women experiencing bulimic episodes. *International Journal of Eating Disorders, 10,* 547–555.

Fairburn, C. G., Kirk, J., O'Connor, M., & Cooper, P. J. (1986). A comparison of two psychological treatments for bulimia nervosa. *Behaviour Research and Therapy, 24,* 629–643.

Fava, M., Copeland, P. M., Schweiger, U., & Herzog, D. B. (1989). Neurochemical abnormalities of anorexia and bulimia nervosa. *American Journal of Psychiatry, 146,* 963–971.

Freeman, C.P.L., Barry, F., Dunkeld-Turnbull, J., & Henderson, A. (1988). Controlled trial of psychotherapy for bulimia nervosa. *British Medical Journal, 296,* 521–525.

Garfinkel, P. E., & Kaplan, A. S. (1985). Starvation based perpetuating mechanisms in anorexia nervosa and bulimia. *International Journal of Eating Disorders, 4,* 651–665.

Garner, D. M., & Bemis, K. M. (1982). A cognitive–behavioral approach to anorexia nervosa. *Cognitive Therapy and Research, 6,* 123–150.

Garner, D. M., & Garfinkel, P. E. (1979). The Eating Attitudes Test: An index of the symptoms of anorexia nervosa. *Psychological Medicine, 9,* 272–279.

Garner, D. M., & Olmstead, M. P. (1984). *Manual for the Eating Attitudes Test (EDI).* Odessa, FL: Psychological Assessment Resources.

Geracioti, T. D., & Liddle, R. A. (1988). Impaired cholecystokinin secretion in bulimia nervosa. *New England Journal of Medicine, 319,* 683–688.

Goodsitt, A. (1985). Self psychology and the treatment of anorexia nervosa. In D. M. Garner & P. E. Garfinkel (Eds.), *Handbook of psychotherapy for anorexia and bulimia* (pp. 307–330). New York: Guilford.

Gull, W. W. (1874). Anorexia nervosa. *Transactions of the Clinical Society of London, 7,* 22–28.

Haaga, D. F., Dyck, M. J., & Ernst, D. (1991). Empirical status of cognitive theory of depression. *Psychological Bulletin, 110,* 215–236.

Halmi, K. A., Eckert, E., LaDu, T. J., & Cohen, J. (1986). Anorexia nervosa: Treatment efficacy of cyproheptadine and amitriptyline. *Archives of General Psychiatry, 43,* 177–181.

Head, S. B., & Williamson, D. A. (1990). Association of family environment and personality disturbances in bulimia nervosa. *International Journal of Eating Disorders, 9,* 667–674.

Heatherton, T. F., & Baumeister, R. F. (1991). Binge eating as escape from self-awareness. *Psychological Bulletin, 110,* 86–108.

Herholz, K., & Emrich, H. M. (1987). Regional cerebral glucose metabolism in anorexia nervosa measured by positron emission tomography. *Biological Psychiatry, 22,* 43–51.

Hinz, L. D., & Williamson, D. A. (1987). Bulimia and depression: A review of the affective variant hypothesis. *Psychological Bulletin, 102,* 150–158.

Horne, R. L., Ferguson, J. M., Pope, H. G., Hudson, J. I., Lineberry, C. G., Ascher, J., & Cato, A. (1988). Treatment of bulimia with bupropion: A multicenter controlled trial. *Journal of Clinical Psychiatry, 49,* 262–266.

Hsu, L.K.G., & Sobkiewicz, T. A. (1989). Body image disturbance: Time to abandon the concept for eating disorders. *International Journal of Eating Disorders, 10,* 15–30.

Hudson, J. I., Pope, H. G., Yurgelun-Todd, D., Jonas, J. M., & Frankenburg, F. R. (1987). A controlled study of lifetime prevalence of affective and other psychiatric disorders in bulimic outpatients. *American Journal of Psychiatry, 144,* 1283–1287.

Hughes, P. L., Wells, L. A., Cunningham, C. J., & Ilstrup, D. M. (1986). Treating bulimia with desipramine. A double-blind, placebo controlled study. *Archives of General Psychiatry, 43,* 182–186.

Humphrey, L. L. (1988). Relationships within subtypes of anorexics, bulimics, and normal families. *Journal of the American Academy of Child and Adolescent Psychiatry, 27,* 544–551.

Jones, D. J., Fox, M. M., Babigian, H. M., & Hutton, H. E. (1980). Epidemiology of anorexia nervosa in Monroe County, new York: 1960–1976. *Psychosomatic Medicine, 42,* 551–558.

Kaye, W. H., Ebert, M. H., Gwirtsman, H. E. (1984). Differences in brain serotonergic metabolism between nonbulimic and bulimic patients with anorexia nervosa. *American Journal of Psychiatry, 141,* 1598–1601.

Kendler, K. S., MacLean, C., Neale, M., Kessler, R., Heath, A., & Eaves, L. (1991). The genetic epidemiology of bulimia nervosa. *American Journal of Psychiatry, 148,* 1627–1637.

Kennedy, S. H., & Garfinkel, P. E. (1989). Patients admitted to a hospital with anorexia nervosa and bulimia nervosa: Psychopathology, weight gain, and attitudes toward treatment. *International Journal of Eating Disorders, 8,* 181–190.

Kirkley, B. G., Schneider, J. A., Agras, W. S., & Bachman, J. A. (1985). Comparison of two group treatments for bulimia. *Journal of Consulting and Clinical, 53,* 43–48.

Lacey, H. (1983). Bulimia nervosa, binge eating, and psychogenic vomiting: A controlled treatment study and long-term outcome. *British Medical Journal, 286,* 1609–1613.

Lee, N. F., & Rush, A. J. (1986). Cognitive–behavioral group therapy for bulimia. *International Journal of Eating Disorders, 5,* 599–615.

Leitenberg, H., Rosen, J. C., Gross, J., Nudelman, S., & Vara, L. S. (1988). Exposure plus response prevention treatment of bulimia nervosa. *Journal of Consulting and Clinical Psychology, 56,* 535–541.

Lerner, H. D. (1983). Contemporary psychoanalytic perspectives on gorge-vomiting: A case illustration. *International Journal of Eating Disorders, 3,* 47–63.

McKenzie, S. J., Williamson, D. A., & Cubic, B. A. (1993). Stable and reactive body image disturbances in bulimia nervosa. *Behavior Therapy, 24,* 195–207.

McNally, R. J. (1990). Psychological approaches to panic disorder: A review. *Psychological Bulletin, 108,* 403–419.

Mitchell, J. E., Pyle, R. L., Eckert, E. D., Hatsukami, D., Pomeroy, C., & Zimmerman, R. (1990). A comparison study of antidepressants and structured intensive group psychotherapy in the treatment of bulimia nervosa. *Archives of General Psychiatry, 47,* 149–157.

Palmer, R., Christie, M., Cordle, C., Davis, D., & Kendrick, J. (1987). The Clinical Eating Disorder Rating Instrument (CEDRI): A preliminary description. *International Journal of Eating Disorders, 6,* 9–16.

Piran, N., Lerner, P., Garfinkel, P. E., Kennedy, S. H., & Brouillete, C. (1988). Personality disorders in anorexic patients. *International Journal of Eating Disorders, 7,* 589–599.

Pope, H. G., Hudson, J. T., Jonas, J. M., & Yurgelun-Todd, D. (1983). Bulimia treated with imipramine: A double-blind placebo-controlled trial. *American Journal of Psychiatry, 140,* 554-558.

Pyle, R. L., Mitchell, J. E., Eckert, E. D., Hatsukami, D., Pomeroy, C., & Zimmerman, R. (1990). Maintenance treatment and 6-month outcome for bulimic patients who respond to initial treatment. *American Journal of Psychiatry, 147,* 871–875.

Rand, C.S.W., & Kuldau, J. M. (1992). Epidemiology of bulimia and symptoms in a general population: Sex, age, race, and socioeconomic status. *International Journal of Eating Disorders, 11,* 37–44.

Rosen, J. C. (1987). A review of behavioral treatment for bulimia nervosa. *Behavior Modification, 11,* 464–486.

Rosen, J. C. (1992). Body image disorder: Definition, development, and contribution to eating disorders. In J. H. Crowther, S. E. Hobfoll, M.A.P. Stephens, & D. L. Tennenbaum (Eds.), *The etiology of bulimia: The individual and family context.* Washington, DC: Hemisphere.

Rosen, J. C., & Leitenberg, H. (1982). Bulimia nervosa: Treatment with exposure and response prevention. *Behavior Therapy, 13,* 117–124.

Ruff, G., & Barrios, B. (1986). Realistic assessment of body image. *Behavioral Assessment, 8,* 237–251.

Schlundt, D. G., & Johnson, W. G. (1990). *Eating disorders: Assessment and treatment.* Needham Heights, MA: Allyn & Bacon.

Schotte, D. E., McNally, R. J., & Turner, M. L. (1990). A dichotic listening analysis of body weight concerns in bulimia nervosa. *International Journal of Eating Disorders, 9,* 109–113.

Scott, D. W. (1986). Anorexia nervosa: A review of possible genetic factors. *International Journal of Eating Disorders, 5,* 1–20.

Slade, P. (1982). Toward a functional analysis of anorexia nervosa. *British Journal of Clinical Psychology, 21,* 167–179.

Slade, P. (1985). A review of body image studies in anorexia and bulimia nervosa. *Journal of Psychiatric Research, 19,* 255–265.

Smith, M. C., & Thelen, M. H. (1984). Development and validation of a test for bulimia. *Journal of Consulting and Clinical Psychology, 52,* 863–872.

Steere, J., Butler, G., & Cooper, P. J. (1990). The anxiety symptoms of bulimia nervosa: A comparative study. *International Journal of Eating Disorders, 9,* 293–301.

Strauss, J., & Ryan, R. M. (1987). Autonomy disturbances in subtypes of anorexia nervosa. *Journal of Abnormal Psychology, 96,* 254–258.

Teusch, R. (1988). Level of ego development and bulimic's conceptualization of their disorder. *International Journal of Eating Disorders, 7,* 115–119.

Thelen, M. H., Farmer, J., Wonderlich, S., & Smith, M. (1991). A revision of the Bulimia Test: The BULIT-R. *Psychological Assessment, 3,* 119–124.

Thompson, J. K. (1992). Body image: Extent of disturbance, associated features, theoretical models, assessment methodologies, intervention strategies, and a proposal for a new DSM-IV diagnostic category-body image disorder. In M. Hersen, R. M. Eisler, & P. M. Miller (Eds.), *Progress in behavior modification* (pp. 3-54). Sycamore, IL: Sycamore.

Touyz, S. W., Beumont, P.J.V., Collins, J. K., McCabe, M. P., & Jupp, J. J. (1984). Body shape perception and its disturbance in anorexia nervosa. *British Journal of Psychiatry, 144,* 167–171.

Vitousek, K. B., & Hollon, S. D. (1990). The investigation of schematic content and processing in eating disorders. *Cognitive Therapy and Research, 14,* 191–214.

Walsh, B. T. (1991). Psychopharmacologic treatment of bulimia nervosa. *Journal of Clinical Psychiatry, 52,* 34–38.

Walsh, B. T., Gladis, M., Roose, S. P., Stewart, J. W., Stetner, F., & Glassman, A. H. (1988). Phenelzine vs. placebo in 50 patients with bulimia. *Archives of General Psychiatry, 45,* 471–475.

Walsh, B. T., Stewart, J. W., Roose, S. P., Gladis, M., & Glassman, A. H. (1984). Treatment of bulimia with phenelzine: A double-blind, placebo controlled study. *Archives of General Psychiatry, 41,* 1105–1109.

Williamson, D. A. (1990). *Assessment of eating disorders: Obesity, anorexia, and bulimia nervosa.* New York: Pergamon.

Williamson, D. A., Barker, S. E., & Norris, L. E. (1993). Etiology and management of eating disorders. In P. B. Sutker & H. E. Adams (Eds.), *Comprehensive handbook of psychopathology* (2nd ed.). New York: Plenum Press.

Williamson, D. A., Davis, C. J., Bennett, S. M., Goreczny, A. J., & Gleaves, D. H. (1989a). Development of a simple procedure for assessing body image disturbances. *Behavioral Assessment, 11,* 433–446.

Williamson, D. A., Davis, C. J., Norris, L., & Van Buren, D. J. (1990, November). *Development of reliability and validity for a new structured interview for diagnosis of eating disorders.* Paper presented at the annual meeting of the Association for the Advancement of Behavior Therapy, San Francisco, CA.

Williamson, D. A., Gleaves, D. H., & Lawson, O. J. (1991). Biased perception of overeating in bulimia nervosa and compulsive binge eating. *Journal of Psychopathology and Behavioral Assessment, 13,* 257–268.

Williamson, D. A., Gleaves, D. H., & Savin, S. S. (1992). Empirical classification of eating disorder not otherwise specified: Support for DSM-IV changes. *Journal of Psychopathology and Behavioral Assessment, 14,* 201–216.

Williamson, D. A., Prather, R. C., Bennett, S. M., Davis, C. J., Watkins, P. C., & Grenier, C. E. (1989b). An uncontrolled evaluation of inpatient and outpatient cognitive-behavior therapy for bulimia nervosa. *Behavior Modification, 13,* 340–360.

Williamson, D. A., Prather, R. C., Goreczny, A. J., Davis, C. J., & McKenzie, S. J. (1989c). A comprehensive model of bulimia nervosa: Empirical evaluation. In W. G. Johnson (Ed.), *Advances in eating disorders* (pp. 137–156). Greenwich, CT: JAI Press.

Williamson, D. A., Prather, R. C., Upton, L., Davis, C. J., Ruggiero, L., & Van Buren D. (1987). Severity of bulimia: Relationship with depression and other psychopathology. *International Journal of Eating Disorders, 6,* 39–47.

Wilson, G. T., Rossiter, E., Kleifield, E. I., & Lindholm, L. (1986). Cognitive–behavioral treatment of bulimia nervosa: A controlled evaluation. *Behaviour Research and Therapy, 24,* 277–288.

Wilson, G. T., & Walsh, B. T. (1991). Eating disorders in the DSM-IV. *Journal of Abnormal Psychology, 100,* 362–365.

Wolchik, S. A., Weiss, L., & Katzman, M. A. (1986). An empirically validated, short-term psychoeducational group treatment for bulimia. *International Journal of Eating Disorders, 5,* 21–34.

Wolf, E. M., & Crowther, J. H. (1992). An evaluation of behavioral and cognitive–behavioral group interventions for the treatment of bulimia nervosa in women. *International Journal of Eating Disorders, 11,* 3–15.

Yates, A. (1989). Current perspectives on the eating disorders: I. History, psychological, and biological aspects. *Journal of the American Academy of Child and Adolescent Psychiatry, 28,* 813–828.

Yates, A. (1990). Current perspectives on the eating disorders: II. Treatment, outcome and research directions. *Journal of the American Academy of Child and Adolescent Psychiatry, 29,* 1–9.

Yates, A. J., & Sambrillo, F. (1984). Bulimia nervosa: A descriptive and therapeutic study. *Behaviour Research and Therapy, 22,* 503–517.

10

Assessment and Modification of Coronary-Prone Behavior
A Transactional View of the Person in Social Context

Timothy W. Smith

INTRODUCTION

The coronary-prone behavior pattern or personality style has been a central focus of the developing fields of health psychology and behavioral medicine for several decades. It has also been the subject of considerable controversy, with opinions ranging from general acceptance (Cooper, Detre, & Weiss, 1981) to outright condemnation (Angell, 1985). One product of this vigorous debate has been a change in the conceptual and empirical description of coronary-prone behavior. Additionally, models of the psychosomatic mechanisms linking behavior and disease have both broadened and become more detailed (Siegman & Dembroski, 1989). During this period of evolution and refinement of issues, important demonstrations of the potential clinical utility of interventions for coronary-prone behavior have appeared (Friedman et al., 1986). Although one must consider these treatment-outcome studies preliminary as they await replication, this intervention research suggests that valuable health-care benefits may accrue from the decades-long investment in research on this concept.

Recent developments in basic research on coronary-prone behavior have many implications for the application of this concept to clinical assessment and intervention. Greater specificity about health risks associated with individual behaviors or personality traits points to refined assessment techniques and more focused treat-

---

Timothy W. Smith • Department of Psychology, University of Utah, Salt Lake City, Utah 84112.
Handbook of Health and Rehabilitation Psychology, edited by Anthony J. Goreczny. Plenum Press, New York, 1995.

ments. At the same time, an emerging view of coronary-prone behavior as embedded in a dynamic social context suggests the potential value of broadening assessments and interventions beyond the traditional focus on individuals to include surrounding interpersonal networks and situations. From this perspective, a primary treatment goal still includes disruption of the hypothesized final common pathway linking coronary-prone behaviors and disease; that is, disrupting the physiological effects of psychological stress. However, this more current social–interactional view also suggests that interventions are likely to be more effective if they also disrupt maladaptive, reciprocal transactions between individuals displaying coronary-prone behavior patterns and unhealthy features of the social environments these individuals inhabit.

In this chapter, I describe recent research and theory on the coronary-prone behavior pattern with an emphasis on its relevance for clinical work with coronary patients and those individuals at risk for cardiovascular disease. The discussion includes a brief review of the literature on the association between these behavioral or personality traits and health, mechanisms underlying this association, and efficacy of related interventions. I also outline the emerging transactional perspective and its implications for clinical assessment and intervention efforts. This review will serve as a guide for future basic and clinical research that is essential to expand our understanding of coronary-prone behavior and its effects.

RECENT THEORY AND RESEARCH

Friedman and Rosenman (1959) originally described the Type A coronary-prone behavior pattern as an "action–emotion complex" consisting of achievement–striving, competitiveness, job-involvement, impatience, and easily provoked hostility. To various degrees, other authors, including Oster (1892) and Dunbar (1943), had anticipated this description of the coronary-prone personality. In the subsequent 35 years, the work of Friedman and Rosenman has stimulated a large amount of research on three general topics: (1) the association between Type A behavior and disease, (2) pathophysiological mechanisms, and (3) clinical interventions. In each area, clear lines of evolution are apparent.

Basic Association with Health Outcomes

The Broadly Defined Type A Pattern

In a review of the first two decades of research on the association between Type A behavior and coronary heart disease (CHD), a panel of experts convened by the American Heart Association concluded that this pattern was indeed a significant risk factor (Cooper et al., 1981). This group suggested that initially healthy Type As were about twice as likely to develop CHD as were more easygoing, soft-spoken, and patient Type Bs.

Since the time of this influential review, several notable failures to replicate the association between the Type A pattern and subsequent CHD have appeared. These have included the results of several large, multicenter studies (e.g., Shekelle, Billings, & Borhani, 1985a; Shekelle, Gale, & Norusis, 1985b) as well as follow-up analyses of the Western Collaborative Group Study (WCGS; Ragland & Brand, 1988), the original prospective study demonstrating a link between Type A behavior and CHD.

Despite these noteworthy studies, the bulk of the evidence still supports the hypothesis that the Type A pattern is a significant CHD risk factor. However, recent meta-analyses of available prospective studies (Matthews, 1988; Miller et al., 1991) found that this is true only for initially healthy populations, and only when assessing the Type A pattern through the structured interview (Rosenman, 1978). The Jenkins Activity Survey (JAS), a widely used questionnaire to assess Type A behavior, did not significantly predict presence of CHD.

Hostility as the Toxic Component

One heuristic consequence of the inconsistent results concerning the broadly defined Type A pattern has been increased attention to individual components of dimensions of the Type A pattern. In one study, Matthews, Glass, Rosenman, and Bortner (1977) examined the association of several Type A components with subsequent CHD over a 4.5-year follow-up of initially healthy WCGS subjects. In this analysis, competitive drive, impatience, and hostility were associated with subsequent disease.

In a refinement and extension of this approach, Hecker, Chesney, Black, and Frautschi (1988) reanalyzed data from the WCGS over an 8.5-year follow-up period. When the investigators separately quantified 14 individual Type A behaviors and considered these behaviors simultaneously in multivariate analyses, only hostility was a significant independent predictor of CHD. Interestingly, when the investigators simultaneously considered hostility and the global rating of Type A versus Type B behavior, both variables significantly related to subsequent CHD. This suggests that hostility does not explain all of the association between the broadly defined Type A pattern and coronary disease.

Nonetheless, recent work by Dembroski, MacDougall, Costa, and Grandits (1989) also supported the importance of hostility. These investigators reexamined structured-interview ratings of Type A behavior in the Multiple Risk-Factor Intervention Trial (MRFIT). It is important to note that global ratings of Type A behavior did not associate with subsequent CHD in the original MRFIT analyses (Shekelle et al., 1985). However, in the Dembroski et al. (1989) analyses, ratings of potential for hostility were associated with subsequent CHD, whereas other aspects of the Type A pattern did not.

A variety of related studies, using several different measures of hostility, have appeared in recent years (for a review, see Smith, 1992). For example, several studies have found that hostility, as assessed by the Cook and Medley (1954) hostility (Ho) scale, relates to increased risk of CHD and/or earlier mortality (e.g., Barefoot et al., 1983; Skekelle, Gale, Ostfeld, & Paul, 1983). However, an equal number of studies using this MMPI-derived, self-report scale have failed to find an effect (e.g., Hearn, Murray, & Luepker, 1989; Leon, Finn, Murray, & Bailey, 1988). Nonetheless, when combined with the studies using interview-based measures of hostility described earlier and other studies of self-reported hostility (e.g., Barefoot et al., 1987; Koskenvuo et al., 1988), prospective evidence generally supports the hypothesis that hostility contributes to subsequent disease (Matthews, 1988; Smith, 1992). This conclusion is supported by the results of another recent meta-analysis in which hostility was a significant predictor of CHD and premature death (Miller et al., 1995).

Are There Other Coronary-Prone Components?

As noted earlier, when considered simultaneously in reanalyses of the WCGS, both hostility and globally defined Type A behavior significantly and independently relate to subsequent CHD (Hecker et al., 1988). This suggests that hostility might not be the sole coronary-prone component of the Type A pattern. In further exploration of this issue, again using reanalyses of the WCGS, Houston, Chesney, Black, Cates, and Hecker (1992) identified two groups of subjects who were at significant risk of subsequent CHD. The first, as expected, primarily evidenced high levels of hostility. The second group evidenced quick interview responses and frequent interruptions of the interviewer but not hostility. Houston et al. (1992) interpreted this latter pattern as reflecting interpersonal dominance and control. Thus, in addition to hostile individuals, those individuals characterized by a socially dominant or interpersonally controlling style might also be at greater risk for CHD.

In this regard, it is interesting to note that socially dominant male monkeys are prone to accelerated development of coronary artery disease when exposed to chronic, recurring threats to their social position or rank (Manuck, Kaplan, Muldoon, Adams, & Clarkson, 1991). Echoing previous suggestions to broaden the search for coronary-prone personality traits beyond the traditional description of Type A behavior (Booth-Kewley & Friedman, 1987), these animal model and human epidemiological findings suggest that social dominance is another possible coronary-prone trait.

Underlying Mechanisms

Researchers have proposed several models to account for the association between coronary-prone behaviors and subsequent health. These models include those applied to the broadly defined Type A pattern (Suls & Sanders, 1989) as well as the more specific trait of hostility (Smith, 1992). The two models that have received the most attention are the psychophysiological reactivity model and the psychosocial vulnerability model. A third theory, the transactional model, provides an integration and extension of the first two approaches. It also serves as a guide to clinical assessment and intervention.

Psychophysiological Reactivity

Several authors have suggested that hostility and the Type A pattern contribute to development of CHD through heightened cardiovascular and neuroendocrine reactivity. Briefly, this model suggests that hostility and/or Type A behavior involves excessive sympathetically mediated increases in blood pressure, heart rate, and stress-related hormones in response to potential stressors. This exaggerated reactivity, in turn, hypothetically initiates and hastens development of coronary atherosclerosis. Among patients with significant coronary artery occlusions, episodes of reactivity might precipitate clinical symptoms of CHD (Houston, 1988; Williams, Barefoot, & Shekelle, 1985). Although the literature documenting a link between physiological reactivity and subsequent disease is somewhat tentative, these cardiovascular and neuroendocrine responses do represent a plausible pathophysiological mechanism (Manuck, 1994; Manuck et al., 1991; Smith & Christensen, 1992).

Many studies have examined cardiovascular and neuroendocrine responses of Type A and Type B subjects to stressful tasks and situations (for reviews, see Harbin, 1989; Houston, 1988). Although not completely consistent, these studies generally do demonstrate the hypothesized differences in reactivity between Type As and Bs. This is particularly evident for blood pressure responses to challenging tasks and primarily when assessing global Type A behavior through structured interviews. Thus, heightened cardiovascular response to environmental challenges and demands is a plausible account of the association between the globally defined Type A pattern and subsequent CHD.

Research using measures of hostility also generally supports the psychophysiological reactivity theory. There are, however, some notable exceptions (Houston, 1994; Smith, 1992; Suls & Wan, 1993). First, when assessing hostility through behavioral ratings from the Type A structured interview, the association with reactivity is somewhat inconsistent. Second, in studies using the Cook and Medley (1954) Ho scale, hostility associates with heightened reactivity only in response to relevant social stressors. For example, subjects with high Ho scores display large increases in blood pressure in response to situations involving interpersonal conflict (Hardy & Smith, 1988; Smith & Allred, 1989), harassment (Suarez & Williams, 1989), and disclosure of personal information (Christensen & Smith, 1993). These findings are consistent with the view of hostile individuals as being mistrusting, easily angered, and quick to see hostile intent in the actions of others. Hostile men are also more physiologically reactive when attempting to influence or control their spouses (Smith & Brown, 1991). This was not true for hostile women, however. Thus, situations involving threats to social dominance or control may also be physiologically taxing for hostile men.

Physiological differences between high- and low-hostility persons are evident outside the laboratory as well. Jamner, Shapiro, Goldstein, and Hug (1991) found that hostile paramedics displayed higher ambulatory levels of blood pressure when compared to their nonhostile counterparts, particularly while at the hospital. These authors suggested that the stressful interpersonal climate of the hospital and associated antagonistic interactions might elicit heightened reactivity in hostile individuals. Similarly, Pope and Smith (1991), assessed cortisol reactivity of high and low cynically hostile men. They found that men high in hostility, as measured by the Ho scale, evidenced a two- to threefold larger increase in urinary cortisol excretion during the period between waking and noon than did men low in hostility. Excessive cortisol reactivity is not only a marker for general adrenal stress response but might also contribute directly to the development of CAD.

Several recent studies have assessed physiological reactivity and its relation to attempts to control or influence others. These studies have demonstrated that subjects who engage in effortful attempts to influence or control others display enhanced cardiovascular reactivity, relative to subjects involved in similar discussions who do not attempt to be controlling or dominant (Brown & Smith, 1992; Smith, Allred, Morrison, & Carlson, 1989; Smith, Baldwin, & Christensen, 1990a). Apparently, this is particularly true for hostile men (Smith & Brown, 1991). These psychophysiological effects of effortful attempts to exert interpersonal control or dominance are interesting in light of the Houston et al. (1992) finding that interpersonally dominant and controlling behaviors are risk factors for CHD. Perhaps this interpersonal style is linked to subsequent CHD, because recurring efforts to exert dominance elicit heightened physiological reactivity. Thus, available evidence suggests that hostility and interpersonal dominance are associated with cardiovascular and neuroendocrine responses that are plausible pathophysiological mechanisms related to coronary problems.

Recent research on the precipitation of acute coronary events is also consistent with the hypothesis that physiological responses to episodes of acute psychological stress might contribute to CHD in coronary-prone persons. For example, the arousal of anger has been found to elicit myocardial ischemia in CHD patients (Ironson et al., 1992). These stress-induced ischemic changes during laboratory tasks are more pronounced among characteristically hostile CHD patients (Burg et al., 1993), and hostile CHD patients display more cardiac ischemia during their daily activities than do nonhostile patients (Helmers et al., 1993). Thus, in the presence of clinically significant coronary artery disease, hostility and other coronary-prone behaviors might increase the likelihood of acute coronary events, such as myocardial infarction or sudden coronary death.

Psychosocial Vulnerability

A second model of the mechanism linking coronary-prone behavior and CHD focuses on associated psychosocial variables. Briefly, this model maintains that individuals with coronary-prone behaviors likely experience a high frequency and severity of stressful life events, significant interpersonal conflict, and low levels of social support. This rather negative psychosocial profile, in turn, would hypothetically confer increased vulnerability to illness.

Research has generally supported the hypothesized association between the globally defined Type A pattern and psychosocial vulnerability. In general, compared to Type Bs, Type A individuals report more frequent and severe life stresses, greater marital conflict, and more job stress (for reviews, see Smith & Anderson, 1986; Suls & Sanders, 1989). However, it is important to note that investigators have conducted most of this research using the JAS. Given that the structural interview generally has greater predictive utility as a CHD risk factor than does the JAS, psychosocial correlates of structured-interview defined Type A behavior are in need of further examination.

Psychosocial correlates of hostility have received considerable attention in recent years (Smith, 1992). High levels of hostility, as assessed by the Ho scale, are associated with low levels of social support and high levels of both major and minor stressful life events (Barefoot, Dahlstrom, & Williams, 1983; Houston & Kelly, 1989; Scherwitz, Perkins, Chesney, & Hughes, 1991; Smith & Frohm, 1985; Smith et al., 1988). High Ho scores are also associated with increased reports and behavioral displays of marital conflict, but this pattern is stronger for men than for women (Houston & Kelly, 1989; Smith et al., 1988; Smith et al., 1990b). This pattern of increased interpersonal conflict and decreased social support is also evident in descriptions of work environments (Smith et al., 1988) and families of origin (Houston & Vavak, 1991; Smith et al., 1988). Although hostility, as measured by the

Ho scale, clearly relates to psychosocial variables, far less is known about psychosocial correlates of interview ratings of hostility.

A large and growing body of research suggests that low levels of social support, high levels of social isolation, interpersonal conflict in several domains, and stressful life events are significant risk factors for CHD and other life-threatening illnesses (for reviews, see Krantz, Contrada, Hill, and Friedler, 1988, and Syme, 1987). Thus, psychosocial correlates of hostility represent a viable mechanism linking this behavioral style to subsequent disease. Of course, some pathophysiological process must still function as a final common pathway linking hostility, stressful circumstances, and disease.

The Transactional Model

Many theorists from many different perspectives have argued that personality traits reciprocally relate to interpersonal environments. Individuals recurrently shape the social contexts they inhabit and the social contexts in turn shape those individuals. Through characteristic thoughts, actions, and choices, individuals influence their social worlds. Once created, the social environment shapes behavior, even the more enduring features and psychological processes commonly associated with personality.

Theorists have applied this transactional view of personality and social relations to Type A behavior (Smith & Anderson, 1986) and hostility (Smith & Pope, 1990). A fundamental tenet of this model is that coronary-prone behavior is stress-engendering behavior (see Smith & Anderson, 1986, for a review). For example, Type As are more likely to prefer challenging and demanding tasks and settings than are Type Bs. Confronted with the same task, Type As are more likely than Type Bs to appraise that task as demanding and set higher self-standards for performance. Type As are also more likely than Type B to evaluate task feedback negatively and to selectively attend to negative rather than positive aspects of feedback. Finally, Type As are more likely than Type Bs to respond to perceived interpersonal challenges and demands with overtly competitive and aggressive behavior. Through these thoughts and actions, Type As recurrently construct a more challenging and demanding proximal environment than do Type Bs. Once created, this environment has two unhealthy consequences. First, it is likely to maintain Type A behavior by creating the perceived necessity of further aggressive striving. Second, this more demanding environment is physiologically taxing because the high levels of perceived and actual challenge elicit heightened cardiovascular and neuroendocrine reactivity.

This general view is also relevant to the specific case of hostility. From this perspective, hostile persons, when compared to nonhostile individuals, not only experience more daily problems and stressors, they also *create* more frequent, severe, and enduring interpersonal conflicts. For example, by anticipating mistreatment and provocation from others, by interpreting actions of others as reflecting hostile intentions, and by treating others in a rude, controlling, and antagonistic manner, hostile individuals are likely to create and maintain high levels of conflict, struggles for dominance and control, low levels of support, and a general sense of isolation. This conflictual and unsupportive environment is, in turn, likely to maintain and exacerbate a hostile worldview and antagonistic interpersonal style. Figure 10.1 depicts this process.

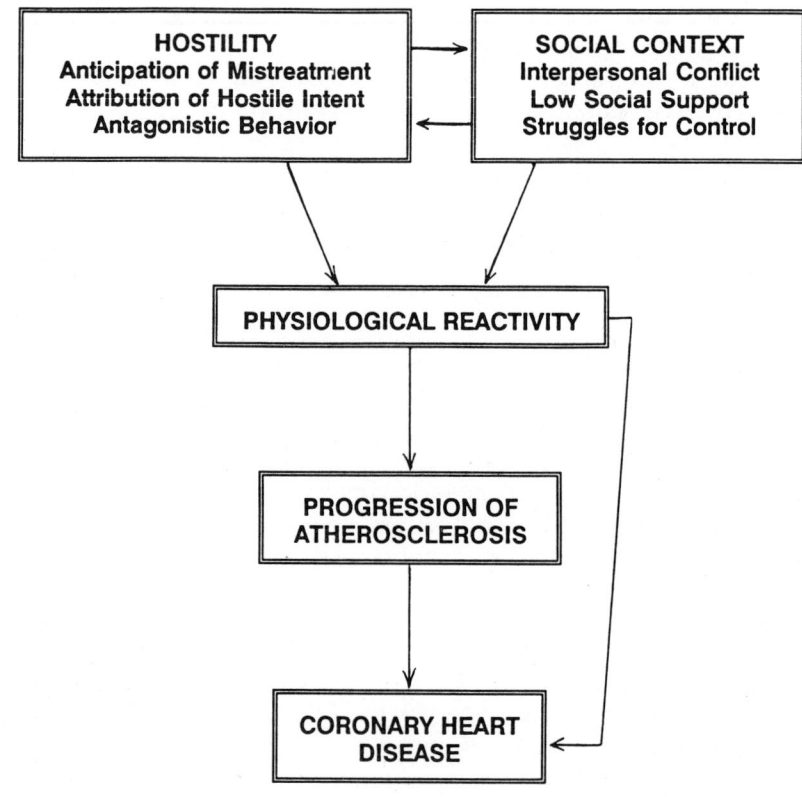

Figure 10.1. The transactional model of hostility, social context, and cardiovascular disease.

From this perspective, the cardiovascular and neuroendocrine reactivity believed to link hostility and cardiovascular disease reflects responses to two classes of situations and events. First, relative to nonhostile individuals, hostile individuals experience more pronounced reactivity to the common daily irritants normally experienced by nearly everyone. Second, hostile individuals experience additional social stressors created by their own characteristic thoughts and actions. The psychosocial vulnerability associated with hostility described earlier reflects the bidirectional impact of hostility and the social environment on one another. The net result of this maladaptive, reciprocal interaction is an increase in the frequency, magnitude, and duration of pathophysiological responses.

In contrast to this stress-engendering process, the far less frequently discussed and rarely studied beneficial effects of nonhostile or agreeable behavior generally reduce exposure to interpersonal stresses and strains. Trust, positive expectations, benign attributions for others' actions, and agreeable overt behavior are likely to have very different effects on the social environment. The end result is likely to be fewer and less severe conflicts and struggles for control, increased support and cooperation, and a general sense of positive social integration. In turn, this environment would have the beneficial effect of maintaining and fostering an agreeable style. In addition, there would be a reduction in the frequency, magnitude, and duration of episodes of pathophysiological reactivity.

One clear and important feature of the transactional model is that it extends the previous focus on the coronary-prone figure to include the surrounding interpersonal ground. From this perspective, comprehensive understanding, assessment, and intervention requires consideration of the individual, social context, and dynamic interactions between person and interpersonal environment.

Psychological Mechanisms Underpinning Unhealthy Behavior

Although researchers have made considerable efforts to explicate the connection between coronary-prone behavior and disease, investigators have given somewhat less attention to the underpinnings of the Type A pattern itself. This is also true of research on hostility. Understanding the psychological, or perhaps even psychobiological, basis of these behavior patterns would be useful in the development and refinement of intervention programs. Theoretical models are necessary to explain why Type As and hostile individuals behave the way they do. To date, only a small number of models exist.

One of the first psychological accounts of Type A behavior was Glass's (1977) view of coronary-prone behavior as a style of responding to perceived threats to one's sense of control over the environment. From this perspective, Type As are quick to perceive threats to their control. Hypothetically, achievement striving, aggressiveness, time urgency, and competitiveness are behavioral methods of maintaining or reestablishing control. Powell (1992) elaborated on this view, suggesting that Type As believe other people and external events are the primary causes of their distress. Furthermore, Powell suggested that Type As believe their sole recourse is to exert control over their surroundings. These convictions, combined with an unrealistic belief in their *ability* to control other people and external events, are core determinants of much of the Type A's actions. As in Glass's (1977) model, Powell (1992) hypothesized that overt Type A behaviors are vigorous attempts to manage other people and environmental situations, with the ultimate goal of obtaining their desired outcomes by firmly controlling external events. From this perspective, appropriate tempering of control beliefs is an important focus of treatment. Examples of such intervention goals include recognition that the external world is not always malleable and use of alternative or secondary control strategies (e.g., finding meaning in aversive events).

A second prominent model also focuses on underlying beliefs. Price (1982) argued that the core assumptions underpinning the overt Type A pattern are that (1) one must constantly prove oneself worthy through continual accomplishments, (2) relevant resources and opportunities to do so are scarce, and (3) no universal moral principles exist to assure that people will behave with a sense of fairness. These underlying beliefs promote insecurity and fears of insufficient self-worth. These beliefs also promote a view that the undersupply of resources to demonstrate self-worth creates the necessity for competition, struggle, and opposition toward others. Price's model clearly implicates beliefs and related cognitive processes as important targets for change.

Given that hostility has only recently become a central focus of the search for coronary-prone behavior, it is perhaps not surprising that there exist fewer models of the underpinnings of hostility than of the Type A behavior pattern. Certainly, it is possible to view anger and hostility as one way of maintaining or reasserting control over the interpersonal environment (Averill, 1982; Smith & Brown, 1991). Furthermore, in Price's (1982) model, hostility is one product of the view that others are untrustworthy and competitors for much needed, yet scarce resources. In a similar vein, Houston and Vavak (1991) suggested that hostility reflects underlying insecurity and an oppositional orientation toward others, resulting from early family interactions. Consistent with their own and others' findings (e.g., McGonigle et al., 1993; Smith et al., 1988; Woodall & Matthews, 1989), these authors suggest that parental behavior, characterized by low levels of genuine acceptance, substantial amounts of hostile control and punitiveness, and high levels of interference with the child's desires are likely to foster hostility. The lingering effects of these parental behaviors are a lack of trust, general expectations of mistreatment at the hands of others, and a low threshold for perceiving intentional interference and attempted domination by others. This low threshold for perceiving interpersonal threat and challenge would, in turn, prompt an antagonistic response style.

Many theoretical perspectives elsewhere in personality and developmental psychology are also relevant to issues regarding development and psychological underpinnings of hostility (for a review, see Thoresen & Pattillo, 1988). The central themes of both the conceptual and empirical literatures converge, however, to underscore the importance of insecure attachment and self-worth, a lack of trust, quickness to view actions of others as controlling and hostile, and a desire to exert control and dominance over others. As discussed by several theorists (e.g., Powell, 1992; Price, 1982; Thoresen & Powell, 1992), these factors are quite plausible underpinnings of hostile, coronary-prone behavior, and they are potentially valuable interpersonal issues in related treatments.

It is important to note that some authors have proposed that an underlying constitutional factor, rather than the psychological processes noted previously, accounts for overt coronary-prone behaviors and their association with disease (Krantz & Durel, 1983). From this psychobiological perspective, individual differences in sympathetic nervous system reactivity may *cause* the overt vocal and interpersonal Type A behaviors. This underlying mechanism, in turn, may also contribute to development of CHD. Thus, the statistical association between behavior and subsequent disease may be an artifact of an underlying, biological third variable as opposed to reflecting a direct causal relationship. Consistent with this view, cardiovascular reactivity (e.g., Smith et al., 1987), hostility (e.g., Smith, McGonigle, Turner, Ford, & Slattery, 1991), and Type A behavior (Matthews, Rosenman, Dembroski, Harris, & MacDougall, 1984) all display at least some genetic variance.

Even if an underlying biological factor, such as sympathetic nervous system reactivity, influences development of hostility and other Type A behaviors, associated psychological and social processes remain relevant to our understanding of the psychosomatic process. As outlined in current developmental theory (e.g., Scarr & McCartney, 1983), genetically influenced behavioral traits are likely to influence the surrounding social environment through the selection of situations and evocation of responses. Thus, as discussed in the transactional model above, hostility is likely to engender a hostile social environment whereas friendliness engenders cooperation and positive connection. Through this reciprocal transaction, effects of genetically influenced behavior on the environment produce further phenotypic differentiation; that is, hostile behavior tends to create a hostile social climate which, in turn, would foster further development and expression of hostility. Genetically influenced agreeable behavior would have an opposite reciprocal association with the social environment.

In addition, as outlined in the discussion of the transactional model, cognitive and behavioral correlates of hostility are likely to influence the pathophysiological process by leading to increased exposure to social stressors. Through their thoughts and actions, constitutionally vulnerable hostile individuals are likely to recurrently become exposed to what is, especially for them, an unhealthy environment. That is, they expose themselves to situations (e.g., competitive interactions) likely to activate their sympathetic diathesis. Thus, even this more basic psychobiological model of the origins and effects of hostility accommodates a focus on the potential cognitive and social processes.

Efficacy of Interventions

In the past decade, clinical researchers have reported many intervention studies. Reviews of this large and growing literature are available in more detail elsewhere (Haaga, 1987; Nunes, Frank, & Kornfeld, 1987; Thoresen & Powell, 1992). However, several important issues and conclusions emerging from this literature are particularly noteworthy. First, it is possible to modify Type A behavior. Although investigators have employed a variety of interventions, relaxation-based stress-management approaches are perhaps the most common. Nonetheless, investigators have also frequently employed cognitive–behavioral therapies, with a focus on modifying self-statements, beliefs, and self-evaluation processes hypothesized to contribute to the overt Type A behaviors of achievement-striving competitiveness, job involvement, impatience, and hostility. In a meta-analysis of treatment outcome studies, Nunes et al. (1987) found that multicomponent interventions were generally more effective than treatments using a single approach (e.g., relaxation therapy or cognitive restructuring alone).

An important limitation of most intervention studies is reliance on self-report methods of assessing Type A behavior. Other limitations of these studies are that they fail to include physiological measures or perform assessments of long-term health outcomes. Thus, while the interventions may reduce Type A behavior, measurement of this change often involves indices that lack clear evidence of an association with subsequent health. Therefore, the majority of these studies offer no direct evidence that changing the Type A pattern has any effect on health. There are important exceptions, however. Several studies have found significant posttreatment therapeutic changes on structured-interview assessments of Type A behavior and/or on physiological outcomes, such as blood pressure (e.g., Bennett, Wallace, Carroll, & Smith, 1991; Gill et al., 1985; Roskies et al., 1986).

The Recurrent Coronary Prevention Project

The most compelling evaluation of the clinical efficacy of modifying Type A behavior is the Recurrent Coronary Prevention Project (RCPP) conducted by Friedman et al. (1986). This large, controlled trial randomly assigned over 1,000 postmyocardial infarction (MI) patients to either a cardiac counseling condition receiving instruction in traditional risk factor change or a Type A group therapy condition. The Type A treatment focused on identification of Type A behaviors, modeling and rehearsal of alternative behaviors, relaxation therapy, and articulation and modification of underlying beliefs. The Type A group therapy condition produced significantly larger decreases in interview-assessed global Type A behavior than did the cardiac counseling control group. The Type A group therapy subjects also evidenced larger decreases in specific components of Type A behavior (e.g., hostility) than did subjects in the control group.

More important, at the end of 4.5 years, the Type A therapy group evidenced significantly fewer cardiac recurrences (i.e., coronary death, nonfatal MI) than the cardiac counseling group, 12.9% versus 21.2%, respectively (Friedman et al., 1986). Further analyses revealed that severity of initial MI related to subsequent cardiac death for members of the therapy group (Powell & Thoresen, 1988). Therapy significantly reduced cardiac deaths among patients with a less severe initial MI, but treatment did not significantly reduce the cardiac death rate for patients with more severe initial disease. These results suggest that therapeutic reduction of Type A behavior is not only possible, but may also have valuable health benefits, depending upon one's pretreatment cardiovascular functioning.

Modification of Anger and Hostility

Reductions in anger and hostility were a secondary focus in several of the Type A intervention studies noted previously. A small number of studies have focused directly on therapeutic modification of anger, outside of the context of the Type A pattern. Relaxation therapies (Hazaleus & Deffenbacher, 1986), social skills training (Deffenbacher, Story, Stark, Hogg, & Brandon, 1987; Moon & Eisler, 1983), and cognitive interventions designed to modify anger-inducing beliefs and self-statements (e.g., Novaco, 1975) have all been at least somewhat effective in reducing anger.

As the coronary-prone behavior literature evolves to focus more explicitly on anger and hostility, the related clinical intervention literature on anger reduction and control will become increasingly relevant and important (for reviews, see Biaggio, 1987 and Deffenbacher, 1994). Targets for these interventions are consistent with general models of Type A behavior, hostility, and the mechanisms linking these behaviors to health. Relaxation-based treatments are potentially useful in modifying the psychophysiological reactivity that accompanies episodes of anger. Cognitive interventions address maladaptive beliefs and appraisals that lead hostile individuals to view others as untrustworthy sources of intentional provocation. Cognitive interventions also attempt to reduce the likelihood that hostile individuals will construe normal daily irritants and frustrations as unfair and representing severe mistreatment. Finally, social skills training is likely to be useful in engendering approaches to interpersonal conflicts and problems that are both effective and less likely to elicit antagonism, mistreatment, and struggles for control from social interaction partners.

Emerging Issues

Several themes are clear in the recent research and theory discussed earlier. First, the association between Type A behavior and CHD is imperfect. Although sufficiently robust as to warrant further research and consideration in patient management, inconsistencies in this literature require alteration of traditional views of the Type A pattern. Several elements within the original description of Type A behavior (e.g., achievement-striving, job involvement) and assessment devices that primarily tap these dimensions (e.g., JAS) are clearly less relevant to cardiovascular health than once believed (Miller et al., 1991). As some elements of the Type A pattern have receded in importance, hostility has emerged as a particularly important trait. Although it is premature to accept hostility as an unquestionable coronary risk factor, evidence is generally supportive (Adler & Matthews, 1994; Miller et al., 1995). However, other related traits, most notably social dominance, might also be important predictors of disease and targets for intervention.

The link between coronary-prone behavior and disease is likely to involve physiological responses to psychological stressors; however, this research has not yet firmly established this. Factors eliciting differential reactivity from hostile and nonhostile individuals identify potentially important targets for intervention. Situations involving interpersonal conflict, provocation, struggles for dominance and control, and opportunities for mistrust are apparently relevant stressors for hostile individuals. Not only do hostile individuals show heightened reactivity to these situations, they also report more of these experiences at home and at work.

Unfortunately, investigators have studied the association between hostility and cardiovascular health, as well as possible underlying mechanisms, far more extensively in men than in women. It is quite possible that there are important gender differences in the correlates and consequences of hostility (Stoney & Engebretson, 1994). Thus, caution is appropriate when considering coronary-prone behaviors among women, and additional research is clearly necessary.

Interventions for coronary-prone behavior have considerable promise. As the focus on hostility and related traits sharpens, previous research and theory on anger management become increasingly relevant. Here again, interpersonal interactions, social skill repertoires, and arousal elicited in specific social situations may be useful targets for change.

Across these topics, the transactional perspective provides a useful model of the psychosomatic process and a guide to develop interventions aimed at interruption of this process. Psychophysiological correlates of recurring cycles in which hostile individuals anticipate, perceive, and exacerbate interpersonal strife are likely to contribute to cardiovascular disease. Spoiled opportunities for stress-dampening supportive relationships may be a further source of vulnerability among hostile individuals. The cognitive and behavioral mechanisms through which hostile individuals recurrently create physiologically taxing social circumstances are important foci for clinical interventions, as are ongoing discordant relationships themselves.

IMPLICATIONS FOR CLINICAL PRACTICE

Although one must consider many conclusions from the research discussed thus far as tentative, relevant evidence is sufficient to justify assessment and modification of coronary-prone behavior in an effort to reduce risk of initial or recurrent coronary events. Certainly, many questions remain unresolved, and additional research is necessary to answer these questions. However, on balance, research supports inclusion of treatments aimed at reducing coronary-prone behavior into cardiovascular disease prevention and management programs. The current review of this literature also permits specific recommendations concerning assessment and intervention targets and techniques. Nonetheless, it is important to place coronary-prone behavior in the context of comprehensive risk-reduction and management programs.

Preliminary Considerations

The relative priority of risk factors and related interventions must guide decisions about the appropriateness of a focus on coronary-prone behavior or personality traits in individual cases. For example, stress management and/or cognitive–behavioral interventions for anger might be poor first-choice treatments for CHD patients who smoke, are inactive, and have severely elevated cholesterol and blood pressure levels. The rigors of smoking cessation, an exercise program, and compliance with what could be a complex medication regimen are likely to present many challenges and demands. Multiple treatments are likely to exhaust most of the patients' and staffs' available time and resources for psychological care. Furthermore, extremely complex and demanding behavioral interventions are likely to be ineffective and could contribute to noncompliance or treatment dropout. Thus, treatment teams must make decisions as to the relative importance of modifying anger, hostility, or other coronary-prone behaviors (e.g., smoking, inactivity).

In making these decisions, there are few firm guidelines. However, a comprehensive evaluation of cardiovascular health status, medical treatment regimens, risk-factor profiles, and psychosocial consequences of existing diseases is necessary. In regard to psychosocial consequences of CHD, clinicians must assess for depression and disability (Smith & Leon, 1992). These factors require direct treatment in some cases. Recent evidence indicating that depression is associated with increased risk of death among CHD patients underscores the importance of considering this aspect of psychological functioning (Frasure-Smith et al., 1993). Brief screening instruments, reviews of patients' records, and clinical interviews can usually provide enough information about priorities for various psychosocial interventions.

The earliest stages of interventions for anger and hostility are particularly important. Angry and hostile patients, not surprisingly, can be defensive, resistant, and quite disagreeable. Often, family members, rather than patients, express concerns about the possible impact of anger and hostility on their family member's (i.e., patients') health. Patients may resist evaluation and treatment. From hostile individuals' externalizing points of view, their personal problems result from undeserved consequences of other people's thoughtless or selfish actions. These patients often vigorously deny that they have any emotional concerns or difficulties other than the burden of having to tolerate the incompetence and hurtful behavior of others. Thus, the earlier stages of clinical services must minimize defensiveness and cultivate participatory and collaborative relationships (Deffenbacher, 1994). A stance that minimizes the therapist's authority and dominance while emphasizing patient involvement and self-control is likely to be the most workable approach.

In the case of CHD patients, treatment team members can lay an important foundation for later work on hostility and related coronary-prone behaviors during phases of care that are not likely to arouse defensiveness. Brief, nonthreatening, supportive contact can facilitate adjustment to and recovery from invasive diagnostic and surgical procedures (for a review, see Smith and Williams, 1992). Therapeutic relationships established during this phase can make entry into more involved therapy much easier.

Assessment

Once the treatment team has identified modification of coronary-prone behavior as part of the overall patients' treatment plan, more detailed assessment is in order. Self-report measures of anger and hostility are important in this regard. Although there exist many scales used for this purpose (see Barefoot and Lipkus, 1994, and Smith, 1992, for reviews), the more widely used measures are the Cook and Medley (1954) Ho scale and the Buss–Durkee (1957) Hostility Inventory (BDHI). The Ho scale is a true–false item measure derived from the MMPI. The BDHI is also a true–false item scale, which assesses two general factors: expression of hostility, and experience of hostility. Interview-based methods of assessing hostility are quite useful, but they require specialized training in administration and scoring (see Barefoot and Lipkus, 1994, for a review).

In choosing between self-report and interview-based assessment procedures, one must be aware of several possible limitations of each approach (Barefoot & Lipkus, 1994). Training, administration, and scoring costs are potentially quite large for interviews. However, the relative ease and inexpense of self-report measures carry with them the problem that some hostile individuals may lack awareness of relevant thoughts and actions, or they may be reluctant to endorse socially undesirable characteristics. During relatively stressful and emotional situations, such as a recent coronary event or impending surgery, patients often cope through denial or minimization of their circumstances. This denial might generalize to emotional processes, such as anger or hostility, making self-reports less accurate.

The transactional approach to coronary-prone behavior and coronary-risk assessment focuses not only on hostility and personality issues; it also identifies other important targets for assessment. Clinicians need to assess frequency and severity of interpersonal conflicts at home and at work, either through existing questionnaires or by careful interviewing. Clinicians must also explore the availability and nature of potentially supportive relationships. Here again, valid questionnaires are widely available, and additional interview assessments are likely to be useful. In the event that spouses become involved in the eventual treatment, treatment team members can obtain additional assessment information from spouses through use of questionnaires and interviews. This information is typically quite important.

Assessment of anger, hostility, and related personality traits, when combined with information about ongoing interpersonal relationships and social situations, can provide a description of the transactional process through which hostility and maladaptive elements of the social environment are related. Additional information is necessary, however, to identify cognitive and behavioral processes underlying these cycles. Overt expressions of hostility and related emotions can take many forms, including sarcasm, condescension, contempt, disgust, and opposition. Thus, the list of overt indicators must go beyond verbal and physical aggressiveness and expressions of anger. Cognitive correlates of hostility are likely to include suspiciousness, cynicism, attributions of hostile intent to others, and the tendency to catastrophize, overgeneralize, and personalize implications of frustrating or otherwise unpleasant events. Discussion of recent or recurring irritating events, conducted carefully, may be able to clarify existing cognitive correlates of chronic anger and hostility. Evaluation of specific cognitive and behavioral correlates of hostility may permit more focused interventions.

Intervention

The transactional model identifies at least three factors that one must consider in comprehensive approaches to modifying coronary-prone behavior. First, therapists must address cognitive and behavioral processes through which hostile individuals increase their exposure to stressful interpersonal circumstances and subsequently undermine their social support. Second, ongoing relationships might be sufficiently dysfunctional as to warrant direct interventions, such as marital therapy or parent training. Finally, although cognitive–behavioral and relationship-focused interventions will likely have important effects on the frequency, duration, and severity of episodes of physiological reactivity, therapists may need to employ specific therapeutic techniques to directly address this final common pathway linking coronary-prone behavior and health.

Cognitive therapy for personality disorders (Beck & Freeman, 1990) and rational-emotive therapy (e.g., Ellis & Grieger, 1986) can readily assist with problems involving chronic anger and hostility. Many of the interventions for coronary-prone behavior discussed previously successfully utilize elements of these approaches. Assertiveness training and problem-solving training are effective approaches that aid in replacing hostile social behaviors with an interactional repertoire that permits appropriate navigation and resolution of interpersonal conflicts as well as effective resolution of other possibly frustrating or provoking circumstances. Several authors have presented integrative approaches to the combination of cognitive and interpersonally focused interventions (e.g., Safran, 1990). These integrative perspectives are consistent with the transactional approach presented here in that they view cognitive and interpersonal interventions as attempts to disrupt ongoing cycles in which recurring social behaviors elicit responses that maintain and exacerbate maladaptive ways of thinking about and behaving toward others.

Also, as noted previously, these maladaptive interaction cycles theoretically have their roots in early family interaction patterns. Thus, conceptual approaches to therapy that view developmental issues as an important context for active interventions intended to disrupt current maladaptive transactional processes (e.g., Strupp & Binder, 1984; Wachtel, 1977) are also consistent with this view. The focus is on disruption of current stress-engendering processes while recognizing that these patterns and their cognitive and motivational underpinnings may relate to early developmental experiences.

Attempts to change individuals' thoughts and behaviors may be very difficult because of the momentum of long-standing, recurring, maladaptive transactions. In such cases, a more direct focus on relationships might be appropriate. Brief marital therapy or communication skills training, for example, might disrupt cycles of conflict and permit more positive changes and transactions to occur. Ewart and his colleagues demonstrated the possible relevance of such techniques to coronary-prone behavior in a study in which they randomly assigned essential hypertensives and their spouses to either a control condition or communication skills training. The communication skills training intervention reduced the degree of cardiovascular reactivity elicited by discussions of marital disagreements and conflicts (Ewart, Taylor, Kraemer, & Agras, 1984). As noted earlier, hostile individuals report greater levels of marital conflict (Smith et al., 1988), display more hostile behavior during discussions of conflict (Smith et al., 1990b), and respond to these interactions with heightened cardiovascular reactivity (Smith & Brown, 1991), relative to nonhostile individuals. Thus, although rarely seen as relevant interventions in behavioral medicine approaches to stress management and modification of coronary-prone behavior, marital or other relationship therapies are clearly worth consideration.

Research evaluating interventions for cardiovascular reactivity remains relatively limited (Jacob & Chesney, 1986). However, various types of relaxation training and related techniques appear promising. Relaxation techniques, as noted, have also been effective in modifying habitual anger, either as a single-component treatment or in combination with other cognitive–behavioral procedures. These techniques are typically effective in producing subjectively pleasing effects quickly and are rarely perceived as threatening. Thus, relaxation procedures can provide an important starting point for otherwise defensive or resistant, hostile clients. It is also important to note that several medications commonly prescribed to CHD patients are likely to dampen reactivity. These medications include propranolol and other beta-adrenergic blocking agents.

From this discussion, it becomes clear that a comprehensive, integrative perspective on coronary-prone behavior can be a valuable framework for identifying relevant treatments, choosing among them, and sequencing their implementation. In this regard, the transactional model is an important aid to patient management.

CONCLUDING COMMENTS

The past three decades have produced important gains in our understanding of coronary-prone behavior. Clearly, much additional research is necessary to evaluate the importance of specific behaviors and personality traits, refine assessment procedures, explicate underlying pathophysiological mechanisms, and evaluate effectiveness of prescribed treatments. This is a large scientific agenda. At the same time, however, enough evidence has accumulated to suggest that general patient-management and risk-reduction efforts might profit from consideration of coronary-prone behavior. Clinical practice and continued research are likely to stimulate and enhance each other. The transactional perspective, by describing the coronary-prone *process* as emerging from active interactions between individuals and their surrounding social contexts, can provide a useful guide to their further evolution.

REFERENCES

Adler, N., & Matthews, K. (1994). Health psychology: Why do some people get sick and some stay well? *Annual Review of Psychology, 45,* 229–259.

Angell, M. (1985). Disease as a reflection of the psyche. *New England Journal of Medicine, 312,* 1570–1572.

Averill, J. R. (1982). *Anger and aggression: An essay on emotion.* New York: Springer-Verlag.

Barefoot, J. C. (1992). Developments in the measurement of hostility. In H. S. Friedman (Ed.), *Hostility, coping, and health* (pp. 13–31). Washington, DC: American Psychological Association.

Barefoot, J. C., Dahlstrom, W. G., & Williams, R. B., Jr. (1983). Hostility, CHD incidence, and total mortality: A 25-year follow-up study of 255 physicians. *Psychosomatic Medicine, 45,* 59–63.

Barefoot, J. C., & Lipkus, I. M. (1994). The assessment of anger and hostility. In A. W. Siegman & T. W. Smith (Eds.), *Anger, hostility, and the heart.* Hillsdale, NJ: Erlbaum.

Barefoot, J. C., Siegler, I. C., Nowlin, J. B., Peterson, B. L., Haney, T. L., & Williams, R. B., Jr. (1987). Suspiciousness, health, and mortality: A follow-up study of 500 older adults. *Psychosomatic Medicine, 49,* 450–457.

Beck, A. T., & Freeman, A. (1990). *Cognitive therapy of personality disorders.* New York: Guilford.

Bennett, P., Wallace, L., Carroll, D., & Smith, N. (1991). Treating type A behaviours and mild hypertension in middle-aged men. *Journal of Psychosomatic Research, 35,* 209–223.

Biaggo, M. K. (1987). Therapeutic management of anger. *Clinical Psychology Review, 7,* 663–675.

Booth-Kewley, S., & Friedman, H. (1987). Psychological predictors of heart disease: A quantitative review. *Psychological Bulletin, 101,* 342–362.

Brown, P. C., & Smith, T. W. (1992). Social influence, marriage, and the heart: Cardiovascular consequences of interpersonal control in husbands and wives. *Health Psychology, 11,* 88–96.

Burg, M., Jain, D., Soufer, R., Kerns, R. D., & Zaret, B. L. (1993). Role of behavioral and psychological factors in mental stress-induced silent left ventricular dysfunction in coronary artery disease. *Journal of the American College of Cardiology, 22,* 440–448.

Buss, A. H., & Durkee, A. (1957). An inventory for assessing different kinds of hostility. *Journal of Consulting Psychology, 21,* 343–349.

Christensen, A. J., & Smith, T. W. (1993). Cyclical hostility and cardiovascular reactivity during self-disclosure. *Psychosomatic Medicine, 55,* 193–202.

Cook, W. W., & Medley, D. M. (1954). Proposed hostility and pharisaic-virtue scales for the MMPI. *Journal of Applied Psychology, 38,* 414–418.

Cooper, T., Detre, T., & Weiss, S. M. (1981). Coronary-prone behavior and coronary heart disease: A critical review. *Circulation, 63,* 1199–1215.

Deffenbacher, J. L. (1994). Anger reduction: Issues, assessment and intervention strategies. In A. W. Siegman & T. W. Smith (Eds.), *Anger, hostility and the heart* (pp. 239–269). Hillsdale, NJ: Erlbaum.

Deffenbacher, J. L., Story, D. A., Stark, R. S., Hogg, J. A., & Brandon, A. D. (1987). Cognitive-relaxation and social skills interventions in the treatment of general anger. *Journal of Counseling Psychology, 34,* 171–176.

Dembroski, T. M., MacDougall, J. M., Costa, P. T., Jr., & Grandits, G. A. (1989). Components of hostility as predictors of sudden death and myocardial infarction in the Multiple Risk Factor Intervention Trial. *Psychosomatic Medicine, 51,* 514–522.

Dunbar, H. F. (1943). *Psychosomatic diagnosis.* New York: Hoeber.

Ellis, A., & Grieger, R. M. (1986). *Handbook of rational-emotive therapy* (vol. 2). New York: Springer.

Ewart, C. K., Taylor, C. B., Kraemer, H. C., & Agras, W. S. (1984). Reducing blood pressure reactivity during interpersonal conflict: Effects of marital communication training. *Behavior Therapy, 15,* 473–484.

Frasure-Smith, N., Lesperance, F., & Talajic, M. (1993). Depression following myocardial infarction: Impact on 6-month survival. *Journal of the American Medical Association, 270,* 1819–1825.

Friedman, M., & Rosenman, R. H. (1959). Association of specific overt behavior pattern with blood and cardiovascular findings. *Journal of the American Medical Association, 169,* 1286–1296.

Friedman, M., Thoresen, C. E., Gill, J. J., Ulmer, D., Powell, L. H., Price, V. A., Brown, B., Thompson, L., Rabin, D. D., Breall, W. S., Bourg, E., Levy, R., Dixon, T. (1986). Alteration of type A behavior and its effects on cardiac recurrences in post myocardial infarction patients: Summary results of the recurrent coronary prevention project. *American Heart Journal, 112,* 653–665.

Gill, J. S., Price, V. A., Friedman, M., Thoresen, C. E., Powell, L. H., Ulmer, D., Brown, B., & Drews, F. R. (1985). Reduction in type A behavior in healthy middle-aged American military officers. *American Heart Journal, 110,* 503–514.

Glass, D. C. (1977). *Behavior patterns, stress, and coronary disease.* Hillsdale, NJ: Erlbaum.

Haaga, D. A. (1987). Treatment for the type A behavior pattern. *Clinical Psychology Review, 7,* 557–574.

Harbin, T. J. (1989). The relationship between type A behavior pattern and physiological responsivity: A quantitative review. *Psychophysiology, 26,* 110–119.

Hardy, J. D., & Smith, T. W. (1988). Cynical hostility and vulnerability to disease: Social support, life stress, and physiological response to conflict. *Health Psychology, 7,* 447–459.

Hazaleus, S. L., Deffenbacher, J. L. (1986). Relaxation and cognitive treatments of anger. *Journal Consulting Clinical Psychology, 54,* 222–226.

Hearn, M. D., Murray, D. M., & Luepker, R. V. (1989). Hostility, coronary heart disease, and total mortality: A 33-year follow-up study of university students. *Journal of Behavioral medicine, 12,* 105–121.

Hecker, M. H. L., Chesney, M. A., Black, G. W., & Frautschi, N. (1988). Coronary-prone behaviors in the Western Collaborative Group Study. *Psychosomatic Medicine, 50,* 153–164.

Helmers, K. F., Krantz, D. S., Howell, R. H., Klein, J., Bairey, N., & Rozanski, A. (1993). Hostility and myocardial ischemia in coronary artery disease patients: Evaluation by gender and ischemic index. *Psychosomatic Medicine, 55,* 29–36.

Houston, B. K. (1988). Cardiovascular and neuroendocrine reactivity, global type A, and components of type A behavior. In B. K. Houston & C. R. Snyder (Eds.), *Type A behavior pattern: Research, theory, and intervention* (pp. 212–253). New York: Wiley.

Houston, B. K. (1994). Anger, hostility, and physiological reactivity. In A. W. Siegman & T. W. Smith (Eds.), *Anger, hostility, and the heart* (pp. 97–115). Hillsdale, NJ: Erlbaum.

Houston, B. K., Chesney, M. A., Black, G. W., Cates, D. S., & Hecker, M.H.L. (1992). Behavioral clusters and coronary heart disease risk. *Psychosomatic Medicine, 54,* 447–461.

Houston, B. K., & Kelly, K. E. (1989). Hostility in employed women: Relation to work and marital experiences, social support, stress, and anger expression. *Personality and Social Psychology Bulletin, 15,* 175–182.

Houston, B. K., & Vavak, C. R. (1991). Hostility: Developmental factors, psychosocial correlates, and health behaviors. *Health Psychology, 10,* 9–17.

Ironson, G., Taylor, C. B., Boltwood, M., Bartzokis, T., Dennis, C., Chesney, M., Spitzer, S., & Segall, G. M. (1992). Effects of anger on left ventricular ejection fraction in coronary artery disease. *American Journal of Cardiology, 70,* 281–285.

Jacob, R. G., & Chesney, M. A. (1986). Psychological and behavioral methods to reduce cardiovascular reactivity. In K. A. Matthews, S. M., Weiss, T. Detre, T. M. Dembroski, B. Falkner, S. B. Manuck, & R. B. Williams, Jr. (Eds.), *Handbook of stress, reactivity, and cardiovascular reactivity* (pp. 417–457). New York: Wiley.

Jamner, L. D., Shapiro, D., Goldstein, I. B., & Hug, R. (1991). Ambulatory blood pressure and heart rate in paramedics: Effects of cynical hostility and defensiveness. *Psychosomatic Medicine, 53,* 393–406.

Koskenvuo, M., Kapiro, J., Rose, R. J., Kesnaiemi, A., Sarnaa, S., Heikkila, K., & Langinvanio, H. (1988). Hostility as a risk factor for mortality and ischemic heart disease in men. *Psychosomatic Medicine, 50,* 330–340.

Krantz, D. S., Contrada, R. J., Hill, R. O., & Friedler, E. (1988). Environmental stress and biobehavioral antecedents of coronary heart disease. *Journal of Consulting and Clinical Psychology, 56,* 333–341.

Krantz, D. S., & Durel, L. A. (1983). Psychobiological substrates of the type A behavior pattern. *Health Psychology, 2,* 393–411.

Leon, G. R., Finn, S. E., Murray, D., & Bailey, J. M. (1988). The inability to predict cardiovascular disease from hostility scores of MMPI items related to type A behavior. *Journal of Consulting and Clinical Psychology, 56,* 597–600.

Manuck, S. B. (1994). Cardiovascular reactivity and cardiovascular disease: "Once more into the breach." *International Journal of Behavioral Medicine, 1,* 4–31.

Manuck, S. B., Kaplan, J. R., Muldoon, M. F., Adams, M. R., & Clarkson, T. B. (1991). The behavioral exacerbation of atherosclerosis and its inhibition by propranolol. In P. M. McCabe, N. Schneiderman, T. M. Field, & J. S. Skyler (Eds.), *Stress, coping, and disease* (pp. 51–72). Hillsdale, NJ: Erlbaum.

Matthews, K. A. (1988). CHD and type A behaviors: Update on and alternative to the Booth-Kewley and Friedman quantitative review. *Psychological Bulletin, 104,* 373–380.

Matthews, K. A., Glass, D. C., Rosenman, R. H., & Bortner, R. W. (1977). Competitive drive, pattern A, and coronary heart disease: A further analysis of some data from the Western Collaborative Group Study. *Journal of Chronic Diseases, 30,* 489–498.

Matthews, K. A., Rosenman, R. H., Dembroski, T. M., Harris, E. L., & MacDougall, J. M. (1984). Familial resemblance in components of the type A behavior pattern: A reanalysis of the California Type A Twin Study. *Psychosomatic Medicine, 46,* 512–522.

McGonigle, M. M., Smith, T. W., Benjamin, L. S., & Turner, C. W. (1993). Hostility and nonshared family environment: A study of monozygotic twins. *Journal of Research in personality, 27,* 23–34.

Miller, T. Q., Turner, C. W., Tindale, R. S., Posavac, E. J., & Dugoni, B. L. (1991). Reasons for the trend toward null findings in research on Type A behavior. *Psychological Bulletin, 110,* 469–485.

Miller, T. Q., Smith, T. W., Turner, C. W., Guijarro, M. L., & Hallet, A. J. (1995). A meta-analytic review of research on hostility and physical health. (Manuscript under review.)

Moon, J. R., Eisler, R. M. (1983). Anger control: An experimental comparison of three behavioral treatments. *Behavioral Therapy, 14,* 493–505.

Novaco, R. (1975). *Anger control: The development and evaluation of an experimental treatment.* Lexington, MA: Heath.

Nunes, E. V., Frank, K. A., Kornfeld, D. S. (1987). Psychologic treatment for the type A behavior pattern and for coronary heart disease: A meta-analysis of the literature. *Psychosomatic Medicine, 48,* 159–173.

Osler, W. (1892). *Lectures on angina pectoris and allied states.* New York: Appleton.

Pope, M. K., & Smith, T. W. (1991). Cortisol excretion in high and low cynically hostile men. *Psychosomatic Medicine, 53,* 386–392.

Powell, L. H. (1992). The cognitive underpinnings of coronary-prone behaviors. *Cognitive Therapy and Research, 16,* 123–142.

Powell, L. H., & Thoresen, C. E. (1988). Effects of type A behavioral counseling and severity of prior acute myocardial infarction on survival. *American Journal of Cardiology, 62,* 1159–1163.

Price, V. A. (1982). *Type A behavior pattern: A model for research and practice.* New York: Academic Press.

Ragland, D. R., & Brand, R. J. (1988). Type A behavior and mortality from coronary heart disease. *New England Journal of Medicine, 318,* 65–69.

Rosenman, R. H. (1978). The interview method of assessment of the coronary-prone behavior pattern. In T. M. Dembroski, S. M. Weiss, J. L. Shields, S. Haynes, & M. Feinleib (Eds.), *Coronary-prone behavior* (pp. 55–69). New York: Springer-Verlag.

Roskies, E., Seraganian, P., Oseasohn, R., Hanley, J. A., Collee, R., Martin, N., & Smilga, C. (1986). The Montreal Type A Intervention Project: Major findings. *Health Psychology, 5,* 45–69.

Safran, J. D. (1990). *Interpersonal process in cognitive therapy.* New York: Basic Books.

Scarr, S., & McCartney, K. (1983). How people make their own environments: A theory of genotype–environment effects. *Child Development, 54,* 424–435.

Scherwitz, L., Perkins, L., Chesney, M., & Hughes, G. (1991). Cook–Medley Hostility Scale scores and subsets: Relationship to demographic and psychosocial characteristics in young adults in the CARDIA study. *Psychosomatic Medicine, 53,* 36–49.

Shekelle, R. B., Billings, J. H., & Borhani, N. O. (1985a). The MRFIT behavior pattern study II. Type A behavior and incidence of coronary heart disease. *American Journal of Epidemiology, 122,* 559–570.

Shekelle, R. B., Gale, M., & Norusis, M. (1985b). Type A score (Jenkins Activity Survey) and risk of recurrent coronary heart disease in the Aspirin Myocardial Infarction Study. *American Journal of Cardiology, 56,* 221–225.

Shekelle, R. B., Gale, M., Ostfeld, A. M., & Paul, O. (1983). Hostility, risk of coronary heart disease, and mortality. *Psychosomatic Medicine, 45,* 109–114.

Siegman, A. W., & Dembroski, T. M. (1989). *In Search of coronary-prone behavior: Beyond type A.* Hillsdale, NJ: Erlbaum.

Smith, T. W. (1992). Hostility and health: Current status of a psychosomatic hypothesis. *Health Psychology, 11,* 139–150.

Smith, T. W., & Allred, K. D. (1989). Blood pressure responses during social interaction in high and low cynically hostile males. *Journal of Behavioral Medicine, 12,* 135–143.

Smith, T. W., Allred, K. D., Morrison, C. A., & Carlson, S. D. (1989). Cardiovascular reactivity and interpersonal influence: Active coping in a social context. *Journal of Personality and Social Psychology, 56,* 209–218.

Smith, T. W., & Anderson, N. B. (1986). Models of personality and disease: An interactional approach to type A behavior and cardiovascular risk. *Journal of Personality and Social Psychology, 50,* 1166–1173.

Smith, T. W., Baldwin, M., & Christensen, A. (1990a). Interpersonal influence as active coping: Effects of task difficulty on cardiovascular reactivity. *Psychophysiology, 27,* 429–437.

Smith, T. W., & Brown, P. (1991). Cynical hostility, attempts to exert social control, and cardiovascular reactivity in married couples. *Journal of Behavioral Medicine, 14,* 579–590.

Smith, T. W., & Christensen, A. J. (1992). Cardiovascular reactivity and interpersonal relations: Psychosomatic processes in social context. *Journal of Social and Clinical Psychology, 11,* 279–301.

Smith, T. W., & Frohm, K. D. (1985). What's so unhealthy about hostility? Construct validity and psychosocial correlates of the Cook and Medley Ho scale. *Health Psychology, 4,* 503–520.

Smith, T. W., & Leon, A. (1992). *Coronary heart disease: A behavioral perspective.* Champaign, IL: Research Press.

Smith, T. W., McGonigle, M., Turner, C. W., Ford, M. H., & Slattery, M. L. (1991). Cynical hostility in adult male twins. *Psychosomatic Medicine, 53,* 684–692.

Smith, T. W., & Pope, M. K. (1990). Cynical hostility as a health risk. Current status and future directions. *Journal of Social Behavior and Personality, 5,* 77–88.

Smith, T. W., Pope, M. K., Sanders, J. D., Allred, K. D., & O'Keeffe, J. L. (1988). Cynical hostility at home and work: Psychosocial vulnerability across domains. *Journal of Research in Personality, 22,* 525–548.

Smith, T. W., Sanders, J. D., & Alexander, J. F. (1990b). What does the cook and Medley Hostility Scale measure? Affect, behavior and attributions in the marital context. *Journal of Personality and Social Psychology, 58,* 699–708.

Smith, T W., Turner, C. W., Ford, M. H., Hunt, S. C., Barlow, G. K., Stults, B. M., & Williams, R. R. (1987). Blood pressure reactivity in adult male twins. *Health Psychology, 6,* 209–220.

Smith, T. W., & Williams, P. G. (1992). Stress reduction in the prevention and management of coronary heart disease. In F. Yanowitz (Ed.), *The prevention of coronary heart disease: A view towards the 21st century* (pp. 427–446). New York: Marcel Dekker.

Stoney, C. M., & Engebretson, T. O. (1994). Anger and hostility: Potential mediators of the gender difference in coronary heart disease. In A. W. Siegman & T. W. Smith (Eds.), *Anger, hostility, and the heart* (pp. 215–238). Hillsdale, NJ: Erlbaum.

Strupp, H. H., & Binder, J. L. (1984). *Psychotherapy in a new key: A guide to time-limited dynamic psychotherapy.* New York: Basic Books.

Suarez, E. C., & Williams, R. B., Jr. (1989). Situational determinants of cardiovascular and emotional reactivity in high and low hostile men. *Psychosomatic Medicine, 51,* 404–418.

Suls, J., & Sanders, G. S. (1989). Why do some behavioral styles place people at coronary risk? In A. W. Siegman & T. M. Dembroski (Eds.), *In search of coronary-prone behavior* (pp. 1–20). Hillsdale, NJ: Erlbaum.

Suls, J., & Wan, C. (1993). The relationship between trait hostility and cardiovascular reactivity: A quantitative review and analysis. *Psychophysiology, 30,* 615–626.

Syme, S. L. (1987). Coronary artery disease: A sociocultural perspective. *Circulation, 76,* 1112–1116.

Thoresen, C. E., & Pattillo, J. R. (1988). Exploring the type A behavior pattern in children and adolescents. In B. K. Houston & C. R. Snyder (Eds.), *Type A behavior pattern: Research, theory, and intervention* (pp. 98–145). New York: Wiley.

Thoresen, C. E., & Powell, L. H. (1992). Type A behavior pattern: New perspectives on theory, assessment and intervention. *Journal of Consulting and Clinical Psychology, 60,* 595–604.

Wachtel, P. L. (1977). *Psychoanalysis and behavior therapy.* New York: Basic Books.

Williams, R. B., Jr., Barefoot, J. C., & Shekelle, R. B. (1985). The health consequences of hostility. In M. A. Chesney & R. H. Rosenman (Eds.), *Anger and hostility in cardiovascular and behavioral disorders* (pp. 173–185). Washington, DC: Hemisphere.

Woodall, K. L., & Matthews, K. A. (1989). Familial environment associated with type A behaviors and psychophysiological responses to stress in children. *Health Psychology, 8,* 403–426.

11

Hypertension

Thomas G. Pickering

The etiology of hypertension remains unknown, but we do know one clearly established fact: No single cause is responsible. High blood pressure is the end result of several factors, both genetic and environmental, that may be quantitatively and qualitatively different for different individuals. It is thus a heterogeneous process. Furthermore, blood pressure distribution is continuous in the population with no clear separation between normal and raised blood pressure. Any definition of hypertension is thus quite arbitrary.

Scientists have, for many years, suspected that psychological factors play a role in development of hypertension, although conclusive evidence is still lacking. Investigators have used three general approaches to identify the potential role of such factors: (1) to study effects of environmental stressors, (2) to look for personality differences between normotensive and hypertensive individuals, and (3) to examine relevance of individual differences in susceptibility (or reactivity) to stress. It seems reasonable to suppose that all three are important and that any effects are likely to be interactive.

Figure 11.1 depicts a convenient model for defining the roles of psychological factors. There are three independent variables in this model. First is the nature of the stressor, which is a characteristic of the environment. Second is perception of the stressor. This depends both on individuals' personalities and previous experiences. What is very stressful for one individual is not necessarily as stressful for another. Effects of perceived stress on blood pressure will, in turn, depend on the third factor, physiological susceptibility. This may depend on genetic and environmental factors (e.g., family history of hypertension, state of sodium balance). We discuss each of these three variables in turn.

Thomas G. Pickering • Cardiovascular Center, The New York Hospital–Cornell University Medical College, New York, New York 10021.
Handbook of Health and Rehabilitation Psychology, edited by Anthony J. Goreczny. Plenum Press, New York, 1995.

BEHAVORIAL FACTORS AND CARDIOVASCULAR DISEASE

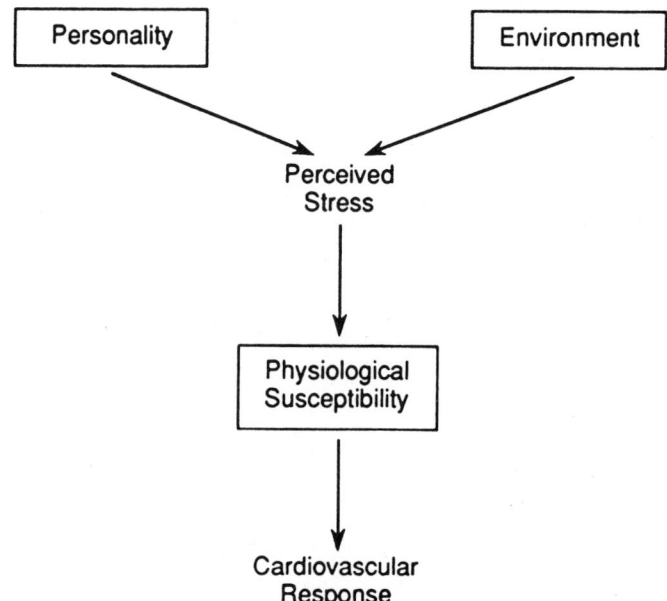

Figure 11.1. Hypothetical interaction of factors that may contribute to behaviorally mediated hypertension.

ENVIRONMENTAL SOURCES OF PSYCHOLOGICAL STRESS

Although blood pressure tends to rise with age, this is not an invariable phenomenon, and there are many known societies in which blood pressure remains low throughout life. Cultural rather than genetic factors appear to determine whether blood pressure changes with age. Timio et al. (1988) provide a good example of this phenomenon with a 20-year observational study of Italian nuns living in a secluded order. Investigators compared the nuns with a control group, both at entry and after 20 years. Blood pressures were the same at entry, but by the end of the study, blood pressures were approximately 30 mmHg higher in controls. Changes in body weight, diet, and childbearing could not explain the differences. The authors concluded that differences were due to the monastic and relatively stress-free environment.

A similar series of observations has occurred utilizing individuals who migrate from a stable traditional society to a westernized one. Studies of the nomadic Samburo in Kenya (Shaper, 1962) and the bushmen of the Kalahari (Kaminer & Lutz, 1960) have shown no increase of blood pressure with age. Bushmen who abandon their traditional lifestyle, however, and become farm laborers, or even prisoners, have blood pressures 15 mmHg higher than the nomads (Turswell, Kennelly, Hansen,

& Lee, 1972). In addition, Samburo warriors who joined the Kenyan army also evidenced an increase of blood pressure (Shaper, Leonard, K. Jones & M. Jones, 1969). Numerous other studies could be quoted that confirm the effects of acculturation from structured traditional societies to contemporary Western life, but the problem with nearly all of them is that it is difficult to know exactly what factors were responsible for the rise of blood pressure. Although stress may be one of the responsible factors, there are also major dietary changes.

One of the most important studies is the Kenyan Luo migration study (Poulter et al., 1990) in which researchers prospectively followed 355 subjects who migrated from rural villages to Nairobi for 2 years after they migrated. The study also included a matched control group that stayed in the villages. Even as soon as 1 month after migrating, the blood pressure distribution curve of migrants had shifted to the right. There were also significant increases in body weight, heart rate, and urinary sodium: potassium ratio. Over the 2-year follow-up period, the differences in blood pressure persisted whereas those of body weight and heart rate did not. The authors suggested that the two factors responsible for the early increase of blood pressure were sodium retention and increased sympathetic nervous system activity occurring in response to the stress of migrating.

The Defense–Defeat Model

The defense reaction is a very fundamental response to challenges in the natural environment and consists of a generalized autonomic arousal, including an increase of blood pressure and cardiac output and increased blood flow to skeletal muscles. Many years ago, Brod, Fencl, Hejl, and Jirka (1959) observed that these changes resemble those seen in young patients with borderline hypertension. Neel (1962) proposed that "diseases of civilization," such as diabetes, may occur as a result of natural selection and that traits that conferred a survival advantage in primitive societies may be detrimental in modern society. Julius, Gudbrandsson, Jamerson, and Andersson (1992) extended this concept to include hypertension, and they proposed that a permanent hemodynamic pattern of the defense reaction would lead to hypertension and insulin resistance.

On the basis of an extensive series of studies of mice housed in colonies designed to promote social interaction and conflict, Henry and Stephens (1977) proposed that two psychophysiological patterns, which they referred to as the *defense* and *defeat reactions,* might determine which individuals become hypertensive and which do not (Figure 11.2). Henry's mice lived in population cages consisting of boxes connected by narrow tubing wide enough to accommodate only one mouse at a time. This promotes development of social hierarchy in which dominant animals develop higher pressures than subordinates. Subsequent work showed that subdominants attempting to achieve control evidenced the highest pressures (160 mmHg); the blood pressure in stable, unchallenged dominants was 145 mmHg, and in subordinates, it was 125 mmHg (Ely, 1981; Henry, Stephens, & Ely, 1986). Using rats, Fokkema (1985) reported results similar to those of Henry and Stephens (1977); subdominant individuals evidenced the highest pressures.

Conceptually, dominant animals display a chronic defense (fight or flight) reaction characterized by activation of the sympathetic nervous system, whereas subor-

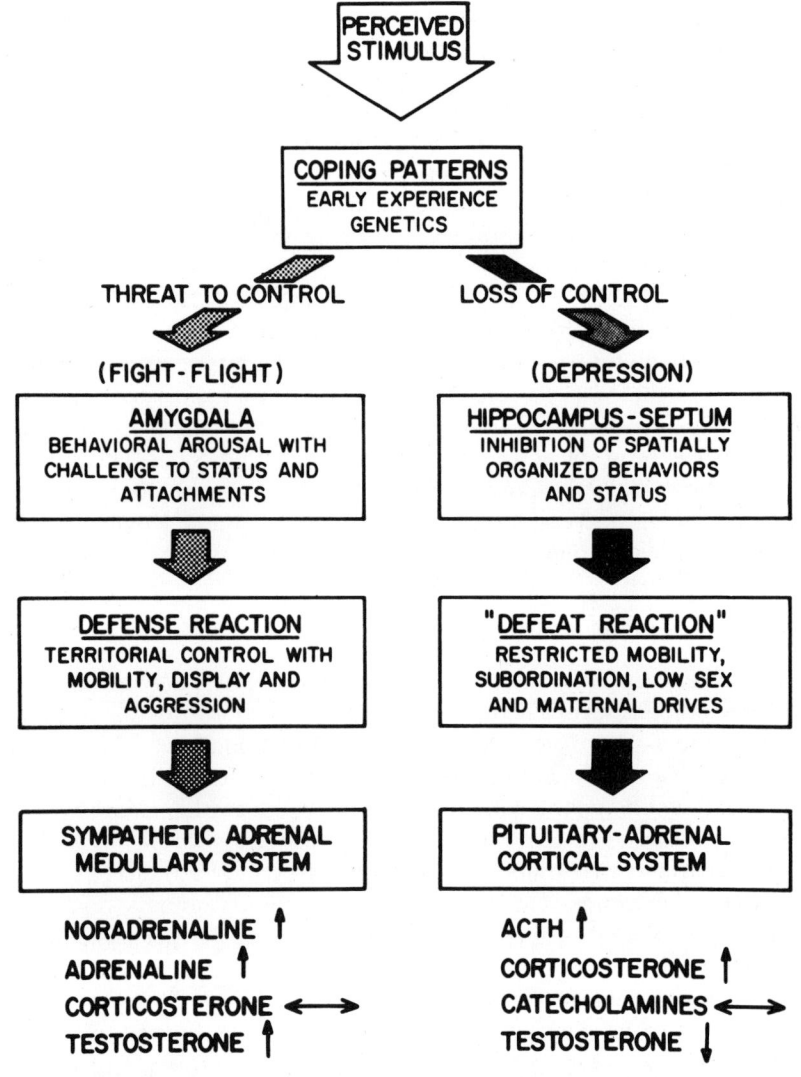

Figure 11.2. The defense–defeat model by Henry. The left-hand arm shows the defense reaction, characterized by sympathetic activation, and the right-hand arm displays the defeat reaction. Reproduced with permission from Henry, Stephens, and Ely (1986).

dinates exhibit the defeat reaction in which there is activation of the pituitary–adrenal cortical axis.

Not surprisingly, comparable studies in man are sparse. D'Atri and Ostfeld (1975), however, reported a situation analogous to the social interaction of mice in population cages; they studied men confined to prison. The systolic blood pressure of men who had lived for several months in a dormitory was 131 mmHg, whereas in men living in single-occupancy cells, it was only 115 mmHg. Furthermore, transfer from a cell to a dormitory caused blood pressure to increase and vice versa (D'Atri,

Fitzgerald, Kasl, & Ostfeld, 1981). Dietary factors were not responsible for these changes because all prisoners ate the same food.

The Demand–Control and Effort–Distress Models

Dominant individuals in the social hierarchy of the defense–defeat model are hypothetically attempting to achieve control. Two models that originated in Sweden and closely resemble each other have some similarity to the model of Henry, Stephens, and Ely (1986). The first is the Job Strain Model of Karasek and Theorell (Karasek, Baker, Marxer, Ahlbohm, & Theorell, 1981), which they specifically designed to assess occupational stress. It has two orthogonal components: (1) psychological demands; and (2) decision latitude, which is equivalent to control (Figure 11.3). The most stressful (or "high strain") jobs are those that, according to individuals' perceptions, combine high demands and low decision latitude. This model has primarily been useful as an aid for studying effects of job strain on development of coronary heart disease (Alfredson, Karasek, & Theorell, 1982; Karasek et al., 1981, 1988), but we have shown that it may also be relevant in the development of hypertension. In a case-control study of men employed in a variety of jobs, we found that hypertensive individuals were approximately three times more likely than normotensive controls to work in high-strain jobs (Schnall et al., 1990). Exposure to job strain was also associated with an increased left ventricular mass, a finding that is consistent with sustained elevation of blood pressure. Subjects in high-strain jobs also had higher ambulatory blood pressures (Schnall, Schwartz, Landsbergis, Warren, & Pickering, 1992). Interestingly, this elevation of pressures was not only seen during subjects' working hours, but also at home and during sleep. An important aspect of these results is that neither of the two components of job strain (i.e., demands and perceived control) were individually associated with any changes of blood pressure; it was only the interaction of high demands and low control that had an effect.

Two interactive effects observed in our study are worth noting. The first was with alcohol intake; the highest blood pressures were observed in subjects who had

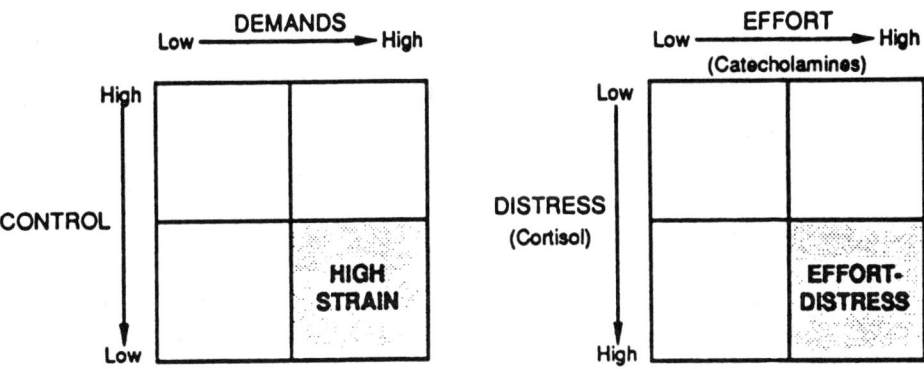

Figure 11.3. Two related models for evaluating effects of stress on blood pressure. On the left, the demand–control model of Karasek, and on the right, the effort–distress model of Frankenhaueser.

high-strain jobs and drank regularly. Alcohol intake had no discernible effect on blood pressure in subjects with low-strain jobs. In the present context, alcohol intake may be another environmental pressor agent, which perhaps relates to personality variables. The second interactive effect was with age; effects of job strain on blood pressure were much greater in older than in younger subjects. This could have at least two explanations: (1) strain effects are cumulative over many years, or (2) physiological susceptibility of older subjects might be greater than susceptibility of younger subjects.

These findings have received support from other studies. Theorell et al. (1991) studied 161 men with borderline hypertension using ambulatory monitoring, and found that job strain (expressed as the ratio between psychological demands and control) was significantly related to diastolic pressure during work and at night. Van Egeren (1992) studied 11 subjects with "high-strain" jobs and 26 subjects with "low-strain" jobs and found that subjects with "high-strain" jobs evidenced higher blood pressures both at work and when at home. There was a less clearcut tendency for sleep pressures to be higher as well.

A closely related model is the effort–distress model of Frankenhaueser (1983). This model also has two orthogonal components (see Figure 11.3): effort and distress. Effort corresponds to demands in the job-strain model, and distress corresponds to control. Effort is conceived as arousing the sympathetic nervous system and distress the adrenocortical system. Lundberg and Frankenhaueser (1980) provide a typical example of this type approach in a study in which normal subjects performed two tasks: the first a monotonous vigilance task perceived to induce effort and distress; and the second a more enjoyable, self-paced reaction-time talk that required effort but was without distress. During the vigilance task, urinary excretion of both epinephrine and cortisol increased, whereas during the reaction-time task, only epinephrine increased. Researchers have not yet related this model to sustained hypertension.

Models of Socioecological Stress

The studies of effects of acculturation briefly reviewed above suggest that there is something about modern society that tends to elevate blood pressure. Waldron, Nowotarski, Freimer, Henry, Post, and Witten (1982) pooled data from 84 different societies and concluded that higher blood pressures were associated with increasing emphasis on a market economy, increased economic competition, and decreased family ties. These associations appear to be independent of salt intake and, in men, obesity.

In a series of studies, Dressler has developed the concept of "lifestyle incongruity," defined as the extent to which a high-status style of life exceeds an individual's occupational class (Dressler, 1982; Dressler, Alfonso, Chavez, & Viteri, 1987a; Dressler, Santos, Gallagher, & Viteri, 1987b). Evaluation of lifestyle incongruity is relatively objective and consists of matching occupation and income on one hand and possession of material goods on the other. Lifestyle incongruity relates to blood pressure not only in developing countries, but also in U.S. blacks.

James and his colleagues used a somewhat similar approach in their development of the concept of John Henryism to investigate effects of socioecological stress in blacks (James, Hartnett, & Kalsbeck, 1983). Individuals who score high on the

John Henryism scale believe that they can control environmental stressors through a combination of hard work and determination. In their first study, they found that men who scored below the sample median on education but above the median on John Henryism had higher blood pressures than men who scored above the median on both measures. In a subsequent study (James, La Croix, Kleinbaum, & Stragatz, 1984), they found that men who had achieved a relatively high level of job success and scored high on John Henryism had higher diastolic pressures than men with similar levels of job success and low John Henryism. Another psychosocial factor that contributed to higher pressures in the more successful men was the perception that being black had hindered their chances of success.

Harburg et al. (1973b) also demonstrated effects of socioecological stress on blood pressure in blacks. These investigators performed a population survey of blood pressure in different neighborhoods of Detroit, defined either as "high stress" or "low stress" according to socioeconomic status of inhabitants (defined by several variables, such as income, home ownership, and education) and instability variables (e.g., crime rate and marital instability). The highest blood pressures were seen in black males under age 40 living in high-stress neighborhoods; black and white males living in low-stress neighborhoods had similar pressures.

INDIVIDUAL PSYCHOLOGICAL FACTORS AND THE PERCEPTION OF STRESS

Two types of factors relevant to individual differences regarding perception of potential stressors are individuals' personalities, which are relatively immutable, and their previous experiences or learning, which obviously are not. Because there is no evidence that hypertension is a learned behavior pattern (although this remains an interesting possibility), this discussion will be restricted to personality variables.

Personality Variables and Hypertension

The idea that there is a "hypertensive personality" has been mooted for many years, but the issue remains unsettled. The concept of a hypertensive personality originated with Alexander (1993) who proposed that hypertensive individuals experience repressed hostility, or "anger-in," which the body channels into the autonomic nervous system resulting in increased blood pressure. Shapiro (1988) renewed this theory. One of the earlier studies reporting this phenomenon, conducted by Wolf and Wolff (1951), evaluated personality measures using both interviews and questionnaires with 103 hypertensive patients, 150 patients with allergies, and 61 normotensive hospitalized patients. They concluded that hypertensives had restrained aggression and excess inner tension. A more recent example of such a finding comes from a study by Perini et al. (1990), who studied younger subjects with borderline hypertension and age-matched normotensive controls with and without family history of hypertension. The hypertensives showed less externalized aggression, more internalized aggression, and more submissiveness. They also demonstrated evidence of increased sympathetic nervous activity, such as faster heart rates and higher plasma catecholamines. A potential problem with such studies is that characteristics such as anger and anxiety, which are frequently associated with hypertension, may be a consequence of making the diagnosis (a "labeling" phenomenon) rather than etiological factors, and there is always a problem of knowing what constitutes an appropriate control group. A more reliable method may be to study a randomly selected population. One such study, conducted by Harburg et al. (1973a), found that in men, "anger-in" correlated with blood pressure.

Although there are many other studies that have reported varying degrees of association between inhibited aggression and blood pressure (reviewed by Cottier, Perini, & Rauchfleisch, 1987), other studies have reported negative or inconsistent results (Ostfeld & Lebovitz, 1959; Steptoe, Melville, & Ross, 1982; Sullivan et al., 1981).

Two other personality variables that have been reported to be characteristic of hypertensive individuals are submissiveness (Esler et al., 1977; Harburg, Julius, McGinn, McLeod, & Hoobler, 1964) and *alexithymia,* defined as inappropriate affect, difficulty expressing emotions, and absence of fantasies (Sifneos, Appel-Savitz, & Frankel, 1977). There is limited evidence, reviewed by Cottier et al. (1987), that both these variables relate to blood pressure.

The Type A behavior pattern, generally regarded as being, at least in part, a personality variable, has been most closely related to coronary heart disease. Most studies, however, have not found any close relationship between the Type A pattern and hypertension (reviewed by Irvine, Garner, Craig, & Logan, 1991), perhaps because most of the studies used only one or two blood pressure measurements. An example was the Western Collaborative Group Study in which 3,524 men were followed for 8 years (Rosenman, Brand, Jenkins, Friedman, Strauss, & Wurm, 1975). Irvine et al. (1991) compared prevalence of Type A in 109 untreated hypertensives and 109 demographically matched controls. The investigators measured blood pressures five times over 5 months and assessed Type A behavior by the structured interviews. The investigators found that Type A behavior was significantly more prevalent in hypertensives (78%) than in normotensives (60%). Hostility, now considered to be one of the most important components of coronary-prone behavior (Dembroski & Williams, 1989), was also higher among hypertensives than normotensives.

Hostility has also been shown to have an interactive effect with occupational stress on blood pressure, at least over the short term. In a study of paramedics who wore ambulatory blood pressure monitors during a workday, Jamner, Shapiro, Goldstein, and Hug (1991) found that subjects who scored high on hostility and defensiveness demonstrated higher diastolic pressures while in the hospital but not while waiting for a call in the ambulance station.

INDIVIDUAL DIFFERENCES IN SUSCEPTIBILITY TO PSYCHOLOGICAL FACTORS

Effects of perceived stress on the cardiovascular system depend to some extent on physiological susceptibility of individuals. In other words, for a given intensity of a stressor, some individuals will be more reactive than others. In practice, it may be difficult to separate physiological and psychological components of reactivity, but conceptually this distinction is important. Of all components of the potential interactions between stress and blood pressure. Reactivity has received much more attention than any other component, and, in my opinion, more than it deserves.

The Reactivity Hypothesis

In its simplest form, the reactivity hypothesis states that individuals who show increased cardiovascular reactivity to psychologically stressful stimuli are at increased risk of developing cardiovascular disease, which is often taken to include hypertension and coronary heart disease as if they were a single entity, which of course they are not. Two forms of the hypothesis, as it relates to hypertension, exist: (1) in the "Recurrent Activation Model," response to laboratory tests is assumed to be correlated with intermittent pressor responses to stress occurring in everyday life, whereas in (2) the "Prevailing State Model," laboratory response predicts average level of blood pressure (Manuck & Krantz, 1986). Folkow (1978) also suggested that stressors initially produce transient elevations of blood pressure by neurohormonal mechanisms and that these elevations may, in turn, induce structural changes in arterial walls that eventually result in sustained increase of vascular resistance and, hence, increased blood pressure. Stimuli that are psychologically stressful hypothetically elicit this mechanism, but there is no clear reason why it need not also apply to physically stressful stimuli, such as exercise.

It must be admitted, however, that direct evidence in support of this mechanism is limited. For example, one recent study demonstrated that neurogenically produced pressor episodes do not, on their own, lead to any sustained increase in basal blood pressure level, although they can produce left ventricular hypertrophy (Julius, Li, Brant, Krause, & Buda, 1989). In addition, exercise training, which certainly produces intermittent neurogenically mediated pressor episodes, results in reduction of resting blood pressure level (Jennings, Nelson, Esler, Leonard, & Korner, 1984).

We have reviewed elsewhere some of the criteria that this hypothesis must satisfy (Pickering & Gerin, 1990). First, degree of reactivity for an individual subject should be stable over time; second, it should to some extent, be generalizable from one type of challenge to another; third, it should be generalizable from the laboratory to the stresses of everyday life; and fourth, reactivity should be an independent predictor of disease.

Several studies have investigated the test–retest reliability of blood pressure changes measured during reactivity testing (Langewitz, Ruddell, Noack, & Wachtarz, 1989; Manuck & Garland, 1980; Manuck & Schaefer, 1978; McKinney et al., 1985; Myrtek, 1985; Parati et al., 1983, 1986; Van Egeren & Sparrow, 1989). Most studies have used noninvasive blood pressure measurements. The interval between tests ranged from 30 minutes to 4 years, and the reported test–retest correlations have varied quite widely, ranging from about 0.4 to 0.7. Thus, the reproducibility is not very good.

Surprisingly few studies have systematically examined extent to which an individual subject's response to one task will predict his or her response to another. Parati et al. (1986) found that responses to two predominantly mental tasks (mental arithmetic and mirror drawing) correlated quite well with each other ($r = 0.78, p < 0.01$), and responses to two predominantly physical tasks (isometric exercise and cold pressor test) also correlated well with each other, but correlations between responses to the mental and physical tasks were not significant. Fredrikson, Dimberg, Frisk-Holmberg, and Strom (1985) examined correlations between change scores for four tasks: an attentional demands task, mental arithmetic, cold pressor test, and isometric exercise. The only significant correlation for systolic pressure was between mental arithmetic and isometric exercise in normotensive subjects; for hypertensives, none of the correlations was significant. In contrast, Turner, Girdler, Sherwood, and Light (1990) found significant correlations between four tasks (two involving speech and two, mental arithmetic) ranging from 0.62 to 0.80 for systolic pressure but considerably lower correlations for diastolic pressure.

These results suggest there is limited evidence for generalizability of reactivity across dissimilar tasks and that characterizing an individual as being generally "hyperactive" has little validity at the present time.

Physiological and Demographic Factors Affecting Reactivity

Several studies have compared blood pressure reactivity in normotensive and hypertensive subjects. We (Pickering & Gerin, 1990) reviewed a selection of these studies, those that gave adequate details of actual blood pressure levels and statistical comparison. The two most extensively studied tests have been mental arithmetic and cold pressor test. We concluded that there is a tendency for hypertensives to show increased reactivity to behavioral tasks but not to physical tasks. Fredrikson and Matthews (1990) performed a formal meta-analysis of studies in the area. They concluded that patients with essential hypertension (blood pressures of at least 165/95 mmHg) showed exaggerated systolic blood pressure responses to passive stressors (including the cold pressor test) in comparison to normotensive controls, although this effect was present in only 31 of 63 studies. Overall, borderline hypertensives showed a significantly greater response to active stressors (in 8 of 25 individual studies).

For mental arithmetic, which is a predominantly behavioral task, there is a fairly consistent tendency for hypertensives to show enhanced responses. This is in contrast to predominantly physical tasks (i.e., cold pressor test, isometric or dynamic exercise) in which there is less convincing evidence of any difference. For the cold pressor test and exercise, there is nonetheless a trend for reactivity to be greater in patients with more severe hypertension. These findings are consistent with increased reactivity being, at least in part, a consequence rather than a cause of hypertension.

The only population-based study, conducted with 169 men and 120 women by Julius et al. (1991) in Tecumseh, Michigan, did not find any correlation between reactivity to mental arithmetic or isometric exercise and resting blood pressure levels. These authors pointed out that one reason for the discrepancy between their findings and those of other studies comparing normotensives and hypertensives was that their subjects were not necessarily aware of which diagnostic group they were in, whereas in most other studies they were. The importance of this is that it has been shown by Rostrup, Kjeldsen, and Eide (1990) demonstrated that labeling subjects as hypertensive increases their blood pressure reactivity.

Several studies have examined influence of family history of hypertension on reactivity, and many of them have dealt with children. The meta-analysis by Fredrikson and Matthews (1990) concluded that 13 of 30 studies demonstrated increased blood pressure or heart rate reactivity in association with positive family history and that overall, this effect was significant in comparison with subjects without family history of hypertension. The difference was more reliable for active than for passive tasks. For example, one study reported that blood pressure responses to dynamic exercise were higher in subjects with family history of hypertension than in those without such history (Molineux & Steptoe, 1988). A more recent study of normotensive young adults found that subjects with positive family history (either one or both parents hypertensive) had higher baseline pressures (measured both in the laboratory and during ambulatory monitoring) but did not show exaggerated blood pressure responses to four different stressors (Ravogli et al., 1990). The Tecumseh study, mentioned previously, did not find any association between blood pressure reactivity and family history (Fredrikson & Matthews, 1990).

Several factors may increase or decrease blood pressure reactivity to stressful stimuli. Caffeine (Lovallo et al., 1989) and sodium (Faulkner, Onesti, & Angelakos, 1981a) both increase it, whereas exercise training (Blumenthal et al., 1990) and a diet high in polyunsaturated fatty acids (Mills, Prkachin, Harvey, & Ward, 1989) tend to reduce it.

Psychological Factors Influencing Differences in Reactivity

As reviewed previously, attempts to relate a specific personality type with hypertension have been, on the whole, disappointing. The picture is a little better with blood pressure reactivity; in a meta-analysis of 71 studies comparing cardiovascular reactivity in Type A and Type B individuals, Harbin concluded that Type A men show consistently greater reactivity of systolic (but not diastolic) pressure and heart rate to cognitive challenges (Harbin, 1989). Parallel with these findings, Weidner et al. (1989) reported that men and women scoring high on tests of hostility have larger blood pressure reactivities, relative to low hostility scorers, when attempting a frustrating task.

With mental-challenge tasks requiring an active response by the subject, subjects' attitudes to the task would be expected to affect the responses. A study by Smith, Allred, Morrison, and Carlson (1989) confirmed this expectation; these investigators found that increases of blood pressure that occur during talking are much greater if the individuals talking are trying to persuade another individual to change his or her opinion about something, relative to subjects who are talking without such attempts at persuasion.

Does Reactivity Measured in the Laboratory Predict Blood Pressure Changes in Everyday Life?

The rationale generally proposed for use of laboratory tests of cardiovascular reactivity is that individuals' responses to such tests may predict how they respond to stressful situations in real life. Until quite recently, it has not been possible to test this assumption, but with introduction of ambulatory monitoring techniques, it can now be attempted.

Four studies have compared responses to laboratory stressors with blood pressure variability measured via the intra-arterial technique of ambulatory monitoring (Floras, Hassan, Jones, & Sleight, 1987; Melville & Raftery, 1981; Parati et al., 1986;

Watson, Stallard, Flinn, & Littler, 1980). Several studies have used noninvasive ambulatory monitoring techniques (Fredrikson, Blumenthal, Evans, Sherwood, & Light, 1989; Fredrikson, Tuonuisto, Lundberg, & Melin, 1990; Harshfield et al., 1988; Ironson et al., 1989; Langewitz, Rüddell, Schächinger, & Schmieder, 1989b; McKinney et al., 1985; Van Egeren & Sparrow, 1989). Because blood pressure recordings occur intermittently rather than continuously by this technique, characterization of blood pressure variability and reactivity is inevitably less precise than with intra-arterial monitoring. All these studies found very low or absent correlations between blood pressure reactivity (measured as change scores) and ambulatory blood pressure.

Viewed as a whole, these studies suggest that if there is an association between reactivity measured in the laboratory and blood pressure variability or reactivity of daily life, it is rather weak, or problems of measurement obscure its detection. Furthermore, this association appears to be quite nonspecific; that is, laboratory challenges demonstrate this association equally well (or badly) both with and without a strong behavioral component. The simplest explanation of findings such as those of Floras et al. (1987) is that there are significant interindividual differences in blood pressure variability that are detectable by both laboratory testing and ambulatory monitoring. As they stand, the results of these studies provide little evidence that the type of reactivity testing commonly used in the laboratory is an ecologically valid representation of the stresses of everyday life. Yet, the assumption of such validity is the basis for much of the work done in this field. It seems clear that a great deal of research must be done in this area before conclusions can be drawn.

It could be argued, however, that it is unreasonable to expect a laboratory task to predict overall blood pressure variability and that it would be more appropriate to look for correlations with blood pressure changes during specific activities of daily life that closely resemble laboratory tasks. Matthews, Manuck, and Saab (1986) used such an approach, and they found a significant correlation between blood pressure changes during a laboratory speaking task and a similar task in the classroom. Turner et al. (1990) used a similar tactic when comparing responses to speaking tasks in the laboratory to a simulated "real-life" speaking task. There were no correlations between reactivity scores for the two types of tasks unless they made adjustments for effects of posture, subjects having performed laboratory tasks while sitting and real-life tasks while standing.

In the Tecumseh population study (Julius et al., 1991) using 169 men and 120 women, the investigators examined the association between two indices of reactivity (mental arithmetic and isometric exercise) and two measures of target-organ damage (left ventricular mass and minimal forearm vascular resistance). Subjects classified as hyperreactors to mental arithmetic did not show any greater signs of vascular damage than those not classified as such.

Prognostic Significance of Blood Pressure Reactivity

Blood pressure is not the only factor used to predict hypertension. A family history of hypertension is also of major importance; in Thomas's prospective study of medical students, subjects who had two hypertensive parents and a high initial clinic systolic pressure (above 125 mmHg) were 12.6 times as likely to become hypertensive over a 30-year follow-up period as subjects without these risk factors (Thomas & Duszyncki, 1982).

If the reactivity hypothesis is correct, increased reactivity would predict future hypertension. Eight studies have used the cold pressor test for evaluating reactivity; investigators followed between 73 and 1,185 subjects for periods ranging from 10 to 45 years (Armstrong & Rafferty, 1960; Barnett, Hines, Schirger, & Gage, 1963; Eich & Jacobsen, 1967; Gillum, Taylor, Anderson, & Blackburn, 1981; Harlan, Obsorne, & Graybiel, 1964; Menkes et al., 1989; Thomas & Duszyncki, 1982; Wood, Sheps, Elvebach, & Schirger, 1984). The results of one study (the Precursors Study of medical students at Johns Hopkins University) appeared in two different analyses (Thomas & Duszyncki, 1982; Menkes et al., 1989). Five of eight studies found no prediction of future hypertension or blood pressure level based on degree of reactivity (Armstrong & Rafferty, 1960; Barnett et al., 1963; Gillum et al., 1981; Harlan et al., 1964; Thomas & Duszyncki, 1982); one other claimed positive predictive results, but only 4 of 207 subjects became hypertensive, 3 of whom had positive family histories (Barnett et al., 1963). Therefore, this study cannot determine whether reactivity would predict hypertension independently of family history, the major predictive factor for hypertension. One other study also reported a significant role of reactivity in 142 individuals followed for 45 years, but the investigators based classification of hyperreactivity on two cold pressor tests performed 27 years apart (Wood et al., 1984).

The most extensive study, and the one that deserves most attention, was the Johns Hopkins Precursors Study. This study involved about 1,000 male medical students followed for up to 35 years. In the first report, published in 1982 (Thomas & Duszyncki, 1982), the cold pressor test failed to predict future hypertension, but a subsequent analysis, published in 1989 and using more sophisticated statistical techniques than the 1982 study (Menkes et al., 1989) found that after adjusting for age, obesity, baseline blood pressure, and smoking, an exaggerated response to the cold pressor test did predict development of hypertension after an interval of 20 years. Without these adjustments, however, there was still no association.

Two studies have reported that reactivity to mental arithmetic, which has more of a psychological component than the cold pressor test, does predict future blood pressure. The first, by Falkner, Onesti, and Hamstra (1981b), followed 80 adolescents with borderline hypertension for up to 5 years. Both a positive family history and exaggerated blood pressure response to mental arithmetic predicted development of hypertension. Unfortunately, the investigators did not evaluate the relative importance of family history versus reactivity. The second study, by Borghi, Costa, Boschi, Mussi, and Ambrosioni (1986), reported that subjects with a positive family history and borderline hypertension showed increased reactivity to both behavioral and physical challenges and that they were more likely to become hypertensive over a 5-year period. Overall, however, evidence that blood pressure reactivity is an independent predictor of future blood pressure status remains unconvincing.

CONCLUSIONS

Attempts to find a "holy grail" of hypertension, a single factor that determines who becomes hypertensive and who does not, have proven universally frustrating. This applies both to psychological and physiological causes. It thus seems plausible that, in any one individual, hypertension may result from the interaction of a variety of contributing factors that may vary in different individuals.

It is well established that blood pressure has social and cultural determinants, but the precise factors responsible for group and individual differences remain elusive. Although dietary habits are undoubtedly important, they cannot explain observed differences, and there is a growing body of evidence to suggest that psychosocial stressors also play a role. Although several different factors and models to explain their effects have been proposed, a common feature to them all is an element of discord between individuals and their social settings. Several examples illustrate this notion. In Henry's defense–defeat model, organisms struggling to maintain a position of social dominance are those with the highest blood pressures, whereas individuals at the lower end of the pecking order who accept "defeat" remain normotensive. In Dressler's model, it is the incongruity between individuals' aspirations and resources that is pathogenic. In the Job Strain, or demand–control model, there is also conflict between demands and control. Thus, most of those models rely on an interaction of two or more factors to produce hypertension rather than postulating any one factor acting on its own. Because human behavior is infinitely complex, these models are not mutually exclusive. We should not necessarily expect a model that predicts hypertension in blacks living in Detroit to have the same predictive ability for Italian nuns living in a convent.

We must also acknowledge that individual factors are important. Personality variables have been the subject of much attention and research studies have produced mixed results. Repressed anger and submissiveness are the two personality variables most frequently invoked, but the findings are inconsistent. In part, this may be a measurement issue because of difficulties quantifying something as nebulous as personality, but it may also mean that we need to focus on subsets of patients (e.g., those with high renin levels) in whom personality variables contribute to blood pressure, perhaps in conjunction with environmental stressors.

The most extensively studied individual factor is blood pressure reactivity, but despite an enormous amount of research on the subject, the relevance of increased cardiovascular reactivity to development and consequences of hypertension remains unclear. There is no consensus as to which test defines reactivity, although most experts express reactivity in terms of the change from a baseline level rather than as the absolute value of blood pressure during the test. Generalization of an individual's responses from one test to another cannot be assumed. Also, hypertensives do tend to show greater reactivity than normotensives, particularly to behavioral challenges, but this may be a consequence rather than a cause of hypertension. This could occur for a variety of reasons, for example, as a labeling phenomenon or from structural changes in arteries. Blood pressure reactivity measured in the laboratory does not provide a good prediction of blood pressure changes that occur during everyday life.

The reactivity hypothesis requires that reactivity should predict the development of hypertension. Attempts to demonstrate this have met with varying success, and in some of the reportedly positive studies, it has not been established that reactivity is independent of other predictors. These considerations lead us to conclude that, on the basis of present evidence, increased blood pressure reactivity to behavioral stimuli is unlikely to play a primary role in development of hypertension. Evidence that chronic exposure to environmental stressors can accelerate development of hypertension, on the other hand, is quite encouraging. Whether such stressors produce a more pronounced effect in particular personality types or individuals who are hyperactive remains unclear, but this area may prove a productive area for future research.

REFERENCES

Alexander, F. (1939). Emotional factors in essential hypertension. *Psychosomatic Medicine, 1,* 173–179.

Alfredsson, L., Karasek, R., & Theorell, T. (1982). Myocardial infarction risk and psychosocial work environment: An analysis of the male Swedish working force. *Social Science and Medicine, 16,* 463–467.

Armstrong, H. G., & Rafferty, J. A. (1960). Cold pressor test: Follow-up study for seven years on 166 officers. *American Heart Journal, 39,* 484–490.

Barnett, P. H. Hines, K. A., Schirger, A., & Gage, R. P. (1963). Blood pressure and vascular reactivity to the cold pressor test. *Journal of the American Medical Association, 183,* 845–848.

Blumenthal, J. A., Fredrikson, M., Kuhn, C. M., Ulmer, R. L., Walsh-Riddle, M., & Appelbaum, M. (1990). Aerobic exercise reduces levels of cardiovascular and sympathodrenal responses to mental stress in subjects without prior evidence of myocardial ischemia. *American Journal of Cardiology, 65,* 93–98.

Borghi, C., Costa, F. V., Boschi, S., Mussi, A., & Ambrosioni, E. (1986). Predictors of stable hypertension in young borderline subjects: A five-year follow-up study. *Journal of Cardiovascular Psychopharmacology, 8*(Suppl. 5), S138–S141.

Brod, J., Fencl, V., Hejl, Z., & Jirka, J. (1959). Circulatory changes underlying blood pressure elevation during acute emotional stress (mental arithmetic) in normotensive and hypertensive subjects. *Clinical Science, 18,* 269–279.

Cottier, C., Perini, C., & Rauchfleisch, U. (1987). Personality traits and hypertension: An overview. In S. Julius & D. R. Bassett (Eds.), *Handbook of hypertension: Vol. 9, Behavioral factors in hypertension* (pp. 123–140). Amsterdam: Elsevier.

D'Atri, D. A., Fitzgerald, E. F., Kasl, S. K., & Ostfeld, A. M. (1981). Crowding in prison: The relationship between changes in housing mode and blood pressure. *Psychosomatic Medicine, 43,* 95–105.

D'Atri, D. A., & Ostfeld, A. M. (1975). Crowding—Its effects on the elevation of blood pressure in prison setting. *Behavioral Medicine, 4,* 550–556.

Dembroski, T. M., & Williams, R. B. (1989). Definition and assessment of coronary-prone behavior. In N. Schneiderman, S. M. Weiss, & P. G. Kaufman (Eds.), *Handbook of research methods in cardiovascular behavioral medicine* (pp. 553–570). New York: Plenum Press.

Dressler, W. W. (1982). *Hypertension and culture change: Acculturation and disease in the West Indies.* South Salem, NY: Redgrave.

Dressler, W. W., Alfonso, M., Chavez, A., & Viteri, F. E. (1987a). Arterial blood pressure and individual modernization in a Mexican community. *Social Science and Medicine, 24,* 679–687.

Dressler, W. W., Santos, I., Gallagher, P. N., & Viteri, F. E. (1987b). Arterial blood pressure and modernization in Brazil. *American Anthropologist, 89,* 389–409.

Eich, R. H., & Jacobsen, E. C. (1967). Vascular reactivity in medical students followed for 10 years. *Journal of Chronic Diseases, 20,* 583–592.

Ely, D. L. (1981). Hypertension, social rank and aortic arteriosclerosis in CBA/J mice. *Physiology and Behavior, 26,* 655–661.

Esler, M. D., Julius, S., Zweifler, A., Randall, O., Harburg, E., Gardiner, H., & De Quattro, V. (1977). Mild high-renin essential hypertension: Neurogenic human hypertension? *New England Journal of Medicine, 296,* 405–411.

Falkner, B., Onesti, G., & Angelakos, E. (1981a). Effect of salt loading on the cardiovascular response to stress in adolescents. *Hypertension, 3*(Suppl. II), II-195–II-199.

Falkner, B., Onesti, G., & Hamstra, B. (1981b). Stress response characteristics of adolescents with high genetic risk for essential hypertension: A five-year follow-up. *Clinical and Experimental Hypertension, 3,* 583–591.

Floras, J. S., Hassan, M. O., Jones, J. V., & Sleight, P. (1987). Pressor responses to laboratory stresses and daytime blood pressure variability. *Journal of Hypertension, 5,* 715–719.

Fokkema, D. S. (1985). *Social behavior and blood pressure (a study of rats).* Unpublished doctoral dissertation. Groningen University, Netherlands.

Folkow, B. (1978). Cardiovascular structural adaptation: Its role in the initiation and maintenance of primary hypertension. *Clinical Science and Molecular Medicine, 55*(Suppl. IV), IV-3–IV-22.

Frankenhaueser, M. (1983). The sympathetic-adrenal and pituitary-adrenal response to challenge: Comparison between the sexes. In T. M. Dembroski, T. H. Schmidt, & G. Blümchen (Eds.), *Biobehavioral bases of coronary heart disease* (pp. 91–105). Basel: Karger.

Fredrikson, M., Blumenthal, J. A., Evans, D. D., Sherwood, A., & Light, K. C. (1989). Cardiovascular responses in the laboratory and in the natural environment: Is blood pressure reactivity to laboratory-induced mental stress related to ambulatory blood pressure during everyday life? *Journal of Psychosomatic Research, 33,* 753–762.

Fredrikson, M., Dimberg, U., Frisk-Holmberg, M., & Strom, G. (1985). Arterial blood pressure and general sympathetic activation in essential hypertension during stimulation. *Acta Medica Scandinavica, 217,* 309–317.

Fredrikson, M., & Matthews, K. A. (1990). Cardiovascular responses to behavioral stress and hypertension: A meta-analytic review. *Annals of Behavioral Medicine, 12,* 30–39.

Fredrikson, M., Tuomisto, M., Lundberg, U., & Melin, B. (1990). Blood pressure in healthy men and women under laboratory and naturalistic conditions. *Journal of Psychosomatic Research, 34,* 675–686.

Gillum, R. F., Taylor, H. L., Anderson, J., & Blackburn, H. (1981). Longitudinal study (32 years) of exercise tolerance, breathing response, blood pressure, and blood lipids in young men. *Arteriosclerosis, 1,* 455–462.

Harbin, T. J. (1989). The relationship between Type A behavior pattern and physiological responsivity: A quantitative review. *Psychophysiology, 26,* 110–119.

Harburg, E., Erfurt, J. C., Chape, C., Hauenstein, L. S., Schull, W. J., & Schork, M. A. (1973a). Socioecological stressor areas and black–white blood pressure: Detroit. *Journal of Chronic Diseases, 26,* 595–611.

Harburg, E., Erfurt, J. C., Hauenstein, L. S., Schull, W. J., & Schork, M. A. (1973b). Socioecological stress, suppressed hostility, skin color, and black–white blood pressure: Detroit. *Psychosomatic Medicine, 35,* 276–296.

Harburg, E., Julius, S., McGinn, N. F., McLeod, J., & Hoobler, S. W. (1964). Personality traits and behavioral patterns associated with systolic blood pressure levels in college males. *Journal of Chronic Diseases, 17,* 405–414.

Harlan, W. R., Osborne, R. K., & Graybiel, A. (1964). Prognostic value of the cold pressor test and the basal blood pressure: Based on an 18-year follow-up study. *American Journal of Cardiology, 13,* 683–687.

Harshfield, G. A., James, G. D., Schlussel, Y., Yee, L. S., Blank, S. G., & Pickering, T. G. (1988). Do laboratory tests of blood pressure reactivity predict blood pressure variability in real life? *American Journal of Hypertension, 1,* 168–174.

Henry, J. P., & Stephens, P. M. (1977). *Stress, health and the social environment: A sociobiologic approach to medicine.* New York: Springer-Verlag.

Henry, J. P., & Stephens, P. M. (1986). Psychosocial hypertension and the defense and defeat reactions. *Journal of Hypertension, 4,* 687–697.

Henry, J. P., Stephens, P. M., & Ely, D. L. (1986). Psychosocial hypertension and the defense and defeat reaction. *Journal of Hypertension, 4,* 687–697.

Ironson, G. H., Gellman, M. D., Spitzer, S. B., Llabre, M. M., DeCarlo, P. R., Weidler, D. J., & Schneiderman, N. (1989). Predicting home and work blood pressure measurements from resting baselines and laboratory reactivity in black and white Americans. *Psychophysiology, 26,* 174–184.

Irvine, J., Garner, D. M., Craig, H. M., & Logan, A. G. (1991). Prevalence of type A behavior in untreated hypertensive individuals. *Hypertension, 18,* 72–78.

James, S. A., Harnett, S. A., & Kalsbeck, W. (1983). John Henryism and blood pressure differences among black men. *Journal of Behavioral Medicine, 6,* 259–278.

James, S. A., La Croix, A. Z., Kleinbaum, D. G., & Stragatz, D. S. (1984). John Henryism and blood pressure differences among black men: II. The role of occupational stressors. *Journal of Behavioral Medicine, 7,* 259–275.

Jamner, L. D., Shapiro, D., Goldstein, I. B., & Hug, R. (1991). Ambulatory blood pressure and heart rate in paramedics: Effects of cynical hostility and defensiveness. *Psychosomatic Medicine, 53,* 393–406.

Jennings, G. J., Nelson, L., Esler, M., Leonard, P., & Korner, P. I. (1984). Effects of changes in physical activity on blood pressure and sympathetic tone. *Journal of Hypertension, 2*(Suppl. 3), 139–141.

Julius, S., Li, Y., Brant, D., Krause, L., & Buda, A. J. (1989). Neurogenic pressor episodes fail to cause hypertension, but do induce cardiac hypertrophy. *Hypertension, 13,* 422–429.

Julius, S., Gudbrandssoin, T., Jamerson, K., & Andersoon, O. (1992). The interconnection between sympathetics, microcirculation and insulin resistance in hypertension. *Blood Pressure, 1,* 9–19.

Julius, S., Jones, K., Schork, N., Johnson, E., Krause, L., Nazzaro, P., & Zemua, A. (1991). Independence of pressure reactivity from pressure levels in Tecumseh, Michigan. *Hypertension, 17*(Suppl. III), III-12–III-21.

Kaminer, B., & Lutz, W. (1960). Blood pressures in Kalahari bushmen. *Circulation, 22,* 289–295.

Karasek, R. A., Baker, D., Marxer, F., Ahlbohm, A., & Theorell, T. (1981). Job decision latitude, job demands, and cardiovascular disease: A prospective study of Swedish men. *American Journal of Public Health, 75,* 694–705.

Karasek, R. A., Theorell, T., Schwartz, J. E., Schnall, P. L., Pieper, C. F., & Michela, J. L. (1988). Job characteristics in relation to the prevalence of myocardial infarction in the U.S. Health Examination Survey (HESS) and the Health and Nutrition Examination Survey (HAINES). *American Journal of Public Health, 78,* 910–918.

Langwitz, W., Rüddel, H., Noack, H., & Wachtarz, K. (1989a). The reliability of psychophysiological examinations under field conditions: Results of repetitive stress testing in middle-aged men. *European Heart Journal, 10,* 657–665.

Langewitz, W., Rüddel, H., Schächinger, H., & Schmieder, R. (1989b). Standardized stress testing in the cardiovascular laboratory: Has it any bearing on ambulatory blood pressure values? *Journal of Hypertension, 7*(Suppl. 3), 541–548.

Lovallo, W. R., Pincomb, G. A., Sung, B. H., Passey, R. B., Sausen, K. P., & Wilson, M. R. (1989). Caffeine may potentiate adrenocortical stress responses in hypertension-prone men. *Hypertension, 14,* 170–176.

Lundberg, U., & Frankenhaeuser, M. (1980). Pituitary-adrenal and sympathetic-adrenal correlates of distress and effort. *Journal of Psychosomatic Research, 24,* 125–130.

Manuck, S. B., & Garland, F. N. (1980). Stability of individual differences in cardiovascular reactivity: A thirteen month follow-up. *Physiology and Behavior, 24,* 621–624.

Manuck, S. B., & Krantz, D. W. (1986). Psychophysiologic reactivity in coronary heart disease and essential hypertension. In K. A. Matthews, S. M. Weiss, T. Detre, T. M. Dembroski, B. Falkner, S. B. Manuck, & R. B. Williams (Eds.), *Handbook of stress, reactivity, and cardiovascular disease.* New York: Wiley.

Manuck, S. B., & Schaefer, D. C. (1978). Stability of individual differences in cardiovascular reactivity. *Physiology and Behavior, 21,* 675–678.

Matthews, K. A., Manuck, S. B., & Saab, P. G. (1986). Cardiovascular responses of adolescents during a naturally occurring stressor and their behavioral and psychophysiological predictors. *Psychophysiology, 23,* 198–209.

McKinney, M. E., Miner, M. H., Ruddell, H., McIlvain, H. E., Witte, H., Buell, J. C., & Eliot, R. S. (1985). The standardized mental stress test protocol: Test–retest reliability and comparison with ambulatory blood pressure monitoring. *Psychophysiology, 22,* 453–463.

Melville, D. I., & Raftery, E. B. (1981). Blood pressure changes during acute mental stress in hypertensive subjects using the Oxford intra-arterial system. *Journal of Psychosomatic Medicine, 24,* 487–497.

Menkes, M. S., Matthews, K. A., Krantz, D. S., Lundberg, U., Mead, L. A., Qaqish, B., Liang, K.-Y., Thomas, C. B., & Pearson, T. A. (1989). Cardiovascular reactivity to the cold pressor test as a predictor of hypertension. *Hypertension, 14,* 524–530.

Mills, D. E., Prkachin, K. M., Harvey, K. A., & Ward, R. P. (1989). Dietary fatty acid supplementation alters stress reactivity and performance in man. *Journal of Human Hypertension, 3,* 111–116.

Molineux, D., & Steptoe, A. (1988). Exaggerated blood pressure responses to submaximal exercise in normotensive adolescents with a family history of hypertension. *Journal of Hypertension, 6,* 361–365.

Myrtek, M. (1985). Adaptation effects and the stability of physiological responses to repeated testing. In A. Steptoe, H. Ruddel, & H. Neus (Eds.), *Clinical and Methodological issues in cardio-vascular psychophysiology.* New York: Springer-Verlag.

Neel, J. V. (1962). Diabetes mellitus: A "thrifty" genotype rendered detrimental by "progress"? *American Journal of Human Genetics, 14,* 353–362.

Ostfeld, A. M., & Lebovitz, B. Z. (1959). Personality factors and pressor mechanisms in renal and essential hypertension. *Archives of Internal Medicine, 104,* 43–52.

Parati, G., Pomidossi, G., Albini, F., Malaspina, D., & Mancia, G. (1987). Relationship of 24-hour blood pressure mean and variability to severity of target-organ damage in hypertension. *Journal of Hypertension, 5,* 93–98.

Parati, G., Pomidossi, G., Casadei, R., Groppelli, A., Ravogli, A., Trazzi, S., Cesana, B., & Mancia, G. (1986).

Limitations of laboratory stress testing in the assessment of subjects' cardiovascular reactivity to stress. *Journal of Hypertension, 4*(Suppl. 6), S51–S53.

Parati, G., Pomidossi, G., Ramirez, A., Guazzi, C., Bertinieri, G., & Manci, G. (1983). Reproducibility of laboratory tests evaluating neural cardiovascular regulation in men. *Journal of Hypertension, 1*(Suppl. 2), 88–90.

Perini, C., Muller, F. B., Rauchfleisch, U., Battegay, R., Hobi, V., & Buhler, F. R. (1990). Psychosomatic factors in borderline hypertensive subjects and offspring of hypertensive patients. *Hypertension, 16,* 627–634.

Pickering, T. G., & Gerin, W. (1990). Reactivity and the role of behavioral factors in hypertension: A critical review. *Annals of Behavioral Medicine, 12,* 3–16.

Poulter, N. R., Khaw, K. T., Hopwood, B.E.C., Mugambi, M., Peart, W. S., Rose, G., & Sever, P. S. (1990). The Kenyan Luo migration study: Observations in the initiation of a rise in blood pressure. *British Medical Journal, 300,* 967–972.

Ravogli, A., Trazzi, S., Villani, A., Mutti, E., Cuspidi, C., Sampieri, L., De Ambroggi, L., Parati, G., Zanchetti, A., & Mancia, G. (1990). Early 24 hour blood pressure elevation in normotensive subjects with parental hypertension. *Hypertension, 16,* 491–497.

Rosenman, R. H., Brand, R. J., Jenkins, C. D., Friedman, M., Strauss, R., & Wurm, M. (1975). Coronary heart disease in the Western Collaborative Group Study, final follow-up experience of $8^{1}/_{2}$ years. *Journal of the American Medical Association, 233,* 872–877.

Rostrup, M., Kjeldsen, S., & Eide, I. K. (1990). Awareness of hypertension increases blood pressure and sympathetic responses to cold pressor test. *American Journal of Hypertension, 3,* 912–917.

Schnall, P. L., Pieper, C., Schwartz, J., Karasek, R., Schlussel, Y., Devereux, R., Ganau, A., Alderman, M., Warren, K., & Pickering, T. G. (1990). The relationship between "job strain," workplace diastolic blood pressure, and left ventricular mass index. *Journal of the American Medical Association, 263,* 1919–1935.

Schnall, P. L., Schwartz, J. E., Landsbergis, P. A., Warren, H., & Pickering, T. G. (1992). Relation between job strain, alcohol, and ambulatory blood pressure. *Hypertension, 19,* 488–494.

Shaper, A. G. (1962). Cardiovascular studies in the Samburo tribe of northern Kenya. *American Heart Journal, 63,* 437–442.

Shaper, A. G., Leonard, P. J., Jones, K. W., & Jones, M. (1969). Environment effects on the body build, blood pressure and blood chemistry of nomadic warriors serving in the army in Kenya. *East African Medical Journal, 46,* 282–289.

Shapiro, A. P. (1988). Psychological factors in hypertension: An overview. *American Heart Journal, 116,* 632–637.

Sifneos, P. E., Appel-Savitz, R., & Frankel, F. H. (1977). The phenomenon of "alexithymia." *Psychotherapy and Psychosomatics, 28,* 47–63.

Smith, T. W., Allred, K. D., Morrison, C. A., & Carlson, S. D. (1989). Cardiovascular reactivity and interpersonal influence: Active coping in a social context. *Journal of Personality and Social Psychology, 56,* 209–218.

Steptoe, A., Melville, D., & Ross, A. (1982). Essential hypertension and psychological functioning: A study of factory workers. *British Journal of Clinical Psychology, 21,* 303–311.

Sullivan, P., Schoentgen, S., De Quattro, V., Procci, W., Levine, D., Van der Meulen, J., & Bornsheimer, J. (1981). Anxiety, anger, and neurogenic tone at rest in a stress with primary hypertension. *Hypertension, 3*(Suppl. II), II-119.

Theorell, T., DeFaire, U., Johnson, J., Hall, E., Perski, A., & Stewart, W. (1991). Job strain and ambulatory blood pressure profiles. *Scandinavian Journal of Work and Environmental Health, 17,* 380–385.

Timio, M., Verdecchia, P., Venanzi, S., Gentili, S., Ronconi, M., Francucci, B., Montanari, M., & Bichisao, E. (1988). Age and blood pressure changes. A 20-year follow-up study in nuns in a secluded order. *Hypertension, 12,* 457–461.

Thomas, C. B., & Duszyncki, K. R. (1982). Blood pressure levels in young adulthood as predictors of hypertension and the fate of the cold pressor test. *John Hopkins Medical Journal, 151,* 93–100.

Turner, J. R., Girdler, S. S., Sherwood, A., & Light, K. C. (1990). Cardiovascular responses to behavioral stressors: Laboratory–field generalization and inter-task consistency. *Journal of Psychosomatic Research, 34,* 581–589.

Turswell, A. M. Kennelly, B. M., Hanson, J.D.L., & Lee, R. B. (1972). Blood pressure of !Kung bushmen in northern Botswana. *American Heart Journal, 84,* 5–12.

Van Egeren, L. F. (1992). The relationship between job strain and blood pressure at work, at home, and during sleep. *Psychosomatic Medicine, 54,* 337–343.

Van Egeren, L. F., & Sparrow, A. W. (1989). Laboratory stress testing to assess real-life cardiovascular reactivity. *Psychosomatic Medicine, 51,* 1–9.

Waldron, I., Nowotarski, M., Freimer, M., Henry, J. P., Post, N., & Witten, C. (1982). Cross-cultural variation in blood pressure: A quantitative analysis of the relationship of blood pressure to cultural characteristics, salt consumption, and body weight. *Social Science and Medicine, 16,* 419–430.

Watson, R. D., Stallard, T. J., Flinn, R. M., & Littler, W. A. (1980). Factors determining direct arterial pressure and its variability in hypertensive men. *Hypertension, 2,* 333–341.

Weidner, G., Friend, R., Ficarrotto, T. J., & Mendell, N. R. (1989). Hostility and cardiovascular reactivity to stress in women and men. *Psychosomatic Medicine, 51,* 36–45.

Wolf, S., & Wolff, H. G. (1951). A summary of experimental evidence relating life stress to the pathogenesis of essential hypertension in man. In E. T. Bell (Ed.), *Hypertension.* Minneapolis: University of Minnesota Press.

Wood, D. L., Sheps, S. G., Elveback, L. R., & Schirger, A. (1984). Cold pressor test as a predictor of hypertension. *Hypertension, 6,* 301–306.

12

Cardiovascular Disorders

Kevin T. Larkin and Elizabeth M. Semenchuk

INTRODUCTION

Diseases of the cardiovascular system, including coronary heart disease, disorders of cardiac rhythm, and cerebrovascular accidents, have been the leading cause of death in most industrialized nations for over 50 years (Jenkins, 1988). Whereas death from these diseases was relatively uncommon in the early 20th century, incidence of cardiac-related deaths increased rapidly, reaching peak mortality rates in the 1950s and 1960s. Since that time, mortality rates have declined substantially, partly due to improved medical interventions for cardiac symptom presentations and partly due to better prevention efforts. Although health practitioners have made significant advances in the prevention and medical management of cardiovascular problems, these illnesses continue to account for approximately 45% of all deaths in the United States (U.S. Bureau of the Census, 1991) with an even greater percentage of persons succumbing to premature mortality (i.e., death prior to age 60). The number of lives affected annually is actually much higher when including survivors of cardiac events, who often face significant difficulties due to decreased work productivity and reduced quality of life.

ETIOLOGICAL CONSIDERATIONS

The majority of diseases of the cardiovascular system result from the reduction (ischemia) or cessation (infarction) of oxygenated blood flow to various organs in the body, including the heart, brain, and kidneys. Most commonly, this compromised

---

Kevin T. Larkin and Elizabeth M. Semenchuk • Department of Psychology, West Virginia University, Morgantown, West Virginia 26506-6040.
Handbook of Health and Rehabilitation Psychology, edited by Anthony J. Goreczny. Plenum Press, New York, 1995.

flow of oxygen results from accumulated deposits of lipoproteins within the arterial wall, a process termed *atherosclerosis*. As lipids accumulate, blood flow to organs become restricted, resulting in clinical symptoms of severe cardiac chest pain (angina pectoris), temporary loss of brain function (transient ischemic attacks), or in some cases, an asymptomatic occurrence of restricted blood flow (silent ischemic attack). This compromised blood flow, if left unattended, often predates total arterial blockage that results from formation of a blood clot (thrombosis) or occlusion by a circulating piece of tissue formed elsewhere in the cardiovascular system (embolism). Through either mechanism, the consequent loss of blood flow results in the degeneration and death of cells distal in circulation to the occluded site. When this occurs in the coronary arteries, the clinical manifestation is a myocardial infarction (heart attack); when it occurs in the cerebrovasculature, the clinical presentation is a stroke.

Although the majority of cardiovascular disturbances are the result of the atherosclerotic process, other problems within the circulatory system can also contribute to clinically relevant cardiac events. Sudden cardiac death, for example, involves a disturbance of the electrical conduction system of the heart (e.g., ventricular fibrillation) that often follows atherogenic blockage. In other cardiac patients, congenital weaknesses in the vasculature may increase risk for ruptures of the circulatory system (e.g., hemorrhages), frequently resulting in immediate death. However, because the preponderance of information pertaining to etiology, identification of risk factors, and intervention and prevention efforts targeting cardiovascular disorders focuses upon those disorders resulting from atherosclerosis (coronary heart disease and stroke), the remainder of this chapter will focus primarily on these disorders.

Standard Risk Factors

Since the 1950s, the major causes of death, including coronary heart disease and stroke, are those diseases that result from the culmination of lifestyles of unhealthy behaviors rather than infectious disease processes. Investigation of etiological factors, then, began not with the identification of causal viral or bacterial agents, but with the discovery of risk factors that precede cardiovascular disease manifestation. Because both biological and behavioral risk factors deserve attention in diseases of "lifestyle," their identification requires a collaborative investigative team consisting of experts in medicine, psychological and behavioral assessment, and epidemiology. A number of major epidemiological studies have confirmed the existence of several prominent risk factors for coronary heart disease (Jenkins, 1988; see Table 12.1).

Risk-Factor Interactions

Findings from these major epidemiological trials suggest that the identified risk factors often interact synergistically in placing a person at risk for cardiovascular disease. For example, data from the Pooling Project (1978) show that male smokers who evidence elevated blood pressure and serum cholesterol levels have six times greater risk for coronary heart disease than men with any single risk factor. In a detailed examination of the complicated interactions among risk factors for coro-

Table 12.1. Risk Factors for Cardiovascular Disease[a]

Biological risk factors
    Family history of heart disease
    Older age
    Male
    Presence of diabetes mellitus
Risk factors affected by behavior
    Smoking
    Elevated serum cholesterol
    Hypertension
    Obesity

---

[a]Adapted from Jenkins (1988).

nary heart disease found in epidemiological trials, Perkins (1989) discovered that a synergistic relative risk (i.e., greater risk than predicted by adding the risk of the two factors) existed for (1) smokers who evidenced elevated serum cholesterol levels and (2) individuals with elevated blood pressure and serum cholesterol levels. There was no synergistic effect between smoking and high blood pressure. These findings led Perkins (1989) to conclude that both smoking and heightened blood pressure may serve as *initiating* factors in facilitating the atherosclerotic process, perhaps by causing arterial wall damage. Elevated serum cholesterol level, then, may act as a *secondary* factor that provides the necessary raw material for atherosclerotic placque development.

The observed interactions among the standard risk factors support the "response-to-injury" hypothesis of atherogenesis that Ross (1979) originally proposed. According to this hypothesis, endothelial cells in the arterial wall receive an injury, either through excessive arterial blood pressure, persistent turbulence of blood flow, or exposure to carbon monoxide (e.g., through smoking cigarettes) or other toxic circulating substances. The cells' adaptive response involves platelet aggregation and adherence at the injured site, resulting in smooth muscle cell proliferation and restoration of the arterial wall. At least two factors appear to disrupt this normal sequence of events causing an exaggerated response-to-injury and increased accumulation of tissue surrounding the site of the injury: recurrent endothelial cell injury and hypercholesterolemia. Regarding the former, if an individual's body has not completed the restorative cycle prior to subsequent injury (e.g., through an additional dose of carbon monoxide or sustained high blood pressure), the regenerative tissue theoretically calcifies rather than returning to its original plasticity. Regarding the latter, chronic hypercholesterolemia causes exaggerated smooth muscle cell proliferation and increased accumulation of lipids at the site of injury (Ross & Harker, 1976).

Despite the accumulation of knowledge pertaining to the involvement of the standard risk factors in atherogenesis, these factors only predict a small proportion of individuals who will develop coronary heart disease or stroke (Rosenman, 1983). In fact, in some studies, it has been shown that patients who smoke and have elevated blood pressure and serum cholesterol levels only exhibit a 10% coronary heart disease incidence over a 10-year period (Marmot & Winklestein, 1975). Also, many patients succumb to coronary heart disease or stroke without exhibiting the risk-factor profile outlined previously.

Psychosocial Risk Factors

The failure of the standard risk factors to predict disease occurrence with confidence provided the impetus toward interdisciplinary investigations with the goal of uncovering additional risk factors. Based upon decades of speculation that psychosocial factors contribute to the onset of cardiovascular disorders, investigators have given a significant amount of attention to the identification of such psychological, emotional, and behavioral characteristics. In one of the first systematic efforts of this nature, Friedman and Rosenman (1959) examined the emotional and behavioral characteristics of their cardiac patients to arrive at the description of the Type A behavior pattern (TABP) or the coronary-prone behavior pattern. The history, measurement, and development of this set of behavioral characteristics have suffered from mixed findings concerning its status as an independent risk factor (see Smith, this volume). Although the initial work was quite promising in establishing TABP as an independent risk factor (Cooper, Detre, & Weiss, 1981), subsequent studies have called into question the generalizability of earlier conclusions (Shekelle, Gale, & Norusis, 1985). In reexamining data from the early investigations, the focus of psychosocial risk-factor research has shifted from global TABP to specific subcomponents of the behavior pattern that pertain to hostility and expression of anger (Hecker, Frautsch, Chesney, Black, & Rosenman, 1985). Findings from investigations of the relation between cynical hostility and cardiovascular disease, for example, have confirmed that males high in hostility have a substantially greater risk for subsequent cardiac-related events than low-hostility males (Barefoot, Dahlstrom, & Williams, 1983). Investigators have also examined other psychosocial factors regarding their potential role as independent risk factors. Such factors include emotional expression (Friedman, 1989), agreeableness (Costa, McCrae, & Dembroski, 1989), and hardiness (Wiebe & McCallum, 1986). Although the exact nature of psychosocial risk factors is not yet known, we can safely conclude that a person's characteristic behavioral profile in some way relates to the onset of coronary heart disease.

Pathophysiological Mechanisms for Psychosocial Risk Factors

A major problem facing the confirmation of behavioral or psychosocial risk factors for coronary heart disease or stroke surrounds the difficulty in explaining how a psychosocial risk factor can result in endothelial cell injury and disrupted cellular restoration following injury. Suls and Sanders (1989) discuss three potential ways that TABP may contribute to damaging cardiovascular changes: (1) TABP is a marker of a genetic propensity for cardiovascular disease, (2) TABP relates to poor cardiovascular health habits (e.g., smoking cigarettes), or (3) TABP predisposes one to manifest exaggerated psychophysiological reactions to environmental stimuli. Based upon limited research and inconsistent findings present in the literature, however, the authors concluded that additional research was necessary to further examine the viability of each of these hypothesized pathophysiological mechanisms.

Extrapolating from speculation regarding how psychosocial risk factors result in cellular damage and findings pertaining to risk-factor interactions and the "response-

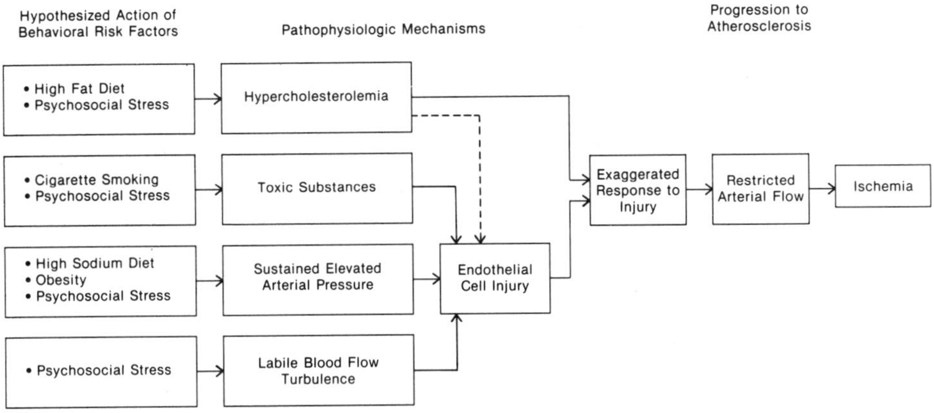

Figure 12.1. A working model outlining hypothesized pathophysiological mechanisms mediating the relationship between psychosocial risk factors and clinical presentations of atherosclerosis.

to-injury" hypothesis, we devised a working model that outlines hypothesized relationships between psychosocial stressors and the atherosclerotic process (see Figure 12.1).

According to this model, each behavioral risk factor relates to a pathophysiological mechanism known to disrupt cellular response to injury. For example, a high-sodium diet may contribute to cell injury indirectly through sustained elevated blood pressure. Cigarette smoking, on the other hand, may augment the atherogenic process by infiltrating the bloodstream with carbon monoxide, a substance known to damage arterial cells.

The relationship between psychosocial stressors and pathophysiological mechanisms, however, is much more complex. In contrast to other behavioral risk factors, psychosocial stressors potentially affect *all* of the pathophysiological mechanisms that may contribute to the progression of atherosclerosis. Therefore, a single psychosocial variable (e.g., job stress) can exert its pathogenic effect in the following ways:

1. Stimulates the release of free fatty acids and triglycerides.
2. Causes the secretion of cortisol or catecholamines which injure endothelial cells.
3. Results in a persistent elevation of blood pressure on the job (e.g., the prevailing state hypothesis).
4. Causes acute exaggerated heart rate or blood pressure responses to environmental challenges (e.g., the recurrent activation hypothesis).
5. Any combination of the aforementioned factors.

In the following paragraphs we discuss each of the possible mechanisms.

Stress and Lipid Function

Lipid metabolism plays a central role in the atherogenic process. Not only do circulating lipoproteins provide the raw material for atherosclerotic plaque development, there is also evidence that excessive free fatty acids can themselves cause endothelial cell injury (Ross & Harker, 1976) or severe cardiac arrhythmias (Kurian

& Oliver, 1966). In addition, plasma concentrations of triglycerides and free fatty acids are higher under stressful conditions, most likely in response to increased concentrations of circulating catecholamines. For example, Taggert and Carruthers (1971) reported increased levels of norepinephrine and free fatty acids before and after an automobile race among drivers and sustained triglyceride levels for several hours after completion of the race. A number of other studies have documented that exposure to a variety of environmental stressors results in a rapid increase in free fatty acids and a more enduring triglyceride response, with the latter most commonly in the form of very low-density lipoproteins (see Herd, 1984). Based upon this evidence, then, we can hypothesize that psychosocial stress precipitates impaired endothelial response to injury through its impact on lipid function.

Neuroendocrine Response to Stress

In addition to the influence that catecholamines have on lipid metabolism, researchers have hypothesized that the presence of the so-called "stress" hormones (i.e., cortisol and catecholamines) can directly injure the endothelium. Although experimental evidence demonstrating such an effect for circulating catecholamines is lacking, studies have demonstrated that the presence of cortisol potentiates atherogenic progression. Sprague, Troxler, Peterson, Schmidt, and Young (1980) compared groups of monkeys fed either a high-cholesterol or controlled diet with or without cortisol supplementation. Results revealed that whereas both groups on high cholesterol diets exhibited elevated serum cholesterol levels, only those on the high-cholesterol diet supplemented with cortisol exhibited advanced atherogenic lesions. Kaplan, Manuck, Clarkson, Lusso, and Taub (1982) replicated these findings using a stressful social-disruption manipulation on monkeys rather than the administration of cortisol. Comparable to the findings of Sprague et al. (1980), both elevated cholesterol levels *and* the presence of stress (and presumably stress hormones) resulted in the most advanced atherogenic lesions. Coupled with convincing data demonstrating a comparable relationship between cortisol and atherosclerosis in humans (Troxler, Sprague, Albanese, Fuchs, & Thompson, 1977), these findings suggest that secretion of cortisol in response to psychosocial stress facilitates the progression of atherosclerosis.

The Prevailing State Hypothesis

The prevailing state hypothesis focuses upon elements of a person's characteristic behavioral response to psychosocial stressors that result in relatively enduring effects on the cardiovascular system (e.g., sustained high blood pressure; Manuck & Krantz, 1984). In a classic example of the prevailing state hypothesis, Julius, Weder, and Hinderliter (1986) discuss the so-called "neurogenic" hypertensive patient who maintains an elevated state of alertness, heightened vigilance to his or her surroundings, and chronic sympathetic nervous system stimulation with elevated catecholamine and plasma renin levels. According to Julius and associates, this prevailing state of sympathetic nervous system arousal results in sustained elevated arterial pressures and subsequent vessel wall hypertrophy. Although scientists have hotly debated the prevalence of neurogenic hypertensive patients, data appear to indicate that at least a subset of individuals conform to this symptom configuration.

The Recurrent Activation Hypothesis

Manuck and Krantz (1984) originally coined the term *recurrent activation hypothesis*. This hypothesis focuses on individual differences in psychophysiological responsivity to environmental stressors. According to this "reactivity" hypothesis, individuals engage in somewhat stable patterns of psychophysiological responding when coping with the variety of daily stressors they encounter. Furthermore, individuals who exhibit exaggerated cardiovascular (i.e., heart rate, blood pressure) responses to daily challenges would hypothetically possess the greatest risk for subsequent cardiovascular complications, including coronary heart disease and essential hypertension.

Evidence to support the "reactivity" hypothesis comes from a variety of sources. For example, several prospective investigations, which have followed individuals for periods of up to 45 years, have shown that subjects who exhibit exaggerated heart rate (HR) or blood pressure responses to standardized laboratory challenges relative to low-reactive counterparts evidenced an increased incidence for myocardial infarction (Keys et al., 1971) and mortality from cardiovascular disease (Loos, Daly, Hickling, & Saco, 1991). The most convincing support for the interaction between exaggerated cardiovascular reactivity to stressors and atherosclerosis hails from a series of investigations upon a colony of cynomolgus macaques (see Manuck, Muldoon, Kaplan, Adams, & Polefrone, 1989). In these studies, high HR-reactive animals exposed to a standard "threat-of-capture" procedure demonstrated increased coronary and carotid artery blockage relative to low HR-reactive animals exposed to the same procedure. Although investigators have not yet delineated the responsible physiological mechanism, one possibility is that exaggerated cardiovascular reactions to stressors result in endothelial cell damage through rapid and excessive alterations in blood flow turbulence.

In addition to findings that support all avenues of psychosocial stressors as risk factors contributing to the atherosclerotic process, there exists evidence linking each pathophysiological route to some of the more promising *behavioral* risk factors. For example, subjects exhibiting characteristics of the TABP in contrast to Type B subjects manifest (1) higher levels of serum cholesterol (Friedman, Byers, Rosenman, & Elevitch, 1970), (2) greater plasma norepinephrine and cortisol responses to stress (Williams et al., 1982), (3) higher prevailing-state blood pressures as indicated by elevated pressures under general anesthesia (Krantz & Durel, 1983), and (4) greater cardiovascular reactions to challenging tasks (Contrada & Krantz, 1988). Although these findings are congruent with the proposed model, they also point out the enormous difficulty researchers face in uncovering specific patterns of psychosocial risk for cardiovascular disease. Most current investigations approach the identification of the pathophysiological mechanism from a unidimensional perspective (i.e., testing a single hypothesis with an identified group at risk for cardiovascular disease). For example, investigators have widely studied differences in cardiovascular reactions to behavioral challenges among Type A and Type B subjects. According to the present model, however, several different mechanisms may put Type A persons at risk for endothelial injury. Such mechanisms include hyperresponsivity to stressors, enhanced cortisol secretion, sustained elevated blood pressures driven by sympathetic overarousal, or any combination of these factors. As long as researchers employ unidimensional approaches, inconsistent findings across experiments will continue to emerge due to the use of different samples. We can hypothesize, then, that a multidimensional approach to the assessment of individual differences in physiological functioning may be necessary to arrive at definitive conclusions pertaining to specific pathogenic avenues of psychosocial risk factors for cardiovascular disease.

HEALTH PROMOTION EFFORTS

Prevention Programs

The Joint World Health Organization/International Society of Hypertension Meeting on the Prevention of Hypertension and Cardiovascular Disease (1992) released a statement that outlines the environmental factors that deserve consideration for intervention. Such factors include body-weight control, increased physical exercise, reduction of alcohol intake, reduction of dietary sodium, increased potassium intake, "prudent diet," and reduction of psychosocial stress. The group of experts at the 1992 meeting recommended targeting both whole (community) and high-risk populations. In response to these recommendations, the scientific and practice-oriented communities have increased their emphasis on the development of primary and secondary prevention efforts to reduce the collective risk for cardiovascular disorders. Elements of most successful cardiovascular "wellness" programs include efforts at smoking cessation (see Chapter 7), the reduction of elevated blood pressures through pharmacological therapy or dietary management (see Chapter 11), the implementation of weight loss and exercise programs (see Chapters 8 and 14), and the modification of coronary-prone behavior (see Chapter 10). Efforts of this nature appear to be at least partly responsible for the annual reduction in cardiac-related mortality that has occurred since the 1960s.

Two recent studies (Alexandrov, Maslennikova, Kulikov, Propirnu, & Perova, 1992; Arbeit et al., 1992) have outlined successful primary prevention efforts. Alexandrov and colleagues showed a greater reduction in cholesterol level, triglycerides, smoking, and blood pressure among 477 high-risk 12-year-old boys in comparison to a control group that did not receive cardiac risk-factor counseling. In the Heart Smart Cardiovascular School Health Promotion program, Arbeit and colleagues (1992) reported participants made healthier lunch selections, increased exercise behaviors, and evidenced higher levels of high-density lipoproteins following implementation of a heart health curriculum. This program consisted of a school lunch program with healthy choices, a physical education program promoting cardiovascular fitness, and a parent outreach effort.

In addition to efforts in primary prevention, it is also important to focus on altering the unhealthy lifestyle habits of patients recovering from cardiac-related hospitalizations. Cardiac rehabilitation programs, designed to increase physical fitness in addition to reducing the standard risk factors for disease, have become a necessary component to the prevention of subsequent problems among cardiac patients (Southard & Broyden, 1990). Data clearly indicate that patients who participate in these cardiac rehabilitation programs, which consist mostly of structured aerobic exercise, have fewer recurrent cardiac events and live longer than nonparticipants (Berra, 1991; Fletcher, 1992).

Reducing Psychosocial Risk for Cardiovascular Disease

Primary and secondary prevention programs have often disregarded psychosocial risk factors and have focused primarily upon reducing the standard risk factors for cardiovascular disease. However, because of the importance of psychological factors in both reducing psychosocial stress and increasing compliance with recommended prevention or rehabilitation programs, health-care practitioners cannot overlook these factors. Several investigations have examined the importance of psychological stress management in cardiac rehabilitation and primary prevention efforts (see Nunes, Frank, & Kornfeld, 1987). In fact, some states require provision of psychological services for certification as a cardiac rehabilitation program (Southard & Broyden, 1990).

As one example, in the Recurrent Coronary Prevention project, Friedman and his colleagues (1986) randomly assigned post-myocardial infarction patients to either a control group, a cardiac counseling group, or both cardiac counseling and Type A behavioral counseling groups. The group receiving the added Type A behavioral-counseling component demonstrated a significant reduction in cardiac morbidity and mortality after the first year. In another study (Ornish et al., 1990), a complete lifestyle-change program, including a low-fat vegetarian diet, moderate aerobic exercise, stress management, and smoking cessation resulted in actual regression of atherosclerosis among coronary patients without any pharmacological intervention. Furthermore, the magnitude of the reduction observed in the atherogenic lesions correlated with extent of lifestyle change.

Despite the increased implementation of stress management programs, their impact upon the pathophysiological mechanisms involved in previously outlined atherogenic progression is unknown. It is unclear, for example, whether an intervention like relaxation training alters free fatty acid and cortisol levels, persistent sympathetic nervous system activation, or cardiovascular responding to stressors. In an effort to specifically target the pathophysiological mechanisms involved in mediating the relationship between psychosocial risk factors and atherosclerotic endpoints, researchers have given increased attention to investigating the effects of standard pharmacological and nonpharmacological interventions upon pathophysiological functioning.

Reducing Cardiovascular Reactivity to Stress

A number of investigations have examined the efficacy of a variety of interventions designed to reduce cardiovascular reactivity to stressors. In one of these studies, Kaplan, Manuck, Adams, Weingand, and Clarkson (1987) demonstrated that a pharmacological intervention aimed at reducing HR reactivity (i.e., propranolol) resulted in decreased coronary artery atherosclerosis among monkeys without affecting social status or dominance. The preponderance of studies using human subjects, however, has focused on nonpharmacological or behavioral interventions. For example, cardiovascular reactions to behavioral challenges have decreased following cognitive interventions in attention diversion (Bloom, Houston, Holmes, & Burish, 1977), training in relaxation or mediation (Lehrer, 1978), and training with biofeedback of cardiovascular parameters (Steptoe, 1977).

Among studies investigating attenuated HR and blood pressure responses to behavioral stressors, demonstrations of reduced cardiovascular reactions most consistently result from training that employs biofeedback of cardiovascular parameters. These findings are particularly impressive when feedback training takes place during the presentation of a behavioral challenge, thereby providing subjects the opportunity to practice lowering HR or blood pressure when most necessary. In fact, a direct comparison of pulse transit-time feedback training conducted during the presentation of a stressor and pulse transit-time feedback training conducted during rest revealed that only subjects who received feedback during stress tasks were capable of reducing cardiovascular reactivity to a posttraining challenge (Bentham & Glaros, 1982). To further support this view, investigations of biofeedback training conducted without exposure to behavioral stressors have less consistently demonstrated significant reductions in cardiovascular stress reactivity (Bouchard & Labelle, 1982; Malcuit & Beaudry, 1980).

Consistent with previous research, we have investigated the reduction in cardiovascular reactivity to behavioral stressors using HR feedback presented *while* the subject actively engages in a challenging task. To facilitate both the maintenance of acceptable task performance and learning to reduce cardiovascular reactivity to that task, we presented both visual HR feedback and a behavioral challenge—a computerized videogame—simultaneously to the subject using a video monitor. The experimental protocols of these studies have involved three phases:

1. A pretreatment assessment of cardiovascular reactivity to the behavioral task(s).
2. A training period during which subjects receive feedback and instructions to decrease HR.
3. A posttreatment assessment of cardiovascular reactivity to the same behavioral task(s) without feedback.

We have conducted several studies employing this experimental HR-feedback protocol.

In the initial study using the experimental HR-feedback–videogame apparatus (Larkin, Manuck, & Kasprowicz, 1989), we measured HRs of 20 HR-reactive males during both a videogame challenge and a preceding baseline period. Ten subjects then participated in a training period in which they received continuous HR feedback during the performance of the videogame. During training, game performance was contingent upon maintaining a lowered HR *and* maintaining acceptable levels of videogame performance. The remaining subjects played the same number of videogames without feedback or instructions to alter HR during training. Results revealed that experimental subjects exhibited a greater reduction in HR reactivity to the posttraining challenge than control subjects (see Figure 12.2). Although game performance did not differ between the two groups at posttraining, performance of feedback subjects was poorer than control subjects during training trials.

Because of the somewhat disconcerting finding of impaired performance associated with reductions in HR during training trials, a second study (Larkin, Manuck, & Kasprowicz, 1990) employed a longer training period to facilitate the learning of both tasks along with inclusion of two additional control groups: an instructions-only control group that received instructions to decrease HR but without any feedback during training and a second feedback group that received instructions to decrease HR with the use of feedback but did not receive the score contingency during training. Blood pressure and HR reactivity assessments showed that only

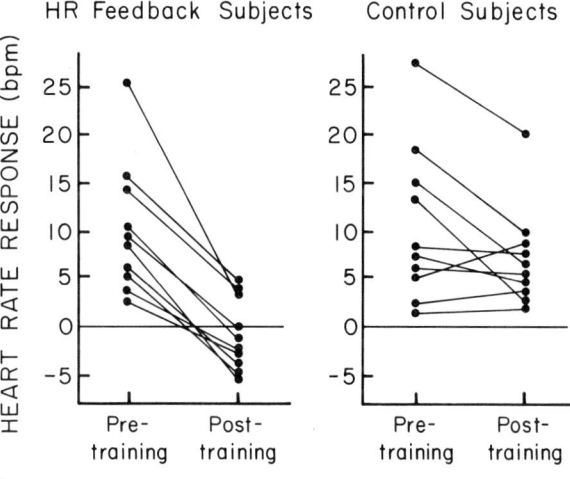

Figure 12.2. Heart rate reactions (change from pretask baseline) of HR feedback and control subjects during pretraining and posttraining presentations of a videogame challenge.

feedback subjects who received instructions to decrease HR *and* operated under the score contingency during training exhibited attenuated HR responses at posttraining relative to pretraining (see Figure 12.3). In contrast to the initial investigation, these reductions in HR were not detrimental to game performance during training and at the posttraining assessment phase. Training with HR feedback did not affect systolic

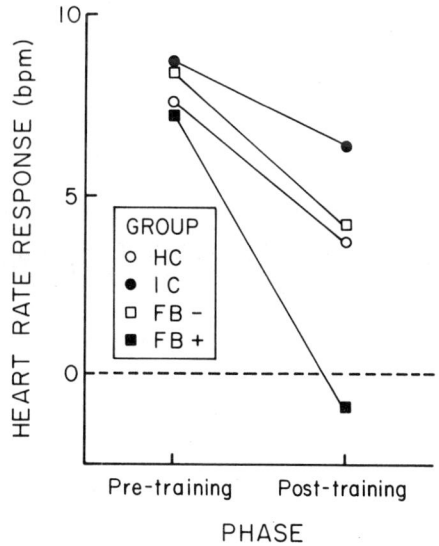

Figure 12.3. Mean heart rate reactions (change from pretask baseline) of HR feedback subjects trained with the score contingency (FB+), HR feedback subjects trained without the contingency (FB−), control subjects instructed to lower HR (IC), and habituation control subjects (HC) during pretraining and posttraining presentations of a videogame challenge.

blood pressure reactivity, but did result in a lower tonic systolic blood pressure at posttraining. Diastolic blood pressure did not change in response to training.

A third study (Larkin, Zayfert, Abel, & Veltum, 1992) examined (1) whether training in HR feedback on the video game generalized to HR reactions to a second behavioral stressor (a mental arithmetic challenge), and (2) whether biofeedback-assisted HR-response reductions were maintained at a follow-up assessment of reactivity 1 week later. Sixteen HR-reactive males underwent assessment of HR reactions during a videogame challenge and a mental arithmetic task. Eight subjects utilized HR feedback in conjunction with the score contingency to reduce HR reactions during the videogame challenge; the remaining 8 subjects received instructions to decrease HR, but they were not provided HR feedback. At the posttreatment assessment, experimental subjects, in contrast to control counterparts, exhibited lower HR reactions to both the training task (videogame) and the mental arithmetic challenge. In addition, experimental subjects maintained lower HR reactions at the follow-up session for both challenges thereby confirming the generalizability of these findings both across task and a 1-week period of time.

A fourth study (Larkin, Zayfert, Veltum, & Abel, 1992) further investigated the importance of the score contingency in demonstrating reduced HR reactions to behavioral challenges. Forty-eight HR-reactive males entered one of four groups: (1) feedback with the score contingency, (2) feedback without the score contingency, (3) no feedback with the score contingency, and (4) no feedback without the score contingency. Results showed that subjects who received training with the score contingency, with or without HR feedback, exhibited reductions in HR reactivity to the posttreatment videogame presentation. Therefore, provision of feedback was not the critical element in training; rather, it appears that making reinforcement contingent upon both improved performance *and* reductions in HR accounts for the observed reductions in HR. As with the previous study, training in HR feedback did not negatively affect game performance. Likewise, reductions in neither systolic nor diastolic blood pressure reactivity accompanied reduction in HR during the posttraining assessment session.

Preliminary investigations of HR-feedback training have provided convincing evidence that heightened HR reactions to behavioral challenges are amenable to treatment in a normal, healthy sample. These reductions can occur without detriment to task performance and do not coincide with a general reduction in blood pressure responsivity. However, investigators have not yet demonstrated these effects convincingly using a clinical sample including borderline essential hypertensive or cardiac rehabilitation patients. In general, investigations of biofeedback-assisted reductions in cardiovascular reactivity have utilized samples of healthy adults. One exception is an investigation in which operant conditioning of HR deceleration occurred in 6 patients diagnosed with angina pectoris (McCroskey, Zagel, Gottlieb, & Lakatta, 1978). These authors reported significant reductions in angina pain associated with HR-feedback training conducted during an exercise stressor. Significant reductions in resting levels of both systolic and diastolic blood pressures have also resulted following HR-feedback training in a sample of essential hypertensive patients (Achmon, Granek, Golomb, & Hart, 1989). Although the evidence is not overwhelming, both studies have demonstrated meaningful reductions in clinically relevant parameters following HR-feedback training (i.e., angina pain, casual blood pressure) lending credence to the utility of this biofeedback-assisted strategy for reducing risk for cardiovascular disease.

CONCLUSIONS AND DIRECTIONS FOR FUTURE RESEARCH

Exciting avenues of interdisciplinary research pertaining to the etiology, prevention, intervention, and rehabilitation of cardiovascular disorders have flourished over the past decade. Augmenting the evidence supporting the role of standard risk factors in all stages of cardiovascular disease, new risk factors have emerged and strategies for measuring psychosocial risk for cardiovascular disease have progressed. More important, identification of these risk factors has made psychological interventions possible. In addition to evaluating the efficacy of interventions targeting psychosocial risk factors, future research must continue to examine the role of psychosocial stress in the development of cardiovascular disorders.

Investigations focusing upon the multidimensional assessment of patterns of pathophysiological functioning of the body's response to stressors represent an important direction for better understanding the physiological processes responsible for the progression of atherosclerosis to clinical disease end points. Due to the abundance of medical technology now available, researchers in this area often find that the development of technology precedes demonstration of its clinical utility. This is clearly the case with the onset of hemodynamic monitoring through impedance cardiography, the noninvasive radionuclide ventricular imaging, ambulatory monitoring of cardiovascular parameters, and continuous blood pressure monitoring. Although these tools are available, increased research is essential in order to establish normative profiles for various populations of interest so that the full clinical utility of these tools can evolve.

Prevention programs have also failed to use newer technology that is available for measuring the impact of the program upon pathophysiological mechanisms hypothetically responsible for the relation between psychosocial stress and atherosclerosis. Additional research needs to examine the impact of available interventions upon the pathophysiological mechanisms hypothesized to link psychosocial stress to atherosclerosis. In addition to the ongoing investigations that are examining the effect of behavioral interventions on cardiovascular response to stress, the impact of treatment procedures upon the modulation of lipid metabolism, sympathetic nervous system activation, and catecholamine and cortisol secretion, deserves further empirical consideration. Studies of this nature also need to employ significant periods of follow-up in order to determine the overall efficacy of such preventive efforts. Outcome investigations of cardiac rehabilitation and prevention programs would benefit from the use of the multidimensional assessment approach, measuring functional capacity, pathophysiological functioning, mental health variables, and quality of life in addition to mortality and morbidity.

Future investigations targeting the reduction of cardiovascular reactivity to stress need to demonstrate the utility of such procedures for clinical and high-risk populations. The empirical questions that McCroskey et al. (1978) and Achmon et al. (1989) began to address with angina and hypertensive patients require replication and extension to other cardiac populations. Further refinement of training procedures are necessary to examine the role of specific reinforcement contingencies employed during training and to determine the nature of pretreatment behavioral characteristics that might predict which patients best benefit through such stress management procedures.

Evidence demonstrating the effectiveness of individual and community interventions on the prevention of risk factors and progression of atherosclerosis is striking. Through the assessment, modification, and evaluation of psychosocial risk factors for cardiovascular disease, behavioral scientists can provide a means for reducing the morbidity and mortality of one of the world's leading causes of death.

REFERENCES

Achmon, J., Granek, M., Golomb, M., & Hart, J. (1989). Behavioral treatment of essential hypertension: A comparison between cognitive therapy and biofeedback of heart rate. *Psychosomatic Medicine, 51,* 152–164.

Alexandrov, A. A., Maslennikova, G. Y., Kulikov, S. M., Propirnu, G. A., & Perova, N. V. (1992). Primary prevention of cardiovascular disease: 3-year intervention results in boys of 12 years of age. *Preventive Medicine, 21,* 53–62.

Arbeit, M. L., Johnson, C. C., Mott, D. S., Harsha, D. W., Nicklas, T. A., Webber, L. S., & Berenson, G. S. (1992). The Heart Smart cardiovascular school health promotion: Behavior correlates of risk factor change. *Preventive Medicine, 21,* 18–32.

Barefoot, J. C., Dahlstrom, W. G., & Williams, R. B. (1983). Hostility, CHD incidence and total mortality: A 25-year follow-up study of 255 physicians. *Psychosomatic Medicine, 45,* 59–63.

Bentham, J. A., & Glaros, A. G. (1982). Self-control of stress-induced cardiovascular change using transit time feedback. *Psychophysiology, 19*(5), 502–505.

Berra, K. (1991). Cardiac and pulmonary rehabilitation: Historical perspectives and future needs. *Journal of Cardiopulmonary Rehabilitation, 11,* 8–15.

Bloom, L. R., Houston, B., Holmes, D. S., & Burish, T. G. (1977). The effectiveness of attentional diversion and situation redefinition for reducing stress due to ambiguous threat. *Journal of Research in Personality, 11,* 83–94.

Bouchard, M. A., & Labelle, J. (1982). Voluntary heart rate deceleration: A critical evaluation. *Biofeedback and Self-Regulation, 7,* 121–137.

Contrada, R. J., & Krantz, D. S. (1988). Stress, reactivity, and Type A behavior: Current status and future directions. *Annals of Behavioral Medicine, 10,* 64–70.

Cooper, T., Detre, T., Weiss, S. M. (1981). Coronary-prone behavior and coronary heart disease: A critical review. *Circulation, 63,* 1199–1215.

Costa, P. T., McCrae, R. R., & Dembroski, T. (1989). Agreeableness versus antagonism: Explication of a potential risk for CHD. In A. W. Seigman & T. Dembroski (Eds.), *In search of coronary-prone behavior* (pp. 41–63). Hillsdale, NJ: Erlbaum.

Fletcher, G. F. (1992). Current status of cardiac rehabilitation. *Current Problems in Cardiology, 17,* 147–203.

Friedman, H. S. (1989). The role of emotional expression in coronary heart disease. In A. W. Seigman & T. Dembroski (Eds.), *In search of coronary-prone behavior* (pp. 149–168). Hillsdale, NJ: Erlbaum.

Friedman, M., Byers, S. O., Rosenman, R. H., & Elevitch, F. R. (1970). Coronary-prone individuals (Type A behavior pattern): Some biochemical characteristics. *Journal of the American Medical Association, 212,* 1030–1037.

Friedman, M., & Rosenman, R. H. (1959). Association of specific overt behavior pattern with increases in blood cholesterol, blood clotting time, incidence of arcus senilis and clinical coronary artery disease. *Journal of the American Medical Association, 169,* 1286–1296.

Friedman, M., Thoresen, C. E. Gill, J. J., Ulmer, D., Powell, L. H., Price, V. A., Brown, B., Thompson, L., Rabin, D. D., Breall, W. S., Bourg, E., Levy, R., & Dixon, T. (1986). Alteration of Type A behavior and its effect on cardiac recurrences in post myocardial infarction patients: Summary results of the recurrent coronary prevention project. *American Heart Journal, 112,* 653–665.

Hecker, M. W., Frautsch, N., Chesney, M., Black, G., & Rosenman, R. H. (1985). Components of Type A behavior and coronary heart disease. *Proceedings of the Sixth Annual Scientific Sessions of the Society of Behavioral Medicine* (p. 42). Rockville, MD: Society of Behavioral Medicine. (Abstract)

Herd, J. A. (1984). Cardiovascular disease and hypertension. In W. D. Gentry (Ed.), *Handbook of behavioral medicine* (pp. 222–281). New York: Guilford.

Jenkins, C. D. (1988). Epidemiology of cardiovascular diseases. *Journal of Consulting and Clinical Psychology, 56,* 324–332.

Joint World Health Organization/International Society of Hypertension Meeting (1992). 1991 guidelines for the prevention of hypertension and associated cardiovascular disease. *Journal of Hypertension, 10,* 97–99.

Julius, S., Weder, A. B., & Hinderliter, A. L. (1986). Does behaviorally induced blood pressure variability lead to hypertension? In K. A. Matthews, S. M. Weiss, T. Detre, T. M. Dembroski, B. Falkner, S. B. Manuck, & R. B. Williams (Eds.), *Handbook of stress, reactivity, and cardiovascular disease* (pp. 71–81). New York: Wiley.

Kaplan, J. R., Manuck, S. B., Adams, M. R., Weingand, K. W., & Clarkson, T. B. (1987). Propranolol inhibits coronary atherosclerosis in behaviorally predisposed monkeys fed an atherogenic diet. *Circulation, 76,* 1364–1372.

Kaplan, J. R., Manuck, S. B., Clarkson, T. B., Lusso, F. M., & Taub, D. M. (1982). Social status, environment, and atherosclerosis in cynomolgus monkeys. *Arteriosclerosis, 2,* 359–368.

Keys, A., Taylor, H. L., Blackburn, H. Y., Brozek, J., Anderson, J., & Simonson, E. (1971). Mortality and coronary heart disease among men studied for 23 years. *Archives of Internal Medicine, 128,* 201–214.

Krantz, D. S., & Durel, L. A. (1983). Psychobiological substates of the Type A behavior pattern. *Health Psychology, 2,* 393–411.

Kurian, V. A., & Oliver, M. F. (1966). Serum-free fatty acids after acute myocardial infarction and cerebral vascular occlusions. *Lancet, 2,* 122–133.

Larkin, K. T., Manuck, S. B., & Kasprowicz, A. L. (1989). Heart rate feedback-assisted reduction in cardiovascular reactivity to a videogame challenge. *The Psychological Record, 39,* 365–371.

Larkin, K. T., Manuck, S. B., & Kasprowicz, A. L. (1990). The effect of feedback-assisted reduction in heart rate reactivity on videogame performance. *Biofeedback and Self-Regulation, 15,* 285–303.

Larkin, K. T., Zayfert, C., Abel, J., & Veltum, L. (1992). Effects of feedback and contingent reinforcement in reducing heart rate response to stress. *Journal of Psychophysiology, 6,* 119–130.

Larkin, K. T., Zayfert, C., Veltum, L., & Abel, J. (1992). Reducing heart rate reactivity to stress with feedback: Generalization across task and time. *Behavior Modification, 16,* 118–131.

Lehrer, P. M. (1978). Psychophysiological effects of progressive relaxation training in anxiety neurotic patients and of progressive relaxation and alpha feedback in nonpatients. *Journal of Consulting and Clinical Psychology, 46,* 389–404.

Loos, W. R., Daly, S. S., Hickling, E. J., & Saco, J. (1991). Mortality and cardiovascular reactivity in male veterans. *Proceedings of the Twelfth Annual Scientific Sessions of the Society of Behavioral Medicine* (p. 94). Rockville, MD: Society of Behavioral Medicine. (Abstract A60)

Malcuit, G., & Beaudry, J. (1980). Voluntary heart rate lowering following a cardiovascular arousing task. *Biological Psychology, 10,* 201–210.

Manuck, S. B., & Krantz, D. S. (1984). Psychophysiologic reactivity in coronary heart disease. *Behavioral Medicine Update, 6,* 11–15.

Manuck, S. B., Muldoon, M. F., Kaplan, J. R., Adams, M. R., & Polefrone, J. M. (1989). Coronary artery atherosclerosis and cardiac response to stress in cynomolgus monkeys. In A. W. Seigman & T. Dembroski (Eds.), *In search of coronary-prone behavior* (pp. 207–227). Hillsdale, NJ: Erlbaum.

Marmot, M. G., & Winklestein, W. (1975). Epidemiological observations on intervention trials for prevention of coronary heart disease. *American Journal of Epidemiology, 101,* 177–181.

McCroskey, J. H., Engel, B. T., Gottlieb, S. M., & Lakatta, E. G. (1978). Operant conditioning of heart rate in patients with angina pectoris. *Psychosomatic Medicine, 40,* 89–90.

Nunes, E. V., Frank, K. A., & Kornfeld, D. S. (1987). Psychologic treatment for the Type A behavior pattern and for coronary heart disease: A meta-analysis of the literature. *Psychosomatic Medicine, 48,* 159–173.

Ornish, D., Brown, S. E., Scherwitz, L. W., Billings, J. H., Armstrong, W. T., Ports, T. A., McLanahan, S. M., Kirkeeide, R. L., Brand, R. J., & Gould, K. L. (1990). Can lifestyle changes reverse coronary heart disease? *Lancet, 336,* 129–133.

Perkins, K. A. (1989). Interactions among coronary heart disease risk factors. *Annals of Behavioral Medicine, 11,* 3–11.

Pooling Project. (1978). Relation of blood pressure, serum cholesterol, smoking habit, relative weight, and ECG abnormalities to incidence of major coronary events: Final report of the Pooling Project. *Journal of Chronic Diseases, 31,* 201–306.

Rosenman, R. H. (1983). Current status of risk factors and Type A behavior pattern in the pathogenesis of ischemic heart disease. In T. M. Dembroski, T. H. Schmidt, & G. Blumchen (Eds.), *Biobehavioral bases of coronary heart disease.* New York: Karger.

Ross, R. (1979). The arterial wall and atherosclerosis. *Annual Review of Medicine, 30,* 1–15.

Ross, R., & Harker, L. (1976). Hyperlipidemia and atherosclerosis. *Science, 193,* 1094–1100.

Shekelle, R. B., Gale, M., & Norusis, M. (1985). Type A score (Jenkins Activity Survey) and risk of recurrent coronary heart disease in the Aspirin Myocardial Infarction Study. *American Journal of Cardiology, 56,* 221–225.

Southard, D. R., & Broyden, R. (1990). Psychosocial services in cardiac rehabilitation: A status report. *Journal of Cardiopulmonary Rehabilitation, 10,* 255–263.

Sprague, E. A., Troxler, R. G., Peterson, D. F., Schmidt, R. E., & Young, J. T. (1980). Effect of cortisol on the development of atherosclerosis in cynomolgus monkeys. In S. S. Kaiter (Ed.), *The use of nonhuman primates in cardiovascular diseases* (pp. 261–264). Austin: University of Texas Press.

Steptoe, A. (1977). Voluntary blood pressure reductions measured with pulse transit time: Training conditions and reactions to mental work. *Psychophysiology, 14,* 492–498.

Suls, J., & Sanders, G. S. (1989). Why do some behavioral styles place people at coronary risk? In A. W. Seigman & T. Dembroski (Eds.), *In search of coronary-prone behavior* (pp. 1–20). Hillsdale, NJ: Erlbaum.

Taggert, P., & Carruthers, M. (1971). Endogenous hyperlipidemia induced by emotional stress of racing driving. *Lancet, 1,* 363–366.

Troxler, R. G., Sprague, E. A., Albanese, R. A., Fuchs, R., & Thompson, A. J. (1977). The association of elevated plasma cortisol and early atherosclerosis as demonstrated by coronary angiography. *Atherosclerosis, 26,* 151–162.

U. S. Bureau of the Census. (1991). *Statistical Abstract of the United States 1991.* Washington, DC: U.S. Department of Commerce.

Wiebe, D. J., & McCallum, D. M. (1986). Health practices and hardiness as mediators in the stress–illness relationship. *Health Psychology, 5,* 425–438.

Williams, R. B., Lane, J. D., Kuhn, C. M., Melosh, W., White, A. D., & Schanberg, S. M. (1982). Type A behavior and elevated physiological and neuroendocrine responses to cognitive tasks. *Science, 218,* 483–495.

13

Exercise and Physical Activity

Patricia M. Dubbert and Barbara A. Stetson

Psychologists working in health promotion and rehabilitation settings can often use their evaluation and intervention skills to help individuals adopt and maintain healthier lifestyles, including increased physical activity. Their expertise in theories and methods of behavior change can also make an important contribution to the design and implementation of specialized exercise and physical activity programs for high-risk groups and even entire communities. We begin this chapter with a brief discussion of physical activity behavior in the United States today and its importance in public health. We describe methods of assessing health-related physical activity and exercise that can be useful in different settings and applications. We briefly describe two behavioral models we believe will lead to improved exercise-promotion interventions. In the final two sections, we briefly present examples of interventions to increase physical activity and discuss physical activity promotion in groups that have until recently received little attention from researchers in this area: minorities, women, and the elderly.

PHYSICAL ACTIVITY AND HEALTH

Increasing exercise and physical activity participation is currently a major health objective in the United States (U.S. Department of Health and Human Services, 1990). People who are active and fit are likely to live longer than those who are not and they are more likely to avoid several debilitating chronic disease conditions. In fact, evidence relating exercise to health now suggests that a larger propor-

---

Patricia M. Dubbert • Department of Psychology, Veterans Affairs Medical Center, and University of Mississippi School of Medicine, Jackson, Mississippi 39216.   **Barbara A. Stetson** • Department of Psychology, Illinois Institute of Technology, Chicago, Illinois 60616.
Handbook of Health and Rehabilitation Psychology, edited by Anthony J. Goreczny. Plenum Press, New York, 1995.

tion of the adult population of the United States has increased risk of disease and early death from a low level of physical activity than from other well-established factors, such as cigarette smoking, high blood cholesterol, obesity, high blood pressure, and family history of heart disease (Blair, Kohl, Gordon, & Paffenbarger, 1992). Available data indicate that appropriate exercise can serve as an effective component of interventions for preventing or treating many highly prevalent health problems, such as obesity, coronary heart disease, diabetes, hypertension, arthritis, chronic pain, and prevention of osteoporosis (Harris, Caspersen, DeFriese, & Estes, 1988). Physical activity also appears related to optimal mental health, although it is less clear that exercise, rather than associated factors, is responsible for the therapeutic effects (Dubbert, 1992). Space does not permit an adequate review of research supporting these exercise effects and their mechanisms of action; interested readers can refer to more specialized sources, such as the edited book *Physical Activity, Fitness, and Health* (Bouchard, Shephard, & Stephens, 1994).

How Much Exercise Is Enough?

Cardiorespiratory fitness improvement generally requires performing endurance-type exercise three to five times per week for 20 to 60 minutes or more at an intensity of 60% to 90% of an individual's maximal heart rate (American College of Sports Medicine, 1990). The American College of Sports Medicine recommendations now also include moderate-intensity strength training (8 to 12 repetitions of exercises for conditioning major muscle groups) at least twice a week. However, in health and rehabilitation settings, it is readily apparent that appropriate exercise prescriptions may differ substantially depending on specific health goals that individuals hope to achieve. Recently published guidelines and objectives (e.g., Blair et al., 1993; Fletcher et al., 1992) acknowledge the uncertainty that still exists about exactly what "dose" of exercise is necessary or optimal for many health benefits. Although vigorous training is the most efficient means to increase cardiorespiratory fitness, it may not be the most effective means of helping most people lose excess weight, reduce their blood pressure, decrease their stress level, or avoid certain cancers. For some health applications, moderate intensities of training may be better, especially if this improves adherence. Many people can benefit significantly from increasing the time they spend in moderate activities, such as walking, gardening, and household- or domestic-type chores. Helping those people who are the most sedentary become a little more active may produce the greatest public health benefits (Blair et al., 1993).

Physical Activity in the United States Today

Americans today are more active than they were two decades ago (Blair, Mulder, & Kohl, 1987; Stephens, 1987), but millions of adults are still sedentary (Pate et al., 1995). Recent surveillance data suggest that physical activity participation has changed little during the past 10–15 years in the United States. Millions of Americans are very inactive or are active only on a sporadic or seasonal basis. Women, people with disabilities, those with low incomes, and the elderly continue to report less vigorous activity than comparison groups (United States Department of Human Services, 1990). The Public Health Service recently established new physical activity and fitness objectives for the year 2000 (United States Department of Health and Human Services, 1990), which reflect both the growing evidence that moderate levels of physical activity are beneficial and the increased appreciation among public health experts for the difficulty of increasing physical activity in our mechanized society.

A series of cross-sectional "snapshot" surveys of activity participation over time can help determine progress toward behavior change in the population, but they give us little information about patterns of physical activity within individuals. In one of the few studies of community exercise, Sallis, Haskell, Fortmann, Vranizan, Taylor, and Solomon (1986) reevaluated adults one year after baseline assessments of physical activity. About 50% of vigorous exercisers and 25–35% of moderate exercisers had stopped exercising during the year. Interestingly, the number of individuals who started exercising during the same period of time kept the net total of exercisers about the same. The investigators did not report reasons why people stopped exercising. Regression analyses showed that maintenance of vigorous activity related to previous levels of activity. Predictors of moderate activity maintenance included health knowledge, exercise knowledge, and education. In a subsequent large mail survey, Sallis et al. (1990) studied adults in San Diego, California. This study found that 40% of respondents who had exercised regularly for 6 months reported a history of at least one 3-month exercise relapse. It is unclear whether these findings are generalizable to populations that are more ethnically and economically diverse than the study population. There exists a great need for increased understanding of physical activity patterns in "natural" settings.

ASSESSMENT OF PHYSICAL ACTIVITY AND EXERCISE

Because one expected contribution of health psychologists is expertise in evaluation and measurement of health promotion and intervention programs, it is important for those working with exercise interventions to develop a good understanding of the advantages and limitations of methods commonly used to assess physical activity. Methodology of activity assessment can significantly impact results of evaluations regarding relationships between exercise and health for individuals and populations. Previous authors have discussed methodological issues in exercise assessment (Caspersen, 1989; Jacobs, Ainsworth, Hartman, & Leon, 1993; LaPorte, Montoye, & Caspersen, 1985; Paffenbarger, Blair, Lee, & Hyde, 1993; Wilson, Paffenbarger, Morris, & Havlik, 1986). According to Caspersen (1989), current literature on exercise and health reflects several difficulties regarding assessment of physical activity:

1. Diverse definitions of activity across studies.
2. Paucity of standardized, valid reliable instruments.
3. Large measurement error of instruments.
4. Inappropriate use of activity measures as part of a research design.
5. Failure of investigators to select an instrument that reflects health-related components of activity.
6. Impracticality of using more precise measures than currently used due to high costs.

In an effort to address some of these difficulties by promoting a consistent definition of exercise, several authors (Blair et al., 1992; Caspersen, Christensen, &

Pollard, 1986) have offered definitions to differentiate among types of exercise reflected in published research. According to these definitions, *physical activity* is movement produced by skeletal muscles, resulting in caloric expenditure. The force generated by the muscle mass producing the movement and by the duration of the muscle contractions are the factors that regulate this energy expenditure. Individuals can perform physical activity as part of work activity, leisure time activity, or household chores. *Exercise* is a subcategory of physical activity, a specific activity that individuals plan, structure, and perform repeatedly. Consistent exercise results in maintenance or improvement of physical fitness. Both physical activity and exercise are observable behaviors. In contrast, *physical fitness* is a set of outcomes or attributes that relates to ability to perform physical activity. Fitness is something that people achieve through consistent activity, such as aerobic power, muscular strength and endurance, flexibility, or a particular body composition.

Methods of physical activity and exercise assessment include both self-report and behavioral observation techniques. We can also estimate levels of activity from physiological measures. We have included a brief overview of some of these assessment methods to provide readers with an understanding of the array of options available.

Behavioral Observation Methods

Several observational systems exist for assessing physical activity. One example is the Fargo Activity Times/Sampling Survey (FATS), used to assess child activity and related parent behavior (Klesges et al., 1984). Using this system, raters code operationally defined behavior in terms of discriminable body movements, with categories rated for intensity. Individuals using the FATS may also record physical and social environmental variables related to body movements. The FATS uses an interval time-sampling procedure. Observer training is time-intensive, but research has indicated high interobserver reliability. Studies using the FATS have consistently found more activity in children who are of normal weight compared to those who are obese.

Baranowski and colleagues (1984) also developed an observational coding system as part of their Family Health Project. In this method, observers record physical activity, social environment, physical location, and foods consumed using time-sampling procedures. Interobserver agreement is good; however, lowest agreements occur during periods of higher activity. One group of investigators recently modified this system for use with college students (Klesges, Eck, Mellon, Fulliton, Somes, & Hanson, 1990). Behavioral observation techniques include direct observation or videotapes. Although ratings do not require much effort on the part of subjects, they may produce reactivity and are costly in terms of time and money for researchers. Studies employing most observational systems typically utilize children, in part because it may be difficult to find a sample of adults who would permit an observer to follow their activities throughout the day (Baranowski, 1988).

Physiological Assessment Methods

Physiological methods of assessing physical activity and fitness offer the advantage of objectivity over self-report methods (Ainsworth, Montoye, & Leon, 1994). Such methods include assessment of flexibility, body composition, and anaerobic and aerobic abilities. Although measures of *flexibility* and *muscular strength per se* do not typically reflect an individual's health status, they may be relevant to current fitness or future health outcomes. Among elderly individuals and those with physical disability, limited range of motion or weak muscles may be primary limiting factors in the ability to perform daily activities and may thereby contribute to sedentary lifestyles. Indirect measures of fitness assessment include evaluations of physiological indicators, such as heart rate (pulse) and body fatness (Paffenbarger, Blair, Lee, & Hyder, 1993). *Body composition* is not a performance measure in itself, but it is an important determinant of fitness and is highly relevant to health, both when individuals are under- or over-fat. Body composition may serve as a dependent measure to assess changes occurring with exercise training (Bar-Or, 1989). *Cardiovascular endurance* frequently serves as an outcome measure in studies examining the relationship of physical activity to health outcomes. Graded exercises tests are the most efficacious and commonly used tests of this type, but heart rate monitors and electronic motion sensors have promise for use with a small number of subjects over short periods of time.

Self-Report Methods

Self-report measures of activity can provide a wealth of information at relatively low cost to both investigators and subjects. Prospective *activity diaries* provide detailed information on activity patterns while avoiding problems of retrospective methods; however, a major difficulty with exercise diaries is reactivity. Investigators usually translate activity diary data to caloric expenditure figures using published values of task-specific energy expenditure. This may be problematic in large samples, given the intraindividual variability in estimates of energy expenditure and the fact that researchers have typically derived such values from studies of male college-aged students rather than populations at risk for chronic disease. Additionally, if patients use diaries for only a few days, there may be problems with the representativeness of the data. Other problems are that sustained record keeping requires a great deal of subject effort and may not be useful with children or adults who are semiliterate. Despite these potential problems, some researchers have successfully employed modified activity diaries with such special populations. For example, Baranowski and colleagues (1984) reported that using segmented forms with time-related cues for the day enhanced children's accuracy in end-of-day record keeping. Logistically, diaries may provide useful data from highly motivated subjects and are more practical for use with small study samples than with larger samples.

Numerous *self-report surveys* exist for assessment of physical activity. These surveys rely on recall of recent activity over the past week, month, or year. Questions typically focus on routine physical activity, structured exercise, and/or leisure-time activity. Unfortunately, investigators developed the majority of these instruments using populations largely comprising white males. Nonetheless, the strengths of self-report surveys are that they are easy to use, inexpensive, and nonreactive. Their chief disadvantages are that they require effort to recall activity information; their utility remains relatively untested with women, ethnic minorities, children, and the elderly; and paper-and-pencil instruments may not be usable in low literacy populations.

Investigators have used self-report survey instruments for assessing physical activity primarily in three general areas of research: (1) large-scale epidemiological studies examining relationships of physical activity to health outcomes, (2) behavior-change studies using self-report instruments as dependent measures when testing interventions aimed at increasing activity, and (3) correlational studies aimed at identifying why some people exercise and others do not (Baranowski, 1988). Examples of some self-report survey instruments appear in Table 13.1. Utility of these various instruments depends greatly on the questions asked. For example, if a health psychologist is evaluating efficacy of a brief-exercise intervention program, a measure assessing exercise patterns over a 1-week period may be preferable to one that assesses habitual exercise patterns over a long period of time. In selecting a particular instrument, users must also consider its appropriateness for special populations. For example, instruments that focus on recreational and leisure-time activity may be irrelevant for low-income, minority, and elderly populations, and those that focus on occupational activity with an emphasis on manual labor may be irrelevant for many female and elderly samples.

In the Study of Activity, Fitness, and Exercise (SAFE), Jacobs, Ainsworth, Hartman, and Leon (1993) simultaneously administered 10 activity questionnaires to evaluate their reliability and validity in adults of varying activity levels. Some questionnaires focused on habitual activity, others on recent activity. The researchers compared questionnaire estimates of energy expenditure to several validation measures of activity, including an accelerometer, graded treadmill exercise test, measures of body fatness, and lung function. They found that most questionnaires, including simple ones, related to performance of heavy-intensity activity and treadmill performance, but few related to performance of moderate or light activity. Measures of occupational activity did not significantly relate to any of the validation measures. These authors concluded that although there appears to be some overlap in what self-report instruments measure, there are also multiple nonoverlapping dimensions of activity reflected in the many validation realms.

A second recent validation study compared physical activity levels, estimated via five activity questionnaires, to an electronic motion sensor (Caltrac) for 7 consecutive days (Miller, Freedson, & Kline, 1994). Results indicated a strong correlation between the accelerometer activity assessments and the 7-day recall questionnaire (.79). Two other measures in Table 13.1 (Godin and Baecke questionnaires) showed moderate correlations (.45 and .40, respectively). Other questionnaires showed relatively low association to the accelerometer measure. These findings suggest that 7-day recall questionnaires may be useful as a measure of moderate activity in large population studies.

Reviews of the current status of self-report measures of physical activity have led to several conclusions. Questionnaires need to be standard and brief, and items need to be clear, with a lack of ambiguity (Paffenbarger et al., 1993). The logic of questionnaire items is likely more important than the detail and length of a questionnaire. For example, Jacobs et al. (1993) reported that the College Alumnus Questionnaire asks only three questions about stair climbing, walking, and sports/recreation, and questions are ambiguous, but scores relate to coronary heart disease (Paffenbarger, Wing, & Hyde, 1978). When evaluating relatively stable activities, such as sleep and heavy-intensity recreational activities, details about the scope of activity may not be critical. Light- and moderate-level activities may be more variable and difficult to define and may need to be assessed with questions that elicit detailed

Table 13.1. Self-Report Activity Surveys

Survey	Activity measured	Time frame	Summary score
Baecke's Netherlands Survey (Baecke, Burema, & Fritters, 1982)	16 items on work, sport and nonsport leisure activity; open-ended questions and 5-point rankings of hours per week, month and year; walking and cycling rated for minutes per day	1 year	Ordinal scale ranging from 16–70
Bouchard Survey (Bouchard et al., 1983)	15-minute by 15-minute blocks of activity recalled for 2 weekdays and 1 weekend day	3 days	Energy expenditure
Canadian Fitness Survey (Stephens & Craig, 1989)	Daily, weekly, monthly, and yearly activities done at home, work, and at leisure; ratings of time and intensity	1 day to 1 year	
Framingham Survey (Kannel & Sorlie, 1979)	Interview of hours per day in sleep, work, and leisure activity; hours weighted for intensities	1 day	Ordinal scale, Ss rank-ordered
Minnesota Leisure Time Physical Activity Questionnaire (Taylor, Jacobs, DeBacker, & Taylor, 1978)	Recall of leisure activity patterns: time per session, months per year, sessions per month; activities chosen from menu	1 year	Energy expenditure
National Health Interview Survey (Bloom, 1982)	Subjects rate their activity level relative to other persons their own age		Population rank-ordered
Paffenbarger Survey (Paffenbarger, Wing, & Hyde, 1978)	Stairs climbed, blocks walked, sports and recreation, hours of intensity per week	1 week	Energy expenditure
7-Day Recall Questionnaire (PAR) (Blair, 1985)	Hours of activity at several levels of intensity	1 week	Energy expenditure
Tecumseh Questionnaire (Montoye, 1989)	Habitual activity, occupational activity, leisure activity	1 year	Energy expenditure
Godin Questionnaire (Godin & Shepard, 1985)	Activities in leisure time, usual activities resulting in sweating, nonleisure light, moderate, and strenuous activities	Usual week	Weighted sum of times per week; sweating frequency

information, address recent versus habitual activity, and provide examples (Jacobs et al., 1993).

PSYCHOLOGICAL MODELS OF PHYSICAL ACTIVITY AND EXERCISE PARTICIPATION

Despite hundreds of studies and increasingly sophisticated assessment methods and statistical models, we still know surprisingly little about who exercises regularly, why, and what determines how long they will continue (Dishman, 1988). Psychological theories and models have contributed to major advances in other areas of health promotion, such as weight loss and smoking cessation. However, these successful applications involve avoiding activities that are immediately pleasurable but have harmful long-term consequences, whereas increasing physical activity requires increasing behavior, which one has avoided, in order to get long-term positive benefits. It is not clear to what extent the models developed for interventions with addictive behaviors are applicable for physical activity promotion (King et al., 1992). There have been several recent reviews of theoretical models and determinants of exercise participation (e.g., Dishman & Sallis, 1994; Dishman, 1988; King et al., 1992). No single model has successfully integrated all the factors known to influence activity participation, and it seems likely that several of the models currently used by researchers will lead to advances in our understanding of this complex set of behaviors. We agree with Dishman (1991) that two models that seem particularly promising at this point in time are the relapse prevention model (Marlatt & Gordon, 1985) and the transtheoretical model (Prochaska, DiClemente, & Norcross, 1992).

Relapse Prevention in Exercise

Developed in the context of the study of relapse in the addictive behaviors, the relapse prevention model suggests an alternative to the view that relapse represents failure of an attempt at behavior change. In this model, relapse is a process, or series of events, which may or may not precede a return to the problem-behavior pattern. Precipitated by exposure to high-risk situations (which can be internal states or external events), outcomes depend on the individuals' coping responses and self-efficacy. Under the best of conditions, high-risk situations present opportunities for learning and may actually result in a decreased probability of relapse because of increased confidence and improved coping skills. However, if coping is ineffective, the episode may lead to lower self-efficacy, an "abstinence violation effect" involving guilt, negative self-attributions, and eventually an increased probability of total relapse.

Failure to exercise during any given period of time is not a single identifiable event analogous to violating an "abstinence" rule in substance-abuse recovery. When does failure to exercise become a "lapse" or "relapse"? What kinds of events (internal or external) are high-risk situations for exercisers vulnerable to relapse? We have explored answers to questions like these by surveying community exercisers (Dubbert et al., 1990; Dubbert, Terre, Rowland, Porzelius, & Krug, 1988). In a series of preliminary studies, we surveyed participants in local fun-runs, walks, and road races about their experiences with exercise relapse and perceptions about associated factors. Demographic characteristics of our sample (primarily middle-class, college-educated, Caucasian men and women 25 to 50 years of age) were similar to those in other studies of exercise relapse (Sallis et al., 1989, 1990). Of our 240 survey participants, 86 men and 85 women responded positively to the question about whether they had ever "started an exercise program and then dropped out for a while." About 30% of the relapsers recalled dropping out within 3 months after starting their previous exercise program, 50% within 6 months, and 90% within 1 year. These results are very consistent with other data indicating that the first 6 months of exercise (or other health-behavior changes) is a time of high vulnerability to relapse (Dishman, 1988).

Although previous researchers (e.g., Sallis et al., 1990) have used 3 months without exercise as an operational definition of exercise relapse, we reasoned that some exercisers might experience the cognitive and behavioral consequences of relapse if they believed they had "dropped out," even if they had not been inactive long enough to become physically deconditioned. We asked our participants how many days or weeks went by without exercise before they felt they had "dropped out" or given up their exercise program. The majority of men (69%) and almost half the women (45%) said they felt they had dropped out after not exercising for 2 weeks; 84% of men and 68% of women said they felt they had dropped out after 1 month without exercise. We also found that exercise experiences significantly related to the period of time without exercise before an individual felt he or she had dropped out. Those who had been exercising for the longest time before their period of inactivity indicated a longer period of time elapsed without exercise before they felt they had dropped out of their program ($p < .01$).

Attributions for reasons for exercise relapse in our participants were consistent with the limited findings available from previous research. Similar to the findings of the survey by Sallis et al. (1990) of San Diego residents, our exercisers reported lack of time, work conflicts, and family demands as the most frequent reasons for dropping their exercise programs. Negative mood states, which are important high-risk situations for relapse in some addictive disorders, were not important contributions to exercise relapse among our participants. Injuries were responsible for 33% of men's and 20% of women's relapses in our survey. Sallis and his colleagues found that injury was the most frequent causes of relapse from vigorous exercise.

Because people appear to drop in and out of regular exercise over time (Sallis et al., 1986), preventing relapse may be a very important means of increasing overall activity participation in some segments of the population, even in the absence of exercise promotion interventions. Teaching exercisers relapse-prevention skills may help promote maintenance of regular activity (e.g., Belisle, Roskies, & Levesque, 1987; King et al., 1992). Prospective studies of high-risk situations for exercise lapse and relapse are necessary to confirm the retrospective data now available. Studies involving minority and elderly populations are also necessary. Health-care providers can then strengthen relapse prevention interventions by incorporating training specifically designed to help exercisers anticipate and cope with such situations.

The Transtheoretical Model and Stages of Exercise Change

The transtheoretical model is also a promising approach for understanding and changing exercise behavior. This model proposes that individuals progress through several *stages of change* as they attempt to overcome problem behaviors. In exercise, as well as the addictive behaviors with which the model has most fully undergone investigation, these stages of change are *precontemplation, contemplation, preparation, action,* and *maintenance* (Prochaska, DiClemente, & Norcross, 1992). This model's reflection of the dynamic nature of health-behavior change appears to be a much better fit to the real world than the static models that dominated early exercise-adherence literature. Much of the early literature consisted of reports comparing people who were currently active or who continued a rehabilitation program with those who had dropped out. Although some of the findings were fairly robust across populations and types of activity, they have not often led to improved interventions for moving people from the inactive to the active categories.

The transtheoretical model proposes not only stages of change through which individuals progress, but also *processes of change* that help facilitate successful modification of behavior. The model describes five experiential and five behavioral-change processes. The experiential processes, such as seeking new information about problem behaviors, reevaluating how behaviors affect the physical and social environment, and increasing awareness of alternatives to current problem lifestyles, are most important in the early stages as individuals become aware of and work through their ambivalence about behavior change. The behavioral processes, such as substituting alternatives for problem behaviors, changing the contingencies that maintain them, or taking control of situations that trigger them, seem most important as individuals actually undergo and attempt to maintain desired behavior changes. People's perceptions of the pros and cons of the behavior also shift as they progress through the stage of change. The decisional balance shifts away from valuing the benefits of problem lifestyles toward valuing the potential benefits of healthier alternative behaviors.

Understanding these processes can help in selection of interventions that will be effective in moving individuals through the stages of change; interventions useful at one stage may not be very effective in another. For example, precontemplators who have no intentions of changing their exercise behavior might receive the most effective assistance in moving toward change by experiential interventions, such as seeing a brief television spot about the benefits of an active lifestyle. On the other hand, those who are ready to make a commitment to increasing activity at home or attending an exercise class might benefit from a behavioral intervention, such as telephone prompts from friends or program staff members. Proponents of the transtheoretical model argue that much of the "resistance" to change results from a mismatch of interventions with an individuals readiness to change. Marcus, Banspach, Lefebvre, Rossi, Carleton, and Abrams (1992) tested interventions matched to stages of change in a community health-promotion study. Their posttest results found that significantly more subjects were physically active after the 6-week intervention than prior to the intervention.

INTERVENTIONS TO INCREASE PHYSICAL ACTIVITY

Several studies reported during the past two decades have shown that interventions based on social learning and other behavioral theories and models can produce at least short-term increases in physical activity (Dishman, 1988; Dubbert, 1992;

King et al., 1992). In this section, we describe examples of interventions tested successfully in a variety of settings. It is important to note that we are providing only a few examples of the application of these strategies; readers interested in more complete or critical reviews can utilize other sources (e.g., Dishman, 1991). Most of the strategies studied in exercise promotion involve what the transtheoretical model describes as behavioral-change processes, but some of the interventions could also be useful with people who have not yet reached the preparation or action stages of exercise.

Stimulus Control and Environmental Prompts

In perhaps the best demonstration of the potential effectiveness of a simple stimulus cue to change physical activity, Brownell, Stunkard, and Albaum (1980) observed commuters' use of escalators versus stairs under conditions in which a sign encouraging use of stairs was present or absent. Stair use increased for men and women, normal weight and obese subjects, when the sign was present. Obese commuters were less likely to use the stairs but responded as well to the sign as the nonobese. The effect diminished rapidly after removal of the sign. Although there seem to have been few systematic studies of this strategy by itself, exercise-promotion interventions often include suggestions to make exercise cues prominent.

Decision Balance Sheet

During a 15-minute phone interview, women who had just enrolled in an exercise class received instructions to write down pros and cons they anticipated from the exercise, including personal benefits and losses, gains and losses to important others, disapproval from self and others and self-approval (Hoyt & Janis, 1975). A second group received instructions to go through the same process but in regard to smoking cessation, and a third group did not go through the interview process. Attendance through the 7-week program was almost twice as high for the exercise balance-sheet groups relative to the other two groups. Assessing decisional balance is important in predicting readiness to change under the transtheoretical model. This kind of intervention can be useful both to facilitate initial adoption of exercise and to assist someone who has relapsed.

Contracting and Lottery

Epstein, Wing, Thompson, and Griffin (1980) studied the effectiveness of behavioral contracting and a lottery for prizes in an exercise program for female college students. Some students contracted to receive money back from a $5 deposit for completing their assigned exercise. Another group's money was used to purchase a lottery prize, and students earned chances to win the prize. Women in the contracting and lottery groups attended the program more regularly than women in groups that did not have these incentives. These kinds of strategies are useful in many health-promotion programs.

Exercise Program Staff Feedback and Goal Setting

Martin et al. (1984) conducted a series of studies with men and women in a community jogging course. In one study, men and women received randomized assignment to groups that set either time or distance goals and received either personalized or general group feedback about progress. Attendance was significantly worse in the group that received general group feedback and distance goals. There were no differences in exercise class attendance among the other three groups. We concluded that the individualized staff attention facilitated adherence, even when exercisers used unpopular time goals.

Self-Monitoring and Phone Call Prompts

In an exercise adoption study, working men and women received individual exercise instructions and a portable heart rate monitor (King, Taylor, Haskell, & DeBusk, 1988). Participants exercised on their own and mailed daily exercise logs to program staff. About 60% of participants also received 10 phone contacts during the 6-month study. The investigators found that women and men made equal fitness gains. Fitness improvement was better for those who received the phone calls. There was no difference in amount of exercise recorded by the two groups. In an exercise-maintenance study reported by the same authors, men and women who had already started exercising received instructions for maintaining their program. About 60% also received phone calls from the program staff to encourage them to maintain their exercise. Maintenance was significantly better in the group that received the phone calls.

Supervised Exercise Testing

Ewart, Taylor, Reese, and DeBusk (1983) evaluated perceived self-efficacy for activity in patients before and after a medically supervised treadmill exercise test. Patients, who were all recovering from a recent myocardial infarction, then received counseling by a physician and nurse. Self-efficacy for physical activity increased after treadmill testing, especially for patients with low self-efficacy before testing. Self-efficacy also increased after the counseling session. The authors reported that patients with greater self-efficacy were more likely to continue physical activity after discharge than were those with less self-efficacy.

"Lifestyle" versus "Programmed" Exercise

Epstein, Wing, Koeske, and Valoski (1985) randomized obese children to one of three exercise conditions: (1) "programmed" exercise requiring aerobic exercise three times per week, (2) "lifestyle" exercise allowing a variety of exercises selected from a menu to equal energy expenditure of the programmed group, or (3) calisthenics involving performance of a set of calisthenics three times per week. Weight changes were similar in all groups for the first year, but during the second year, children in the "lifestyle" exercise group maintained their weight changes, whereas those in the other two groups gained weight back. Only the programmed-aerobic-exercise group showed improved fitness.

Cognitive Distraction and Goal Setting

In another of our exercise study series, Martin et al. (1984) randomized men and women in a community jogging course to one of two groups: one attending to internal body sensations and setting high standards for exercise performance, and the other attending to pleasant external stimuli and setting flexible and realistic exercise standards. Those taught to attend to external stimuli and set flexible realistic goals had significantly better class attendance.

Cognitive Modification, Goal Setting, and Contracting

Atkins, Kaplan, Timms, Reinsch, and Lofbach (1984) randomly assigned chronic obstructive pulmonary disease patients to several intervention groups, including (1) behavior modification, (2) cognition modification, and (3) combined behavior and cognitive modification. In the behavior modification group, patients received requests to contract to make highly probable behaviors contingent on walking, and there was also a discussion about scheduling exercise. In the cognitive modification group, patients received encouragement to monitor for and substitute goal-oriented self-statements for self-defeating ones and also to monitor and praise themselves for partial goal attainment. The combination cognitive and behavioral modification group received both interventions. The combination group achieved the most total time walking during the study; nonetheless, the other two intervention groups did better than patients given no intervention or an intervention unrelated to exercise.

Relapse Prevention

Belisle, Roskies, and Levesque (1987) assigned participants in a university-based sports center program to receive either the standard training or an experimental one, including discussion of obstacles to exercise and means of coping with these obstacles. Experimental-condition participants showed better adherence and maintenance of exercise to 3-month follow-up in two studies.

Stage of Change-Matched Interventions to Increase Activity

In a study mentioned earlier, community adults, assessed by questionnaire to determine stage of readiness for exercise, received a stage-matched manual (based on responses to the questionnaire) for exercise adoption and maintenance (Marcus et al., 1992). Participants were significantly more active after the 6-week program than they were prior to the program. Sixty-two percent of participants in the contemplation stage became more active, as did 61% of those in the preparation stage.

Group/Facility versus Individual/Home-Based Exercise

At least some of the recent experimental intervention studies have involved unsupervised, "home-based" exercise of moderate intensity and utilized inexpensive interventions requiring minimal program contact. One particularly noteworthy recent trial making use of such strategies to enhance adherence (King, Haskell, Taylor, Kraemer, & DeBusk, 1991) compared two formats (group classes versus home-based exercise) and two intensities (higher versus lower) in 50- to 65-year-old men and women. Fitness change data showed that all exercise intervention groups improved relative to assessment-only controls, and home-based exercise participants had better adherence than group-class participants. Long-term adherence for home-based exercise in this study (about 70% at 1 year) compared favorably with many earlier studies in which dropout typically reached 50% by 6 months.

EXERCISE PROMOTION IN SPECIAL POPULATIONS

Much of the early exercise adherence literature involved studies of cardiac rehabilitation patients in highly structured and monitored programs. During the past 10 years, researchers have increasingly recognized and worked to begin to fill the large gaps in our knowledge about physical activity participation/adherence in populations other than middle-aged males.

Ethnic Minorities

Few studies have systematically examined physical activity and health in minority populations, and available data generally do not allow conclusions about which of the observed differences are due to economic, educational, cultural, and other factors. However, some interesting findings suggesting the kinds of difference that may exist have already emerged.

Several epidemiological studies have found differences in physical activity of black and white Americans. The 1985 National Health Interview Survey, for example, revealed an interesting pattern of physical activity differences by race and gender (DiPietro & Caspersen, 1991). Black women and men reported more minutes per day of walking than white, and black men also reported more minutes per day of vigorous team-sports play (8 minutes per day) than white men (3 minutes per day). White men, however, reported about twice as much average time in gardening activity (10 minutes per day) as black men (5 minutes per day). Women of both racial groups reported very little time in vigorous team-sports play and about half as much time gardening relative to men (6 minutes for white women, and 3 minutes for black women). Behavioral risk-factor surveillance data from 1988 (Merritt, Caspersen, Heath, & Yaeger, 1990) also showed racial differences in leisure-time activity, particularly among minority women. Although 27% of white men, 31% of nonwhite men, and 30% of white women reported sedentary lifestyles, 40% of nonwhite women were inactive. Nine percent of white women, but only 4% of nonwhite women, reported regular vigorous activity.

In an analysis of data from the Healthy Women Study, Wing et al. (1989) examined subjects' responses to the Paffenbarger Activity Questionnaire and found that African-American women reported significantly less physical activity than Caucasian women. Racial differences in activity remained constant even when controlling for education. It is important to note that nearly all of the studies relied on self-report methods emphasizing leisure-time activity and sports as measures of physical activity and exercise. The extent to which these questions are relevant to minority and blue-collar populations is questionable and may have strongly impacted the studies' findings.

Although there has been recent implementation of community-level cardiovascular risk-modification intervention programs for low-income populations, few have focused on specific needs of black communities. Baranowski et al. (1990) described a comprehensive, center-based program to improve diet and increase aerobic activity in blue-collar African-American families. The investigators actively recruited participants from the community and conducted educational sessions in a convenient building that was important within the participants' community. Activity sessions took place in a modern fitness center. Incentives included free transportation, baby-sitters, and reminders to promote attendance. The investigators obtained regular input from an advisor group of African-American community leaders and informal dialogue with members of the African-American community, and components of the intervention underwent a pretesting. In spite of these careful preparations, participation was extremely low, with only 20% of 94 families participating in the fitness sessions by the end of the program. Postprogram interviews revealed that high frequency of changes in job status (e.g., from unemployed to employed status, employed to unemployed looking for work, and switching from day to evening shifts) substantially impacted subjects' abilities to attend evening sessions. There were higher participation rates among daytime employed adults. In their discussion of this intervention effort, the authors underscored the importance of considering the unique social and economic characteristics, and needs of the target population before beginning an intervention program.

Women

All of the elements of health-related activity and fitness, including flexibility, body composition, muscular strength and endurance, and aerobic activity, appear to be independent of gender and are equally important for both women and men (Drinkwater, 1989). Unfortunately, in recent history, women did not receive encouragement to participate in physical activities until the past two decades (Drinkwater, 1989; Dubbert & Martin, 1988), and women today, particularly those who are middle-aged and elderly, still exercise substantially less than their male counterparts (Lee, 1991).

When women exercise on their own, there appear to be differences in their activity patterns compared to men. For example, low intensity activity, such as walking, appears to be more prevalent among women than among men. In a prospective study of activity patterns of a small sample of community exercisers, we found that, although men and women exercised a comparable number of days per week, women omitted more planned exercise days than men (Dubbert, Stetson, & Corrigan, 1991). There have been only a few well-controlled exercise intervention studies conducted with women. Those that have statistically controlled for exercise frequency and intensity in samples of men and women indicate that women experience cardiovascular benefits from exercise that are similar to those obtained by men of similar age (Getchell & Moore, 1975; Jette, Sidney, & Campbell, 1988; Lee, 1991). It is still unclear which types of exercise regimens provide optimal health benefits to women of various ages. Although premenopausal women experience benefits from vigorous aerobic activity, some research has shown that low-intensity exercise produces substantial increases in fitness for elderly women (e.g., Foster, Hume, Byrnes, Dickinson, & Chatfield, 1989). This is particularly promising because, as a group, older women engage in less frequent and lower intensity activities than men, and such an intervention approach may be more realistic for them. There is a great need for research on intervention strategies for women at all stages of the life cycle.

The Elderly

Eighty percent of elderly persons have at least one chronic health problem, such as diabetes, hypertension, cardiovascular problems, or arthritis, that could substantially impact on individual levels of physical activity (King, 1991). The importance of each of the aspects of health-related fitness previously discussed becomes increasingly obvious as individuals age. Strength, flexibility, and ability to balance are all critical to attempts to move about and carry out daily activities. Lack of strength may lead to frailty and loss of functional capacity. Without sufficient cardiovascular capacity, simple daily tasks, such as bathing, may require substantial effort or even supportive, structured care. With significant declines in skeletal structure, fractures may occur, further reducing abilities to ambulate and function independently (Buschner & de Lateur, 1991; Smith & Gilligan, 1989).

In the general population, health-related fitness begins to decline in many body systems after about age 35. Our elderly population is largely sedentary, and it is difficult to separate influences of genetic and environmental factors on these declines in activity and health-related fitness (Smith & Gilligan, 1989). McAvoy (1976) found that adults over age 65 had a low self-concept of their ability to exercise regularly. Sidney and Shephard (1977) reported that city-dwelling elderly persons had physical fitness levels that were average or below average, yet perceived themselves as engaging in sufficient activity. These studies suggest that although elderly persons underestimate their abilities to engage in exercise, they remain largely satisfied with their fitness levels. Buskirk (1990) expressed concern that a lack of willingness to engage in activities that require strength may reflect an inaccurate self-perception of weakness.

Data from the National Health Interview Survey indicate that people between the ages of 65 to 75 spend less time in vigorous, conditioning activities but more time walking, and considerably more time gardening and performing home-repair activities than their younger cohorts. At age 75, all activities tend to decline (Caspersen, Pollard, & Pratt, 1987). For the active elderly, walking may be the most likely source of activity of sufficient duration and intensity to promote good health. Gardening and household activities may promote strength and flexibility and contribute substantially to caloric expenditure if done consistently. These less intensive activities may be more realistic physical activity goals compared to more vigorous, structured activities for elderly persons who have been sedentary (Caspersen et al., 1987; Haskell, Montoye, & Orenstein, 1985).

CONCLUDING COMMENTS

The public health significance of exercise promotion has now received wide recognition and the *Healthy People 2000* physical activity objectives have already stimulated increased interest among many health professionals and researchers. The National Institutes of Health have sponsored a variety of projects that will improve understanding of how best to increase activity in different populations at risk. Public health and other experts are turning to health psychologists and other behavioral scientists for guidance in achieving physical activity health objectives. At present, we still know surprisingly little about exercise behavior in natural settings and less than we need to know about the physical, cognitive, and emotional effects of exercise conducted under carefully controlled conditions. It seems likely that we can successfully adapt some of the theories and methods developed in other areas of psychological practice to the problems of physical activity assessment and behavior change. Health psychologists interested in physical activity promotion and research will find that this field offers many challenges and potential rewards.

REFERENCES

Ainsworth, B. E., Montoye, H. J., & Leon, A. S. (1994). Methods of assessing physical activity during leisure and work. In C. Bouchard, R. J. Shephard, & T. Stephens (Eds.), *Physical activity, fitness, and health* (pp. 146–159). Champaign, IL: Human Kinetics Press.

American College of Sports Medicine. (1990). The recommended quantity and quality of exercise for developing and maintaining cardiorespiratory and muscular fitness in healthy adults. *Medicine and Science in Sports and Exercise, 22,* 265–274.

Atkins, C. J., Kaplan, R. M., Timms, R. M., Reinsch, S., & Lofback, K. (1984). Behavioral exercise programs in the management of chronic obstructive pulmonary disease. *Journal of Consulting and Clinical Psychology, 52,* 591–603.

Bar-Or, O. (1989). Fitness and activity assessment of children and adolescents. In *Assessing Physical Fitness and Physical Activity in Population-based Surveys* (DHHS Publication No. PHS 89-1253). Hyattsville, MD: U.S. Department of Health and Human Services.

Baranowski, T. (1988). Validity and reliability of self-report measures of physical activity: An information processing perspective. *Research Quarterly for Exercise and Sport, 59,* 314–327.

Baranowski, T., Dworkin, R., Cieslik, C. J., Hooks, P., Clearman, D. R., Ray, L., Dunn, J. K., & Nader, P. R. (1984). Reliability and validity of self-report of aerobic activity: Family Health Project. *Research Quarterly for Exercise and Sport, 55,* 309–317.

Baranowski, T., Simms-Morton, B., Hooks, P., Henske, J., Tiernan, K., Dunn, J. K., Burkhalter, H., Harper, J., & Palmer, J. (1990). A center-based program for exercise change among black-American families. *Health Education Quarterly, 17,* 179–196.

Belisle, M., Roskies, E., & Levesque, J. M. (1987). Improving adherence to physical activity. *Health Psychology, 6,* 159–172.

Blair, S. N., Kohl, H. W., Gordon, N., & Paffenbarger, R. S., Jr. (1992). How much physical activity is good for health? *Annual Review of Public Health 13,* 99–126.

Blair, S. N., Mulder, R. T., & Kohl, H. W. (1987). Reaction to "Secular trends in adult physical activity: Exercise boom or bust?" *Research Quarterly for Exercise and Sport, 58,* 106–110.

Blair, S. N., Powell, K. E., Bazzarre, T. L., Early, J. L., Epstein, L. H., Green, L. W., Harris, S. S., Haskell, W. L., King, A. C., Koplan, J., Marcus, B., Paffenbarger, R. S., Yeager, K. K. (1993). Physical inactivity. *Circulation, 88,* 1402–1405.

Bouchard, C., Shephard, R. J., & Stephens, T. (1994). *Physical activity, fitness, and health.* Champaign, IL: Human Kinetics Press.

Brownell, K. D., Stunkard, A. J., & Album, J. M. (1980). Evaluation and modification of exercise patterns in the natural environment. *American Journal of Psychiatry, 137,* 1540–1545.

Buschner, D. M., & de Lateur, B. J. (1991). The importance of skeletal muscle strength to physical function in older adults. *Annals of Behavioral Medicine, 13,* 133–140.

Buskirk, E. R. (1990). Exercise, fitness and aging. In C. Bouchard, R. J. Shepard, T. Stephens, J. R. Sutton, & B. D. McPherson (Eds.), *Exercise, fitness and health: A consensus of current knowledge.* Champaign, IL: Human Kinetics Books.

Caspersen, C. J. (1989). Physical activity epidemiology: Concepts, methods, and applications to exercise science. *Exercise and Sports Sciences Reviews, 17,* 423–473.

Caspersen, C. J., Christenson, G. M., & Pollard, R. A. (1986). Status of the 1990 physical fitness and exercise objectives—Evidence from NHIS 1985. *Public Health Reports, 101,* 587–592.

Caspersen, C. J., Pollard, R. A., & Pratt, S. O. (1987). Scoring physical activity data with special consideration for elderly populations. In *Proceedings of the 1987 Public Health Conference on Records and Statistics: Data for an aging population, July 13–15, 1987* (DHHS Publication No. PHS 88-1214 pp. 30–34). Washington, DC: U.S. Department of Health and Human Services.

Dishman, R. K. (Ed.). (1988). *Exercise adherence: Its impact on public health.* Campaign, IL: Human Kinetics Press.

Dishman, R. K. (1991). Increasing and maintaining exercise and physical activity. *Behavior Therapy, 22,* 345–378.

Dishman, R. K., & Sallis, J. F. (1994). Determinants and interventions for physical activity and exercise. In C. Bouchard, R. J. Shephard, & T. Stephens (Eds.), *Physical activity, fitness, and health* (pp. 214–238). Champaign, IL: Human Kinetics Press.

Drinkwater, B. L. (1989). Assessing fitness and activity patterns of women in general population studies. In *Assessing physical fitness and physical activity in population-based surveys.* (DHHS Publication No. PHS 89-1253. Hyattsville, MD: U.S. Department of Health and Human Services.

Dubbert, P. M. (1992). Exercise in behavioral medicine. *Journal of Consulting and Clinical Psychology, 60,* 613–618.

Dubbert, P. M., Corrigan, S., Wittrock, D., Stetson, B., Caddell, J., Hinkle, L., & Liggett, M. V. (1990, April). *Relapse in exercise: Study II.* Presentation at the Society of Behavioral Medicine, Chicago, IL.

Dubbert, P. M., & Martin, J. E. (1988). Exercise. In E. A. Blechman & K. D. Brownell (Eds.), *Behavioral medicine for women* (pp. 291–304). New York: Pergamon.

Dubbert, P. M., Stetson, B. A., & Corrigan, S. A. (1991, August). *Predictors of exercise maintenance in community women.* Presentation at the American Psychology Association Annual Meeting, San Francisco, CA.

Dubbert, P. M., Terre, L., Rowland, A. K., Porzelius, J., & Krug, L. M. (1988, April). *Relapse in exercise.* Presentation at the Society of Behavioral Medicine, Boston, MA.

Epstein, L. H., Wing, R. R., Koeske, R., & Valoski, A. (1985). A comparison of lifestyle exercise, aerobic exercise, and calisthenics on weight loss in obese children. *Behavior Therapy, 16,* 345–356.

Epstein, L. H., Wing, R. R., Thompson, J. K., & Griffin, W. (1980). Attendance and fitness in aerobics exercise. *Behavior Modification, 4*(4), 465–479.

Ewart, C. K., Taylor, C. B., Reese, L. B., & DeBusk, R. F. (1983). Effects of early postmyocardial infarction exercise testing on self-perception and subsequent physical activity. *American Journal of Cardiology, 51,* 1076–1080.

Fletcher, C. J., Blair, S. N., Blumenthal, J., Caspersen, C., Chaitman, B., Epstein, S., Falls, H., Froelicher, E.S.S., Froelicher, V. F., & Pina, I. L. (1992). Benefits and recommendations for physical activity programs for all Americans: A statement for health professionals by the Committee on Exercise and Cardiac Rehabilitation of the Council on Clinical Cardiology, American Heart Association. *Circulation, 86,* 340–344.

Foster, V. L., Hume, G.J.E., Byrnes, W. C., Dickinson, A. L., & Chatfield, S. J. (1989). Endurance training for elderly women: Moderate vs. low intensity. *Journal of Gerontology: Medical Sciences, 44,* M184–M178.

Getchell, L. H., & Moore, J. C. (1975). Physical training: Comparative responses of middle-aged adults. *Archives of Physical Medicine and Rehabilitation, 56,* 250–254.

Harris, S. S., Caspersen, C. J., DeFriese, G. H., & Estes, E. H. (1989). Physical activity counseling for healthy adults as a primary preventive intervention in the clinical setting. *Journal of the American Medical Association, 261,* 3590–3598.

Haskell, W. L., Montoye, H. J., & Orenstein, D. (1985). Physical activity and exercise to achieve health-related physical fitness components. *Public Health Reports, 100,* 202–212.

Hoyt, M. F., & Janis, I. L. (1975). Increasing adherence to a stressful decision via a motivational balance-sheet procedure: A field experiment. *Journal of Personality and Social Psychology, 31,* 833–839.

Jacobs, D., Ainsworth, B., Hartman, T., & Leon, A. (1993). A simultaneous evaluation of 10 commonly used physical activity questionnaires. *Medicine and Science in Sports and Exercise, 25,* 81–91.

Jette, M., Sidney, K., & Campbell, J. (1988). Effects of a twelve-week program on maximal and submaximal work output indices in sedentary middle-aged men and women. *Journal of Sports Medicine and Physical Fitness, 28,* 59–66.

King, A. C. (1991). Physical activity and health enhancement in older adults: Current status and future prospects. *Annals of Behavioral Medicine, 13,* 87–90.

King, A. C., Bild, D., Dishman, R. K., Dubbert, P. M., Marcus, B. M., Oldridge, N., Paffenbarger, R. S., Jr., Powell, K. E., Yaeger, K., & Blair, S. N. (1992). Determinants of physical activity and interventions in adults. *Medicine and Science in Sports and Exercise, 24,* S221–S236.

King, A. C., Haskell, W. L., Taylor, B., Kraemer, H. C., & DeBusk, R. F. (1991). Group- vs. home-based exercise training in healthy older men and women. *Journal of the American Medical Association, 266,* 1535–1542.

King, A. C., Taylor, C. B., Haskell, W. L., & DeBusk, R. F. (1988). Strategies for increasing early adherence to and long-term maintenance of home-based exercise training in healthy middle-aged men and women. *American Journal of Cardiology, 61,* 628–632.

Klesges, R. C., Coates, T. J., Moldenhauer-Klesges, L. M., Holzer, B., Gustavson, J., & Barnes, J. (1984). The FATS: An observational system for assessing physical activity in children and associated parent behavior. *Behavioral Assessment, 6,* 333–345.

Klesges, R. C., Eck, L. H., Mellon, M. W., Fulliton, W., Somes, G. W., & Hanson, C. (1990). The accuracy of self-reports of physical activity. *Medicine and Science in Sports and Exercise, 22,* 690–697.

LaPorte, R. E., Montoye, H. J., & Caspersen, C. J. (1985). Assessment of physical activity in epidemiologic research: Problems and prospects. *Public Health Reports, 100,* 131–146.

Lee, C. (1991). Women and aerobic exercise: Directions for research development. *Annals of Behavioral Medicine, 13,* 133–140.

Marcus, B. H., Banspach, S. W., Lefebvre, R. C., Rossi, J. S., Carleton, R. A., & Abrams, D. (1992). Increasing the adoption of physical activity among community participants. *American Journal of Health Promotion, 6,* 424–429.

Marlatt, G. A., & Gordon, J. R. (1985). *Relapse prevention.* New York: Guilford.

Martin, J. E., Dubbert, P. M., Katell, A. D., Thompson, J. K., Raczynski, J. R., Lake, M., Smith, P. O., Webster, J. S., Sikora, T., & Cohen, R. E. (1984). Behavioral control of exercise in sedentary adults: Studies 1 through 6. *Journal of Consulting and Clinical Psychology, 52,* 795–811.

McAvoy, L. H. (1976). *Recreation preferences of the elderly persons in Minnesota.* Unpublished doctoral dissertation, University of Minnesota, Minneapolis.

Merritt, R. K., Caspersen, C. J., Heath, C. W., & Yaeger, K. (1990). Physical activity in white versus nonwhite men and women. *Medicine and Science in Sports and Exercise, 22,* S-46.

Miller, D., Freedson, P., & Kline, G. (1994). Comparison of activity levels using the Caltrac accelerometer and five questionnaires (1994). *Medicine and Science in Sports and Exercise, 26,* 376–382.

Paffenbarger, R., Blair, S., Lee, I., & Hyde, R. (1993). Measurement of physical activity to assess health effects in free-living populations. *Medicine and Science in Sports and Exercise, 25,* 60–70.

Paffenbarger, R. S., Wing, A. L., & Hyde, R. T. (1978). Physical activity as an index of heart attack risk in college alumni. *American Journal of Epidemiology, 108,* 161–175.

Pate, R. R., Pratt, M., Blair, S. N., Haskell, W. L., Macera, C. A., Bouchard, C., Buchner, D., Ettinger, W., Heath, G. W., King, A. C., Kriska, A., Leon, A. S., Marcus, B. H., Morris, J., Paffenbarger, R. S., Jr., Patrick, K., Pollock, M. L., Rippe, J. M., Sallis, J., & Wilmore, J. H. (1995). Physical activity and health. *Journal of the American Medical Association, 273,* 402–407.

Prochaska, J. O., DiClemente, C. C., & Norcross, J. C. (1992). In search of how people change. *American Psychologist, 47,* 1102–1114.

Sallis, J. F., Haskell, W. L., Fortmann, S. P., Vranizan, K. M., Taylor, C. B., & Solomon, D. S. (1986). Predictors of adoption and maintenance of physical activity in a community sample. *Preventive Medicine, 15,* 331–341.

Sallis, J. F., Hovell, M. F., Hofstetter, C. R., Elder, J. P., Faucher, P., Spry, V. M., Barrington, E., & Hackley, M. (1990). Lifetime history of relapse from exercise. *Addictive Behaviors, 15,* 573–579.

Sallis, J. F., Hovell, M. F., Hofstetter, C. R., Faucher, P., Elder, J. P., Blanchard, J., Caspersen, C. J., Powell, K. E., & Christenson, G. M. (1989). A multivariate study of determinants of vigorous exercise in a community sample. *Preventive Medicine, 18,* 20–34.

Sidney, K. H., & Shephard, R. J. (1977). Activity patterns of elderly men and women. *Journal of Gerontology, 32,* 25–32.

Smith, E. L., & Gilligan, C. (1989). Health-related fitness of the older adult. In *Assessing physical fitness and physical activity in population-based surveys.* DHHS Publication No. PHS 89-1253. Hyattsville, MD: U.S. Department of Health and Human Services.

Stephens, T. (1987). Secular trends in adult physical activity: Exercise boom or bust? *Research Quarterly for Exercise and Sport, 58,* 94–105.

U.S. Department of Health and Human Services, Public Health Service (1990). *Healthy people 2000.* Washington, DC: U.S. Government Printing Office.

Wilson, P.W.F., Paffenbarger, R. S., Morris, J. N., & Havlik, R. J. (1986). Assessment methods for physical activity and physical fitness in populations studies: Report of a NHLBI workshop. *American Heart Journal, 111,* 1177–1192.

Wing, R. R., Killer, L. H., Bunker, C., Matthews, K., Caggiula, A., Meihlan, E., & Kelsey, S. (1989). Obesity, obesity-related behaviors and coronary heart disease risk factors in black and white premenopausal women. *International Journal of Obesity, 13,* 511–519.

14

Stress and Stress Management

Phillip J. Brantley and Bradley T. Thomason

HISTORY OF STRESS

The origins of stress date back to antiquity. In the 14th century, the term *stress* described social hardship and economic adversity prevalent at the time. The concept of *stress* remained relatively obscure until physical science adopted the term. Inspired by the work of Robert Hooke, 18th-century physicist Thomas Young defined *stress* as the "ratio of force within the elastic body, which balances an external applied force, to the area over which the force acts" (Engel, 1985).

The notion of stress as a physical phenomenon grew in popularity over the next one hundred years. The conceptualization of stress expanded into other scientific disciplines, most notably physiology. By the end of the 19th century, European physiologists, such as Bernard (1879), Pfluger (1877), and Fredericq (1885) offered similar explanations of stress phenomenology. These scientists referred to stress as a dynamic challenge presented to a living organism, disrupting its attempt to maintain a stable, internal environment (Selye, 1982).

Interest in stress physiology quickly spread to the United States during the early 1900s. William Cannon's (1939) research on biobehavioral survival mechanisms resulted in his theory of "fight or flight." Shadowing the work of European physiologists, he coined the term *homeostasis* and defined it as "the coordinated physiological process which maintains . . . steady states in the organism."

In the early 20th century, Hans Selye, a medical student in Prague, Czechoslovakia, began his pioneer research. Eventually Selye's work paved the way for the systematic study of stress (Everly, 1989). As a result of Selye's endeavors, professionals in many scientific disciplines began to recognize the importance of behavioral factors in the study of stress. Selye (1936) posited that a "general adaptation syndrome" (GAS) occurs within an organism when confronted by "diverse nocuous agents." This GAS or "biologic stress syndrome" occurs in three discrete stages: alarm, resistance, and exhaustion. Selye reformulated his concept of stress for nearly half a century. Contemporary theorists continue to include Selye's GAS among the most highly regarded descriptions of the stress response.

The current conceptualization of stress did not entirely evolve from scientific and scholarly endeavors. The notoriety of stress grew, in part, due to effects of world conflicts, especially the Korean conflict and World Wars I and II. In 1945, Grinker and Spiegel authored the book *Men Under Stress*. This literary work depicted the psychological sequelae of soldiers during and following military combat. As a result of these and other writings, terms such as "shell shock" and "war neurosis" developed (Mott, 1919).

Building on foundations created by physics and biology, social scientists became interested in the stress concept. Social scientists, mainly sociologists, adopted the term *stress* to describe social demands and disruptions (Lazarus & Folkman, 1984). Within psychology, interest in stress grew exponentially. Lazarus (1966) considered stress a subdiscipline within psychology, similar to that of motivation or learning. The *Diagnostic and Statistical Manual of Mental Disorders* (American Psychiatric Association, 1968) gave attention to stress as a contributing factor in psychosomatic diseases. Journals dedicated to the study of stress emerged, including the *Journal of Human Stress, Psychophysiology,* and the *Journal of Traumatic Stress*.

Stress has become a household term over the past 25 years. In 1969, the U.S. Surgeon General helped popularize the notion of stress by cautioning the general public about ill effects of stress on health (Everly, 1989). As a result of global interest in stress, the 1980s became known as the "Age of Stress" (Selye, 1982).

Lazarus and Folkman (1984) attributed the vast interest in stress to five contemporary developments in social sciences. First, research examining *individual differences* uncovered important intermediate variables, such as coping and motivation. Second, *renewed interest in psychosomatics* provided support for a multidisciplinary approach to medicine and led to the emergence of specialty fields, such as psychoneuroimmunology. A third influence was the evolution of *behavior therapy*. This genre of psychotherapy placed a great deal of emphasis on managing stress. Certain behavioral approaches (e.g., stress inoculation training) considered stress the central target element (Meichenbaum & Jaremko, 1983). The *life course developmental perspective* focused on social changes and the stress of lifetime transitions, providing a fourth important influence on modern interest in stress. Finally, concern over effects of the *environment* on personal and social functioning heightened attention to stressology as a modern scientific discipline.

DEFINITION AND NATURE OF STRESS

The evolution of stress has met with scrutiny. Disagreements concerning the definition of stress have created factions among stress researchers, preventing stress from becoming a universally accepted construct. Critics maintain that the concept of stress is too broad and ambiguous to adequately define (Engel, 1985). Ader (1980) urged researchers to discard *stress* as a descriptive label and focus efforts toward uncovering mechanisms subsumed under "stress."

Despite criticism, investigators have attempted to explain and define the nature of stress. The primary source of conflict concerns the stimulus versus response debate. Stress researchers have quarreled over the issue of whether the term *stress* indicates a stimulus, a response, or perhaps an interaction between the two.

Stimulus Theories

Cannon's (1939) research on homeostasis first identified stress as a stimulus. He referred to *stress* as any emotionally laden event that readied the organism for the "fight or flight" response. Researchers have heralded the stimulus approach to stress as objective and tangible and have applied the term *stressor* to the stimulus label of stress. Subsequent investigators have regarded stressors as internal or external (Lazarus & Folkman, 1984) and psychosocial or biogenic (Everly, 1989). Considering stimulus properties (i.e., frequency, intensity, and duration) of the stressor, Elliott and Eisdorfer (1982) described four types of stress: (1) acute, time-limited (e.g., surgery); (2) stressor sequences (e.g., divorce); (3) chronic, intermittent (e.g., sexual difficulty); and (4) chronic (e.g., job stress). Stimulus definitions provide useful taxonomies, but researchers acknowledge that individual differences in stress appraisal are important considerations as well (Lazarus & Folkman, 1984).

Life-events research branched directly from the stress–stimulus approach. Influenced by Cannon, researchers have provided data suggesting stressful life events impact certain illnesses (Brown & Harris, 1989). Holmes and Masuda (1974), however, did not limit the context of life events to physical illness, but stated that an event is noteworthy if it brings about change in an individual's life structure.

Important distinctions about the nature of stressful life events have emerged from life-events research. One distinction concerns the differential effects of major versus minor life events. Traditionally, stress research has focused on major life events (e.g., death of a loved one, job loss). More contemporary stress theorists have begun to study the impact of minor life events (e.g., argument with spouse, late for work), frequently referred to as *daily stressors* or *hassles,* on health and behavior (Brantley & Jones, 1989; Delongis, Coyne, Dakof, Folkman, & Lazarus, 1982). Data have indicated the effect of minor stressors may be greater than that of major stressors on progression of physical and psychological disorders (Brantley & Jones, 1993; Delongis et al., 1982).

Another important point is that most individuals typically consider stress a negative phenomenon. Consistent with this, research indicates that the degree of subjective unpleasantness associated with a stressor may be the most significant factor governing the impact of stress (Brown, Sklair, Harris, & Birley, 1973). As such, the notion of positive stress, occasionally labeled *eustress* (Selye, 1974), has received less attention in stress literature. However, according to Selye, achieving the "optimal stress level" requires a delicate balance between eustress and distress.

Response Theories

Vis-à-vis the stimulus approach, some stress theorists have defined stress in a response context. Selye (1974) contended that stress is the "*nonspecific* response of the body to any demand" (p. 27). In a similar vein, Everly (1989) discussed the stress response in a biological framework, defining *stress* as a "physiological response that serves as a mechanism of mediation, linking any given stressor to its target-organ effect or arousal" (p. 7). However, unlike Selye, Everly and Lacey (1950) noted the importance of *specificity* in the response mechanism. *Specificity* refers to the notion that different individuals will respond to the same stressor with physiological reactions in different domains (e.g., cardiovascular versus muscular).

Physiological representation of the stress response is prevalent throughout the literature (e.g., Weiner, Floren, Murison, & Hellhammer, 1989). The primary hypothesis is that the sympatho–adrenomedullary (SAM) and hypothalamo–pituitary–adrenocortical (HPAC) systems mediate stress responses. When an individual possesses the resources to actively cope with a stressor, electrochemical changes in the brain stem mobilize the SAM axis to release catecholamines (namely epinephrine and norepinephrine) via the adrenal medulla (Jemmott & Locke, 1984). These neurochemical events ready the individual for the "fight or flight" response that Cannon (1939) originally described. Selye (1982) referred to this type of response, during which increased metabolic activity enables the organism to attack the stressor, as *catatoxic*. If no coping resources are available to the individual, a *syntoxic* response occurs (Selye, 1982). During the syntoxic response, a state of passive tolerance results. Hypervigilance and withdrawal characterize this type of response. These behaviors activate the HPAC pathways, resulting in corticosteroid (mainly cortisol) release by the adrenal cortex (Jemmott & Locke, 1984).

This cascade of neuroendocrine events parallels the biobehavioral responses (alarm, resistance, exhaustion) Selye (1936) originally described as the GAS. During the *alarm* phase, anxiety alerts the body's physiological defenses, thus arousing the sympathetic nervous and HPAC systems. Hyperarousal of these systems occurs during the *resistance* phase, and the body's homeostatic mechanisms and defenses engage. Finally, if the organism is unsuccessful warding off the stressor, the *exhaustion* phase takes over. Both psychological (depression) and physiological (disease of vulnerable target organs) exhaustion become apparent, with death as the possible final result (Everly, 1989; Selye, 1982).

Interaction Theories

Investigators have criticized *stimulus* and *response* definitions on several levels. A major criticism of both camps is the paucity of attention to individual differences. Addressing the importance of individual differences, theorists have offered *interaction* definitions of the stress experience. Wolff (1953) first pointed out that stress is a "dynamic" state dependent on the interaction between an organism and its aversive external environment.

Lazarus (1966) expanded the interactionist theory, creating a *transactional* model of stress. In the transactional model, *stress* is the "particular relationship between the person and environment that is appraised by the person as . . . exceeding his or her resources and endangering his or her well-being" (Lazarus & Folkman, 1984). Two critical mediators determine the existence of stress among different individuals. *Cognitive appraisal*, the individual's subjective evaluation of the transaction between self and the environment, is the first important mediator. The second mediator, following appraisal of the situation, is the person's *coping* ability, which determines whether he or she can successfully manage the presenting stressor (Lazarus & Folkman, 1984).

MEASUREMENT OF STRESS

It is not surprising that differences over stress semantics have extended into the measurement domain. With no uniform definition of stress, psychometricians have encountered difficulty reaching a consensus about appropriate stress measurements. Traditionally, researchers have utilized laboratory methods to assess the effects of stress (Baum, Grunberg, & Singer, 1982). For example, laboratory technicians may administer noxious physical stimuli (e.g., electric shock) or frustrating psychological tasks (e.g., mental arithmetic) to human or animal subjects. Following application of the stressor, the technician codes physiological reactions (e.g., heart rate, skin conductance) and ratings of observed psychological distress as stress responses. Laboratory procedures have limited generalizability because they can only stimulate, not replicate, naturally occurring stress. Moreover, they are fraught with methodological and ethical concerns (Baum et al., 1982; Brantley & Jones, 1993).

As previously described, certain biochemical events characterize the stress response. Corticosteroid and catecholamine levels provide useful indices of the biochemical events associated with stress. Researchers often employ blood and urinary assays to assess corticosteroid and catecholamine levels in naturalistic or laboratory settings (Baum et al., 1982; Feverstein, Labbe, & Kuczmierczyk, 1986). When used in conjunction with other stress measures, biochemical indices may improve the validity of stress assessment (Baum et al., 1982; Brantley, Dietz, McKnight, Jones, & Tulley, 1988). However, the authors caution against use of biochemical measures alone, because they are susceptible to several confounding events outside the realm of stress (e.g., caffeine ingestion, exercise; Baum et al., 1982).

Life-events research has provided the most consistent point of reference in stress measurement. However, dissent among life events investigators and criticisms of existing indices are evident. Thomas Holmes pioneered life events research by constructing the Schedule of Recent Experiences in the mid-1950s (Hawkins, Davies, & Holmes, 1957). Soon thereafter, Holmes and Rahe (1967) set the standard for life-events scales with the Social Readjustment Rating Scale (SRRS).

The SRRS is a 43-item self-report questionnaire providing an index of amount of change or readjustment associated with recent, major life events. Each item receives an assigned, *a priori* rating according to the amount of readjustment associated with the event. These weightings, commonly referred to as *life change units* (LCUs), derived form a series of scaling studies on a sample of 394 subjects with a wide demographic range. Subject ratings yielded a significant degree of concordance (Holmes & Rahe, 1967). Modifications over the years have broadened utility of the SRRS (e.g., Coddington, 1972), and other life-events researchers have adopted the LCU approach (Paykel, Prusoff, & Uhlenhuth, 1971).

Investigators have both praised and criticized LCU measures. Horowitz, Schaefer, Hiroto, Wilner, and Levin (1977) reviewed the advantages and disadvantages of the SRRS and similar LCU measures. These authors recognized good face validity and complimented the simplicity of the SRRS. They also acknowledged that the highly concordant ratings from a heterogenous sample make the SRRS a generalizable assessment tool. In addition, the SRRS is highly predictive of psychiatric and physical illnesses (Horowitz et al., 1977; Miller, 1989).

Critics have voiced concern over psychometric properties of LCU scales. The temporal nature of LCU measures has raised questions about their stability over time. The length of time between event occurrence and administration of the scale may be a noteworthy consideration. Some researchers have suggested that the formula for calculating LCUs needs to include temporal remoteness (Horowitz et al., 1977). Also, there is concern that time since occurrence of the event affects ability to recall the event and can therefore compromise stability (test–retest reliability) of LCU scores (Horowitz, 1977; Monroe, 1982).

Explication of life-events assessment raises two additional issues: weighted versus subjective ratings of life change, and the desirability (or pleasantness) of events. Sarason, Johnson, and Siegel (1978) addressed these issues in construction of the Life Experiences Survey (LES). This 57-item scale instructs subjects to rate items' desirability and degree of impact on a 7-point Likert-type scale ranging from *Extremely negative* (-3) to *Extremely positive* ($+3$). The scale renders three scores: positive, negative, and total.

The subjective nature of the LES and other life-event indices has fueled disputes regarding stress assessment. Brown (1989) cited the possibility of response biases creating, exaggerating, or attenuating associations between stress and relevant outcome variables. Additionally, others have debated whether stress measures employing subjective ratings have greater predictive power than measures with weighted ratings (Brown, 1989; Rahe, 1974).

Regardless of criticism, life-events measures continue to be among the most widely used psychological assessment tools (Brown, 1989; Monroe, 1982). A current trend among stress researchers is to attempt to discern the theoretical distinction between major life events (or major stressors) and minor life events (or minor stressors; Brantley & Jones, 1989; Kanner, Coyne, Schaefer, & Lazarus, 1981; Zautra, Guarnaccia, & Dohrenwend, 1986).

Kanner et al. (1981) first directed attention to minor stressors with the Hassles Scale, a 117-item questionnaire measuring severity and frequency of minor stressors (e.g., misplacing an item, owing money). Subjects rate the impact of undesirable items occurring over the past month on 3-point Likert-type scale. Similarly, Kanner et al. constructed the Uplifts Scale, an index of desirable minor life events nearly identical in format to the Hassles Scale. Extending the focus on minor stressors, Brantley, Waggoner, Jones, and Rappaport (1987) published the Daily Stress Inventory. Minimizing the problem of temporal remoteness, this 58-item questionnaire measures the frequency and impact of minor stressors likely to occur on a daily basis.

Researchers and clinicians have used stress measures with a variety of psychiatric and medical populations. As previously mentioned, data have indicated that minor life events exert a greater influence on health status than major life events (Brantley & Jones, 1989; Delongis et al., 1982). However, critics maintain that minor life-events scales contain measures of physical symptoms and psychological distress, thereby confounding studies that investigate the relationship between minor life events and health (B. S. Dohrenwend, B. P. Dohrenwend, Dodson, & Shrout, 1984; Dohrenwend & Shrout, 1985).

Dissatisfied with event-specific measures, a group of researchers constructed the Perceived Stress Scale (PSS) (Cohen, Kamarck, & Mermelstein, 1983). The PSS is consistent with cognitive-based, interactionist stress theories and measures a respondent's appraisal of global stress level in his or her life. The developers have reported the PSS has adequate reliability and validity, and an abbreviated phone-interview version is available. Additionally, the authors purported that the predictive power of the PSS is greater than life-events scores. However, opponents of this approach have indicated that the PSS contains confounds with outcome measures that are greater than the confounds associated with minor life-event scales (Lazarus, DeLongis, Folkman, & Gruen, 1985).

FUTURE DIRECTIONS IN STRESS RESEARCH

Although dissension regarding the nature and measurement of stress abounds, empirical interest in stress continues to grow. Schafer (1990) reviewed methodological concerns in stress research and provided three main suggestions for directions of future investigations. First, for stress research to be theory-driven and for scientists to be able to replicated studies in this area, researchers must first clarify terminology in present models. Investigators must also avoid overlapping and unoperationalized terms. Second, stress measures need closer scrutiny. Researchers need to avoid developing scales that present confusion between predictor and outcome variables. Authors of stress measures must provide extensive validity data to assure that they are truly measuring the "stress" construct. Third, investigators must carefully select appropriate research designs and statistical analyses. Designs need to fit proposed models, and investigators must be cautious to avoid experimenter bias (Schafer, 1990).

STRESS MANAGEMENT

Whereas stress researchers and psychometricians have battled over semantics and stress measurement, clinicians have accepted the earnest task of developing treatment strategies countering effects of stress. *Stress management* has echoed the popularity of *stress* as a theoretical notion. Applications of stress management techniques have proven successful in research arenas, clinical settings, and the marketplace.

According to Cotton (1990), the purpose of stress management is to achieve a balance between the amount of external stress an individual experiences and his or her capacity to deal with it. Balance is a key concept because too much stress can lead to hyperarousal and a deprivation of stress can manifest in apathy. Therefore, eliminating stress totally is not the goal. Teaching stress tolerance and alternative, healthy expressions of stress to individuals is paramount.

Clinicians can implement a myriad of psychotherapeutic approaches to stress management. However, when tailoring a stress management program, clinicians must address and take into account client characteristics, such as personality variables, lifestyle, motivation, level and type of distress, and methods of coping (Cotton, 1990; Hillenberg & DiLorenzo, 1987). Approaches may differ (e.g., group vs. individual), but the overall goals of attenuating the negative impact of stress and empowering individuals to better cope remain constant.

After choosing the appropriate format for intervention, there are a few guidelines regarding the therapist–client relationship that clinicians need to consider. A therapeutic contract is an effective way to establish such guidelines and strengthen the therapist–client relationship. Among the topics addressed in the contractual agreement are monetary obligations, responsibilities and rights of client and therapist, treatment targets and goals, sources of assessment and treatment, and estimated length of therapy (Cotton, 1990).

Stress manifests in various ways. Emotional distress, impaired cognitive processes, maladaptive behaviors, and pathophysiology constitute a few potential effects of stress. As previously mentioned, a number of clinical approaches selectively target these differing stress elements. It is possible to delineate three categories that match the nature of stress effects to the clinical strategies employed: biology, behavior, and cognition.

Biology

Researchers have provided substantial documentation regarding the impact of stress on biological functioning. Physiological hyperarousal is one of the most common consequences of excessive stress. Clinically, hyperarousal is clearly evident in somatic and psychiatric disorders (Brown & Harris, 1989). Several biological mechanisms are susceptible to pathognomic effects of stress-induced hyperarousal. These mechanisms include any combination of neuronal, endocrine, cardiopulmonary, and muscular pathways.

Relaxation is a well-established treatment strategy for combating hyperarousal and muscular tension. In the late 1930s, Jacobson developed progressive relaxation training (PRT). PRT involves teaching patients to tense and relax various isolated muscle groups. Therapists monitor patients in-session to ensure proper technique and encourage clients to self-practice. The goal is for patients to recognize excessive muscular tension and reduce it with relaxation skills. Over the past 50 years, researchers have restructured and abbreviated PRT (Jacobson, 1964; Bernstein & Borkovec, 1973) making it a widely accepted treatment strategy with broad clinical utility.

In addition to PRT, a variety of other relaxation approaches are available to consumers. Relaxation procedures have proven efficacious as a stress prophylactic (Girdano, Everly, & Dusek, 1990) and as a treatment for many stress-related conditions (see Everly, 1989). Although researchers have consistently documented the efficacy of relaxation procedures, such procedures may promote untoward side effects in approximately 3–4% of those treated. Precautionary populations include thyroid patients, psychotic individuals, "fragile egos," individuals with major affective disorders, and pharmacotherapy patients (Everly, 1989).

Biofeedback adds an element of medical technology to relaxation principles and assists patients in establishing and maintaining self-control over biological functions. For stress-related psychophysiological profiles, electromyography (EMG) is the biofeedback approach typically employed (Olton & Noonberg, 1980). EMG involves attaching electrodes to the skin surface of various muscle groups and recording the electrical activity. Patients receive visual or auditory feedback regarding the monitored physiological processes. Feedback signals help the patient decrease muscular tension and autonomic reactivity, thereby promoting a relaxation response. Inducing stress during biofeedback may enable patients to overcome resultant biological changes. In addition to EMG, common forms of biofeedback include: skin temperature (thermal), brain wave or electroencephalography (EEG), blood pressure or constant cuff method, and galvanic skin response (GSR; Olton & Noonberg, 1980).

Meditative procedures are perhaps the oldest relaxation category. Eastern religions and cultures have advocated meditation for thousands of years. Meditation not only promotes relaxation but also provides a means to transcendence. Yoga and transcendental meditation (TM) are two prominent meditation procedures. Therapists have not traditionally utilized meditation procedures in clinical settings, but research has supported the benefits of such procedures for reducing the effects of stress (see Woolfolk & Lehrer, 1984).

A more conventional clinical approach closely associated with meditation is Benson's relaxation response (Benson, 1975). With the goal of decreasing psychophysiological arousal, Benson's approach eliminates the religious themes of TM but combines meditation, controlled breathing, and relaxation principles. The relaxation response is easy and inexpensive to master. In addition, clinical studies have supported its efficacy in ameliorating affective distress and autonomic hyperarousal (Benson & Friedman, 1985).

Behavior

Stress can lead to maladaptive behavioral patterns that result in an unhealthy lifestyle. Moreover, maintaining healthy behaviors can deter negative effects of stress (Girdano, Everly, & Dusek, 1990). promoting wellness has become a popular theme among various health and fitness programs, including stress management programs (Schafer, 1983). Brownell (1982) posited that the increase in obesity and stress-related disorders over the past century has resulted from sedentary lifestyles. A renewed interest in exercise during the past decade has paralleled research that suggests physical fitness is a significant stress moderator (Brandon & Loftin, 1991; Roth & Holmes, 1985). Moreover, Everly (1989) contends that exercise, more than any other stress management strategy, prevents disease by ventilating the pathophysiological changes associated with the stress response.

To attain a salubrious lifestyle, eliminating health-risk behaviors may be the initial step. Smoking cessation can comprise an important element of stress management. Smoking is often a maladaptive response to stressful situations, and stress can maintain the habit (Best, Wainwright, Mills, & Kirkland, 1988; Feverstein et al., 1986). Nicotine potentiates sympathetic arousal (Trap-Jensen, 1988), and smoking compromises physiological systems (e.g., cardiopulmonary and immune) susceptible to stress (McGill, 1988). Smoking cessation programs frequently include behavioral strategies (e.g., self-management, aversives, and satiation), and research has proven such strategies produce successful results (Kamarck & Lichtenstein, 1985).

Millions of individuals also use alcohol to negate stress and tension (Williams, Stinson, Parker, Harford, & Noble, 1987). Evidence suggests that stress may be an important cofactor in predicting alcoholism (Brantley & Garrett, 1993). Additionally, individuals who become alcoholics may lack stress management skills necessary to avoid alcoholism (Cotton, 1990). If alcoholism is a target problem, substance-abuse treatment typically precludes standard stress management procedures.

In addition to addressing lifestyle factors, a primary stress management objective is to eliminate behaviors that precede or follow stress. The ability to regulate stress-related behaviors is an important skill for clients to learn. Self-regulation (Kanfer & Goldstein, 1986) is a clinical approach that provides clients with behavioral strategies to avoid or lessen the impact of stress. Using a problem-focused, therapeutic framework, therapists teach clients three phases of action: self-monitoring, self-evaluation, and self-reinforcement. Specific behavioral techniques employed include behavioral analysis, shaping, modeling, behavioral rehearsal, flooding, role playing, reinforcement, and negative practice (Cotton, 1990).

For both clinical and nonclinical populations, therapists frequently incorporate additional behavioral strategies within the stress management context. Assertiveness training, time management, and leisure planning benefit virtually anyone. Assertiveness-training programs minimize stress by providing individuals with a sense of behavioral control (Alberti & Emmons, 1982). Establishing priorities and scheduling time effectively are especially useful strategies in occupational settings for managing stress overload (Murphy & Schoenborn, 1989). Additionally, planning nonstressful leisure time with fulfilling and enjoyable activities keeps stress levels balanced and enhances overall quality of life (Iso-Ahola, 1980).

Cognition

According to the principle of "cognitive primacy," cognition precedes emotional expression (Arnold, 1960; Lazarus, 1982). Many theorists argue that *appraisal* of a stressful event is the most important factor dictating affective distress. Lazarus and Folkman (1984) described two types of cognitive appraisal. *Primary appraisal* is the initial process whereby individuals determine whether an event is stressful. When individuals characterize an event as stressful, secondary appraisal follows. During *secondary appraisal,* individuals determine if they possess the necessary coping resources to confront the presenting stressor. Although some researchers deny the importance of cognitive elements (e.g., Zajonc, 1984), many view the appraisal process as an important factor in stress management.

Beck (1984) offered a model explaining cognitive components of the stress reaction. Cognitive structuring and appraisal of stressful situations mobilize organisms for action and result in behavioral inclinations and affective expression. When stress becomes intense, cognitions become distorted and disrupted. Consequently, maladaptive behavioral patterns and emotions develop. Cognitive therapy aims to break this aberrant cycle of cognition, behavior, and affect. Cognitive applications in stress management programs have become more sophisticated in recent years with the matching of idiosyncratic elements of stress to appropriate therapies (Pretzer, Beck, & Newman, 1989).

The general objective of cognitive therapy is to alter distorted cognitions. Treatment begins with providing a rationale and defining problem areas with clients. Goals are to increase clients' objectivity and perspectives of stressful situations. The first treatment step is to change individuals' cognitive sets by manipulating the environment, creating diversion, and employing relaxation. Second, therapists help clients identify, restructure, and correct dysfunctional cognitions. In addition to addressing specific stressful events, therapists may focus on changing the overall structure of clients' characteristic cognitive sets. They can accomplish this by fostering "nonegocentric" modes of thinking, identifying and challenging irrational rules, and eliminating specific cognitive vulnerabilities (Beck, 1984; Pretzer, Beck, & Newman, 1989).

Stress inoculation training (SIT; Meichenbaum & Jaremko, 1983; Meichenbaum & Deffenbacher, 1988), another cognitive treatment approach, teaches clients skills to manage stress-related anxiety. The SIT clinical framework strongly aligns with the transactional model of stress (Cameron & Meichenbaum, 1982; Lazarus, 1966). The scope of SIT application has expanded during recent years with reported success in treating several stress-related problems, including pain, psychophysiological disorders, Type A behavior, and surgical anxiety (see Meichenbaum & Deffenbacher, 1988).

SIT consists of three phases: (1) Conceptualization, (2) Skill Acquisition and Rehearsal, and (3) Application and Follow Through. In the first phase, *Conceptualization,* therapists assess clients' skills via interview, image-based reconstruction of stressful experiences, behavioral observation and generation, and self-monitoring. Together, clients and therapists integrate the data and form a treatment plan. Throughout assessment, therapists coach clients to self-assess problem situations in a manner that is more sophisticated and functional than their normal manner (Meichenbaum & Cameron, 1983).

During the second phase, *Skills Acquisition and Rehearsal,* therapists teach clients specific coping skills. Clients learn that coping can be *instrumental* (altering the stressful event) or *palliative* (adapting to unavoidable stress when altering the stressor is not possible). Problem solving, communication, and time management constitute important instrumental coping skills. Palliative strategies include perspective taking and diversion. Therapists model these skills, and clients rehearse them. The goal of the Rehearsal phase is for clients to successfully generate positive self-statements and use self-instruction of learned skills in stressful encounters (Meichenbaum & Cameron, 1983).

The purpose of the final phase, *Application and Follow Through,* is to ensure that clients have incorporated sufficient stress management skills and that they implement these skills appropriately. Therapists use imaginal exposure and role playing to test clients' skills. Once the skills are satisfactory, clients attempt *in vivo* exposure. To ascertain skill maintenance, it is important for therapists to obtain routine follow-up information for at least 1 year (Meichenbaum & Cameron, 1983).

EMERGING TRENDS AND FUTURE DIRECTIONS IN STRESS MANAGEMENT

Knowledge and application of stress management principles have increased greatly during the past decade (Ivancevich, Matteson, Freedman, & Phillips, 1990). The recent success of stress management is evident in a miscellany of settings and populations, including psychiatric patients (Courtney & Escobedo, 1990), migraine patients (Lascelles, Cunningham, McGrath, & Sullivan, 1989), military personnel (White & Cruz, 1991), caregivers of elderly individuals (Gregory, 1991), cardiac patients (Frasure-Smith & Prince, 1989), the worksite (Ivancevich et al., 1990), and hypertensive individuals (Bosley & Allen, 1989). Contemporary experts advocate use of multimethod (i.e., educative, physiological, behavioral, and cognitive) stress management programs (Everly, 1989; Meichenbaum & Turk, 1987) and encourage their continued application in a wide variety of settings (Romano, 1988). Several authors have offered their descriptions of comprehensive stress management programs. These authors include Everly (1989), Cotton (1990), Courtney and Escobedo (1990), Girdano, Everly, and Dusek (1990), and Ivancevich et al. (1990).

Bernier and Gaston (1989) reviewed stress management effectiveness and concluded that most programs significantly reduce physical and cognitive consequences of stress while increasing work and academic performance. These authors reported that no particular therapeutic strategy proved superior relative to others. However, experts agree that future studies need to assess the long-term benefits of stress management within a theoretical framework (Bernier & Gaston, 1989; Ivancevich et al., 1990).

CONCLUSION

As a result of rigorous research efforts in psychosocial and medical arenas, stressology has evolved into an important scientific subdiscipline. In addition, lay literature and the media have heightened public awareness of stress in recent years. Despite the ubiquitous nature of stress, controversy persists regarding a uniform definition and appropriate avenues of assessment. Fortunately, although the battle among stress experts continues, increased knowledge about the nature of stress has resulted in positive endeavors. Stress management has become a universally accepted form of health intervention and has improved the quality of life for many individuals.

REFERENCES

Ader, R. (1980). Psychosomatic and psychoimmunological research. Presidential Address. *Psychosomatic Medicine, 42,* 307–321.

Alberti, R., & Emmons, M. (1982). *Your perfect right: A guide to assertive behavior* (4th ed.). San Luis Opispo, CA: Impact.

American Psychiatric Association (1968). *Diagnostic and statistical manual of mental disorders* (2nd ed.). Washington, DC: Author.

Arnold, M. B. (1960). *Emotion and personality* (2 vols.). New York: Columbia University Press.

Baum, A., Grunberg, N. E., & Singer, J. E. (1982). The use of psychological and neuroendocrinological measurements in the study of stress. *Health Psychology, 1,* 217–236.

Beck, A. (1984). Cognitive approaches to stress. In R. Woolfolk & P. Lehrer (Eds.), *Principles and practice of stress management* (pp. 255–305). New York: Guilford Press.

Benson, H. (1975). *The relaxation response.* New York: Morrow.

Benson, H., & Friedman, R. (1985). A rebuttal to the conclusions of David S. Holmes' article: Meditation and somatic arousal reduction. *American Psychologist, 40,* 725–728.

Bernard, C. (1879). *Lecons sur phenomenes de la vie commune aux animaux et aux vegetaux* (vol. 2). Paris: Bailliere.

Bernier, D., & Gaston, L. (1989). Stress management: A review. *Canada's Mental Health, 37,* 15–19.

Bernstein, D., & Borkovec, T. (1973). *Progressive relaxation training: A manual for the helping professions.* Champaign, IL: Research Press.

Best, J. A., Wainwright, P. E., Mills, D. E., & Kirkland, S. A. (1988). Biobehavioral approaches to smoking control. In W. Linden (Ed.), *Biological barriers in behavioral medicine* (pp. 63–99). New York: Plenum Press.

Bosley, F., & Allen, T. W. (1989). Stress management training for hypertensives: Cognitive and physiological effects. *Journal of Behavioral Medicine, 12,* 77–89.

Brandon, J. E., & Loftin, J. M. (1991). Relationship of fitness to depression, state and trait anxiety, internal health locus of control, and self-control. *Perpetual and Motor Skills, 73,* 563–568.

Brantley, P. J., Dietz, L. S., McKnight, G. T., Jones, G. N., & Tulley, R. (1988). Convergence between the daily stress inventory and endocrine measures of stress. *Journal of Consulting and Clinical Psychology, 56,* 549–551.

Brantley, P. J., & Garrett, V. D. (1993). Psychobiological approaches to health and disease. In P. Sutker & H. Adams (Eds.), *Comprehensive handbook of psychopathology.* New York: Plenum.

Brantley, P. J., & Jones, G. N. (1989). *Daily stress inventory: Professional manual.* Odessa, FL: Psychological Assessment Resources.

Brantley, P. J., & Jones, G. N. (1993). Daily stress and stress-related disorders. *Annals of Behavioral Medicine.*

Brantley, P. J., Waggoner, C. D., Jones, G. N., & Rappaport, N. (1987). A daily stress inventory: Development, reliability, and validity. *Journal of Behavioral Medicine, 10,* 61–73.

Brown, G. W. (1989). Life events and measurement. In G. W. Brown & T. O. Harris (Eds.), *Life events and illness* (pp. 3–45). New York: Guilford.

Brown, G. W., & Harris, T. O. (Eds.). (1989). *Life events and illness.* New York: Guilford.

Brown, G. W., Sklair, F., Harris, T. O., & Birley, J. L. (1973). Life events and psychiatric disorders: Some methodological issues. *Psychological Medicine, 3,* 74–78.

Brownell, K. (1982). Obesity: Understanding and treating a serious, prevalent and refractory disorder. *Journal of Consulting and Clinical Psychology, 50,* 820–840.

Cameron, R., & Meichenbaum, D. (1982). The nature of effective coping and the treatment of stress related problems: A cognitive–behavioral perspective. In L. Goldberger & S. Breznitz (Eds.), *Handbook of stress: Theoretical and clinical aspects* (pp. 695–710). New York: Free Press.

Cannon, W. B. (1939). *The wisdom of the body* (2nd ed.). New York: Norton.

Coddington, R. D. (1972). The significance of life events as etiologic factors in the diseases of children: Part 1. A survey of professional workers. *Journal of Psychosomatic Research, 16,* 7–18.

Cohen, S., Kamarck, T., & Mermelstein, R. (1983). A global measure of perceived stress. *Journal of Health and Social Behavior, 24,* 385–396.

Cotton, D. H. (1990). *Stress management.* New York: Brunner/Mazel.

Courtney, C., & Escobedo, B. (1990). A stress management program: Inpatient to outpatient continuity. *American Journal of Occupational Therapy, 44,* 306–310.

DeLongis, A., Coyne, J. C., Dakof, G., Folkman, S., & Lazarus, R. S. (1982). Relationship of daily hassles, uplifts, and major life events to health status. *Health Psychology, 1,* 119–146.

Dohrenwend, B. S., Dohrenwend, B. P., Dodson, M., & Shrout, P. E. (1984). Symptoms, hassles, social supports, and life events: Problem of confounded measures. *Journal of Abnormal Psychology, 93,* 222–230.

Dohrenwend, B. P., & Shrout, P. E. (1985). "Hassles" in the conceptualization and measurement of life stress variables. *American Psychologist, 40,* 780–785.

Elliott, G. R., & Eisdorfer, C. (1982). *Stress and health.* New York: Springer.

Engel, B. T. (1985). Stress is a noun! No, a verb! No, an adjective! In T. M. Field, P. M. McCabe, & N. Schneiderman (Eds.), *Stress and coping* (pp. 3–12). Hillsdale, NJ: Erlbaum.

Everly, G. S. (1989). *A clinical guide to the treatment of the human stress response.* New York: Plenum Press.

Feverstein, M., Labbe, E. E., & Kuczmierczyk, A. R. (1986). *Health psychology: A psychobiological perspective.* New York: Plenum Press.

Field, T. M., McCabe, P. M., & Schneiderman, N. (Eds.). (1985). *Stress and coping.* Hillsdale, NJ: Erlbaum.

Flach, F. (Ed.). (1989). *Stress and its management.* New York: Norton.

Frasure-Smith, N., & Prince, R. (1989). Long-term follow-up of the ischemic heart disease life stress monitoring program. *Psychosomatic Medicine, 51,* 485–513.

Fredericq, L. (1985). Influence du milieu ambiant sur la compsoition du sang des animaux aquatiques. *Archives de Zoologie Experimental et Generale, 3,* 34.

Girdano, D. A., Everly, G. S., & Dusek, D. E. (1990). *Controlling stress and tension: A holistic approach.* Englewood Cliffs, NJ: Prentice-Hall.

Goldberger, L., & Breznitz, S. (Eds.). (1982). *Handbook of stress: Theoretical and clinical aspects*. New York: Free Press.

Gregory, S. (1991). Stress management for careers. *British Journal of Occupational Therapy, 54,* 427–429.

Grinker, R. R., & Spiegel, J. P. (1945). *Men under stress*. Philadelphia: Blakiston.

Hawkins, N. G., Davis, W. G., & Holmes, T. H. (1957). Evidence of psychosocial factors in the development of pulmonary tuberculosis. *American Review of Tuberculosis and Pulmonary Diseases, 75,* 768–780.

Hillenberg, J. B., & DiLorenzo, T. M. (1987). Stress management training in health psychology practice: Critical clinical issues. *Professional Psychology: Research and Practice, 18,* 402–404.

Holmes, T. H., & Masuda, M. (1974). Life changes and illness susceptibility. In B. S. Dohrenwend & B. P. Dohrenwend (Eds.), *Stressful life events: Their nature and effects* (pp. 45–72). New York: Wiley.

Holmes, T. H., & Rahe, R. H. (1967). The social readjustment rating scale. *Journal of Psychosomatic Research, 11,* 213–218.

Horowitz, M., Schaefer, C., Hiroto, D., Wilner, N., & Levin, B. (1977). Life event questionnaires for measuring presumptive stress. *Psychosomatic Medicine, 39,* 413–430.

Iso-Ahola, S. (1980). *The social psychology of leisure and recreation*. Dubuque, IA: Brown.

Ivancevich, J. M., Matteson, M. T., Freedman, S. M., & Phillips, J. S. (1990). Worksite stress management interventions. *American Psychologist, 45,* 252–261.

Jacobson, E. (1964). *Self operations control*. Chicago: National Foundation for Progressive Relaxation.

Jemmott, J. B., & Locke, S. E. (1984). Psychosocial factors, immunologic mediation, and human susceptibility to infectious diseases: How much do we know? *Psychological Bulletin, 95,* 78–108.

Kamarck, M. S., & Lichtenstein, E. (1985). Current trends in clinic-based smoking control. *Annals of Behavioral Medicine, 7,* 19–23.

Kanfer, F. H., & Goldstein, A. P. (Eds.). (1986). *Helping people change: A textbook of methods* (3rd ed.). New York: Pergamon.

Kanner, A. D., Coyne, J. C., Schaefer, C., & Lazarus, R. S. (1981). Comparison of two modes of measurement: Daily hassles and uplifts versus major life events. *Journal of Behavioral Medicine, 4,* 1–39.

Lacey, J. I. (1950). Individual differences in somatic response patterns. *Journal of Comparative and Physiological Psychology, 43,* 338–350.

Lascelles, M. A., Cunningham, S. J., McGrath, P. J., & Sullivan, M. J. (1989). Teaching coping strategies to adolescents with migraine. *Journal of Pain and Symptom Management, 4,* 135–145.

Lazarus, R. S. (1966). *Psychological stress and the coping process*. New York: McGraw-Hill.

Lazarus, R. S. (1982). Thoughts on the relation between emotions and cognition. *American Psychologist, 37,* 1019–1024.

Lazarus, R. S., DeLongis, A., Folkman, S., & Gruen, R. (1985). Stress and adaptational outcomes: The problem of confounded measures. *American Psychologist, 40,* 770–779.

Lazarus, R. S., & Folkman, S. (1984). *Stress, appraisal, and coping*. New York: Springer.

McGill, H. C. (1988). The cardiovascular pathology of smoking. *American Heart Journal, 115,* 250–257.

Meichenbaum, D. H., & Cameron, R. (1983). Stress inoculation training: Toward a general paradigm for training coping skills. In D. H. Meichenbaum & M. E. Jaremko (Eds.), *Stress reduction and prevention* (pp. 115–154). New York: Plenum Press.

Meichenbaum, D. H., & Deffenbacher, J. L. (1988). Stress inoculation training. *Counseling Psychologist, 16,* 69–90.

Meichenbaum, D. H., & Jaremko, M. E. (Eds.). (1983). *Stress reduction and prevention*. New York: Plenum Press.

Meichenbaum, D. H., & Turk, D. (1987). *Facilitating treatment adherence: A practitioner's guidebook*. New York: Plenum Press.

Miller, T. W. (Ed.). (1989). *Stressful life events*. Madison, CT: International Universities Press.

Monroe, S. M. (1982). Life events assessment: Current practices, emerging trends. *Clinical Psychology Review, 2,* 435–453.

Mott, F. (1919). *War neurosis and shell shock*. London: Oxford Medical Publications.

Murphy, L. R., & Schoenborn, T. F. (Eds.). (1989). *Stress management in work settings*. New York: Praeger.

Olton, D. S., & Noonberg, A. R. (1980). *Biofeedback: Clinical applications in behavioral medicine*. Englewood Cliffs, NJ: Prentice-Hall.

Paykel, E. S., Prusoff, B. A., & Uhlenhuth, E. H. (1971). Scaling of life events. *Archives of General Psychiatry, 25,* 340–347.

Pfluger, E. (1877). Die teleologische mechanik der lebendigen. *Natur. Pfluger's Archiv fur die gesamte Physiologie des menschen umd der tiere, 15,* 57.

Pretzer, J. L., Beck, A. T., & Newman, C. F. (1989). Stress and stress management: A cognitive view. *Journal of Cognitive Psychotherapy, 3,* 163–179.

Rahe, R. H. (1974). Predictions of near-future health change from subjects' preceding life changes. *Journal of Psychosomatic Research, 13,* 72–177.

Romano, J. L. (1988). Stress management counseling: From crisis to prevention. *Counseling Psychology Quarterly, 1,* 211–219.

Roth, D. L., & Holmes, D. S. (1985). Influence of physical fitness in determining the impact of stressful life events on physical and psychological health. *Psychosomatic Medicine, 47,* 164–173.

Sarason, I. G., Johnson, J. H., & Siegel, J. M. (1978). Assessing the impact of life changes: Development of the life experiences survey. *Journal of Consulting and Clinical Psychology, 46,* 348–349.

Schafer, J. (1990, April). Issues of methodology, design, and analytic procedure in psychological research on stress. Poster presented at the 11th Annual Meeting of the Society of Behavioral Medicine, Chicago, IL.

Schafer, W. (1983). *Wellness through stress management.* Davis, CA: International Dialogue Press.

Selye, H. (1936). A syndrome produced by diverse nocuous agents. *Nature, 138,* 32.

Selye, H. (1974). *Stress without distress.* Philadelphia: Lippincott.

Selye, H. (1982). History and present status of the stress concept. In L. Goldberger & S. Breznitz (Eds.), *Handbook of stress: Theoretical and clinical aspects* (pp. 7–17). New York: The Free Press.

Trap-Jensen, J. (1988). Effects of smoking on the heart and peripheral circulation. *American Heart Journal, 115,* 263–267.

Weiner, H., Florin, I., Murison, R., & Hellhammer, D. (Eds.). (1989). *Frontier of stress research.* Toronto: Hans Huber.

White, L. S., & Cruz, J. D. (1991). A model program: Stress management unit: A clinic run by army nurses. *Military Medicine, 156,* 599–602.

Williams, G. D., Stinson, F. S., Parker, D. A., Harford, T. C., & Noble, J. (1987). Demographic trends, alcohol abuse, and alcoholism, 1985–1995. *Alcohol Health and Research World, 11,* 80–83.

Wolff, H. G. (1953). *Stress and disease.* Springfield, IL: Thomas.

Woolfolk, R. L., & Lehrer, P. M. (Eds.). (1984). *Principles and practice of stress management.* New York: Guilford.

Zajonc, R. B. (1984). On the primacy of emotion. *American Psychologist, 39,* 117–123.

Zautra, A. J., Guarnaccia, C. A., & Dohrenwend, B. P. (1986). Measuring small life events. *American Journal of Community Psychology, 14,* 629–655.

15

Preparation for Surgery

Steve Webne

> Those who practice [surgery] should . . . comfort the patient by gentle actions, soft words, agreeable and proper, and promise him cure in all cases even though they are hopeless; and the operating physician himself remains convinced that there is no chance for health in such an infirmity. . . . For the mind of the patient derives, from such discourse and promises, a secret influence and a great disposition by which nature acquires vigor and resistance against disease. That is why there will result an action more powerful than that which can be produced by all the efforts of the physician with his instruments and even his medicines, an action such that it routs the illness.
> —William of Salicet, *Surgery*

Preoperative psychological preparation of patients for surgery has existed in some form from the time stone knife first pressed against flesh. It is an integral part of the process of surgery that investigators have systematically studied only over the last 35 years. During that time, researchers have empirically established that patients who receive psychological preparation prior to surgery demonstrate less distress, fewer medical complications, and shorter stays in hospital than patients who do not receive such preparation (Alberts, Lyons, Moretti, & Erickson, 1989; Anderson & Masur, 1983; Devine & Cook, 1983; Hathaway, 1986; Horne, Vatmanidis, & Careri, 1994; Mumford, Schlesinger, & Glass, 1982; Rogers & Reich, 1986; Suls & Wan, 1989).

This chapter introduces and critiques the major theoretical considerations regarding surgical preparation and addresses ways in which clinicians apply and practice such preparation. In addition, this chapter highlights methodological concerns and gives special attention to emerging trends and innovations in the area.

Steve Webne • Mental Health Association, 2401 21st Avenue South, Nashville, Tennessee 37212.
Handbook of Health and Rehabilitation Psychology, edited by Anthony J. Goreczny. Plenum Press, New York, 1995.

THEORETICAL CONSIDERATIONS

Historical Models

Current theories designed to explain the relationship between preoperative intervention and postoperative outcome can trace their origins to Janis (1958). He postulated that a curvilinear relationship exists between preoperative anxiety and postoperative patient adjustment. He measured self-reported anger, emotional disturbance, and complaints about staff and concluded that patients who demonstrated a moderate amount of anticipatory anxiety had the best postoperative adjustment, whereas those with low or high preoperative anxiety showed a relatively larger amount of postoperative distress. Janis hypothesized that a moderate level of preoperative anxiety is adaptive because it helps initiate an emotional inoculation process called the "work of worrying." With too little or too much preoperative anxiety, patients do not initiate this process. This emotional inoculation includes three steps. First, the patient obtains information about the upcoming stressful event. That stimulates fear. Second, mental rehearsal of the event leads to accurate expectations. Third, the patient generates and applies coping techniques and becomes assured of successfully completing the stressful event. Researchers found little support for Janis's curvilinear model. In fact, there is evidence for an inverse linear relationship between level of preoperative anxiety and postoperative well-being of patients (Auerbach, 1973; Cohen & Lazarus, 1973; Sime, 1976). However, the components of Janis's theory are the forerunners of several hypotheses currently considered important in explaining the effect of preoperative preparation on surgical outcome. Current theoretical models contain an emphasis on information, cognitive processes, such as rehearsal, and coping techniques.

Current Models

Current models generally fall into one of two broad categories: consistency theories and control theories. Consistency models explain the relationship between preparation and outcome as a function of matching some element of intervention employed with some element of the patient or surgical situation. For example, researchers have established that some patients characteristically seek information under highly stressful conditions, whereas others prefer to avoid information. Information seekers provided with high levels of information generally have more positive postoperative outcomes than do those who avoid or distract themselves from preoperative information (Auerbach, Martelli, & Mercuri, 1983; Martelli, Auerbach, Alexander, & Mercuri, 1987; Miller & Mangan, 1983).

Another consistency model applicable to preoperative preparation is the self-regulation theory (Johnson, Lauver, & Nail, 1989; Leventhal & Johnson, 1983). This theory posits that patients organize, store, and retrieve preoperative information according to their own schemata. Concrete, objective information, such as physical sensations or sequence of events associated with a given procedure hypothetically shape these schemata. In turn, these schemata influence how patients process new and stored information, guide attention, and implement goal-directed behavior. Expectations associated with such schemata that are consistent with one's experience enhance postoperative outcome.

Wilson (1981) found support for self-regulation theory. He studied 70 elective cholecystectomy and hysterectomy patients stratified by type of surgery and randomly assigned to one of four groups: control, information, relaxation, and combined information–relaxation groups. Control group members received routine hospital care. Patients in the information group listened to a 9-minute tape that described sensations and procedures they were about to undergo. Relaxation training group members received taped instructions on deep muscle relaxation. The fourth group was a combined information–relaxation group whose members received both tapes. Four outcome indices provided measures of therapeutic efficacy. These indices included length of hospital stay, analgesics used, in-hospital recovery (including self-ratings of mood, pain, and ambulation), and epinephrine–norepinephrine levels. Self-regulation theory predicts that information group patients would benefit because their intervention encourages schemata changes and the other interventions do not. Results were consistent with the prediction. Patients who receive preoperative information discharge from the hospital significantly sooner than controls. Also in support of self-regulation theory is earlier work that has demonstrated preoperative interventions based on information about sensations reduce distress and length of hospital stay for surgical patients (Johnson, 1975; Johnson, Fuller, Endress, & Rice, 1978; Johnson, Rice, Fuller, & Endress, 1978).

Self-regulation theory strongly implies a dynamic equilibrium between expectations and experience that occurs across time. Early studies, and some recent ones (e.g., Lynch, 1994), although generally supportive of the self-regulation model, were methodologically unable to capture the theory's essence, because each dealt with surgery as a stressor that occurred at a single point in time. In an important departure from these studies, Johnson et al. (1989) studied 84 men undergoing a series of radiation treatments for prostate cancer. These authors used six taped messages of concrete objective information about radiation therapy designed to describe what individuals were likely to experience at each of six successive points during the course of treatment. Compared to a group controlled for amount of staff-contact time, experimental group members demonstrated significantly less disruption in recreation and pastime activities, both during the course of radiation treatments and at 3-month follow-up. Furthermore, this effect was a function of degree of self-reported, perceived similarities between expectations and treatment experience, as well as a function of self-reported comprehension of the procedures that the patients experienced. This outcome affords strong support for self-regulation theory because patient self-reports allowed the investigators to obtain data regarding the process of self-regulation as they measured the effects of self-regulation repeatedly across time. Whereas this study marks several important methodological and theoretical advances, additional challenges to development and validation of self-regulation theory remain. Primary among these is need for a clearer demonstration of the theory's basic premise: that schemata, such as those described, exist. It is also crucial to demonstrate that these schemata function to guide the organization and retrieval of information as postulated. Given the necessarily abstract nature of such cognitive schemata, these are formidable challenges. Johnson et al. (1989) attempted such demonstration by measuring process variables in the form of patients' self-report about degree to which patients' expectations matched experiences as well as self-report regarding patients' level of understanding. Additional efforts in these same areas could provide further confirmation of self-regulation theory. For example, for a given procedure, self-regulation theory predicts that patients who have previously undergone the same or similar procedure will have a more developed schemata than those with little or no previous experience. Thus, tests of patients assigned to groups by level of previous procedural experience would be valuable. Also useful would be additional demonstrations that the relationship between procedural schemata and interventions influences postoperative outcome.

Suls and Wan (1989) developed another theory to explain the relationship between preoperative intervention and postoperative outcome. It is called the Dual Process Preparation Hypothesis and is another example of a consistency model. The basic tenet of this hypothesis is that clinicians can provide two types of information preoperatively to patients: (1) sensory information, which describes sensations one is about to experience; and (2) procedural information, which emphasizes the sequence of specific events about to take place. In a meta-analytic review of 21 studies that evaluated whether sensory, procedural, or combined sensory–procedural information was the most effective form of intervention, Suls and Wan found no difference in effectiveness between procedural information alone and no information. Sensory information was more effective than no information. Combined sensory–procedural information was the most effective. The authors hypothesized that combined information interventions were maximally effective because the sensory information component has an emotionally reassuring effect, and the procedural information component provides specific events to which individuals can apply such reassurance: thus, the dual process.

Although this hypothesis has immediate appeal, its basic tenets stem from studies that share two important methodological and conceptual vulnerabilities. First, the database used by Suls and Wan (1989) included studies that were devoid of process checks. As a result, it is not known if, for example, sensory-information interventions actually had the desired impact on a given patient or group of patients. Second, researchers ignored individual differences as well as the process of surgery in most of these studies. For example, the studies in this dataset typically prepared patients at a single point in time for surgery in a manner that did not account for individual features, such as previous experience and age, that investigators have shown affects coping (Melamed, Dearborn, & Hermecz, 1983). Third, some of the Suls and Wan database involved studies biased by measuring outcome across short time frames, thus not allowing for detection of potentially important postsurgery data. As a result, problems in internal validity and generalizability are a concern for some studies in this analysis.

Consistency theories have been instrumental in focusing on a clearer and broader appreciation of complexity involved in surgery preparation. This has led to a scrutiny of individual patient differences, surgery type, and environmental features. At the same time, consistency theories have yet to clearly identify specific parameters that need to be consistent in order to enhance outcome. Nor have these theories identified the standard by which researchers are to measure consistency among parameters. As a result, opportunities exist for tautological explanations of outcome. This is especially the case in studies that involve only pre- and postintervention measures with no intervention checks or other process data. For example, if intervention enhances postoperative outcome, then researchers hypothesize that information included in the intervention is consistent with features of the patients. If intervention does not enhance outcome, then the hypothesis is that such consistency is lacking. This tautological set represents internal methodological problems in some studies. Continued efforts to collect process data would help minimize these concerns. In addition, studies that compare individuals or groups for whom consistency exists with individuals or groups for whom consistency does not exist would help clarify the significance of this construct.

Control theories are another group of models that researchers have used to explain the relationship between preoperative preparation and postsurgical outcome. Thompson (1981) defined *control* as "the belief that one has at one's disposal a response that can influence the aversiveness of an event" (p. 89). This belief is an intrinsic part of the cognitive appraisal model of stress and coping (Janis, 1958; Lazarus, 1966; Lazarus & Folkman, 1984). This model posits that coping responses depend on the meaning one assigns to a potentially stressful event (primary appraisal) and judgments made about available coping options (secondary appraisal). These judgments and the concepts of control as defined here are similar concepts. *Coping* refers to managing demands that arise from the confluence of stressful events and the judgments made about them. There are two general types of coping: problem-focused and emotion-focused. Problem-focused coping involves efforts to alter the stressful event itself. An example of problem-focused coping is asking an anesthesiologist to induce anesthesia intravenously if one is fearful of masks. Emotion-focused coping includes efforts to regulate one's emotional response to stress. One example of emotion-focused coping is accepting a mask induction even though one is fearful of it but wishing the experience to be over soon.

For stressors appraised as uncontrollable, control theories predict that emotion-focused coping more greatly enhances outcome than does problem-focused coping. For stressors appraised as controllable, problem-focused coping is more efficacious than emotion-focused coping. Researchers have not always succeeded in their attempts to demonstrate such relationships. For example, Felton and Revenson (1984) evaluated the role of wish-fulfilling fantasy, considered an emotion-focused form of coping, and information seeking, considered a problem-focused coping form, in the psychological adjustment of 151 middle-aged and older adults with one or more illnesses. Patients judged two illnesses, rheumatoid arthritis and systemic blood cancer, as relatively less controllable and two other illnesses, hypertension and diabetes, as relatively more controllable. Measures of illness acceptance and affective state showed that information seeking predicted better adjustment whereas wish-fulfilling fantasy predicted poorer adjustment. Remarkably, illness controllability did not modify these results.

More recently, however, several studies have demonstrated that improved outcome occurs when patients perceive a stressor is controllable and employ problem-focused coping strategies, or when they perceive a stressor is not controllable and employ emotion-focused coping strategies. For example, Compas, Malcarne, and Fondacoro (1988) studied how children and adolescents cope with academic and interpersonal stressors and found that mismatches between problem-focused coping strategies and perceived control yielded significantly more behavioral problems than did matches. In a sample of college undergraduates, Forsythe and Compas (1987) investigated the relationship among perceived control, coping style, and symptoms of distress for stressors considered "daily hassles," such as receiving a low mark on a paper versus major life events, such as the death of a family member. For major life events, distress symptom scores were low for individuals who employed problem-focused coping in situations they perceived as controllable and emotion-focused coping for events they perceived as not controllable relative to individuals who employed a coping style inconsistent with the perceived controllability of the stressor. This interaction was not significant for events considered "daily hassles." Vitaliano, DeWolfe, Maiuro, Russo, and Katon (1990) studied the relationship among perceived control, coping strategies, and depression in a population with psychiatric, physical health, work, or family problems. Except for those individuals with psychiatric problems, problem-focused coping and depressed mood negatively related when individuals appraised a stressor as controllable but did not relate when individuals perceived a stressor as uncontrollable. Also, except for the psychiatric group, emotion-focused coping positively related to depression when individuals appraised a stressor as controllable. Finally, in studies of distress among those about to donate blood, presumably a low-control situation, problem-focused coping was relatively ineffective (Kaloupek & Stoupakis, 1985; Kaloupek, White, & Wong, 1984). Thus, researchers have established the relationship between coping strategies and perceived control as an important element in the processing of coping across several populations.

Nonetheless, investigators have rarely conducted studies designed to evaluate the relationship between perceived control and coping type with surgery patients. This obviously limits conclusions that clinicians can make regarding applicability of such studies to surgery situations. Furthermore, recent advances have begun to embrace a more complex conceptualization of coping. Rather than viewing problem-focused and emotion-focused coping as distinct forms, some studies have blended them. Researchers have recently identified combinations of these coping modes and termed them *mixed-focused* coping models (e.g., Martelli et al., 1987). However, more clearly identifying the parameters of these models and other forms of coping would lend precision to control models. Finally, an important strength of control models is the demand they place for a detailed account of a variety of features inherent in surgery situations. These features include individual differences that affect perception of a stressor, situational variables that contribute to quality of the stressor itself, and other factors. These factors constitute determinants of complexity that theorists have recently begun to detail and incorporate into both consistency and control models.

DETERMINANTS OF COMPLEXITY

Individual Differences

Age, previous hospital experience, gender, and predispositional coping style comprise the individual differences most frequently studied to date.

Developmental trends in surgery preparation across the life span are not yet mapped out in detail. In particular, there is a dearth of specific information regarding developmental aspects of surgery preparation for patients in the early through middle-adult years. Ironically, this is the range most frequently studied in surgery preparation research. However, authors of such studies almost never explicitly identify developmental features. Conversely, researchers have assembled a considerable literature regarding surgery preparation among the very young and the very old.

Melamed et al. (1983) studied 58 children aged 4 to 17 who viewed either a surgery-relevant or irrelevant film prior to their surgery. The hospital-relevant film sensitized participants who had previous hospital experience if they were under age 8. This was not the case for children older than age 8. Faust and Melamed (1984) also found age differences among pediatric surgery patients with respect to amount of information retained from viewing a surgery-relevant film. Older children retained more of the information than did younger children. Melamed, Meyer, Gee, and Soule (1976) discovered that older children could benefit from preparatory information presented a week prior to surgery, whereas younger children required preparation the night prior to surgery. In a sample of younger and older children undergoing cardiac catheterization, Caire and Erickson (1986) found that taped nursery rhymes reduced crying during the procedure in infants, but older children did not evidence widespread salubrious effects from either relaxation or rock music tapes. Further studies need to identify details of differential effects of interventions across developmental periods. However, extant findings underscore the importance of developmental considerations in determining the effect of preparatory interventions on surgery outcome.

Individuals over age 65 undergo twice as many surgeries than those in any other age group (American College of Surgeons, 1987). Furthermore, surgery patients in this age group may be more vulnerable to postsurgical psychological complications and respond differently to preoperative preparations than those of other ages (Johnson & Leventhal, 1974; Keyes, Bisnow, Richardson, & Marston, 1987; Leventhal & Prohaska, 1986; Liston, 1982). To address these features and take advantage of other characteristics more likely associated with elderly patients, Rybarczyk and Auerbach (1990) conducted reminiscence interviews as a form of preoperative intervention with 104 male surgery patients. The mean age of the subjects was 65.7 years. The reminiscence interviews involved prompting patients to recall and relate, in detail, positive events from the first half of their lives. The authors especially encouraged recall of childhood, school, family, and social experiences. There were three interview types: (1) standard reminiscence interviews, as described; (2) challenge interviews, during which patients focused on successfully met challenges they had previously faced; and (3) present-focused interviews during which patients discussed their current lives. The latter condition served as an attention placebo. The investigators also employed a no-treatment control condition and utilized same-aged peers versus younger researchers as interviews. Dependent measures consisted of state anxiety and coping (self-reported ratings of fear, positive attitude, determination, and courage). The standard and challenge interview conditions reduced state anxiety and enhanced coping relative to the attention placebo and no-treatment control conditions. In addition, relative to interviews conducted by younger researchers, peer administered challenge interviews resulted in significantly higher (i.e., enhanced) coping scores. Subsequent work confirmed the effectiveness of same-aged peers in conducting reminiscence interviews as a form of preoperative preparation of elderly surgery patients (Rybarczyk, Jorn, Lofland, Perlman, & Auerbach, 1992).

Previous hospital experience appears to serve as a moderator variable for young surgery patients. Melamed et al. (1984) showed that a hospital relevant preparatory film sensitized children under age 8 who had previously been in a hospital but did not sensitize children without such experience. Prior hospital experience may have a twofold effect. First, it provides information to patients and is thus similar to many preoperative interventions. Second, it can influence patients' appraisals of current circumstances depending on their perception regarding how they negotiated the course of previous surgery. Further investigations regarding effects of previous hospital experience could help identify whether experienced patients benefit from further preoperative preparation and, if so, how such interventions could best meet patients' needs.

Gender issues in surgery preparation have received relatively little attention. Except for studies of gender-specific procedures, such as gynecological colposcopy (Miller & Mangan, 1983), researchers have rarely isolated gender as a variable of interest in surgery preparation research. Although there are data to show that women anticipate surgery with greater anxiety than men do (Auerbach & Kendall, 1978; Johnston, 1986; Volicer & Burns, 1977), the question remains whether there is a need for differential preparation of patients for surgery based on gender and whether different forms of preparation produce gender-specific benefits. In addition, investigators need to cautiously interpret studies involving non-gender-specific surgery and be careful not to generalize from studies involving patients of one gender to populations involving the other gender.

A number of studies have attempted to investigate the relationship among patient coping style, preparatory intervention, and postoperative outcome (see Schultheis, Peterson, and Selby, 1987, and Salmon, 1992, for detailed reviews). Nonetheless, such studies have not clearly established the existence of characteristic coping styles. Early studies tended to identify people as either repressors (i.e., "avoiders" or "deniers") or sensitizers (i.e., "vigilant" or "information seekers"). These studies did not utilize a standard method to identify coping styles, characteristically failed to perform process checks in order to determine whether participants designated as sensitizers or repressors in fact acted that way postintervention, and did not standardize the nature of the stressor studied. As a result, this literature has poor internal consistency. There is evidence, however, that sensitizers given higher levels of preoperative information have better postoperative outcomes than do repressors, and repressors who can avoid or distract themselves from preoperative information have better postoperative outcome than do sensitizers having a similar level of preoperative stimulus input (Andrew, 1970; Delong, 1970; Shipley, Butt, & Horowitz, 1979). Subsequent studies (Auerbach et al., 1983; Martelli et al., 1987) have demonstrated the utility of a situation-specific measure to determine the amount of preoperative information an individual patient desires at the point of intervention. When clinicians give patients the level of information indicated by the Krantz Health Opinion Survey (Krantz, Baum, & Wideman, 1980), patients generally exhibit enhanced postoperative outcome. This relationship has proven more consistent and more practical than efforts to determine characteristic patient coping style when attempting to enhance postoperative outcome.

Situational Variables

Situational variables have included surgery type, illness severity, and other diagnosis-related features. Researchers have typically addressed surgery type more as a function of convenience or investigator preference rather than as a function of theoretical need. Patients undergoing cardiac surgery, hysterectomy, dental procedures, or cholecystectomy typically served as the primary subjects of study. A notable systematic exception to the way researchers typically treat surgery type is a large study of 12 different procedures (O'Hara, Ghoneim, Hinrichs, Metha, & Wright, 1989). The investigators assessed 1,420 patients about to undergo a surgical procedure of either the digestive, musculoskeletal, integumentary, urinary, endocrine, respiratory, nervous, hemic and lymphatic systems, female genital organs, male genital organs, or nose, mouth, and pharynx. They found that surgery type did not predict level of postoperative distress. Similarly, patient's self-report of postoperative memory change revealed no significant effect for surgery type. Fiefel, Strack, and Nagy (1987) studied a group of 223 men with either life-threatening illness (cancer or myocardial infarction) or non-life-threatening illness (rheumatoid arthritis or orthopedic disability). They found that relative to men experiencing a non-life-threatening illness, those experiencing a life-threatening illness engaged in more problem-focused coping, such as seeking information, talking with others about the illness, and becoming actively involved in treatment. Finally, Felton and Revenson (1984) asked 151 middle-aged and older adults to rate the degree of control they had over their illness. Patients rated two of the illnesses studied, rheumatoid arthritis and systemic blood cancers, as relatively less controllable and two others, hypertension and diabetes, as relatively more controllable. Patients with less controllable illnesses experienced less positive affect and were less accepting of their illness than patients with more controllable illnesses.

These studies demonstrate that under certain conditions, patients are reactive to situational variables in a manner that influences coping. However, the relationships between situational variables and coping are not clear. Categorizing such relationships would be an important, but exceedingly complex, undertaking. Not only are situational features numerous, they may influence coping as a function of patients' perceptions rather than actual existence (Gil, 1984).

Timing and Time

Researchers in the area of surgery preparation have studied timing with respect to when, relative to a given procedure, clinicians intervene. *Time* implies the process of coping throughout the span of existence of a stressor.

Faust and Melamed (1984) found that a hospital-relevant film was an effective means of preparing children if they entered the hospital the night before elective surgery, but not if they entered on the day of surgery. For those admitted the same day of surgery, a distracting, hospital-irrelevant presentation was most effective. The authors suggested that same-day admissions involve a level of arousal that is too great to allow utilization of information for effective problem-focused coping. Levesque, Grenier, Kerouac, and Reidy (1984) compared two groups of adult cholecystectomy patients: One group received surgery preparation the night before surgery; and the other received the intervention prior to admission. The investigators found no postoperative difference between the two groups. Few other studies have examined the effects of timing (e.g., Wolfer & Visintainer, 1975). This area requires further study to better understand when, during the course of a medical procedure, a given intervention is likely to have its greatest effect.

Timing as an indicator of the process of coping has served as the focus of several studies. Some studies indicate high levels of stress exist both pre- and postoperatively and, therefore, patients may benefit from interventions at several points during the surgery process (Johnston, 1980). Other work shows that in order to remain effective, coping strategies must shift to meet demands that change as patients progress through events (Auerbach, 1989; Cohen & Lazarus, 1979; Johnson et al., 1989). For example, emotion-focused approaches, such as denial, may be effective forms of coping in situations in which arousal is high and potential for control through direct action is low. An example of such a situation is when a patient is told she has breast cancer and needs a mastectomy. These same coping strategies may prove ineffective at a later time, such as when demands to adhere to medical regimens, diet, and exercise routines in order to recover and prevent the spread or recurrence of cancer become a focus. Thompson (1981) has provided a four-period framework within which temporal features related to coping may necessitate different interventions: an anticipatory period, impact period, immediate postevent period, and a long-term period. There is a need for systematic longitudinal research, perhaps utilizing such frameworks, to answer two questions: (1) Can researchers and clinicians reliably identify temporally related patterns of coping or adaptive functioning for particular medical procedures across diverse populations? (2) If such patterns exist, what characterizes them?

Further theoretical development is necessary in order to clarify the effects of preoperative intervention on postsurgical outcome. In particular, further development of both consistency and control models demands additional study of individual differences, such as the nature of schemata, primary and secondary appraisal, and other internal representations of the stressor complex. Moreover, researchers in this area need to integrate predispositional individual differences, such as age, gender, and level of anxiety into future theory development. The stressor complex itself requires additional conceptual refinement. What features of that complex influence outcome? Is this influence direct or is it the impact these features have on patient perception that affects outcome?

Theory in this area will also advance as clinicians conduct additional intervention studies. However, the usefulness of such studies depends upon the degree to which they account for both distal (i.e., postoperative) and proximal (i.e., immediate postintervention) outcomes. Process measures can be helpful in this regard. They can also help to account for changes in the stressor complex and patient response to it across time within a given procedure. Additionally, greater specificity of the nature of the stressor complex itself, as well as how patients perceive it, would help clarify the impact of interventions on outcome. Finally, investigators in the area of surgery preparation need to make efforts to standardize research methodologies, especially dependent measures, so that internal consistency and generalizability increase. Until this occurs, existing methodological inconsistencies will hamper efforts to integrate findings across studies.

PRACTICAL APPLICATIONS

How therapists actually perform preoperative preparation in clinical situations is largely unknown. Use of such preparation at nonchronic-care pediatric facilities in the United States is high (74%), but less than half of eligible patients receive interventions at these facilities (Peterson & Ridley-Johnson, 1980). Questions remain regarding the criteria that practitioners use to select patients for intervention, the nature, cost, and effectiveness of such preparation, and its use in adult populations.

Research findings suggest the following helpful guidelines for shaping clinical application of preoperative preparations.

Target Interventions for Select Groups

Individuals at high risk for postoperative complications who may benefit from effective preoperative preparation include anxious individuals and those under age 8 or over 65. Whereas many others may also obtain significant benefits from preoperative interventions, high-risk individuals merit particular attention.

Tailor Interventions for Each Recipient

Minimally, clinicians need to know the following information about each individual who is to receive a preoperative preparatory intervention: (1) the coping demands made upon or experienced by the patient at a particular point in time; (2) how the patient previously addressed these or similar demands; (3) how the patient is currently addressing the demands; (4) how much control the patient perceives him- or herself to have over these demands; (5) how anxious the patient is; (6) how much information the patient desires regarding these demands; and (7) the patient's gender, age, and previous hospital or procedural experience.

This information would allow staff to tailor an intervention to meet individual patients' needs more effectively than would be the case without such information.

Intervene Early and Intervene Late

There are at least two reasons to intervene several days before surgery takes place. First, certain forms of intervention that are effective when administered a day or two prior to surgery are not effective when administered immediately before surgery (Faust & Melamed, 1984). Second, especially with the increasingly common use of day surgery, early, preadmission interventions may be the only practical preoperative form available.

There are several reasons to intervene late (i.e., postoperatively). First, there are no data to indicate that the postoperative period is less stressful than the preoperative period. In fact, the postoperative period may be particularly stressful for procedures that result in, or fail to correct, noticeable disfigurement (e.g., skin grafts to repair a burn), that involve a major lifestyle change (e.g., colectomy/colostomy), that are highly emotionally laden because of prognosis (e.g., only partial resection of a malignant tumor), or for which there was very little time to prepare preoperatively (e.g., trauma injury repair). Second, as is the case for emergency surgery, postoperative interventions may be the only form of intervention that is practical.

Evaluate Outcome with Care

Assessment of outcome involves evaluating effects of interventions on the coping skills an individual uses to manage demands posed by a stressor complex at specific points in time. Process checks can help determine immediate effects of interventions and can assist in interpretation of traditional outcome measures. Clinicians assessing outcome need to carefully analyze the effects of time for at least two reasons. First, patients experience a stressor complex that is likely to change across time, and outcome measures must be sensitive to such changes, and second, using time itself as an outcome measure (i.e., in the form of postoperative days to discharge) may no longer demonstrate the effectiveness of interventions because of a ceiling effect introduced by diagnostically related groups or other administrative constraints (Rothrock, 1989).

Collect Data

Research has not yet fully addressed the issues of whether, for whom, with which stressors, and at what point in time preoperative interventions improve unaided coping (Auerbach, 1989). Until practitioners understand these issues, clinical applications or preoperative interventions need to include data-collection procedures to help address the issues.

Research literature is replete with other findings that can influence practice in any given case. The five guidelines discussed above have wide applicability. Several other findings, although not as well established, represent the latest trends and innovations in the field.

EMERGING TRENDS

Researchers have traditionally measured the effectiveness of preoperative interventions to prepare people for surgery via postoperative assessments. There have been few attempts to evaluate impact of interventions shortly after administration of the intervention and prior to surgery (e.g., Johnson et al., 1989). Thus, intervention effect can be measured both preoperatively and postoperatively. A very small number of studies have begun to also explore intraoperative effects. Bennett, Benson, and Kuiken (1986), for example, randomly assigned ninety-two 11- to 69-year-old elective spinal surgery patients to either a no-treatment control, relaxation training, or a blood shunting group. Patients in the blood shunting group received preoperative instructions that "the blood will move away" from the operative site during the procedure and will subsequently return to the area. All patients received general anesthesia. The study utilized a single-blind design. The investigators measured blood loss during the procedure from the suction reservoir of an autotransfusion machine and obtained estimates of blood loss from sponges. Patients in the blood shunting group lost significantly less blood than did those in the other two groups. Such findings have implications regarding need for transfusions and other complications during and after surgery. Thus, this study demonstrated an important intraoperative effect of preoperative preparations. There is need for further exploration of intraoperative effects of preoperative preparation.

There is growing recognition that surgery affects more people than just the patient. Campbell, Clark, and Kirkpatrick (1986) studied twenty-six 16- to 17-year-olds and their parents. The pediatric patients were about to undergo cardiac catheterization. The investigators randomly assigned patients to a treatment or attention placebo group. Patients and parents assigned to the treatment group received an extensive intervention of relaxation training, biofeedback, guided imagery, deep breathing techniques, counseling, cognitive reframing, and self-hypnosis. The attention placebo group received a hospital brochure. Children in the experimental group cooperated with the procedure more than children in the control group. In addition, experimental-group parents reported less stress than control-group parents. Similarly, Wolfer and Visintainer (1979) examined the effect of preoperative preparation for both pediatric tonsillectomy patients and their parents. Finally, Jay and Elliott (1990) studied parents of pediatric leukemia patients by assigning parents to either a child-focused intervention group or stress inoculation group. Parents in the child-focus group observed their children undergoing a cognitive–behavioral therapy program in preparation for bone marrow aspiration or lumbar puncture. Parents who received stress inoculation reported lower anxiety and more positive self-statement scores than parents in the child-focused intervention. Finally, Faust, Olson, and Rodriguez (1991) speculated on the impact on mothers of a preoperative participant modeling procedure indicating that caretaker–child interactions require further study.

This small literature is provocative in at least two ways. First, there is virtually no information on the effects of surgery preparation for family members of adult patients. Could spouses, siblings, and offspring of adult patients benefit from such intervention? Second, clinicians generally consider the effects of preoperative interventions typically to reside within the recipient. There is, however, some speculation that parents who observe their children receiving preoperative training, or who know that their children have received such training, also obtain salubrious effects (Jay & Elliott, 1990). Research has not yet confirmed this speculation. However, such speculation suggests that interventions may also have an impact on systems and not just individuals. Although clinical researchers have not conducted studies of preoperative interventions on family systems, there is a study of the impact of such intervention on members of the health-care team. Hinshaw, Gerber, Atwood, and Allen (1983) demonstrated that the amount of patient information known by the perioperative nurse was greater for patients who received preoperative teaching relative to control patients who did not. Additionally, postanesthesia care unit staff received more patient information about prepared patients than control patients. Staff judged care delivered to prepared patients as safer than that delivered to control patients, and nurse ratings of overall care was higher for prepared patients than for control patients. Furthermore, preoperatively prepared patients expressed greater satisfaction with care, less anxiety, more effective coping, and greater ability relative to self-care control patients. Thus, there is preliminary evidence that preoperative preparation not only affects patients who receive it, but that it also has systemic effects involving patients' families and the health-care team. Further study is necessary to confirm these findings and to discover how the systemic aspects of preoperative intervention can further enhance care.

Preoperative preparation for surgery combines a well-established beneficial clinical effect with a body of theory that is emerging. As findings regarding intraoperative and systemic effects of preoperative interventions demonstrate, boundaries of the effects and influences of preoperative preparation have yet to be established. The challenge in discovering these boundaries is to further develop a clinical and theoretical sensitivity to the complexity of surgery as it is experienced. Then the secret influence identified by William of Salicet will have been revealed and the action he thought more powerful than instruments or medicines fulfilled.

REFERENCES

Alberts, M. S., Lyons, J. S., Moretti, R. J., & Erickson, J. L. (1989). Psychological interventions in the presurgical period. *International Journal of Psychiatry in Medicine, 19,* 91–106.

American College of Surgeons. (1987). *Socio-economic textbook for surgery.* New York: Author.

Anderson, K. D., & Masur, F. T. (1983). Psychological preparation for invasive medical and dental procedures. *Journal of Behavioral Medicine, 6,* 1–40.

Andrew, J. M. (1970). Recovery from surgery with or without preparatory instructions for three coping styles. *Journal of Personality and Social Psychology, 15,* 223–236.

Auerbach, S. M. (1973). Trait–state anxiety and adjustment to surgery. *Journal of Consulting and Clinical Psychology, 40,* 264–271.

Auerbach, S. M. (1989). Stress management and coping research in the health care setting: An overview and methodological commentary. *Journal of Consulting and Clinical Psychology, 57,* 388–395.

Auerbach, S. M., & Kendall, P. C. (1978). Sex differences in anxiety response and adjustment to dental surgery: Effects of general versus specific preoperative information. *Journal of Clinical Psychiatry, 34,* 309–313.

Auerbach, S. M., Kendall, P. C., Cuttler, H. F., & Levitt, N. R. (1976). Anxiety, locus of control, type of preparatory information and adjustment to dental surgery. *Journal of Consulting and Clinical Psychology, 44,* 809–818.

Auerbach, S. M., Martelli, M. F., & Mercuri, L. G. (1983). Anxiety, information, interpersonal impacts, and adjustment to a stressful health care situation. *Journal of Personality and Social Psychology, 44,* 1284–1296.

Bennett, H. L., Benson, D. R., & Kuiken, D. A. (1986). Preoperative instructions for decreased bleeding during spine surgery. *Anesthesiology, 85,* A245.

Caire, J. B., & Erickson, S. (1986). Reducing distress in pediatric patients undergoing cardiac catheterization. *Children's Health Care, 14,* 146–152.

Campbell, L., Clark, M., & Kirkpatrick, S. E. (1986). Stress management training for parents and their children undergoing cardiac catheterization. *American Journal of Orthopsychiatry, 56,* 234–243.

Cohen, F., & Lazarus, R. S. (1973). Active coping processes, coping dispositions, and recovery from surgery. *Psychosomatic Medicine, 35,* 375–389.

Cohen, F., & Lazarus, R. S. (1979). Coping with the stresses of illness. In G. C. Stone, F. Cohen, & N. E. Adler (Eds.), *Health psychology* (pp. 217–254). San Francisco: Jossey-Bass.

Compas, B. E., Malcarne, V. L., & Fondacoro, K. M. (1988). Coping with stressful events in older children and young adolescents. *Journal of Consulting and Clinical Psychology, 56,* 405–411.

Delong, D. R. (1970). Individual differences in patterns of anxiety arousal, stress-relevant information, and recovery from surgery. Unpublished doctoral dissertation, University of California, Los Angeles.

Devine, E. C., & Cook, T. D. (1983). A meta-analytic analysis of effects of psychoeducational interventions on length of postsurgical hospital stay. *Nursing Research, 32,* 267–274.

Faust, J., & Melamed, B. G. (1984). The influence of arousal, previous experience, and age on surgery preparation of same-day and in-hospital pediatric patients. *Journal of Consulting and Clinical Psychology, 52,* 359–365.

Faust, J., Olson, R., & Rodriguez, H. (1991). Same-day surgery preparation: Reduction of pediatric patient arousal and distress through participant modeling. *Journal of Consulting and Clinical Psychology, 59,* 475–478.

Feifel, H., Strack, S., & Nagy, V. T. (1987). Degree of life-threat and differential use of coping modes. *Journal of Psychosomatic Research, 31,* 91–99.

Felton, B. J., & Revenson, T. A. (1984). Coping with chronic illness: A study of illness controllability and the influence of coping strategies on psychological adjustment. *Journal of Consulting and Clinical Psychology, 52,* 343–353.

Forsythe, C. J., & Compas, B. E. (1987). Interaction of cognitive appraisals of stressful events and coping: Testing the goodness of fit hypothesis. *Cognitive Therapy and Research, 11,* 473–485.

Gil, K. (1984). Coping effectively with invasive medical procedures. *Clinical Psychology Review, 4,* 339–362.

Hathaway, D. (1986). Effect of preoperative instruction on postoperative outcomes: A meta-analysis. *Nursing Research, 32,* 267–274.

Hinshaw, A. S., Gerber, R. M., Atwood, J. R., & Allen, J. R. (1983). The use of predictive modeling to test nursing practice outcomes. *Nursing Research, 32,* 36–42.

Horne, D. J., Vatmanidis, P., & Careri, A. (1994). Preparing patients for invasive medical and surgical procedures 1: Adding behavioral and cognitive interventions. *Behavioral Medicine, 20,* 5–13.

Janis, I. L. (1958). *Psychological stress.* New York: Wiley.

Jay, S. M., & Elliott, C. H. (1990). A stress inoculation program for parents whose children are undergoing painful medical procedures. *Journal of Consulting and Clinical Psychology, 58,* 799–804.

Johnson, J. E. (1975). Stress reduction through sensation information. In J. G. Sarason & C. D. Spielberger (Eds.), *Stress and anxiety* (Vol. 2, pp. 361–378). New York: Wiley.

Johnson, J. E., Fuller, S. S., Endress, M. P., & Rice, V. H. (1978). Altering patients' responses to surgery: An extension and replication. *Research in Nursing and Health, 1,* 111–121.

Johnson, J. E., Lauver, D. R., & Nail, L. M. (1989). Process of coping with radiation therapy. *Journal of Consulting and Clinical Psychology, 57,* 358–365.

Johnson, J. E., & Leventhal, H. (1974). Effects of accurate expectations and behavioral instructions on reactions during a noxious medical examination. *Journal of Personality and Social Psychology, 29,* 710–718.

Johnson, J. E., Rice, V. H., Fuller, S. S., & Endress, M. P. (1978). Sensory information instruction in a coping strategy and recovery from surgery. *Research in Nursing Health, 1,* 4–17.

Johnston, M. (1980). Anxiety in surgical patients. *Psychological Medicine, 10,* 142–152.

Johnston, M. (1986). Preoperative emotional states and postoperative recovery. *Advances in Psychosomatic Medicine, 15,* 1–22.

Kaloupek, D. G., & Stoupakis, T. (1985). Coping with a stressful medical procedure: Further investigation with volunteer blood donors. *Journal of Behavioral Medicine, 8,* 131–148.

Kaloupek, D. G., White, H., & Wong, M. (1984). Multiple assessment of coping strategies used by volunteer blood donors. *Journal of Behavioral Medicine, 7,* 35–60.

Keyes, K., Bisnow, B., Richardson, J., & Marston, A. (1987). Age differences in coping, behavioral dysfunction and depression following colostomy surgery. *The Gerontologist, 27,* 182–184.

Krantz, D. S., Baum, A., & Wideman, M. (1980). Assessment of preferences for self-treatment and information in health care. *Journal of Personality and Social Psychology, 39,* 977–990.

Lazarus, R. S. (1966). *Psychological stress and the coping process.* New York: McGraw-Hill.

Lazarus, R. S., & Folkman, S. (1984). *Stress, appraisal, and coping.* New York: Springer.

Leventhal, E. A., & Prohaska, T. R. (1986). Age, symptom interpretation, and health behavior. *Journal of the American Geriatrics Society, 34,* 185–191.

Leventhal, H., & Johnson, J. E. (1983). Laboratory and field experimentation: Development of a theory of self-regulation. In P. J. Woolridge, M. H. Schmitt, J. U. Skipper, Jr., & R. C. Leonard (Eds.), *Behavioral science and nursing theory* (pp. 189–262). St. Louis: Mosby.

Levesque, L., Grenier, R., Kerouac, S., & Reidy, M. (1984). Evaluation of a presurgical group program given at two different times. *Research in Nursing and Health, 7,* 227–236.

Liston, E. H. (1982). Delirium and the aged. *Pediatric Clinics of North America, 5,* 49–66.

Lynch, M. (1994). Preparing children for day surgery. *Children's Health Care, 23,* 75–85.

Martelli, M. F., Auerbach, S. M., Alexander, J., & Mercuri, L. G. (1987). Stress management in the health care setting: Matching interventions with patient coping styles. *Journal of Consulting and Clinical Psychology, 56,* 201–207.

Melamed, B. G., Dearborn, M., & Hermecz, A. A. (1983). Necessary considerations for surgery preparation: Age and previous experience. *Psychosomatic Medicine, 45,* 517–525.

Melamed, B. G., Meyer, R., Gee, C., & Soule, L. (1976). The influence of time and type of preparation on children's adjustment to hospitalization. *Journal of Pediatric Psychology, 1,* 31–37.

Miller, S. M., & Mangan, C. E. (1983). Interacting effects of information and coping style in adapting to gynecologic stress: Should the doctor tell all? *Journal of Personality and Social Psychology, 45,* 226–236.

Mumford, E., Schlesinger, H. J., & Glass, G. V. (1982). The effects of psychological intervention on recovery from surgery and heart attacks: An analysis of the literature. *American Journal of Public Health, 72,* 141–151.

O'Hara, M. W., Ghoneim, M. M., Hinrichs, J. V., Mehta, M. P., & Wright, E. J. (1989). Psychological consequences of surgery. *Psychosomatic Medicine, 51,* 356–370.

Peterson, L., & Ridley-Johnson, R. (1980). Pediatric hospital response to survey on prehospital preparation for children. *Journal of Pediatric Psychology, 5,* 1–7.

Rogers, M., & Reich, P. (1986). Psychological intervention with surgical patients: Evaluation outcome. *Advances in Psychosomatic Medicine, 15,* 23–50.

Rothrock, J. C. (1989). Perioperative nursing: Part I: Preoperative psychoeducational interventions. *Association of Registered Nurses Journal, 49,* 597–619.

Rybarczyk, B. D., & Auerbach, S. M. (1990). Reminiscence interviews as stress management intervention for older patients undergoing surgery. *The Gerontologist, 30,* 523–528.

Rybarczyk, B. D., Jorn, M., Lofland, K., Perlman, M., & Auerbach, S. M. (1992). The reminiscence interview: Using volunteers to help older patients cope with stressful medical procedures. Symposium submission to Gerontological Society of America Annual Convention. Washington, D. C.

Schultheis, K., Peterson, L., & Selby, V. (1987). Preparation for stressful medical procedures and person X treatment interactions. *Clinical Psychology Review, 7,* 329–352.

Shipley, R., Butt, J. H., & Horowitz, B. (1979). Preparation to reexperience a stressful medical examination: Effect of repetitious videotape exposure and coping style. *Journal of Consulting and Clinical Psychology, 47,* 485–492.

Sime, A. M. (1976). Relationship of pre-operative fear, type of coping and information received about surgery to recovery from surgery. *Journal of Personality and Social Psychology, 34,* 716–724.

Suls, J., & Wan, C. K. (1989). Effects of sensory and procedural information on coping with stressful medical procedures and pain: A meta-analysis. *Journal of Consulting and Clinical Psychology, 57,* 372–379.

Thompson, S. C. (1981). Will it hurt if I can control it? A complex answer to a simple question. *Psychological Bulletin, 90,* 90–101.

Vitaliano, P. P., DeWolfe, D. J., Maiuro, R. D., Russo, J., & Katon, W. (1990). Appraised changeability of a stressor as a modifier of the relationship between coping and depression: A test of the hypothesis of fit. *Journal of Personality and Social Psychology, 59,* 582–592.

Volicer, B. J., & Burns, M. W. (1977). Preexisting correlates of hospital stress. *Nursing Research, 26,* 408–415.

Wilson, J. F. (1981). Behavioral preparation for surgery: Benefit or harm? *Journal of Behavioral Medicine, 4,* 79–102.

Wolfer, J. A., & Visintainer, M. (1976). Pediatric surgical patients' and parents' stress responses and adjustment as a function of psychologic preparation and stress point nursing care. *Nursing Research, 24,* 244–255.

Wolfer, J. A., & Visintainer, M. A. (1979). Prehospital psychological preparation for tonsillectomy patients: Effects on children's and parents' adjustment. *Pediatrics, 64,* 646–655.

16

Relapse Prevention

Cheza W. Collier and G. Alan Marlatt

This chapter discusses relapse prevention (RP) as it pertains to health behavior change, particularly in the addictions. RP is a cognitive–behavioral approach to treatment of habitual problem behaviors and maintenance of alternative coping behaviors. It is particularly applicable during the maintenance stage of behavior change when patients are most likely to lose their motivation for change and are at risk for reverting back to old, undesirable habits (e.g., smoking, overeating, excessive drinking, or other substance abuse).

Thus, the general goals of relapse prevention are (1) maintain behavior change (e.g., abstinence in the case of severe alcohol dependence, or moderation in the case of eating disorders or less severe alcohol abuse); (2) increase confidence or self-efficacy in individuals' abilities to successfully cope with high-risk situations for relapse; and (3) reduce harmful effects if a lapse or relapse occurs and motivate renewed efforts at behavior change.

In this chapter, we present theoretical underpinnings of the notion of relapse prevention based primarily on the work of Marlatt and Gordon (1985). We discuss assessment, treatment, lifestyle, and cultural issues relevant to treating addictive behaviors and using relapse prevention as a maintenance strategy.

THE RELAPSE PREVENTION APPROACH

Our approach to relapse prevention is a biopsychosocial one (Donovan & Marlatt, 1988; Marlatt, 1992) based on social learning and self-efficacy theory (Bandura,

---

Cheza W. Collier and G. Alan Marlatt • Addictive Behaviors Research Center, Department of Psychology, University of Washington, Seattle, Washington 98195.
Handbook of Health and Rehabilitation Psychology, edited by Anthony J. Goreczny. Plenum Press, New York, 1995.

1977, 1978, 1986). Addictive behaviors hypothetically develop from multiple determinants that are biological, psychological, and social–environmental in nature. Learning theorists hypothesize that high-risk individuals learn maladaptive ways to cope by engaging in behaviors that become habitual, or addictive, through reinforcement and other higher level learning processes (e.g., expectancy). Individuals' degrees of self-efficacy (i.e., confidence in their ability to change target behaviors) greatly influence motivation, performance, and outcome.

Biological factors include genetic and neuropsychological characteristics (Cloninger, 1987; Goodwin, 1990; Parsons, 1989). Studies show that family history of alcoholism increases risk of drinking problems and that this predisposition is more prevalent in sons of alcoholic fathers (Goodwin, 1990; Newlin & Thompson, 1991). It is also clear that long-term alcohol and other drug abuse may lead to impaired brain functioning (Parsons, 1989) and the associated need for specific cognitive deficit training (Forsberg & Goldman, 1987). Persons with a family history of problems with addictive behaviors are not only at a higher risk of developing similar problems, but may also have greater difficulty maintaining goals of moderation or abstinence.

Psychological factors include emotional and cognitive experiences associated with addictive behaviors. These experiences help determine whether, and in what circumstances, individuals are likely to engage in target behaviors. Positive outcome expectancies play a major role in development of addictive behaviors (Marlatt & Gordon, 1985). Expectancies exert strong influence over perceptions and consequent behavior of individuals (Connors & Maisto, 1988). If individuals have expectancies of positive or negative reinforcement, they are more likely to engage in the behavior. This is true in the case of alcohol consumption, even when individuals are given a nonalcoholic drink or placebo but expect to receive alcohol (Marlatt & Rohsenow, 1980; Rohsenow & Marlatt, 1981).

Social and environmental factors include societal beliefs, which vary among different cultures; observation of others modeling target behaviors; peer influences in adolescence and adulthood; and societal portrayals of effects of certain behaviors (Hover & Gaffney, 1988; Oetting & Beauvais, 1987; Stein, Newcomb, & Bentler, 1987). Both print and film media often portray drinking and drug-taking models. For example, alcohol advertisements contain numerous implications that individuals who drink a certain type of alcohol become more attractive to the opposite sex, more "hip," more "cool," and more socially acceptable. This has strong appeal for adolescents and young adults who rely on maladaptive drinking, gambling, or smoking crack/cocaine to help them deal with life's stresses. Relapse prevention helps individuals create a new social environment and lifestyle and assess the previous one more realistically.

CONDITIONING FACTORS IN ADDICTION AND RELAPSE

Both classical and operant conditioning have strong roles in establishing and maintaining addictive behaviors (Donovan & Marlatt, 1988; George & Marlatt, 1983; Marlatt & Gordon, 1985; Wallace, 1991). We are all familiar with Pavlov's dog, conditioned to salivate at the sound of a bell after repeated pairing of the bell with the presentation of meat. A similar process occurs when former addicts experience anticipatory cravings as they come into contact with cues repeatedly associated with rewarding drug use.

Take the example of Bob, a college student who attends weekly football, basketball, and baseball games during their respective seasons. Every week, Bob drinks five or six 16-ounce glasses of beer during the game. By the end of the game, he is drunk and often gets into a fight or becomes involved in some other disruptive or potentially dangerous behavior. For Bob, sports events, football and baseball fields, basketball courts, balls and other equipment for those sports, crowds sitting in the stands, crowds cheering, buzzers and referee whistles, and 16-ounce plastic glasses all become conditioned stimuli to which he responds by desiring and anticipating the effects of beer. These previously neutral stimuli in the environment have elicited positive outcome expectancies for him to drink. When Bob decides to cut down or abstain from drinking, he finds it very difficult to refuse a few beers while watching a game, even though he knows the consequences will be negative for him.

Operant conditioning maintains established behaviors. Both positive and negative reinforcement are at work here. In the example of drug abusers initial euphoric sensations positively reinforce use of particular substances; individuals then continue consumption of the substance in order to prolong the high. Negative reinforcement occurs when individuals use the drug to cope with unwanted feelings, such as anxiety, depression, or unpleasant withdrawal symptoms. Once those feelings are gone (escape response), individuals are likely to continue to use the drug repeatedly in order to keep unwanted feelings from returning (avoidance response). When abusers use a drug, such as cocaine, for self-medication purposes, they are able to successfully avoid dealing with painful feelings. In anticipating potential for relapse after treatment, the former drug abusers must learn alternative means of successfully coping with such negative emotional states.

RELAPSE PREVENTION AND MODELS OF HELPING AND COPING

The biopsychosocial habit model contrasts with the moral, medical, and spiritual or enlightenment models of addiction. Each of these four models ascribes responsibility for problems and subsequent solutions to different sources (Brickman et al., 1982).

The moral model views individuals as responsible for development of problems and solutions. This model considers addicted patients to be morally flawed individuals who must exercise greater willpower in order to return from a fallen state.

The medical or disease model does not hold clients responsible for either the cause or solution of the problems. Instead, this model considers biological factors as the root of problem behaviors. Onset of the disorder and its progressive course is due to genetic and physiological factors beyond the individuals' control, and solutions lie in the expertise of professional, usually medical, providers (e.g., inpatient treatment).

The enlightenment or spiritual model views clients as responsible for their problems but not for the solutions. According to this model, clients find solutions to problems in God through prayer and teachings of religious leaders and similar others.

The biopsychosocial habit (or compensatory model) considers clients responsible for both finding and implementing solutions to their problems but not for the initial cause of the problems. Because future addicts are hypothetically born with biological predispositions toward addiction and may mature in an environment that fosters development of addictive behaviors, addiction problems according to this model, are not the personal fault of affected individuals. However, it is clear in this model that changes in behavior cannot occur without full commitment and initiative of addicted clients. This model helps to relieve clients of guilt associated with the moral and spiritual models. In comparison with the medical model, the biopsychosocial-habit model allows clients to assume greater responsibility and power in the process of recovery in order to better cope with the likelihood of a lapse or relapse.

USING RELAPSE PREVENTION

One goal of RP is to influence beliefs and expectancies of clients and to help them clearly recognize their own roles in establishing new behaviors. It may be necessary to challenge clients' traditional notions of relapse in order to create a reframe that allows individuals to exercise more choices, thereby enhancing personal power and self-efficacy in the change process.

Webster (1984) defined relapse as follows: "Relapse—1. To fall back or revert to an earlier state. 2. To regress after partial recovery from illness. 3. To slip back into bad ways: *BACKSLIDE. n.* An act, instance, or result of relapsing."

This definition provides a simple way of understanding what happens during the relapse process. When we think of relapse, we usually think of completely returning to undesirable behaviors. An example of this idea is the saying used among Alcoholics Anonymous (AA) members: "One drink is a drunk." This implies that anytime individuals slip from complete abstinence, they will experience loss of control and go on a binge of intoxication.

Relapse is a complex process mediated by cognitive and emotional reactions and by individuals' coping skills. The relapse prevention model encourages clients who experience a lapse to view the "slip" as a temporary setback that commonly happens during attempts to establish new behavior patterns. Clients learn to plan for these slips by developing coping strategies for use in high-risk situations. RP allows individuals to maintain their dignity and responsibility by reassuring them that lapsing from desired behaviors does not mean that they are total failures; rather, RP views the lapse as an opportunity for individuals to learn more about their unique process of recovery.

Consider the following definition of lapse: "Lapse—*vi.* 1.a. To fall from one level to a different, usu. less desirable one: *BACKSLIDE.—n.* 1.a. A slip, error, or failure, esp. a slight or unimportant one [a lapse of judgment]" (Webster, 1984).

The term *lapse* serves to better delineate the slips in behavior that frequently occur among those who are in the process of changing an addictive behavior. A single lapse does not indicate a devastating turn for the worse but rather a milder error from which one may recover more easily if appropriate coping strategies are in place. A full relapse then, would be a more complete return of undesired behaviors, repeatedly, and over a longer period of time.

Lapses and relapses are a normal part of the recovery stage of maintenance.

Hence, rather than defining *relapse* as a sign of treatment failure, the real problem is keeping individuals involved in the change process (i.e., preventing treatment dropout and motivational collapse). The objective is to help clients persevere despite lapse or relapse experiences.

RELAPSE ASSESSMENT

Self-Monitoring

The purpose of self-monitoring is to encourage clients to take a closer look at their daily problem-behavior patterns. Both clients and therapists can then use these dairy records to assess the context and extent of problems and to identify potential high-risk situations for relapse. For alcohol abusers, Marlatt and Gordon (1985) suggest using a Daily Drinking Diary to record information about drinking, such as time, duration, setting, antecedents, amount consumed, and consequences of drinking. This type of information is helpful in planning for later situations in which clients will encounter urges to drink. A thorough familiarity with one's own drinking style and patterns allows for development of individualized coping plans for high-risk situations.

Identifying High-Risk Situations

An essential ingredient in the RP approach is identification of situations in which clients are likely at high risk of engaging in the addictive behavior. These can be "... any situation that poses a threat to the individual's sense of control and increases the risk of potential relapse" (Marlatt & Gordon, 1985, p. 37). In order to assess, document, and plan for these situations, specific assessment tools, in addition to self-monitoring records, are available. Annis (1990; Annis & Davis, 1989) has developed the Inventory of Drinking Situations (IDS) and the Situational Confidence Questionnaire (SCQ-39). The IDS provides an individualized list of high-risk drinking situations for each client. Annis designed the SCQ-39 to "assess drinking-related self-efficacy" by having clients rate the likelihood of resisting drinking excessively in a given situation. A measure that assesses coping responses in high-risk situations is the Situational Competency Test (Chaney, O'Leary, & Marlatt, 1978), designed to assess inpatient alcoholics' level of skill in coping with a variety of difficult situations.

Negative Emotional States or "The Temple of Doom"

Consider examples of problem drinkers and binge eaters, each of whom usually feels depressed and lonely when not drinking or eating. When angry, they may turn to food or drink instead of expressing their anger directly. Social skills deficits and low self-esteem play major roles in maintaining maladaptive behaviors in these examples. When feeling anxious, insecure, lonely, depressed, or angry, the substance of choice helps them temporarily to feel better.

These negative emotional states often associate with high-risk situations for relapse. Cummings, Gordon, and Marlatt (1980) reported that individuals experienced negative emotional states in 35% of described relapses. Interpersonal conflict was another trigger for relapse (16% of relapses). Both categories involve negative emotions, such as depression, anger, anxiety, and frustration. When combined, they accounted for 51% of the relapses in this particular sample. RP attempts to provide strategies to help unlock the doors to this figurative "Temple of Doom" by increasing coping skills and self-efficacy for handling situations in which these negative emotions may occur.

Social Pressure

Social pressure is the other large category of high-risk relapse situations. The pressure can be direct (e.g., urging someone to have a drink) or it can be subtle (e.g., a social environment in which everyone appears to be drinking alcohol). Consider the case of Jane, a woman trying to kick the cocaine habit. Jane tends to live a drug-free life except when in the company of a favorite cousin who lives in the same city. When the two get together, they inevitably do "a few lines" of cocaine or smoke a few "rocks." Jane knows that this usually leads to a weekend binge that takes her until the middle of the next week to overcome and results in subsequent neglect of work and home obligations. For Jane, the high-risk situation is social influence in the presence of this cousin. Because Jane is a member of a very close family system, close proximity to her cousin may occur in any family gathering and at many social events. When she thinks about avoiding this cousin, she has great difficulty because, after all, they grew up together, and they are family.

Relapse Fantasies

In assessing potential for relapse, it is often useful to explore clients' fantasies about relapse (Sandberg & Marlatt, 1989). Under what circumstances do they think relapse is most likely to happen? Where and with whom will they be? What would be their emotional state? Would there have been recent events that they think might precipitate a relapse? Assessment of relapse fantasies allows clinicians to learn more about clients' high-risk situations, coping skills, and perceptions of self-efficacy in these situations.

RELAPSE PREVENTION STRATEGIES

Coping Skills Training

Most clinical approaches to relapse prevention utilize an educational skills training group format (Annis & Davis, 1989; Daley, 1989; Marlatt & Gordon, 1985; Wallace, 1991). These coed groups tend to incorporate a combination of psycho-educational instruction, modeling of new skills, coaching, rehearsal of new skills, and group processes. Groups help provide social support for members, an opportunity for rehearsal of new skills in the form of role play, and feedback on progress.

RP coping strategies are helpful for use in high-risk situations. Clients develop a repertoire of strategies to use in such situations and they receive encouragement to choose appropriate strategies for given situations. As an example, for a recovering alcoholic, this repertoire might include substituting nonalcoholic drinks; avoiding drinking cues, such as certain places and people; traveling different daily routes in order to avoid these cues; engaging in distracting activities, such as hobbies, exercise, or social events where alcohol is not available; and refusal of drinks and invitations where drinking might occur. In addition to new repertoires of behavior, clients need to learn skills required to practice these new behaviors.

Problem Solving

An initial step in relapse prevention skills training, problem solving skills help clients feel more in control of their lives. Steps to good problem solving include: assessing one's orientation to the problem, defining the problem, brainstorming potential solutions to the problem, and determining effectiveness of proposed solutions. When first learning problem solving, it is best to start with simple problems (proximal goal-setting). As clients become proficient in using these steps, clinicians need to encourage clients to move on to using these newly developed skills with more complex, difficult problems.

Assertiveness Training

Many clients lack motivation or skills to refuse drinks or ask for nonalcoholic drinks at a social event. Assertiveness training and role playing assist in making this task easier. Clients must learn to identify their tendency to be passive in a variety of situations and practice more assertive responses. They learn the differences between passivity, assertiveness, and aggressiveness and the role of each in their lives. Successful assertive behavior can lead to increased self-efficacy and self-esteem.

Anger Management

Anger management training is also useful in working with some of the negative emotions associated with relapse, including exploration of extent of anger problems, styles of coping with anger, and more adaptive coping and conflict management. A common tendency is to hold anger in rather than to express it directly and appropriately. Individuals may be afraid of letting the anger build up until they explode. When this happens, addicted individuals often feel out of control and turn to their substance of choice to alleviate this emotional tension.

Relaxation and Meditation

Relaxation skills relate to stress management and can help addicted individuals control urges to engage in problem behaviors. Because people respond differently to different methods, it is best to teach a variety of forms of relaxation. Progressive muscle relaxation is popular and allows individuals to feel the contrast between tensed and relaxed muscle groups. A simpler method is to focus on breathing using a simple mental device, such as the word *one,* to evoke the relaxation response (Benson, 1975). This method relates to meditation techniques that use a mantra to induce a rhythmic breathing pattern and a deeply relaxed state. Some individuals prefer meditation techniques into which they can incorporate religious practices, such as prayer. Others do not like including the suggestion of religious practice. In any case, there are numerous techniques from which to choose, including utilization of tape-recorded music or other sounds, and visual and other sensory images that are available in local variety stores.

Communication and Social Skills

Addictive behaviors often have their roots in deficits of interpersonal relations. Feelings of low self-esteem and lack of practice interacting with others without influence of drugs, particularly in dating situations, may be part of the problem. Clients need to receive opportunities to practice expressing themselves in a supportive environment. They also need to learn to listen to and paraphrase others and to switch their focus from their own thoughts and insecurities to the interaction in which they are participating.

Handling Urges and Cravings

In order to cope effectively with cravings, it is important for clients to understand that urges to indulge in addictive behaviors are a normal part of the recovery process and that environmental cues usually trigger the urges. When this inevitable experience occurs, clients must be ready to use positive self-talk to get through it. It is helpful to be able to say to oneself, "I know what this is, I expected this craving, I know what to do, I can wait it out, I know I can get through this." The "urge surfing" analogy helps clients understand the task of dealing with urges. An urge is like an ocean wave that rises, crests, and falls. The client must learn to "ride out the urge wave and to maintain balance without wiping out" (George, 1989).

It is also helpful to develop a sense of detachment from the craving process so as to allow individuals to explore what is going on without panicking and losing emotional control. Normalizing cravings as an aspect of recovery that all ex-addicts go through helps foster this detachment.

Cue exposure is one way of facilitating extinction of cravings (Blakey & Baker, 1980; Childress, McLellan, & O'Brien, 1986; Cooney, Gillespie, Baker, & Kaplan, 1987). Clients undergo exposure to both conditioned and unconditioned drug stimuli so that they experience urges and learn active coping strategies. As clients become skilled in using coping strategies in response to urges, urges begin to subside in the presence of those environmental cues and clients begin to experience these cues as neutral again. Eventually, these cues no longer trigger urges to engage in the addictive behavior (Marlatt, 1990).

Dealing with Lapses

For clients motivated to maintain abstinence, the first response to an actual lapse is likely to be a feeling of despair with subsequent feelings of guilt and a sense of failure. These and similar cognitive-emotional responses constitute the abstinence violation effect (AVE; Curry, Marlatt, & Gordon, 1987) or goal violation effect (GVE). The GVE can be severe enough to destroy feelings of self-efficacy and propel individuals into mind-sets that lead to a full-blown relapse.

Cognitive reframes, such as the earlier discussion of relapse and lapse definitions, are helpful in de-escalating the GVE. One way of viewing a lapse is similar to the way the Chinese interpret the word *crisis*. *Crisis* signifies both danger and opportunity in Chinese culture. It is an occasion to stop, reassess, and seize the opportunity to learn something new.

In case of a lapse, clients must learn to initiate the following six "emergency" steps:

1. *Stop* the behavior.
2. *Look* and listen to what is going on in the situation.
3. Remain *calm* and remember that one slip does not mean the end of the show.
4. *Renew* one's *commitment* to the goal of behavior change.
5. *Review antecedents* to the current situation (e.g., time, place, mood) and avoid excessive self-blame.
6. Make an *immediate plan for recovery,* call for help or support, take a time-out and leave the scene, find a distraction, and do a good deed.

Therapists and clients may also want to make a relapse contract that delineates the commitment to change and outlines consequences for a lapse. Components of the contract may include agreement to delay engaging in the addictive behavior after first experiencing a craving, to allow time for the GVE to pass, and to instigate coping strategies.

An important component in managing a lapse is ability to confront one's motivational difficulties and denial. To this end, clients in RP programs learn to explore ways in which they may engage in covert planning and set themselves up for relapse to occur. When examining antecedents of a lapse, therapists encourage clients to identify the "apparently irrelevant decisions" that led to the lapse. When recognized, these minidecisions can be early warning signs that one is off the main road and on a path toward relapse. In-depth restructuring of events leading to the lapse can highlight these apparently irrelevant decisions and provide information to help prepare clients for future occasions.

LIFESTYLE MODIFICATION AND BALANCE

Lifestyle modification is a necessary ingredient for a successful RP strategy. Because many substance abusers have histories of family dysfunction, it is not surprising that this dysfunction may be carried from one generation to the next (Wallace, 1991). When a dysfunctional history does not exist, individuals battling with addiction have likely develop some maladaptive behavior patterns and belief systems that must change in order to maintain new goals. Thus, those recovering from maladaptive addictions can benefit from therapy designed to assist in development of personal growth and improved overall health.

One prescription from Marlatt and Gordon (1985) for a healthier lifestyle is to balance number of obligations in one's life with number of leisure or work activities one does for pleasure or satisfaction. Obligations are "shoulds," and activities done for pleasure or other benefit are "wants."

To assess this balance, clients can complete a list of daily "wants" and "shoulds" for work and vacation days. Marlatt described the Daily Want–Should Tally Form designed for this purpose (Marlatt & Gordon, 1985). When "shoulds" are in great excess of "wants," individuals may experience too much stress and may feel exhausted, frustrated, and resentful. They may return to alcohol consumption or other addictive behaviors to cope with these feelings and restore a superficial sense of balance. An appropriate balance between "wants" and "shoulds" is one in which there is perception of optimal engagement in both kinds of activities.

Marlatt and Gordon (1985) encourage development of positive addictions, such as exercise or meditation. These are behaviors that are reinforcing and become habitual, but are generally healthy. Whereas maladaptive addictive behaviors provide an initial feeling of euphoria and well-being with negative after-effects, positive addictions tend to have negative initial effects, such as soreness with exercise, but positive effects in the long term. Chiauzzi (1991) warned against other compensatory habits, including excessive exercise, spending, or sexual behavior that may become maladaptive.

Other aspects of lifestyle change include establishing and maintaining good nutrition habits. A regular exercise program helps individuals achieve greater balance and feel better overall (Murphy, Pagano, & Marlatt, 1986). It is also essential to find a way to relax deeply without assistance of old addictive behaviors. Social activities also provide an outlet for stress, and supportive friends can be a source of social support when recovery becomes difficult and a lapse seems imminent.

The idea of maintaining a sense of balance is pivotal to healthy modification of a lifestyle pattern. A seesaw metaphor provides useful visual imagery regarding balance. One end of a giant seesaw represents "shoulds," while the other end represents "wants." Characterizing the ends of the seesaw are opposing forces, such as "work" and "relaxation," "salad" and "ice cream," or "responsible sobriety" and "irresponsible drug binge." Without a sense of balance, individuals may find themselves running on this giant seesaw from one end to the other in a volatile, out-of-control manner, trying to keep either end from bottoming out. When one pictures sitting in the center of the seesaw with the ends suspended evenly, one can imagine a more serene, less stressful existence that incorporates these opposing forces into one whole.

Relearning Joy, or "Re-Joyment"

Cognitive and environmental factors related to quality of life influence relapse. Sensation seekers may become bored without their previous "unbalanced" lifestyle (Chiauzzi, 1991). Others may feel they have lost or given up something and need to continually remind themselves of benefits of their new lifestyles (Marlatt & Gordon, 1985). Still others may be dealing with drug-abusing partners or otherwise dysfunctional relationships that require yet another layer of change (Daley, 1989; Wallace, 1991). For these people, use of drugs, gambling, or compulsive eating may have been their joy.

Marlatt's prescription for balancing "wants" and "shoulds" helps to address this issue. Zackon (1989) explored this more directly and urged clinicians to go beyond attempts to heal psychological pain and provide general encouragement to engage in fun activities. He asserted that pleasure must be relearned, thus, his term "re-joyment." He stated that the "ex-addict must allow for a lowering of his so-called 'pleasure threshold'" in order to find pleasure in less intense stimulation of the everyday drug-free world. He called for incorporation of activities geared toward re-joyment into therapeutic programs. In this way, clients can begin the pleasure relearning process at the same time they begin to learn to live without their addiction. Then they have a basis from which to continue this relearning process in creative ways in their new lifestyles.

RELAPSE PREVENTION APPLICATIONS IN BEHAVIORAL MEDICINE

As mentioned previously, relapse prevention is useful with a variety of addictive behaviors in addition to substance abuse. These include smoking, eating disorders, compulsive gambling, anger dyscontrol, and sexual aggression (Laws, 1989; Loberg, Miller, Nathan, & Marlatt, 1989; Marlatt & Gordon, 1985). The current applications may also address family-system functioning (Marlatt & Barrett, 1994). In addition, the principles of RP may aid maintenance of other health behavior change efforts.

For example, recent research (Collier-Phillips, 1992) used relapse prevention counseling with hypertension patients to promote a period of abstinence from alcohol. The same principles would be useful with these patients to facilitate their adherence to a low-salt, low-fat dietary regimen, regular exercise routine or to encourage medication compliance in the interest of maintaining a lower blood pressure.

Consider the example of a pregnant diabetic patient who must adhere to a special diet, take daily insulin, increase her rest, and avoid stressful situations for the safety of herself and her unborn baby. She may feel more confident if she can identify situations in which she would be at high risk to violate this regimen and can plan ahead to avoid such violations. Once a minor violation occurs, she might benefit from the ability to explore minidecisions that led to the violation in order to choose a different path next time.

Therapists can extrapolate RP strategies to circumstances of cancer patients, chronic pain patients, and injury rehabilitation patients. Indeed, treatment teams can apply RP strategies to any patients for whom long-term lifestyle adjustments are necessary for positive health outcomes.

CULTURAL ISSUES IN RELAPSE PREVENTION

It is essential to consider the roles of ethnicity, culture, and social class in an approach to behavior change in American society. Although necessary, this is not a simple notion. On the one hand, there are many similarities among various groups in our society, and some treatment and prevention approaches that have worked with middle- and upper-class Caucasians (i.e., the mainstream) may also work with some individuals from different ethnic and social-class groups. However, critical differences exist in belief systems, cultural and religious practices, health behaviors, and access to services among diverse cultural groups. These differences indicate that some treatment and prevention approaches applied to middle- and upper-class Caucasians are *not* likely to work with some individuals from different ethnic and social-class groups (Weibel-Orlando, 1987; Weiner, Wallen, & Zankowski, 1990).

Approaches may or may not work with different populations, because groups are heterogeneous within each culture. Because there are varying levels of acculturation and assimilation among members of ethnic groups, therapists must assess each client individually regarding the client's cultural needs in treatment and aftercare. It is important to avoid using general stereotypes to determine what kind of approach to take with clients from nonmaintstream environments. It is equally important to have culture-specific approaches available to treat those clients for whom cultural issues are salient.

Weibel-Orlando (1987) provided a discussion of these issues and focused on cultural relevance of alcoholism treatment for Native Americans. The approach that seems likely to accommodate needs of many Native Americans is called the *syncretic* model because it blends traditional Native American healing practices with standard mainstream approaches to alcoholism treatment. Unfortunately, there are barriers to making these kinds of services available on a widespread basis.

Some researchers have found that alcohol and other drug abuse is less prevalent among African-Americans than among Caucasians (Brannock, Schandler, & Oncley, 1990), but this may reverse as the population in each group grows older (Robbins & Clayton, 1989). According to Weibel-Orlando (1987) and Harper (1983), there is inadequate literature about drinking practices of African-Americans. In fact, Graham (1992) asserted that there is a dearth of empirical data about African-Americans in psychological literature in general. From what we do know, a treatment approach that incorporates extended family, school, and/or church involvement might be most useful for some African-Americans (Weibel-Orlando, 1987). For others, more acculturated to the mainstream culture, mainstream services may suffice. In any case, treatment approaches must recognize and include knowledge regarding the "long history of oppression and discrimination" toward African-Americans that may affect their drinking habits (Watts & Wright, 1983).

Clinicians need to individually assess cultural influences among Asians and Latinos because of large variations in heritage. Clients may be first-generation immigrants from several different countries with different cultures and beliefs, or their families may have been in the United States for several generations with members of those families having fully assimilated to Western culture.

Self-Efficacy and Social Marginalization

Bandura's discussion of self-efficacy (1978) provides interesting food for thought when contemplating relapse prevention for individuals who have traditionally lived outside mainstream American culture, especially those who may also be struggling with poverty. Bandura stressed that self-efficacy refers to individuals' confidence that they can perform a certain behavior, not their confidence regarding outcome of that behavior once performed.

One might surmise that among poor and ethnic groups that have typically been outside of mainstream American culture, the concepts of self-efficacy and helplessness intertwine. Low self-efficacy implies that individuals feel unable to do what it would take to achieve a particular goal. High self-efficacy implies that individuals believe themselves competent to do what it takes to achieve a goal. Learned helplessness implies that individuals believe that even if they could perform behaviors necessary to achieve a goal, the achievement would not occur due to some other, usually environmental, reason.

In an atmosphere of race, class, and gender discrimination and prejudice, it seems reasonable to speculate that even if individuals approach goals with high beliefs of self-efficacy but experience feelings of helplessness in an unresponsive environment, those individuals may eventually lose their confidence regarding their ability to perform behaviors necessary to achieve their goals. They may then abandon their efforts, thereby losing practice with the behaviors, and/or they may doubt that they ever performed the behaviors properly in the first place.

Consider, for example, Denise, a student who does a project for a classroom assignment in which it was necessary for her to perform the research and produce a model product. The work produced is equivalent to that of any other student who receives a grade of "A" for the assignment. However, because the instructor does not believe students of Denise's race and social class can do well on this type of work, she received a "C." She may begin to doubt her ability to do the required work and stop trying. This would be especially likely after repeated attempts produced similar outcomes. thus, Denise's confidence is undermined in both her ability to perform appropriate behaviors and effect desired outcomes. Unfortunately, it is probable that discrimination need not be as obvious as in the example of Denise to have this type of effect.

An example more relevant to relapse prevention might be the case of Bill, an alcohol-dependent African-American man assigned to a Caucasian counselor who happens to be "color-blind." The "color-blind" counselor views race and ethnicity as unimportant and irrelevant to treatment and may avoid appropriate confrontation with the client (Bell & Evans, 1983). Even though the counselor may have good intentions, Bill is left feeling that the counselor discounted an important part of who Bill is. It may be that his racial heritage plays an important role in both his reasons for drinking and his self-concept. For such a client, it may be difficult to develop confidence in his abilities to perform behaviors necessary to maintain treatment goals, partly due to his emotional reactions to the treatment process itself. (See Bell & Evans, 1983, for further discussion on counseling African-American clients.)

Addicted individuals who are poor and/or from ethnic minority groups often have low self-esteem related to both statuses; many are likely to have grown up in dysfunctional family systems due to substance abuse (Wallace, 1991; Weibel-Orlando, 1987). It is also difficult for poor clients to avoid environments in which drugs are readily available. In particular are the perils of homelessness, as discussed by Wallace (1991) in reference to crack smokers who become homeless due to their drug use. Once undomiciled, they tend to use shelters where crack use and availability are flagrant.

Wallace contended that we live in a dysfunctional society. She postulated that in a society that views women and ethnic minorities through negative images and expects them to be low achievers, "narcissistic injuries" to the self occur. These injuries can be so painful that the perpetuate a self-fulfilling prophecy of underachievement and even antisocial behaviors, including substance abuse and other addictions. This also leads to alienation from figures of authority, including mistrust of clinicians whom they view as representatives of society and who often seem to take a "blame the victim" position. Wallace urged that clinicians must be ". . . sensitive to these societal dynamics that affect women and minorities and must structure treatment facilities and programs in such a way that they do not duplicate the subtle projection of low and negative expectations for these groups" (p. 116).

REFERENCES

Annis, H. M. (1990). Relapse to substance abuse: Empirical findings within a cognitive-social learning approach. *Journal of Psychoactive Drugs, 22*(2), 117–123.

Annis, H. M., & Davis, C. S. (1989). Relapse prevention training: A cognitive-behavioral approach based on self-efficacy theory. *Journal of Chemical Dependency Treatment, 2*(2), 81–103.

Bandura, A. (1977). Self-efficacy: Toward a unifying theory of behavior change. *Psychological Review, 84,* 191–215.

Bandura, A. (1978). Reflections on self-efficacy. *Advances in Behaviour Research and Therapy, 1,* 237–269.

Bandura, A. (1986). *Social foundations of thought and action: A social cognitive theory.* Englewood Cliffs, NJ: Prentice-Hall.

Bell, P., & Evans, J. (1983). Counseling the Black alcoholic client. In T. D. Watts & R. Wright, Jr., (Eds.), *Black alcoholism: Toward a comprehensive understanding.* Springfield, IL: Thomas.

Benson, H. (1975). *The relaxation response.* New York: Morrow.

Blakey, R., & Baker, T. (1980). An exposure approach to alcohol abuse. *Behavior Research and Therapy, 18,* 319-325.

Brannock, J. C., Schandler, S. L., & Oncley, Jr., P. R. (1990). Cross-cultural and cognitive factors examined in groups of adolescent drinkers. *Journal of Drug Issues, 20,* 427–442.

Brickman, P., Rabinowitz, V. C., Karuza, Jr., J., Coates, D., Cohn, E., & Kidder, L. (1982). Models of helping and coping. *American Psychologist, 37,* 368–384.

Chaney, E. F., O'Leary, M. R., & Marlatt, G. A. (1978). Skill training with alcoholics. *Journal of Consulting and Clinical Psychology, 46,* 1092–1104.

Chiauzzi, E. J. (1991). *Preventing relapse in the addictions: A biopsychosocial approach.* Elmsford, NY: Pergamon.

Childress, R. F., McLellan, A. T., & O'Brien, C. P. (1986). Role of conditioning factors in the development of drug dependence. *Psychiatric Clinics of North America, 9,* 413–425.

Cloninger, C. R. (1987). Neurogenetic adaptive mechanisms in alcoholism. *Science, 236,* 410–416.

Collier-Phillips, W. C. (1992). *Alcohol and hypertension: A lifestyle connection.* Unpublished manuscript, University of Washington, Seattle, WA.

Connors, G. J., & Maisto, S. A. (1988). The alcohol expectancy construct: Overview and clinical applications. *Cognitive Therapy and Research, 12,* 487–504.

Cooney, N. L., Gillespie, R. A., Baker, L. H., & Kaplan, R. F. (1987). Cognitive changes after alcohol cue exposure. *Journal of Consulting and Clinical Psychology, 55,* 150–155.

Cummings, C., Gordon, J. R., & Marlatt, G. A. (1980). Relapse: Strategies of prevention and prediction. In W. R. Miller (Ed.), *The addictive behaviors: Treatment of alcoholism, drug abuse, smoking and obesity* (pp. 291–321). Oxford, UK: Pergamon.

Curry, S., Marlatt, G. A., & Gordon, J. R. (1987). Abstinence violation effect: Validation of an attributional construct with smoking cessation. *Journal of Consulting and Clinical Psychology, 55,* 145–149.

Daley, D. C. (1989). A psychoeducational approach to relapse prevention. *Journal of Chemical Dependency Treatment, 2*(2), 105–124.

Donovan, D. M., & Marlatt, G. A. (Eds.). (1988). *Assessment of addictive behaviors.* New York: Guilford.

Forsberg, L. K., & Goldman, M. S. (1987). Experience-dependent recovery of cognitive deficits in alcoholics: Extended transfer of training. *Journal of Abnormal Psychology, 96*(4), 345–353.

George, W. H. (1989). Marlatt and Gordon's relapse prevention model: A cognitive–behavioral approach to understanding and preventing relapse. *Journal of Chemical Dependency Treatment, 2*(2), 125–152.

George, W. H., & Marlatt, G. A. (1983). Alcoholism: The evolution of a behavioral perspective. In M. Galanter (Ed.), *Recent developments in alcoholism,* (Vol. 1, pp. 105–138). New York: Plenum Press.

Goodwin, D. W. (1990). Genetic determinants of reinforcement from alcohol. In W. M. Cox (Ed.), *Why people drink* (pp. 37–50). New York: Gardner.

Graham, S. (1992). "Most of the subjects were white and middle class": Trends in published research on African Americans in selected APA journals, 1970–1989. *American Psychologist, 47,* 629–639.

Harper, F. D. (1983). Alcohol use and alcoholism among Black Americans: A review. In T. D. Watts & R. Wright, Jr. (Eds.), *Black alcoholism: Toward a comprehensive understanding.* Springfield, IL: Thomas.

Hover, S. J., & Gaffney, L. R. (1988). Factors associated with smoking behavior in adolescent girls. *Addictive Behaviors, 13,* 139–145.

Laws, R. (1989). *Relapse prevention with sex offenders.* New York: Guilford.

Loberg, T., Miller, W. R., Nathan, P. E., & Marlatt, G. A. (Eds.). (1989). *Addictive behaviors: Prevention and early intervention.* Amsterdam: Swets & Zeitlinger.

Marlatt, G. A. (1990). Cue exposure and relapse prevention in the treatment of addictive behaviors. *Addictive Behaviors, 15,* 395–399.

Marlatt, G. A. (1992). Substance abuse: Implications of a biopsychosocial model for prevention, treatment, and relapse prevention. In J. Grabowski & G. R. VandenBos (Eds.), *Psychopharmacology: Basic mechanisms and applied intervention* (pp. 127–162). Washington, DC: American Psychological Association.

Marlatt, G. A., & Barrett, K. (1994). Relapse prevention in the treatment of substance abuse. In M. Galanter & H. D. Kleber (Eds.), *The treatment of substance abuse* (pp. 285–299). New York: American Psychiatric Press.

Marlatt, G. A., & Gordon, J. R. (1985). *Relapse prevention.* New York: Guilford.

Marlatt, G. A., & Rohsenow, D. R. (1980). Cognitive processes in alcohol use: Expectancy and the balanced placebo design. In N. K. Mello (Ed.), *Advances in substance abuse* (vol. 1, pp. 159–199). Greenwich, CT: JAI Press.

Murphy, T. J., Pagano, R. R., & Marlatt, G. A. (1986). Lifestyle modification with heavy alcohol drinkers: Effects of aerobic exercise and meditation. *Addictive Behaviors, 11,* 175–186.

Newlin, D. B., & Thompson, J. B. (1991). Chronic tolerance and sensitization to alcohol in sons of alcoholics. *Alcoholism: Clinical and Experimental Research, 15,* 399–405.

Oetting, E. R., & Beauvais, F. (1987). Common elements in youth drug abuse: Peer clusters and other psychosocial factors. *Journal of Drug Issues, 17,* 133–151.

Parsons, O. A. (1989). Impairment in sober alcoholics' cognitive functioning: The search for determinants. In T. Loberg, W. R. Miller, P. E. Nathan, & G. A. Marlatt, (Eds.), *Addictive behaviors: Prevention and early intervention* (pp. 101–116). Amsterdam: Swets & Zeitlinger.

Robbins, C., & Clayton, R. R. (1989). Gender-related differences in psychoactive drug use among older adults. *Journal of Drug Issues, 19,* 207–219.

Rohsenow, D. J., & Marlatt, G. A. (1981). The balanced placebo design: Methodological considerations. *Addictive Behaviors, 6,* 107–122.

Sandberg, G. G., & Marlatt, G. A. (1989). Relapse fantasies. In R. Laws, (Ed.), *Relapse prevention with sex offenders* (pp. 147–151). New York: Guilford.

Stein, J. A., Newcomb, M. D., & Bentler, P. M. (1987). An 8-year study of multiple influences on drug use and drug use consequences. *Journal of Personality and Social Psychology, 53,* 1094–1105.

Wallace, B. C. (1991). *Crack cocaine: A practical treatment approach for the chemically dependent.* New York: Brunner/Mazel.

Watts, T. D., & Wright, R., Jr. (Eds.). (1983). *Black alcoholism: Toward a comprehensive understandings.* Springfield, IL: Thomas.

Webster's II: New Riverside University Dictionary. (1984). New York: Riverside.

Weibel-Orlando, J. (1987). Culture-specific treatment modalities: Assessing client-to-treatment fit in Indian alcoholism programs. In W. M. Cox (Ed.), *Treatment and prevention of alcohol problems: A resource manual* (pp. 261–283). Orlando, FL: Academic Press.

Weiner, H. D., Wallen, M. C., & Zankowski, G. L. (1990). Culture and social class as intervening variables in relapse prevention with chemically dependent women. *Journal of Psychoactive Drugs, 22*(2), 239–248.

Zackon, F. N. (1989). Relapse and "re-joyment": Observations and reflections. *Journal of Chemical Dependency Treatment, 2*(2), 67–77.

III
REHABILITATION

17

Toward an Integrative Diathesis–Stress Model of Chronic Pain

Robert D. Kerns and Mary Casey Jacob

INTRODUCTION

The devastating problem of chronic pain exemplifies the need for innovation in conceptualizing health problems and the importance of developing alternative health-care delivery systems. First, there is probably no greater source of stress and human suffering than the experience of pain. Researchers have estimated that one third of Americans suffer from persistent and recurrent pain (Bonica, 1981) with 35 million people suffering from low back pain alone (Bonica, 1980). In a survey of subscribers to a large community health maintenance organization, Von Korff, Dworkin, LeResche, and Kruger (1988) reported that 41% had suffered low back pain in the last 6 months. In the same sample, 26% had recurrent headaches, 18% reported abdominal pain, 12% had chest pain, and 12% had facial pain. The economic costs of chronic pain are equally staggering due to both direct health-care costs, including the purchase of prescribed and over-the-counter medications, and the indirect financial burden of underemployment, lost productivity, and disability compensation. As one example, Stone (1984) estimated the lifetime economic costs of rheumatoid arthritis to exceed $20,000 per patient in 1977 dollars!

Traditional difficulties in defining pain and categorizing clinical pain problems

---

Robert D. Kerns • Psychology Service, West Haven Veterans Administration Medical Center, and Departments of Psychiatry, Neurology, and Psychology, Yale University, West Haven, Connecticut 06516. **Mary Casey Jacob** • Departments of Psychiatry (Psychology), and Obstetrics and Gynecology, University of Connecticut Health Center, Farmington, Connecticut 06030.

Handbook of Health and Rehabilitation Psychology, edited by Anthony J. Goreczny. Plenum Press, New York, 1995.

further contribute to the need for alternative perspectives. "Somatic" models of pain that hypothesize a relatively linear, one-to-one relationship between structural tissue damage and pain intensity remain as the primary neurophysiological theories of pain (Mountcastle, 1974). These models, although important in outlining basic somatic sensory processes, are inadequate because lay phenomenology of the experience of pain and common anecdotes acknowledge the apparent influence of a range of psychological and environmental variables. Among these variables are personality attributes (Timmerans & Sternbach, 1974), attentional focus (Beers & Karoly, 1979; McCaul & Malott, 1984), the relevance of cognitive appraisal and coping (Jensen, Turner, Romano, & Karoly, 1991; Turk & Rudy, 1986), affective state (Haythornthwaite, Seiber, & Kerns, 1991; Sachem, Dar, & Cleeland, 1984), and gender and age (Kashima & McCreary, 1987; Melding, 1992). In the case of chronic pain, somatic models are also unsatisfactory because of the exclusion of frequent concomitant clinical and social problems, including depression, alcohol, and substance abuse (Atkinson, Slater, Patterson, Grant, & Garfin, 1991), marital and family dysfunction (Flor, Turk, & Scholz, 1987; Thomas & Roy, 1989), and unemployment and underemployment (Gervais, Dupuis, Veronneau, Bergeron, Millette, & Avard, 1991), as well as other factors.

A National Institutes of Health Consensus Report (1986) titled "An Integrative Approach to the Management of Pain" strongly supported what many clinicians and researchers have come to know: The complexity and multidimensional nature of most clinical pain problems require an integrative theoretical perspective, a broadband approach to assessment, and the development of comprehensive, interdisciplinary, and individually tailored plans for its management. Despite continued lack of agreement on such central issues as what pain is or how it is best measured, there is increasing appreciation of the far-reaching impact of the experience of chronic pain and the need to apply intervention strategies that focus on the *patient* with persistent pain rather than on the problem of *pain, per se* (Fordyce, 1988). The thoughtful and creative integration of alternative, but compatible, viewpoints now permeates both the empirical and clinical realms. The expanding availability of interdisciplinary pain management programs and services and increasing evidence of meaningful clinical outcomes are evidence that such integration is having a substantial impact (Flor, Fydrich, & Turk, 1992).

THEORIES OF CHRONIC PAIN

A central question in the field concerns the etiology of persistent or chronic pain; that is, what are the primary contributors to the perpetuation of the painful experience? Corollaries of this question relate to the frequent development of functional disability (Turk & Rudy, 1991) and associated symptoms of affective distress, particularly depression (Romano & Turner, 1985), among individuals who experience chronic pain. In the following section, we briefly describe several of the most frequently cited models of chronic pain and provide a summary of the evidence that supports these models.

Peripheral Neural Mechanisms

The perspective clinicians most frequently imply in the assessment and treatment of chronic pain is one that emphasizes the role of continued nociception at the site of structural pathology. Continued nociception may relate to a progressive and deteriorating disease process (e.g., osteoarthritis, painful neuropathy), residual pathology following trauma or surgery, or an unresolved acute disease process (postherpetic neuralgia). This model most closely represents historical sensory models of pain, acute or chronic. Researchers are beginning to better understand basic peripheral neural mechanisms of nociception and the common classes of events mediating the relationship between tissue damage and nociceptive stimulation (Campbell et al., 1989). However, practitioners in the field of chronic pain have limited knowledge of peripheral mechanisms responsible for the perpetuation of chronic musculoskeletal pain, a condition that accounts for a relatively large proportion of chronic pain problems (Simons & Travell, 1989).

Efforts to identify the source of peripheral nociception and treat the underlying pathology continue as the primary goal of most physicians. The inadequacy of clinical efforts limited by this perspective is well established, however (Flor & Turk, 1984; White & Sweet, 1969). These shortcomings apparently relate to the lack of reliable relationships between evidence of structural pathology and either pain or impairment (e.g., Boden, Davis, Dina, Patronis, & Wiesel, 1990). Ultimately, reliance on a peripheral model of chronic pain is unsatisfactory because of its failure to consider the more complex role of central mechanisms in the experience of pain.

Central Models

In its simplest form, a centralist view of chronic pain emphasizes the roles that the central nervous system and psychological factors play in the modulation, or in the case of chronic pain, the perpetuation, of peripheral nociception. Generally speaking, these models incorporate a role of peripheral nociception but emphasize the role that central factors play in determining the extent of pain, disability, and distress. Central models range from those that are primarily neurophysiological or neurochemical to those that are distinctly psychological or behavioral.

Gate Control Theory of Pain

One particularly comprehensive central model, known as the "gate control theory" of pain (Melzack & Wall, 1965), has provided heuristic value in fostering a multidimensional perspective of chronic pain. Melzack and Wall postulated a neural gating system in the dorsal horn of the spinal cord, the section of the spinal cord that receives afferent impulses from the peripheral nervous system. According to the model, inhibitory mechanisms within the central nervous system are brought to bear on the functioning of the "gate," thus acting to modulate the pain experience. These impulses primarily travel along descending pathways from the brain and exert their inhibitory influence at the spinal cord level. Although researchers have criticized the postulated physiological and anatomical bases of gate-control theory (Kerr, 1975; Nathan, 1976), researchers have amassed substantial support for the multidimensional perspective represented by this model (E. Hilgard & J. Hilgard, 1975).

Neurotransmitter Models

At the level of brain neurochemistry, considerable evidence now links endogenous opioids to nociception; low opioid levels may predispose one to exhibit low pain thresholds (Noel & Nemeroff, 1988). Similarly, researchers have shown that brain monoamines also play an important role in pain perception (Cain, Nemeroff, Banki, France, & Krishnan, 1988; Gershon, 1986). However, it remains unclear how these transmitter systems either alone, or in concert, influence the development of a chronic pain problem. Hypothesized roles of these neurotransmitters in the regulation of emotion and motivation provide one possible clue (e.g., Burger & Nemeroff, 1987; DeLeon-Jones, 1982). Sternbach (1976), for example, hypothesized that persistent pain depletes brain serotonin, and that low serotonin turnover leads to a hypersensitivity to both pain and depression. In support of this widely examined serotonergic hypothesis, several investigators have found that drugs that block serotonin reuptake are sometimes effective in the treatment of chronic pain (e.g., Goodkin & Guillion, 1989; Goodman & Charney, 1985). To date, however, there are few testable hypotheses about the relationships between these neurochemical systems and chronic pain and limited empirical data available that offer support to these hypotheses (Kraemer, Kerns, & Robohm, 1992).

Personality Models

Several primarily psychological models of chronic pain have proposed that internalization of negative affect and depression is a significant etiological factor in chronic pain. Engel (1959) described pain-prone patients as individuals who protect themselves from frank depression through the experience of pain as a alternative psychic mechanism. Blumer and Heilbronn (1982) proposed that chronic pain is best characterized as a variant of depressive disease. These authors cite a broad range of clinical, psychodynamic, biographical, and genetic features of chronic pain patients to support their hypothesis. According to the model, chronic pain patients without a clear somatic basis for their pain manifest a muted depressive state, or masked depression, that is similar psychobiologically to other patients with depressive disorder. Although the model has considerable intuitive and clinical appeal, the hypothesis has only limited empirical support, and some authors have critically challenged the basic premise of the model (Turk & Salovey, 1984).

Beutler, Engle, Oro'-Beutler, Daldrup, and Meredith (1986) proposed that chronic pain develops as a function of a pervasive inability to express intense negative emotions. This tendency, according to Beutler, leads to suppression of immune and endogenous opioid functioning and, in the face of acute nociception, leads to the development of chronic pain. Recent studies provide empirical support for a relationship between experiences of anger and anger inhibition and pain intensity among chronic pain patients (Kerns, Rosenberg, & Jacob, 1994).

Operant/Behavioral Model

As early as 1968, Wilbert Fordyce (Fordyce, Fowler, & DeLateur, 1968) proposed that chronic pain is a behavioral disorder in which a set of observable "pain behaviors" serve as the primary identifying criteria. These behaviors include excessive time spent reclining, excessive use of pain medication, verbal complaints of pain, and protective behaviors, such as limping and bracing. Fordyce (1976) suggested that, although patients express these behaviors in direct relationship to acute pain, over time, as a function of social contingencies (e.g., attention from family members, escape from aversive work situations), environmental consequences rather than structural pathology and continued nociceptive stimulation maintain the pain behaviors. Fordyce and his colleagues have provided the initial demonstrations regarding the efficacy of an intervention that applied behavioral strategies to alter environmental consequences of pain (Fordyce et al., 1968; Fordyce et al., 1973). These reports documented dramatic recoveries in previously treatment-refractory chronic pain patients. A well-controlled outcome study supported these initial findings (Turner & Clancy, 1988).

Cognitive–Behavioral Model

Theorists extended and elaborated on Fordyce's operant model by incorporating cognitive–social learning theory and cognitive–behavioral intervention perspectives (Hanson & Gerber, 1990; Turk, Meichenbaum, & Genest, 1983). Additionally, Turk and his colleagues have encouraged an integrative biobehavioral model of persistent pain and disability (Turk & Rudy, 1991). Of central importance in the model is the dynamic role that patients' idiosyncratic beliefs, attitudes, and coping resources play in determining pain, disability, and distress. Turk suggests that patients' maladaptive appraisals of their situation and their personal efficacy directly contribute to the persistence of the pain experience. Within this perspective, cognitive appraisal and developing beliefs interact with environmental (e.g., social responses) and biomedical (e.g., structural pathology and nociception) factors in contributing to a range of negative outcomes common among chronic pain patients. These negative effects hypothetically contribute to additional dysfunctional cognition that, through a dynamic and cyclical process, further extend the pain experience over time (Turk & Rudy, 1991). Evaluations of the efficacy of treatment efforts based on the cognitive–behavioral perspective have produced encouraging results (Kerns, Turk, Holzman, & Rudy, 1986; Turner, 1982; Turner & Clancy, 1988). Keefe, Dunsmore, and Burnett (1992) provided an updated review that highlights some of the recent advances as well as future clinical and research directions from behavioral and cognitive–behavioral perspectives of chronic pain.

An Integrative Diathesis–Stress Model of Chronic Pain

Despite the presence of multiple explanatory models for the development of chronic pain, there are surprisingly few empirically derived data to directly support any of them. For example, there has yet to appear a substantial theory-driven longitudinal study with direct etiological implications. Furthermore, despite the increasingly widespread acceptance of the multidimensional nature of the pain experience, theorists have not provided a model of the development of chronic pain that takes into account an integration of contemporary neurobiological and psychosocial perspectives.

Karoly (1985) emphasized that, in the case of chronic pain, researchers and clinicians need to view the *context* of the pain experience as the primary unit of inquiry or investigation. This context includes both peripheral and central nervous system factors as well as a host of psychological and social variables that interact with one another to determine the experience of chronic pain. It is important to recognize that this dynamic interaction has a temporal context as well. This context is explicit in psychodynamic models of the etiology of chronic pain that emphasize the role of those preexisting personality features that place individuals at risk for developing chronic pain. Most other models emphasize changes in neurobiological and psychosocial functioning that follow the onset of acute pain but continue over time and serve to perpetuate and extend the deleterious effects of the pain experience.

Despite a stated appreciation of this temporal context, most research in the area has been cross-sectional in design. Furthermore, participants in these studies are typically patients with chronic pain of several years' duration. It is true that these studies contribute to a growing body of knowledge about neurobiological and psychosocial *correlates* of the experience of chronic pain as well as the *relationships* among these variables. Researchers have postulated causal inferences about the role of neurobiological and psychosocial variables and their interrelationships as support for one or more of the explanatory models of chronic pain described previously. Unfortunately, with few exceptions, investigators have failed to demonstrate an appreciation of the historical context in which their observations occur and therefore interpret their data largely on the basis of speculation and unsubstantiated theory. For example, recent research has identified reliable relationships between chronic pain and psychological variables, such as maladaptive cognitive coping (Jensen et al., 1991) and depression and affective distress (Haythornthwaite et al., 1991), as well as neurobiological variables, such as low serotonin turnover (Magni et al., 1987). However, in these studies it is unclear whether the identified problems or deficits occur secondary to the experience of chronic pain or precede and possibly contribute to the development of the disorder.

The concept that individuals who develop chronic pain have preexisting vulnerabilities placing them at risk for the development of the syndrome is not new. However, researchers and clinicians have not fully explicated or appreciated the complexity of this vulnerability across biological, psychological, and social domains, nor have scientists clarified the possible mechanisms by which these vulnerabilities become clinically manifest. Our current state of knowledge regarding chronic pain and the associated factors does, however, permit the development of a model that incorporates this concept of multiple possible vulnerabilities.

In addition to these multiple potential *vulnerabilities,* the experience of acute pain typically includes multiple *challenges* to the individual across the domains of biological, psychological, interpersonal, and social functioning. These include physical impairment, activation of central monoamine and endorphin systems, anxiety, and fear. It is reasonable to hypothesize that individuals in whom there is a congruence between a preexisting vulnerability to develop chronic pain and a specific challenge or stress represented by the pain problem may experience persistent pain, disability, and distress.

Researchers have proposed similar *diathesis–stress* models to account for observations involving the diagnoses of schizophrenia (Bleuler, 1963; Meehl, 1962; Rosenthal, 1963) and depression (Abramson, Metalsky, & Alloy, 1989; Monroe & Simons, 1991; Robins & Block, 1989). Those individuals interested in an integration or accommodation of both biogenetic and psychosocial models of the etiology of psychopathology favor such models. Central to these models, and the model of chronic pain proposed herein, is the notion that stress activates a diathesis resulting in the clinical manifestation of the vulnerability.

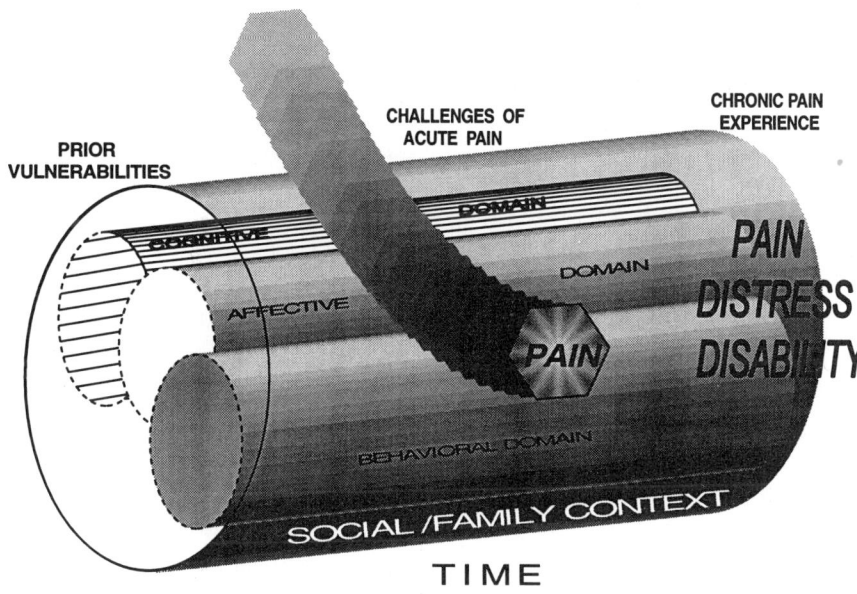

Figure 17.1. Schematic representation of the diathesis–stress model of chronic pain.

Further delineation of some of the preexisting vulnerabilities and the stressful or challenging aspects of the experience of acute nociception may help clarify this diathesis–stress model of chronic pain development. These factors represent several interrelated and broad domains, including cognitive, affective, behavioral, and family/social domains. Figure 17.1 schematically represents the proposed model.

The Cognitive Domain

Turk and his colleagues (Flor & Turk, 1988; Turk et al., 1983; Turk & Rudy, 1986) have emphasized the common cognitive challenges patients associate with the pain experience. The challenge to individuals' perceptions of control and efficacy with regard to their pain and their lives in general is salient. Perceptions of helplessness and hopelessness commonly result from the continued failure of personal efforts and from an inability of medical professionals to alleviate pain. These negative appraisals reinforce behavioral avoidance, declines in constructive coping and problem solving, and a growing negative affective experience, which, in turn, hypothetically extend secondary peripheral effects (e.g., muscle tension and atrophy; Ahern, Follick, Council, Laser-Wolston, & Litchman, 1988) and functional disability (Turk & Rudy, 1991).

According to Turk, this constellation of dysfunctional information processing and associated pervasive negative self-statements and beliefs underlies development of the chronic pain condition. However, it is clear that not all individuals with chronic pain manifest dysfunctional thinking. Turk's own work has identified a subclass of patients who seek treatment yet continue to report relatively high levels of perceived self-control; Turk labeled these individuals "adaptive copers" (Turk & Rudy, 1988, 1990). It is therefore incumbent on a plausible etiological model to account for these apparent individual differences. In addition, the model must accept the likelihood that other variables contribute to chronic pain development among other subsets of patients.

At least two possibilities exist to explain the variation in degree to which chronic pain patients manifest dysfunctional thinking. One possibility is that declines in perceptions of self-control occur in conjunction with a unique set of circumstances that only a subset of individuals who develop persistent pain experience. More appealing is a model that takes into account individual differences in information processing style, skill, and existing perceptions of personal control and efficacy prior to the onset of pain. Development of pain-specific perceptions of low self-control and personal mastery may have a higher probability of occurring among individuals with a preexisting negative style and deficient coping skills. These perceptions may even develop among individuals who had previously succeeded in multiple domains of their lives despite this preexisting "cognitive vulnerability." In these cases, the vulnerability only becomes manifest in the face of a specific set of challenges that tax the individuals' cognitive resources. Conversely, individuals with well-developed and flexible styles of coping may more likely face the challenges the pain experience represents with continued mastery and confidence. Thus, researchers in the area of chronic pain must consider alternative explanations for the continued pain experience among such individuals.

The Affective Domain

A second domain in which interactions between prior vulnerabilities and sequelae to pain may exist is the area of affective distress. In this domain, both depression and anxiety/fear may have potentially important roles in the maintenance of chronic pain, and they represent important coexisting clinical problems in their own right. In the case of depression, research has demonstrated a positive relationship with both pain intensity and pain behavior frequency (Keefe, Wilkins, Cook, Crisson, & Muhlbaier, 1986). Although depression appears to occur most frequently as a sequelae to the development of the pain problem (Atkinson et al., 1991; Brown, 1990), considerable evidence supports the possibility of a prior psychobiological or biogenetic vulnerability to depression among chronic pain patients (e.g., Blumer & Heilbronn, 1982).

One potential link between chronic pain and depression is the serotonin system. This brain neurotransmitter appears to have a significant role in affective disorders (DeLeon-Jones, 1982) and in pain perception (Gershon, 1986). Sternbach, Janowsky, Huey, and Segal (1976) hypothesized that pain depletes the level of available serotonin in the brain and that low serotonin then leads to a hypersensitivity to both chronic pain and depression. This challenge to serotonin regulation may activate a prior biogenetic vulnerability in the serotonin system. Both the noradrenergic system (Max et al., 1992) and the endogenous opiate systems (Ward, 1990) may respond in ways similar to the serotonergic system, or they may interact with one another in the etiology of these disorders.

Anxiety and fear of pain or further damage may play a significant role in the perpetuation of pain, functional impairment, and disability (Lethem, Slade, Troup, & Bentley, 1983; McCracken, Zayfert, & Gross, 1992). Laboratory analogue research has demonstrated that pain-related anxiety increases reports of pain intensity (Al Absi & Rokke, 1991; Weisenberg, Aviram, Wolf, & Raphaeli, 1984) and directs attention to pain (Arntz, Dreessen, & Merckelbach, 1991). Lethem et al. (1983) hypothesized that patients' fear of pain and further injury contributes to behavioral avoidance and increased pain behavior. Within a diathesis–stress framework, one would hypothesize that pain-related anxiety and its deleterious effects are more likely to occur among individuals who experience trait anxiety (Spielberger, Gorsuch, & Luschene, 1970) and have an avoidant style of problem solving (Heppner & Peterson, 1982) as preexisting characteristics.

The Behavioral Domain

Also characteristic of chronic pain patients are declines in functional activity, including work-related, avocational, and social/recreational activities. Such declines may directly relate to structural pathology and neurologically associated impairments. Less direct contributors to activity declines may include fear of pain and further physical harm, social reinforcement of the "sick role," and medication side effects. Researchers have hypothesized that behavioral inhibition and associated deconditioning effects contribute to the perpetuation of pain and disability in several ways. Within a behavioral perspective, broad declines in instrumental behavior and associated decreases in social reinforcement may increase the salience of social reinforcement contingent upon demonstrations of pain, thus further increasing the frequency of pain behaviors. From a psychophysiological perspective, deconditioning may increase musculoskeletal contributions to the pain experience. In addition, Kerns and colleagues have demonstrated that pain patients who manifest a low level of activity or a high degree of perceived interference of pain in the performance of functional activity are more likely to be depressed (Kerns & Haythornthwaite, 1988; Rudy, Kerns, & Turk, 1988).

Deficits in instrumental behavior may more likely occur among individuals with premorbid instrumental-skill deficits. These existing deficits may reduce the individual flexibility necessary to cope behaviorally with the challenges that structural pathology and related physical impairments present. Alternatively, individuals with a preexisting restricted repertoire of behaviors may suffer greater losses due to the limitations that follow the onset of pain. In either case, knowledge of patients' behavioral skill repertoires prior to the onset of pain may aid in understanding the reported changes in functioning that individuals associate with the chronic pain condition.

The Family/Social Domain

The proposed model places central importance on the social, and particularly the family, context of the pain experience. The model emphasizes the role of social interactions in mediating changes in cognitive, affective, and behavioral functioning that relate to the perpetuation of pain over time. The proposed primary mechanism by which the social context exerts its effects, either adaptive or maladaptive, is via instrumental learning. Within the model, social interactions play a direct role in the development of the deleterious effects and perpetuation of pain (e.g., reinforcement of pain behaviors and disability) and an indirect role by causing negative changes in functioning that result in additional negative effects (e.g., reinforcement of declines in activity that secondarily result in deconditioning and further muscle-tension-mediated peripheral nociception). Social interactions can have mixed effects, as in the case in which spousal support may inadvertently reinforce pain behaviors while exerting a moderating or buffering effect on the development of depression (e.g., Goldberg, Kerns, & Rosenberg, 1993). Finally, the effects of the social context may be specific (as in the examples provided earlier) or global (e.g., in the case of marital satisfaction or depression; Kerns & Turk, 1984).

As we already noted, the operant conditioning or behavioral model of the etiology of chronic pain emphasizes the role of social reinforcement or pain behaviors (Fordyce, 1976). A recent study supported this model by demonstrating statistical relationships between reported disability and observed solicitous spousal behavior that was contingent upon patients' demonstrations of pain (Romano et al., 1992). These data extend the findings of other researchers demonstrating relationships between perceived spousal response to pain and reports of pain, pain-behavior frequency, disability, and affective distress (Flor, Kerns, & Turk, 1987; Flor, Turk, & Rudy, 1989; Kerns, Haythornthwaite, Southwick, & Giller, 1990; Kerns et al., 1991). To date, however, no studies have examined the possible role of social interaction in the development or exacerbation of cognitive deficits that hypothetically contribute to chronic pain development.

In the case of social interaction, some researchers have hypothesized that pain-contingent reward is a powerful reinforcer of pain behaviors among patients that have an otherwise limited range of social reinforcement available to them (Goldberg et al., 1993; Kerns & Turk, 1984). Thus, preexisting deficits in instrumental skill and associated sources of social reward may place the individual at an increased vulnerability for the development of operantly based chronic pain. The model also suggests that acute pain and related challenge in one domain (e.g., social interaction) may activate a preexisting vulnerability in another domain (e.g., instrumental skill). There exist numerous interactive possibilities.

Chronic illness models must also consider the positive aspects of social interaction and support. According to the proposed diathesis–stress model, positive social support moderates the experience of pain and the likelihood of disability and distress. Continued support and encouragement of positive coping with pain and productive activity will hypothetically have broad positive effects. In a similar manner, relative strengths in any one domain may "buffer" or moderate the negative effects of prior vulnerabilities or challenges associated with another domain.

In summary, the diathesis–stress model of chronic pain integrates contemporary centralist perspectives on the etiology of chronic pain by suggesting that any of several important factors may contribute to the perpetuation of the pain experience. The model emphasizes the temporal and social contexts in which this development occurs. It elaborates on notions of preexisting vulnerabilities that place individuals at increased risk for chronic pain and associated disability and distress. The model is explicit in hypothesizing that these prior vulnerabilities may manifest in the face of specific challenges to the individual that the experience of acute pain poses. Specific vulnerabilities may become activated by either direct challenges (e.g., difficult personal problems resulting from acute pain and impairment in an individual who evidenced prior problem-solving skill deficits) or indirect effects (e.g., increased pain-contingent attention from the spouse in an individual with a prior restricted range of instrumental skill can activate the individual's specific vulnerabilities). Finally, the model emphasizes the likely moderating role of social support and other affective, behavioral, or cognitive strengths of the individual.

CLINICAL IMPLICATIONS

The concept that a rational theory should drive clinical decision making is most important. The proposed diathesis–stress model of chronic pain has several important specific implications. To the extent that available research has informed development of the model, it is not surprising that many of these implications are already largely in place in clinical practice.

The model encourages adoption of broadly conceived, multidimensional clinical program formats, particularly those that are multidisciplinary in their organization. The model encourages attention to possible sources of peripheral nociception, hence the active involvement of physicians, physical therapists, and others who can evaluate and treat the biomedical aspects of the problem. Experts who can focus on the neuropharmacological and psychosocial aspects of the problem are also critical team members. Ultimately, an evaluation and treatment plan that represents an integration of the perspectives of these professionals are the principle goals of the program.

The model encourages that the clinical team utilize a hypothesis-generation and testing approach. The model challenges clinicians to hypothesize possible mechanisms that contribute to the development and maintenance of the pain experience and associated clinical problems. These hypotheses further drive assessment and treatment efforts that, in turn, serve to test the working hypotheses.

Assessment efforts begin with a broadband approach that scans for both historical and current vulnerabilities and strengths across affective, behavioral, cognitive, and interpersonal domains (Kerns & Jacob, 1992). This process should become increasingly specific in order to identify possible targets for intervention.

Plans for intervention should be theory-driven and continue this hypothesis-testing approach. Clinicians need to develop broadly conceived and individualized plans for intervention that target multiple problem areas and consider preexisting vulnerabilities and strengths. Contemporary cognitive–behavioral (Turk et al., 1983) and self-management approaches (Hanson & Gerber, 1990) to the treatment of chronic pain are most consistent with the proposed diathesis–stress model. The model particularly encourages treatment that emphasizes the family and broader social context and the role of social interactions in the development and maintenance of pain and concurrent disability and distress. Aspects of interpersonal therapy approaches (Klerman, Weissman, Rounsaville, & Chevron, 1984) and cognitive–behavioral marital therapy (Fincham & Bradbury, 1990; Jacobson & Margolin, 1979) are particularly likely to help in the treatment process. Ongoing monitoring and evaluation of the intervention is critical in testing hypotheses about the underlying contributors to the chronic pain condition. Ideally, clinicians will incorporate long-term follow-up and opportunities for program reentry.

RESEARCH IMPLICATIONS

Ultimately it will be critical to conduct studies in which researchers longitudinally assess individuals at risk for the development of chronic pain until the research team identifies a large enough cohort of individuals who convert from a state of acute pain to chronic pain. From such a sample, the researchers can then attempt to identify variables that discriminate individuals who develop a chronic condition from those who do not. Recent work by Dworkin et al. (1992) and by Gervais and his colleagues (Gervais et al., 1991) represent steps in this direction. Unfortunately, a lack of theoretical clarity, not to mention the high cost of such studies, currently preclude the elaborate designs necessary to truly explore developmental and explanatory hypotheses.

In the short run, clinicians and researchers alike need to make efforts to retrospectively assess preexisting vulnerabilities as best they can. Interviews with family members may provide relatively reliable historical information of relevance. Investigators can then incorporate statistical control of important exogenous, prior vulnerabilities in tests of theory-based, longitudinal causal models. Although the ideal test is one that incorporates all aspects of the proposed model simultaneously, research efforts can also focus on more specific testing of discrete links or interactions that investigators hypothesize as contributing to the development of chronic pain, disability, and distress. For example, researchers who have examined the putative role of social interaction in the development of chronic pain have focused their attention on the behavioral/disability domain (e.g., Romano et al., 1992) and, to a lesser extent, depression (Kerns et al., 1991). The role of social interaction in the development of maladaptive cognition associated with chronic pain is an equally viable target for investigation.

Finally, collaborations between neurobiological and behavioral scientists are encouraged by the model. Genetic predispositions, such as to depression or alcohol abuse, are worthy of consideration. Investigations focused on possible interactions between the challenges of pain and impairment and such prior vulnerabilities would generate particularly productive information.

SUMMARY

Clinical and experimental work in the area of chronic pain increasingly demands theoretical refinement and integration. The proposed diathesis–stress model of chronic pain is an attempt to integrate contemporary social-learning-based models. In addition, the proposed model draws attention to possible preexisting vulnerabilities that place the individual at risk for the development of chronic pain, disability, and distress in the face of the challenges that ongoing nociceptive stimulation pose for pain patients. We hope that this formulation will encourage future refinements in the theory and stimulate theory-based investigation and the continued integration of science in the practice of pain management.

REFERENCES

Abramson, L. Y., Metalsky, G. I., & Alloy, L. B. (1989). Hopelessness depression: A theory-based subtype of depression. *Psychological Review, 96,* 358–372.

Ahern, D. K., Follick, M. J., Council, J. R., Laser-Wolston, N., & Litchman, H. (1988). Comparison of lumbar paravertebral EMG patterns in chronic low back pain. *Pain, 34,* 153–160.

Al Absi, M., & Rokke, P. D. (1991). Can anxiety help us tolerate pain? *Pain, 46,* 43–51.

Arntz, A., Dreessen, L., & Merckelbach, H. (1991). Attention, not anxiety, influences pain. *Behaviour Research and Therapy, 29,* 41–50.

Atkinson, J. H., Slater, M. A., Patterson, T. L., Grant, I., & Garfin, S. R. (1991). Prevalence, onset, and risk of psychiatric disorders in men with chronic low back pain: A controlled study. *Pain, 45,* 111–121.

Beers, T. M., & Karoly, P. (1979). Cognitive strategies, expectancy, and coping style in the control of pain. *Journal of Consulting and Clinical Psychology, 47,* 179–180.

Beutler, L. E., Engle, D., Oro'-Beutler, M. E., Daldrup, R., & Meredith, K. (1986). Inability to express intense affect: A common link between depression and pain? *Journal of Consulting and Clinical Psychology, 54,* 752–759.

Bleuler, M. (1963). Conception of schizophrenia within the last fifty years and today. *Proceedings of the Royal Society of Medicine, 56,* 945–952.

Blumer, D., & Heilbronn, M. (1982). Chronic pain and a variant of depressive disease: The pain-prone disorder. *Journal of Nervous and Mental Diseases, 170,* 381–394.

Boden, S. D., Davis, D. O., Dina, T. S., Patronis, N. J., & Wiesel, S. W. (1990). Abnormal magnetic-resonance scans of the lumbar spine in asymptomatic subjects. *The Journal of Bone and Joint Surgery, 72-A,* 403–408.

Bonica, J. J. (1980). Pain research and therapy: Past and current status and future needs. In L.K.Y. Ng & J. J. Bonica (Eds.), *Pain, discomfort, and humanitarian care* (pp. 1–46). New York: Elsevier.

Bonica, J. J. (1981). Preface. In L.K.Y. Ng (Ed.), *New approaches to treatment of chronic pain: A review of multidisciplinary pain clinics and pain centers* (pp. vii–x). Rockville, MD: Alcohol, Drug Abuse, & Mental Health Administration.

Brown, G. K. (1990). A causal analysis of chronic pain and depression. *Journal of Abnormal Psychology, 99,* 121–137.

Burger, P. A., & Nemeroff, C. B. (1987). Opioid peptides in affective disorders. In H. Y. Meltzer (Ed.), *Psychopharmacology: The third generation of progress* (pp. 636–646). New York: Raven.

Cain, S. T., Nemeroff, C. B., Banki, M. B., France, R. D., & Krishnan, K.R.R. (1988). Catecholamines and indolamines: Role in nociception and chronic pain. In R. D. France & K.R.R. Krishnan (Eds.), *Chronic pain* (pp. 42–53). Washington, DC: American Psychiatric Press.

Campbell, J. N., Raja, S. N., Cohen, R. H., Manning, D. C., Khan, A. A., & Meyer, R. A. (1989). Peripheral neural mechanisms of nociception. In P. D. Wall & R. Melzack (Eds.), *Textbook of pain* (pp. 22–45). New York: Churchill Livingstone.

DeLeon-Jones, F. A. (1982). Biochemical aspects of affective disorders. In E. R. Val, F. M. Gaviria, & J. A. Flaherty (Eds.), *Affective disorders: Psychopathology and treatment* (pp. 117–136). Chicago: Yearbook Medical Publishers.

Dworkin, R. H., Hartstein, G., Rosner, H. L., Walther, R. R., Sweeney, E. W., & Brand, L. (1992). A high-risk method for studying psychosocial antecedents of chronic pain: The prospective investigation of herpes zoster. *Journal of Abnormal Psychology, 101,* 200–205.

Engel, G. L. (1959). "Psychogenic" pain and the pain-prone patient. *American Journal of Medicine, 26,* 899–918.

Fincham, F. D., & Bradbury, T. N. (1990). *The psychology of marriage: Basic issues and applications.* New York: Guilford.

Flor, H., Fydrich, T., & Turk, D. C. (1992). Efficacy of multidisciplinary pain treatment centers: A meta-analytic review. *Pain, 49,* 221–230.

Flor, H., Kerns, R. D., & Turk, D. C. (1987). The perceived role of spouse reinforcement, perceived pain, and activity levels of chronic pain patients. *Journal of Psychosomatic Research, 31,* 251–259.

Flor, H., & Turk, D. C. (1984). Etiological theories and treatments for chronic low back pain: I. Somatic models and interventions. *Pain, 19,* 105–121.

Flor, H., & Turk, D. C. (1988). Chronic back pain and rheumatoid arthritis: Predicting pain and disability from cognitive variables. *Journal of Behavioral Medicine, 11,* 151–165.

Flor, H., Turk, D. C., & Rudy, T. E. (1989). Relationship of pain impact and significant other reinforcement of pain behaviors: The mediating role of gender, marital status and marital satisfaction. *Pain, 38,* 45–50.

Flor, H., Turk, D. C., & Scholz, O. B. (1987). Impact of chronic pain on the spouse: Marital, emotional and physical consequences. *Journal of Psychosomatic Research, 31,* 63–71.

Fordyce, W. E. (1976). *Behavioral methods for chronic pain and illness.* St. Louis, MO: Mosby.

Fordyce, W. E. (1988). Pain and suffering: A reappraisal. *American Psychologist, 43,* 276–283.

Fordyce, W. E., Fowler, R. S., & DeLateur, B. (1968). An application of behavior modification technique to a problem of chronic pain. *Behavior Research and Therapy, 6,* 105–107.

Fordyce, W. E., Fowler, R. S., Lehmann, J. F., DeLateur, B. J., Sand, P. L., & Trieschmann, R. B. (1973).

Operant conditioning in the treatment of chronic pain. *Archives of Physical Medicine and Rehabilitation, 54,* 399–408.

Gershon, S. (1986). Chronic pain: Hypothesized mechanism and rationale for treatment. *Neuropsychobiology, 15*(Suppl. 1), 22–27.

Gervais, S., Dupuis, G., Veronneau, F., Bergeron, Y., Millette, D., & Avard, J. (1991). Predictive model to determine cost/benefit of early detection and intervention in occupational low back pain. *Journal of Occupational Rehabilitation, 1,* 113–131.

Goldberg, G. M., Kerns, R. D., & Rosenberg, M. S. (1993). Pain relevant support as a buffer from depression among chronic pain patients low in instrumental activity. *Clinical Journal of Pain, 9,* 34–40.

Goodkin, K., & Gullion, C. M. (1989). Antidepressants for the relief of chronic pain: Do they work? *Annals of Behavioral Medicine, 11,* 83–101.

Goodman, W. K., & Charney, D. S. (1985). Therapeutic applications and mechanisms of action of monoamine oxidase inhibitor and heterocyclic antidepressant drugs. *Journal of Clinical Psychiatry, 46,* 6–22.

Hanson, R. W., & Gerber, K. E. (1990). *Coping with chronic pain: A guide to patient self-management.* New York: Guilford.

Haythornthwaite, J. A., Sieber, W. J., & Kerns, R. D. (1991). Depression and the chronic pain experience. *Pain, 46,* 177–184.

Heppner, P. P., & Peterson, C. H. (1982). The development and implications of a personal problem-solving inventory. *Journal of Counseling Psychology, 29,* 66–75.

Hilgard, E. R., & Hilgard, J. R. (1975). *Hypnosis in the relief of chronic pain.* Los Altos, CA: Kaufman.

Jacobson, N. S., & Margolin, G. (1979). *Marital therapy.* New York: Brunner/Mazel.

Jensen, M. P., Turner, J. A., Romano, J. M., & Karoly, P. (1991). Coping with chronic pain: A critical review of the literature. *Pain, 47,* 249–283.

Karoly, P. (1985). The assessment of pain: Concepts and procedures. In P. Karoly (Ed.), *Measurement strategies in health psychology* (pp. 461–515). New York: Wiley.

Kashima, K. J., & McCreary, C. P. (1987, August). *Sex differences in chronic low back pain patients.* Paper presented at the annual meeting of the American Psychological Association, New York, NY.

Keefe, F. J., Dunsmore, J., & Burnett, R. (1992). Behavioral and cognitive–behavioral approaches to chronic pain: Recent advances and future directions. *Journal of Consulting and Clinical Psychology, 60,* 528–536.

Keefe, F. J., Wilkins, R. H., Cook, W. A., Jr., Crisson, J. E., & Muhlbaier, L. H. (1986). Depression, pain, and pain behavior. *Journal of Consulting and Clinical Psychology, 54,* 665–669.

Kerns, R. D., & Haythornthwaite, J. (1988). Depression among chronic pain patients: Cognitive–behavioral analysis and effect on rehabilitation outcome. *Journal of Consulting and Clinical Psychology, 56,* 870–876.

Kerns, R. D., Haythornthwaite, J., Southwick, S., & Giller, E. L., Jr. (1990). The role of marital interaction in chronic pain and depressive symptom severity. *Journal of Psychosomatic Research, 34,* 401–408.

Kerns, R. D., & Jacob, M. C. (1992). Assessment of the psychosocial context in the experience of chronic pain. In D. C. Turk & R. Melzack (Eds.), *Handbook of pain assessment* (pp. 235–256). New York: Guilford.

Kerns, R. D., Rosenberg, R., & Jacob, M. C. (1994). Anger expression and chronic pain. *Journal of Behavioral Medicine, 17,* 57–67.

Kerns, R. D., Southwick, S., Giller, E. L., Haythornthwaite, J., Jacob, M. C., & Rosenberg, R. (1991). The relationship between reports of pain-related social interactions and expressions of pain and affective distress. *Behavior Therapy, 22,* 101–111.

Kerns, R. D., & Turk, D. C. (1984). Depression, marital satisfaction, and perceived support among chronic pain patients and their spouses. *Journal of Marriage and the Family, 46,* 845–852.

Kerns, R. D., Turk, D. C., Holzman, A. D., & Rudy, T. E. (1986). Comparison of cognitive–behavioral and behavioral approaches to the outpatient treatment of chronic pain. *Clinical Journal of Pain, 1,* 195–203.

Kerr, F.W.L. (1975). Pain: A central inhibitory balance theory. *Mayo Clinic Proceedings, 50,* 685–690.

Klerman, G., Weissman, M., Rounsaville, B., & Chevron, E. (1984). *Interpersonal psychotherapy of depression.* New York: Basic Books.

Kraemer, D. T., Kerns, R. D., & Robohm, J. (1992). Chronic pain and depression: A literature review of biological data. Unpublished manuscript.

Lethem, J., Slade, P. D., Troup, J.D.G., & Bentley, G. (1983). Outline of a fear-avoidance model of exaggerated pain perception—I. *Behavior Research and Therapy, 21,* 401–408.

Magni, G., Andreoli, F., Arduino, C., Arsie, D., Ceccherelli, F., Ambrosio, F., & Eandi, M. (1987). Modifications of 3H-imipramine binding sites in platelets of chronic pain patients treated with mianserin. *Pain, 30,* 311–320.

Max, M. B., Lynch, S. A., Muir, J., Shoaf, S. E., Smoller, B., & Dubner, R. (1992). Effects of desipramine, amitriptyline, and fluoxetine on pain in diabetic neuropathy. *New England Journal of Medicine, 326,* 1250–1256.

McCaul, K. D., & Malott, J. M. (1984). Distraction and coping with pain. *Psychological Bulletin, 95,* 516–533.

McCracken, L. M., Zayfert, C., & Gross, R. T. (1992). The Pain Anxiety Symptoms Scale: Development and validation of a scale to measure fear of pain. *Pain, 50,* 67–73.

Meehl, P. E. (1962). Schizotaxia, schizotypy, schizophrenia. *American Psychologist, 17,* 827–838.

Melding, P. S. (1992, January/February). Psychosocial aspects of chronic pain and the elderly. *IASP Newsletter,* pp. 2–4.

Melzack, R., & Wall, P. D. (1965). Pain mechanisms: A new theory. *Science, 50,* 971–979.

Monroe, S. M., & Simons, A. D. (1991). Diathesis–stress theories in the context of life stress research: Implications for the depressive disorders. *Psychological Bulletin, 110,* 406–425.

Mountcastle, V. B. (Ed.). (1974). *Medical physiology.* St. Louis, MO: Mosby.

Nathan, P. W. (1976). The gate-control theory of pain: A critical review. *Brain, 99,* 123–158.

National Institutes of Health. (1986). An integrative approach to the management of pain. *Connecticut Medicine, 50,* 677–682.

Noel, M., & Nemeroff, C. B. (1988). Endogenous opiates in chronic pain. In R. D. France & K.R.R. Krishnan (Eds.), *Chronic pain* (pp. 54–65). Washington, DC: American Psychiatric Press.

Robins, C. J., & Block, P. (1989). Cognitive theories of depression viewed from a diathesis–stress perspective: Evaluations of the models of Beck and of Abramson, Seligman, and Teasdale. *Cognitive Therapy and Research, 13,* 297–313.

Romano, J. M., & Turner, J. A. (1985). Chronic pain and depression: Does the evidence support a relationship? *Psychological Bulletin, 97,* 18–34.

Romano, J. M., Turner, J. A., Friedman, L. S., Bulcroft, R. A., Jensen, M. P., Hops, H., & Wright, S. F. (1992). Sequential analysis of chronic pain behaviors and spouse responses. *Journal of Consulting and Clinical Psychology, 60,* 777–782.

Rosenthal, D. (1963). A suggested conceptual framework. In D. Rosenthal (Ed.), *The Genain quadruplets* (pp. 505–516). New York: Basic Books.

Rudy, T. E., Kerns, R. D., & Turk, D. C. (1988). Chronic pain and depression: Toward a cognitive–behavioral mediation model. *Pain, 35,* 129–140.

Sachem, S., Dar, R., & Cleeland, C. S. (1984). The relationship of mood state to the severity of clinical pain. *Pain, 18,* 187–197.

Simons, D. G., & Travell, J. G. (1989). Myofascial pain syndromes. In R. D. Wall & R. Melzack (Eds.), *Textbook of pain* (2nd ed., pp. 368–385). New York: Churchill Livingstone.

Spielberger, C., Gorsuch, R., & Luchene, R. (1970). *STAI: Manual for the State–Trait Anxiety Inventory.* Palo Alto, CA: Consulting Psychologists Press.

Sternbach, R. A. (1976). The need for an animal model of pain. *Pain, 2,* 2–4.

Sternbach, R. A., Janowsky, D. S., Huey, L. Y., & Segal, D. S. (1976). Effects of altering brain serotonin activity on human chronic pain. In J. J. Bonica & D. G. Albe-Fessard (Eds.), *Advances in pain research and therapy. Vol. I, Proceedings of the First World Congress on Pain* (pp. 601–606). New York: Raven Press.

Stone, C. E. (1984). The lifetime economic costs of rheumatoid arthritis. *Journal of Rheumatology, 11,* 819–827.

Thomas, M., & Roy, R. (1989). Pain patients and marital relations. *Clinical Journal of Pain, 5,* 255–259.

Timmerans, G., & Sternbach, R. A. (1974). Factors of human chronic pain: An analysis of personality and pain reaction variables. *Science, 184,* 806–808.

Turk, D. C., Meichenbaum, D., & Genest, M. (1983). *Pain and behavioral medicine: A cognitive–behavioral perspective.* New York: Guilford.

Turk, D. C., & Rudy, T. E. (1986). Assessment of cognitive factors in chronic pain: A worthwhile enterprise? *Journal of Consulting and Clinical Psychology, 54,* 760–768.

Turk, D. C., & Rudy, T. E. (1988). Toward an empirically derived taxonomy of chronic pain patients: Integration of psychological assessment data. *Journal of Consulting and Clinical Psychology, 56,* 233–238.

Turk, D. C., & Rudy, T. E. (1990). The robustness of an empirically derived taxonomy of chronic pain patients. *Pain, 43,* 27–35.

Turk, D. C., & Rudy, T. E. (1991). Neglected topics in the treatment of chronic pain patients—Relapse, noncompliance, and adherence enhancement. *Pain, 44,* 5–28.

Turk, D. C., & Salovey, P. (1984). Chronic pain as a variant of depressive disease: A critical reappraisal. *Journal of Nervous and Mental Disease, 172,* 1–7.

Turner, J. A. (1982). Comparison of group progressive-relaxation training and cognitive–behavioral group therapy for chronic low back pain. *Journal of Consulting and Clinical Psychology, 50,* 757–765.

Turner, J. A., & Clancy, S. (1988). Comparison of operant–behavioral and cognitive–behavioral group treatment for chronic low back pain. *Journal of Consulting and Clinical Psychology, 56,* 261–266.

Von Korff, M., Dworkin, S. F., LeResche, L., & Kruger, A. (1988). An epidemiologic comparison of pain complaints. *Pain, 32,* 173–183.

Ward, N. G. (1990). Pain and depression. In J. J. Bonica (Ed.), *The management of pain* (Vol. 1, pp. 310–319). Philadelphia: Lea & Febiger.

Weisenberg, M., Aviram, D., Wolf, Y., & Raphael, I. N. (1984). Relevant and irrelevant anxiety in the reaction to pain. *Pain, 20,* 371–385.

White, J. C., & Sweet, W. H. (1969). *Pain and the neurosurgeon: A forty-year experience.* Springfield, IL: Thomas.

18

Spinal Cord Injury

Allen W. Heinemann

INTRODUCTION

Spinal cord injury resulting in permanent paralysis and loss of sensation may appear to many individuals as one of the most devastating experiences imaginable. Emptying one's bladder with a catheter, using a wheelchair, having difficulty entering one's home and public buildings, being unable to participate in enjoyed activities, and disrupted sexual expression may seem to the outsider a life not worth living. Yet the experience of most persons who live with spinal cord injury (SCI) is quite different. Advances in acute care and rehabilitation practices have reduced morbidity and mortality dramatically over the past 10 years (Brown, 1992; DeVivo, Stover, & Black, 1992). People who sustain SCI do live independent and fulfilling lives. The process by which they deal with disability-related limitations and attain a meaningful quality of life is the focus of this chapter.

This chapter summarizes recent advances in our understanding of psychological and social aspects of SCI. In doing so, it reviews theoretical formulations of how SCI affects people, examines research evidence, and explores implications for psychological interventions. This chapter also provides a context for integrating psychological and social theory by first reviewing current data on quality of life and community reintegration following SCI.

QUALITY OF LIFE AND COMMUNITY REINTEGRATION

Although enhanced quality of life as a goal of rehabilitation has emerged as an important topic (Anderson, 1982; Crewe, 1980), few studies have examined this

---

Allen W. Heinemann • Department of Physical Medicine and Rehabilitation, Northwestern University Medical School, and Rehabilitation Institute of Chicago, Chicago, Illinois 60657.
Handbook of Health and Rehabilitation Psychology, edited by Anthony J. Goreczny. Plenum Press, New York, 1995.

subject explicitly. One source of information related to this topic is the National Spinal Cord Injury Statistical Center, which maintains a database on persons nationwide who have received care from the model SCI care system. DeVivo and Richards (1992) reported information on residence, employment, and marital status from this database. They reported that almost everyone (94%) who completes rehabilitation returns to a private residence; 10 years after rehabilitation, 98% of persons with SCI who completed rehabilitation reside in a private residence. As in the able-bodied population, nursing home residence is more likely for persons with SCI as they age. While less than 2% of persons between 16 and 30 years of age reside in nursing homes, 22% of those over age 75 do so. Competitive employment for individuals 16 to 59 years of age increases from 13% two years after injury to 38% twelve years after injury. Employment rates relate to specific demographic factors. Employment is more likely for persons who are male, white, and have employment histories prior to injury. In addition, relative to unemployed persons with SCI, individuals with a SCI who are employed are likely to be younger and have greater education, higher motivation, and greater functional ability. Disincentives to employment include disability payments and health insurance that are available only to those with low incomes. Krause (1992) reported similar results for individuals receiving outpatient services at a urology clinic. Employed persons are more likely than unemployed persons to be younger and have paraplegia, to have sustained injuries longer ago, and to have completed more years of education. A separate analysis of this sample (Krause, 1990) found that employed individuals reported higher levels of overall adjustment compared with unemployed individuals, whereas those working in unpaid productive activities reported intermediate levels of satisfaction. Injury level was not related to level of productivity, but persons with quadriplegia spent fewer hours working per week than their nonquadriplegic cohorts. Time elapsed since injury related to productivity, with employed persons having the longest period of disability (15 years) followed by unemployed persons (14 years) and patients who remain productive but unemployed (12 years).

SCI affects the opportunity for marriage among single persons. Only 12% of never-married persons with SCI marry within 5 years of injury, whereas the expected rate of marriage for able-bodied peers is nearly three times the rate of persons with SCI. The impact of SCI on marriage is smaller. Five years after SCI, 81% of married persons remained married, whereas the comparable rate for able-bodied individuals is 88%. Finally, 56% of postinjury marriages continued for 8 years compared to an expected rate of 77% in demographically similar, able-bodied adults. Divorce rates are higher for individuals who are relatively young, females, African-Americans, and those who are nonambulatory, have no children or a history of prior divorce.

Quality of life also reflects the extent to which one is able to direct or independently carry out activities of daily living. Yarkony, Roth, Heinemann, Lovell, and Wu (1988) described the functional status of persons discharged from a model SCI care system over 3 years after rehabilitation. They reported that patients attain a relatively independent level of functioning in self-care and ambulation that they usually maintain or improve. Level of injury (quadriplegia vs. paraplegia) and completeness of lesion (partial vs. total paralysis and sensory loss) relate to independent functioning in an expected manner: Persons with incomplete lesions and those with paraplegia require less assistance.

A national survey of 719 community-dwelling veterans with SCI also provides information on quality of life (Saltz, Eisenberg, Fillenbaum, & George, 1991). The investigators of this study collected information about impairment in five areas of functioning: social and economic resources, mental and physical health, and activities of daily living. They concluded that quality of life enjoyed by young and old veterans with SCIs is relatively good, and quality of life of older veterans with SCIs is better than for able-bodied men of a similar age. Disorders that limited activities of daily living include chronic pain, urinary tract disorders, and skin infections. The veterans group generally found the quality of medical and other services, which they primarily received from Veterans Administration hospitals, satisfactory.

Life satisfaction was the focus of a study (Krause & Dawis, 1992) in which 286 urology-clinic patients completed a questionnaire describing activities and satisfaction with specific life domains. The average age of the sample was 42 years; an average of 19 years elapsed from injury to study participation. Study participants completed the Multidimensional Personality Questionnaire from which measures of positive and negative affect and constraint derive. Persons who reported experiencing less emotional distress, less dependency (defined as family conflicts and lack of transportation, income, and control), fewer health problems, and greater positive affect also reported greater life satisfaction. Information gathered 4 years earlier also predicted current life satisfaction; persons who earlier reported higher levels of adjustment and activity level, fewer health problems, and less dependency reported greater general life satisfaction at the second time period. In contrast, dependency and employment were the best predictors of economic satisfaction both concurrently and from data collected 4 years earlier. Demographic characteristics did not relate to satisfaction. These results illustrate the distinct nature of satisfaction in general and economic-specific domains.

With this functional and community-living information providing a background, we are better able to ask what affects postinjury adjustment and identify the characteristics of persons who attain favorable outcomes.

THEORETICAL CONCEPTS IN SPINAL CORD INJURY ADJUSTMENT

SCI is a relatively low-incidence impairment with about 8 thousand people annually sustaining injury that results in permanent disability and a total population of 250 thousand persons with SCI in the United States (Stover & Fine, 1986). Consequently, investigators have developed few unique theoretical approaches specifically related to spinal injury. Instead, psychologists have, for the most part, borrowed theoretical models and approaches developed to explain health behaviors generally. Nonetheless, several recurring questions have focused on specific concerns of rehabilitation professionals in dealing with persons who sustain spinal cord injury. Trieschmann (1992) identified key clinical questions that emerge in light of life expectancies that approach those of able-bodied peers and increasing opportunities for employment and community living: "How do we teach people to cope more effectively with this disability?" (p. 58); "How can we facilitate better communication among professionals and people with SCI to enhance independent functioning within the hospital and community environment?" (p. 59); "What are the best methods of promoting wellness in the SCI community?" (p. 59); and "How do we teach coping skills to [persons with] new SCI with a history of alcohol and drug abuse?" (p. 60). Asking the right questions allows theory to relate usefully to experiences of individuals with SCI.

Early theorists drew on their clinical experience and tended to focus on patients' emotional responses immediately after injury and the life disruption following SCI. Implicit in these models were several questions: How do people cope with SCI-related limitations? Are there predictable stages by which persons with SCI attain adjustment? Is depression a necessary reaction to injury? What kinds of people attain favorable adjustment? Early reports on postinjury adjustment often focused on describing emotional consequences and psychopathological reactions (Hohmann, 1975; Mueller & Thompson, 1950; Shontz, 1965; Siller, 1969; Stewart, 1978). This focus reflected the fact that rehabilitation hospitalization could extend up to a year, life expectancies were relatively short, and community accommodation of persons with disabilities was uncommon.

Dembo, Leviton, and Wright (1956) described an early model of disability acceptance that has influenced thinking about spinal injury reactions, and Wright (1960, 1983) later elaborated on this model, which developed out of extensive interviews with veterans who sustained amputations. A model of value changes emerged by which the authors defined a concept they termed *disability acceptance*. From this model, the investigators identified several central value changes required of individuals with disabilities to perceive themselves in nondevaluing terms. These changes included enlarging their scope of values, containing disability effects, emphasizing self-evaluation with asset values rather than deriving self worth by comparing themselves with others, and subordinating the importance of physique and physical appearance. The authors based these concepts on Kurt Lewin's (1935) field-theoretical approach to personality and a focus on intrapsychic processes. However, the authors did not describe the process by which these value changes occur.

Trieschmann (1988) recently described an influential theoretical model of spinal injury adjustment. She based her model on the assumption that disability adjustment is synonymous with balance in life, and that persons are integral, mind–body systems. She described a systems model in which one's psychological resources, biological–organic state, and the environment determine behavior, health, and adjustment. Within this model, she defined rehabilitation as "the process of teaching people to live with their disability in their own environment" (p. 26). Rehabilitation, and hence life, is a dynamic process; hence, no specific end point of adjustment or rehabilitation is possible or desirable.

Shontz (1982) highlighted the apparent paradox that exists when an individual successfully completes psychological adaptation to an unchangeable condition, such as disability. The disability exists only when adaptation is in process, yet outsiders still react to visible signs of disability and often treat the person as having a handicap even when adaptation is complete. Extending Dembo's (1969) distinction between insiders (those with a condition) and outsiders, Shontz argues that from the perspective of individuals who have successfully dealt with chronic illness or disability, they no longer adapt to illness or disability because the condition no longer exists. Instead,

> Like everyone else, they adapt to the full array of possibilities and limitations that are afforded by the complete panorama of their biological states and their social and physical environments. . . . The question [for psychology] is how they come to satisfactory and satisfying terms with the same world in which everyone lives. (p. 155)

Like Trieschmann, he proposed that signs of psychological adjustment are no different for people with disabilities than for anyone else. Implicit in this perspective is that clinicians and researchers need no special psychology of disability. Instead, satisfactory adaptation is evident when disability is no longer the dominant issue in a person's life space. The next section examines models that describe how this adaptive process occurs.

MODELS OF ADAPTATION

The belief that persons sustaining SCI experience a more or less predictable sequence of reactions to less accompanying injury has appeared at length in the rehabilitation literature (Dunn, 1975; Gunther, 1969; Kerr, 1961). George Hohmann's (1975) experiences dealing with SCI—his description of denial, withdrawal, hostility, and reactions against dependence—parallel those of writers who describe reactions to terminal illness and other health crises (Kubler-Ross, 1969; Parkes, 1972). The possibility of sequential phases of adaptation has had an allure for rehabilitation professionals. For example, investigators have described intervention plans for nurses based on anticipated patient reactions (French & Phillips, 1991).

Fink (1967) described one model with heuristic value, on which Shontz (1965) later elaborated. This model describes a disability, such as SCI, as a crisis-inducing event that results in four stages of adjustment: shock, defensive retreat, acknowledgment, and adaptation. Investigators have focused several studies on examination of the consequences of progressing, or failing to progress, through these hypothesized stages. One early researcher (Dinardo, 1971) found that persons who experienced depression after SCI attained poorer long-term adjustment, whereas denial of depression associated with better adjustment. Kalb (1971) highlighted the importance of socioeconomic factors, revealing that income was associated with depression, cooperation during hospitalization, and long-term adjustment. However, for middle-income men, cooperation with nurses did not predict rehabilitation success, and depression did not relate to outcome. For low-income men, denial of depression appeared to work best. Neither of these early studies found evidence to support a process model of adaptation.

Researchers have criticized stage models of adjustment for their lack of empirical evidence (Trieschmann, 1988) and for failing to account for variability in individuals' responses to life disruption (Silver & Wortman, 1980). For example, one would expect that time since injury would be a crude marker of the adjustment process. Krause and Crewe (1991) examined the effects of age, time since injury, and time of measurement on post-SCI adjustment. Two groups of subjects, recruited in 1974 and 1985 from patients seeking services at a renal clinic, entered one of five cohorts, based on age and time since injury. The group, originally recruited in 1974, underwent assessment again in 1985; both groups averaged about 10 years postinjury. Indices of activity, medical stability, adjustment, interpersonal satisfaction, and economic satisfaction derived from a Life Satisfaction Questionnaire. They found that the nature of SCI-related changes depended on the nature of adjustment considered. Activities more strongly related with chronological age, whereas medical problems more strongly related to time since injury. Both age and time since injury related to psychological indices of adjustment, such as life satisfaction and self-rated adjustment. Older persons, relative to younger persons in the study, reported less activity, as measured by sitting tolerance and frequency of leaving one's home, and older persons also reported less rewarding lives, as measured by number of weekly visitors, satisfaction with sex life, and self-rated adjustment. However, older individuals indicated they found their living arrangements and employment more satisfactory and worked more hours per week than younger persons in the study. Time since injury related to enhanced psychological functioning, measured by satisfaction with living arrangements and employment, self-rated adjustment, number of hours working per week, and medical adjustment. These findings suggest that age and time since injury work in opposite directions. Persons injured at younger ages not only have greater opportunity to deal with consequences of injury, but they may also be dealing with different developmental issues in their lives. These results illustrate the outcomes of a developmental process, the phases or turning points of which are not yet clear.

Antonak and Livneh (1991) approached the issue of disability adaptation from a developmental perspective in which acceptance of changes to body, self, and social interactions gradually occur. They reported evidence for a hierarchy of reactions to disability. Using an ordering-theoretical data analysis procedure on a sample of 118 adults who sustained disabilities an average of 8 years earlier, the investigators found support for a nonlinear, multidimensional process. In addition to SCI patients, the sample included persons who sustained stroke, myocardial infarction, amputation, sensory impairment, and degenerative conditions. The investigators used the Reactions to Impairment and Disability Inventory to assess 8 emotional states: shock, anxiety, denial, depression, internalized anger, externalized hostility, acknowledgment, and adjustment. A pattern of nonlinear, empirical contingencies emerged among this set of reactions in which 5 of the 6 nonadapted responses were prerequisites for the 2 adapted responses (acknowledgment and adjustment). Anxiety, depression, internalized anger, and externalized hostility were prerequisite to adaptation. However, there was considerable variability in the sequence of these reactions. These results are consistent with the observation that people sometimes regress to earlier phases or bypass phases because of their life situations or capacities to cope effectively. The experience of shock was a prerequisite of depression and internalized anger, which, in turn, were prerequisites of acknowledgment and adaptation. Only denial was independent of the two sets of reactions. This result is consistent with Wright's (1983) position that years may pass before a person is able to realize the full implications of a disability. This model allows persons to acknowledge a disability without attaining full adjustment. The statistical method in this study is noteworthy because it allows researchers to examine contingent relationships in a cross-sectional design.

Heinemann and Shontz (1984, 1985) conducted a personological investigation of emotional and cognitive experiences following SCI to illustrate another approach to understanding adaptation. They studied two carefully selected persons as a means of evaluating a process model of adaptation. The goal of this representative case study was to determine the extent to which adjustment proceeds in a sequential fashion and the extent to which adjustment follows patterns that are characteristic of the individual before injury. Both persons were 24 years old and had sustained quadriplegia as the result of traumatic injuries more than 2 years prior to the study. The subjects were similar in socioeconomic (middle-income), religious (Roman Catholic), and educational (postbaccalaureate) backgrounds. They differed in terms of gender, the extent to which they were the perpetrator (hang-gliding crash) or victim (passenger in an auto crash), and previously established coping style (emotionally expressive vs. reserved).

The study participants completed several nomothetic measures of intelligence, depression, disability acceptance, and personality. Idiographic measures included Kelly's (1955) Role Repertory Technique to identify personal constructs related to disability acceptance and a Q-sort designed to tap stages of reaction to crisis (Fink, 1967). The investigators used a modification of Flanagan's (1954) Critical Incident Technique to obtain course-of-life landmarks before and after injury.

The two participants provided strikingly different data. One participant, Deirdre, provided data that supported a model of sequential emotional reactions and value changes, while the other participant, Craig, did not. Deirdre reported experiencing a period of depression prior to adjustment, although the sequence of stages was not in the expected order. Instead, her reactions strongly related to external events in her family and rehabilitation. In contrast, Craig, who had attempted suicide earlier as a self-reported means of restoring control over his life, never consciously mourned his loss but, instead, quickly assumed a position of doing the best he could. Congruence with preinjury coping styles was apparent in both cases: Deirdre used intellectualizing, fantasy, and obsessive patterns of thinking as mechanisms to cope with stress; and Craig avoided introspection and attempted to master his body and physical environment. Both achieved academic success despite their different pattern of adjustment, disability-related value changes, and coping styles.

Deirdre's readiness to mourn her lost abilities provides a notable contrast with Craig's tendency to focus on physical values and tackle rehabilitation tasks without attending to his emotional reactions. No single, common underlying process of adjustment was illustrated by these two cases. Instead, they illustrate two different solutions to life problems that seem similar because of similar impairment. These results show that symbolic integration of loss was more complete in the person who experienced a sequence of reactions than in the person who did not. Who experiences injury, the meaning of the loss, the person's established means of dealing with life disruption, and the context within which the person undergoes rehabilitation and community reentry affect the way persons experience emotional and behavioral reactions.

Adopting a developmental perspective that considers life course before SCI, identity established before injury, and commitments made, allows us to understand how SCI affects psychological well-being. More recently, reports have focused on effective problem-solving and coping strategies, the role of social support in enhancing adjustment, the value of caregiver roles and peer support, substance abuse as a maladaptive coping strategy, and quality of life. The next sections cover these topics.

APPLICATIONS OF STRESS AND COPING MODELS

Several clinicians have used the cognitive–phenomenological perspective of Lazarus and Folkman (1984) to describe the experiences of persons undergoing rehabilitation. Stress and coping theory allows us to view adverse life events as experiences that tax adaptive resources, threaten well-being, and place individuals at risk for stress-related dysfunction and psychopathology.

One set of investigators applied social–psychological theory to understand adjustment of persons with SCI. Bulman and Wortman (1977) examined the short-term adjustment of 29 persons with SCI during initial rehabilitation hospitalization. They found that persons who blamed themselves for causing their injury and perceived the injury as unavoidable coped better with disability as rated by rehabilitation staff. All subjects had questioned why the injury occurred, and all but one developed answers to explain why. A need for meaning was implicit in this process. Although criticized for small sample size, use of staff-rated coping and an outsider's perspective of problem-selection and interpretation (Shontz, 1982), this study illuminates what may be a universal process when misfortune occurs: the attempt to ascribe meaning to the event. This study did not find better outcomes associated with specific types of meaning. Instead, many persons whom staff voted as coping effectively provided several different meanings.

Nielson and MacDonald (1988) reported on the longer term relationship between self-blame and adjustment. In a sample of community residents, they found results quite different from those of Bulman and Wortman: self-blame was negatively associated with adjustment, sociability, pessimism, hostility, and dysphoria. Furthermore, they found that perceiving injury as avoidable positively related to coping and adjustment. They concluded that self-blame is maladaptive after community reentry.

Heinemann, Bulka, and Smetak (1988) conducted a replication and extension of these studies with a sample of 52 community residents with quadriplegia. Although these subjects were similar to Bulman and Wortman's sample in terms of age at injury, gender, and injury etiology, subjects from the Heinemann et al. study completed more years of education and employment. In addition, both groups reported equivalent levels of self-blame, perceived avoidability, and present happiness, but subjects in the Bulman and Wortman study rated SCI significantly more negatively. Greater disability acceptance related to younger age, greater time since injury, and absence of maladaptive coping efforts, such as drinking. Like Bulman and Wortman's sample, nearly all (94%) had asked themselves why their injuries occurred; in contrast, 65% of those asking the question reported no specific answer. Neither specific attributions for injury nor satisfaction with the answer related to greater disability acceptance. However, perceiving some good as coming from injury positively related to disability acceptance. This study also provided support for the notion that adaptation is a developmental process evincing a relationship between time since injury and disability acceptance; greater time since injury related to stronger endorsement of the value changes described by Wright (1983). Although self-blame and specific attributions for injury may be adaptive shortly after injury, they do not appear to serve this function with greater time. The passage of time appears to allow people to reframe their experience of injury and disability in ways that promote greater self-valuation. Whereas the question "Why me?" is compelling shortly after injury and some reasonably satisfactory answer appears to be important, it is the resolution of the question that allows persons to redirect psychological energy to the external world, relationships, and important goals.

Researchers have also explored the effects of individual differences in coping styles on psychological distress and depression in order to clarify the process by which adaptation occurs. Frank et al. (1987) used cluster analysis to identify two subgroups of persons with recent SCI based on scores from the Ways of Coping

Checklist and the Millon Health Locus-of-Control Scale. One subgroup more strongly endorsed all coping factors and relied less on internal attributions of beliefs than did the second subgroup. They also differed on measures of depression, negative life events, and general distress. The first group experienced higher (although not clinically significant) depression, more negative life stress, and more negative life events in the previous year. Persons in the two subgroups did not differ in terms of level of injury, age, time since injury, or positive life stressors during the past year. Although the cross-sectional nature of this study does not allow identification of causal relationships, the authors speculate that coping efforts of persons in the first subgroup were less effective. The authors interpreted their results to suggest that an external health locus of control relates to greater distress and depression and that external events may be important in affecting mood and attributional styles. Consistent with Wright's emphasis on value changes that allow positive self-valuation, Frank and associates support the clinical practice of helping people with SCI come to value their internal resources.

The same group of investigators also reported a relationship between coping styles and psychological distress in 57 inpatients with SCI who were undergoing rehabilitation a median of 3.6 months after injury (Buckelew, Baumstark, Frank, & Hewett, 1990). In this cross-sectional study, only 26% of the sample reported high levels of distress as measured by the Symptom Checklist (T-score greater than 70). When divided into three, equal-sized groups defined by distress level, individuals experiencing high distress also reported they were more likely to use coping strategies that included self-blame, wish-fulfilling fantasy, emotional expression, and threat minimization relative to persons with moderate and low levels of distress. Groups of patients defined by SCL scores did not differ on age, time since injury, gender, level of injury, or marital status. However, self-blame strongly correlated with distress, suggesting this coping strategy is maladaptive. Correlational analyses involving time since injury did not provide evidence in support of a developmental process of adaptation. These results built on a related study (Frank & Elliott, 1987) in which psychological distress as measured by the SCL related to life events independent of time since injury. This study demonstrated that external events can disrupt an individual's well-being whether injuries occurred recently or in the more distant past. The authors note that frequent use of coping strategies is not necessarily a successful means of managing psychological distress and may instead reflect characteristic (and ineffective) efforts to deal with stress.

It is clear that external factors, such as rehabilitation practices, affect well-being above and beyond the effect of cognitive and affective processes. Buckelew, Hanson, and Frank (1991) explored the effects of developmental factors and changes in rehabilitation practices on psychological well-being. They compared two samples of 53 persons who sustained SCI between 1981 and 1982 or between 1984 and 1986 and averaged 3.6 and 1.7 years postinjury, respectively. Dependent measures included measures of health locus of control and psychological distress. Age and time since injury did not relate to health beliefs or psychological distress. However, the group with more recent injuries reported more anxiety, phobic anxiety, psychoticism, and hostility than the first group. Shorter lengths of stay and earlier transfers to rehabilitation also distinguished the groups. This study illustrates important consequences of rehabilitation practices that reflect recent efforts to contain health-care costs. In such an economic climate, the questions of who experiences greater levels of well-being, how adaptation proceeds, and how clinicians can support adaptation attain even more importance.

SOCIAL SUPPORT AND ADJUSTMENT

Research and clinical interest regarding the effect of social support on adjustment after SCI has increased parallel to theoretical developments in this field. Overlapping and unclear definitions of social support have limited understanding in this area of inquiry, beginning with Cobb's (1976) landmark article that described the benefits of social support. However, investigators have attempted to define and clarify the concept of social support. Barrera (1986) contributed to conceptual clarity by distinguishing between social embeddedness, perceived social support, and enacted support as three major categories of social support. Sarason, Shearin, Pierce, and Sarason (1987) concluded that, despite distinctions between support concepts, most measures of social support assess a sense of feeling accepted, loved, and involved in relationships where open communication exists.

Cohen and Wills (1985) reviewed studies that evaluated two hypothesized mechanisms through which social support benefits health: (1) global benefits of support and (2) social support as a buffer against the impact of stressful life events. They concluded that empirical evidence supports both models. Heller, Swindle, and Dusenbury (1986) noted that the way social ties provide health-protective effects are unclear even though many studies demonstrate a correlation between social support and physical and psychological outcomes. Broadhead and associates (1983) summarized social support and health relationships. They noted 11 characteristics of social support, including temporal, strength, consistency, and dynamics of social support. They reviewed evidence that poor social support precedes adverse psychological outcomes; consistently relates to outcomes across various groups defined by age, sex, racial, ethnic, and illness characteristics; and is dependent on life events.

Schulz and Decker (1985) examined the effects of social support on long-term adjustment of persons with SCI in a cross-sectional study. They studied 100 middle-aged and older community residents who average 20-years postinjury. They found level of self-reported well-being was only slightly lower than that of nondisabled peers. High levels of social support, satisfaction with social contacts, and perceived control over one's well-being related to higher levels of well-being after statistically controlling for health and income. In contrast to Bulman and Wortman's (1977) results in which self-blame and staff-rated coping strongly correlated, Schulz and Decker found only a modest correlation between self-blame and life satisfaction. They interpreted their results by emphasizing that participants appeared to attain favorable self-perceptions by selectively focusing on attributes in which they had an advantage, by ascribing meaning to injury, and by defining standards of adjustment in which they could excel. This coping process illustrates how Wright's (1983) value changes that define disability acceptance can proceed. In Wright's terms, favorable coping was achieved by subordination of physique and employing asset values.

Rintala, Young, Hart, Clearman, and Fuhrer (1992) replicated and extended the work of Shulz and Decker by selecting a more representative community sample that over-sampled women and objectively measuring health status and secondary medical complications (e.g., urinary tract infections, pressure ulcers) that might affect well-being. The sample of 140 individuals averaged 10.6-years postinjury. Using Schulz and Decker's (1985) questionnaire, they found that greater levels of social support related to greater life satisfaction, better self-assessed physical health, and absence of urinary tract infections. Greater satisfaction with one's social support related to lower levels of depression and greater life satisfaction; however, the secondary medical complications did not relate to satisfaction with support. The association between social support and life satisfaction was about twice as strong for men as for women. The authors speculated about the mechanisms that underlie the correlation between physical health and social support; these mechanisms may include influence by significant others to engage in health maintenance activities, reduction of stress, or provision of goods or services by others that enhance health. Alternately, healthy persons may attract the support of others or be more likely to seek support from others.

Coca (1991) reported further evidence for a relationship between social support and long-term adjustment in a sample of 80 men who sustained injuries an average of 17 years prior to the study and who received outpatient services at a Veterans Administration hospital. Perceived social support from family and friends strongly associated with disability acceptance and psychological distress, such that persons perceiving greater support from family and friends reported greater disability acceptance and lower levels of psychological distress. Income and social support from friends were the best predictors of disability acceptance. Friends' support positively correlated with coping efforts that involved planful problem solving and seeking social support, whereas it negatively correlated with self-controlled coping efforts and escape/avoidance.

Elliott, Herrick, Witty, Godshall, and Spruell (1992) investigated the relationship between social support and depression in a sample of 182 patients who sustained their injuries an average of 8 years prior to the study. Persons who reported lower levels of depressive symptomatology also reported stronger support in the form of relationships that reassured self-worth and a sense of social integration. Time since injury related modestly to depression, such that persons with more recent injuries tended to report higher levels of depression. Time since injury did not relate to any of the social support measures. Although researchers need to conduct a longitudinal design to clarify causal relationships, available empirical results suggest that people who are able to solicit social support experience better mental health. One context in which some people socialize and experience social support involves drinking alcohol. The relationship between alcohol and other drug use and SCI is the focus of the next section.

SUBSTANCE ABUSE AND SPINAL CORD INJURY

Problems resulting from alcohol and other drug abuse provide another example of how issues in the mainstream of health psychology extend to persons with spinal cord injuries. The prevalence of substance abuse problems in persons who incur traumatic SCI has emerged as an important issue for psychologists in rehabilitation settings. Alcohol and other drug abuse contributes to onset of disability by increasing risk taking among intoxicated individuals, limits rehabilitation gains by impairing learning, and hampers rehabilitation outcomes by contributing to increased morbidity and mortality. This section describes our knowledge about (1) prevalence of alcohol and other drug use by individuals with SCI, (2) rate at which SCI persons obtain treatment for substance-use problems, (3) effects of substance use on rehabilitation, and (4) effects of alcohol and other drug use on rehabilitation outcome.

Prevalence of Alcohol and Other Drug Use

Several investigators have recognized intoxication as a frequent contributor to SCI onset. O'Donnell, Cooper, Gessner, Shehan, and Ashley (1981–1982) reported a 68% rate of self-reported alcohol use at SCI onset with 68% resuming drinking during hospitalization. Depending on site and sample, the rate of intoxication for persons incurring traumatic injury varies between 17% and 49% (Frisbie & Tun, 1984; Fullerton, Harvey, Klein, & Howell, 1981; Galbraith, Murray, Patel, & Knitt-Jones, 1976; Gale, Dikmen, Wyler, Temkin, & McClean, 1983; Heinemann, Goranson, Ginsburg, & Schnoll, 1989). Intoxication resulting in impaired judgment appears responsible for increased risk taking that results in many injuries.

Several studies have reported the prevalence of alcohol use and abuse following initial care for traumatic disability. Johnson (1985) reported that vocational rehabilitation and independent living center clients with SCI exhibited a rate of moderate or heavy drinking that was nearly twice the rate reported in the general population (46% vs. 25%), and the rate of alcoholic symptoms varies from 49% of individuals with recent SCI (Heinemann, Donohue, Keen, & Schnoll, 1988) to 62% of vocational rehabilitation facility clients (Rasmussen & DeBoer, 1980). However, one study of primarily older veterans with SCI highlighted age-related differences in drinking problems (Kirubakaran, Kumar, Powell, Tyler, & Armatas, 1986). This study revealed that alcohol and drug use among older veterans was less than the rate reported in the National Institute on Drug Abuse's National Household Survey (1988). These findings support the conclusion that age-related differences in rate of alcohol and other drug abuse among the able-bodied population also exist among persons with SCI.

One study examined prevalence of intoxication at injury onset among a sample of 88 cases admitted to an acute SCI center (Heinemann, Schnoll, Brandt, Maltz, & Keen, 1988). Serum ethanol greater than 50 mg/dl was present in 40% of the cases. Urinalysis also revealed evidence of other substance use, including cocaine (14%), cannabinoids (8%), benzodiazepines (5%), and opiates (4%). Overall, 35% of the sample had evidence of substances with abuse potential in their urine. A total of 62% had either serum ethanol greater than 50 mg/dl or a positive urinalysis. These results do not provide compelling evidence of chemical dependence because false-positive results may reflect occasional or low-dose use of substances with abuse potential.

Another recent study addressed chronicity of substance use by assessing histories of 103 persons with recent SCI (Heinemann et al., 1988). Inclusion criteria included age between 13 and 65 years at injury, absence of cognitive impairment that would limit self-report, injury within the past year, and ability to speak English. The mean age of the sample was 28 years; 75% were men. Lifetime exposure to and recent use of several substances with abuse potential were greater in this sample than for a like-age national sample. Compared with a national sample collected by the National Institute on Drug Abuse (NIDA, 1988), the SCI sample of 18- to 25-year-olds reported significantly greater exposure to amphetamines, marijuana, cocaine, and hallucinogens. This age group also reported recent use of alcohol, amphetamines, marijuana, cocaine, and hallucinogens at a rate significantly greater than a like-aged national sample. The SCI group that was 26 years of age and older reported significantly greater exposure to narcotic analgesics and tranquilizers than did the national sample. They also reported recent use of tobacco, alcohol, amphetamines, and marijuana that was at least 10 percentage points greater than the national sample. Finally, larger proportions of the SCI sample in the 18- to 25-year-old and 26 years and older groups reported greater recent use of 9 of 10 substance categories relative to the national sample.

Within the SCI sample, young adults (18- to 25-year-olds) reported greater recent use of marijuana before injury and greater cocaine exposure than the 26 years and older group. However, the 26 years and older group reported greater tobacco exposure than the 18- to 25-year-olds. Intoxication at time of injury was an important marker for prior substance use. Thirty-nine percent reported that, at the time of injury, they were under the influence of intoxicating substances. These persons were more likely than persons who denied such intoxication to report greater exposure to tobacco, amphetamines, marijuana, hallucinogens, tranquilizers, and sedatives, along with recent use of tobacco, alcohol, amphetamines, cocaine, and hallucinogens.

These results suggest that persons incurring SCI are more likely to use and abuse alcohol and other drugs than are persons in the general population. However, before classifying persons that incur SCI as probable drug abusers and further enhancing their stigma, several methodological considerations warrant discussion when interpreting these comparisons. Although the methodologies in both the Heinemann et al. (1988) study and the National Household Survey were essentially the same, minor differences in definitions of recent use require mention. For instance, NIDA's recent use of criteria of one or more times during the past month versus the Heinemann et al. criteria of three or more times during the past 6 months may not assess substance use in a comparable manner. Despite complications in interpreting the results, these findings highlight a previously undocumented fact: Substance use and abuse among SCI patients occurs frequently, may complicate the rehabilitation process, and may limit long-term outcomes and capacity for independent living.

Intoxication at SCI onset appears to be a marker of preinjury substance use, and thus, it is important to screen for substance abuse in persons who incur traumatic injury. Implications for clinicians are apparent because the lifetime exposure to and recent use of substances reported by this sample indicates that many persons with SCI are at risk for substance abuse. Studies that report a relationship between previous substance use and subsequent use of other drugs underscore such risk (Dembo, Blount, Schmeidler, & Burgos, 1985). Substance use is not necessarily substance abuse or dependence, nor does use necessarily result in specific problems. However, it is important to understand the context, expectancies, and motives for use. For example, substance use may be a means of reestablishing social relationships or managing stress, or it may represent escalating pattern of addiction. Clinicians need to take note of substance use and observe whether it relates to other problems. These results highlight the importance of assessing alcohol and drug-abuse–related problems so that clinicians identify and treat a potential dual disability in a timely fashion.

Other investigators have examined the possibility that intoxication at injury may relate to individual differences, such as sensation seeking. Mawson, Jacobs, Winchester, and Biundo (1988) reported that persons who scored high on a measure of sensation seeking were younger and more likely to be using substances at the time of injury. In contrast, Rohe and Basford (1989) found that only elevated MacAndrew Alcoholism Scale scores of the Minnesota Multiphasic Personality Inventory scale distinguished patients with positive blood alcohol concentrations from patients with negative blood alcohol concentrations and a normative sample. Further research needs to clarify this issue.

Treatment for Substance-Use Problems

One study also examined the rate of self-reported alcohol problems, perceived need for treatment, and receipt of treatment by persons with recent SCI (Heinemann, Doll, & Schnoll, 1989). Participants in this study reported alcohol-use information across three time periods: 6 months before injury, the first 6 months after injury, and the next 12 months after injury. Ninety-three percent of participants reported drinking on three or more occasions at one or more of the assessment periods whereas 71% reported experiencing one or more drinking problems across the three assessment periods. Of the entire sample, only 15% reported perceiving a need for treatment of alcohol abuse, and 11% actually received treatment. Postinjury alcohol abuse in persons who did not experience preinjury abuse appears to occur infrequently; 65% reported having had drinking problems before injury, whereas only 6% reported that drinking problems began after injury. Longer term follow-up needs to verify this impression because the researchers obtained data regarding participants for only 18 months. Even though the incidence of self-recognized alcohol problems may be low, the total number of persons affected by alcohol problems may be substantial. Routine assessment of substance abuse and provision of treatment services to persons with traumatic SCI may help prevent a potential dual disability.

Effects of Alcohol and Other Drug Use on the Rehabilitation Process

One study (Heinemann et al., 1989a) investigated a sample of persons with recent SCI to determine their activity patterns during an inpatient rehabilitation stay. They described their activities using the Activity Pattern Indicators time-line format during a structured interview. More drinking before injury and more family drinking problems predicted a greater number of drinking problems after injury. In turn, those who reported more drinking problems reported spending less time in quiet activities, such as sleeping and resting during rehabilitation, but more time in quiet recreation activities, such as watching television and reading. Of greatest concern, persons who drank more before injury spent less time in productive activities, such as rehabilitation therapies. These relationships are of concern because the often fast paced and increasingly short rehabilitation stays may limit rehabilitation outcomes. Although further study needs to determine consequences of drinking on long-term rehabilitation outcome, these results suggest that heavy preinjury drinking may relate to a constellation of psychological factors that impact rehabilitation adversely.

Effects of Substance Use on Rehabilitation Outcome

The ways that changes in employment, substance use, depression, and disability acceptance may relate were the subject of a study using a sample of community residents following SCI (Heinemann, Kiley, Schnoll, & Yarkony, 1989b). These persons each completed the Beck Depression Inventory and the Linkowski Acceptance of Disability Scale, and the investigators used Hollingshead and Redlich's Social Position Index (SPI, 1958) to code social status. Twenty-one percent of the sample worked at the same status as before injury; 16% had higher job status; 23% began gainful employment; 18% lost their jobs; and 22% remained unemployed. Use of diazepam (Valium), alcohol, marijuana, and cocaine was lower among employed persons. Persons who were unemployed at injury and later became employed, as well as individuals who evidenced an increase in SPI score between injury and interview reported greater disability acceptance than other groups. Finally, persons who used prescription medications, either as prescribed or in a nonprescribed manner, evidenced more depression and less acceptance of their disability than persons who did not use prescription medications. These results reveal substance use can affect long-term rehabilitation outcomes, even when the substances are medically sanctioned prescriptions. The clinical team needs to examine reasons underlying prescription use, whether for management of spasticity, chronic pain, or other problems. These are issues that rehabilitation and health psychologists can address as members of a team.

IMPLICATIONS FOR CLINICAL INTERVENTIONS

Rehabilitation and health psychologists are coming to realize that the literature does not support the expectation that persons with SCI will experience predictable emotional reactions in a specific sequence or develop clinical depression, and such expectations may be potentially harmful (Frank, Elliott, Corcoran, & Wonderlich, 1987). Even though the rate of suicide may be two to six times greater among persons with SCI than for able-bodied peers (Charlifue & Gerhart, 1991), specific characteristics appear to place people at risk. These characteristics include pre- and postinjury despondency, a sense of shame, apathy, hopelessness, family disruption before injury, alcohol abuse, active involvement in SCI etiology, and antisocial behavior. Based on a review of case histories, Judd and Brown (1992) added to this list schizoid, depressive, and narcissistic personality characteristics, postinjury depression, and having important others view death as a preferred option to living with SCI. Depression, particularly severe depression in which the person considers suicide, may be an understandable but maladaptive reaction to crisis. The psychological structure and life experiences of some individuals may place them at risk for negative reactions. Understanding these personal characteristics and the meaning individuals ascribe to the experience of injury is necessary before intervention. The observation that rehabilitation staff frequently overestimate the level of depression patients experience illustrates the importance of this approach (Cushman & Dijkers, 1990).

This appreciation for individual differences in adaptation following SCI is evident in Hammell's (1992) statement:

> The rehabilitation team will need to become more flexible in recognizing the heterogeneity of the life values of the individual.... The lifelong process of adjustment to disability and to interacting with society and the environment is not complete at discharge from an inpatient facility. Rather, this is when true adjustment and adaptation begins. (p. 324)

Livneh (1986) described intervention strategies that reflect sensitivity to individuals' experiences of coping with crisis. He proposed that timing of psychotherapeutic strategies (e.g., supportive, insight-oriented, cognitive, and behavioral) consider the experience and needs of clients.

In addition to psychological and social needs, substance abuse issues are often important during rehabilitation. Unfortunately, clinicians in rehabilitation settings have often overlooked these issues. This oversight results from staff who do not know how to recognize substance abuse problems and consequently are unlikely to intervene in a timely and effective manner and from rehabilitation programs that have not recognized substance abuse treatment as part of their mission. However, it is clear that early identification of persons with SCI who abuse or are dependent on substances should minimize incidence of secondary complications, decrease cost of rehabilitation, and improve rehabilitation outcome. Specific suggestions regarding assessment and management of substance abuse also emerge from this literature review. Assessment of alcohol use and alcoholism need to become a routine part of inpatient screenings in acute care and rehabilitation programs for persons incurring SCI. A variety of team members could assume responsibility for this screening, but, rehabilitation and health psychologists are in a unique position to appreciate the interplay of medical, functional, psychological, and social forces in a developmental context. Continuing education to recognize alcohol abuse may be necessary in order to allow these professionals to provide this assessment. Consultation with alcoholism and other drug-abuse treatment-program professionals may aid in the acquisition of such knowledge. Relationships with substance-abuse treatment providers are also necessary in order to address problems before patients develop dual disabilities. Establishing these links is likely to require educating substance-abuse treatment counselors about the special needs of individuals with SCI. Not only are disability-related issues, such as architectural accessibility and functional abilities, important to address, but so are attitudes toward individuals with disabling conditions, because such attitudes may limit program access. In larger communities, chemical-dependence treatment programs designed specifically for individuals with physical disabilities are another treatment alternative (Anderson, 1980–1981; Lowenthal & Anderson, 1980–1981; Sweeney & Foote, 1982).

SUMMARY

The process by which people make sense of a major life disruption, such as SCI, emerges as a critical concern for psychologists working in rehabilitation settings. Investigators originally described this in terms of a series of stages of emotional reactions. Theorists and clinicians differed in how they described the order and rigidity of this process. More recently, researchers have applied a stress-and-coping model and have studied the importance of social support in achieving successful outcomes. Making sense of injury is an early task in rehabilitation. "Why did this happen to me?" is a question many people ask themselves during and shortly after rehabilitation. Finding an answer appears to be important, although the particular attribution the person makes does not appear to be critical. In dealing with disability, it is helpful to regard the adaptive task as involving not just the specific functional and behavioral limitations resulting from impairment, but rather the full array of life options, some of which the disability may seem to have abridged. No best route to adaptation is evident in our current understanding of this process. In fact, respect for and sensitivity to individual differences has emerged as a key principle in helping people make sense of their experience. In addition, researchers have identified some barriers to long-term adjustment, such as handicapping attitudes, employment biases, lack of social support, and alcohol and other drug abuse. Research investigating means of enhancing the process by which persons with SCIs achieve favorable long-term adjustment is necessary in order to assist this population more effectively.

REFERENCES

Anderson, P. (1980–1981). Alcoholism and the spinal cord disabled: A model program. *Alcohol Health and Research World, 5,* 37–41.

Anderson, T. P. (1982). Quality of life of the individual with a disability. *Archives of Physical Medicine and Rehabilitation, 63,* 65.

Antonak, R. F., & Livneh, H. (1991). A hierarchy of reactions to disability. *International Journal of Rehabilitation Research, 14,* 13–24.

Barrera, M. (1986). Distinctions between social support concepts, measures and models. *American Journal of Community Psychology, 14,* 413–445.

Beck, A. (1967). *Depression: Causes and treatment.* Philadelphia: University of Pennsylvania Press.

Broadhead, W. E., Kaplan, B. H., James, S. A., Wagner, E. H., Schoenbach, V. J., Grimson, R., Heyden, S., Tibblin, G., & Gehlbach, S. H. (1983). The epidemiologic evidence for a relationship between social support and health. *American Journal of Epidemiology, 117,* 521–537.

Brown, D. J. (1992). Spinal cord injuries: The last decade and the next. *Paraplegia, 30,* 77–82.

Buckelew, S. P., Baumstark, K. E., Frank, R. G., & Hewett, J. E. (1990). Adjustment following spinal cord injury. *Rehabilitation Psychology, 35,* 101–109.

Buckelew, S. P., Frank, R. G., Elliott, T. R., Chaney, M. A., & Hewett, J. (1991). Adjustment to spinal cord injury: Stage theory revisited. *Paraplegia, 29,* 125–130.

Buckelew, S. P., Hanson, S., & Frank, R. G. (1991). Psychological factors and adjustment to spinal cord injury. *NeuroRehabilitation, 4,* 36–45.

Bulman, R., & Wortman, C. (1977). Attributions of blame and coping in the "real world": Severe accident victims react to their lot. *Journal of Personality and Social Psychology, 35,* 351–363.

Charlifue, S. W., & Gerhart, K. A. (1991). Behavioral and demographic predictors of suicide after traumatic spinal cord injury. *Archives of Physical Medicine and Rehabilitation, 72,* 488–492.

Cobb, S. (1976). Social support as a moderator of life stress. *Psychosomatic Medicine, 38,* 300–314.

Coca, B. (1991, August). *Coping, social support and acceptance of disability among persons with SCI.* Paper presented at the 99th Annual Convention of the American Psychological Association, San Francisco.

Cohen, S., & Wills, T. A. (1985). Stress, social support, and the buffering hypothesis. *Psychological Bulletin, 98,* 310–357.

Crewe, N. (1980). Quality of life: The ultimate goal in rehabilitation. *Minerva Medica, 63,* 586–589.

Cushman, L. A., & Dijkers, M. P. (1990). Depressed mood in spinal cord injured patients: Staff perceptions and patient realities. *Archives of Physical Medicine and Rehabilitation, 71,* 191–196.

Dembo, T. (1969). Rehabilitation psychology and its immediate future: A problem of utilization of psychological knowledge. *Rehabilitation Psychology (Psychological Aspects of Disability), 16,* 63–72.

Dembo, T., Blount, W., Schmeidler, J., & Burgos, W. (1985). Methodological and substantive issues involved in using the concept of risk in research into the etiology of drug use among adolescents. *Journal of Drug Issues, 4,* 537–553.

Dembo, T., Leviton, G., & Wright, B. A. (1956). Adjustment to misfortune: A problem in social–psychological rehabilitation. *Artificial Limbs, 3,* 4–62.

DeVivo, M. J., & Richards, J. S. (1992). Community reintegration and quality of life following spinal cord injury. *Paraplegia, 30,* 108–112.

DeVivo, M. J., Stover, S. L., & Black, K. J. (1992). Prognostic factors for 12-year survival after spinal cord injury. *Archives of Physical Medicine and Rehabilitation, 73,* 156–162.

Dinardo, G. (1971). Psychological adjustment to spinal cord injury. *Dissertation Abstracts International, 32,* 4206B–4207B.

Dunn, M. (1975). Psychological intervention in a spinal cord injury center: An introduction. *Rehabilitation Psychology, 22,* 165–178.

Elliott, T. R., Herrick, S. M., Witty, T. E., Godshall, F., & Spruell, M. (1992). Social support and depression following spinal cord injury. *Rehabilitation Psychology, 37,* 37–48.

Fink, S. (1967). Crisis and motivation: A theoretical model. *Archives of Physical Medicine and Rehabilitation, 48,* 592–597.

Flanagan, J. (1954). The critical incident technique. *Psychological Bulletin, 51,* 327–358.

Frank, R. G., & Elliott, T. R. (1987). Life stress and psychologic adjustment following spinal cord injury. *Archives of Physical Medicine and Rehabilitation, 68,* 344–347.

Frank, R. G., Elliott, T. R., Corcoran, J. R., & Wonderlich, S. A. (1987). Depression after spinal cord injury: Is it necessary? *Clinical Psychology Review, 7,* 611–630.

Frank, R. G., Umlauf, R. L., Wonderlich, S. A., Askanazi, G. S., Buckelew, S. P., & Elliott, T. R. (1987). Differences in coping styles among persons with spinal cord injury: A cluster-analytic approach. *Journal of Consulting and Clinical Psychology, 55,* 727–731.

French, J. K., & Phillips, J. A. (1991). Shattered images: Recovery for the SCI client. *Rehabilitation Nursing, 16,* 134–136.

Frisbie, J. H., & Tun, C. G. (1984). Drinking and spinal cord injury. *Journal of the American Paraplegia Society, 7,* 71–73.

Fullerton, D. T., Harvey, R. F., Klein, M. H., & Howell, T. (1981). Psychiatric disorders in patients with spinal cord injuries. *Archives of General Psychiatry, 38,* 1369–1371.

Galbraith, S., Murray, W. R., Patel, A. R., & Knitt-Jones, R. (1976). The relationship between alcohol and head injury and its effects on the conscious level. *British Journal of Surgery, 63,* 128–130.

Gale, J. L., Dikmen, S., Wyler, A., Temkin, N., & McClean, A. (1983). Head injury in the Pacific Northwest. *Neurosurgery, 12,* 487–491.

Gunther, M. (1969). Emotional aspects. In D. Ruge (Ed.), *Spinal cord injuries* (pp. 93–108). Springfield, IL: Thomas.

Hammel, K.R.W. (1992). Psychological and sociological theories concerning adjustment to traumatic spinal cord injury: The implications for rehabilitation. *Paraplegia, 30,* 317–326.

Heinemann, A. W., Bulka, M., & Smetak, S. (1988). Attributions and disability acceptance following traumatic injury: A replication and extension. *Rehabilitation Psychology, 33,* 195–206.

Heinemann, A. W., Doll, M., & Schnoll, S. (1989). Treatment of alcohol abuse in persons with recent spinal cord injuries. *Alcohol Health and Research World, 13,* 110–117.

Heinemann, A. W., Donohue, R., Keen, M., & Schnoll, S. (1988). Alcohol use by persons with recent spinal cord injuries. *Archives of Physical Medicine and Rehabilitation, 69,* 619–624.

Heinemann, A. W., Goranson, N., Ginsburg, K., & Schnoll, S. (1989a). Alcohol use and activity patterns following spinal cord injury. *Rehabilitation Psychology, 34,* 191–206.

Heinemann, A. W., Kiley, D., Schnoll, S., & Yarkony, G. (1989b, November). Effects of substance use on vocational outcome following spinal cord injury. Paper presented at American Congress of Rehabilitation Medicine, San Antonio, TX.

Heinemann, A. W., Schnoll, S., Brandt, M., Maltz, R., & Keen, M. (1988). Toxicology screening in acute spinal cord injury. *Alcoholism: Clinical and Experimental Research, 12,* 815–819.

Heinemann, A. W., & Shontz, F. C. (1984). Adjustment following disability: Representative case studies. *Rehabilitation Counseling Bulletin, 28,* 3–14.

Heinemann, A. W., & Shontz, F. C. (1985). Methods of studying persons. *The Counseling Psychologist, 13,* 111–125.

Heller, K., Swindle, R. W., & Dusenbury, L. (1986). Component social support processes: Comments and integration. *Journal of Consulting and Clinical Psychology, 54,* 466–470.

Hohmann, G. (1975). Psychological aspects of treatment and rehabilitation of the spinal injured person. *Clinical Orthopedics, 112,* 81–88.
Hollingshead, A., & Redlich, F. (1958). *Social class and mental illness.* New York: Wiley.
Johnson, D. C. (1985). *Alcohol use by persons with disabilities.* Madison: Wisconsin Department of Health and Social Services.
Judd, F. K., & Brown, D. J. (1992). Suicide following acute traumatic spinal cord injury. *Paraplegia, 30,* 173–177.
Kalb, M. (1971). An examination of the relationship between hospital ward behaviors and post-discharge behaviors in spinal cord injury patients. *Dissertation Abstracts International, 32,* 3005B–3006B.
Kelly, G. (1955). *A theory of personality: The psychology of personal constructs.* New York: Norton.
Kerr, N. (1961). Understanding the process of adjustment in disability. *Journal of Rehabilitation, 27,* 16–18.
Kirubakaran, V. R., Kumar, V. N., Powell, B. J., Tyler, A. J., & Armatas, P. J. (1986). Survey of alcohol and drug misuse in spinal cord injured veterans. *Journal of Studies on Alcohol, 47,* 223–227.
Krause, J. S. (1990). The relationship between productivity and adjustment following spinal cord injury. *Rehabilitation Counseling Bulletin, 33,* 188–199.
Krause, J. S. (1992). Employment after spinal cord injury. *Archives of Physical Medicine and Rehabilitation, 73,* 163–169.
Krause, J. S., & Crewe, N. M. (1991). Chronologic age, time since injury, and time of measurement: Effect on adjustment after spinal cord injury. *Archives of Physical Medicine and Rehabilitation, 72,* 91–100.
Krause, J. S., & Dawis, R. V. (1992). Prediction of life satisfaction after spinal cord injury. *Rehabilitation Psychology, 37,* 49–60.
Kübler-Ross, E. (1969). *On death and dying.* New York: Macmillan.
Lazarus, R., & Folkman, S. (1984). *Stress, appraisal and coping.* New York: Springer.
Lewin, K. (1935). *A dynamic theory of personality.* New York: McGraw-Hill.
Lindowski, G. (1971). A scale to measure acceptance of disability. *Rehabilitation Counseling Bulletin, 4,* 236–244.
Livneh, H. (1986). A unified approach to existing models of adaptation to disability: Part II—Intervention strategies. *Journal of Applied Rehabilitation Counseling, 17,* 6–10.
Lowenthal, A., & Anderson, P. (1980–1981). Network development: Linking the disabled community to alcoholism and drug abuse programs. *Alcohol Health and Research World, 5,* 16–19.
Mawson, A. R., Jacobs, K. W., Winchester, Y., & Biundo, J. J. (1988). Sensation-seeking and traumatic spinal cord injury: Case-control study. *Archives of Physical Medicine and Rehabilitation, 69,* 1039–1043.
National Institute on Drug Abuse. (1988). *National Household Survey on Drug Abuse: Main findings.* Rockville, MD: Author.
Nielson, W. R., & MacDonald, M. R. (1988). Attributions of blame and coping following spinal cord injury: Is self-blame adaptive? *Journal of Social and Clinical Psychology, 4,* 163–175.
Mueller, A., & Thompson, C. E. (1950). Personality problems of the spinal cord injured. *Journal of Consulting Psychology, 4,* 89–892.
O'Donnell, J. J., Cooper, J. E., Gessner, J. E., Shehan, I., & Ashley, J. (1981–1982). Alcohol, drugs and spinal cord injury. *Alcohol Health and Research World, 6,* 27–29.
Parkes, C. (1972). *Bereavement: Studies in grief in adult life.* New York: International Universities Press.
Rasmussen, G. A., & DeBoer, R. P. (1980). Alcohol and drug use among clients at a residential vocational rehabilitation facility. *Alcohol Health and Research World, 5,* 48–56.
Rintala, D. H., Young, M. E., Hart, K. A., Clearman, R. R., & Fuhrer, M. J. (1992). Social support and the well-being of persons with spinal cord injury living in the community. *Rehabilitation Psychology, 37,* 155–164.
Rohe, D. E., & Basford, J. R. (1990). Traumatic spinal cord injury, alcohol, and the Minnesota Multiphasic Personality Inventory. *Rehabilitation Psychology, 34,* 25–32.
Saltz, C. C., Eisenberg, M. G., Fillenbaum, G., & George, L. K. (1991). Functional status and service use among community-based spinal cord injured male veterans. *NeuroRehabilitation, 4,* 25–35.
Sarason, B. R., Shearin, E. N., Pierce, G. R., & Sarason, I. G. (1987). Interrelations of social support measures: Theoretical and practical implications. *Journal of Personality and Social Support, 52,* 813–832.
Schulz, R., & Decker, S. (1985). Long-term adjustment to physical disability: The role of social support, perceived control and self-blame. *Journal of Personality and Social Psychology, 48,* 1162–1172.
Shontz, F. C. (1965). Reactions to crisis. *Volta Review, 67,* 364–370.

Shontz, F. C. (1982). Adaptation to chronic illness and disability. In T. Millon, C. Green, & R. Meagher (Eds.), *Handbook of clinical health psychology* (pp. 153–172). New York: Plenum Press.

Siller, J. (1969). Psychological situation of the disabled with spinal cord injuries. *Rehabilitation Literature, 30,* 290–296.

Silver, R., & Wortman, C. (1980). Coping with undesirable life events. In J. Garber & N. Seligman (Eds.), *Human helplessness: Theory and applications* (pp. 279–339). New York: Academic Press.

Stewart, T. D. (1978). Coping behavior and the moratorium following spinal cord injury. *Paraplegia, 15,* 338–342.

Stover, S. L., & Fine, P. R. (1986). *Spinal cord injury: The facts and figures.* Birmingham, AL: University of Alabama at Birmingham.

Sweeney, T. T., & Foote, J. E. (1982). Treatment of drug and alcohol abuse in spinal cord injury veterans. *International Journal of the Addictions, 17,* 897–904.

Trieschmann, R. B. (1988). *Spinal cord injuries: Psychological, social, and vocational rehabilitation* (2nd ed.). New York: Demos.

Trieschmann, R. B. (1992). Psychosocial research in spinal cord injury: The state of the art. *Paraplegia, 30,* 58–60.

Wright, B. A. (1960). *Physical disability: A psychological approach.* New York: Harper & Row.

Wright, B. A. (1983). *Physical disability: A psychosocial approach.* New York: Harper & Row.

Yarkony, G., Roth, E., Heinemann, A. W., Lovell, L., & Wu, Y. (1988). Functional skills after spinal cord injury rehabilitation: Three-year longitudinal follow-up. *Archives of Physical Medicine and Rehabilitation, 69,* 111–114.

19

Assessment and Conservative Treatment of Occupational Musculoskeletal Disability

Terence E. Fitzgerald and Nomita Sonty

INTRODUCTION

An epidemic of chronic work disability secondary to benign musculoskeletal trauma has presented industrialized societies with a multifaceted dilemma that has no clear solution. The incidence of sustained low back pain and, more recently, functional impairment secondary to upper extremity cumulative trauma disorder (UECTD) has increased dramatically during the latter half of the 20th century. The pervasive impact and refractory nature of work disability have necessitated infusion of expertise from diverse fields, such as sports medicine, occupational health psychology and behavioral medicine, ergonomics, exercise physiology, finance, law, and vocational rehabilitation, and has spawned new specialties, such as disability management. No longer the sole domain of independent provider or passive modality efforts, conservative care now reflects interdisciplinary participation in prevention, assessment, and treatment of these disorders.

The purpose of this chapter is to present a concise review of scope and determinants of work disability and articulate a holistic approach to nonoperative treatment based on an evolving biopsychosocial conceptual framework of functional restoration. Finally, we discuss controversies and trends regarding rehabilitation of injured workers.

Terence E. Fitzgerald • Occupational Health Institute, Blue Ridge Rehabilitation Medicine, Asheville, North Carolina 28801.   **Nomita Sonty** • Department of Psychology, National Rehabilitation Hospital, Washington, DC 20010.

Handbook of Health and Rehabilitation Psychology, edited by Anthony J. Goreczny. Plenum Press, New York, 1995.

MAGNITUDE OF THE PROBLEM

Musculoskeletal impairment and attendant pain represent a major cause of work disability, occasioning untold opportunity cost in terms of economic productivity, societal resources, and human potential. Occupational injuries currently affect 11 million American workers annually, reducing the extant labor pool by 10% at any given time (U.S. Public Health Service, 1988). Low back pain is the most prevalent cause of disability among workers under age 45, impairing some 5 million Americans, half of whom become permanently disabled (Kelsey, 1982; LaPlante, 1988). Although the majority of workers report transient low back discomfort at some point in their lives, prolonged functional impairment is much less common.

Cross-sectional and prospective surveys have articulated a fairly consistent natural history of occupational low back pain. Despite an estimated 1.4% annual incidence of work absence related to back strain or injury, 70% of injured individuals return to work within 1 month (acute course), and greater than 90% return within 4 months (subacute course) following first report of symptoms. The 5–7% of workers whose pain-related disability persists for longer than 4 months (chronic course) account for over 75% of compensation-related expenses (Abenhaim & Suissa, 1987; Spitzer, LeBlanc, & Dupuis, 1987). The majority of this chronically disabled subset of workers present with little or no objective evidence of structural or nerve root pathology that would account for their signs, symptoms, and limitations. Complicating matters further, associations between radiological and bone scan findings and pain-related disability remain equivocal. In addition, well-controlled analyses of CAT scan and MRI data suggest "pathogenic" findings for over one third of asymptomatic individuals (Boden, Davis, Dina, Patronas, & Wiesel, 1990; Murphy, E. Sperr, & S. Sperr, 1986; Wiesel, Tsourmas, Feffer, Citrin, & Patronas, 1984). Thus, there are no reliable objective measures that would permit quick, accurate dispensation of compensation claims.

Direct and indirect costs of prolonged musculoskeletal disability are staggering; annual projections exceed $16 billion (Holbrook, Grazier, Kelsey, & Stauffer, 1984). Research indicates that over 60% of these payments are for lost wages, and the remainder are for diagnostics, medical and surgical treatments, and rehabilitation (Federspiel, Guy, Kane, & Spengler, 1989). In 1986, total average workers' compensation for low back pain was $6,807 with a median payment of $391 (Webster & Snook, 1990); this further supports the finding that a small minority of claimants account for the great majority of costs. A recent regional survey found that upper extremity disorders involving overuse and repetitive stress resulted in total average claims of $5,606, even though these injuries do not engender comparable rates of total permanent work disability often associated with injuries to the low back (Fletcher, 1990). An analysis of closed Workers' Compensation cases in New York State for the period 1981–1987 revealed that, while number of upper extremity injury claims declined slightly, indemnity-related costs increased by 50% (Feuerstein, 1991).

Clearly, prolonged musculoskeletal impairment creates a financial burden that is socially disabling, a burden that is increasing at a rate that grossly exceeds population growth and changes in occupational injury prevalence. Projections of compensation payments, health-care expenditures, legal fees, lost productivity, and retraining or replacement of injured workers, however, do not meaningfully reflect psychosocial impact of chronic work disability. Although research has not prospectively examined specific consequences of pain-related musculoskeletal disability, several studies have attempted to isolate effects of involuntary job loss on workers and their families. Such research has suggested a causal relationship between unemployment and increased somatic complaints, utilization of health-care providers, anxiety, depression, and interpersonal conflict (Broman, Hamilton, & Hoffman, 1990; Kessler, Turner, & House, 1987; Linn, Sandifer, & Stein, 1985). Conversely, timely reemployment often reverses signs of psychological distress, most likely through enhanced financial stability and social affiliation mechanisms (Vinoker, Van Ryn, Gramlich, & Price, 1991).

Despite these compelling findings, it may be tempting to postpone or forego expenditures associated with comprehensive assessment and rehabilitation of chronic musculoskeletal pain and work disability. Unfortunately, time delays created by lengthy medical observation, multiple specialist consultations, and inefficient coordination of disability-related services appear to exacerbate the natural course of this complex problem. Data from an early study of industrial workers with nonspecific low back pain suggest that work reentry is, indeed, time contingent. Absenteeism greater than 6 months occasioned a 50% return-to-work rate. Those out of work greater than 1 year had a 25% chance of return to work, and a 2-year absence generally eliminated the possibility of gainful employment for this cohort (McGill, 1968). Alternatively, time-sensitive management of rehabilitation efforts focused on return to work has potential for saving as much as $30 for each dollar spent (cf. Roberts, 1989).

DETERMINANTS OF OCCUPATIONAL DISABILITY

Occupational disability research has long suffered from inconsistent selection of predictor and outcome measures along with reliance on cross-sectional and retrospective designs, which do not permit determination of causality. Although researchers have theorized that sciatica, claudication, and degenerative changes associated with age are primary causes of chronic low back pain, correlations between these predictors and treatment criteria (e.g., strength, range of motion, and aerobic capacity) and outcome measures (e.g., percentage returning to work) are weak (Frymoyer, 1991). Additionally, investigators have only rarely examined influences of activity-specific changes in postural loading on soft tissues. Contemporary multivariate studies (e.g., Frymoyer & Cats-Baril, 1987; Gervais, Dupuis, Veronneau, Bergeron, Millette, & Avard, 1991), however, appear to hold promise for clarifying recursive relationships among primary (preinjury) and secondary (prechronicity) predictors of disability.

The following review addresses several acknowledged determinants of chronic work disability: (1) pain-related deconditioning, (2) demographics, (3) psychological distress, (4) perceptions about work environments, and (5) biomechanical risk factors.

Pain-Related Deconditioning

We can conceptualize pain simply as the centralized integration and interpretation of multiple inputs, such as aversive peripheral stimuli, changes in brain neuromodulators, emotional state, contextual factors, and past experience. This transactional view receives support from research that demonstrates pain perception can occur in absence of overt nociception or pathophysiology, such as in anesthesia dolorosa (Bouckoms, 1985). *Persistent pain,* by definition, implies a complicated learning history whereby cognitive processes may reciprocally affect pain perception and behavior (Turk, Meichenbaum, & Genest, 1983). Avoidance of activities that patients believe exacerbate pain and increase risk of reinjury (i.e., "hurt equals harm") frequently sets the stage for unnecessary progression from a subacute course to a chronic course maintained by muscular and aerobic deconditioning, posture and gait abnormalities, spasm, psychological distress, and aversive cognitive appraisals. Stress-related thoughts may directly foster muscular tension that, in turn, may precipitate increased pain perception (Flor, Turk, & Birbaumer, 1985).

Functional impairment and work disability are natural consequences of this progressive, downward spiral of physical deconditioning. A significant body of research has demonstrated that gross inactivity and disuse, excessive mechanical stress and postural loading, and neurologically altered muscle tone exacerbate any deconditioning that may have occurred (cf. Mayer & Gatchel, 1988). Specifically, research has linked the deconditioning process to decreased cardiovascular function, soft tissue homeostasis, weak scar tissue formation, impaired disc nutrition, protein loss, delayed collagen maturation, muscle atrophy, and loss of muscle and bone mass (Bortz, 1982, 1984; Videman, 1987). Secondary functional consequences of deconditioning may include decrements in proprioception, agility, and physical capacity, and increased likelihood of injury and prolonged disability.

Demographics

Work absence following musculoskeletal injury or strain most notably relates with age, educational history, transferable job skills, economic climate, and level of replacement income, all of which presumably contribute additively to personal vulnerability to chronic disability. Just as prevalence and annual incidence of low back complaints increase with age, peaking at age 50 (Frymoyer, 1991), work disability demonstrates a stable age-related association. For workers between ages 35 and 44 years, average prevalence of work disability is 7.3%, increasing to 11.7% for the 45- to 54-year-old cohort and to 23.2% for the 55- to 64-year-old preretirement group (Kraus & Stoddard, 1989; McNeil, 1982).

Some researchers have advanced a theoretical link between age, pathophysiological changes, and increased risk for musculoskeletal impairment (e.g., Biering-Sorenson, 1982); however, age-related physiological changes are similar to many of the previously noted signs of prolonged inactivity and disuse. Although we cannot discount the influence of progressive spinal degeneration, there exists no evidence supportive of an inevitable age-related physical decline (Matheson, MacIntyre, Taunton, Clement, & Lloyd-Smith, 1989; McPherson, 1984; Shephard, 1978).

Level of education and, relatedly, transferable job skills following occupational injury are strong predictors of return to work. Anecdotal clinical evidence suggests that low back injuries affect young, male blue-collar workers with 12 years or less of formal schooling. This subgroup may be particularly vulnerable to prolonged disability due to ancillary factors, such as poor adherence to functional restoration recommendations during the subacute phase, limited comprehension skills, personal attitudes toward accepting indemnity compensation, and vagaries of the American workers' compensation system. Large-scale survey data have consistently shown that lower educational level significantly correlates with increased limitation of activity, bedrest, and work absence (Deyo & Tsui-Wu, 1987; Frymoyer & Cats-Baril, 1987).

Although individuals frequently cite availability and level of Workers' Compensation indemnity payments (i.e., replacement income) as the primary contributor to unnecessary disability, research does not unequivocally support this contention (Yelin, 1986). As Greenwood (1991) noted in her comprehensive review of so-called "compensation neurosis," macrolevel social factors, such as regional economic projections, unemployment rate, prevalence of food stamp use, and relative tendency of federal and state disability programs to respond to economic downturns with increased awards, also enhance likelihood of personal disability. Also of significance is the (perceived) adversarial stance of Workers' Compensation systems, which generally require proof of "work relatedness" of injuries.

The vast bureaucracy of the system occasions inevitable confusion and time delays in referral and treatment that may, in and of themselves, promote a chronic disability course. The latter observation suggests a potential bias in treatment-outcome research that compares compensated versus noncompensated groups who may receive more timely interventions.

Psychological Distress

Some research has linked mood-related appraisals and overlearned, maladaptive behaviors to chronic pain, inadequate coping, and unnecessary disability, although it remains unknown whether negative affective states, such as anger, anxiety, and depression, are primarily reactive, concomitant, or dispositional (Romano & Turner, 1985; Fishbain, Cutler, R. S. Rosomoff, & H. L. Rosomoff, 1994). Anxiety (generalized anxiety disorder, adjustment disorder with anxious mood, phobic-like avoidance behavior) is frequently observed in work-disabled pain patients although this relationship has not been well investigated. Depression (major depressive disorder, dysthymia, or adjustment disorder with depressed mood) frequently occurs in chronic pain populations, with incidence rates as high as 87% (Lindsay & Wyckoff, 1981; Magni, 1987). In the most recent revision of psychiatric nosological classification, *Diagnostic and Statistical Manual, DSM-IV* (American Psychiatric Association, 1994), a previous criterion excluding major depressive symptoms "due to a physical condition" has been eliminated. Given the often observed overlap between symptoms of chronic pain and major depression (e.g., sleep disturbance, weight and appetite changes, anhedonia, fatigue, and concentration difficulties), the current ability to offer a putative link between the two disorders may serve to clarify these complex etiological relationships (Fishbain, 1995). These data suggest several common mechanisms for pain-related musculoskeletal disability and frank mood disturbance.

First, neurovegetative signs, especially sleep disturbance, appear to link chronic pain and mood disorders. Heterocyclic antidepressants, such as doxepin and amitriptyline, that block reuptake of central nervous system (CNS) serotonin also increase pain tolerance, relax skeletal musculature, and enhance sleep regulation in low doses and ameliorate mood disturbance at higher doses (e.g., Goodkin & Gullion, 1989). Interestingly, anecdotal clinical evidence suggests that highly selective serotonin reuptake blockers such as fluoxetine are relatively ineffective in the amelioration of pain, muscle tension, and neurovegetative disturbance, whereas less selective antidepressants that block both serotonin and norepinephrine reuptake are effective.

Second, researchers have identified patterns of cognitive distortion associated with onset and maintenance of depression in chronic pain patients with and without affective distress (Lefebvre, 1981; Smith, Aberger, Follick, & Ahern, 1986). So-called pain beliefs regarding blame, biomedical causation, and projected duration of symptoms relate to psychological distress, somatization, disability behaviors, subjective pain intensity, multidisciplinary treatment compliance, self-esteem, and locus of control (Dolce, 1987; Williams & Thorn, 1989). These findings correspond to those of other investigations involving self-efficacy and cognitive and behavioral coping with acute and chronic medical stressors (e.g., Fitzgerald, Tennen, Affleck, & Pransky, 1993; Gattuso, Litt, & Fitzgerald, 1992).

Third, dispositional styles may underlie pain-related disability and other chronic health complaints (Barsky & Klerman, 1983; Watson & Pennebaker, 1989). Specifically, trait-negative affectivity and amplification of body sensations may be responsible for abnormal illness behavior, disease conviction, and overutilization of medical services. These factors may, in turn, affect information processing and confound validity of evaluation and treatment efforts, especially with older workers (Mital, 1994). For a comprehensive review of biopsychosocial explanatory models of pain-related disability, refer to Fitzgerald (1992).

Perceptions about Work Environment

Whereas secondary predictors of disability mediate probability of progression from injury to impairment and chronic work absence, job-related appraisals and biomechanical factors may contribute to both initial risk of injury and relative likelihood of safe return to former job tasks following musculoskeletal trauma. A series of longitudinal, prospective investigations involving 3,020 factory employees at the Boeing Company underscored importance of work environment perceptions as primary predictors of injury. With the exception of back pain report at baseline, level of job satisfaction had greater predictive power than all physical (e.g., cardiovascular, lifting strength, spinal flexibility, anthropometrics) and nonphysical measures (e.g., demographics, Minnesota Multiphasic Personality Inventory (MMPI) scales, psychosocial data) over the course of 4-year follow-up periods (Battie et al., 1989; Battie et al., 1990; Bigos et al., 1991). Similarly, validated secondary, or prechronicity, predictors of work disability include job satisfaction, employment stability, relations with supervisors, and perceptions of job tasks as boring, monotonous, or highly repetitive (Frymoyer & Cats-Baril, 1987; Linton & Kamwendo, 1989).

Biomechanical Risk Factors

For purposes of this discussion, biomechanical factors comprise personal resources, such as strength/maximum voluntary contraction (MVC), the greatest amount of effort an individual may exert. Typically, this involves concentration of effort on a single muscle or joint (Basmajian & DeLuca, 1985). Additional personal resources (i.e., biomechanical factors) include aerobic capacity (maximum oxygen uptake), anthropometric considerations, occupational task demands (mechanical stressors), work style, and interactions among these elements. An example that illustrates the interactive nature of biomechanical factors is the case of some UECTDs in which extreme postural deviations in combination with highly repetitive application of submaximal loads without adequate rest may result in damage to collagen tissue and resultant inflammation and discomfort.

Some research has linked personal resources, such as level of physical fitness, age, and gender, to aerobic capacity and whole body fatigue (Rodgers, 1988). Generally, to avoid muscular fatigue, a worker's rate of energy expenditure (kcal/min) must not exceed one third of aerobic capacity over an 8-hour shift. When task demands necessitate 60% of maximum strength or aerobic capacity, time required for muscle recovery is greater than time for task completion. Prior to returning to work, assessment of job-specific sustained metabolic demands, therefore, may be particularly important in determination of occupational rehabilitation goals, initial work tolerances, and work–rest cycles.

In addition to personal resources, clinicians have implicated anthropometric factors, such as height, weight, postural scoliosis, excessive kyphosis or lordosis of the spine, and spinal canal dimensions, as causal agents in low back pain disability; these associations have generally not withstood objective analyses and more precise radiographic assessments (Frymoyer, 1991). This is not to say that human body dimensions do not contribute to biomechanical risk, only that we cannot measure such influences in isolation from other factors. Ergonomic job analyses may reveal pathnogmic interactions between individual anthropometrics (e.g., height and weight in the upper fifth quintile) and recognized occupational risk factors, such as forceful/repetitive exertions, heavy lifting, awkward postures, static mechanical stresses, vibration, and temperature variability (Armstrong, Fine, Goldstein, Lifshitz, & Silverstein, 1987; Frymoyer, Pope, Clements, Wilder, MacPherson, & Ashikaga, 1983; Keyserling, Armstrong, & Punnett, 1991).

Recent research has identified work styles characterized by heightened behavioral expressivity as a potential risk factor for development, exacerbation, and maintenance of work-related musculoskeletal disability. Feuerstein and Fitzgerald (1992) examined biomechanical differences in job-task behaviors in an analog case-control study of professional sign language interpreters employed in a university setting. Subjects working with concomitant pain and/or fatigue demonstrated fewer rest breaks, more frequent hand/wrist deviations from a neutral posture, more frequent lateral excursions from an optimal work envelope, and more frequent interpretive finger/hand movements than pain-free controls. The work style construct appears to hold promise as a heuristic for better understanding interactions among multiple determinants of occupational disability.

EVALUATION COMPONENTS

Increasingly, treatment teams select evaluation and treatment options for workers with activity-related musculoskeletal disorders on the basis of algorithms generated by epidemiological and treatment-outcome research. Perhaps the most influential and widely used of these algorithm-driven approaches is the one outlined in the Report of the Quebec Task Force (QTF) on Spinal Disorders (Spitzer, LeBlanc, & Dupuis, 1987). This report recommended adoption of a parsimonious four-tier sys-

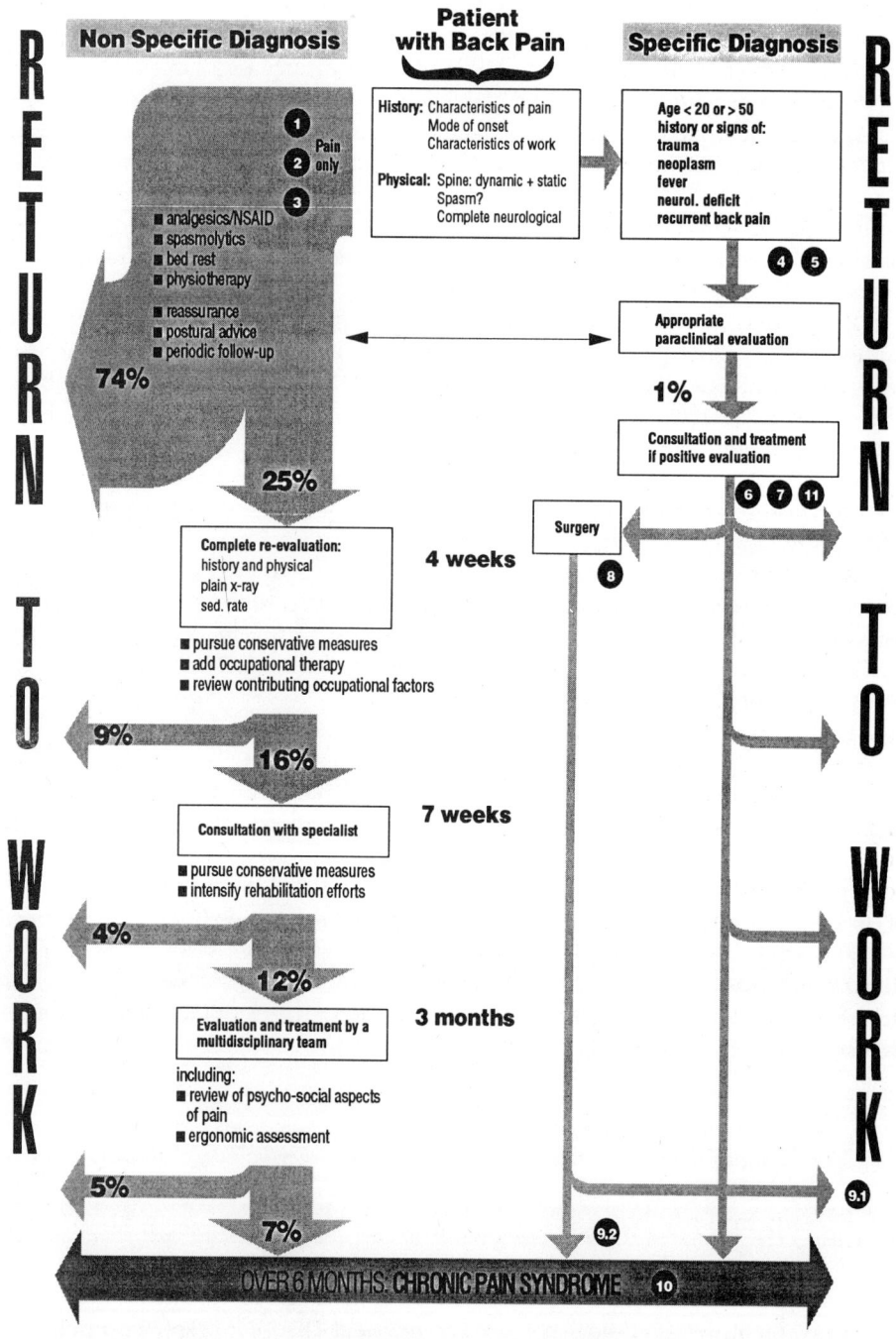

Figure 19.1. Quebec Task Force algorithm: A time-sensitive referral pathway for occupational rehabilitation (Spitzer, LeBlanc, & Depuis, 1987).

tem of classification for nonspecific mechanical spine problems based on lumbar, dorsal, or cervical pain distributions: (1) pain without radiation beyond the gluteal fold or shoulder (absent neurologic signs); (2) pain with proximal radiation (may be neurogenic, but absent neurological signs); (3) pain with distal radiation beyond the knee or elbow (may be radicular, but absent neurological signs); and (4) pain with radiation to a limb in the presence of focal neurological signs, such as loss of bowel, bladder, or sexual function or dermatome-specific sensory loss.

The time-sensitive QTF system involves physician management by "critical pathway" as illustrated in Figure 19.1. As indicated in this figure, 74% of workers with activity-related, nonspecific spinal problems will return to work within 4 weeks after onset of disability. After 7 weeks, 16% will remain out of work, justifying referral for consultation with a specialist, such as an orthopedic surgeon, neurosurgeon, occupational medical consultant, or physiatrist. If a worker remains disabled after 12 weeks of conservative care and specialist consultation, gatekeeper physicians need to consider consultation with a multidisciplinary team of chronic pain specialists. The nature of subsequent functional restorative services depends on updated physical exams, medical and surgical histories, radiographic and bone scan findings, clinical outcomes at low-intensive treatment levels, and presumed underlying determinants of occupational disability. Numerous naturalistic and clinical investigations have upheld the logic of a stepwise, conservative approach to evaluation and treatment of these disorders (cf. Frymoyer, 1991; J. A. Saal & J. S. Saal, 1989).

A recent meta-analytic review (Flor, Fydrich, & Turk, 1992) of 65 chronic low back pain treatment-efficacy studies demonstrated superiority of multidisciplinary approaches over no treatment, waiting-list, and single-discipline interventions (e.g., medical or physical therapy). Effects of holistic treatments include not only pain relief but also include increased function; timely return to work; regulation of mood, sleep, and activity level; decreased utilization of the health-care system; and decreased medical and compensation costs. These effects appear to be stable over time. In a recent review of prospective studies of return-to-work outcomes following multidisciplinary rehabilitation efforts (average duration of work disability = 16 months), 71% of injured workers were working or were involved in formal vocational rehabilitation at 12-month posttreatment follow-up in contrast to 44% of nontreated controls (Feuerstein, Menz, Zastowny, & Barron, 1994).

Following medical clearance for participation in a multidisciplinary occupational rehabilitation program and determination of cardiovascular and physical restrictions, if any, workers generally participate in some or all of the following evaluations:

1. Functional capacity, as conducted by a physical therapist, occupational therapist, or exercise physiologist.
2. Psychophysiological status, including assessment of risk factors to include neurovegetative interference and autonomic and muscular reactivity, as measured by a psychologist.
3. Job description and/or review of ergonomic job demands performed at the worksite.

Based on integration of findings from these evaluations, treatment teams formulate individualized treatment plans in context of a vocational/case-management model.

Functional Capacity

The functional capacity evaluation (FCE) involves quantification of function through use of systematic, comprehensive, objective measurements of individuals' maximal (demonstrated) work abilities (Tramposh, 1991). Physical measures of human performance must be physiologically relevant, valid, and reproducible. In order to enhance clinical utility of FCEs, assessors need to include measures that identify submaximal efforts (Polatin & Mayer, 1992). Such measures may include, but are not limited to, multiple-trial grip and pinch strength, Waddell signs, pain behavior ratings/abnormal illness behavior, and dynamometer assessment of nonphysiological indicators.

Examiners may use differing protocols that include various combinations of data (generic, work-specific), muscle strength methodologies (isometric, isotonic, isokinetic, isoinertial), and applied technologies (manual, computer-assisted) to obtain measures of functional capacity. Each assessment protocol has relative merits in terms of reliability, validity, access to normative databases, complexity, cost, and time demands. Clinicians may collect objective data (i.e., range of motion, level of lumbar stabilization, dynamic postural control, trunk strength, endurance, and coordination) in isolation as generic treatment-outcome measures or compared with actual task requirements/work envelopes. Job-specific data may include demonstrated tolerances for repetitive lifting, forceful exertions, carrying, pushing, pulling, reaching, bending, twisting, sitting and standing, crouching, climbing, gripping, or a variety of other behavioral movements.

Muscle strength plays a key role in individuals' performances during FCEs. By definition, *muscle strength* is the maximum force that a muscle can exert in a single maximum contraction. Typically, these contractions may be either concentric or eccentric. Concentric contractions are frequently necessary in sports activities, such as weight lifting and hitting a baseball. In such a contraction, increase in tension correlates with shortening of the muscle and overcoming resistance applied to it. Eccentric contractions are those in which external resistance overcomes power exerted by the muscle. In this case, the muscle lengthens while maintaining a certain amount of tension.

Contractions may also be static or dynamic. Static, or isometric, contractions are those in which there is no associated joint movement, and such contractions occur when static strength involves increases in muscle tension without corresponding changes in muscle length (internal force is equal to external resistance). Dynamic contractions involve joint movement and may be isotonic or isokinetic. Isotonic contractions occur when muscles shorten as they respond to constant internal force or torque. Isokinetic contractions involve application of force across a preset velocity, distance, or range of motion, thereby permitting measurement of changes in resistance. Finally, isoinertial contractions occur against constant loads with torque exceeding resistance, thereby facilitating measurement of changes in torque and velocity, factors that remain uncontrolled. Although the four methodological options for quantifying strength relate to type of muscle contraction, there is no consensus as to which type best predicts functional recovery in real-life work situations (Saal, Lerman, & Keane, 1990).

Neuromuscular fatigue may affect performance on FCEs, and contribute to individuals' submaximal performances. Ordet and Grand (1992) outlined the following types of fatigue: (1) nutrient fatigue, which occurs as a result of submaximal exercise; (2) anaerobic fatigue, which occurs after short-term maximal exercise; and (3) neural fatigue, which occurs after a variable period of time, thereby suggesting reduction in neural activity. The latter classification remains controversial.

Historically, FCEs have changed focus over the years and have included not only vocational aspects of assessment (e.g., WEST—Work Evaluation Systems Technology, Huntington Beach, CA; Valpar—Valpar International Corporation, Tucson, AZ; and Singer—New Concepts Corporation, Tucson, AZ) but also various multidisciplinary assessment approaches as well (e.g., Blankenship FCE—American Therapeutics, Macon, GA; Key Functional Assessments, Minneapolis, MN; Functional Capacity Assessments—Polinsky Medical Center, Duluth, MN; and the Functionally Fit for Work Analysis—FFWA, Work Capacity, Inc., Lenexa, KS). Similar systems, developed more recently, include Isernhagen Work Systems—Isernhagen and Associates, Duluth, MN; SWEAT Functional Evaluation—Bi-State Medical, Kansas City, MO; and Ergos Work Simulator—Work Recovery Systems, Tucson, AZ. Unfortunately, review of these systems is beyond the scope of this chapter, but interested readers may obtain information from the referenced organizations.

Technological applications used in FCEs have also changed over the years and have included not only so-called low-tech devices, such as simple goniometers, inclinometers, and the Progressive Isoinertial Lifting Evaluation free lifting test (Mayer et al., 1988) to high-tech dynamometers, such as the B200 (Isotechnologies, Hillsborough, NC), that can simultaneously measure changes in torque and velocity across frontal, sagittal, and transverse planes of motion. Although low-tech approaches may consist of low intra- and interrater reliability and external validity, computer-assisted measurement of range using the EDI-320 (Cybex, Ronkonkoma, NY), for example, has enhanced simple assessment of true lumbar parameters by factoring out movement of the hip–pelvic segment (Mayer, Tencer, Kristofferson, & Mooney, 1984). Difficulties with anatomical isolation have plagued high-tech evaluations as well, but new developments appear to address this concern. In particular, the lumbar extension machine from MedX (Ocala, FL) offers potential for testing and rehabilitation applications by isolating lumbar isometric strength from the rest of the anatomy through a range of motions (Graves et al., 1990a, 1990b).

Although the FCE approach excels in articulating a range of salient factors mediating return to work, methodological problems (e.g., poor predictive validity, inadequate norms) undermine utility of FCEs. Recognizing vagaries of the FCE maximal-function testing model, some researchers have attempted to use an alternative framework: Acceptable Maximal Effort (AME) (Khalil et al., 1987). This approach consists of an ergonomic test battery that quantifies functional abilities in context of a psychophysical static testing model. It assumes that there is a critical interaction between actual physical capabilities and perceived capabilities, the latter referring to maximal voluntary effort without onset of unacceptably adverse pain. The AME protocol has demonstrated reliability coefficients above .90 for all strength measures.

As with the AME heuristic, ongoing psychophysiological monitoring may facilitate interpretation of FCE results. Surface electromyography (sEMG) is a useful technique to facilitate identification of fatigue onset in individuals and distinguish between psychological fatigue, secondary to boredom, or fear of reinjury from physiological fatigue, which is a consequence of prolonged activity. Sophisticated analyses of muscle activity during periods of sustained, static contraction have demonstrated fatigue-induced increases in sEMG signals. Although no unequivocal explanation has emerged, some investigators have speculated that there may be changes in motor unit recruitment, motor unit synchronization (i.e., tendency for motor units to discharge at nearly the same time), and muscle fiber conduction velocity (Barnes & Williams, 1987). Ongoing research that addresses questions such as quantification of muscle strength, fatigue, and endurance, and the effects of intermittent isometric exercise on muscle fatigue and recovery will increase our understanding of how muscles function in pathological states (Milner-Brown, Mellenthin, & Miller, 1986; Rodriguez & Agre, 1991).

Psychophysiological Data

Patterns of abnormal muscle use, gross postural deviations, and autonomic nervous system hyperarousal are frequent in individuals with musculoskeletal pain. A compensatory posture may account for these patterns and contribute to chronic overuse of some muscles and avoidance/underuse of others (Yeh, Gonyea, Lemke, & Volpe, 1985). Several investigators have reported increased incidence of pain in individuals with severe postural abnormalities (e.g., Dolan, Adams, & Hutton, 1988; Griegel-Morris, Larson, Mueller-Klaus, & Oatis, 1992) with implications regarding development of secondary pain sites. Systematic observations have suggested that compensatory postures and muscular bracing secondary to low back pain may contribute to upper back pain and headaches (e.g., Ahern, Iezzi, Hursey, & Follick, 1988). Furthermore, individuals with chronic pain demonstrate significantly enhanced muscle tension (Flor, Schugens, & Birbaumer, 1992). Taking into consideration the major role played by primary or secondary muscle involvement in painful musculoskeletal conditions, pain management centers have historically employed sEMG assessment in treatment of pain conditions, especially chronic low-back pain (Ng, 1981).

Electromyographic Data

Hagberg and Kvarnstrom (1984) demonstrated the validity of sEMG assessment in a study of industrial workers diagnosed with cumulative trauma disorders; these investigators documented that submaximal performance was due to decreased endurance resulting from increased physiological fatigability. In addition to its use as an assessment tool, sEMG with a feedback component is a useful adjunct in treatment, especially in exercise regimens for increasing muscle strength (Asfour, Khalil, Waly, Goldberg, Rosomoff, & Rosomoff, 1990; Croce, 1986; Lucca & Recciuti, 1983).

Numerous evaluation protocols for sEMG scanning have emerged since the seminal work of Cram and Steger (1983). Such evaluations may determine muscle activity at rest (static), during movement (dynamic), or under variable conditions. A typical plan for assessment ("muscle scan") may include observations at rest; with or without feedback; with our without diversions of attention from the task at hand; during MVC; and during recovery after sustained contractions. Assessments, therefore, involve measurements taken at rest (resting baseline), on amplitude during contraction, and on return to baseline (recovery). Ancillary systematic observations may include range of motion, symmetry in muscle use, pain tolerance as measured with an algometer (Schiffman, Fricton, Haley, & Tylka, 1988), observation of pain behaviors, and compensatory postural changes. Clinicians interpret sEMG evaluations using all of the aforementioned information, bearing in mind that research has not clearly established the association between sEMG measurement and pain-related functional impairment. It is therefore important to consider sEMG data as valuable for planning treatment and as objective measures of an individual's muscle status, particularly in the assessment of work/rest cycles.

With the rapid growth of information on sEMG, both as a research and clinical tool, controversies with regard to validity of sEMG normative data have arisen (Iacono, 1991). Several variables may confound sEMG data: type of electrodes (surface vs. indwelling electrode); size of electrodes; preparation of recording sites; interelectrode spaces; electrode location (unilateral vs. bilateral); documentation (pen recording vs. oscilloscope and FM storage tape); and finally, methods of quantifying EMG signal (observation of action potentials vs. analog to digital conversion; Soderberg, 1992; L. Wolf, Segal, S. Wolf, & Nyberg, 1991). Furthermore, utilizing one to two sites may not adequately represent the complex muscular hyper- and hypoactive states associated with antalgic postures. In addition, individual differences in subcutaneous fat and muscle geometry may compromise intersubject comparisons. Finally, inadequacies in use of appropriate control groups and analytical and statistical methods used with raw sEMG data also may affect outcome and interpretation of findings. In an attempt to eliminate some of the aforementioned confounds, researchers have recommended (1) a transformation/normalization process to allow for comparison between subjects (Soderberg, 1992), (2) use of an ipsative versus nomothetic approach (Iacono, 1991), and (3) use of MVC versus effort-based methodologies to understand dysfunctional muscle use.

Various models of sEMG equipment are available. One example of instrumentation is J&J model M57 with IP-5 EMG channels and a D200 integrator (Biomedical Instruments, Warren, MI). The same company also markets I-330, which is a modular interface for an IBM PC-type EGA/VG color computer. This instrument has capability for up to 12 plug-in modalities (sEMG, temperature, dermograph, pneumograph, EEG, blood pressure, and pulse rate). Another computerized instrumentation that includes sEMG capabilities is Davicon (American Biotech Corporation, Ossining, NY). Personal-sized, portable versions are also available from Thought Technologies, Inc. (Montreal, Canada) and others. With advancement in technology, these computer-interfaced programs have potential to do multisite assessments, provide data graphically with good visual and auditory feedback, and collect data on patients' responses to treatment over sessions. Some of them are compatible with various types of statistical software, allowing for data collection and analysis. For example, Davicon has a utility program that can convert data files to ASCII format for subsequent use by some statistical software packages. Despite these advantages, Iacono (1991) warned users of systematic errors that can arise from interpreting sEMG findings based on fixed norms as generated by some computer software. Recent advances in so-called static imaging software (SIS) and dynamic assessment and treatment protocols for cervical, upper quarter, and low back applications appear to address concerns regarding data transformations, postural muscle tone, and normative and ipsative comparisons (SIS; Clinical Resources, Nevada City, CA).

A manual examination of specific muscle sites can be a useful addition to sEMG assessment. An important component of this evaluation is muscle palpation, done either by hand or with help of an algometer, allowing examiners to note evidence of muscle irritation or tenderness not directly observable via sEMG. It is a fairly standard technique used by physical therapists in their assessment of tenderness/pain on palpation, range of motion, behavioral response to palpation, and increased muscle tension.

Specialists have developed separate evaluation protocols for sites involving facial pain, head and neck pain, and low back pain. The general rule during palpation is to make sure that clinicians apply constant pressure of about 3–4 pounds while examining key muscles. One such procedure, described by Duckro et al. (1992), involves three primary steps:

1. Assess cervical and mandibular range of motion.
2. Palpate the following muscles: masseter, anterior temporalis, frontalis, cervical paraspinals, scalenes, sternocleidomastoid (SCM), levator scapula, and upper fibers of the trapezius and suprascapular.
3. For each muscle group, rate the patient's response to palpation, with 0 = *No Pain*, 1 = *Some Pain Reported*, and 2 = *Flinch Response*. Figure 19.2 illustrates the location of relevant muscle groups (scan sites) palpated during manual and sEMG examinations.

Therapists can also perform a similar examination to assess the aforementioned variables at the upper and low back. For this purpose, therapists may palpate the following muscles: cervical paraspinals, SCM, scalenes, upper and lower fibers of the trapezius, intrascapular region, levator scapula, lumbar paraspinals, and symmetry of hip. Clinicians may also evaluate cervical and lumbar range of motion.

Autonomic Data

Individuals differ with regard to intensity of stress response, type of stressors to which they react, and physiological systems through which they react. Autonomic nervous system(ANS)-mediated stress responses often lead to changes in peripheral skin temperature, heart rate or pulse rate, skin conductance, and blood pressure. Some clinical conditions that frequently manifest the aforementioned cardiovascular symptoms are migraine headaches, Raynaud's disease, and other stress disorders. In these conditions, it is useful to evaluate individuals' reactivities and incorporate results into treatment plans. Cardiovascular measures include blood flow, digital skin temperature, blood pressure, and heart rate. Although these measures may play a significant role regarding onset, exacerbation, and maintenance of vascular pain problems, they may be of little use for management of soft tissue injuries. Skin conductance measurement, including both tonic and phasic responses, may serve as general indicators of hyperreactivity, which is sometimes found with injuries resulting in causalgia or reflex sympathetic dystrophy.

Multimodal assessment protocols may help capture individual stress responses not easily identified in analogue settings. One such protocol employed at the Biobehavioral Treatment Center at St. Louis University Medical Center exposes each patient to three standard stressors of differing quality: (1) mental arithmetic (passive coping, achievement task), (2) video game (active coping, competitive), and (3) cold pressor (physiological stressor, pain tolerance measure). The assessment involves measurement of a variety of peripheral systems: sEMG at frontal and upper back sites, digital skin temperature, skin conductance, pulse rate, breathing rate, and systolic and diastolic blood pressure. Recordings of all observations occur during baseline, stressor, and recovery periods, with inclusion of a postassessment sampling of the relaxation response. Clinicians review the data to obtain information regard-

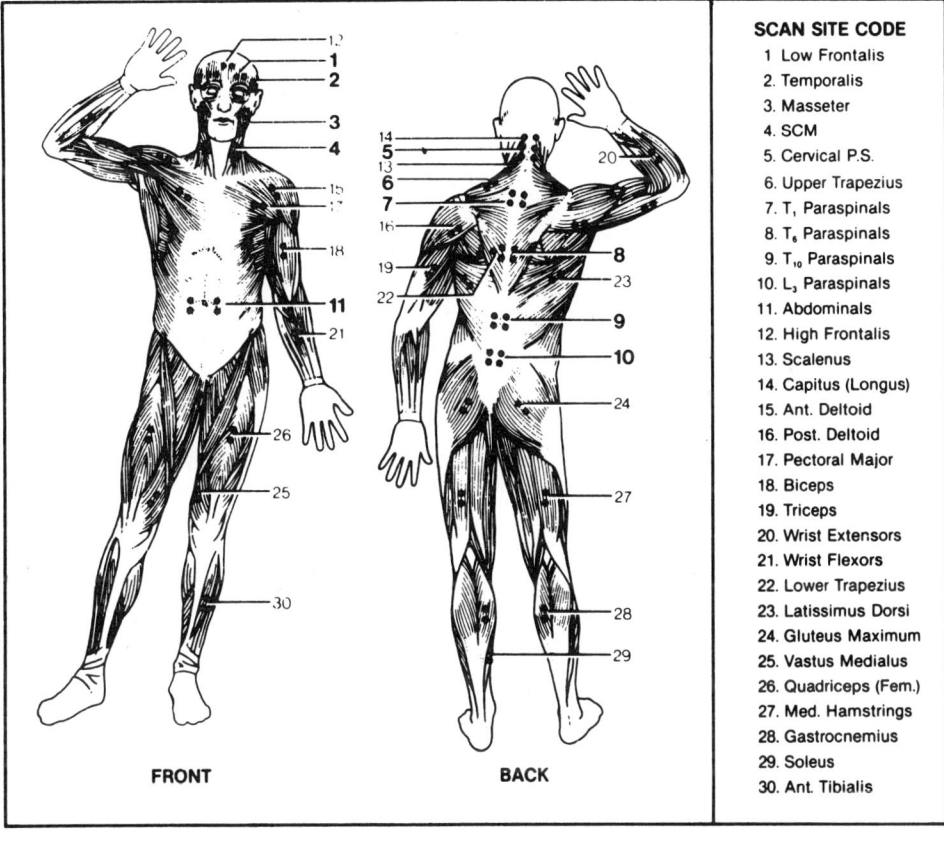

Figure 19.2. Scan sites for EMG assessment and muscle palpation (Cram & Steger, 1983).

ing overall arousal, behavioral observations, most significant stressor, and most reactive systems. As indicated by assessment data, laboratory technicians may substitute other stressors, including personalized stressors. Although the ANS lends itself to assessment, it is a fairly unstable system that is reactive to most stimuli. It is therefore useful as a clinical tool but requires cautious interpretation, especially when used in research.

Pain Self-Report

In order to assess subjective pain reports of patients, clinicians often utilize standardized assessments to supplement information obtained during comprehensive clinical interviews. Some of the more frequently used measures include pain drawings, pain rating scales, and disability impact indexes. Psychologists often utilize objective assessments of depression, anxiety, anger, personality, and assertiveness to measure pain-related problems. An exhaustive review of pain assessment strategies is beyond the scope of this chapter, nor does pain self-report *per se* account for the majority of variance in return-to-work outcomes. We encourage the interested reader to refer to Kerns and Jacob's chapter on pain heuristics in this handbook and to an excellent review of objective pain assessment edited by Turk and Melzack (1992).

Use of pain drawings (i.e., topographical pain representations) is a nonverbal method of identifying pain sites, severity, and subjectively perceived characteristics of pain. Mooney, Cairns, and Robertson (1976) were the first group to use this method to identify psychogenic "magnification" of pain. Subsequently, other investigators have made several attempts to quantify pain drawings with a numerical scoring system or grid scoring system (Ransford, Cairns, & Mooney, 1976). With regard to administration of pain drawings, patients typically receive simple diagrams of the human body, as seen from the front and back, on which they mark areas of pain with different symbols for "burning," "stabbing," "aching," "numbness," "pins and needles," and "cramping."

Pain experts have developed, used, and discarded numerous pain rating scales over the years. One of the more frequently employed scales is the McGill–Melzack Pain Questionnaire (MMPQ). The originators developed this instrument to provide a quantitative measure of the subjective experience of clinical pain that clinicians and researchers could statistically analyze (Melzack, 1975). Twenty word groups describing pain cluster into three categories, including an additional miscellaneous category. Patients refer to their present pain experience and pick one word from each of the 20 groups that best describes their pain. Patients also complete a pain drawing and rate their pain intensity on a scale of 1 to 5 (*Mild* to *Excruciating*). Other rating scales include simple numeric scales ranging from a 0–5 or 1–10 ratings, or visual analogue scales (VAS) that require patients to mark a point on a 10-cm line, the lower end representing mild pain and the top end, severe pain.

Some self-report scales obtain information from patients regarding perception of pain, emotional state, functional limitations, attitudes about pain, and so-called illness behavior. A frequently used self-rating scale is the Pain Disability Index (PDI) Standardized by Tait, Pollard, Margolis, Duckro, and Krause (1987). The scale assesses overall impact of pain on a 10-point scale ranging from 0 (*No Disability*) to 10 (*Total Disability*) across several focal areas: family/home responsibility, recreation, social activity, occupation, sexual behavior, self-care, and life-support activities.

Job-Task Analysis

On-site job-task analysis, sometimes referred to as ergonomic job analysis (EJA), serves a focal role in returning employees to work, particularly when occupational demands (i.e., job description) require clarification or when job tasks require modification to meet workers' current tolerances. In light of recent mandates from the Americans with Disabilities Act (ADA) of 1990, companies are likely to perform job-task analyses more frequently than in the past as companies attempt to determine appropriate accommodations for injured employees and reduce future ergonomic risk. Company representatives can compare occupational demands documented in EJAs to workers' current physical capabilities as determined during FCEs; treatment team members can subsequently address functional discrepancies via individualized work reconditioning protocols.

Evaluation of work requirements for manual materials-handling jobs may include use of direct/videotaped observation, National Institute for Occupation Safety and Health (NIOSH, 1981) lifting guidelines, physical stress checklists, and analyses of posture and psychophysiological strength. NIOSH guidelines have established two lifting standards, maximum permissible limit (MPL) and action limit (AL) for use in job task design and redesign.

MPL is a lift that produces an L5–S1 disc compression of 1,430 pounds and a 5.0 kcal/min metabolic load. MPL is within strength capabilities of 25% of men and virtually no women. AL defines job tasks that are presumably safe (low overexertion injury risk) for most workers according to the following three conditions: (1) maximum of 770 pounds of disc compression, (2) 3.5 kcal/min energy expenditure or less, and (3) does not exceed strength capabilities of 75% of female workers (NIOSH, 1981). Development of slide rule lifting calculation devices (National Safety Council, Chicago, IL) and computer-assisted biomechanical modeling, which predicts forces produced in various postures (Chaffin, 1988), have enhanced application of NIOSH guidelines.

Physical stress measures, such as the Michigan Checklist for upper extremity cumulative trauma disorders (Lifshitz & Armstrong, 1986), assess risk factors for reinjury (e.g., force, postural deviations, workstation dimensions, repetitive motions, and tool design). Self-report measures of physical stress have also demonstrated validity as components of EJA. Examples of such measures include the Rating of Perceived Exertion (RPE) scale (Borg, 1985) and the Nordic Questionnaires (Kuorinka, Kilbom, Nilsson, Andersson, & Bjurvald, 1987). Finally, posture-analysis methodologies range from accessible, low-tech observer-rating systems, such as the Ovaco Working Posture Analysis System (OWPAS) (Heinsalimi, 1984), to three-dimensional modeling techniques utilizing postural-deviation-recording LED suits (Samuelson, Wangenheim, & Wos, 1987).

For a survey of representative EJA protocols, refer to Feuerstein and Hickey (1992). Detailed information on ergonomic methodologies may be found in publications from the UAW-Ford Ergonomics Process (University of Michigan, 1988) and Taylor and Francis, Inc. (e.g., Ayoub & Mital, 1989; Fraser, 1989; Wilson & Corlett, 1990).

TREATMENT COMPONENTS

Guided by evaluation data, workers presenting with chronic musculoskeletal impairment may receive rehabilitation services in the context of a wide range of treatment components as supervised by teams representing many different combinations of professional disciplines. Simply put, there are a multitude of treatment/discipline permutations that may be highly effective depending on how well they address local rehabilitation exigencies (e.g., "Who," "What," "When," "Where," and "How"). *Who* pertains to level of complexity of presenting complaint(s), demographics, and patient-mix characteristics. Relatedly, *What* refers to treatment needs of the population served. As previously stated, patients differ with respect to experience with pain-related deconditioning, psychological distress, perceptions about work environment, endorsement of biomechanical risk factors, and appropriateness of return-to-work facilitation. *When* addresses the all-important time dimension in clinical referral patterns. Some rehabilitation centers treat patients with acute, subacute, and chronic pain, whereas others focus only on complex, refractory conditions. *Where* details relevant aspects of the local environment, such as type of facility (inpatient, freestanding outpatient, combined); program focus (musculoskeletal only, or in combination with programs for stroke, spinal cord injury, and traumatic brain injury); and state laws and regulations as they impact workers' compensation and health insurance practices related to adjudication of responsibility for injury indemnity, referral process and program approval, provider participation, and reimbursement. Finally, *How* reflects the process of enacting mechanisms of therapeutic change (e.g., multidisciplinary vs. interdisciplinary, modality-driven vs. integrative, and medical model vs. rehabilitation model focus). Subsequent sections on treatment components are suggestive, not prescriptive.

Physical Reconditioning

An integral part of the treatment regimen for injured workers is some form of fitness activity that enhances level of cardiovascular functioning, energy reserves, performance, and well-being and decreases risk of reinjury. Endurance, a measure of fitness, is the ability to work for prolonged periods of time and resist fatigue. Rehabilitation programs include various exercise regimens in the treatment of injured workers; such exercise regimens may focus on aerobic capacity, isotonic weight training, and isokinetic strengthening, endurance, mobility, or skill. The American College of Sports Medicine (1980) recommended that providers structure the following five factors for optimal functional outcomes: (1) type/mode of activity, (2) intensity, (3) duration, (4) frequency, and (5) rate of progression. Research on association between aerobic conditioning and incidence of back injury is sparse. However, one group of investigators reported a preventive value from increasing levels of physical fitness. They also demonstrated a 25% decrease in workers' compensation costs related to improvements in cardiovascular fitness and initiation of a policy permitting a more rapid return to work (Cady, Thomas, & Karwasky, 1985).

Therapists must tailor exercise prescriptions and daily quotas to specific needs of injured workers across all treatment modalities (e.g., one-on-one physical therapy or relatively independent activities, such as use of aerobic equipment in a gym setting, at work, or at home). Ideally, all regimens will additively contribute to overall reduction of the baseline discrepancy between demonstrated physical capabilities and required work tolerances. Relatedly, fitness levels at time of program discharge must be sufficient to guarantee that workers' capabilities upon return to work will sustain prolonged, taxing physical demands (i.e., MVC and maximum oxygen uptake) and repetitive application of submaximal loads without required rest (Feuerstein & Fitzgerald, 1992).

Generally, aggressive pain control is a prerequisite for most subacute- and chronic-course rehabilitation programs. Individuals need to receive training in a sequence of self-management strategies, such as the FISH-R approach (i.e., *f*ocused abdominal breathing, *i*ce massage, *s*tretching, moist *h*eat, and *r*elaxation/neuromuscular control). Treatment providers may employ adjunctive pain-control methods through selective use of epidural, intra-articular facet, or nerve root injections, transcutaneous nerve stimulation, acupuncture, and nonnarcotic analgesics, tricyclic antidepressants, and nonsteroidal anti-inflammatory drugs (NSAIDs), as needed. Following maximal alleviation of inflammation and pain, treatment team members can institute a program of dynamic postural control/lumbar stabilization exercises focusing on definition and maintenance of neutral pelvic and head posture. As clarified by J. A. Saal and J. S. Saal (1989), neutral position does not require zero degrees of lordosis, but rather the least painful spine position that minimizes segmental biomechanical stress and radicular discomfort. Following mastery of technique through coordinated repetition of static exercises under close supervision, patients may graduate to a more advanced program of dynamic exercises in context of a gym or water-based program. Typically, advanced programs include, but are not restricted to, the following: (1) dynamic abdominal bracing, (2) trunk raises, (3) bridging movements progressing to balancing with a gym ball, (4) quadruped exercises, (5) knee stabilization, (6) wall-slide quadricep technique, and (7) advanced postural control during transitions between complex activities (J. A. Saal & J. S. Saal, 1989, 1991). As with reconditioning protocols (e.g., McKenzie extension exercises, Williams flexion exercises) utilized during the acute phase of treatment for so-called postural dysfunction, or derangement syndromes, dynamic stabilization programs are predicated on the belief that exercise sequences establish automatic, cortically activated multimuscular movement patterns or engrams that can be subsequently enacted without conscious control or direct supervision by rehabilitation professionals.

Work Reconditioning

A fundamental theme of the return-to-work-readiness approach is the notion that early return to work favors the relationship between employer, worker, and work environment and facilitates "occupational bonding" (Lacerte & Wright, 1992). The return-to-work process typically has four phases, most of which can proceed concurrently: evaluation, analysis and planning, interventions, and resolution. Work reconditioning programs (i.e., work "hardening" or work "simulation" activities) came into existence in order to meet complex needs of injured workers and decrease unnecessary work disability.

As previously mentioned, work-related injuries are notorious for increasing absenteeism from work. They not only cause physical debilitation and deconditioning but also may promote aversive conditioning to work sites and reinforce fear of reinjury. Given the formidable nature of these risk factors for occupational disability, work hardening programs must effectively address concerns pertaining to productivity, safety, physical tolerances, interpersonal relationships, and work behaviors while providing manageable transition between various levels of care (acute to chronic) and from treatment to return to work.

Commercially available work-reconditioning programs offer standardized workstations and well-defined simulated activities in order to demonstrate proficiency in the job tasks that individuals will be performing. Although this approach is relatively capital-intensive, its standardization and ease of norm-based evaluation of performance may offer considerable utility, even when simulated tasks are not identical to actual job demands. Work reconditioning programs attempt to replicate job tasks via therapeutic projects designed to increase specific tolerances, analogue work simulations; actual work-situation assignments (light duty), and transitions in which a worker "ramps ups" to full-time work through graded, same-day participation in the rehabilitation program and, *in vivo,* at work.

The primary issue of controversy with regard to application of work reconditioning technology pertains to the relative necessity of screening patients for such therapy. According to the Committee for Accreditation of Rehabilitation Facilities (CARF) definition, individuals in transition between acute care and return to work are suitable for work simulation therapy. Proponents of various reconditioning models differ on this issue and recommend work therapy from as early as day-1 postinjury to much later in the chronic disability progression. Lichter (1991) noted that work therapy is not for everyone, and medical professionals must recommend work therapy judiciously in order to prevent physical injuries from premature therapy and psychological "trauma" from frustration and inability to achieve program goals. Some work reconditioning programs require administration of a "feasibility screen" to assess patient appropriateness and motivation. In contrast, other programs have demonstrated that most postacute patients are eligible for work reconditioning provided that therapists individualize treatment within patients' baseline capacities (Mitchell & Carmen, 1990).

Employers and health-care providers are finding themselves in a dilemma when confronted with disability issues in the case of injured workers. Changes in disability costs and utilization have led to development of various models of disability management. One such example is the WorkAbility (CORE Management, Inc., Burlington, MA) system developed to facilitate clinical decisions about employees' treatments, disability durations, and return-to-work options. For a description of the WorkAbility system, refer to Carpenter (1992). More recently, proactive employers are developing on-site work-return transition programs in order to prevent lengthy absenteeism, promote safe and timely return to work, and accommodate disabled workers (Shrey & Olsheski, 1992).

Behavioral Self-Regulation Training

For many injured workers, successful functional restoration may require both assumption of personal responsibility for change (perceived control) and the sense that one has capabilities to perform certain behaviors that will produce desirable outcomes (self-efficacy). Interestingly, psychoeducational approaches to coping enhancement, such as those reviewed in the subsequent discussion of so-called "back schools," primarily focus on development and refinement of instrumental responses, cognitive/information control strategies, and decision-making skills. Recent cognitive–

behavioral technologies, such as self-change and self-efficacy enhancement models, however, appear to foster maintenance of health-related behaviors and avoidance of relapse.

Back School and Body Mechanics Coaching

Frequently employed as a formal adjunct to physical or work reconditioning efforts, back school educational modules help injured workers in acute and subacute phases of recovery develop skills to increase function. Although content and organization of back schools have varied considerably since their formal inception in Sweden in 1970, a core curriculum generally includes information on safe body mechanics; anatomy and physiology; generic pain and stress-management-skill acquisition; and rationale for graded enhancement of strength, flexibility, and endurance (Linton & Kimwendo, 1987). Typically taught by physical therapists or occupational therapists, course-work consists of practical information and application strategies that help individuals appropriately improve their performances on activities of daily living and job tasks and increase adherence to safe body mechanics and home-based exercise and fitness regimens.

When integrated with other aspects of individualized rehabilitation protocols (e.g., results of FCEs and ergonomic job analyses), generic educational modules appear to be efficacious components of primary- and secondary-prevention programs. Mandates from federal and state Occupational Safety and Health Administration (OSHA) offices, the recent Americans with Disabilities Act, state ergonomic standards, safe work practice regulations, and efficacy research in industrial settings have all advanced back school and body mechanics approaches (Caruso, D. Chan, & A. Chan, 1987; Hurri, 1989; Morris & Randolph, 1984). Similar to other individual treatment components, however, there exist no well-controlled, prospective studies that support incremental utility and universal application of this methodology across the varied populations and clinical settings that constitute occupational rehabilitation.

Self-Efficacy Enhancement Technologies

Numerous researchers have demonstrated the important role of the self-efficacy construct (Bandura, 1977, 1986) in enhancing performance and/or reducing disability and pain-related behaviors in several areas, including exercise compliance and workload performance (e.g., Ewart, Taylor, Reese, & DeBusk, 1983; Kaplan, Atkins, & Reinsch, 1984), muscular endurance (Gould & Weiss, 1981), motor skills (Feltz, Landers, & Raeder, 1979), mood-related performance deficits (Davies & Yates, 1982), and pain tolerance (e.g., Bandura, O'Leary, Taylor, Gauthier, & Gossard, 1987; Litt, 1988).

Recent advances regarding clinical enhancement of self-efficacy in an aversive medical situation (Gattuso et al., 1992) suggest that this approach has potential for improving functional capabilities in individuals with complex, chronic musculoskeletal disabilities (e.g., those with some combination of pain-related deconditioning, affective distress, fear of reinjury, and communication-skill deficits). Relatedly, Fitzgerald and Feuerstein (1992) developed the Physical Capabilities Scale (PCS), a validated, 8-item scale for rating expected performance during a standardized evaluation of isokinetic strength, range of motion, and endurance, as measured by a computer-interfaced dynamometer. This methodology appears to hold promise for use as an adjunct to psychophysiological assessment and biofeedback applications as well.

Finally, incorporation of constructs from other health-behavior change technologies, particularly those from well-validated addictive behavior models, may improve clinical protocols for disability risk reduction and adherence enhancement (Fitzgerald, 1992). In particular, the stage-specific "self-change" and relapse prevention training models (e.g., Fitzgerald & Prochaska, 1990, 1991; Marlatt & Gordon, 1985; Prochaska & DiClemente, 1983, 1985) appear to have considerable utility in prevention and management of work-related musculoskeletal disability, but neither framework has undergone empirical investigation within this context.

CONTROVERSIES AND TRENDS IN OCCUPATIONAL REHABILITATION

Despite dynamic changes that have recently taken place in the field of occupational rehabilitation, resolution of four focal issues may enhance cost-effectiveness and treatment outcomes. First, there exists a natural tension in the process of transition from a single provider to a multidisciplinary team approach and from a multidisciplinary to an interdisciplinary or transdisciplinary approach. Although few researchers would argue against advantages of interdisciplinary evaluation and treatment of chronic musculoskeletal disorders, external mandates (e.g., educational and licensing standards, third-party payor requirements) may serve to reinforce unnecessary barriers among clinical disciplines. Such barriers may, in turn, impede both development of a common lexicon and holistic strategies for prevention and management of work-related disability.

Second, although some clinical researchers have advanced sophisticated disability management algorithms, unnecessary time delays and redundant or inappropriate interventions can neutralize even the most centralized referral control and tracking mechanisms. Time-sensitive guidelines for assessment, referral, and treatment, such as those proposed by the QTF and the Colorado Division for Workers' Compensation appear to address a wide range of service delivery problems raised by epidemiological research.

Third, impact of the ADA on worker's compensation systems and individual workers has not yet become totally discernible. Preliminary data from the Equal Employment Opportunity Commission, however, suggest that occupationally injured workers will be the primary beneficiaries of the Act, specifically with respect to worksite accommodations (Bell, 1993). Yet another complicating factor is the prospective impact of likely national health-care reform.

Finally, there is a pressing need for funding of relevant empirical investigation, such as that provided by the National Institute for Disability and Rehabilitation Research and other agencies. Development of normative databases for work tolerances and psychophysiological measures across occupational groups, gender, and age, may facilitate treatment and return-to-work planning. Additionally, outcome research in context of randomized clinical trials may contribute to an understanding of efficacy of current treatment approaches, individually and additively, and articulate alternative pathways for risk reduction in the workplace.

ACKNOWLEDGMENT

The authors extend their appreciation to Marge Elliott for her thoughtful contributions to the typing and editing of the manuscript for this chapter.

REFERENCES

Abenhaim, L., & Suissa, S. (1987). Importance and economic burden of occupational back pain: A study of 2,500 cases representative of Quebec. *Journal of Occupational Medicine, 29,* 670–674.

Ahern, D. K., Iezzi, A., Hursey, K., & Follick, M. J. (1988). The co-occurrence of chronic low back pain and headache: Prevalence, neuroticism, and treatment outcome. *Clinical Journal of Pain, 4,* 27–31.

American College of Sports Medicine. (1980). *Guidelines for graded exercise testing and exercise prescription.* Philadelphia: Lea & Febiger.

American Psychiatric Association. (1994). *Diagnostic and statistical manual of mental disorders, 4th ed.* (DSM-IV). Washington, DC: Author.

Armstrong, T. J., Fine, L. J., Goldstein, S. A., Lifshitz, Y. R., & Silverstein, B. A. (1987). Ergonomic considerations in hand and wrist tendinitis. *Journal of Hand Surgery, 12A,* 830–837.

Asfour, S. S., Khalil, T. M., Waly, S. M., Goldberg, M. L., Rosomoff, R. S., & Rosomoff, H. L. (1990). Biofeedback in back muscle strengthening. *Spine, 15,* 510–513.

Ayoub, M. M., & Mital, A. (1989). *Manual material handling.* Philadelphia: Taylor & Francis.

Bandura, A. (1997). Self-efficacy: Toward a unifying theory of behavioral change. *Psychological Review, 84,* 191–215.

Bandura, A. (1986). *Social foundations of thought and action: A social cognitive theory.* Englewood Cliffs, NJ: Prentice-Hall.

Bandura, A., O'Leary, A., Taylor, C. B., Gauthier, J., & Gossard, D. (1987). Perceived self-efficacy and pain control: Opioid and nonopioid mechanisms. *Journal of Personality and Social Psychology, 53,* 563–571.

Barnes, W. S., & Williams, J. H. (1987). Effects of myoelectrical signal characteristics during rest and recovery from static work. *American Journal of Physical Medicine, 66,* 249–263.

Barsky, A. J., & Klerman, G. L. (1983). Overview: Hypochondriasis, bodily complaints, and somatic styles. *American Journal of Psychiatry, 140,* 273–283.

Basmajian, J. V., & DeLuca, C. J. (1985). *Muscles alive: Their functions revealed by electromyography.* Baltimore, MD: Williams & Wilkins.

Battie, M. C., Bigos, S. J., Fisher, L. D., Hansson, T. H., Nachemson, A. L., Spengler, D. M., Wortley, M. D., & Zeh, J. (1989). A prospective study of the role of cardiovascular risk factors and fitness in industrial back pain complaints. *Spine, 14,* 141–147.

Battie, M. C., Bigos, S. J., Fisher, L. D., Spengler, D. M., Hansson, T. H., Nachemson, A. L., & Wortley, M. D. (1990). The role of spinal flexibility in back pain complaints within industry: A prospective study. *Spine, 15,* 768–773.

Bell, C. G. (1993). The Americans with Disabilities Act and injured workers: Implications for rehabilitation professionals and the Worker's Compensation system. *Rehabilitation Psychology, 38,* 103–115.

Biering-Sorenson, F. (1982). Low back trouble in a general population of 30-, 40-, 50-, and 60-year-old men and women. *Danish Medical Bulletin, 29,* 289–299.

Bigos, S. J., Battie, M. C., Spengler, D. M., Fisher, L. D., Fordyce, W. E., Hansson, T. H., Nachemson, A. L., & Wortley, M. D. (1991). A prospective study of work perceptions and psychosocial factors affecting the report of back injury. *Spine, 16,* 1–6.

Boden, S. D., Davis, D. O., Dina, T. S., Patronas, N. J., & Wiesel, S. W. (1990). Abnormal magnetic-resonance scans of the lumbar spine in asymptomatic subjects. *Journal of Bone and Joint Surgery, 72-A,* 403–408.

Borg, G. (1985). *An introduction to Borg's RPE-Scale.* Ithaca, NY: Movement Publications.

Bortz, W. M. (1982). Disuse and aging. *Journal of the American Medical Association, 248,* 1203–1208.

Bortz, W. M. (1984). The disuse syndrome. *Western Journal of Medicine, 141,* 691–694.

Bouckoms, A. (1985). Recent developments in the classification of pain. *Psychosomatics, 26,* 637–645.

Broman, C. L., Hamilton, V. L., & Hoffman, W. S. (1990). Unemployment and its effects on families: Evidence from a plant closing study. *American Journal of Community Psychology, 18,* 643–659.

Cady, L. D., Thomas, P. C., & Karwasky, R. J. (1985). Program for increasing health and physical fitness of fire fighters. *Journal of Occupational Medicine, 2,* 111–114.

Carpenter, G. C. (1992). Disabilities management strategies: The WorkAbility system. *Physical Medicine and Rehabilitation: State of the Art Reviews, 6,* 273–281.

Caruso, L., Chan, D., & Chan, A. (1987). The management of work related back pain. *American Journal of Occupational Therapy, 41,* 112–117.

Chaffin, D. B. (1988). A biomechanical strength model for use in industry. *Applied Industrial Hygiene, 3,* 79–85.

Cram, J. R., & Steger, J. C. (1983). EMG scanning in the diagnosis of chronic pain. *Biofeedback and Self-Regulation, 8,* 229–241.

Croce, R. V. (1986). The effects of EMG biofeedback on strength acquisition. *Biofeedback and Self-Regulation, 11,* 299–310.

Davies, F. W., & Yates, B. T. (1982). Self-efficacy expectancies versus outcome expectancies as determinants of performance deficits and depressive affect. *Cognitive Therapy and Research, 6,* 23–35.

Deyo, R. A., & Tsui-Wu, Y. J. (1987). Functional disability due to back pain: A population-based study indicating the importance of socioeconomic factors. *Arthritis and Rheumatology, 30,* 1247–1254.

Dolan, P., Adams, M. A., & Hutton, W. C. (1988). Commonly adopted postures and their effect on the lumbar spine. *Spine, 13,* 197–201.

Dolce, J. J. (1987). Self-efficacy and disability beliefs in behavioral treatment of pain. *Behavior Research and Therapy, 25,* 289–299.

Duckro, P. N., Greenberg, M., Schultz, K. T., Burton, S. M., Tait, R. C., Deshields, T. L., & Richardson, W. D. (1992). Clinical features of chronic post-traumatic headache. *Headaches Quarterly, Current Treatment and Research, 3,* 295–308.

Ewart, C. K., Taylor, C. B., Reese, L. B., & DeBusk, R. F. (1983). Effects of early post-myocardial infarction exercise testing on self-perception and subsequent physical activity. *American Journal of Cardiology, 51,* 1076–1080.

Federspiel, C. F., Guy, D., Kane, D., & Spengler, D. (1989). Expenditures for nonspecific back injuries in the workplace. *Journal of Occupational Medicine, 31,* 919–924.

Feltz, D. L., Landers, D. M., & Raeder, U. (1979). Enhancing self-efficacy in high avoidance motor tasks: A comparison of modeling techniques. *Journal of Sport Psychology, 1,* 112–122.

Feuerstein, M. (1991). A multidisciplinary approach to the prevention, evaluation, and management of work disability. *Journal of Occupational Rehabilitation, 1,* 5–12.

Feuerstein, M., & Fitzgerald, T. E. (1992). Biomechanical factors affecting upper extremity cumulative trauma disorders in sign language interpreters. *Journal of Occupational Medicine, 34,* 257–264.

Feuerstein, M., & Hickey, P. F. (1992). Ergonomic approaches in the clinical assessment of occupational musculoskeletal disorders. In D. C. Turk & R. Melzack (Eds.), *Handbook of pain assessment* (pp. 71–99). New York: Guilford.

Feuerstein, M., Menz, L., Zastowny, T., & Barron, B. (1994). Chronic back pain and work disability: Vocational outcomes following multidisciplinary rehabilitation. *Journal of Occupational Rehabilitation, 4,* 229–251.

Fishbain, D. A. (1995). DSM-IV: Implications for the pain clinician. *American Pain Society Bulletin, 5,* 6–18.

Fishbain, D. A., Cutler, R. B., Rosomoff, R. S., & Rosomoff, H. L. (1994). The problem-oriented psychiatric examination of the chronic pain patient and its application to the litigation consultation. *Clinical Journal of Pain, 10,* 28–51.

Fitzgerald, T. E. (1992). Psychosocial aspects of work-related musculoskeletal disability. In J. C. Quick, L. R. Murphy, & J. J. Hurrell, Jr. (Eds.), *Stress and well-being at work: Assessments and interventions for occupational mental health* (pp. 117–133). Washington, DC: American Psychological Association.

Fitzgerald, T. E., & Feuerstein, M. (1992, March). *Self-efficacy, physical performance, and pain behaviors following musculoskeletal injury.* Paper presented at the meeting of the Society of Behavioral Medicine, New York, NY.

Fitzgerald, T. E., & Prochaska, J. O. (1990). Nonprogressing profiles in smoking cessation: What keeps people refractory to self-change? *Journal of Substance Abuse, 2,* 87–105.

Fitzgerald, T. E., & Prochaska, J. O. (1991). Longitudinal typologies of self-change of smoking behavior: Implications for intervention and education. In R. H. Feldman & J. H. Humphrey (Eds.), *Advances in health education: Current research* (Vol. 3, pp. 1–25). New York: AMS Press.

Fitzgerald, T. E., Tennen, H., Affleck, G., & Pransky, G. S. (1993). The relative importance of dispositional optimism and control appraisals in quality of life after coronary artery bypass surgery. *Journal of Behavioral Medicine, 16,* 25–43.

Fletcher, M. (1990, September 10). Cumulative trauma disorders: Repetitive motion cases cost billions annually. *Business Insurance,* pp. 3–6.

Flor, H., Frydrich, T., & Turk, D. C. (1992). Efficacy of multidisciplinary pain treatment centers: A meta-analytic review. *Pain, 49,* 221–230.

Flor, H., Schugens, M. M., & Birbaumer, N. (1992). Discrimination of muscle tension in chronic pain patients and healthy controls. *Biofeedback and Self-Regulation, 17,* 165–177.

Flor, H., Turk, D. C., & Birbaumer, N. (1985). Assessment of stress-related psychophysiological responses in chronic back pain patients. *Journal of Consulting and Clinical Psychology, 53,* 354–364.

Fraser, T. (1989). *The worker at work.* Philadelphia: Taylor & Francis.

Frymoyer, J. W. (1991). Epidemiology of spinal diseases. In T. G. Meyer, V. Mooney, & R. J. Gatchel (Eds.), *Contemporary conservative care for painful spinal disorders* (pp. 10–23). Philadelphia: Lea & Febiger.

Frymoyer, J., & Cats-Baril, W. (1987). Predictors of low back pain disability. *Clinical Orthopedics, 221,* 89–98.

Frymoyer, J. W., Pope, M. H., Clements, J. H., Wilder, D. G., MacPherson, B., & Ashikaga, T. (1983). Risk factors in low back pain: An epidemiological survey. *Journal of Bone and Joint Surgery, 65A,* 213–218.

Gattuso, S. M., Litt, M. D., & Fitzgerald, T. E. (1992). Coping with gastrointestinal endoscopy: Self-efficacy enhancement and coping style. *Journal of Consulting and Clinical Psychology, 60,* 133–139.

Gervais, S., Dupuis, G., Veronneau, F., Bergeron, Y., Millette, D., & Avard, J. (1991). Predictive model to determine cost/benefit of early detection and intervention in occupational low back pain. *Journal of Occupational Rehabilitation, 1,* 113–131.

Goodkin, K., & Gullion, C. M. (1989). Anti-depressants for the relief of chronic pain: Do they work? *Annals of Behavioral Medicine, 11,* 83–101.

Gould, D., & Weiss, M. (1981). Effect of model similarity and model self-talk on self-efficacy in muscular endurance. *Journal of Sport Psychology, 3,* 17–29.

Graves, J. E., Pollock, M. L., Carpenter, D. M., Leggett, S. H., Jones, A., MacMillan, M., & Fulton, M. (1990a). Quantitative assessment of full range-of-motion isometric lumbar extension strength. *Spine, 15,* 289–294.

Graves, J. E., Pollock, M. L., Foster, D., Leggett, S. H., Carpenter, D. M., Vuoso, R., & Jones, A. (1990b). Effect of training frequency and specificity on isometric lumbar extension strength. *Spine, 15,* 504–509.

Greenwood, J. (1991). Socioeconomic factors in back pain and compensation systems. In T. G. Meyer, V. Mooney, & R. J. Gatchel (Eds.), *Contemporary conservative care for painful spinal disorders* (pp. 155–166). Philadelphia: Lea & Febiger.

Griegel-Morris, P., Larson, K., Mueller-Klause, K., & Oatis, C. A. (1992). Incidence of common postural abnormalities in the cervical, shoulder, and thoracic regions and their association with pain in two age groups of healthy subjects. *Physical Therapy, 72,* 425–431.

Hagberg, M., & Kvarnstrom, S. (1984). Muscular endurance and electromyographic fatigue in myofascial shoulder pain. *Archives of Physical Medicine and Rehabilitation, 65,* 522–525.

Hatch, J. P., Prihoda, T. J., & Moore, P. J. (1992). The application of generalizability theory to surface electromyographic measurements during psychophysiological stress testing: How many measurements are needed? *Biofeedback and Self-Regulation, 17,* 17–39.

Heinsalimi, P. (1984). Method to measure working posture loads at working sites (OWPAs). In E. N. Cortlett (Ed.), *Ergonomics of working postures* (pp. 100–104). London: Taylor & Francis.

Holbrook, T. L., Grazier, K., Kelsey, J., & Stauffer, R. (1984). *The frequency of occurrence, impact, and cost of selected musculoskeletal conditions in the United States.* Chicago: American Academy of Orthopaedic Surgeons.

Hurri, H. (1989). The Swedish back school in chronic low back pain. Part I: Benefits. *Scandinavian Journal of Rehabilitation Medicine, 21,* 33–40.

Iacono, C. U. (1991). EMG scanning norms: Caveat emptor. *Biofeedback and Self Regulation, 16,* 227–241.

Kaplan, R. M., Atkins, C. J., & Reinch, S. (1984). Specific efficacy expectations mediate exercise compliance in patients with COPD. *Health Psychology, 3,* 223–242.

Kelsey, J. L. (1982). *Epidemiology of musculoskeletal disorders.* New York: Oxford University Press.

Kessler, R. C., Turner, J. B., & House, J. S. (1987). Intervening processes in the relationship between unemployment and health. *Psychological Medicine, 17,* 949–961.

Keyserling, W. M., Armstrong, T. J., & Punnett, L. (1991). Ergonomic job analysis: A structured approach for identifying risk factors associated with overexertion injuries and disorders. *Applied Occupational Environmental Hygiene, 6,* 353–363.

Khalil, T. M., Goldberg, M. L., Asfour, S. S., Moty, E. A., Rosomoff, R. S., & Rosomoff, H. L. (1987). Acceptable maximum effort (AME): A psychophysical measure of strength in back pain patients. *Spine, 12,* 372–376.

Kraus, L. E., & Stoddard, S. (1989). *Chartbook on disability in the United States: An info use report.* Washington, DC: National Institute on Disability and Rehabilitation Research.

Kuorinka, I., Kilbom, A., Nilsson, B., Andersson, R., & Bjurvald, M. (1987). Standardised Nordic questionnaires for the analysis of musculoskeletal symptoms. *Applied Ergonomics, 18,* 233–237.

Lacerte, M., & Wright, G. R. (1992). Return to work determination. *Physical Medicine and Rehabilitation: State of the Art Reviews, 6,* 283–302.

LaPlante, M. P. (1988). *Data on disability from the National Health Interview Survey, 1983–85.* Washington, DC: National Institute on Disability and Rehabilitation Research.

Lefebvre, M. (1981). Cognitive distortion and cognitive errors in depressed psychiatric and low back pain patients. *Journal of Consulting and Clinical Psychology, 49,* 517–525.

Liang, M., & Komaroff, A. (1982). Roentgenograms in primary care patients with acute low back pain: A cost effective analysis. *Archives of Internal Medicine, 142,* 1108–1112.

Lichter, R. (1991). Work simulation: Putting training to work. *Spine: State of the Art Reviews, 5,* 449–462.

Lifshitz, Y., & Armstrong, T. (1986). A design checklist for control and prediction of cumulative trauma disorders in hand intensive manual jobs. *Proceedings of the 30th Annual Meeting of Human Factors Society, 1,* 837–841.

Lindsay, P., & Wyckoff, M. (1981). The depression–pain syndrome and its response to antidepressants. *Psychosomatics, 22,* 571–577.

Linn, M. W., Sandifer, R., & Stein, S. (1985). Effects of unemployment on mental and physical health. *American Journal of Public Health, 75,* 502–506.

Linton, S. J., & Kamwendo, K. (1987). Low back schools: A critical review. *Physical Therapy, 67,* 1375–1383.

Linton, S. J., & Kamwendo, D. (1989). Risk factors in the psychological work environment for neck and shoulder pain in secretaries. *Journal of Occupational Medicine, 31,* 609–613.

Litt, M. D. (1988). Self-efficacy and perceived control: Cognitive mediators of pain tolerance. *Journal of Personality and Social Psychology, 54,* 143–160.

Lucca, J. A., & Recciuti, S. J. (1983). Effect of electromyographic biofeedback on an isometric strengthening program. *Physical Therapy, 63,* 200–203.

Magni, G. (1987). On the relationship between chronic pain and depression when there is no organic lesion. *Pain, 31,* 1–21.

Marlatt, G. A., & Gordon, J. R. (Eds.). (1985). *Relapse prevention: Maintenance strategies in the treatment of addictive behaviors.* New York: Guilford.

Matheson, G. O., MacIntyre, J. G., Taunton, J. E., Clement, D. B., & Lloyd-Smith, R. (1989). Musculoskeletal injuries associated with physical activity in older adults. *Medicine and Science in Sport and Exercise, 21,* 379–385.

Mayer, T. G., & Gatchel, R. J. (1988). *Functional restoration for spinal disorders: The sports medicine approach.* Philadelphia: Lea & Febiger.

Mayer, T. G., Kishing, N. D., Nichols, G., Gatchel, R. J., Mayer, H., & Mooney, V. (1988). Progressive isoinertial lifting evaluation: I. A standardized protocol and normative database. *Spine, 13,* 993–997.

Mayer, T. G., Tencer, A., Kristofferson, S., & Mooney, V. (1984). Use of noninvasive techniques for quantification of spinal range of motion in normal subjects and chronic low back dysfunction patients. *Spine, 9,* 588–595.

McGill, C. (1968). Industrial back problems: A control program. *Journal of Occupational Medicine, 10,* 174–178.

McNeil, J. M. (1982). *Labor force status and other characteristics of persons with a work disability.* Washington, DC: U.S. Government Printing Office.

McPherson, B. D. (1984). Sport, health, well-being, and aging: Some conceptual and methodological questions for sport scientists. In *The 1984 Olympic Scientific Congress Proceedings* (Vol. 5, pp. 3–24). Champaign, IL: Human Kinetics.

Melzack, R. (1975). The McGill Pain Questionnaire: Major properties and scoring methods. *Pain, 1,* 277–299.

Middaugh, S. J., & Kee, W. G. (1987). Advances in electromyographic monitoring and biofeedback in treatment of chronic cervical and low back pain. In M. G. Eisenberg & R. C. Grzesiak (Eds.), *Advances in clinical rehabilitation* (pp. 137–172). New York: Springer.

Milner-Brown, H. S., Mellenthin, M., & Miller, R. G. (1986). Quantifying human muscle strength, endurance, and fatigue. *Archives of Physical Medicine and Rehabilitation, 67,* 530–535.

Mital, A. (1994). Issues and concerns in accommodating the elderly in the workplace. *Journal of Occupational Rehabilitation, 4,* 253–268.

Mitchell, R. I., & Carmen, G. M. (1990). Results of a multicenter trial using an intensive active exercise program for the treatment of acute soft tissue and back injuries. *Spine, 15,* 514–521.

Mooney, V., Cairns, D., & Robertson, J. (1976). A system of evaluating and treating chronic back disability. *Western Journal of Medicine, 124,* 370–376.

Morris, A., & Randolph, J. (1984). Back rehabilitation programs speed recovery of injured workers. *Occupational Health and Safety, 53,* 64–68.

Murphy, J. K., Sperr, E. V., & Sperr, S. J. (1986). Chronic pain: An investigation of assessment instruments. *Journal of Psychosomatic Research, 30,* 289–296.

National Institute of Occupational Safety and Health. (1981). *Work practices guide for manual lifting* (Report No. 81-22). Cincinnati, OH: U.S. Department of Health and Human Services.

Ng, L. K. Y. (1981). *New approaches to treatment of chronic pain: Review of multidisciplinary pain centers.* (NIDA Research Monograph Series No. 36.) Rockville, MD: U.S. Department of Health and Human Services.

Ogden-Neimeyer, L., & Jacobs, K. (1989). *Work hardening: State of the art.* Thorofare, NJ: Slack.

Ordet, S. M., & Grand, L. S. (1992). *Dynamics of clinical rehabilitative exercise.* Baltimore, MD: Williams & Wilkins.

Polatin, P. B., & Mayer, T. G. (1992). Quantification of function in chronic low back pain. In D. C. Turk & R. Melzack (Eds.), *Handbook of pain assessment* (pp. 37–48). New York: Guilford.

Prochaska, J. O., & DiClemente, C. C. (1983). Stages and processes of self-change of smoking: Toward an integrative model of change. *Journal of Consulting and Clinical Psychology, 51,* 390–395.

Prochaska, J. O., & DiClemente, C. C. (1985). Common processes of change for smoking, weight control, and psychological distress. In S. Shiffman & T. Wills (Eds.), *Coping and substance use* (pp. 345–363). San Diego, CA: Academic Press.

Ransford, A. O., Cairns, D., & Mooney, V. (1976). The pain drawing as an aid to the psychologic evaluation of patients with low back pain. *Spine, 1,* 127–134.

Roberts, B. (1989). Vocational rehabilitation of the industrially injured worker: A new approach. *NARPPS News, 10,* 6.

Rodgers, S. H. (1988). Job evaluation in worker fitness determination. *Occupational Medicine: State of the Art Reviews, 3,* 219–239.

Rodriquez, A. A., & Agre, J. C. (1991). Electrophysiological study of the quadriceps muscles during fatiguing exercise and recovery: A comparison of symptomatic and asymptomatic postpolio patients and controls. *Archives of Physical Medicine and Rehabilitation, 72,* 993–997.

Romano, J. M., & Turner, J. A. (1985). Chronic pain and depression: Does the evidence support a relationship? *Psychological Bulletin, 97,* 18–34.

Saal, J. A., & Saal, J. S. (1989). Nonoperative treatment of herniated lumbar intervertebral disc with radiculopathy: An outcome study. *Spine, 14,* 431–437.

Saal, J. A., & Saal, J. S. (1991). Later stage management of lumbar spine problems. In S. A. Herring (Ed.), *Physical medicine and rehabilitation clinics of North America* (pp. 205–221). Philadelphia: Saunders.

Saal, J. S., Lerman, R. M., & Keane, G. P. (1990). Objective assessment of lumbar spine function. *Critical Reviews in Physical Medicine and Rehabilitation, 2,* 25–38.

Samuelson, B., Wangenheim, M., & Wos, H. (1987). A device for three-dimensional registration of human movement. *Ergonomics, 30,* 1655–1670.

Schiffman, E., Fricton, J., Haley, D., & Tylka, D. (1988). A pressure algometer for myofascial pain syndrome: Reliability and validity testing. In R. Dubner, G. F. Gebhart, & M. R. Bond (Eds.), *Proceedings of the 5th World Congress on Pain* (pp. 407–413). Amsterdam: Elsevier.

Shephard, R. J. (1978). *Physical activity and aging.* Chicago: Year Book Medical Publishers.

Shrey, D. E., & Olesheski, J. A. (1992). Disability management and industry-based return transition programs. *Physical Medicine and Rehabilitation: State of the Art Reviews, 6,* 303–313.

Smith, T. W., Aberger, E. W., Follick, M. J., & Ahern, D. K. (1986). Cognitive distortion and psychological distress in chronic low back pain. *Journal of Consulting and Clinical Psychology, 54,* 573–575.

Soderberg, G. (1992). *Selected topics in surface electromyography for use in the occupational setting: Expert perspectives.* (NIOSH Publication 91-100.) Washington, DC: U.S. Department of Health and Human Services.

Spitzer, W. O., LeBlanc, F. E., & Dupuis, M. (1987). Scientific approach to the assessment and management of activity-related spinal disorders: A monograph for clinicians. Report of the Quebec Task Force on spinal disorders. *Spine, 12* (7S), 3–59.

Tait, R. C., Pollard, A., Margolis, R. B., Duckro, P. N., & Krause, S. J. (1987). The pain disability index: Psychometric and validity data. *Archives of Physical Medicine and Rehabilitation, 68,* 438–441.

Tramposh, A. K. (1991). The functional capacity evaluation: Measuring maximal work abilities. *Spine: State of the Art Reviews, 5,* 437–448.

Turk, D. C., Meichenbaum, D., & Genest, M. (1983). *Pain and behavioral medicine: A cognitive-behavioral perspective.* New York: Guilford.

Turk, D. C., & Melzack, R. (1992). *Handbook of pain assessment.* New York: Guilford.

U.S. Public Health Service. (1988). *National health survey.* Washington, DC: Author.

University of Michigan Center for Ergonomics. (1988). *UAW-Ford Ergonomics Process Job Improvement Guide.* Ann Arbor, MI: Author.

Videman, T. (1987). Connective tissue and immobilization: Key factors in musculoskeletal degeneration. *Clinical Orthopedics, 221,* 6–32.

Vinokur, A. D., Van Ryn, M., Gramlich, E. M., & Price, R. H. (1991). Long-term follow-up and benefit/cost analysis of the Jobs Project: A preventive intervention for the unemployed. *Journal of Applied Psychology, 76,* 1–7.

Watson, D., & Pennebaker, J. W. (1989). Health complaints, stress, and distress: Exploring the central role of negative effectivity. *Psychological Review, 96,* 234–254.

Webster, B. S., & Snook, S. H. (1990). The cost of compensable low back pain. *Journal of Occupational Medicine, 32,* 13–15.

Wiesel, S. W., Tsourmas, N., Feffer, H. L., Citrin, C. M., & Patronas, N. (1984). A study of computer-assisted tomography: 1. The incidence of positive CAT scans in an asymptomatic group of patients. *Spine, 9,* 549–551.

Williams, D. A., & Thorn, B. E. (1989). An empirical assessment of pain beliefs. *Pain, 36,* 351–358.

Wilson, J. R., & Corlett, E. N. (Eds.), (1990). *Evaluation of human work: A practical ergonomics methodology.* Philadelphia: Taylor & Francis.

Wolf, L. B., Segal, R. L., Wolf, S. L., & Nyberg, R. (1991). Quantitative analysis of surface and percutaneous electromyographic activity in lumbar erector spinae of normal young women. *Spine, 16,* 155–161.

Yeh, C., Gonyea, M., Lemke, J., & Volpe, M. (1985). Physical therapy: Evaluation and treatment of chronic pain. In G. M. Aronoff (Ed.), *Evaluation and treatment of chronic pain* (pp. 251–261). Baltimore, MD: Urban & Schwarzenberg.

Yelin, E. (1986). The myth of malingering: Why individuals withdraw from work in the presence of illness. *Milbank Quarterly, 64,* 622–649.

20

Assessment and Treatment of Multiple Sclerosis

Daniel N. Allen and Anthony J. Goreczny

INTRODUCTION

Multiple sclerosis (MS) affects approximately 250 thousand individuals living in the United States or about 50 to 60 individuals per 100 thousand (Maloney, 1985; National Institutes of Health, 1984). The majority of individuals with MS are between the ages of 15 and 50 and typically experience initial symptoms of the disorder between the ages of 25 and 35. Females have a disproportionately higher rate of MS than do males; some reports indicate that approximately twice as many women as men have a diagnosis of MS (Kurtzke, 1983a; Sibley, Bamford, & Clark, 1984). MS also appears related to race; for example, there is a lower frequency of the disorder in Japanese-Americans and in Japan (Kurtzke, 1983a).

MS is somewhat unusual because it has an uneven geographical distribution, with the highest incidence of the disorder reported between 65° and 45° latitude in the Northern and Southern hemispheres (Kurtzke, 1983a). However, it appears that this geographical risk factor interacts with age such that individuals younger than 13–15 years of age living between these latitudes are the most susceptible to developing MS. As such, individuals older than 13–15 years who move from a location outside the 65th and 45th latitudes to a location between the 65th and 45th latitudes have the same susceptibility to MS as do those individuals living outside these latitudes. Familial and twin studies have demonstrated that there also appears to be a

---

Daniel N. Allen • Department of Psychology, Highland Drive Veterans Affairs Medical Center, Pittsburgh, Pennsylvania 15206.   **Anthony J. Goreczny** • Highland Drive Veterans Affairs Medical Center and University of Pittsburgh School of Medicine, Pittsburgh, Pennsylvania 15206.
Handbook of Health and Rehabilitation Psychology, edited by Anthony J. Goreczny. Plenum Press, New York, 1995.

genetic factor. Reitan and Wolfson (1985) noted that the chances of acquiring MS are 12 times higher than normal if a parent has MS, whereas the chances are 20 times higher if a sibling has MS (Batchelor, 1985; Ellison, Visscher, Graves, & Fahey, 1984; National Institutes of Health, 1984).

Many authors have speculated that MS is the result of an immunological response to some type of slowly progressive viral infection (Batchelor, 1985; McFarland & Dhib-Jalbut, 1989; Narod, Johnson-Lussenburg, Zheng, & Nelson, 1985; Sibley, 1988; Sibley et al., 1984), although the susceptibility to MS may have genetic determinants. Several lines of evidence converge to support this general theory. First, the aforementioned risk factors (geographic distribution, race, familial link, and critical age) all suggest that a viral agent present in the environment could be a common cause. This viral agent could infect individuals during a susceptible period (childhood) and subsequently infect other family members. A second line of evidence includes studies reporting epidemic-like outbreaks of MS that have occurred in relatively isolated populations. These epidemics are also suggestive of a common environmental mechanism. Third, the inflammation noted during formation of MS lesions suggests an underlying immunological response, possibly in reaction to a virus. However, at this time researchers have not identified any virus that produces the effects seen in MS.

NEUROLOGICAL PROCESSES UNDERLYING MS

In order to adequately understand the neuropathological process of MS, some basic knowledge of the human nervous system is essential. Because of this, we first provide a brief and basic summary of pertinent information on this topic. The human nervous system consists of three subdivisions, which include the central nervous system (CNS), the peripheral nervous system (PNS), and the autonomic nervous system (ANS). The CNS consists of the brain and spinal cord and is primarily responsible for overall regulation of functions of various parts of the human body. The PNS includes cranial and spinal nerves. It communicates motor commands from the brain to muscles and glands, and relays both internal and external sensory information from the environment to the brain. The ANS regulates automatic functions of the vital organs (e.g., the heart, lungs, and blood vessels).

Each of these nervous systems contains two types of cells, known as neurons and neuroglia. Neurons conduct nerve impulses and thus serve as pathways of communication to and from the three divisions of the nervous system. Neurons consist of a cell body, dendrites, and an axon. Of primary importance to the current discussion are axons, which are responsible for carrying impulses away from neurons to adjacent neurons. The second type of cells, neuroglia, perform several important functions, including provision of structural support to neurons, repair of insults to the CNS, and production of a fatty substance known as *myelin*. Myelin, produced by neuroglia, forms sheaths around axons of neurons. These sheaths serve as insulators, thereby allowing quick and efficient communication of nerve impulses between neurons. In the CNS, cells called oligodendrocytes produce myelin, while Schwann cells produce myelin in the PNS. The fatty insulating sheaths produced by oligodendrocytes form when the cytoplasms of the oligodendrocytes wrap around neuron axons in a spiraling manner. The myelin sheath consists of many concentric layers of lipids and proteins, although the majority (70%) of myelin is lipids and the rest is proteins. One oligodendrocyte can produce as many as 50 myelin sheaths. As a result, loss of one of these cells can negatively impact functioning of multiple neurons.

MS is highly specific in its attack on the nervous system; MS attacks only the myelin produced by oligodendrocytes within the CNS. Destruction of myelin sheaths and oligodendrocytes is a process known as *demyelinization*. Although the exact cause of this demyelinization remains unknown, it appears that the process begins when a breach occurs in the blood–brain barrier (BBB). The BBB typically separates immune system cells from CNS cells. Raine (1985, 1990) has suggested that when immune system cells breach the BBB and enter the CNS, they misidentify elements of the CNS and, as a result, attack these elements. Attack on the CNS produces scarring (or sclerosis) of involved CNS cells by causing swelling and accumulation of fluid within the myelin sheath which, in turn, causes loosening and/or separation of the typically tightly wrapped layers of myelin. These scars, also known as *plaques,* cause a "short circuit" of nerve impulses that normally travel down axons to adjacent nerve cells. Raine (1990) and Lampert (1983) have provided excellent discussions of the neuropathology of MS, and interested readers may wish to refer to these sources for a more in-depth review of the topic.

The plaques noted in MS can be located anywhere in the white matter of the CNS, although Cobble, Dietz, Grigsby, and Kennedy (1993) indicate that MS plaques occur more often in specific white matter regions, including the optic nerves, periventricular white matter, frontal white matter, cervical spinal cord, brain stem, cerebellum, and basal ganglia. Because of its widespread attack on the CNS, those nerve tracts that are the longest have the greatest probability of becoming damaged as the disease progresses. As a result, many individuals with MS experience initial symptoms in the lower extremities. In addition to white matter structures, gray matter can also experience adverse effects, primarily due to plaques that occur in the white matter at the tips of gyri. Destruction of white matter caused by these plaques can spill over into adjacent gray matter (see Raine, 1990).

DIAGNOSIS

Because of its extensive attack on the CNS, MS produces a wide variety of symptoms. This, along with other factors, can lead to difficulty diagnosing the disorder when symptoms initially occur. However, two sets of criteria exist to aid in diagnosis of MS. In 1965, Schumacher and colleagues suggested that clinicians could diagnose patients with "clinically definite" MS if patients exhibited the following four criteria:

1. Abnormal neurological findings.
2. Evidence indicating that two separate lesions have developed, with at least 30 days separating development of the two lesions.
3. Symptoms that last at least 24 hours and are suggestive of white matter lesions (for patients within the typical age range).
4. No alternate explanation for the symptoms.

Since formulation of these diagnostic criteria, there has been an attempt to update them in accord with advancing medical technology.

Poser et al. (1983) revised these criteria to include four possible diagnostic categories of MS, including clinically definite MS, laboratory-supported definite MS, clinically probable MS, and laboratory-supported probable MS. It is beyond the scope of the current discussion to describe these categories in depth; however, addition of the "laboratory-supported" categories probably reflects the most significant change in diagnostic criteria since the original diagnostic formulation by Schumacher et al. (1965). Poser and colleagues suggested that clinicians need not rely solely on neurological examination for detection of white matter lesions, but could also use laboratory tests, such as magnetic resonance imaging (MRI), computer-aided tomography (CAT), evoked potential studies, and cerebrospinal fluid examinations to help confirm the presence of white matter lesions. Of these techniques, MRI is especially sensitive to white matter lesions. In fact, some authors have suggested that MRI is 10 times more effective at detecting white matter lesions than CAT scans (Young et al., 1981). As MRI technology continues to progress, it is quite likely that this technique will become an integral part of the diagnostic process.

However, some caution is warranted when utilizing results of MRI scans in the diagnosis of MS. This is because MRI hyperintensities, commonly observed in scans of patients with MS and indicative of compromised brain tissue, often do not relate to neurological dysfunction and neuropathological processes. In fact, Coffey, Figiel, Djang, and Weiner (1990) along with others (Bradley, 1984) have noted presence of hyperintensities in subcortical white matter in their samples of normal elderly individuals. Presence of these hyperintensities in many individuals remains unexplained (Brown, Lewine, Hudgins, & Risch, 1992). With this caution in mind, the diagnostic approach advocated by Sibley (1990) seems warranted. Sibley suggested that although all of the aforementioned laboratory tests may be useful, there is a relative order of importance: the history, the neurological examination, imaging techniques (particularly MRI), evoked potentials, and cerebrospinal fluid studies.

Although these diagnostic criteria may appear straightforward, actual diagnosis of MS as it presents in its initial stages is often problematic. This fact is evident from studies that report a significant time lapse between onset of the first symptoms and formal diagnosis. For example, in a recent study, Rao, Leo, Bernardin, and Unverzagt (1991a) reported that, on average, their group of 100 individuals with MS experienced their first symptoms 14.2 years earlier but received formal diagnosis of MS only 9.5 years prior to the study. As one can imagine, this delay can cause increased frustration and stress for individuals with MS; they may often feel certain that there is a problem but are unable to obtain a medical diagnosis that would confirm their impressions.

The delay that often occurs between symptom onset and formal diagnosis appears to be due to several factors. First, initial symptoms are often transitory and/or relatively mild in nature. As a result, some individuals do not seek medical attention when these mild symptoms occur but wait until more severe symptomology is present. Second, individuals with MS may initially seek treatment for affective disturbances, such as depression; such disturbances precede onset of symptoms typically associated with neurological dysfunction as much as 20% of the time (Schiffer & Babigian, 1984). Third, clinicians may overlook the diagnosis of MS because some diagnosticians, in an attempt to explain their patients' neurological symptoms, may misdiagnose their patients as suffering from psychiatric disorders, such as hysterical neuroses or conversion disorders. K. Skegg, Corwin, and D. Skegg

(1988) reported that out of 91 patients identified as having MS from a group of 112 thousand individuals, 9% had received psychiatric diagnoses after referral to psychiatrists, even though clear neurological symptoms were present. Common diagnoses included depression and hysterical personality/conversion disorder. However, Skegg et al. concluded that their finding of 9% is probably an underestimate of the total number of individuals with MS who initially received psychiatric diagnoses. There is some confirmation of their conclusion from other studies. For example, Tissenbaum, Harter, and Friedman (1951) reported that of 395 Veterans Administration patients diagnosed with neurological disorders, 30 had diagnoses of MS. Of these 30, ten had initially received psychiatric diagnoses. Disease course in MS can also influence diagnosis because some types of MS, relative to others, are more obvious from the onset. However, there is little literature that addresses incidence of diagnosis or misdiagnosis based on disease course.

DISEASE COURSE

MS patients typically experience periods of exacerbation and remission. During periods of exacerbation, symptoms that are already present may become more severe and/or new symptoms may become apparent. Sibley (1990) reported that exacerbations occur at a rate of between 0.5 to 1.0 time over the course of a year. During periods of remission, some resolution of symptoms may occur or, at least, symptoms will appear to become stable with no further increase in severity. During exacerbations of MS, any number of symptoms may develop, and these can continue from 1–2 days up to 4–12 weeks (Matthews, 1985a; Sibley, 1990). Symptoms usually remit at some point during this time period, and remission of symptoms may last several months to many years. During remission, there is often improvement in symptomatology, although many individuals never experience full recovery of lost functions. Researchers have offered several reasons to explain the recovery of function sometimes seen following exacerbations. These include decreased inflammation and edema, partial remyelinization, and/or conduction of nerve impulses through alternate neural pathways (Prineas et al., 1989). Although there can be great diversity in the symptomatology of MS, there does appear to be at least two general categories of disease course: relapsing–remitting MS and chronic–progressive MS.

Relapsing–Remitting Disease Course

In a relapsing–remitting (RR) course, individuals with MS experience acute exacerbations often manifested by clinically significant symptomatology. Separating these periods of acute exacerbation are periods during which the disease course appears to be relatively stable. Approximately 85% of individuals with MS exhibit a RR course (Sibley, 1990). Schapiro, van der Noort, and Scheinberg (1984; Schapiro, 1990) identified several subtypes of MS that present with a RR course. First, the term *benign sensory* MS describes a disease course in which numbness in a specific body part or some other symptom is present. This symptom may or may not remit but, in either case, the disease does not appear to progress. This disease course accounts for about 10% of MS cases. A second category is *benign relapsing–remitting* MS. In these cases, individuals experience mild symptoms that wax and wane but do not produce significant levels of disability. This disease course accounts for approximately 20–30% of MS cases. A third subcategory of RR MS is a *chronic relapsing–progressive* course. In these patients, a chronic downhill progression of increasingly severe symptomatology is present, but this downhill progression fluctuates over the course of time. Approximately 50–60% of individuals with MS manifest symptoms consistent with this disease course.

There is one final category of disease course that seems most consistent with the RR category. Gilbert and Sadler (1983) reported instances in which individuals received diagnoses of MS after autopsy revealed the presence of MS plaques. Prior to autopsy, these individuals exhibited no clinically significant symptoms that would indicate presence of MS. It appears that these individuals account for a small proportion of MS cases.

Chronic–Progressive Disease Course

The second general category of disease course is chronic–progressive (CP) MS in which neurological deficits produced by MS plaques progress steadily without periods of remission. Sibley (1990) suggested that approximately 15–20% of individuals who have MS experience CP disease courses. Schapiro and colleagues (1984; Schapiro, 1990) suggested that two subcategories of CP MS exist. The first subcategory, termed *chronic progressive,* involves symptoms that proceed gradually without remission, finally leading to disability. This subtype affects about 10% of individuals with MS. The second subcategory, termed *acute–rapid progressive,* includes individuals with MS that progresses rapidly from onset of initial symptoms, eventually leading to death and affects about 10% of individuals with CP MS. RR MS can progress into CP MS as length of time between exacerbations decreases.

As one would expect, disease course relates to development of plaques. MRI studies have indicated that individuals identified as having CP disease courses develop approximately six new lesions each year (Koopmans et al., 1989), whereas patients with RR courses develop approximately three new lesions per year (Willoughby et al., 1989). Also, in addition to differences in levels of physical disability among these groups, several investigators have reported that cognitive deficits that accompany CP MS are more severe than those accompanying RR MS (W. Beatty, Goodkin, Monson, & P. Beatty, 1989a; Heaton, Nelson, Thompson, Burks, & Franklin, 1985). There is also some evidence that would suggest the etiology of RR MS that progresses to a CP course and the etiology of CP MS may be different (Thompson et al., 1991).

MULTIPLE SCLEROSIS SYMPTOMATOLOGY

The distribution of plaques throughout the CNS, noted in both RR and CP forms of MS cause a wide array of symptoms. Schapiro et al. (1984) suggested classification of these symptoms as: (1) *primary,* or symptoms that result directly from MS; (2) *secondary,* or symptoms that are the result of complications produced by primary symptomatology; and (3) *tertiary,* or symptoms that are psychosocial in nature.

Table 20.1 presents many of the more common symptoms noted in individuals with MS. Although it is easy to classify some of the symptoms into one of these three symptom categories, appropriate classification of others is more difficult. For exam-

Table 20.1. Disorders Resulting from Multiple Sclerosis[a]

Sensory and perceptual dysfunction	Sexual dysfunction
Trigeminal neuralgia	Erectile dysfunction
Dysethesias	Delayed ejaculation
Parathesias	Loss of genital sensation
Low back pain	Decreased (typical) or increased
Numbness	(atypical) libido
Cold feet	Decreased vaginal lubrication
Optic neuritis	Diminished orgasm intensity
Diplopia	Motor dysfunction
Nystagmus	Spasticity
Vertigo	Tremor
Impaired hearing	Weakness
Impaired taste	Ataxia
Bowel dysfunction	Dysarthria
Constipation	Dysphagia
Diarrhea	Cognitive dysfunction
Incontinence	Decreased information-processing
Bladder dysfunction	speed
Incontinence	Impaired memory
Hesitancy	Decreased motor speed
Frequency	Decreased simple and complex
Urgency	attention
Dribbling	Aphasia
Other disorders	Dementia
Fatigue	Psychiatric disorders
Weight gain	Depression
Decubiti	Euphoria
Edema	Bipolar disorder
Pathological laughing or weeping	Psychosis

[a]Adapted from Allen, D. N., Landis, R. K. B., & Schramke, C. J. (1995). The role of psychologists in the treatment of multiple sclerosis. *International Journal of Rehabilitation and Health, 1,* 97–123.

ple, it is unclear whether the affective disorders that often occur belong in the primary or tertiary classes, because there is evidence that would support classification in either one or both of these categories. On the face of it, making this type of distinction may seem picayune. However, proper understanding of the etiology of MS symptoms can have a significant impact on the type of intervention used to treat it. Going back to our example, if depression were primarily psychosocial in nature, one might choose to intervene using traditional psychological techniques. On the other hand, if affective disorders are a primary symptom of MS caused by damage to white matter structures integral to regulation of emotions, they may not be amenable to standard psychotherapeutic treatments.

Probably the most remarkable piece of information that Table 20.1 conveys is the multitude of ways in which MS can negatively impact functioning of individuals. MS seemingly spares no area of functioning as the disease progresses. Because of the plethora of symptoms caused by MS, in the following sections we discuss only those that most frequently require psychological intervention. The following discussion is not exhaustive but rather provides clinicians with a working knowledge of the etiology, prevalence, and possible treatment modalities for specific problems.

Physical Symptoms

Table 20.1 lists many of the physical symptoms experienced by individuals with MS. Because there are several other chapters and texts devoted to discussion of treatment and physical rehabilitation of such symptoms (Cobble et al., 1993; Maloney, Burks, & Ringel, 1985; Schapiro, 1987) we will not be discuss them further except to say that some of the most common physical symptoms are optic neuritis, bladder dysfunction, gait disturbance, affective disturbances, and numbness or parethesia. These symptoms relate to the structures primarily and most often affected by MS.

Sexual Dysfunction

Sexual dysfunction is quite common in individuals with MS. Some authors have reported that as many as 90% of males and 70% of females experience negative changes in sexual functioning following onset of the disorder (Harowski, Harris, Nager, & Schapiro, 1987). These percentages include reports that indicate 63–80% of males with MS experience erectile dysfunction, and 44–77% of males report some type of orgasm phase dysfunction (Goldstein, Siroky, Sax, & Kane, 1982; Lilius, Baltonen, & Wilkström, 1976; Minderhoud, Leemhius, Kremer, Laban, & Smits, 1984; Valleroy & Kraft, 1984). Valleroy and Kraft surveyed 217 individuals with MS (149 females and 68 males) in an attempt to determine types of sexual dysfunction experienced as well as factors that contributed to sexual dysfunction. They found that 56% of all females and 75% of all males reported some type of sexual dysfunction. The problems that males most commonly reported were difficulty achieving erections (63%), decreased sensation (55%), and difficulty maintaining erections (52%). The most prevalent problems among the female respondents were fatigue (68%), decreased sensation (48%), and decreased libido (41%).

Valleroy and Kraft (1984) also reported that bladder dysfunction and spasticity tended to be the symptoms most highly associated with sexual dysfunction. Depression, fatigue, motor weakness, and changes in sensation were not more prevalent in those individuals who reported sexual dysfunction than in those who reported no such dysfunction. In light of this pattern of symptoms, Valleroy and Kraft concluded that lesion location may be the most important factor regarding development of sexual dysfunction. Harowski and co-workers (1987) echoed this conclusion when they stated, "Given the complexity of the sexual response in terms of the neuromuscular transmissions involved, it is no surprise that sexual difficulties are often encountered in MS" (p. 45). However, Harowski et al. also indicated that there is often a psychological overlay to many of the difficulties individuals with MS experience in regard to sexual functioning. Issues of a nonneurological nature that often interfere with sexual functioning include poor body image, decreased self-esteem, and dysphoric emotions (e.g., guilt, anxiety, and depression).

Psychological Disorders

Etiology

Depression, anxiety, bipolar disorder, euphoria, emotional lability, and psychosis may all occur in individuals with MS, as may a variety of other psychiatric disorders (Minden, Orav, & Reich, 1987). Charcot (1877, 1881) noted that affective disturbances were quite common in his MS patients. He viewed these emotional disturbances as cardinal features of MS and as a direct result of the underlying neuropathological process. Other investigators, such as Cottrell and Wilson (1926) supported Charcot's conclusion; Cottrell and Wilson, for example, reported disturbances of affect in all of the 100 MS patients they interviewed. Because Charcot proposed his original neural dysfunction account of emotional disturbances in this patient group, there has been some debate as to whether these affective disturbances are (1) the direct result of damage to the CNS, (2) precipitants (along with stressful life events) of MS and future exacerbations of the disorder, (3) normal reactions to a chronic debilitative disease, or (4) some combination of all three of these factors (Mei-Tal, Meyerowitz, & Engel, 1970; Rabins, 1990; Rabins et al., 1986; Ron & Logsdail, 1989; Schiffer, 1990; S. Warren, Greenhill, & K. Warren, 1982; S. Warren, K. Warren, & Cockerill, 1991). Research supports the contention that all of these factors may somehow play a role in the increased prevalence of affective disturbances.

However, there is mounting evidence that suggests a disruption of the neural pathways responsible for regulation of emotions is a powerful contributor to the occurrence of psychiatric disorders. For example, one MRI study of 46 inpatients experiencing acute MS exacerbations (Reischies, Baum, Bräu, Hedde, & Schwindt, 1988) indicated that periventricular and nonperiventricular frontal white matter lesions were the only type of lesions that significantly correlated with psychopathology (i.e., depression, euphoria, irritability, lability, drive reduction, and impaired judgment). Other studies have reported significant correlations between elation and widespread MRI abnormalities (Ron & Logsdail, 1989). Ron and Logsdail also reported that symptoms associated with psychosis (e.g., flattened affect, delusions, and thought disorder) significantly related to temporoparietal lesions. Similarly, Honer, Hurwitz, Li, Palmer, and Paty (1987) found that a small group of MS patients with diagnosed psychiatric disorders had more plaques in the temporal lobes than a matched MS control group, even though there was no apparent difference between the two groups in the total number of plaques. Finally, studies using CAT scans and clinical evaluations (Rabins et al., 1986) have also indicated that patients who score higher on measures of depression also tend to have fewer spinal cord lesions and more cerebral lesions.

In addition to imaging studies, Ron and Logsdail (1989) reported that incidence of psychiatric disorders was not significantly related to severity of physical disability, while Schiffer and Wineman (1990) reported that severity of depression was only weakly correlated with severity of physical disability. If the psychiatric (and particularly affective) disorders noted in these individuals were reactions to a chronic debilitating illness, one might expect that level of distress would increase as physical disability increases. This does not appear to be the case. Finally, a recent study suggested that incidence of psychological distress (and particularly depression) relates to immune system dysregulation (Foley et al., 1992). Therefore, psychiatric disturbances evidenced by MS patients appear primarily due to the pathophysiological processes present in MS.

Incidence

There have been several investigations that have examined incidence of psychiatric disorders in individuals with MS. Depression and euphoria/bipolar disorder have received the most attention in the literature. Incidence of depression in individuals with MS appears to be higher than among normal controls (Baldwin, 1952) and individuals with other neurological disorders (Pratt, 1951). Depression will affect approximately 40–60% of individuals diagnosed with MS over the course of their lifetimes. As many as one third of these individuals experience depressive symptomology that is severe enough to meet criteria for major depression over the course of a year (Minden et al., 1987; Minden & Schiffer, 1990; Schiffer & Babigian, 1984). In contrast, the lifetime frequency rate for depression in the general population is 9.7%, and the rate in patient groups with chronic medical disorders other than MS is 12.9% (Wells, Golding, & Burnam, 1988). Depression also occurs more frequently in individuals with MS than in other groups with neurological disorders (Whitlock & Siskind, 1980).

Studies using self-report measures of depression have confirmed higher rates of depression among MS patients than other groups of individuals. Rao et al. (1991a) reported that when compared to a control group that was similar in age, education, gender, premorbid intelligence, and premorbid occupational status, MS patients had significantly higher Zung Self-Rating Depression Scale (Zung, 1965) scores. Minden et al. (1987) reported results similar to Rao et al. (1991a) when using the Beck Depression Inventory (BDI; Beck, Ward, Mendelson, Mock, & Erbaugh, 1961) to compare MS patients' scores to the scores of other groups of medical patients.

The relationship between suicidal behavior and depression in MS patients is unclear. However, as with depression, the prevalence rate of completed suicides among individuals with MS is significantly higher than for the general population or other individuals with chronic medical disorders (Sadovnick, Eisen, Ebers, & Paty, 1991). Suicide was the cause of death in 15.1% of the cases among a group of individuals representative of the MS population in Canada who were followed over a 16-year period; an additional 1.7% of the deaths appeared to be suicides, but suicide was not the official cause of death. For this same group, among individuals who did not die of the direct effects of MS, the percentage of deaths due to suicide was between 28.6% and 31.7%. Sadovnick et al. reported that those individuals who died from suicide were younger, experienced less disability, and had shorter disease duration compared to other individuals in their sample. Kahan, Leibowitz, and Alter (1971) reported percentages similar to Sadovnick et al. (1991). Kahan et al. found that suicide accounted for 17% of the deaths in a group of individuals with MS they followed over the course of 6 years. To put these percentages in perspective, Mackenzie and Popkin (1987) noted that the rates reported by Kahan et al. (1971) translate into a death rate of 400/100,000 for individuals with MS, which is in sharp contrast to the overall national suicide rate of about 11.9/100,000.

There have been several investigations that have reported a higher incidence of bipolar disorder among individuals with MS than among nonneurologically and other neurologically impaired groups. Schiffer, Wineman, and Weitkamp (1986) reported that bipolar disorder was twice as prevalent in individuals with MS when compared to nonneurologically impaired groups. Joffe, Lippert, Gray, Sawa, and Horvath (1987) found that of a sample of 100 individuals diagnosed with definite MS, 13 met RDC criteria for bipolar disorder at some time in their lives. In a recent review of the literature, Garland and Zis (1991) concluded that bipolar disorder occurs at a higher incidence among MS patients than one would expect in the general population of individuals without family backgrounds that would predispose them to develop manic–depression. It is important to distinguish bipolar disorder from pathological laughing or pseudobulbar affect, in which individuals exhibit outbursts of emotion (typically laughing or weeping) in the obvious lack of presence of stimuli that would elicit such an emotion. Often, individuals report that on these occasions they are not subjectively experiencing any strong emotion. This type of emotional disconnection may relate to damage of the subcortical forebrain structures. As a result, individuals with MS may be susceptible to this condition.

Neuropsychological Deficits

Cognitive deficits caused by demyelinization within the CNS are quite prevalent in individuals with MS. However, there is currently some question as to the percentage of individuals with MS who have concurrent cognitive deficits. Estimates of prevalence rates range between 43% and 72% (Heaton et al., 1985; Klonoff, Clark, Oger, Paty, & Li, 1991; McIntosh-Michaelis et al., 1991; Rao et al., 1991a). Much of the discrepancy appears due to type of patients under investigation, duration of MS symptoms, and the course of MS in the patient groups studied. In this regard, Rao and colleagues (1991a) indicated that many of the studies that have reported high incident rates studied patients selected from listings of university-based hospitals. These patients often exhibit significantly more impairment than the typical or more general MS population (Nelson et al., 1988).

In an attempt to determine prevalence of cognitive dysfunction in the general MS population, Rao and colleagues (1991a) randomly selected individuals from a listing of individuals with MS that they obtained from a society for MS patients. Of the 730 individuals initially selected, 299 expressed interest in participating in the investigation. Of these 299 prospective subjects, 199 did not meet inclusion and/or exclusion criteria. Some of these exclusion criteria included history of alcohol/drug abuse, coexisting neurological conditions in addition to MS, severe visual and/or motor impairment, and previous neuropsychological evaluation at the investigators' center. Of the remaining 100 individuals, 39 had relapsing–remitting MS, 19 had chronic–progressive MS, and 42 had chronic-stable MS. All 100 individuals underwent extensive neuropsychological evaluation, which included tests of verbal intelligence, memory (immediate, recent, and remote), abstracting abilities, attention/concentration, language abilities, and visuospatial abilities. On the average, this group reported that they had experienced their first symptoms 14.2 years ($SD = 10.0$) earlier and had received formal MS diagnosis 9.5 years ($SD = 9.0$) prior to the study. Their average age was 45.7 years ($SD = 11.3$), and their average level of education was 13.2 years ($SD = 2.4$). The average premorbid IQ for the group, calculated utilizing demographic variables, was 106.8 ($SD = 7.3$).

Results of the cognitive evaluations indicated that this group of MS patients failed significantly more of the neuropsychological tests than did a control group. Out of 31 test indices, the MS group failed an average of 4.64 ($SD = 4.9$) tests, and the control group failed 1.13 ($SD = 1.8$) tests. Forty-eight individuals (48%) from the MS group became classified as cognitively impaired based on the criteria of four or more test indices failed. Investigators determined the true frequency rate of cognitive impairment was 43% because 5% of the individuals in the control group also failed four or more of the tests. In regard to type of tasks failed, those requiring recent memory were the most sensitive; 31% of the MS patients failed tests requiring this ability. About 25% of the MS group failed tests requiring sustained attention and verbal fluency, and about 20% exhibited impaired performance on tests requiring visuospatial perception and conceptual reasoning. Between 15% and 21% of the MS group obtained impaired scores on the Verbal IQ composite and/or the four verbal subtests. This estimate is somewhat lower than previous reports and may be due to the authors' attempts to sample a more general and less severely impaired population than previous studies. The authors indicated that their inclusion–exclusion criteria may have excluded the more severely impaired patients, which may have decreased the level of overall impairment in their group.

However, the pattern of results obtained by Rao et al. (1991a) is similar to those reported by other authors (Beatty & Gange, 1977; W. Beatty, Goodkin, P. Beatty, & Monson, 1989; W. Beatty, Goodkin, Monson, P. Beatty, & Hertsgaard, 1988; Heaton et al., 1985; Kessler, Cohen, Lauer, & Kausch, 1992; Rao, Hammeke, McQuillen, Khatri, & Lloyd, 1984; van den Burg, van Zomeren, Minderhoud, Prange, & Meijer, 1987). Klonoff and co-workers (1991) compared performances of 86 individuals with mild MS to performances of 46 age, education, gender, marital status, and occupational status matched controls. Out of 42 test indices, there were 21 significant differences between performances of these two groups. Eight of these differences were on tests requiring "pure motor functions" (p. 130). An additional 6 required some type of motor ability. Given the nature of MS, authors expected impairment on tests of motor functions. However, individuals with MS also performed more poorly than controls on the Wechsler Adult Intelligence Scale-Revised (WAIS-R) Similarities subtest, Speech Perception test, Word Fluency test, Memory for Objects test, and last, two "hard" trials of the Wechsler Memory Scale (WMS) Paired Associates Learning test. These differences were present despite the fact that there was not a significant difference between the two groups on their WAIS-R Verbal IQ (VIQ) scores.

Because of the pattern of cognitive deficits observed in individuals with MS, some authors have suggested that MS can cause subcortical dementia. Although the distinction between subcortical and cortical dementia has been somewhat controversial (Mayeaux, Stern, Rosen, & Benson, 1983; Whitehouse, 1986), the concept of subcortical dementias has received greater acceptance than in the past because research has begun to indicate that there do appear to be significant cognitive and neurological differences between individuals with diseases that affect primarily the cortex as opposed to diseases that affect primarily white matter structures (Cummings, 1986; Huber, Shuttleworth, Paulson, Bellchambers, & Clapp, 1986). Other authors have extensively described differentiation between cortical and subcortical dementias (Cummings, 1990; Cummings & Benson, 1992; Mahler & Benson, 1990). Therefore, we discuss it here only briefly.

Cortical dementias are a group of disorders that are characterized by degeneration of the cerebral cortex. The most common and most well-known cortical dementia is senile dementia of the Alzheimer's type. The cognitive deficits produced by cortical dementias include impairment of intellect and memory. In addition, aphasia, agnosia, apraxia, and visuospatial and constructional deficits are often present. Personality, gait, and other motor functions are characteristically unaffected by cortical dementia (Cummings & Benson, 1992). In contrast, subcortical dementia is a condition characterized by ". . . mental slowness, inertia and lack of initiative, forgetfulness, dilapidation of cognition, . . . mood disturbance . . . [and] movement disorders" (p. 95). Diseases that cause this group of dementias affect primarily white matter structures that form the frontosubcortical system. The primary structures that compose this system include the frontal cortex, frontal subcortical connections, basal ganglia, brain stem, and thalamus. There are several disorders that affect different components of the frontosubcortical system. For example, Parkinson's disease affects the cerebrum in a diffuse manner so that atrophy of the frontal lobes, putamen, and caudate nucleus often occur. The rationale for classifying such an apparently broad group of disorders as subcortical dementias stems largely from the observation that damage to any part of the frontosubcortical system produces, in a fairly consistent manner, the aforementioned pattern of deficits (Alexander, DeLong, & Strik, 1986).

From the discussion of course and progression of MS, along with the discussion of cognitive deficits and mood disturbances common to the disorder, it is apparent that MS could easily fall within the rubric of subcortical dementia. However, there is still some question as to the number of individuals with MS that actually meet diagnostic criteria for dementia. Given that the cognitive deficits noted in these individuals runs the gamut from mild to severe, clinicians must answer the question of whether individuals suffer from dementia on a case-by-case basis. In order to do this, clinicians must perform careful assessment of cognitive deficits and functional impairment.

It is important to note that the percentage of individuals with MS who have dementia is not clear at this time. It is likely, however, that the course of the disorder has a direct impact on the prevalence rate of dementia among MS patients. Individuals with RR MS who experience only one or two exacerbations over the course of their lives would be much less likely to develop cognitive deficits that are severe enough to warrant diagnoses of dementia than would be individuals with CP disease courses. Individuals with CP disease courses would be more likely to develop dementia as their disease progresses because they sustain more damage than individuals with RR disease courses. Although studies that have attempted to document cognitive and functional deficits in MS patients have suggested that 43–72% of MS patients have cognitive deficits of one type or another, it is likely that diagnosable dementia occurs in only a portion of MS patients. Because of these factors, it appears that although the cognitive deficits caused by MS can have a significant impact on cognitive, functional, and emotional status, clinicians must be careful not to assume that dementia is present in all individuals with MS. It is important that clinicians make this diagnosis only after careful assessment.

Another issue that is of interest here is proper differential diagnosis of dementia caused by MS as opposed to other types of dementia, particularly in older individuals. Fox and colleagues (1989) reported on three cases referred to Rush Alzheimer's Disease Center by physicians who thought that the patients might have Alzheimer's disease. These three individuals were older, and two of them had previously received diagnoses of MS. However, because the course of their disease had been rather stable and asymptomatic for quite some time, the physicians apparently did not suspect that MS could have been the cause of the suspected dementia. Physical examinations, MRI scans, cerebrospinal fluid analyses, and evoked responses of these three individuals all yielded results that were consistent with MS. The authors concluded, "We should stress that multiple sclerosis should be considered when clinically appropriate in any patient with progressive dementia, regardless of age" (p. 1269).

The relationship between physical disability and degree of cognitive impairment in MS patients is not totally clear at this time, but there are a growing number of studies that suggest degree of cognitive impairment and physical impairment do not correlate highly (Peyser, Edwards, Poser, & Filskov, 1980; Rao et al., 1984, Rao et al., 1991a; Ron, Callanan, & Warrington, 1991; van den Burg et al., 1987). Similarly, Baumhefner et al. (1990) demonstrated weak correlations between neurological signs, as determined through neurological examination, and abnormalities present on cerebral MRIs. Furthermore, Rao et al. (1991a) indicated that although the number of cognitive tests failed significantly correlates with tests of disability, this correlation accounts for only 6% of the variance. In regard to duration of illness, Rao et al. also reported no significant relationship between duration of disease and cognitive dysfunction. Finally, Rao et al. reported that individuals with RR MS failed significantly fewer cognitive tests ($X = 3.3$) than those individuals with CP MS ($X = 5.6$) or chronic–stable MS ($X = 5.7$). Similarly, Beatty and colleagues (1988, 1989a,b) found that individuals with CP MS experience more severe cognitive deficits than individuals with RR MS. For instance, they reported that relative to individuals without MS and individuals with RR MS, individuals with CP MS suffered deficits in naming abilities in addition to the typical deficits in abilities associated with subcortical dementias.

Although it does not appear that cognitive dysfunction relates to physical disability, cognitive dysfunction does significantly impact social and vocational functioning. Rao et al. (1991b) studied impact of cognitive impairment on psychosocial functioning of 100 individuals with MS. Of this group, 48 evidenced cognitive impairment. The impaired and unimpaired groups were similar in level of physical disability and duration of illness. However, relative to individuals in the cognitively intact group, individuals in the cognitively impaired group were significantly less likely to have gainful employment, were less likely to participate in social activities, required greater physical assistance, exhibited more problems maintaining personal hygiene and activities of daily living, and were less able to follow a simple recipe when cooking.

In a more recent study, Kessler et al. (1992) attempted to examine the relationships between memory deficits and level of disability assessed by a broad spectrum of functional abilities, including mobility, communication, personal care, domestic activities, education, employment, and social activities. Fifty-six individuals with MS received a variety of tests that assessed cognitive abilities (and, in particular, memory abilities) and levels of physical and functional disability. Because they regarded half of their sample as "relatively unimpaired" in regard to functional impairment, they divided the sample into two groups. Individuals in the group with high levels of functional impairment scored significantly lower on tests requiring memory ability and motor ability (finger tapping and grooved Peg-Board). No statistically significant differences between the groups on other measures of cognitive abilities were present, but the group with the highest level of functional impairment tended to receive lower scores on tests of cognitive abilities. These results are consistent with those reported by Rao et al. (1991b). However, the Kessler et al. study also suggests that impaired memory and motor abilities may more adversely affect functional status than would impairment of other cognitive abilities.

We can draw several conclusions from the literature that has examined incidence and effect of cognitive deficits in individuals with MS. First, it is likely that the actual prevalence rate of cognitive impairment for the general MS population is somewhere between 43% and 72%. Second, cognitive deficits caused by MS can present as a subcortical dementia and, as such, deficits in recent memory, sustained attention, information processing speed, and motor abilities, along with significant psychiatric disturbances (particularly affective disorders) are common. Third, cognitive deficits produced by MS can vary widely from one patient to the next. Fourth, cognitive dysfunction does not relate to physical disability. However, cognitive deficits resulting from MS can significantly interfere with functional abilities, including employability, social functioning, and activities of daily living. It also appears that impairment of some abilities, such as memory and motor abilities, may more adversely affect functional status than would impairment of other abilities. Because of the impact that cognitive dysfunction can have on the well-being of individuals with MS, careful assessment of this area is essential.

ASSESSMENT

Because of the wide range of symptoms produced by MS, there currently exists a large body of literature discussing assessment of these concomitant symptoms. In the current discussion we place emphasis on assessment of sexual dysfunction, cognitive deficits, and psychological disorders because these are the most commonly encountered areas requiring assessment by psychologists. However, we also provide a brief presentation of instruments used to assess physical disability and functional status, because authors frequently refer to these instruments in the literature and clinicians sometimes use them in clinical practice. With regard to neuropsychological assessment, we have limited our discussion to efficacy of brief to intermediate length screening devices because a review of full neuropsychological assessment of MS falls outside the purview of this chapter.

Physical Disabilities

There are several of scales used to assess the level of physical disability and impairment of functional status in patients with MS. Probably the most popular of these is Kurtzke's Expanded Disability Status Scale (EDSS; Kurtzke, 1983b). The EDSS, based on data derived from neurological examinations, assess eight functional systems, including pyramidal, cerebellar, brain stem, sensory, bowel and bladder, visual, and cerebral functions. Patients receive ratings from 0 (normal neurological results) to 5 or 6 (indicative of significant impairment) depending on the specific area of functioning. The eighth category is entitled "other" (i.e., miscellaneous) functions and ranges from 0 (none) to 1 (other neurological findings caused by MS). Clinicians then use scores from each of these eight functional systems to derive an overall rating of physical disability, which ranges from 0 (normal neurological examination) to 10 (death due to MS). Ratings increase by 0.5 point increments so that, for example, an EDSS score of 2.0 equates with minimal disability in one functional system; a score of 2.5 equates with minimal disability in two functional systems; and a score of 8.5 is indicative of being restricted to bed much of the day. Other scales reported to assess a variety of functional ability areas include Kurtzke's Functional Systems Scale (FS; Kurtzke, 1983b), Incapacity Status Scale (ISS; Granger, 1981), and

Environmental Status Scale (ESS; Mellerup et al., 1981). The EDSS, FS, ISS, and ESS combine to form a Minimal Record of Disability (MRD; Holland, Francadandera, & Wiesel-Levison, 1986; Kurtzke, 1981). The MRD has the advantage of providing a broader sampling of functional behaviors than any one of the scales by themselves.

A final scale used to assess functional status is the Activities of Daily Living Scale (ADLS; Staples & Lincoln, 1979). It consists of 42 items on which individuals who have MS receive ratings on a 1- to 3-point scale across seven major areas of functioning. The functional abilities that the ADLS assess include communication, mobility, personal care, domestic activities, education, employment, and social activities. Lower scores on the ADLS are indicative of lower levels of impairment. The ADLS is useful both as a self-report measure and as a rating scale completed by an individual adequately acquainted with a patient's functional abilities. The ADLS has several advantages, including the fact that it is relatively quick to administer, requires no special training to administer, provides a sampling of a broad range of functional behaviors, and appears to be sensitive to the ways in which cognitive deficits can affect level of functioning (Kessler et al., 1992). However, its use is not as widely reported in the literature as is use of the scales composing the MRD.

Assessment of Sexual Dysfunction

Because of the physiological and psychological nature of sexual dysfunction in these individuals, Schapiro et al. (1984) suggested that assessment focus on answering the following three questions:

1. What are the psychological effects on the MS person? 2. What are the physical effects? 3. What are the psychological effects on the spouse (partner)? (p. 432)

In addition to these general suggestion by Schapiro et al., it is important to obtain a thorough history of sexual functioning as well as explore current sexual practices. Two excellent sources that provide information on important aspects of interviewing patients regarding their sexual history and practices are works by Kaplan (1974) and J. LoPiccolo and L. LoPiccolo (1978). Personality assessment measures, such as the Minnesota Multiphasic Personality Inventory (MMPI; Hathaway & McKinley, 1943) and BDI (Beck et al., 1961), may help rule out psychological causes of sexual dysfunction, such as depression or substance abuse. However, as noted in the following section on assessment of affective disorders, some caution is necessary when employing standard psychological tests, such as the MMPI, to assess individuals with MS. It is also important for clinicians to remember that the goal of psychosocial evaluations is to understand patients' current levels of sexual adjustment (i.e., patients' levels of satisfaction regarding expression of their sexuality). As a result, focus of evaluation is not to determine whether a specific patient is engaging in a specific sexual behavior (e.g., intercourse) but, rather, to determine if clients perceive their sexual behaviors as satisfactory and fulfilling. In this light, Ducharme, Gill, Biener-Bergman, and Fertitta (1993) emphasize that sexual adjustment may or may not include genital stimulation. With a clear understanding of what clients find fulfilling or need in their sexual lives, clinicians are then able to treat the sexual dysfunction of individuals with MS.

Thorough physical examinations are also an essential part of sexual dysfunction assessments. Ducharme et al. (1993) provided recommendations for physical examinations that take into account the special needs of individuals with physical disabilities. In addition, they noted that other medical evaluations worth consideration when assessing sexual dysfunctions in physical disabled populations include "blood chemistry, hormonal assays, sensory threshold of the genital area, vascular assessment, neurological evaluation of male sexual dysfunction, and nocturnal penile tumescence monitoring" (p. 765). Finally, because prescription and nonprescription medications can contribute to many types of sexual dysfunction, thorough evaluation of current medications is necessary. Ducharme et al. (1993), Lieberman (1988), and Halstead (1985) provide information regarding possible side effects various medications can have on sexual functioning, and interested readers can refer to these sources for more information.

Psychological Disorders

Given the prevalence of psychiatric disorders in individuals who have MS, psychological assessment is often of great importance when evaluating overall functioning of individuals. Any number of a variety of techniques, including structured interviews, self-report assessment scales, behavioral rating scales, and clinical interviews can assist in diagnosing psychiatric disorders in this group. Presence of physical symptoms, however, can complicate diagnosis, particularly when using self-report measures that contain items reflecting somatic complaints that can accompany psychological disorders.

Minnesota Multiphasic Personality Inventory

There have been several studies that have examined MMPI (Hathaway & McKinley, 1943) profiles of individuals with MS in an attempt to determine what effect, if any, physical symptoms of the disorder have on scale elevations (Marsh, Hirsch, & Leung, 1982; Meyerink, Reitan, & Selz, 1988; Mueller & Girace, 1988; Peyser et al., 1980). There has been the contention that MS patients appear more emotionally or psychologically distressed than they actually are because items that contribute to some of the MMPI scales (most notably Scales 1, 2, 3, and 8) reflect actual physical symptoms produced by MS rather than psychosomatic symptoms that a nonneurologically impaired population exhibits. Because of this, several investigators have removed items from the MMPI thought to reflect common symptomology produced by MS in an attempt to provide a more accurate picture of the psychological functioning of these patients (Baldwin, 1952; Marsh et al., 1982). However, the studies by Baldwin and Marsh et al. did not employ control groups, so the authors were unable to determine what effect the item deletion strategy would have when used with a nonneurologically impaired population.

Studies employing similar methodology (Meyerink et al., 1988; Mueller & Girace, 1988), however, have employed control groups. Mueller and Girace compared MMPI profiles of 26 individuals with MS to profiles of 26 individuals without MS after deletion of 22 MMPI items. The deleted items were those that four qualified raters had rated as moderately related, greatly related, or exactly related to MS symptomology. The authors selected the 26 individuals in the control group from a population of prison inmates with the intent of matching their MMPI profiles to those of the individuals with MS; the authors matched patients on Scales 1, 3, and 8, because previous research has reported MS symptomology most significantly affects these scales. After selection of the groups, the authors removed the items identified as representing MS symptomology. Significant differences were present between the MS group and control group on Scales 1 and 8 after removal of the items, with the MS groups receiving lower t-scores than the control group (53.65 vs. 58.73 for Scale 1, and 59.00 vs. 65.38 for Scale 8).

In a similar study, Meyerink et al. (1988) examined the impact of deleting MMPI items reflecting MS symptoms in 83 individuals with MS. They selected a control group matched for gender from the individuals who served as the adult normative group for the MMPI. Two neurologists selected 30 MMPI items they thought reflected MS symptomology. The authors examined scales that contained five or more of these items (Scales 1, 2, 3, 7, and 8) and found that individuals with MS endorsed more items reflecting MS symptomology than did individuals in the control group, whereas both groups endorsed items that did not reflect MS symptoms about equally. The effect of this endorsement pattern was to elevate scores of the MS group on Scales 1, 2, 3, and 8. Scale 1 increased 12–15 t-score points; Scale 2 increased 3–4 t-score points; Scale 3 increased 5–6 t-score points; and Scale 8 increased 5–7 t-score points.

Results of these studies suggest that individuals with MS receive artificially inflated MMPI t-score elevations, particularly on Scales 1 and 8 and possibly on Scales 2 and 3, due to endorsement of MMPI items that are consistent with their MS symptomatology. Furthermore, after removing items reflecting MS symptomatology, their MMPI code types changed significantly. For example, Mueller and Girace (1988) reported that after removal of MS items, the MS group profile changed from an 8/1 to a 2/4. This change in code type has significant interpretive implications. It is not yet certain which of these two code types more accurately reflects the psychological sequelae produced by MS, but Mueller and Girace indicated that they are actively investigating this question. These findings indicate that clinicians must use some caution when interpreting MMPI profiles of individuals with MS and might want to consider inspecting items that contribute to Scales 1, 2, 3, and 8. Research has yet to determine if the findings reported for the MMPI will also hold true for the MMPI-2 (Butcher, Dahlstrom, Graham, Tellegen, & Kaemmer, 1989).

Depression Screening Instruments

Other studies have employed briefer measure of emotional functioning, such as the State–Trait Anxiety Inventory (STAI; Spielberger, 1983), and the BDI (Beck et al., 1961). It does not appear that researcher have systematically investigated possible affects that MS symptomatology might have on scores of these briefer measures. However, this is a potential concern, because research has shown that some of the measures currently available are susceptible to effects of physical dysfunction. For example, several studies have attempted to determine if somatic symptoms that occur as a result of aging artificially inflate scores on self-report measures of depression (Berry, Storandt, & Coyne, 1984; Blumenthal, 1975; Downes, Davies, & Copeland, 1988; Hertzog, VanAlstine, Usala, Hultsch, & Dixon, 1990; Steuer, Bank, Olsen, & Jarvik, 1980). Some of these studies have indicated that some depression scales are susceptible to somatic complaints associated with aging, thereby making elderly individuals look more depressed than they actually are. One could expect that MS will produce some of these same concerns. However, researchers have not yet addressed the concern about whether somatic complaints noted in MS appreciably increase scores on measures of depression and anxiety in an empirical fashion. Therefore, when performing assessments of individuals with MS, clinicians must use caution interpreting scores of brief inventories and take special care to determine which endorsed items may be due to MS symptomology rather than the emotional disorder under consideration. In order to do this, clinicians can discuss questionable items with individual patients, who can shed light on why they endorsed particular items.

Assessment of Cognitive Disabilities

Neuropsychological deficits commonly observed among MS patients sometimes go undetected by health-care providers. For example, one report indicated that clinical neurologists fail to detect cognitive dysfunction in 50% of patients they evaluate (Peyser et al., 1980). This may happen for several different reasons:

1. Cognitive deficits do not relate to degree of physical disability.
2. Cognitive deficits can occur in early stages of the disease.
3. Cognitive deficits can occur in cases that appear to be mild.
4. Patients may not be aware of the nature or severity of their cognitive deficits.
5. Cognitive deficits typically manifest as discrete problems affecting one or two specific abilities rather than as global deficiencies.
6. Any profile of cognitive deficits can occur in this group. (Beatty & Monson, 1991; Franklin, Nelson, Filley, & Heaton, 1989; Jennekens-Schinkel, van der Velde, Sanders, & Lanser, 1989; Klonoff et al., 1991; Taylor, 1990; van den Burg et al., 1987)

However, as already discussed, cognitive impairment can significantly impact the functional status of individuals with MS. These cognitive deficits may also interfere with patients' abilities to take advantage of therapy, create false expectations on the part of family members with regard to functional abilities and employability of patients, and impede treatment compliance. Even though these deficits may be significantly disabling, unless detected, individuals will not be able to obtain disability benefits. Therefore, it is beneficial to perform some type of cognitive assessment on all individuals with MS.

Cognitive assessment can entail short or intermediate cognitive screening methods or full neuropsychological assessments. However, because neuropsychological evaluation is time- and resource-intensive and requires a certain expertise that is often not available, it is often impractical to provide each patient who has MS with a full neuropsychological evaluation. This does not mean that possible cognitive deficits need go undetected. One solution is to use some type of cognitive screening procedure with each MS patient. Ideally, this procedure would not require highly specialized training, yet have a high enough degree of specificity and sensitively to accurately identify patients with cognitive deficits. There are several brief, cognitive screening procedures currently available that clinicians could use for this purpose, but not all procedures have undergone evaluation with MS patients. Typically, cutoffs for these short screening instruments do exist, such that scores below the cutoff are indicative of significant cognitive impairment.

The following section discusses sensitivity and specificity of brief and intermediate-length cognitive screens. We do not review research regarding administration of full neuropsychological batteries, however, because that is beyond the scope of the current discussion. Interested readers may consult texts by Lezak (1976) and Reitan and Davison (1974) for information on the most popular neuropsychological tests and philosophies of assessment.

Brief Cognitive Screening

One of the best known cognitive screening instruments is the Mini-Mental State Examination (MMSE; M. Folstein, S. Folstein, & McHugh, 1975). The Cognitive Capacity Screening Examination (CCSE; Jacobs, Bernhard, Delgado, & Strain, 1977) is similar to the MMSE; it too is a brief screening instrument devised to detect cognitive impairment. There are several recent reports in the literature regarding use of both these instruments with individuals diagnosed with clinically definite MS (Beatty & Goodkin, 1990; Franklin et al., 1988; Heaton, Thompson, Nelson, Filley, & Franklin, 1990; Rao et al., 1991a).

Rao et al. (1991a) reported that the MMSE successfully classified 11 individuals as cognitively impaired out of a group of 100. However, more extensive neuropsychological assessment indicated that 43 of these same individuals exhibited cognitive impairment. Thus, in their sample, the MMSE had a specificity rate of 98%, but a sensitivity rate of only 23%, a rate which the authors viewed as "unacceptable" (p. 690). Rao and co-workers did not use the standard cutoff of 21 when classifying individuals as impaired in their study, but considered any score below the fifth percentile of the control group's scores as impaired. Heaton et al. (1990) reported that in a group of 40 individuals with clinically definite MS, of whom 55% exhibited cognitive impairment based on Halstead–Reitan Neuropsychological Battery (HRNB; Reitan & Davison, 1974) performance, the MMSE failed to classify any of the individuals as cognitively impaired when using the standard cutoff score of less than 21. When using MMSE scores more than 1 SD below the mean, the MMSE classified 22.5% of the MS group and 12.2% of the control group ($N = 90$) as impaired. These classification percentages yield a sensitivity rate of 0.36 and a specificity rate of 0.94, given consideration of the cognitive impairment (i.e., exclusion of performances on tests requiring sensorimotor abilities) of the samples. Finally, MMSE scores correlated -0.33 with average impairment ratings of the HRNB. Similar to both preceding studies, Swirsky-Sacchetti et al. (1992) reported that sensitivity of the MMSE to cognitive impairment in 56 individuals with definite MS was low and did not correlate well with total lesion area calculated from MRI scans. This finding was in contrast to the high correlations observed between more thorough neuropsychological tests and total lesion area.

Efforts are currently underway to modify the MMSE so that it will be more sensitive to cognitive deficits produced by MS. Beatty and Goodkin (1990) suggested that, with some modifications, the MMSE might be much more sensitive to focal cognitive deficits while retaining its utility as a brief, easily administered screening instrument. They investigated 42 patients with RR MS and 43 patients with CP MS. In these groups, they defined *dementia* as performance below the fifth percentile (relative to age- and education-matched controls) on cognitive tests assessing three of four ability areas: confrontational naming, problem solving, information processing speed, and memory. They found that when using cutoff scores of 27 and below, the MMSE was insufficiently sensitive to identify patients in the MS groups who had dementia. Cutoff scores of 28 and below tended to misclassify too many (16%) nonimpaired control group members. They suggested replacing the MMSE naming items (two items) with the Boston Naming Test (60 items; Kaplan, Goodglass, & Weintraub, 1983). They also recommended changing the three verbal free-recall items to seven items, as anterograde verbal memory was a good predictor of MS-type dementia. Finally, they suggested including the Symbol Digit Modalities Test (Smith, 1973) when assessing the cognitive functioning of individuals with MS because it is quick and easy to administer (usually requiring less than 3 minutes) and quite sensitive to the decreases in information processing speed that are often some of the earliest signs of cognitive decline among MS patients.

Heaton et al. (1990) reported on use of the CCSE and MS patients. Using a standard cutoff score of less than 20, the CCSE did not classify any individuals with MS as cognitively impaired. When using scores that fell 1 *SD* below the mean to determine cognitive impairment, the CCSE classified 22.5% of the MS group and 10% of the control group as impaired. The sensitivity and specificity of the CCSE to cognitive impairment was 0.41 and 0.94, respectively. CCSE scores correlated -0.70 with HRNB impairment ratings in the MS group. These studies suggest that although the CCSE has a higher degree of specificity and sensitivity than the MMSE in detecting cognitive deficits that result from MS, neither of these brief screening instruments is adequate, primarily due to low sensitivity. This is not surprising given the sometimes subtle nature of deficits noted in individuals with MS and the relatively easy tasks required by these screening instruments. Because of this, two brief screening instruments do not appear sensitive to deficits noted in individuals with MS, and efficacy of their use with this population is highly questionable. However, there has been at least one attempt to modify the MMSE so that it will be more sensitive when used with this population (Beatty & Goodkin, 1990). Initial results of these modifications did not appear to increase sensitivity of the MMSE significantly.

Intermediate-Length Cognitive Screening

Alternates to brief cognitive screening examinations are intermediate-length screening batteries. Several published screening batteries for cognitive impairment exist, and include the Neurobehavioral Cognitive Status Examination (NCSE; Kiernan, Mueller, Langston, & Van Dyke, 1987), the Dementia Rating Scale (DRS; Mattis, 1988), and Middlesex Elderly Assessment of Mental State (MEAMS; Golding, 1989). Developers specifically designed two of these three (DRS and MEAMS) for use with elderly populations to detect dementia as well as other types of cognitive dysfunction. The NCSE is a relatively new instrument that clinicians can use with individuals of various ages and with various types of cognitive deficits. Although these instruments have the advantages of requiring relatively little time to administer (about 20 or fewer minutes in most cases) and relatively little training to administer properly, there exist no published studies using these instruments with individuals who have MS. As a result, it is not currently possible to judge the efficacy of these instruments in detecting often mild and specific cognitive deficits produced by MS.

Some authors have attempted to develop intermediate-length cognitive screening batteries that are sensitive to cognitive deficits that often accompany MS. However, it is important to remember that because there is no specific pattern of cognitive deficits characteristic of all individuals with MS, developing these types of screening batteries is a difficult undertaking. With this in mind, several authors have attempted to establish a group of tests that are effective in differentiating individuals with MS from individuals without MS. They have reported that certain instruments appear more sensitive to cognitive dysfunction in individuals with MS than other instruments. For example, Rao et al. (1991a) reported that, in a sample of 100 individuals with MS who underwent extensive neuropsychological evaluation, out of 31 cognitive test scores, four indices were more sensitive than the others in detecting cognitive deficits in the MS group. These four tests included the consistent long-term retrieval from the Selective Reminding Test (Buschke & Fuld, 1974), 7/24 Spatial Recall Test (Barbizet & Cany, 1968), Controlled Oral Word Association Test (Benton & Hamsher, 1976), and Paced Auditory Serial Addition Test (Gronwall, 1977). When they used a liberal cutoff (i.e., failure of one or more of these four test indices), sensitivity of the brief screening procedure was 0.90 and specificity was 0.77. When they raised the cutoff to two or more of these four tests, they achieved a sensitivity rate of 0.71 and a specificity rate of 0.94. As previously mentioned, in this sample, the MMSE identified only 11% of the MS patients as experiencing cognitive dysfunction.

Heaton et al. also described use of an intermediate-length cognitive screening battery composed of 18 brief tests that clinicians can administer in about 45 minutes (for an in-depth description of these tests, see Heaton et al., 1990). Clinicians can obtain scores for each of the instruments that compose this brief battery. In addition, they can calculate a Total Summary Score (TSS; i.e., includes tests of sensorimotor and cognitive abilities) and a Cognitive Summary Score (CSS; i.e., includes only tests of cognitive abilities). Sensitivity of the TSS to detect cognitive impairment was 0.77, and specificity was 0.56. Sensitivity and specificity of this brief battery when using the CSS to detect cognitive impairment were 0.55 and 0.94, respectively. Although the CSS and TSS performed better than brief cognitive screens (MMSE and CCSE) administered by Heaton et al., the sensitivity of both scores is relatively low. Heaton et al. suggest that use of a summary score may obscure cognitive deficits present in individuals with MS, thereby lowering the sensitivity of their intermediate-length battery. Based on this observation, it is expected that examination of individual test scores may increase the battery's sensitivity. However, the veracity of this conclusion awaits further empirical investigation.

Based on these studies, it appears that although the use of brief cognitive screening instruments like the MMSE and CCSE may provide some benefit in detecting cognitive deficits produced by MS, they are not adequately sensitive to cognitive deficits in their present forms. Of the two, the CCSE appears to be the better choice, because it is somewhat more sensitive than the MMSE yet retains about the same level of specificity. However, it is important that individuals who administer screening instruments be cognizant of the fact that patients may score above the cutoff and still have cognitive deficits. In fact, previously reviewed studies indicate that it is quite likely that individuals with MS who have cognitive deficits will "pass" these screening instruments. To conclude that no deficits are present based on a score above the cutoff would do a great disservice to individuals with MS if they truly have cognitive deficits.

Intermediate-length screening batteries appear to hold more promise because they tend to have higher sensitivity and specificity than the MMSE and CCSE. However, clinicians must use similar caution when interpreting "normal" performances on these batteries because they still tend to incorrectly classify many impaired individuals as normal. Advantages that these intermediate-length batteries have over shorter screens is that they provide a profile of patients' cognitive strengths and weaknesses based on abilities tapped by the various tests, and they are more sensitive than brief screens.

If, based on results of cognitive screening, cognitive deficits appear to be present, referral for full neuropsychological assessment is in order. Based on results of more thorough neuropsychological assessment, patients can learn the nature and severity of their deficits and obtain information regarding how these deficits may affect daily functioning. In addition, treatment team members can make referrals for vocational rehabilitation or to lawyers to begin the process of obtaining disability benefits in the case of severe deficits, educate family members and adjust expectations, and implement strategies to help patients compensate for cognitive deficits (e.g., keeping daily planners to help patients with memory deficits remember important appointments and dates).

TREATMENTS

Treatment is particularly important for MS patients because approximately 85% of individuals with MS have normal life expectancies (Cobble et al., 1993). Other studies indicate that many individuals (20–30%) continue to work for 25 years after symptom onset and never become severely disabled (Bauer & Firnhaber, 1965; MacKay & Hirano, 1967). The primary focus of this section is on psychological interventions reported in the literature. However, we also provide a brief review of the comprehensive care model of treatment, treatments for physical disorders that often accompany MS, and chemotherapeutic treatments.

Five general categories of treatment for medical disorders include prophylactic, curative, restorative, symptomatic, and rehabilitative treatments (Cobble et al., 1993). For individuals with MS, treatments currently available are primarily symptomatic and rehabilitative in nature because risk factors associated with MS do not appear to be highly amenable to preventive efforts (prophylaxis), there is currently no cure for the disorder (curative), and we do not currently know how to adequately restore damaged myelin and neurons (restorative). Schapiro (1987) noted that treatment of multiple sclerosis focuses on two broad areas, which include "shortening exacerbations and slowing the progress of the disease, and . . . control [of] specific symptoms, such as spasticity, bowel and bladder problems, or fatigue" (p. 7). These areas are important, but it is essential to emphasize that, in the treatment process, treatment team members intervene in other ways as well.

Comprehensive Care Model of Treatment

Because MS can produce such a broad spectrum of symptoms that require treatment by multiple disciplines, advisory panels have long suggested that treatment facilities use a model of Comprehensive Care (CC) in the treatment and rehabilitation of patients with this disorder (National Advisory Commission on Multiple

Sclerosis, 1975). Since the Commission's suggestion, there have been several articles and volumes that describe such programs (Cobble et al., 1993; Hartings, Pavlou, & Davis, 1976; LaRocca, 1990; Maloney et al., 1985; Marsh, Ellison, & Strite, 1983; Schapiro, 1987; Schapiro et al., 1984; Scheinberg, Holland, Kirschenbaum, Oaklander, & Geronemus, 1981). Although variations exist among CC programs, the major components are quite similar.

To summarize, CC rehabilitation programs emphasize importance of interdisciplinary teams to adequately meet needs of patients. These teams can include psychologists, psychiatrists, physiatrists, neurologists, nurses, physical therapists, occupational therapists, and lawyers (to secure disability benefits when necessary). Core team members are responsible for developing treatment plans based on information generated through initial interviews with patients and, often times, significant others; appropriate diagnostic testing; and thorough review of pertinent medical records. With this information in hand, team members usually meet, discuss each case, and develop treatment plans. Following development of treatment plans, team members discuss plans and recommendations with patients and family members (when appropriate) and often make referrals to appropriate specialties. Patients typically receive the majority of these services from institutions carrying interdisciplinary team affiliations, but team members can also make referrals to outside resources, particularly if this proves more convenient for patients. Team members follow progress of patients by scheduling routine periodic follow-up visits. Depending on patients' needs, inpatient treatment may be necessary, but this is rarely the case. Team members can often make this determination at the time of the intake evaluations.

Services that psychologists provide within the framework of the CC model vary substantially. For example, LaRocca (1990) suggested that as integral members of interdisciplinary teams, psychologists are often responsible for provision of psychological assessment, psychodiagnostics, clarification for the individuals and family members, creation of realistic expectations in treatment plans, therapeutic interventions, individual and group counseling and psychotherapy, orientation groups, cognitive retraining, consulting expertise, and conducting research. These categories comprise four major areas: (1) assessment and psychodiagnosis, (2) psychotherapy and education, (3) consultation, and (4) research.

Chemotherapeutic Treatments

General Symptoms of MS

Cobble et al. (1993) provide an extensive listing of symptoms, medications, usual dosages, side effects, and benefits expected from possible chemotherapeutic treatment strategies that one can utilize to ameliorate the symptoms produced by MS. Spasticity, cerebellar incoordination, pain, paroxysmal symptoms, pseudobulbar palsy, bladder hyperactivity, fatigue, vertigo, nausea, depression, mania, organic brain syndrome, and orgasm phase dysfunction are some of the various symptoms reported to be responsive to chemotherapeutic treatments (Kahn, Stevenson, & Douglas, 1988; Peselow, Fieve, Deutsch, & Kaufman, 1981; Schiffer & Wineman, 1990; Schover, Thomas, Lakin, Montague, & Fischer, 1988).

In addition to alleviating and controlling specific symptoms produced by MS, there have also been attempts to manage MS by decreasing the duration of exacerbations and slowing its progress (curative treatments) by using corticosteroids (e.g., prednisone, dexamethasone, and adrenocorticotropic hormone) and immunosuppressants (e.g., azathiaprine and cyclophosphamide). Corticosteroids can reduce the swelling that occurs during exacerbations, thereby shortening duration of attacks. The rationale for utilizing drugs that suppress immune system activity has its basis in the observation that much of the damage caused during MS exacerbations results from the immune system's erroneous recognition of myelin as a foreign agent. There have been several excellent reviews of the use of these drugs in MS patients and interested readers may refer to these sources for more information (Matthews, 1985b; Schapiro et al., 1984; Thompson et al., 1989; Weiner & Hafler, 1988). It is important to note that corticosteroids can cause affective disturbances and psychosis in some individuals undergoing treatment. In fact, some authors have suggested that the increased incidence of depression and bipolar affective disorder noted among MS patients group may be partially the result of corticosteroid treatments. We discuss this issue further in the following section on treatment of mood disorders.

Mood Disorders

As previously mentioned, there have been several reports suggesting the mood disorders that often accompany MS are amenable to chemotherapeutic treatments. These reports have focused on two major affective disturbances: mania and depression.

Mania. In regard to chemotherapeutic treatment of mania, most of the reports are relatively old and involve reporting a single case (Falk, Mahnke, & Poskanzer, 1979; Kemp, Lion, & Magram, 1977; Mehta, 1976; Peselow et al., 1981; Solomon, 1978). Outcome measures in these reports are generally absent. However, one retrospective study (Falk et al., 1979) did compare incidence of psychosis in a group of MS patients undergoing treatment with corticotropin. One group ($n = 27$) received lithium during corticotropin treatment, whereas the other group ($n = 44$) did not. In the group that did not receive lithium, six patients experienced mania or depression that was severe enough to prematurely end corticotropin treatment. Two other individuals experienced mild depressive disorders while undergoing treatment. In the group that received lithium, there were no moderate or severe mood disorders or psychosis. This difference was statistically significant and appears to indicate that lithium alleviates manic and depressive episodes associated with corticotropin therapy.

Results of the study by Falk et al. (1979) are consistent with reports of other authors who generally report that lithium can be an effective treatment of manic episodes, even when these episodes may have results from corticosteroid treatments. One author does caution that the fact that lithium toxicity may masquerade as an exacerbation of MS presents a concern when instituting lithium therapy (Solomon, 1978). Also, some patients can become toxic on lithium before they reach typical therapeutic doses (Falk et al.). Reduction of lithium in these patients, however, does not appear to adversely alter beneficial effects of the medication.

Depression. To date, there appears to be only one controlled study that examined effects that antidepressant medications have on depression in MS patients

(Schiffer & Wineman, 1990). Schiffer and Wineman reported results of a double-blind study that compared effects of desipramine combined with psychotherapy to effects of placebo combined with psychotherapy in ameliorating depression in 28 individuals with MS. The investigators made diagnoses of major depressive disorder (RDC criteria) using the Schedule for Affective Disorders and Schizophrenia. After subjects agreed to participate in the study, they completed the Hamilton Depression Rating Scale (HDRS; Hamilton, 1960), the BDI (Beck et al., 1961), and the DSS (Kurtzke, 1983b). Subjects then received assignment to either placebo plus psychotherapy or desipramine plus psychotherapy conditions. The authors described the psychotherapy as being "supportive and medical in orientation, interpersonal and social in orientation, or insight oriented" (p. 1494). Therapy occurred in 45-minute weekly sessions over the course of 5 weeks. Patients completed the BDI and HDRS on a weekly basis. However, the primary outcome measure was a clinical assessment of improvement by the primary therapist. The authors judged improvement to have occurred if depressive symptomatology decreased to the extent that primary therapist noted an improvement in psychosocial functioning.

At the end of the 5-week treatment, 11 of 13 patients in the desipramine plus psychotherapy group had improved significantly, whereas only 6 of 14 patients in the placebo plus psychotherapy group had improved. Differential rates of improvement between the two groups were statistically significant. Also, the authors noted significant decreases in HDRS scores at the end of 5 weeks in the desipramine group but not in the placebo group. On the BDI, there were no statistically significant differences in pre- and posttest scores of either group, but the desipramine group's posttherapy scores were lower than the placebos group's scores (11.4 vs. 15.5, respectively). Side effects to the medication occurred in 12 individuals in the desipramine group, such that 7 of the individuals could not receive typical therapeutic dosages. However, 6 of these 7 individuals exhibited significant improvement, as did 6 of the remaining individuals whose serum levels indicated they had obtained therapeutic doses.

There has also been a case report in which a 41-year-old female patient with RR MS received treatment with fluoxetine (Shafey, 1992). Shafey reported that fluoxetine improved mood and cognitive functioning of this patient after a 2-month course of therapy. Fluoxetine was superior to the doxepin hydrochloride in this patient; the latter had relatively little effect on the patient's depression, even after 9 months of treatment. Fewer anticholinergic side effects were reported by the patient after changing from doxepin hydrochloride to fluoxetine.

Treatment of Sexual Dysfunction

There do not appear to be any empirical investigations that examine effectiveness of various sex therapies when used with individuals who have MS. However, there is a significant literature that provides information on treating sexual dysfunction in individuals who have become disabled due to neurological or medical conditions (Schover & Jensen, 1988) as well as several works that provide suggestions for treatment of individuals with MS (Ducharme et al., 1993; Halstead, 1985; Harowski et al., 1987). Several themes regarding treatment of individuals with MS are present in each of these works, and the following section summarizes these themes.

Ducharme et al. (1993) suggested there is a process of adjustment that individuals with acquired disabilities go through after becoming disabled; that process includes learning to accept the disability, grieving loss of functioning, and learning how to meet new challenges in daily living resulting from the disability. Therapists can facilitate effective coping by helping their clients acquire a new repertoire of behaviors and develop existing preserved strengths. Sexual functioning is one area in which this adjustment process may occur. Psychological intervention may be necessary at each stage of the adjustment process. Ducharme et al. suggested that individual and couple psychotherapy may be particularly beneficial in helping individuals adjust to physical disabilities and sexual dysfunctions caused by MS.

Halstead (1985) provided a general treatment program for disabled individuals with MS that consists of four stages:

1. Giving patients permission to engage in sexual behavior and experiment with new or alternative sexual techniques.
2. Providing patients with educational information about their sexual dysfunction and functioning following onset of MS.
3. Giving practical and specific suggestions for sexual techniques and aids that may help individuals adjust to their physical disabilities and sexual dysfunctions.
4. Referring patients who do not appear to benefit from the first three stages of treatment to therapists who specialize in the treatment of sexual dysfunctions.

Therapists can conduct individual and couple therapy within this four-phase treatment program.

Common intrapersonal themes that often need to be addressed following acquired disability include issues of self-esteem, identity, comfort with a disabled/changed body, and dysphoric emotions, such as depression and anxiety. Also, the individual therapy setting may be the appropriate place to help individuals overcome "myths" about sexual functioning in disabled individuals. Common myths include the ideas that: (1) a perfect body is essential in order for individuals to have satisfactory sexual relationships, (2) the goal of sexual expression is intercourse or orgasm, (3) disabled individuals do not maintain an interest in having sexual relations, and (4) individuals with disabilities may hurt themselves if they engage in sexual activities (Ducharme et al., 1993; Halstead, 1985; Harowski et al., 1987).

Couple therapy can help deal with issues that affect interpersonal functioning between individuals with MS and their significant others. As one would expect, acquisition of a disability causes changes in the roles of both individuals. Because of this, each partner may need basic education regarding the sexual dysfunction and functioning of the disabled individual. Also, therapists working with disabled individuals will often need to emphasize the importance of increasing communication about the issue of sexual expression. Exploration of alternative sexual behaviors may be necessary in order to circumvent difficulties produced by MS. Ducharme et al. (1993) noted that *sensate focus* techniques to improve intimacy and overcome sexual dysfunction are the same for able-bodied and disabled individuals. These techniques typically begin with an exploration of each partners' attitudes about sex followed by engaging in sexual self-exploration in order to learn about his or her own sexual responses. Clients then share information gained through these exercises with their partners. Following an understanding of the others' needs, clients and their partners initiate massage and caressing of nongenital areas. This caressing progresses toward genital caressing, which may or may not lead to intercourse.

Halstead (1985) and others (Ducharme et al., 1993; Harowski et al., 1987) have provided several specific and practical suggestions that may help individuals compensate and/or overcome problems in sexual functioning produced by MS symptomatology, such as bladder dysfunction, erectile dysfunction, and spasticity. Patients can manage incontinence by limiting intake of fluids 2–3 hours prior to sexual activity and emptying their bladders through catheterization immediately before sexual activity. These procedures do not totally eliminate the possibility of incontinence during sexual activity; however, taking steps to stop incontinence can relieve anxiety about the possibility of its occurrence. Also, acknowledging the possibility can help decrease anxiety and embarrassment surrounding episodes of incontinence. Male patients can manage the inconvenience caused by indwelling catheters by folding the catheter over, taping it to the penis, and then placing a condom over the penis and catheter. Females can tape indwelling catheters to their abdomens. K-Y jelly can help patients who experience decreased vaginal lubrication. Halstead (1985) also suggested changes in position that can be helpful in circumventing problems caused by spasticity, decreased mobility, limited range of movement, and decreased strength. Men with MS who suffer from erectile dysfunction, including inability to obtain and/or maintain erections can receive penile prostheses, papaverine injections, or use vacuum constrictive devices. Finally, experimentation with alternative methods of stimulation other than intercourse can prove helpful; these include masturbation and oral sex. Also, aids, such as vibrators, can be helpful in cases of decreased genital sensation.

Despite the relatively high incidence of sexual dysfunction among patients with MS, there remain few controlled outcome studies specifically assessing efficacy of sex therapies with these individuals. Although clinicians may choose to use standard sex therapy treatments, complications resulting from neurological impairment may impede treatment progress. As such, researchers must establish efficacy of these therapies with MS patients.

Psychotherapy

Group Psychotherapy

Several authors have advocated use of various forms of group therapy to treat psychological disorders in patients with MS. Clinician researchers have employed five types of treatments, including insight-oriented psychotherapy groups (Crawford & McIvor, 1985), psychoanalytic psychotherapy groups (M. Day, E. Day, & Herrmann, 1953), cognitive–behavioral psychotherapy groups (Larcombe & Wilson, 1984), stress management therapy groups (Crawford & McIvor, 1987), supportive psychotherapy groups (Bolding, 1960; Marsh et al., 1983; Schneiber, 1983; Spiegelberg, 1980; Surridge, 1969), and educational/orientation groups (Hartings et al., 1976; LaRocca, Kalb, & Kaplan, 1987; LaRocca, 1990; Pavlou, Johnson, Davis, & Lefebvre, 1979). However, there have been very few studies that have empirically examined efficacy of these treatments by employing control groups and/or by utilizing outcome measures. Of the aforementioned studies, only Larcombe and Wilson (1984) and Crawford and McIvor (1985, 1987) have employed control groups and pre- and postintervention outcome measures. The results of these three studies are encouraging because all three reported that, relative to control groups, treatment groups exhibited significant decreases in depression.

Cognitive–Behavioral Group Therapy. Larcombe and Wilson (1984) randomly assigned 19 depressed individuals with MS into two cognitive–behavioral therapy groups ($n = 4$ and $n = 5$) or two waiting-list control groups ($n = 5$ for both groups). Pre- and posttherapy evaluations utilized the BDI (Beck et al., 1961), HDRS (Hamilton, 1960), self-reported daily mood ratings, and ratings by significant others. The treatment group met once a week for a total of six 1½ hour sessions. Therapy consisted of a combination of behavioral and cognitive procedures based largely on the work of Lewinsohn (1975) and colleagues Lewinsohn, Biglan, and Zeiss (1976) and Beck, Rush, Shaw, and Emery (1979). At the end of therapy, individuals in the treatment group exhibited significant improvement on all measures, whereas subjects in the waiting-list control did not improve on any of the measures. The investigators performed 1-month follow-up assessments on the two therapy groups using all of the original outcome measures except the HDRS. No significant differences were present between posttreatment and follow-up evaluation scores on any of the three measures. These results provide initial support for use of cognitive–behavioral group psychotherapy with individuals who have MS, and the changes caused by this therapy appear to persist at least 1 month after treatment ends. It is important to note that Larcombe and Wilson (1984) used a paired-associates learning task to screen out individuals with suspected verbal learning deficits. Therefore, it is unclear whether individuals with verbal learning deficits could benefit from the cognitive–behavioral therapy approach employed in this study.

Insight-Oriented Group Therapy. Crawford and McIvor (1985) attempted to investigate effects of insight-oriented group psychotherapy on depression, anxiety, locus of control, and self-concept. These authors divided 32 patients into three groups: a traditional psychotherapy group, a current events group, and a no-treatment group (the investigators did not specify number of individuals in each group). The authors described the insight-oriented psychotherapy group as follows: "Patients were actively encouraged to verbalize and confront issues of conflict" (p. 811). The current events group discussed current issues in the news, and the no-treatment group received no treatment during the course of the study. The insight-oriented and current events groups participated in fifty 1-hour sessions over the course of 25 weeks. The investigators composed triads of individuals matched according to gender, duration of illness, and pretest scores and then randomly assigned each member of the triads to one of the three groups. Pre- and posttest measures included the Minnesota Multiphasic Personality Inventory Depression-30 Scale (D-30; Dempsey, 1964), Ability-Testing Anxiety Scale Questionnaire (ASQ; Krug, Scheier, & Cattell, 1976), Adult Nowicki-Strickland Internal–External Control Scale (IECS; Nowicki & Duke, 1974), and Rosenberg Self-Esteem Scale (RSES; Silber & Tippett, 1965). At the end of 50 sessions, there were no differences between the three groups on the ASQ and RSES. The current events group and psychotherapy group both differed from the no-treatment group on the IECS, with both groups reporting increased internal locus of control relative to changes for the no-treatment group. Finally, scores of psychotherapy group members on the D-30 suggested that they felt significantly less depressed than members of the other two groups. The authors suggested that the lack of difference between the groups on the measure of anxiety may have resulted from the fact that posttesting coincided with termination of group therapy. This may have had the effect of raising the level of anxiety of all individuals in the study. Again, it is important to note that the only patients included in this study supposedly had no serious cognitive impairment. Also, the investigators did not describe the nature of the therapy groups adequately, thereby making replication of this study and application of their results in clinical settings difficult.

Stress Management Group Therapy. Crawford and McIvor (1987) also conducted another study that attempted to use a group psychotherapeutic approach in the treatment of affective disorders among MS patients. The authors applied stress management in a group setting to inpatients with MS. A total of 55 inpatients participated in the study; 34 patients participated in stress management and the remaining 21 received assignment to a no-treatment control condition. The authors did not match treatment and control subjects, but no significant differences were present between the groups on age, length of illness, or degree of physical disability. Treatment groups consisted of 8 or 9 individuals per group, and the authors conducted four groups. Patients received treatment once per week for 10 weeks along with three follow-up sessions 6 weeks after the end of the 10-week treatment. Treatment primarily focused on teaching relaxation, cognitive, and behavioral techniques to reduce stress. Of the original 34 subjects in the stress management groups, 23 completed all 13 sessions. Subjects in the stress management groups completed the Profile of Mood States (POMS; McNair, Lorr, & Droppleman, 1971) prior to each treatment session. The POMS yielded measures of tension–anxiety, depression–dejection, vigor–activity, and fatigue–inertia. At posttest, the control group's POMS indicated increased depression–dejection and fatigue–inertia, decreased vigor–activity, and no change in tension–anxiety. In contrast, the treatment groups exhibited significant decreases in depression–dejection and tension–anxiety, significant increases in vigor–activity, and no significant change in fatigue–inertia.

From these three studies, it appears that individuals with MS can benefit from cognitive–behavioral psychotherapy, insight-oriented psychotherapy, or stress management programs. However, research studies to date have consistently demonstrated only positive effects on feelings of depression. Also, relative efficacy of insight-oriented psychotherapy versus cognitive–behavioral psychotherapy remains unknown. Finally, with the exception of the 1-month follow-up reported in the study by Larcombe and Wilson (1984), there is a conspicuous lack of information on the robustness of these treatment effects. The 1-month follow-up included in the Larcombe and Wilson study is a step in the right direction, but 1 month is a relatively short time period for follow-up, especially with a disorder such as MS, which has periods of relapse and remission. Three-, 6-, and 12-month follow-ups are necessary. Further research is essential if we are to determine which of these approaches is more efficacious and whether group approaches to treatment can also consistently reduce the level of dysphoric mood states other than depression.

Individual Psychotherapy

Different investigators have recommended treating individuals who have MS with any of a variety of individual psychotherapeutic approaches, including psychoanalytic psychotherapy (Stern, 1988), psychodynamic psychotherapy (Day et al., 1953), supportive psychotherapy (Hamburg & Adams, 1967), hypnotherapy (Brunn,

1966), chemotherapy plus brief psychotherapy (Schiffer, & Wineman, 1990), stress inoculation training (Foley, Bedell, LaRocca, Scheinberg, & Reznikoff, 1987), and biofeedback (Becker & Liebermeister, 1986; Sims, Remler, & Cox, 1987).

Many of these reports are relatively old case studies that did not employ pre- and posttherapy outcome measures. Rather, the authors judged improvement based on opinions of clinicians. For example, Stern (1988) reported using psychoanalysis on a 35-year-old female to deal with physical pain caused by MS. During analysis, issues surfaced and resulted in discussion included marital conflict, feelings of anger, and occupational changes. At the end of therapy, Stern suggested that the patient's condition had improved by stating, "Her body, even in its mutiny, propagated self-trust, and this has been the result of her therapy" (p. 11).

Similarly, Bates, Burns, and Moorey (1989) reported the case of a 42-year-old male diagnosed with MS who became anxious and depressed subsequent to diagnosis. The authors used procedures described by Beck et al. (1979) to help the patient restructure cognitive distortions centered around how others might view him after finding out that he suffered from MS. The authors mentioned the issue of evaluating depression through the use of the BDI (Beck et al., 1961). However, the authors did not provide any objective measures to indicate presence (or absence) of improvement in the patient's mood, but they did imply that his condition improved as a result of treatment. Although these types of report do suggest that therapists are attempting to deal with problematic issues common in MS patients through application of psychotherapy, these types of single case report do not provide objective evidence that individual therapy is actually an effective treatment.

There appear to be only two controlled studies that have examined effects of individual psychotherapy on psychiatric sequelae of MS. These include the studies by Schiffer and Wineman (1990) and Foley et al. (1987). The study by Schiffer and Wineman, previously reviewed, had as its primary purpose to evaluate impact of desipramine on depression in MS. However, they did report that 6 of 14 individuals who participated in the psychotherapy, only the control group improved by the end of therapy. Because of this, they stated that "the magnitude of psychopharmacologic response to antidepression in these patients was not vastly greater than their response to the standardized psychotherapy" (p. 1497). This statement appears to support the impression of other investigators who have reported case studies in which individuals with MS benefited from individual psychotherapy.

Foley et al. (1987), in their study of stress inoculation training with MS patients, also confirmed the impression that MS patients can benefit from individual therapy. Foley and colleagues described the stress inoculation training (SIT) as involving cognitive–behavioral psychotherapy and progressive deep muscle relaxation. It is important to note that the authors adapted relaxation techniques for individuals with MS. Subjects in the study had confirmed MS, were free from significant cognitive deficits, and exhibited no more disability than being wheelchair bound. The control group received standard services/current available care (CAC) offered by the hospital. Instruments used to evaluate the individuals at pretest, posttest, and 6-month follow-up included the BDI (Beck et al., 1961), STAI (Spielberger, 1983), Hassles Scale (Kanner, Coyne, Schaefer, & Lazarus, 1981), Internal–External Locus-of-Control Scale (LCS; Rotter, 1966), and Ways of Coping Checklist (WCC; Folkman, & Lazarus, 1980). Thirty-six individuals met inclusion criteria for the study and received random assignment to either SIT ($n = 20$) or CAC ($n = 16$) groups. The SIT group met for six sessions over a 5-week period.

The results of the study indicated that there were no significant differences between the groups at pretreatment. However, at posttreatment, individuals in the SIT group exhibited decreased depression, more effective coping with daily stressors/hassles, increased problem-focused coping, and decreased state anxiety relative to pretreatment and the control group. A 6-month follow-up conducted on 10 of the SIT group members suggested that the only significant change from posttreatment scores was on the WCC, which indicated that these individuals were utilizing problem-focused coping strategies less often at 6-month follow-up than they had at the end of therapy. On the other hand, individuals receiving CAC treatment showed no significant improvements on any of the measures at posttreatment. No changes were evident in the SIT group's STAI or LOC scores at posttreatment. Therefore, although it appears that individual psychotherapy may be beneficial in treating individuals with MS, there are currently no controlled studies that compare a specific psychotherapeutic technique with no-treatment. However, the results of the studies by Foley et al. (1987) and Schiffer and Wineman (1990) are promising, as they appear to indicate that significant improvement in mood can occur in patients with MS who participate in individual psychotherapy.

Biofeedback

Some clinicians have also used biofeedback in the treatment of MS-related symptomatology. Sims et al. (1987) used biofeedback to treat fecal incontinence and retention in a 46-year-old paraplegic female with a 15-year history of MS. The goal of treatment was to help her gain control over sphincter and abdominal muscles. The technique utilized by Sims et al. was somewhat different than techniques previously employed for incontinence; these investigators used external rather than internal electrodes to train muscle control. They used two sets of EMG electrodes placed as follows: the first set was

> anterior to and bilateral of the anal opening with the ground electrode on the anterior superior iliac crest . . . [and the] second set of electrodes were attached to the lower part of the patient's abdomen, over the urinary bladder region, with the ground on the patients coccyx. (p. 117)

The investigators conducted four biofeedback sessions at 1, 4, 6, and 9 weeks. The patient received instructions to practice contractions 50 times per day between sessions. By the 20th week, the patient reported a 74% reduction in time spent on the toilet, a treatment effect attributed to improved bowel control. These results remained unchanged 6 months after initiation of treatment. These results occurred despite the fact that the causes of the fecal incontinence and retention were paraplegia and rectosphincter spasticity.

Becker and Liebermeister (1986) used biofeedback to treat postural instability in a 27-year-old female with a 3-year history of MS, for whom ataxia was a major symptom of the disorder. In order to teach postural stability, Becker and Liebermeister developed a strength pickup plate that enabled individuals standing on the plate to receive feedback regarding shifts in load. The investigators conducted 35 daily biofeedback session. During the course of biofeedback training, the patient also engaged in standard physical therapy exercises intended to increase postural stability. At the end of treatment, the authors reported that postural instability, as assessed by the strength pickup plate, decreased, but they did not indicate specific significance levels. Becker and Liebermeister, however, noted that such improvement is "rare" and that many individuals with postural instability do not benefit from this type of training. Because of this, efficacy of using the strength pickup plate in ataxic individuals who have MS is questionable. Although clinical researchers have only rarely used biofeedback as a treatment for MS, the two studies reviewed here indicate positive therapeutic effectiveness. Nonetheless, future work in this area is essential before we can draw any firm conclusions regarding efficacy of biofeedback with MS patients.

SUMMARY AND RECOMMENDATIONS

Because of the prevalence of MS, it would not be uncommon for psychologists in many settings to come into contact with individuals who have MS. Psychologists can offer a wide array of services to individuals with MS; however, because of the breadth of symptomatology produced by MS, treatment teams can most efficiently conduct treatment through an interdisciplinary CC approach. Psychologists can be an integral part of treatment teams whose focus is to assist individuals with MS to deal more effectively with challenges that MS symptomatology presents to daily living. Clinical services that psychologists can provide include assessment of psychopathological conditions and cognitive deficits, and individual and group psychotherapy. Clinical practice and literature suggest that these services are effective and invaluable to the treatment of individuals with MS. For example, within the field of health psychology, there have been several articles that suggest health psychologists can provide services in many areas, including assessment and treatment of sexual dysfunction, stress inoculation and/or stress management training, biofeedback for incontinence and poor balance, and cognitive restructuring. Health psychologists may be particularly adept at treating this patient group because of their awareness of how physical functioning can affect psychological status and vice versa. Outside the scope of a comprehensive care program, psychologists can continue to offer similar types of services to individuals with MS. However, psychologists operating independent of CC programs will need to spend more time coordinating treatment efforts with other professionals.

In addition to clinical services, LaRocca (1990) pointed out that psychologists are often the only individuals on interdisciplinary teams who have had formal training in research methods and design. Therefore, as one might expect, psychologists have conducted much of the research that has examined various aspects of MS symptomatology. Psychologists can continue to contribute to this body of research in several areas.

For example, further research is necessary within the areas of psychological and cognitive assessment of patients with MS. Current standard psychological-assessment instruments, such as the MMPI, may not accurately reflect psychological profiles of individuals with MS because symptomatology produced by the disorder artificially inflates some of the scales. Because of this, studies that more thoroughly assess the impact that MS symptomatology has on assessment of mood and other psychiatric disorders are necessary. With regard to cognitive assessment, there is a need to develop short and intermediate-length screening batteries for individuals with MS. Although there is a relatively large body of literature that describes the prevalence and type of cognitive dysfunction that occurs in individuals with MS, detection of these deficits remains problematic; only full neuropsychological evaluations, which are often impractical, provide reasonably accurate assessment of cognitive functioning and detection of cognitive deficits.

Further research is also necessary to more thoroughly assess efficacy of individual and group psychotherapies with individuals who have MS. Results of initial studies that have examined use of cognitive–behavioral therapy, insight-oriented psychotherapy, stress management, stress inoculation training, and chemotherapeutic treatments of affective disorders, particularly depression, are promising in that MS patients who received these treatments did exhibit improvements. However, researchers have not examined the relative efficacy of these treatments, and therefore, it is unclear if one of these treatments is more effective than the others. Also, the majority of these studies excluded individuals who had cognitive dysfunction. Because the incidence of cognitive dysfunction in this patient group is quite high, exclusion of individuals with cognitive dysfunction from the aforementioned treatment studies significantly limits the generalizability of the findings. Research has not yet shown whether individuals with cognitive dysfunction caused by MS can benefit from standard psychotherapies.

Another area that is lacking in treatment studies, and particularly group-treatment studies, is long-term outcome data. Only one of the investigations reviewed employed a follow-up period and this was only 1 month. Outside of typical considerations for treatment of individuals without progressive neurological disorders, follow-up seems particularly important for patients with MS because they experience periods of exacerbation and remission that can affect cognitive, physical, and emotional functioning. With this in mind, it is of the utmost importance to determine if the gains made while in therapy last beyond the duration of treatment and if these gains remain stable following exacerbations of the disorder.

There is also a need to more thoroughly explore use of biofeedback with this patient group. Initial studies indicate that biofeedback can successfully alleviate fecal retention and incontinence and, in some cases, postural instability. There may be broader applications of biofeedback in the area of urinary incontinence, which is much more prevalent among this group that fecal incontinence. In treating urinary incontinence, clinical researchers could develop techniques for treatment of urinary incontinence similar to those developed for the treatment of fecal incontinence. If biofeedback for urinary incontinence using external electrode placements proves beneficial, clinicians could easily begin to implement treatment, because instrumentation is commonly available in many settings where practitioners use biofeedback.

Finally, one area that remains unexplored is efficacy of cognitive rehabilitation in this patient group. Cognitive rehabilitation includes both compensatory rehabilitative techniques, wherein individuals learn how to compensate for their cognitive deficits using an external aid, and retraining techniques, whereby patients regain lost cognitive abilities by engaging in activities designed specifically to retrain lost skills. One author (LaRocca, 1990) indicated that examination of this issue is currently underway, although there does not appear to be any published account examining these cognitive rehabilitative techniques in individuals with MS.

REFERENCES

Alexander, F. G., DeLong, M. R., & Strik, P. L. (1986). Parallel organization of functionally segregated circuits linking basal ganglia and cortex. *Annual Review of Neuroscience, 9,* 357–381.

Baldwin, M. V. (1952). A clinico-experimental investigation into the psychologic aspects of multiple sclerosis. *Journal of Nervous and Mental Disease, 115,* 299–343.

Barbizet, J., & Cany, E. (1968). Clinical and psychometrical study of a patient with memory disturbances. *International Journal of Neurology, 7,* 44–54.

Batchelor, J. R. (1985). Immunological and genetic aspects of multiple sclerosis. In W. B. Matthews (Ed.), *McAlpine's multiple sclerosis* (pp. 281–300). Edinburgh: Churchill Livingstone.

Bates, A., Burns, D. D., & Moorey, S. (1989). Medical illness and the acceptance of suffering. *International Journal of Psychiatry in Medicine, 19,* 269–280.

Baumhefner, R. W., Tourtellote, W. W., Syndulko, K., Waluch, V., Ellison, G. W., Meyers, L. W., Cohen, S. N., Osborne, M., & Shapsak, P. (1990). Quantitative multiple sclerosis plaque assessment with magnetic resonance imaging: Its correlation with clinical parameters, evoked potentials, and intra-blood-brain barrier IgG synthesis. *Archives of Neurology, 47,* 19–26.

Baur, J. J., & Firnhaber, W. (1965). Prognostic criteria in multiple sclerosis. *Annals of the New York Academy of Science, 122,* 542–551.

Beatty, D., & Gange, J. (1977). Neuropsychological aspects of multiple sclerosis. *Journal of Nervous and Mental Disease, 164,* 42–50.

Beatty, W. W., & Goodkin, D. E. (1990). Screening for cognitive impairment in multiple sclerosis: An evaluation of the Mini-Mental State Examination. *Archives of Neurology, 47,* 297–301.

Beatty, W. W., Goodkin, D. E., Beatty, P. A., & Monson, N. (1989b). Frontal lobe dysfunction and memory impairment in patients with chronic progressive multiple sclerosis. *Brain and Cognition, 11,* 73–86.

Beatty, W. W., Goodkin, D. E., Monson, N., & Beatty, P. A. (1989a). Cognitive disturbances in patients with relapsing remitting multiple sclerosis. *Archives of Neurology, 46,* 1113–1119.

Beatty, W. W., Goodkin, D. E., Monson, N., Beatty, P. A., & Hertsgaard, D. (1988). Anterograde and retrograde amnesia in patients with chronic progressive multiple sclerosis. *Archives of Neurology, 45,* 611–619.

Beatty, W. W., & Monson, N. (1991). Metamemory in multiple sclerosis. *Journal of Clinical and Experimental Neuropsychology, 13,* 309–327.

Beck, A. T., Rush, A. J., Shaw, B. F., & Emery, G. (1979). *Cognitive therapy of depression.* New York: Guilford.

Beck, A. T., Ward, C. H., Mendelson, M., Mock, J. E., & Erbaugh, J. K. (1961). An inventory for measuring depression. *Archives of General Psychiatry, 4,* 561–571.

Becker, R., & Liebermeister, R. (1986). Biofeedback with the strength pickup plate. *Clinical Biofeedback and Health, 9,* 81–84.

Benton, A. L., & Hamsher, K. de S. (1976). *Multilingual Aphasia Examination.* Iowa City, IA: University of Iowa Press.

Berry, J. M., Storandt, M., & Coyne, A. (1984). Age and sex differences in somatic complaints associated with depression. *Journal of Gerontology, 39,* 465–467.

Blumenthal, M. D. (1975). Measuring depressive symptomology in a general population. *Archives of General Psychiatry, 32,* 971–978.

Bolding, H. (1960). Psychotherapeutic aspects in management of patients with multiple sclerosis. *Diseases of the Nervous System, 21,* 24–26.

Bradley, W. G. (1984). Patchy periventricular white matter lesions in the elderly: A common observation during NMR imaging. *Non-Invasive Medical Imaging, 1,* 35–41.

Brown, F. W., Lewine, R. J., Hudgins, P. A., & Risch, S. C. (1992). White matter hyperintensity signals in psychiatric and nonpsychiatric subjects. *American Journal of Psychiatry, 149,* 620–625.

Brunn, J. T. (1966). Hypnosis and neurological disease: A case report. *American Journal of Clinical Hypnosis, 8,* 312–320.

Buschke, H., & Fuld, P. A. (1974). Evaluating storage, retention, and retrieval in disordered memory and learning. *Neurology, 24,* 1019–1025.

Butcher, J. N., Dahlstrom, W. G., Graham, J. R., Tellegen, A. M., & Kaemmer, B. (1989). *MMPI-2; Minnesota Multiphasic Personality Inventory-2. Manual for Administration and Scoring.* Minneapolis: University of Minnesota Press.

Charcot, S. M. (1877). *Lectures on diseases of the nervous system* (G. Sigerson, Trans.). London: New Sydenham Society. [Cited by N. P. Dalos, P. V. Rabins, & P. O'Donnell (1983). Disease activity and emotional state in multiple sclerosis. *Annals of Neurology, 13,* 573–577.]

Charcot, S. M. (1881). *Lectures on diseases of the nervous system delivered at La Salpetrier.* London: New Sydenham Society 2. [Cited by R. B. Schiffer (1990). Disturbances of affect. In S. A. Rao

(Ed.), *Neurobehavioral aspects of multiple sclerosis* (pp. 187–195). New York: Oxford University Press.]

Cobble, N. D., Dietz, M. A., Grigsby, J., & Kennedy, P. M. (1993). Rehabilitation of the patient with multiple sclerosis. In J. A. DeLisa & B. M. Gans (Eds.), *Rehabilitation medicine: Principles and practice* (2nd ed., pp. 861–885). Philadelphia: Lippincott.

Coffey, C. E., Figiel, G. S., Djang, W. T., & Weiner, R. D. (1990). Subcortical hyperintensity on magnetic resonance imaging: A comparison of normal and depressed elderly subjects. *American Journal of Psychiatry, 147,* 187–189.

Cottrell, S. S., & Wilson, S. A. K. (1926). The affective symptomology of disseminated sclerosis: A study of 100 cases. *Journal of Neurological Psychopathology, 7,* 1–30. [Cited by R. B. Schiffer & N. M. Wineman (1990). Antidepressant pharmacotherapy of depression associated with multiple sclerosis. *American Journal of Psychiatry, 147,* 1493–1497.]

Crawford, J. D., & McIvor, G. P. (1985). Group psychotherapy: Benefit in multiple sclerosis. *Archives of Physical Medicine and Rehabilitation, 66,* 810–813.

Crawford, J. D., & McIvor, G. P. (1987). Stress management for multiple sclerosis patients. *Psychological Reports, 61,* 423–429.

Cummings, J. L. (1986). Subcortical dementia: Neuropsychology, neuropsychiatry, and pathophysiology. *British Review of Psychiatry, 149,* 682–697.

Cummings, J. L. (1990). *Subcortical dementias.* Oxford University Press: New York.

Cummings, J. L., & Benson, D. F. (1992). *Dementia: A clinical approach* (2nd ed.). Boston: Buttersworth-Heinemann.

Day, M., Day, E., & Hermann, R. (1953). Groups therapy in patients with multiple sclerosis. *Archives of Neurology and Psychiatry, 69,* 193–201.

Dempsey, P. (1964). Unidimensional depression scale for MMPI. *Journal of Consulting Psychology, 28,* 364–370.

Downes, J. J., Davies, A. D. M., & Copeland, J. R. M. (1988). Organization of depressive symptoms in the elderly population: Hierarchical patterns and the Guttman scales. *Psychology and Aging, 3,* 367–374.

Ducharme, S., Gill, K. M., Biener-Bergman, S., & Fertitta, L. C. (1993). Sexual functioning: Medical and psychological aspects. In J. A. Delisa (Ed.), *Rehabilitation medicine: Principles and practice* (2nd ed., pp. 763–781). Philadelphia: Lippincott.

Ellison, G. W., Visscher, B. R., Graves, M. C., & Fahey, J. L. (1984). Multiple sclerosis. *Annals of Internal Medicine, 101,* 514–526.

Falk, W. E., Mahnke, M. W., & Poskanzer, D. D. (1979). Lithium prophylaxis of corticotropin-induced psychosis. *Journal of the American Medical Association, 241,* 1011–1012.

Foley, F. W., Bedell, J. R., LaRocca, N. G., Scheinberg, L. C., & Reznikoff, M. (1987). Efficacy of stress-inoculation training in coping with multiple sclerosis. *Journal of Consulting and Clinical Psychology, 55,* 919–922.

Foley, F. W., Traugott, U., LaRocca, N. G., Smith, C. R., Perlman, K. R., Caruso, L. S., & Scheinberg, L. C. (1992). A prospective study of depression and immune dysregulation in multiple sclerosis. *Archives of Neurology, 49,* 238–244.

Folkman, S., & Lazarus, R. (1980). An analysis of coping in a middle-aged community sample. *Journal of Health and Social Behavior, 21,* 219–239.

Folstein, M. F., Folstein, S. E., & McHugh, P. R. (1975). Mini-mental state: A practical method for grading the cognitive state of patients for the clinician. *Journal of Psychiatric Research, 12,* 189–198.

Fox, J. H., Bernard, B., Gilley, D., Stebbins, G. T., Wilson, R. S., & Huckman, M. S. (1989). Multiple sclerosis: An unexpected cause of senile dementia. *Archives of Neurology, 46,* 1269.

Franklin, G. M., Heaton, R. K., Nelson, L. M., Filley, C. M., & Seibert, C. (1988). Correlation of neuropsychological and MRI findings in chronic/progressive multiple sclerosis. *Neurology, 38,* 1826–1829.

Franklin, G. M., Nelson, L. M., Filley, C. M., & Heaton, R. K. (1989). Cognitive loss in multiple sclerosis: Case reports and review of the literature. *Archives of Neurology, 46,* 162–167.

Garland, E. J., & Zis, A. P. (1991). Multiple sclerosis and affective disorders. *Canadian Journal of Psychiatry, 36,* 112–117.

Gilbert, J. J., & Sadler, M. (1983). Unsuspected multiple sclerosis. *Archives of Neurology, 40,* 533–536.

Golding, E. (1989). *MEAMS: The Middlesex Elderly Assessment of Mental State description and validation.* Fareham, UK: Thames Valley Test Company.

Goldstein, I., Siroky, M. B., Sax, D. S., & Kane, R. J. (1982). Neurologic abnormalities in multiple sclerosis. *Journal of Urology, 128,* 541–545.

Granger, C. V. (1981). Assessment of functional status: A model for multiple sclerosis. *Acta Neurologica Scandinavica, 64,* 40–47.

Gronwall, D. M. A. (1977). Paced auditory serial-addition task: A measure of recovery from concussion. *Perceptual and Motor Skills, 44,* 367–373.

Halstead, L. S. (1985). Sexuality and disability. In L. S. Halstead, M. Grabois, & C. A. Howland (Eds.), *Medical rehabilitation* (pp. 325–333). New York: Raven.

Hamburg, D. A., & Adams, J. E. (1967). A perspective on coping: Seeking and utilizing information in major transitions. *Archives of General Psychiatry, 17,* 277–284.

Hamilton, M. A. (1960). A rating scale for depression. *Journal of Neurology, Neurosurgery and Psychiatry, 23,* 56–62.

Harowski, K., Harris, L., Nager, E., & Schapiro, R. T. (1987). Sexuality. In R. T. Schapiro (Ed.), *Symptom management in multiple sclerosis* (pp. 43–47). New York: Demos.

Hartings, M. F., Pavlou, M. M., & Davis, F. A. (1976). Groups counseling of MS patients in a program of comprehensive care. *Journal of Chronic Disease, 29,* 65–73.

Hathaway, S. R., & McKinley, J. C. (1943). *Booklet for the Minnesota Multiphasic Personality Inventory.* New York: Psychological Corporation.

Heaton, R., Nelson, L., Thompson, D. S., Burks, J. S., & Franklin, G. M. (1985). Neuropsychological findings in relapsing–remitting and chronic–progressive multiple sclerosis. *Journal of Consulting and Clinical Psychology, 53,* 103–110.

Heaton, R., Thompson, L. L., Nelson, L. M., Filley, C. M., & Franklin, G. M. (1990). Brief and intermediate-length screening of neuropsychological impairment in multiple sclerosis. In S. A. Rao (Ed.), *Neurobehavioral aspects of multiple sclerosis* (pp. 149–160). New York: Oxford University Press.

Hertzog, C., VanAlstine, J., Usala, P. D., Hultsch, D. F., & Dixon, R. (1990). Measurement properties of the Center for Epidemiological Studies depression scale (CES-D) in older populations. *Psychological Assessment: A Journal of Consulting and Clinical Psychology, 2,* 64–72.

Holland, N. J., Francadandera, F., & Wiesel-Levison, P. (1986). International scale for assessment of disability in multiple sclerosis. *Journal of Neurosciences Nursing, 18,* 39–44.

Honer, W. G., Hurwitz, T., Li, D. K. B., Palmer, M., & Paty, D. W. (1987). Temporal lobe involvement in multiple sclerosis patients with psychiatric disorders. *Archives of Neurology, 44,* 187–190.

Huber, S. J., Shuttleworth, E. C., Paulson, G. W., Bellchambers, M. J. G., & Clapp, L. E. (1986). Cortical vs. subcortical dementia: Neuropsychological differences. *Archives of Neurology, 43,* 392–394.

Jacobs, J. W., Bernhard, M. R., Delgado, A., & Strain, J. J. (1977). Screening for organic mental syndromes in the medically ill. *Annals of Internal Medicine, 86,* 40–46.

Jennekens-Schinkel, A., van der Velde, E. A., Sanders, E. A. C. M., & Lanser, J. B. K. (1989). Visuospatial problem solving, conceptual reasoning and sorting behaviour in multiple sclerosis out-patients. *Journal of the Neurological Sciences, 90,* 187–201.

Joffe, R. T., Lippert, G. P., Gray, T. A., Sawa, G., & Horvath, Z. (1987). Mood disorder and multiple sclerosis. *Archives of Neurology, 44,* 376–378.

Kahan, E., Leibowitz, U., & Alter, M. (1971). Cerebral multiple sclerosis. *Neurology, 21,* 1179–1185.

Kahn, D., Stevenson, E., & Douglas, C. J. (1988). Effect of sodium valproate in three patients with organic brain syndromes. *American Journal of Psychiatry, 145,* 1010–1011.

Kanner, A., Coyne, J., Schaefer, C., & Lazarus, R. (1981). Comparisons of two modes of stress measurement: Daily hassles and uplifts versus major life events. *Journal of Behavioral Medicine, 4,* 1–39.

Kaplan, E., Goodglass, H., & Weintraub, S. (1983). *Boston Naming Test.* Philadelphia: Lea & Febiger.

Kaplan, H. S. (1974). *The new sex therapy: Active treatment of sexual dysfunctions.* New York: Brunner/Mazel.

Kemp, K., Lion, J. R., & Magram, G. (1977). Lithium in the treatment of a manic patient with multiple sclerosis: A case report. *Diseases of the Nervous System, 38,* 210–211.

Kessler, H. R., Cohen, R. A., Lauer, K., & Kausch, D. F. (1992). The relationship between disability and memory dysfunction in multiple sclerosis. International Journal of Neuroscience, 62, 17–34.

Kiernan, R. J., Mueller, J., Langston, J. W., & Van Dyke, C. (1987). The Neurobehavioral Cognitive Status Examination: A brief but differentiated approach to cognitive assessment. *Annals of Internal Medicine, 107,* 481–485.

Klonoff, H., Clark, C., Oger, J., Paty, D., & Li, D. (1991). Neuropsychological performance in patients with mild multiple sclerosis. *The Journal of Nervous and Mental Disease, 179,* 127–131.

Koopmans, R. A., Li, D. K. B., Oger, J. J. F., Kastrukoff, L. F., Jardine, C., Costley, L., Hall, S., Grochowski,

E. W., & Paty, D. W. (1989). Chronic progressive multiple sclerosis: Serial magnetic resonance brain imaging over six months. *Annals of Neurology, 26,* 248–256.

Krug, S. E., Scheier, I. H., & Cattell, R. B. (1976). *Handbook for the IPAT Anxiety Scale.* Champaign, IL: Institute for Personality and Ability Testing.

Kurtzke, J. F. (1981). A proposal for a uniform minimal record of disability in multiple sclerosis. *Acta Neurologica Scandinavica, 64,* 110–129.

Kurtzke, J. F. (1983a). Epidemiology of multiple sclerosis. In J. F. Hallpike, C. W. M. Adams, & W. W. Tourtellotte (Eds.), *Multiple sclerosis: Pathology, diagnosis, and management* (pp. 47–95). Baltimore, MD: Williams & Wilkins.

Kurtzke, J. F. (1938b). Rating neurological impairment in multiple sclerosis: An expanded disability status scale (EDSS). *Neurology, 33,* 1444–1452.

Lampert, P. N. (1983). Fine structure of the demyelinating process. In J. F. Hallpike, C. W. M. Adams, & W. W. Tourtellotte (Eds.), *Multiple sclerosis: Pathology, diagnosis, and management* (pp. 29–46). Baltimore, MD: Williams & wilkins.

Larcombe, N. A., & Wilson, P. H. (1984). An evaluation of cognitive behavior therapy for depression in patients with multiple sclerosis. *British Journal of Psychiatry, 145,* 366–371.

LaRocca, N. G. (1990). A rehabilitation perspective. In S. A. Rao (Ed.), *Neurobehavioral aspects of multiple sclerosis* (pp. 215–229). New York: Oxford University Press.

LaRocca, N. G., Kalb, R. C., & Kaplan, S. R. (1987). Psychological issues. In L. C. Scheinberg, & N. J. Hollands (Eds.), *Multiple sclerosis: A guide for patients and their families* (2nd ed., pp. 197–213). New York: Raven.

Lewinsohn, P. M. (1975). The behavioral study and treatment of depression. In M. Hersen, R. M. Eisler, & P. M. Miller (Eds.), *Progress in behavior modification* (Vol. 1) (pp. 19–64). New York: Academic Press.

Lewinsohn, P. M., Biglan, A., & Zeiss, A. M. (1976). Behavioral treatment of depression. In P. O. Davison (Ed.), *The behavioral management of anxiety, depression, and pain* (pp. 91–146). New York: Brunner/Mazel.

Lezak, M. D. (1976). *Neuropsychological assessment,* 2nd ed. New York: Oxford University Press.

Lieberman, M. L. (1988). *The sexual pharmacy: The complete guide to drugs with sexual side effects.* New York: New American Library.

Lilius, H. G., Baltonen, E. J., & Wilkström, J. (1976). Sexual problems in patients suffering from multiple sclerosis. *Journal of Chronic Diseases, 29,* 643–647.

LoPiccolo, J., & LoPiccolo, L. (Eds.), (1978). *Handbook of sex therapy.* New York: Plenum Press.

MacKay, R. P., & Hirano, A. (1967). Forms of benign multiple sclerosis. *Archives of Neurology, 17,* 588–592.

Mackenzie, T. B., & Popkin, M. K. (1987). Suicide in the medical patient. *International Journal of Psychiatry in Medicine, 17,* 3–22.

Mahler, M. E., & Benson, D. F. (1990). Cognitive dysfunction in multiple sclerosis: A subcortical dementia? In S. M. Rao (Ed.), *Neurobehavioral aspects of multiple sclerosis* (pp. 89–101). New York: Oxford University Press.

Maloney, F. P. (1985). Rehabilitation of patients with progressive and remitting disorders. In F. P. Maloney, J. S. Burks, & S. P. Ringel (Eds.). *Interdisciplinary rehabilitation of multiple sclerosis and neuromuscular disorders* (pp. 3–8). Philadelphia: Lippincott.

Maloney, F. P., Burks, J. S., & Ringel, S. P. (Eds.). (1985). Interdisciplinary rehabilitation of multiple sclerosis and neuromuscular disorders. Philadelphia: Lippincott.

Marsh, G. Ellison, G. W., & Strite, C. (1983). Psychosocial and vocational rehabilitation approaches to multiple sclerosis. *Annual Review of Rehabilitation, 3,* 242–267.

Marsh, G., Hirsch, S. H., & Leung, G. (1982). Use and misuse of the MMPI in multiple sclerosis. *Psychological Reports, 51,* 1127–1134.

Matthews, W. B. (1985a). Some aspects of the natural history. In W. B. Matthews (Ed.), *McAlpine's multiple sclerosis* (pp. 73–95). Edinburgh: Churchill Livingstone.

Matthews, W. B. (1985b). Treatment. In W. B. Matthews (Ed.), *McAlpine's multiple sclerosis* (pp. 233–278). Edinburgh: Churchill Livingstone.

Mattis, S. (1988). *DRS: Dementia Rating Scale professional manual.* Odessa, FL: Psychological Assessment Resources.

Mayeaux, R., Stern, Y., Rosen, J., & Benson, D. F. (1983). Is "subcortical dementia" a recognizable clinical entity? *Annals of Neurology, 14,* 278–283.

McFarland, H. F., & Dhib-Jalbut, S. (1989). Multiple sclerosis: Possible immunological mechanisms. *Clinical Immunology and Immunopathology, 50,* 96–105.

McIntosh-Michaelis, S. M., Roberts, M. H., Wilkinson, S. M., Diamond, I. D., McLellan, D. L., Martin, J. P., & Spackman, A. J. (1991). The prevalence of cognitive impairment in a community survey of multiple sclerosis. *British Journal of Clinical Psychology, 30,* 333–348.

McNair, D. M., Lorr, M., & Droppleman, L. F. (1971). *Manual for the Profile of Mood States.* Anaheim, CA: Educational and Industrial Testing Service.

Mehta, D. B. (1976). Lithium and affective disorders associated with organic brain impairment [Letter to the editor]. *American Journal of Psychiatry, 133,* 236.

Mei-Tal, V., Meyerowitz, S., & Engel, G. L. (1970). The role of psychological process in a somatic disorder: Multiple sclerosis. *Psychosomatic Medicine, 32,* 67–86.

Mellerup, E., Fog, T., Raun, N., Colville, P., de Rham, B., Hannah, B., & Kurtzke, J. (1981). The socioeconomic scale. *Acta Neurologica Scandinavica, 64,* 130–138.

Meyerink, L. H., Reitan, R. M., & Selz, M. (1988). The validity of the MMPI with multiple sclerosis patients. *Journal of Clinical Psychology, 44,* 764–769.

Minden, S. L., Orav, J., & Reich, P. (1987). Depression in multiple sclerosis. *General Hospital Psychiatry, 9,* 426–434.

Minden, S. L., & Schiffer, R. B. (1990). Affective disorders in multiple sclerosis. Review and recommendations for clinical research. *Archives of Neurology, 47,* 98–104.

Minderhoud, J. M., Leemhius, J. G., Kremer, J., Laban, E., & Smits, P. M. L. (1984). Sexual disturbances arising from multiple sclerosis. *Acta Neurologica Scandinavica, 70,* 299–306.

Mueller, S. R., & Girace, M. (1988). Use and misuse of the MMPI, a reconsideration. *Psychological Reports, 63,* 483–491.

Narod, S., Johnson-Lussenburg, C. M., Zheng, Q., & Nelson, R. (1985). Viral infections and M.S. *Lancet, 2,* 165.

National Advisory Commission on Multiple Sclerosis. (1975). *Report and recommendations* (vol. 2, pp. 147–148). Washington, DC: Department of Health, Education, and Welfare.

National Institutes of Health. (1984). *Multiple sclerosis: A national survey* (NIH Publication No. 84-2479). Washington, DC: U.S. Government Printing Office.

Nelson, L. M., Franklin, G. M., Hamman, R. F., Boteler, D. L., Baum, H. M., & Burks, J. S. (1988). Referral bias in multiple sclerosis research. *Journal of Clinical Epidemiology, 41,* 187–192.

Nowicki, S., & Duke, M. P. (1974). Locus of control scale for noncollege as well as college adults. *Journal of Personality Assessment, 38,* 136–137.

Pavlou, M., Johnson, P., Davis, F. A., & Lefebvre, K. (1979). Program of psychological service delivery in multiple sclerosis center. *Professional Psychology, 10,* 503–510.

Peselow, E. D., Fieve, R. R., Deutsch, S. I., & Kaufman, M. (1981). Coexistent manic symptoms and multiple sclerosis. *Psychosomatics, 22,* 824–825.

Peyser, J. M., Edwards, K. R., Poser, C. M., & Filskov, S. B. (1980). Cognitive function in patients with multiple sclerosis. *Archives of Neurology, 37,* 577–579.

Poser, C. M., Paty, D. W., Scheinberg, L., McDonald, W. I., Davis, F. A., Ebers, G. C., Johnson, K. P., Sibley, W. A., Silberberg, D. H., & Tourtellotte, W. W. (1983). New diagnostic criteria for multiple sclerosis. *Annals of Neurology, 13,* 227–231.

Pratt, R. T. C. (1951). An investigation of the psychiatric aspects of disseminated sclerosis. *Journal of Neurology, Neurosurgery, and Psychiatry, 14,* 326, 335.

Prineas, J. W., Kwon, E. E., Goldenberg, P. Z., Ilyas, A. A., Quarles, R. H., Benjamins, J. A., & Sprinkle, T. J. (1989). Multiple sclerosis: Oligodendrocyte proliferation and differentiation in fresh lesions. *Laboratory Investigation, 61,* 489–503.

Rabins, P. V. (1990). Euphoria in multiple sclerosis. In S. A. Rao (Ed.), *Neurobehavioral aspects of multiple sclerosis* (pp. 180–185). New York: Oxford University Press.

Rabins, P. V., Brooks, B. R., O'Donnell, P., Pearlson, G. D., Moberg, P., Jubelt, B., Boyle, P., Dalos, N., & Folstein, M. F. (1986). Structural brain correlates of emotional disorder in multiple sclerosis. *Brain, 109,* 585–597.

Radloff, L. S. (1977). The CES-D scale: A self-report depression scale for research in the general population. *Applied Psychological Measurement, 1,* 385–401.

Raine, C. S. (1985). Experimental allergic encephalomyelitis and experimental ailergic neuritis. In J. C. Koetsier (Ed.), *Handbook of clinical neurology, Vol. 3: Demyelinating diseases* (pp. 429–466). Amsterdam: Elsevier.

Raine, C. S. (1990). Neuropathology. In S. A. Rao (Ed.), *Neurobehavioral aspects of multiple sclerosis* (pp. 15–36). New York: Oxford University Press.

Rao, S. M., Hammeke, T., McQuillen, M. P., Khatri, B. O., & Lloyd, D. (1984). Memory disturbance in chronic progressive multiple sclerosis. *Archives of Neurology, 41,* 625–631.

Rao, S. M., Leo, G. J., Bernardin, L., & Unverzagt, F. (1991a),. Cognitive dysfunction in multiple sclerosis. I. Frequency, patterns, and prediction. *Neurology, 21,* 685–691.

Rao, S. M., Leo, G. J., Ellington, L., Nauertz, T., Bernardin, L., & Unverzagt, F. (1991b). Cognitive dysfunction in multiple sclerosis. II. Impact on employment and social functioning. *Neurology, 21,* 692–696.

Reischies, F. M., Baum, K., Bräu, H., Hedde, J. P., & Schwindt, G. (1988). Cerebral magnetic resonance imaging findings in multiple sclerosis: Relation to disturbance of affect, drive, and cognition. *Archives of Neurology, 45,* 1114–1116.

Reitan, R. M., & Davison, L. A. (1974). *Clinical neuropsychology: Current status and applications.* Washington DC: Winston.

Reitan, R. M., & Wolfson, D. (1985). *Neuroanatomy and neuropathology: A clinical guide for neuropsychologists.* Tucson, AZ: Neuropsychology Press.

Ron, M. A., Callanan, M. M., & Warrington, E. K. (1991). Cognitive abnormalities in multiple sclerosis: A psychometric and MRI study. *Psychological Medicine, 21,* 59–68.

Ron, M. A., & Logsdail, S. J. (1989). Psychiatric morbidity in multiple sclerosis: A clinical and MRI study. *Psychological Medicine, 19,* 887–895.

Rotter, J. (1966). Generalized expectations for internal versus external control of reinforcement. *Psychological Monographs, 80,* 1–28.

Sadovnick, A. D., Eisen, K., Ebers, G. C., & Paty, D. W. (1991). Cause of death in patients attending multiple sclerosis clinics. *Neurology, 41,* 1193–1196.

Schapiro, R. T. (1987). *Symptom management in multiple sclerosis.* New York: Demos.

Schapiro, R. T. (1990). The rehabilitation of multiple sclerosis. *Journal of Neurological Rehabilitation, 4,* 215–217.

Schapiro, R. T., van der Noort, S., & Scheinberg, L. (1984). The current management of multiple sclerosis. *Annals of the New York Academy of Sciences, 436,* 425–434.

Scheinberg, L., Holland, N. J., Kirschenbaum, M., Oaklander, A., & Geronemus, D. F. (1981). Comprehensive long-term care of patients with multiple sclerosis. *Neurology, 31,* 1121–1123.

Schiffer, R. B. (1990). Disturbances of affect. In S. A. Rao (Ed.), *Neurobehavioral aspects of multiple sclerosis* (pp. 186–195). New York: Oxford University Press.

Schiffer, R. B., & Babigian, H. M. (1984). Behavioral disorders in multiple sclerosis, temporal lobe epilepsy, and amyotrophic lateral sclerosis: An epidemiologic study. *Archives of Neurology, 41,* 1067–1069.

Schiffer, R. B., & Wineman, N. M. (1990). Antidepressant pharmacotherapy of depression associated with multiple sclerosis. *American Journal of Psychiatry, 147,* 1493–1497.

Schiffer, R. B., Wineman, N. M., & Weitkamp, L. R. (1986). Association between bipolar affective disorder and multiple sclerosis. *American Journal of Psychiatry, 143,* 94–95.

Schneiber, L. C. (Ed.). (1983). *Multiple sclerosis: A guide for patients and their families.* New York: Raven.

Schover, L. R., & Jensen, S. B. (1988). *Sexuality and chronic illness: A comprehensive approach.* New York: Guilford.

Schover, L. R., Thomas, A. J., Lakin, M. M., Montague, D. K., & Fischer, J. (1988). Orgasm phase dysfunction in multiple sclerosis. *Journal of Sex Research, 25,* 548–554.

Schumacher, G. A., Beebe, G., Kibler, R. F., Kurland, L. T., Kurtzke, J. F., McDowell, F., Nagler, B., Sibley, W. A., Tourtellotte, W. W., & Willmon, T. F. (1965). Problems of experimental trials of therapy in multiple sclerosis: Report by the panel on the evaluation of experimental trials of therapy in multiple sclerosis. *Annals of the New York Academy of Science, 122,* 552–556.

Shafey, H. (1992). The effect of fluoxetine in depression associated with multiple sclerosis. *Canadian Journal of Psychiatry, 37,* 147–148.

Sibley, W. A. (1988). Risk factors in multiple sclerosis—Implications for pathogenesis. In G. Crescenzi (Ed.), *A multidisciplinary approach to myelin diseases* (pp. 227–232). New York: Plenum Press.

Sibley, W. A. (1990). Diagnosis and course of multiple sclerosis. In S. M. Rao (Ed.), *Neurobehavioral aspects of multiple sclerosis* (pp. 5–14). New York: Oxford University Press.

Sibley, W. A., Bamford, C. R., & Clark, K. (1984). Triggering factors in multiple sclerosis. In C. Poser (Ed.), *Diagnosis of multiple sclerosis* (pp. 14–24). New York: Thieme-Stratton.

Silber, E., & Tippett, J. S. (1965). Self-esteem: Clinical assessment and measurement validation. *Psychological Reports, 16,* 1017–1071.

Sims, C. G., Remler, H., & Cox, D. J. (1987). Biofeedback and behavioral treatment of elimination disorders. *Clinical Biofeedback and Health, 10,* 115–122.

Skegg, K., Corwin, P. A., & Skegg, D. C. G. (1988). How often is multiple sclerosis mistaken for a psychiatric disorder? *Psychological Medicine, 18,* 733–736.

Smith, A. A. (1973). *Symbol Digit Modalities Test Manual.* Palo Alto, CA: Western Psychological Services.

Solomon, J. G. (1978). Multiple sclerosis masquerading as lithium toxicity. *Journal of Nervous and Mental Disease, 166,* 663–665.

Spiegelberg, N. (1980). Support groups improves quality of life. *Rehabilitation Nursing, 5,* 9–11.

Spielberger, C. (1983). *Manual for the State-Trait Anxiety Inventory* (rev. ed.). Palo Alto, CA: Consulting Psychologists Press.

Staples, D., & Lincoln, N. B. (1979). Intellectual impairment in multiple sclerosis and its relation to functional abilities. *Rheumatology and Rehabilitation, 18,* 153–160.

Stern, E. M. (1988). Pain and the endurance of the soul. *Psychotherapy Patient, 4,* 3–11.

Steuer, J., Bank, L., Olsen, E. J., & Jarvik, L. F. (1980). Depression, physical health, and somatic complaints in the elderly: A study of the Zung Self-Rating Scale. *Journal of Gerontology, 35,* 683–688.

Surridge, D. (1969). An investigation into some psychiatric aspects of multiple sclerosis. *British Journal of Psychiatry, 140,* 728–733.

Swirsky-Sacchetti, T., Field, H. L., Mitchell, D. R., Seward, J., Lublin, F. D., Knobler, R. L., & Gonzalez, C. F. (1992). The sensitivity of the mini-mental state exam in the white matter dementia of multiple sclerosis. *Journal of Clinical Psychology, 48,* 779–786.

Taylor, R. (1990). Relationships between cognitive test performance and everyday cognitive difficulties in multiple sclerosis. *British Journal of Clinical Psychology, 29,* 251–252.

Thompson, A. J., Kennard, C., Swash, M., Summers, B., Yuill, G. M., Shepherd, D. I., Roche, S., Perkin, G. D., Loizou, L. A., Ferner, R., Hughes, R. A. C., Thompson, M., & Hand, J. (1989). Relative efficacy of intravenous methylprednisolone in the treatment of acute relapse in M.S. *Neurology, 39,* 969–971.

Thompson, A. J., Kermode, A. G., Wicks, D., MacManus, D. G., Kendall, B. E., Kingsley, D. P. E., & McDonald, W. I. (1991). Major differences in the dynamics of primary and secondary progressive multiple sclerosis. *Annals of Neurology, 29,* 53–62.

Tissenbaum, M. J., Harter, H. M., & Friedman, A. P. (1951). Organic neurological syndromes diagnosed as functional disorders. *Journal of the American Medical Association, 147,* 1519–1521.

Valleroy, M. L., & Kraft, G. H. (1984). Sexual dysfunction in multiple sclerosis. *Archives of Physical Medicine and Rehabilitation, 65,* 125–128.

van den Burg, W., van Zomeren, A. H., Minderhoud, J. M., Prange, A. J. A., & Meijer, N. S. A. (1987). Cognitive impairment in patients with multiple sclerosis and mild physical disability. *Archives of Neurology, 44,* 494–501.

Warren, S., Greenhill, S., & Warren, K. G. (1982). Emotional stress and the development of multiple sclerosis: Case-control evidence of a relationship. *Journal of Chronic Diseases, 35,* 821–831.

Warren, S., Warren, K. G., & Cockerill, R. (1991). Emotional stress and coping in multiple sclerosis (MS) exacerbations. *Journal of Psychosomatic Research, 35,* 37–47.

Weiner, H. L., & Hafler, D. A. (1988). Immunotherapy of multiple sclerosis. *Annals of Neurology, 23,* 211–222.

Wells, K. B., Golding, J. A., & Burnam, M. A. (1988). Psychiatric disorder in a sample of the general population with and without chronic medical conditions. *American Journal of Psychiatry, 145,* 976–981.

Whitehouse, P. J. (1986). The concept of subcortical and cortical dementia: Another look. *Annals of Neurology, 19,* 1–6.

Whitlock, F. A., & Siskind, M. M. (1980). Depression as a major symptom of multiple sclerosis. *Journal of Neurology, Neurosurgery, and Psychiatry, 43,* 861–865.

Willoughby, E. W., Grochowski, E., Li, D. B. K., Oger, J. J. F., Kastrukoff, L. F., & Paty, D. W. (1989). Serial magnetic resonance scanning in multiple sclerosis: A second prospective study in relapsing patients. *Annals of Neurology, 25,* 43–49.

Young, I. R., Hall, A. S., Pallis, C. A., Legg, N. J., Bydder, G. M., & Steiner, R. E. (1981). Nuclear magnetic resonance imaging of the brain in multiple sclerosis. *Lancet, 2,* 1063–1066.

Zung, W. W. K. (1965). A self-rating depression scale. *Archives of General Psychiatry, 12,* 63–70.

21

Traumatic Brain Injury

Eleanor B. Callon and Warren T. Jackson

INTRODUCTION

Medical scientists recognized and described traumatic brain injury (TBI) as early as 3000 B.C. (Walsh, 1978). Over the past two decades, advances in trauma evaluation (Collicott, 1991), neuroimaging (Bigler, Yeo, & Turkheimer, 1989), and neurosurgery (Adams & Victor, 1989) have greatly increased survival rates for TBI patients. Rehabilitation utilizing combined knowledge and cooperative efforts of medicine, physical therapy, occupational therapy, speech pathology, therapeutic recreation, rehabilitation psychology, neuropsychology, and social work has improved quality of lives of those survivors. Yet, our understanding of the brain and how it recovers is still in early development, and we have much to learn.

Excellent texts and reviews detail each aspect of related literature. We reference many of them in this chapter. Present space limitations dictate a brief review of this broad subject. Because of particular susceptibility of the anterior brain to damage in TBI, we focus most of the chapter on the study of the frontal lobes. First, we review anatomy and sequelae of injury. Next, we describe three tiers of assessment and note the emphasis within each tier. The next section summarizes treatment approaches, ranging from initial rehabilitation efforts to community reintegration. The chapter concludes with a look toward the future of this very exciting field.

EPIDEMIOLOGIC AND DEMOGRAPHIC CHARACTERISTICS

Traumatic brain injury is a major public health problem in industrialized countries; incidence rates range from approximately 300 to 450 new cases per 100

Eleanor B. Callon • Department of Family Medicine, Louisiana State University Medical Center, Baton Rouge, Louisiana 70805. **Warren T. Jackson** • Department of Psychology, Louisiana State University, Baton Rouge, Louisiana 70803.
Handbook of Health and Rehabilitation Psychology, edited by Anthony J. Goreczny. Plenum Press, New York, 1995.

thousand population each year (Kolb & Whishaw, 1990). In the United States, current incidence rates fall between 500 thousand and 1.5 million new cases each year. Between 50 thousand and 70 thousand of these cases range in classification from moderate to severe (Brandstater, Bontke, Cobble, & Horn, 1991). There is substantial variability among estimated incidence rates across studies, however. Several factors may contribute to this variability: (1) underreporting of mild head injuries; (2) overreporting of severe head injuries, possibly by counting patients more than once as they move from one level of care to another; (3) failure to count those who died before reaching primary care (Alexander, 1982); (4) lack of uniformly accepted diagnostic standards that define TBI; and (5) variable classification protocols for determining severity (Russell, 1932; Teasdale & Jennett, 1974). Sorenson and Kraus (1991) summarized studies of eight communities in the United States. They concluded that 200 per 100 thousand population each year is a good estimate regarding the number of new brain injuries in the typical American community.

The highest incidence of TBI occurs between ages 15 and 25. Beyond age 25, rates decline until the late middle age, but begin to rise again between the ages of 60 and 70. Males are two to three times more likely to have head injuries than females within each age group (Sorenson & Kraus, 1991). Motor vehicle accidents are the leading cause of TBI, followed by falls. In urban areas, firearms and assaults are the third leading cause. Individuals with brain damage from TBI tend to be single and of lower socioeconomic status.

PATHOPHYSIOLOGY

Types of Traumatic Brain Injury

TBIs generally consist of two categories: open head injuries and closed head injuries. Open head injuries occur when an object, such as a bullet, penetrates the skull or when skull fragments impinge upon brain tissue, as in compound fractures. Significant tissue damage tends to concentrate along paths of penetrating objects, but shock waves and pressure effects can cause diffuse damage (Newcombe, 1969). Surgical debridement of wounds is necessary to remove debris, bone fragments, and damaged brain tissue, leaving the rest of the brain intact. Open head injuries typically result in focal lesions and relatively circumscribed neuropsychological sequelae (Lezak, 1983).

A closed head injury results from a blow to the head. The skull may fracture, but the brain suffers no external penetration. Three biomechanical phenomena are important in understanding closed head injury. First, the blow molds the skull inward (regardless of fracture) compacting brain tissue medial to the point of impact resulting in a *coup* lesion. Second, the force vector that causes coup damage may push the brain against the other side of the skull producing a contusion (bruise) in the area opposite the blow. This *contrecoup* damage results from translation of the force vector through soft brain tissue that rests on a flexible brain stem surrounded by cerebrospinal fluid (Gurdjian, 1975). Third, shearing forces within the brain result from combined impact force and rotational acceleration of the brain within the skull. Rapid deceleration, coupled with impact force, as in motor vehicle accidents, also cause this shearing effect (Ommaya & Gennarelli, 1974). Shearing is maximal at the level of the cortex and minimal at the level of the brain stem. Importantly, shearing may produce diffuse microscopic lesions that affect major fiber tracts in the brain. Strong shearing forces may radiate back from the cortex to the diencephalon (affecting the corpus collosum) and even to the brain stem in more severe cases (Long, 1991). Such diffuse axonal injury relates to wide-ranging neuropsychological impairment (Lezak, 1983; Oppenheimer, 1968).

Secondary Brain Damage

Macroscopic and microscopic primary brain injuries sustained upon impact often give rise to complicating secondary mechanisms of brain injury. Compounded damage to the brain can result from each of the following processes: (1) intracranial hemorrhage and subsequent hematoma, (2) edema in white matter adjacent to focal mass lesions, (3) diffuse brain swelling, (4) ischemic damage, (5) increased intracranial pressure, and (6) brain shift and herniation (Levin, Benton, & Grossman, 1982). TBI can result in physiological changes, such as decreased brain glucose utilization, suppression of sensory evoked potentials, and reduced forebrain electroencephalograph (EEG) activity. Other delayed effects of primary brain injury include dysfunction of cerebrospinal fluid flow and white matter degeneration (Kolb & Whishaw, 1990).

Primary brain damage also affects levels of important brain neurotransmitters. Hayes, Lyeth, and Jenkins (1989) reviewed neurochemical mechanisms of mild and moderate head injuries. They presented evidence that temporary traumatic unconsciousness may result from increased activity within endogenous, inhibitory neural systems, such as the muscarinic cholinergic system of the rostral pons. Long-term behavioral deficits may result from diffuse hyperexcitation of neurons produced by excessive acetylcholine release following concussion. Recent studies that show delayed tissue death in cases of oxygen deprivation support such a hyperexcitation hypothesis (Kolb & Whishaw, 1990). Neuron hypoxia hypothetically causes release of glutamate that overexcites and kills cells. Primary brain injury affects other neurotransmitter systems as well. Serotonin increases in the cerebral cortex, hypothalamus, hippocampus, pons, and cerebrospinal fluid in response to brain injury (Osterholm, Bell, Meyer, & Pyenson, 1969). In addition, brain injuries may result in chronic decreases in the synthesis of dopamine and norepinephrine (Bakay, Sweeney, & Wood, 1986).

Susceptibility of the Anterior Brain to Traumatic Damage

Not all areas of the brain are equally susceptible to traumatic damage. Focal lesions occur at a higher rate in the frontal and temporal lobes relative to other brain regions (Kolb & Whishaw, 1990). Two main reasons may explain this differential susceptibility. The first reason is ergonomic (external), and the second, biomechanic (internal). The high incidence of traumatic head injury caused by motor vehicle accidents is important. Accidents necessarily associate with anterior bodily injury due to the ergonomic design of motor vehicles. It follows that motor vehicle accidents damage anterior brain regions at a high rate, however, further explanation is necessary.

Damage to the frontal and temporal lobes occurs at a high rate even when the initial blow is not directly anterior (Grubb & Coxe, 1978). When a force is strong enough to move the brain within the skull, the inferior frontal lobe and the anterior temporal lobes may strike the bony falx cerebri and wings of the sphenoid bones (Brandstater et al., 1991). Tissue lacerations can occur in addition to shearing tissue damage that shows an affinity for these anterior regions (Walsh, 1978). The phenomenon of differential susceptibility to traumatic injury in the anterior brain necessitates the detailed study of this region. It is from this assertion that the review proceeds.

THE FRONTAL LOBES

Anatomy

Researchers have extensively reviewed the structure of the frontal lobes (Damasio, 1985; Fuster, 1989; Stuss & Benson, 1986). In the following section, we outline only the crucial aspects of frontal lobe structure. In gross anatomical terms, the frontal lobes comprise all of the cortical tissue anterior to the central sulcus and above the lateral sulcus (Sylvian fissure). The frontal cortex consists of three anatomical regions: (1) primary motor cortex; (2) premotor and supplementary motor, or secondary, cortex; and (3) prefrontal, or tertiary, cortex. Figure 21.1 depicts the gross anatomy of the left cerebral cortex, including approximate boundaries of the four cortical lobes and functional regions within the frontal lobe.

Within the frontal lobes, the primary motor cortex is adjacent to the central sulcus. The premotor cortex is anterior to the primary motor cortex and inferior to

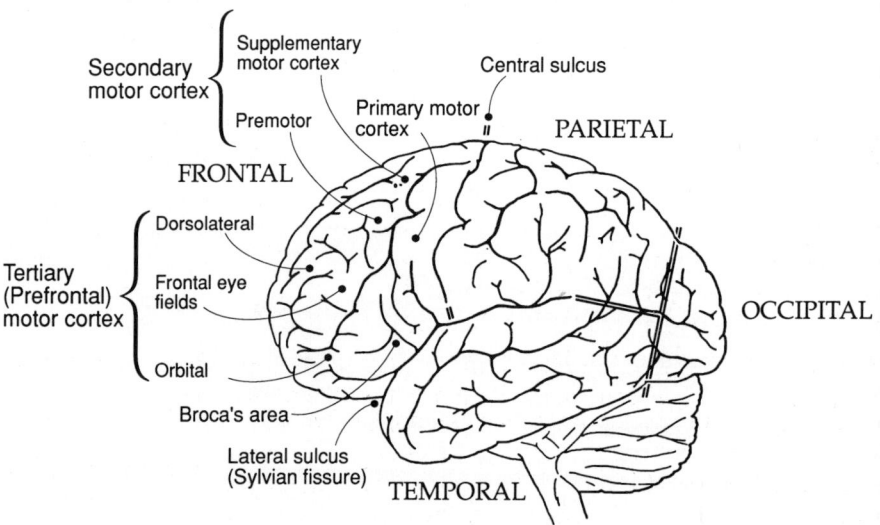

Figure 21.1. Gross anatomical regions of the left (language-dominant) cerebral cortex and approximate functional areas within the frontal lobe.

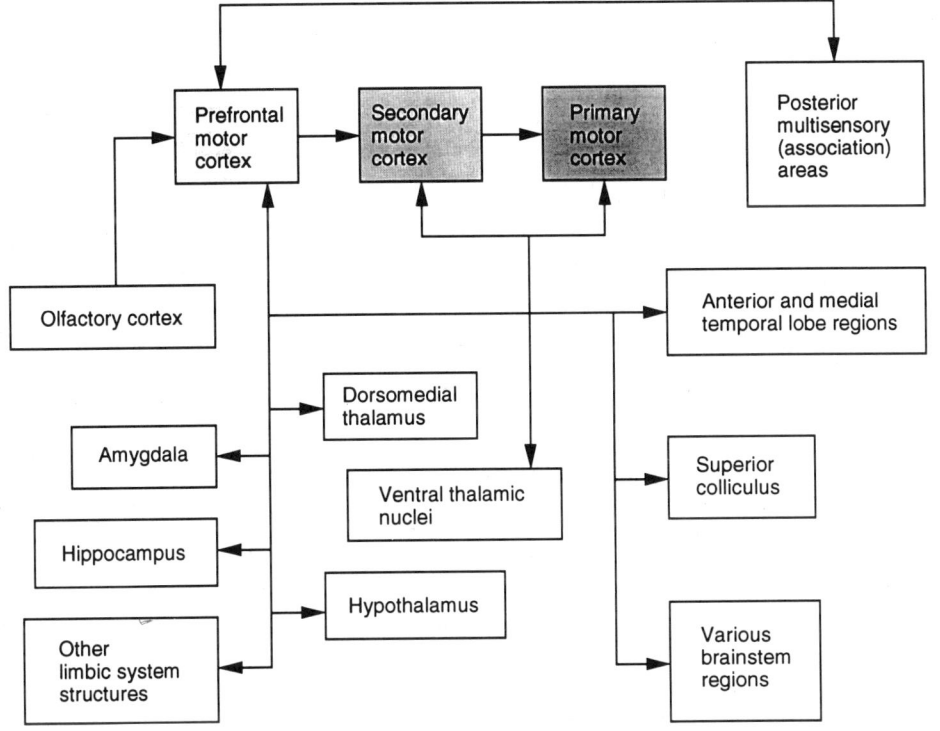

Figure 21.2. Diagrammatic representation of the connections between the frontal lobes and other brain structures.

the supplementary motor cortex that wraps onto the superior medial cortex (not pictured). Associated with the premotor cortex and supplementary motor cortex is Broca's area (involved in language production), usually found in the inferior portion of the premotor region in the language-dominant hemisphere. The prefrontal cortex is the most anterior region of the frontal cortex. A widely accepted model separates the prefrontal cortex into three divisions: (1) orbital, inferior; (2) dorsolateral, superior; and (3) frontal eye fields, medial (Kolb & Whishaw, 1990).

Connections of the frontal lobes to other brain regions are broad and complex. In fact, the prefrontal cortex has rich connections with most parts of the central nervous system (Stuss & Benson, 1986). Figure 21.2 depicts a simplified diagrammatic representation of this complex system. Major cortical connections exist within the frontal lobes (from prefrontal, to secondary, to primary motor cortex); between prefrontal regions and multisensory (association) areas in the temporal, parietal, and occipital lobes; and between the orbital prefrontal regions and the anterior and medial regions of the temporal lobes. Major subcortical connections exist between the frontal lobes and the thalamus (prefrontal cortex with dorsomedial thalamus, primary and secondary cortex with ventral thalamic nuclei), amygdala, hippocampus, superior colliculus, hypothalamus, and various brain stem areas. In addition, the frontal lobes project to other limbic system structures and receive projections from the olfactory cortex (Damasio, 1985).

Function

The various theories of frontal lobe function suggest an inextricable link between the anterior cerebral cortex and the most complex human behaviors. Early investigators based their theories on studies of tumor patients and frontal lobotomy patients. These populations do not provide an adequate model of patients with traumatic frontal lesions because TBI pathophysiology, although similar in some respects, is not identical. Tumors often cause widespread pressure effects within the brain (Kolb & Whishaw, 1990), and psychiatric patients show impairment on neuropsychological tests prior to any surgical intervention (Saykin et al., 1991). Recent work has clarified earlier research inconsistencies, making possible a unified explanation of frontal lobe function (Teuber, 1964). According to current neuropsychological theory, the frontal lobes mediate the highest forms of cerebral activity, including abstract reasoning, conceptual abilities, and creativity (Mattson & Levin, 1990; Milner & Petrides, 1984; Stuss & Benson, 1986).

Luria (1966, 1973) greatly advanced understanding of the frontal lobes. He built his theory on earlier findings that (1) the anterior cortex has more involvement in motor functions than does the posterior cortex, and (2) we can divide the cortex into primary sensory and motor zones, secondary sensory and motor zones, and tertiary association zones. Luria divided the cortex into two functional units: (1) the posterior sensory unit, made up of the temporal, parietal, and occipital lobes; and (2) the anterior motor unit, made up of the frontal lobes. According to basic Lurian theory, the sensory unit receives raw multisensory information (primary zones), translates the information into a form for further processing (secondary zones), and synthesizes a unified meaningful perception (tertiary zones). The synthesized information is then sent to the hippocampus for memory processing and to the amygdala for assessment of its emotional value. The sensory unit tertiary zones also send this information to the motor unit, where the frontal lobes formulate subsequent intentions (tertiary zones), organize those intentions into programs of action (secondary zones), and then execute the planned actions (primary zones).

Kolb and Whishaw (1990) criticized Luria's formulation on three main points: (1) oversimplification of the organization of sensory and motor representation, (2) overreliance on the notion of fixed sequential processing between zones in the sensor and motor units, and (3) weaknesses in the explanation regarding integration of perceptions. Incorporating more recent findings, Kolb and Whishaw offered a revised description of the functional organization of the frontal lobes. They hypothesized three levels of motor function in the frontal system that roughly correspond to the Lurian motor unit zones and the anatomical regions reviewed previously. The first level of motor function consists of neurons in the primary motor cortex that synapse directly on spinal motor neurons and cranial nerve motor nuclei. This level controls fine hand, finger, and facial movements. The second level consists of neurons in the primary motor cortex, premotor cortex, and supplementary motor cortex (along with associated neurons in the posterior parietal cortex). These neurons control limb, body, and eye movements.

The third level of frontal motor function is not understood as well as the first and second levels. The third level comprises neurons in the prefrontal cortex. These neurons have a nonspecific influence on movement, but a common theoretical theme in the literature contends that the prefrontal cortex has substantial involvement in the temporal organization of behavior (Fuster, 1989). Temporal memory, mediation of internal and external stimuli, inhibition and excitation of motor impulses to produce appropriate behavior sequences, and control of context-dependent behavior are theoretical functions of the prefrontal cortex (Kolb & Whishaw, 1990). Theoretically, the prefrontal cortex is also involved in executive functions (i.e., formulating goals, planning, carrying out goal-directed behavior, and performing effectively; Hecaen & Albert, 1978; Lezak, 1983; Shallice & Burgess, 1991).

A brief note is in order concerning frontal lobe laterality of function. Researchers have documented the principles of cerebral asymmetry for quite a long time (Hecaen, 1962; Zangwill, 1960). Functional organization of the frontal lobes is consistent with these principles. The left frontal lobe controls movement primarily related to language, whereas the right frontal lobe controls movement primarily related to nonverbal abilities; however, this asymmetry is relative rather than absolute. Milner (1974) reviewed studies documenting the role of the frontal lobes in almost all aspects of human behavior, emphasizing that the most anterior regions of the frontal lobes are the least asymmetrical in function.

SEQUELAE OF TRAUMATIC BRAIN INJURY

Variables Affecting Expression of Deficits

No two TBIs are exactly alike, even among those limited to the frontal lobes. Lezak (1983) reviewed factors that influence how effects of brain damage manifest. Lesion characteristics that affect deficit expression include site, type of damage (i.e., focal or diffuse), and severity. Of these factors, lesion severity is the most important variable in predicting patients' ultimate levels of improvement (Gilchrist & Wilkinson, 1979). Reliance on lesion site alone to predict effects is inadequate because normal intraindividual variability in brain organization can produce different sequelae in patients with similar lesion sites. Time since injury is another important determinant. Bond (1979) noted that patients make the greatest cognitive gains within the first 6 months after injury. In addition, several patient variables affect deficit expression. Age, sex, lateral dominance, and premorbid intellectual and psychosocial functioning are important variables. If one holds lesion variables constant, the individual with the best functional prognosis after frontal lobe damage is theoretically young, female, left-handed, intelligent, vivacious, and psychosocially well-adjusted (Sawicki, 1990).

Medical Sequelae

Posttraumatic Epilepsy. Approximately 5% of patients with closed head injuries and about 50% of those whose trauma involved compound skull fractures and brain injury will develop posttraumatic epilepsy (PTE) (Adams & Victor, 1989). Early PTE (seizures within the first week) occur within 4–5% of hospitalized TBI patients. Factors that increase probability of late PTE (onset after the first week) include early PTE, dural tearing, signs of focal neurologic deficit (e.g., hemiparesis), posttraumatic amnesia of longer than 24 hours (Bontke, 1989), and parietal or posterior frontal lesions (Adams & Victor, 1989). Bontke (1989) discussed the controversy regarding prophylactic anticonvulsant therapy which may prevent development of seizure activity, but one must weigh risk for PTE against possibility of medication side effects.

Posttraumatic Hydrocephalus. Intermittent headaches, vomiting, confusion, and drowsiness, followed by mental dullness, apathy, and psychomotor retardation may indicate posttraumatic hydrocephalus (PTH; Adams & Victor, 1989). Bontke (1989) added dementia, ataxia and incontinence as possible manifestations of PTH.

Headaches and the Postconcussion Syndrome. Goldstein (1991) discussed two types of headaches that TBI patients experience. The International Headache Society classified these as acute traumatic headaches and posttraumatic headaches. Both types of headaches have associated lapse of consciousness, posttraumatic amnesia of longer than 15 minutes, and/or relevant abnormality on any of a variety of neurodiagnostic and neuropsychological tests. Onset of these headaches is usually less than 14 days after patients regain consciousness. The difference between the two types is that acute traumatic headaches usually disappear within 8 weeks, whereas posttraumatic headaches persist. The character of these headaches may be that of muscle contraction or migraine and they frequently have associated dizziness, irritability, decreased concentration, and intolerance to alcohol. The latter symptoms comprise the postconcussion syndrome.

Nonneurologic Sequelae. Bontke (1989) indicated that TBI can result in numerous medical complications that can affect diverse physiological systems, including musculoskeletal, cardiovascular, respiratory, gastrointestinal, genitourinary, hematologic, dermatologic, endocrine, and/or autonomic systems.

Behavioral Sequelae

Exhaustive review of findings from observational and experimental studies is beyond the scope of this chapter (see Damasio, 1985; Kolb & Whishaw, 1990, and Mattson and Levin, 1990, for reviews). The following is a brief outline of major behavioral sequelae associated with TBI. Where firm evidence for localization is available, the specific frontal lobe region follows the impaired function in parentheses.

Motor Functions. Disturbances of motor function following frontal lobe damage include loss of fine movements (primary motor cortex; Kuypers, 1981), loss of strength (primary motor, supplementary motor, and dorsolateral prefrontal cortex; Leonard, Jones, & Milner, 1988), impaired movement programming (supplementary motor cortex; Kolb & Milner, 1981; Roland, Larsen, Lassen, & Skinhoj, 1980), and poor voluntary eye gaze (dorsolateral prefrontal cortex and frontal eye fields; Guitton, Buchtel, & Douglas, 1982). In addition, Damasio (1985) reported evidence for abnormal reflexes and muscle tone, abnormal gait and posture, and changes in sphincter control.

Memory. Several studies have reported poor temporal memory in patients with frontal lobe damage. Experimental paradigms have found impairment in recency memory (Milner, 1974), frequency estimation (Smith & Milner, 1984), and sequencing (Petrides & Milner, 1982) associated with damage to the dorsolateral prefrontal cortex. Patients with frontal lobe lesions also show reliable impairment on tasks of delayed response and delayed alternation (dorsolateral prefrontal cortex; Freedman & Oscar-Berman, 1986).

Divergent Reasoning. Patients with frontal lobe damage consistently show impaired verbal fluency (left prefrontal cortex; Benton, 1968; Miller, 1984b; Milner, 1964; Perret, 1974). Jones-Gotman and Milner (1977) documented an associated impairment phenomenon in design fluency (right prefrontal cortex).

Executive Functions and Regulation of Behavior. Lezak (1983) described a set of behavioral disturbances associated with damage to the prefrontal cortex: (1) problems starting, (2) difficulties making mental or behavioral shifts, (3) problems stopping, (4) deficient self-awareness, and (5) a concrete attitude. Problems starting involve decreased rates at which patients emit behavior; this manifests as decreased spontaneity, loss of productivity, lack of initiative, and difficulty carrying out plans or completing projects. Problems of starting that are more severe than those described include apathy, mutism, and general unresponsiveness.

Difficulties making mental or behavioral shifts involve many areas of function, including attention and concentration, movement, verbal output, and expression of attitudes. Perseveration and rigidity are common in patients with prefrontal cortex damage. These behaviors relate to impaired social behavior (Blumer & Benson, 1975) and inability to form or shift mental sets in neuropsychological testing (Cicerone, Lazar, & Shapiro, 1983; Drewe, 1974; Nelson, 1976). Problems stopping manifest as impulsivity, disinhibition, and hypersensitivity to environmental stimuli. Miller (1985) also reported increased risk taking and rule breaking among patients with prefrontal cortex damage. Patients with frontal lobe damage also show increased susceptibility to distraction and interference (left prefrontal cortex; Perret, 1974; Stuss et al., 1982).

Deficient self-awareness following frontal lobe damage results in impaired perception of performance errors and functional limitations, difficulty responding appropriately to environmental cues about behavior (i.e., "feedback"), and problems analyzing social situations. Milner (1964, 1965) also observed that patients with frontal damage exhibit an inability to use knowledge or verbal mediation to regulate behavior. Lezak's (1983) description of concrete attitude among these individuals encompasses changes in goal-oriented behavior (Damasio, 1985) along with impaired planning and strategy formation, organization, and problem-solving abilities (prefrontal cortex; Corkin, 1965; Shallice & Evans, 1978).

Language. Damage to the left frontal lobe involving Broca's area results in a well-documented disturbance of expressive language known as *Broca's aphasia* (Kolb & Whishaw, 1990). This nonfluent aphasia consists of very slow, deliberate speech and oversimplified grammatical structure. Patients with Broca's aphasia continue to understand speech despite difficulty producing it. Severity of Broca's aphasia ranges from speechlessness to presence of recurring utterances, to a slight, but obvious, articulation disorder involving paraphasia, dysnomia, and/or altered prosody. As noted, impaired verbal fluency is often present in patients with damage to the left prefrontal cortex (Benton, 1968; Miller, 1984b; Milner, 1964; Perret, 1974).

Transcortical motor aphasia is another form of nonfluent language impairment associated with anterior cortical lesions. This form of aphasia manifests as lack of verbal initiative without compromise of articulation. Perseveration and echolalia may also be present. Confrontation naming of objects is intact relative to production of spontaneous speech and verbal narrative. Frequently, patients with transcortical motor aphasia are unable to comprehend words despite adequate repetition ability (Mazzocchi & Vignolo, 1979).

Sexual Behavior. Effects of traumatic head injury on sexual behavior have begun to receive more attention recently (Blackerby, 1990). Reports specific to frontal lobe dysfunction, however, are anecdotal rather than empirically based (Kolb & Whishaw, 1990). Generally, two patterns of abnormal sexual behavior emerge after frontal lobe damage (Walker & Blumer, 1975). The first pattern manifests as disinhibition of sexual drive characterized by inappropriate sexual advances and display (orbital prefrontal cortex). The second pattern involves decreased sexual desire, but performance remains intact (dorsolateral prefrontal cortex).

Olfaction. Recent findings show that olfactory deficits (dysosmia) are present in 20% to 30% of severe head injuries (Costanzo & Zasler, 1992). Levin, High, and Eisenberg (1985) reported low incidence of complete anosmia after traumatic head injury, but relatively high incidence of impaired olfactory naming and recognition (33%). Potter and Butters (1980) reported findings specific to patients with prefrontal cortex damage: Olfactory detection was intact, whereas olfactory discrimination ability evidenced severe impairment.

Secondary Psychopathology

Patients with frontal lobe dysfunction often show changes in affect and regulation of emotional responses (Damasio, 1985; Hecaen, 1964). Blumer and Benson (1975) described two distinct personality patterns that manifest after frontal lobe damage. The "pseudodepressed" personality consists of behavioral slowness, outward display of apathy and indifference, loss of initiative, reduced sexual interest, blunted affect, and little or no verbal output (dorsolateral prefrontal cortex). In contrast, patients with "pseudopsychopathic" personality exhibit poor impulse control, irritability, hyperkinesis, inappropriate sexual behavior, and general impairment of social skills (orbital prefrontal cortex). Investigation of relationships between lesion laterality and regulation of emotional responses has documented increased anxiety and depression in patients with right-sided lesions (orbital prefrontal cortex). Some investigators have reported increased anger and hostility in patients with left-sided damage (dorsolateral prefrontal cortex; Grafman, Vance, Weingartner, Salazar, & Amin, 1986).

At the current time, there is very little research regarding depression and anxiety following traumatic head injury (Kolb & Whishaw, 1990). Alexander (1982) noted that diagnosis of depression in patients with traumatic brain injuries is difficult. Certainly, various behavioral sequelae of frontal lobe dysfunction can complicate the diagnostic picture and make estimates of incidence unreliable. Therefore, much more research in this area is essential.

The Family

Lezak (1978, 1986, 1988) published a series of articles that document difficulties experienced by families of patients with behavioral disturbances and personality alterations. Several behaviors were specifically linked to family problems (Lezak, 1988). The problem behaviors resulting directly from a TBI include (1) impaired social perception and social awareness; (2) impaired control; (3) dependency; (4) inability to learn from experience; and (5) specific emotional alterations, such as apathy or lability. Anxiety, paranoia, and depression are often indirect consequences of TBI that also contribute to family adjustment difficulties. Manifestation of any of these behaviors often present difficulties that family members are unprepared to manage. Researchers have taken an increased interest in studying these problems empirically (Hendryx, 1989; Willer, Allen, Liss, & Zicht, 1991).

Empirical studies have not only documented problems experienced by families of TBI patients but have also identified important differences between patients' and family members' perceptions of problems. For instance, Hendryx (1989) found that adult TBI patients tend to rate their cognitive difficulties as their most extreme problems, whereas family members rated emotional changes as most problematic. This finding reflects both different perceptions within the family unit and the complexity of cognitive and emotional interactions that influence human interpersonal behavior. These issues evince the necessary involvement of family in the entire rehabilitation process.

ASSESSMENT

Approaches to assessment of dysfunction following TBI arrange into three tiers. The first tier includes basic neurological evaluations conducted by attending neurologists and all relevant neurodiagnostic procedures (e.g., skull X-ray, CAT scan, MRI). Second-tier assessment consists of interview, direct behavioral observation, mental status examination, and neuropsychological assessment. Evaluations conducted by other members of the interdisciplinary team (e.g., physical therapy, occupational therapy, speech therapy, and recreational therapy) also occur in the second tier. Standardized self-report inventories, self-monitoring, and family interview/evaluation are third-tier assessment approaches. Table 21.1 summarizes appropriate assessment approaches for each phase of patient care. As seen in Table 21.1, some assessment approaches found in each tier are applicable at each phase of treatment. The difference lies in emphasis of approaches at each phase. Tier 1 is most important in the acute phase. Tier 2 grows in importance in the rehabilitation phase. Finally, postdischarge, Tiers 2 and 3 provide the most pertinent information about level of patient recovery.

Medical/Neurological Evaluation

Nearly 80% of TBI patients first receive evaluations by general physicians, and fewer than 20% ever require neurosurgery (Adams & Victor, 1989). For those first seen by trauma teams, initial evaluations follow standardized guidelines (Collicott, 1991). Treatment teams simultaneously identify and treat conditions crucial to survival. Clinicians must establish an adequate respiratory exchange while protect-

Table 21.1. Assessment of the TBI Patient: Acute Care through Recovery

Phase of treatment	Tier 1 assessment	Tier 2 assessment	Tier 3 assessment
Acute	Neurological exam Clinical tests	Select interdisciplinary team evaluations Patient interview Behavioral observation Mental status exam	Family interview
Rehab	Neurological exam Clinical tests	Interdisciplinary team evaluations Patient interview Behavioral observation Mental status exam Neuropsychological	Family interview/evaluation Self-report inventories
Outpatient	Neurological exam Clinical tests	Select interdisciplinary team evaluations Patient interview Behavioral observation Neuropsychological	Family interview/evaluation Self-report inventories Self-monitoring

ing the cervical spine; they must also control hemorrhages and maintain peripheral vascular circulation. Team members can then begin preliminary neurological evaluation and diagnostic tests, which they repeat at frequent intervals. Results of neurological examinations are the basis of management decisions. Neuroimaging, essential in early care, will typically consist of computerized axial tomography (CAT) rather than magnetic resonance imagery (MRI) for two reasons. First, patients often require metal support equipment that would interfere with MRI. Second, patients often cannot hold still for any length of time (Ruff, Cullum, & Luerssen, 1989). Other tests may include skull X-rays, evoked potentials, spinal fluid examinations, and vestibular function tests (Goldstein, 1991). Neurologists and/or neurosurgeons serve as consultants on an as-needed basis. Reassessment continues throughout hospitalization to identify conditions that may not have been evident initially and to monitor any changes in patients' conditions.

Mental Status Examination

In the acute stage after traumatic head injury, patient interviews and direct behavioral observations are part of mental status exams (Berg, Franzen, & Wedding, 1987; Strub & Black, 1985). Two important functions of mental status exams are (1) to measure depth and duration of coma, and (2) to define the parameters of amnesia. The Glasgow Coma Scale (Teasdale & Jennett, 1974) helps objectify coma assessment. Rappaport, Hall, Hopkins, Belleza, and Cope (1982) expanded design of the Glasgow Coma Scale to make it more sensitive than the earlier version in detecting and measuring clinical changes in patients with severe head injury. Researchers and clinicians widely use both scales.

Recent literature reviews have concluded that duration of posttraumatic amnesia (PTA) is a better predictor of recovery than duration of coma (Bond, 1983; Levin et al., 1982; Russell, 1971). PTA often lasts much longer than coma following head injury. Thus, ongoing mental status examination is essential to clearly document severity and duration of PTA. Two behavioral rating instruments help assess PTA and related behavioral disturbances: the Neurobehavioral Rating Scale (Levin et al., 1987), and the Cognitive-Behavior Rating Scale (Williams, 1987). Initial reliability data are good, but both instruments are still in the validation process.

Neuropsychological Assessment

In the postacute stage of recovery, patients with frontal lobe damage become appropriate for standardized neuropsychological testing once they stabilize medically and their PTA begins to resolve.

Motor Functions

In the absence of dense hemiplegia, clinicians can obtain measures of grip strength (hand dynamometer; Reitan & Davison, 1974) and finger dexterity (Finger Tapping Test; Reitan, 1969). Both measures are well-normed and have demonstrated adequate reliability and validity.

Intelligence

The Wechsler Adult Intelligence Scale-Revised (WAIS-R; Wechsler, 1981) is the most well-established and thoroughly researched instrument for measuring intellectual functioning (Bigler, 1987). It is a fundamental component of the Halstead–Reitan Neuropsychological Test Battery. Frontal lobe damage typically affects intellectual functioning in some manner (Damasio, 1985); however, well-learned behaviors are often resistant to frontal lobe damage. Russell (1979) reviewed the differential sensitivity to brain damage among the subtests of the WAIS. He concluded that Block Design, Digit Span, and Digit Symbol are the most prone to brain damage, whereas Information and Vocabulary are usually the least sensitive to brain damage. It is on tests of adaptive intelligence (e.g, new learning ability, abstract reasoning), rather than on tests of well-learned abilities, that patients with frontal lobe dysfunction perform most poorly (Bigler, 1987).

Executive Functions and the Regulation of Behavior

A few standardized neuropsychological tests are useful for assessing anterior frontal lobe function. Currently, the best measure for assessing dorsolateral prefrontal cortex function is the Wisconsin Card Sorting Test (WCST; Heaton, 1981). The WCST assessed ability to form abstract concepts and to shift or maintain a behavioral set. The Controlled Oral Word Association Test (i.e., Word Fluency or FAS-Test) requires spontaneous production of words beginning with a given letter within a limited amount of time (Spreen & Strauss, 1991; Thurstone, 1938). Both tests are well-normed and have demonstrated adequate psychometric properties. Bigler (1987) noted that several other tests have utility in assessing frontal lobe function, including the Halstead Category Test (Halstead, 1947; Reitan & Davison, 1974), the Raven Progressive Matrices (Raven, 1962), and variations of the Stroop Word Color Test (Stroop, 1935; Trenerry, Crosson, DeBoe, & Leber, 1989). These tests hypothetically measure concept generalization, abstract reasoning, and complex problem solving; however, each test has yielded less experimental evidence for frontal lobe specificity than the WCST and the Controlled Oral Word Association test. Lezak (1993) summarized recent developments in the neuropsychological assessment of frontal lobe executive functions. Additional research is necessary to confirm validity of these measures; however, they represent a hopeful trend toward better evaluation of subtle executive processes that affect TBI patients' success in life after rehabilitation.

Language

It is often difficult to lateralize frontal lobe damage based on neuropsychological test results without presence of language deficits (Kolb & Whishaw, 1990). Thus, evaluation of language skills is essential. The Reitan–Indiana Aphasia Screening Test (Reitan, 1984) is an aphasia screening tool that clinicians can quickly administer. The Revised Token Test (McNeil & Prescott, 1978) helps assess verbal comprehension of increasingly complex commands. Psychometric properties of the Revised Token Test have improved substantially over those of the original version (DeRenzi & Vignolo, 1962).

Self-Report Inventories and Self-Monitoring

Various sequelae of frontal lobe injury often make application of standardized self-report inventories unreliable and attempts at self-monitoring impossible, at least in the acute stage and often well into the postacute stage. Clinicians must therefore interpret standardized self-report measures with caution. Postacute assessment must rely on corroborative behavioral assessment by other members of the interdisciplinary treatment team and patients' significant others.

The Behavior Change Inventory (Hartlage, 1989) and the Change Assessment Questionnaire (Lam, McMahon, Priddy, & Gehred-Schultz, 1988) are self-report inventories developed to measure personality change and "readiness to change," respectively, among traumatically brain-injured individuals. Much more research is necessary to verify validity of these measures; however, both instruments can help identify target behaviors for intervention. More research is also essential for development of sound techniques for assessing secondary psychopathology in TBI survivors. The assessment strategies detailed in handbooks (e.g., Bellack & Hersen, 1988) offer the most empirically sound approaches.

The Family

Information about premorbid functioning assists in predicting outcome. Family and significant others are essential sources of such information. They can often obtain important documents that verify level of premorbid functioning (e.g., school records, standardized testing, work evaluations, prior psychiatric evaluations, premorbid work samples). Clinicians must also closely monitor the identified primary caregivers for signs of psychological distress, as described by Novack, Bergquist, Bennet, and Gouvier (1991). In addition, evaluation of family functioning is an important part of discharge and long-term care planning. The Family Environment Scale (R. Moos & B. Moos, 1981) and the McMaster Family Assessment Device (Epstein, Baldwin, & Bishop, 1983) represent well-established measures of family functioning.

TREATMENT

Recovery of Function

Several trends in recovery of function following brain damage have surfaced in the animal literature (Finger, 1978; LeVere, Davis, & Gonder, 1979):

1. The functional recovery curve tends to be regular and consistent.
2. Younger subjects show less behavioral impairment and better recovery relative to older subjects with comparable lesions.
3. Highly overlearned skills tend to recover best and suffer least after brain injury.
4. Remotely acquired skills usually suffer less impairment and recover more quickly than recently acquired skills.
5. Severe lesions tend to affect behavior more profoundly and result in slower and more limited recovery than less severe lesions.
6. Better recovery and less severe deficits are more common with slowly progressive lesions than with other types of brain dysfunction.
7. Experience after brain damage can influence recovery of function.
8. Interventions that influence recovery of function tend to be most effective when performed proximally to time of injury rather than at some distant time.

Rehabilitation

Interdisciplinary Team Approach

In a recent review, Cobble, Bontke, Brandstater, and Horn (1991) summarized the importance of interdisciplinary intervention strategies in managing patients with brain disorders. Barry and O'Leary (1989) noted that psychologists on TBI rehabilitation teams serve important specific roles. Little has been published about specific treatment of frontal lobe dysfunction; however, other than one recent review regarding management of executive dysfunction (Sohlberg, Mateer, & Stuss, 1993) there has been relatively little information about specific treatment of frontal lobe dysfunction and the roles of interdisciplinary team members. Nonetheless, given the susceptibility of the anterior cortex to damage after traumatic head injury, interventions applied to heterogeneous brain-damaged patients appear germane.

Pharmacological Interventions

Rose (1988) reported drugs having a small but vital role in treatment of patients with brain damage secondary to traumatic head injury, particularly in management of posttraumatic epilepsy (Willmore, 1990). Pharmacological interventions are also available for use in clinical management of behavior disorders. In a recent review, however, Rose (1988) called for physicians to exercise restraint in prescribing sedative medication for agitated, confused, or disinhibited patients. Environmental interventions and behavior management plans serve as the preferred frontline treatments for TBI patients; however, real-world situations arise in which a pharmacological adjunct is necessary, such as when a patient becomes dangerous to self or others. Pharmacological treatment of active behavior disorders has included both benzodiazepines and neuroleptics, but amnestic and sedating properties of these medications limit their desirability. Carbamazepine (Tegretol), propranolol (Inderal), and lithium have helped manage impulsive and overactive TBI patients with minimal, documented adverse side effects relative to those of benzodiazepines and neuroleptics (Rose, 1988). Massagli (1991), however, in a review of the neurobehavioral effects of anticonvulsants on patients with TBI, concluded that carbamazepine, phenytoin (Dilantin), and valproic acid (Depakene, Depakote) may all compromise cognitive functioning, especially at higher plasma levels. Rose (1988) indicated that lithium and amitriptyline (Elavil, Endep) may help manage emotional lability that often accompanies post-TBI mood disturbance. Unfortunately, amitriptyline may also lower seizure threshold in patients already at risk for posttraumatic epilepsy. There is currently no drug of choice for treatment of depression following traumatic brain injury (Glenn & Wroblewski, 1989).

In summary, use of pharmacological interventions in treatment of TBI patients is often necessary but difficult to implement successfully. Conservative use of these agents as carefully planned, data-driven supplements to treatment is preferable to cursory application as "antibehavior" agents for unmanageable situations. There is clearly a need for much more research in this area.

Cognitive Rehabilitation

Since the late 1970s, there has been a proliferation of cognitive retraining techniques and cognitive rehabilitation programs for patients with traumatic brain damage (Boake, 1989). For instance, Craine (1982) reported a case study involving cognitive retraining of a traumatic frontal-lobe-dysfunction patient in which specific treatment effects generalized well to the naturalistic domain. In contrast, Gouvier, Webster, and Blanton (1986) conducted a review of cognitive retraining techniques and concluded that cognitive retraining is a "fledgling therapy technique," and its external validity needs cautious interpretation. More rigorous applications of single-case experimental designs may be appropriate for cognitive rehabilitation research (Franzen & Iverson, 1990).

Nonetheless, recent work with specific focus on retraining executive-system dysfunction is quite promising. Ylvisaker and Szekeres (1989) indicated that several content domains are potential targets for intervention with patients who have mild to moderate residual cognitive impairment or specific executive problems following TBI. Self-awareness of strengths and weaknesses may be increased by guiding patients through a sequence of therapist-planned tasks that reveal deficits gently (i.e., "self-discovery") rather than by potentially overwhelming and/or adversarial confrontations. Teaching realistic goal setting and planning also requires thoughtful therapist guidance. Involving patients as active participants in setting their own short- and long-term goals is important. Patients and clinicians must carefully discuss with each other successes and failures that patients experience as they attempt to reach goals so that they receive realistic feedback about effects of their choices. In addition, executive-system treatment plans must include self-control strategies to manage patient initiation, inhibition, and evaluation (self-monitoring). It is important to note that these treatment strategies have received little empirical support; however, Sohlberg et al. (1993) recently offered a conceptual model of executive-system functions that may improve matching of treatment options to patient needs. This is a ripe area for future research.

Behavioral Approaches

A growing literature seeks to develop an interface between neuropsychology and behavior therapy (Horton & Miller, 1985; Lawson-Kerr, Smith, & Beck, 1990). Efficacy of behavioral interventions with brain-damaged patients is gaining increased support in this literature (Boake, 1991; Franzen, 1991; Ince, 1976; Seron, 1987; Webster & Scott, 1988). McGlynn (1990) noted there has been successful application of behavioral interventions to six categories of target behaviors: (1) inappropriate social behavior, (2) attention and motivation, (3) unawareness of deficits, (4) memory, (5) language and speech, and (6) motor disturbances. At this time, single-case experimental design is the most valid methodology for evaluating behavioral treatment of patients with frontal lobe dysfunction.

Among the few group-outcome studies that have used behavioral treatments, social skills training and problem-solving skills training have received the most empirically rigorous attention. Brotherton, Thomas, Wisotzek, and Milan (1988) used a multiple baseline single-case experimental design in their treatment of four TBI patients with social skills deficits. The treatment package comprised five components: (1) instruction/education, (2) modeling, (3) behavior rehearsal, (4) videotape feedback, and (5) social reinforcement. In order to assess effectiveness of treatment, the investigators collected ratings of six operationally defined target behaviors include distracting hand/arm movements, posture, speech dysfluency, conversational focus on other person, showing interest, and making positive statements; the ratings occurred during confederate-assisted enactments of social "problem situations" that clinicians had developed for each subject from a initial social skills assessments. Clear treatment effects evolved in 3 of the 4 patients' target behaviors (1 patient had poor motivation and was resistant to intervention). Positive treatment effects generalized across problem situations and maintained at 1-year follow-up. Simple motoric target behaviors were more responsive to intervention than more complex verbal target behaviors.

In another small group study, Foxx, Martella, and Marchand-Martella (1989) used a nonrandomized pretest-posttest control group experimental design to evaluate a program for teaching a problem-solving strategy to three young adults with TBI. The investigators targeted four functional domains for training: (1) community awareness and transportation; (2) medication, alcohol, and drugs; (3) stating one's rights; and (4) emergencies, injuries, and safety. The training program incorporated cue cards, response-specific feedback, modeling, self-monitoring, positive reinforcement, response practice, self-correction, and individualized performance criterion levels. Therapists presented subjects with problem-solving situations printed on 4″

× 6" index cards and recorded subjects' responses to four criterion questions (e.g., "Where would you look for help?") during pretest assessment, baseline, probe, and two training conditions (with and without cue cards). Testing of generalization effects transpired during posttest interviews and in staged interactions conducted in the natural environment. A control group of 3 additional young adult TBI survivors received only pretest and posttest assessments. Results showed that control group scores changed little from pretest to posttest, whereas experimental group scores improved substantially and generalized well at posttest. In fact, experimental group scores were comparable to a group of normal individuals who also underwent the training program. These results are quite encouraging; however, future research must focus on generalization of verbal problem solving and responses to staged interactions and, ultimately, to actual performance in uncontrolled situations. Foxx and Bittle (1989) published a revised version of the training package used in this study under the title *Thinking It Through*.

These two studies represent an encouraging trend in experimental investigation of treatment outcome for TBI patients. Although one limitation of these studies is the small sample size employed, both studies do a very good job of using existing technology in single-case experimental design to control for the many variables at play regarding social behavior of brain-damaged persons. This area needs more work of such high caliber. An emphasis on predicting generalization of acquired compensatory skills to the naturalistic domain is especially important.

The Family

Various problems of TBI patients directly affect psychological states of family members. Rosenthal and Geckler (1986) outlined TBI sequelae that most affect family functioning: presence of cognitive deficits, disorders of communication, emotional regression, frontal lobe behavior, withdrawal from social contacts, inappropriate social behavior, depression, and inability to resume premorbid role within the family. Just as cognitive and behavioral impairment of TBI patients affects family members, functioning of family members has a reciprocal effect on patients' continuing rehabilitation outcomes. Thus, successful treatment of patients must involve appropriate family-based interventions (Jackson & Gouvier, 1992). Fortunately, a growing body of information has developed during the last few years that will likely aid interdisciplinary teams in providing adequate interventions to family members in need (Kreutzer, Zasler, Camplair, & Leininger, 1990; Rosenthal & Geckler, 1986; Williams & Kay, 1991).

Health-care providers can implement three levels of intervention with families of TBI patients: (1) education, (2) counseling/support, and (3) therapy. The first level of intervention is education. Education of family members about the nature of TBI and relevant behavior-management strategies is an integral part of patient care throughout the entire rehabilitation process. In the acute setting, education is the frontline strategy for orienting families to policies and procedures of the rehabilitation center, personnel that comprise the interdisciplinary treatment team, and the broad goals of rehabilitation. Establishing an information base early in patients' hospitalizations is important in helping family members develop realistic expectations for patients' recovery of function and potential adaptations in family functioning that may be necessary upon discharge. Education also includes patient advocacy and making families aware of community resources that they can explore, even while the patient is still hospitalized.

Counseling and support are the second level of family intervention. Family counseling promotes adaptive adjustment to the stressful reintegration of TBI patients into family systems. Even the most intelligent and resourceful families will feel overwhelmed at times, especially in the early phases of rehabilitation when extent of residual impairment is still not clear. Support from psychosocial personnel (e.g., clinical psychologist, social worker, rehabilitation counselor) assists in the adjustment process. A primary intervention that is often useful in the acute setting involves helping family members, especially spouses, to shift focus from TBI patients to themselves. By the time most TBI patients enter rehabilitation, family members feel exhausted. They may have spent most of their time at the hospital with the patient and neglected other responsibilities, such as jobs, routine finances, and other family members. Families need encouragement to take breaks from the hospital so that they can tend to these other responsibilities and try to rest. Rest is very important at this stage because once TBI patients return to previous home environments, caregiving demands increase markedly.

Another important function of counseling and support involves management of emotional reactions, such as frustration, anger, and grief. Denial is another feature of family adjustment that clinicians must address. Management of denial involves the careful balancing of hopeful wishes with awareness of problem areas and implications for change. Consistent, accurate communication of initial assessment findings and weekly patient progress are very important in helping family members maintain this adaptive balance between hope and despair. Family conferences at which family members can sit down with the entire treatment team and ask questions about patients' progress and prognosis have been quite helpful in clinical practice. Such a group setting is a good place to report poor progress and make concrete recommendations about caring for severely compromised TBI patients at home. More support is available from the team than from any one therapist. Similarly, family members often respond well to peer support groups on the rehabilitation unit or in the community. Peer support groups afford families that are newer to TBI the coping perspective of "seasoned veteran" families. Sometimes, family members are able to make coping adjustments with peer support that were previously unsuccessful with staff counseling alone.

The third and final level of intervention involves formalized family therapy. Because this form of intervention is the most time consuming, family therapy is most often effective after acute inpatient rehabilitation, when family members fully realize what residual deficits remain and family system feels stressed in the absence of multiple supportive rehabilitation personnel. Rosenthal and Geckler (1986) asserted that the primary goal of family therapy is to "alter maladaptive communication and interaction patterns within the family system" (p. 339). Family therapy with TBI patients is especially challenging. Premorbid dysfunction in family communications and interactions, maladaptive patient behaviors, and adjustment difficulties, interact in the now very unstable family system. Therapists can utilize this period of instability and frustration to change otherwise stubborn, long-standing family behaviors by encouraging open communication about feelings and beliefs, teaching improved methods of communication and problem solving, and renegotiating roles and responsibilities within family systems. An important consideration is whether to include TBI patients in family therapy sessions. In general, therapists must exercise judgment to determine the answer to a fundamental question: Will this TBI patient benefit in a meaningful way? Cognitive level alone cannot guide this decision. TBI patients also need to have core executive functions as well as adequate language abilities and behavioral controls so that they do not disrupt therapy sessions.

In summary, family therapy is a necessary and useful intervention that often reaches peak effectiveness once rehabilitation gains have slowed and TBI patients have returned home. Education, counseling, and support are most effective during inpatient rehabilitation, when the patient is making rapid gains. Formal family therapy requires commitment of time and effort that most families simply cannot make while the patient is still hospitalized. We base these summary statements largely on years of clinical experience in treating families of TBI patients at various stages of the rehabilitation process. Further research is essential if we are to learn how better to match level of need with appropriate interventions and to study utilization patterns of family education, counseling/support, and therapy for program development and optimal treatment outcome.

Community Reintegration

Recent passage of the Americans with Disabilities Act (1990) calls attention to the need to provide continuing care after discharge from postacute inpatient rehabilitation. TBI patients, their families, the allied health professions, advocacy groups (e.g., National Head Injury Foundation), and governmental agencies (e.g., Rehabilitation Services Administration and the National Institute on Disability and Rehabilitation Research) are intensifying their reviews of needs and proposed solutions. Obvious shortcomings to postdischarge rehabilitation efforts are clear; patients leave postacute settings and return home where they encounter extensive obstacles to regaining their premorbid quality of life. Effective long-term rehabilitation is necessary.

Increased efforts to provide a unified approach to meeting such long-term needs are currently under development. Continued emphasis on the interdisciplinary team approach is essential. Lewis, Burke, and Carrillo (1987) outlined a model for postacute care of TBI patients; such care needs to integrate ongoing individualized treatment of specific cognitive, behavioral, and social skills deficits addressed during inpatient rehabilitation with physical conditioning, activities of daily-living training, and vocational retraining. Vocational programs attempt to prepare TBI patients for competitive employment by providing training through a progression from transitional employment at training facilities, to volunteer community placements, to supported employment in the community under close supervision of vocational specialists. The final step is for TBI patients to gain competitive employment in the community.

A recent article by West and associates (1991) reported average costs for one TBI patient to participate in a supported employment program and achieve job stabilization: 237.8 hours of staff intervention at a cost of $6,896. Continuing follow-up after job stabilization averaged 1.64 staff hours per week at a cost of $47.56 for each TBI patient. These figures are staggering when one considers total national incidence rates of TBI. Using one of the more conservative estimates of TBI incidence (500 thousand new cases each year), costs of supported employment programs alone would be over $3 billion. This figure does not include costs of acute care, rehabilitation, or outpatient follow-up. Problems regarding community reintegration for TBI patients are far from being solved.

SUMMARY AND FUTURE DIRECTIONS

TBI is a common event with profound consequences. Technological advances and knowledge have resulted in a greatly increased proportion of survivors. Survival, however, has its costs to both TBI patients and their families. The allied health fields that comprise the interdisciplinary treatment team must extend their responsibility into the postacute phase of rehabilitation: Survival is not sufficient. Increased efforts toward providing an acceptable quality of life for TBI survivors and their families now requires a unified team of health-care providers, citizen advocates, and government agencies.

Despite recent growth in knowledge about TBI, there remains much that we must learn using rigorous basic, applied, and programmatic research. Certainly, this will post tough methodological challenges. Careful design and statistical control of numerous interacting variables will help determine ways to maximize treatment efficacy with optimal economic efficiency. Large, carefully designed correlational studies will assist in identifying variables that account for significant variance in the rehabilitation equation. Once identified, researchers can experimentally manipulate these sources of variance in efforts to compare and evaluate different treatment methods. Health-care providers need to apply single-case experimental design methodology in the treatment of individual TBI patients while results of larger correlational studies are pending. Finally, TBI researchers need to apply longitudinal design technology more often than in the past and work to increase funding for these very expensive projects. We hope that, in the next 10 years, rehabilitation of TBI patients will operate from a more sophisticated empirical base than is currently available. TBI survivors, their families, and society as a whole will be the beneficiaries.

REFERENCES

Adams, R. D., & Victor, M. (1989). *Principles of neurology* (4th ed.). New York: McGraw-Hill.
Alexander, M. P. (1982). Traumatic brain injury. In D. F. Benson & D. Blumer (Eds.), *Psychiatric aspects of neurologic disease* (Vol. 2, pp. 219–249). New York: Grune & Stratton.
Americans with Disabilities Act. (1990). P.L. 101–336, 104 Stat. 327 (July 26, 1990).
Bakay, R.A.E., Sweeney, K. M., & Wood, J. H. (1986). Pathophysiology of cerebrospinal fluid in head injury. Part 1. *Neurosurgery, 18,* 234–243.
Barry, P., & O'Leary, J. (1989). Roles of the psychologist on a traumatic brain injury rehabilitation team. *Rehabilitation Psychology, 34*(2), 83–92.
Bellack, A. S., & Hersen, M. (Eds.). (1988). *Behavioral assessment: A practical handbook* (3rd ed.). New York: Pergamon.
Benton, A. L. (1968). Differential behavioral effects in frontal lobe disease. *Neuropsychologia, 6,* 53–60.
Berg, R., Franzen, M., & Wedding, D. (1987). *Screening for brain impairment: A manual for mental health practice.* New York: Springer.
Bigler, E. D. (1987). Assessment of cortical functions. In L. C. Hartlage, M. J. Asken, & J. L. Hornsby (Eds.), *Essentials of neuropsychological assessment.* (pp. 46–70). New York: Springer.
Bigler, E. D., Yeo, R. A., & Turkheimer, E. (Eds.). (1989). *Neuropsychological function and brain imaging.* New York: Plenum Press.

Blackerby, W. F. (1990). A treatment model for sexuality disturbance following brain injury. *The Journal of Head Trauma Rehabilitation, 5*(2), 73–82.

Blumer, D., & Benson, D. G. (1975). Personality changes with frontal and temporal lobe lesions. In D. F. Benson & D. Blumer (Eds.), *Psychiatric aspects of neurologic disease* (pp. 151–170). New York: Grune & Stratton.

Boake, C. (1989). A history of cognitive rehabilitation of head-injured patients, 1915–1980. *The Journal of Head Trauma Rehabilitation, 4*(3), 1–8.

Boake, C. (1991). Social skills training following head injury. In J. S. Kreutzer & P. H. Wehman (Eds.), *Cognitive rehabilitation for persons with traumatic brain injury: A functional approach* (pp. 181–189). Baltimore, MD: Brookes.

Bond, M. R. (1979). The stages of recovery from severe head injury with special reference to late outcome. *International Rehabilitation Medicine, 1,* 155–159.

Bond, M. R. (1983). Standardized methods of assessing and predicting outcome. In M. Rosenthal, E. Griffith, M. Bond, & J. Miller (Eds.), *Rehabilitation of the head injured adult* (pp. 97–113). Philadelphia: Davis.

Bontke, C. F. (1989). Medical complications related to traumatic brain injury. *Physical Medicine and Rehabilitation: State of the Art Reviews, 3*(1), 43–59.

Brandstater, M. E., Bontke, C. F., Cobble, N. D., & Horn, L. J. (1991). Rehabilitation in brain disorders: 4. Specific Disorders. *Archives of Physical Medicine and Rehabilitation, 72,* S332–S340.

Brotherton, F. A., Thomas, L. L., Wisotzek, I. E., & Milan, M. A. (1988). Social skills training in rehabilitation of patients with traumatic closed head injury. *Archives of Physical Medicine and Rehabilitation, 69,* 827–832.

Cicerone, K. D., Lazar, R. M., & Shapiro, W. R. (1983). Effects of frontal lobe lesions on hypothesis sampling during concept formation. *Neuropsychologia, 21,* 513–524.

Cobble, N. D., Bontke, C. F., Brandstater, M. E., & Horn, L. J. (1991). Rehabilitation in brain disorders: 3. Intervention strategies. *Archives of Physical Medicine and Rehabilitation, 72,* S324–S331.

Collicott, P. E. (1991). Initial assessment of the trauma patient. In E. E. Moore, K. L. Mattox, & D. V. Feliciano (Eds.), *Trauma* (2nd ed., pp. 109–125). Norwalk, CT: Appleton & Lange.

Corkin, S. (1965). Tactually-guided maze learning in man: Effects of unilateral cortical excisions and bilateral hippocampal lesions. *Neuropsychologia, 3,* 339–351.

Costanzo, R. M., & Zasler, N. D. (1992). Epidemiology and pathophysiology of olfactory and gustatory dysfunction in head trauma. *Journal of Head Trauma Rehabilitation, 7*(1), 15–24.

Craine, J. F. (1982). The retraining of frontal lobe dysfunction. In L. E. Trexler (Ed.), *Cognitive rehabilitation: Conceptualization and intervention* (pp. 239–262). New York: Plenum Press.

Damasio, A. R. (1985). The frontal lobes. In K. M. Heilman & E. Valenstein (Eds.), *Clinical neuropsychology* (2nd ed., pp. 339–375). New York: Oxford University Press.

DeRenzi, E., & Vignolo, L. (1962). The Token Test: A sensitive test to detect receptive disturbances in aphasics. *Brain, 85,* 665–678.

Drewe, E. A. (1974). The effect of type and area of brain lesion on Wisconsin Card Sorting Test performance. *Cortex, 10,* 159–170.

Epstein, N. B., Baldwin, L. M., & Bishop, D. S. (1983). McMaster family assessment device. *Journal of Marital and Family Therapy, 8,* 171–180.

Finger, S. (Ed.). (1978). *Recovery from brain damage: Research and theory.* New York: Plenum Press.

Foxx, R. M., & Bittle, R. (1989). *Thinking it through: Teaching a problem-solving strategy for community living.* Champaign, IL: Research Press.

Foxx, R. M., Martella, R. C., & Marchand-Martella, N. E. (1989). The acquisition, maintenance, and generalization of problem-solving skills by closed head-injured adults. *Behavior Therapy, 20,* 61–76.

Franzen, M. D. (1991). Behavioral assessment and treatment of brain-impaired individuals. In M. Hersen, R. M. Eisler, & P. M. Miller (Eds.), *Progress in behavior modification* (Vol. 27, pp. 56–85). London: Sage.

Franzen, M. D., & Iverson, G. L. (1990). Applications of single subject design to cognitive rehabilitation. In A. M. Horton, Jr. (Ed.), *Neuropsychology across the life-span: Assessment and treatment* (pp. 155–174). New York: Springer.

Freedman, M., & Oscar-Berman, M. (1986). Bilateral frontal lobe disease and selective delayed response deficits in humans. *Behavioral Neuroscience, 100,* 337–342.

Fuster, J. M. (1989). *The prefrontal cortex: Anatomy, physiology and neuropsychology of the frontal lobe* (2nd ed.). New York: Raven.

Gilchrist, E., & Wilkinson, M. (1979). Some factors determining prognosis in young people with severe head injuries. *Archives of Neurology, 36,* 355–359.

Glenn, M. B., & Wroblewski, B. (1989). The choice of antidepressants in depressed survivors of traumatic brain injury. *Journal of Head Trauma Rehabilitation, 4*(3), 85–88.

Goldstein, J. (1991). Posttraumatic headache and the postconcussion syndrome. *Medical Clinics of North America, 75*(3), 641–651.

Gouvier, W. D., Webster, J. S., & Blanton, P. D. (1986). Cognitive retraining with brain-damaged patients. In D. Wedding, A. M. Horton, Jr., & J. Webster (Eds.), *The neuropsychology handbook: Behavioral and clinical perspectives.* (pp. 278–324). New York: Springer.

Grafman, J., Vance, S. C., Weingartner, H., Salazar, A. M., & Amin, D. (1986). The effects of lateralized frontal lesions on mood regulation. *Brain, 109,* 1127–1148.

Grubb, R. L., & Coxe, W. S. (1978). Central nervous system trauma; Cranial. In S. G. Eliasson, A. L. Prensky, & W. B. Hardin, Jr. (Eds.), *Neurological pathophysiology* (2nd ed., pp. 329–347). New York: Oxford University Press.

Guitton, D., Buchtel, H. A., & Douglas, R. M. (1982). Disturbances of voluntary saccadic eye-movement mechanisms following discrete unilateral frontal-lobe removals. In G. Lennerstrand, D. S. Lee, & E. L. Keller (Eds.), *Functional basis of ocular motility disorders* (pp. 497–499). Oxford: Pergamon.

Gurdjian, E. S. (1975). Recent developments in biomechanics, management, and mitigation of head injuries. In D. B. Tower (Ed.), *The nervous system. Vol. 2: The clinical neurosciences* (pp. 407–420). New York: Raven Press.

Halstead, W. C. (1947). *Brain and intelligence.* Chicago: University of Chicago Press.

Hartlage, L. C. (1989). *Behavior Change Inventory.* Brandon, VT: Clinical Psychology Publishing.

Hayes, R. L., Lyeth, B. G., & Jenkins, L. W. (1989). Neurochemical mechanisms of mild and moderate head injury: Implications for treatment. In H. S. Levin, H. M. Eisenberg, & A. L. Benton (Eds.), *Mild head injury* (pp. 54–79). New York: Oxford University Press.

Heaton, R. K. (1981). *Wisconsin Card Sorting Test Manual.* Odessa, FL: Psychological Assessment Resources.

Hecaen, H. (1962). Clinical symptomology in right and left hemisphere lesions. In V. B. Mountcastle (Ed.), *Interhemispheric relations and cerebral dominance* (pp. 215–243). Baltimore, MD: Johns Hopkins University Press.

Hecaen, H. (1964). Mental symptoms associated with tumors of the frontal lobe. In J. M. Warren & K. Akert (Eds.), *The frontal granular cortex and behavior* (pp. 335–352). New York: McGraw-Hill.

Hecaen, H., & Albert, M. L. (1978). *Human neuropsychology.* New York: Wiley.

Hendryx, P. M. (1989). Psychosocial changes perceived by closed-head-injured adults and their families. *Archives of Physical Medicine and Rehabilitation, 70,* 526–530.

Horton, A. M., & Miller, W. G. (1985). Neuropsychology and behavior therapy. In M. Hersen, R. M. Eisler, & P. M. Miller (Eds.), *Progress in behavior modification* (Vol. 19, pp. 1–55). Orlando, FL: Academic Press.

Ince, L. P. (1976). *Behavior modification in rehabilitation medicine.* Springfield, IL: Thomas.

Jackson, W. T., & Gouvier, W. D. (1992). Group psychotherapy with brain-damaged patients and their families. In C. J. Long & L. K. Ross (Eds.), *Handbook of head trauma: Acute care to recovery* (pp. 309–327). New York: Plenum Press.

Jones-Gotman, M., & Milner, B. (1977). Design fluency: The invention of nonsense drawings after focal cortical lesions. *Neuropsychologia, 15,* 653–674.

Kolb, B., & Milner, B. (1981). Performance of complex arm and facial movements after focal brain lesions. *Neuropsychologia, 19,* 505–514.

Kolb, B., & Whishaw, I. Q. (1990). *Fundamentals of human neuropsychology* (3rd ed.). New York: Freeman.

Kreutzer, J. S., Zasler, N. D., Camplair, P. S., & Leininger, B. E. (1990). A practical guide to family intervention following adult traumatic brain injury. In J. S. Kreutzer & P. Wehman (Eds.), *Community integration following traumatic brain injury* (pp. 249–273). Baltimore, MD: Brookes.

Kuypers, H.G.J.M. (1981). Anatomy of the descending pathways. In V. B. Brooks (Ed.), *Handbook of physiology: Vol. 2. The nervous system.* Baltimore, MD: Williams & Wilkins.

Lam, C. S., McMahon, B. T., Priddy, D. A., & Gehred-Schultz, M. A. (1988). Deficit awareness and treatment performance among traumatic head injury adults. *Brain Injury, 2,* 235–242.

Lawson-Kerr, K., Smith, S., & Beck, D. (1990). The interface between neuropsychology and behavior therapy. In A. M. Horton, Jr. (Ed.), *Neuropsychology across the life-span: Assessment and treatment* (pp. 103–131). New York: Springer.

Leonard, G., Jones, L., & Milner, B. (1988). Residual impairment in handgrip strength after unilateral frontal-lobe lesions. *Neuropsychologia, 26,* 555–564.

LeVere, T. E., Davis, N., & Gonder, L. (1979). Recovery of function after brain damage: Toward understanding the deficit. *Physiological Psychology, 7,* 317–326.

Levin, H. S., Benton, A. L., & Grossman, R. G. (1982). *Neurobehavioral consequences of closed head injury.* New York: Oxford University Press.

Levin, H. S., High, W. M., & Eisenberg, H. M. (1985). Impairment of olfactory recognition after closed head injury. *Brain, 108,* 579–591.

Levin, H. S., High, W. M., Goethe, K. E., Sisson, R. A., Overall, J. E., Rhoades, H. M., Eisenberg, H. M., Kalisky, Z., & Gary, H. E. (1987). The neurobehavioral rating scale: Assessment of behavioral sequelae of head injury by the clinician. *Journal of Neurology, Neurosurgery and Psychiatry, 50,* 183–193.

Lewis, F. D., Burke, W. H., & Carrillo, R. (1987). Model for rehabilitation of head injured adults in the post acute care setting. *Journal of Applied Rehabilitation Counseling, 18*(2), 39–45.

Lezak, M. D. (1978). Living with the characterologically altered brain injured patient. *Journal of Clinical Psychiatry, 39,* 592–598.

Lezak, M. D. (1983). *Neuropsychological assessment* (2nd ed.). New York: Oxford University Press.

Lezak, M. D. (1986). Psychological implications of traumatic brain damage for the patient's family. *Rehabilitation Psychology, 31*(4), 241–250.

Lezak, M. D. (1988). Brain damage is a family affair. *Journal of Clinical and Experimental Neuropsychology, 10*(1), 111–123.

Lezak, M. D. (1993). Newer contributions to the neuropsychological assessment of executive functions. *Journal of Head Trauma Rehabilitation, 8*(1), 24–31.

Long, C. J. (1991). A model of recovery to maximize the rehabilitation of individuals with head trauma. *Journal of Head Injury, 2*(3), 18–28.

Luria, A. R. (1966). *Higher cortical functions in man* (B. Haigh, Trans.). New York: Basic Books.

Luria, A. R. (1973). *The working brain: An introduction to neuropsychology* (B. Haigh, Trans.). New York: Basic Books.

Massagli, T. L. (1991). Neurobehavioral effects of phenytoin, carbamazepine, and valproic acid: Implications for use in traumatic brain injury. *Archives of Physical Medicine and Rehabilitation, 72,* 219–226.

Mattson, A. J., & Levin, H. S. (1990). Frontal lobe dysfunction following closed head injury: A review of the literature. *Journal of Nervous and Mental Disease, 178*(5), 282–291.

Mazzocchi, F., & Vignolo, L. A. (1979). Localization of lesions in aphasia: Clinical-CT scan correlations in stroke patients. *Cortex, 15,* 627–654.

McGlynn, S. (1990). Behavioral approaches to neuropsychological rehabilitation. *Psychological Bulletin, 108*(3), 420–441.

McNeil, M. R., & Prescott, T. E. (1978). *Revised Token Test Manual.* Austin, TX: PRO-ED.

Miller, E. (1984a). *Recovery and management of neuropsychological impairments.* New York: Wiley.

Miller, E. (1984b). Verbal influency as a function of a measure of verbal intelligence in relation to different types of cerebral pathology. *British Journal of Clinical Psychology, 23,* 53–57.

Miller, L. (1985). Cognitive risk taking after frontal or temporal lobectomy. I. The synthesis of fragmented visual information. *Neuropsychologia, 23,* 359–369.

Milner, B. (1964). Some effects of frontal lobectomy in man. In J. M. Warren & K. Akert (Eds.), *The frontal granular cortex and behavior* (pp. 313–334). New York: McGraw-Hill.

Milner, B. (1965). Visually guided maze learning in man: Effects of bilateral hippocampal, bilateral frontal, and unilateral cerebral lesions. *Neuropsychologia, 3,* 317–338.

Milner, B. (1974). Hemispheric specialization: Scope and limits. In F. O. Schmitt & F. G. Worden (Eds.), *The neurosciences: Third study program* (pp. 75–89). Cambridge, MA: MIT Press.

Milner, B., & Petrides, M. (1984). Behavioral effects of frontal-lobe lesions in man. *Trends in Neurosciences, 7,* 403–407.

Moos, R. H., & Moos, B. S. (1981). *Family Environmental Scale manual.* Palo Alto, CA: Consulting Psychologists Press.

Nelson, H. E. (1976). A modified card sorting test sensitive to frontal lobe deficits. *Cortex, 12,* 312–324.

Newcombe, F. (1969). *Missile wounds of the brain.* London: Oxford University Press.

Novack, T. A., Bergquist, T. F., Bennett, G., & Gouvier, W. D. (1991). Primary caregiver distress following severe head injury. *Journal of Head Trauma Rehabilitation, 6*(4), 69–77.

Ommaya, A., & Gennarelli, T. (1974). Cerebral concussion and traumatic unconsciousness: Correlation of experimental and clinical observations on blunt head injuries. *Brain, 97,* 633–654.

Oppenheimer, D. R. (1968). Microscopic lesions in the brain following head injury. *Journal of Neurology, Neurosurgery, and Psychiatry, 31,* 299–306.

Osterholm, J. L., Bell, J., Meyer, R., & Pyenson, J. (1969). Experimental effects of free serotonin on the brain and its relation to brain injury. *Journal of Neurosurgery, 31,* 408–421.

Perret, E. (1974). The left frontal lobe of man and the suppression of habitual responses in verbal categorical behavior. *Neuropsychologia, 12,* 323–330.

Petrides, M., & Milner, B. (1982). Deficits on subject ordered tasks after frontal- and temporal-lobe lesions in man. *Neuropsychologia, 20,* 249–262.

Potter, H., & Butters, N. (1980). An assessment of olfactory deficits in patients with damage to prefrontal cortex. *Neuropsychologia, 18,* 621–628.

Rappaport, M., Hall, K. M., Hopkins, K., Belleza, T., Cope, D. N. (1982). Disability Rating Scale for severe head trauma: Coma to community. *Archives of Physical Medicine and Rehabilitation, 63,* 118–123.

Raven, J. C. (1962). *Coloured Progressive Matrices.* London: E. T. Heron.

Reitan, R. M. (1969). *Manual for administration of neuropsychological test batteries for adults and children.* Unpublished manuscript, Indianapolis University Medical Center.

Reitan, R. M. (1984). *Aphasia and sensory-perceptual deficits in adults.* Tucson, AZ: Reitan Neuropsychological Laboratories.

Reitan, R. M., & Davison, L. A. (1974). *Clinical neuropsychology: Current status and applications.* Washington, DC: V. H. Winston.

Roland, P. E., Larsen, B., Lassen, N. A., & Skinhoj, E. (1980). Supplementary motor area and other cortical areas in organization of voluntary movements in man. *Journal of Neurophysiology, 43,* 118–136.

Rosenthal, M., & Geckler, C. (1986). Family therapy issues in neuropsychology. In D. Wedding, A. M. Horton, Jr., & J. Webster (Eds.), *The neuropsychology handbook: Behavioral and clinical perspectives* (pp. 325–344). New York: Springer.

Rose, M. (1988). The place of drugs in the management of behavior disorders after traumatic brain injury. *Journal of Head Trauma Rehabilitation, 3*(3), 7–13.

Ruff, R. M., Cullum, C. M., & Luerssen, T. G. (1989). Brain imaging and neuropsychological outcome in traumatic brain injury. In E. D. Bigler, R. A. Yeo, & E. Turkheimer (Eds.), *Neuropsychological function and brain imaging* (pp. 161–183). New York: Plenum Press.

Russell, E. W. (1979). Three patterns of brain damage on the WAIS. *Journal of Clinical Psychology, 35,* 611–620.

Russell, W. R. (1932). Cerebral involvement in head injury: A study based on the examination of 200 cases. *Brain, 55,* 549–603.

Russell, W. R. (1971). *The traumatic amnesias.* New York: Oxford University Press.

Sawicki, R. (1990, March). Recovery curves from head injury. In J. Samuels (Chair), *Planning issues in head injury recovery.* Symposium conducted at Our Lady of the Lake Regional Medical Center, Baton Rouge, LA.

Saykin, A. J., Gur, R. C., Gur, R. E., Mozley, P. D., Mozley, L. H., Resnick, S. M., Kester, B., & Stafiniak, P. (1991). Neuropsychological function in schizophrenia: Selective impairment in memory and learning. *Archives of General Psychiatry, 48,* 618–624.

Seron, X. (1987). Operant procedures and neuropsychological rehabilitation. In M. J. Meier, A. L. Benton, & L. Diller (Eds.), *Neuropsychological rehabilitation* (pp. 132–161). New York: Guilford Press.

Shallice, T., & Burgess, P. W. (1991). Deficits in strategy application following frontal lobe damage in man. *Brain, 114,* 727–741.

Shallice, T., & Evans, M. E. (1978). The involvement of the frontal lobes in cognitive estimation. *Cortex, 4,* 294–303.

Smith, M. L., & Milner, B. (1984). Differential effects of frontal-lobe lesions on cognitive estimation and spatial memory. *Neuropsychologia, 22,* 697–705.

Sohlberg, M. M., Mateer, C. A., & Stuss, D. T. (1993). Contemporary approaches to the management of executive control dysfunction. *The Journal of Head Trauma Rehabilitation, 8*(1), 45–58.

Sorenson, S. B., & Kraus, J. F. (1991). Occurrence, severity, and outcome of brain injury. *Journal of Head Trauma Rehabilitation, 6*(2), 1–10.

Spreen, O., & Strauss, E. (1991). *A compendium of neuropsychological tests: Administration, norms, and commentary.* New York: Oxford University Press.

Stroop, J. R. (1935). Studies of interference in serial verbal reactions. *Journal of Experimental Psychology, 18,* 643–662.

Strub, R. L., & Black, F. W. (1985). *The mental status examination in neurology* (2nd ed.). Philadelphia: Davis.

Stuss, D. T., & Benson, D. F. (1986). *The frontal lobes.* New York: Raven.

Stuss, D. T., Kaplan, E. F., Benson, D. F., Weir, W. S., Chiulli, S., & Sarazin, F. F. (1982). Evidence for the involvement of orbitofrontal cortex in memory functions: An interference effect. *Journal of Comparative and Physiological Psychology, 96,* 913–925.

Teasdale, G., & Jennett, B. (1974). Assessment of coma and impaired consciousness: A practical scale. *Lancet, 2,* 81–84.

Teuber, H.-L. (1964). The riddle of frontal lobe function in man. In J. M. Warren & K. Akert (Eds.), *The frontal granular cortex and behavior* (pp. 410–444). New York: McGraw-Hill.

Thurstone, L. L. (1938). *Primary mental abilities.* Chicago: University of Chicago Press.

Trenerry, M. R., Crosson, B., DeBoe, J., & Leber, W. R. (1989). *Stroop Neuropsychological Screening Test manual.* Odessa, FL: Psychological Assessment Resources.

Walker, E. A., & Blumer, D. (1975). The localization of sex in the brain. In K. J. Zulch, O. Creutzfeldt, & G. C. Galbraith (Eds.), *Cerebral localization* (pp. 184–199). New York: Springer-Verlag.

Walsh, K. W. (1978). *Neuropsychology: A clinical approach.* New York: Churchill Livingstone.

Webster, J. S., & Scott, R. R. (1988). Behavioral assessment and treatment of the brain-injured patient. In M. Hersen, R. M. Eisler, & P. M. Miller (Eds.), *Progress in behavior modification* (Vol. 22, pp. 48–87). Orlando, FL: Academic Press.

Wechsler, D. (1981). *Wechsler Adult Intelligence Scale-Revised manual.* Cleveland, OH: The Psychological Corporation.

West, M., Wehman, P., Kregel, J., Kreutzer, J., Sherron, P., & Zasler, N. (1991). Costs of operating a supported work program for traumatically brain-injured individuals. *Archives of Physical Medicine and Rehabilitation, 72,* 127–131.

Willer, B. S., Allen, K. M., Liss, M., & Zicht, M. S. (1991). Problems and coping strategies of individuals with traumatic brain injury and their spouses. *Archives of Physical Medicine and Rehabilitation, 72,* 460–464.

Williams, J. M. (1987). *Cognitive Behavior Rating Scale manual: Research edition.* Odessa, FL: Psychological Assessment Resources.

Williams, J. M., & Kay, T. (Eds.). (1991). *Head injury: A family matter.* Baltimore, MD: Brookes.

Ylvisaker, M., & Szekeres, S. F. (1989). Metacognitive and executive impairments in head-injured children and adults. *Topics in Language Disorders, 9*(2), 34–49.

Zangwill, O. L. (1960). *Cerebral dominance and its relation to psychological function.* Springfield, IL: Thomas.

22

Cancer Rehabilitation
Concepts and Interventions

James C. Gilchrist and Blaine L. Block

INTRODUCTION

The number of individuals who receive cancer diagnoses continues to increase each year. In 1986, there were approximately 930 thousand new cases of cancer (Kurtzman, Gardner, & Kellner, 1988). The estimated number of new cancer patients in 1995 is expected to be about 1,252,000 (Wingo, Tona, & Bolden, 1995). Although research data continue to show a trend of a steadily increasing number of individuals diagnosed with cancer, there has also been an increase in the number of individuals expected to survive 5 years or more. The increase in the number of cancer survivors is a result of early diagnosis and ongoing improvements in available treatment modalities (Loescher, Welch-McCaffrey, Leigh, Hoffman, & Meyskens, 1989). At this time, approximately 50% of patients diagnosed with cancer will survive at least 5 years. In contrast, in 1960, about one patient in three survived 5 years or more (Wingo et al., 1995; Ganz, 1990).

It is apparent that cancer constitutes a problem of significant magnitude. The American Cancer Society (1983) reports that cancer will affect one out of four Americans and three out of every four families. As cancer research and improvements in treatment modalities continue, there will be an ever increasing number of cancer survivors. Presently there are about 6 million cancer survivors in the United States; 3 million of these individuals have lived 5 years past the termination of treatment (Ganz, 1990). As a result, issues and concerns that relate to survivors will likely become an area of increasing focus and attention. Although the survival and

---

James C. Gilchrist • St. Elizabeth Rehabilitation Center, St. Elizabeth Medical Center, Dayton, Ohio 45408.   **Blaine L. Block** • St. Elizabeth Regional Cancer Center, Dayton, Ohio 45408.
Handbook of Health and Rehabilitation Psychology, edited by Anthony J. Goreczny. Plenum Press, New York, 1995.

life expectancy of cancer patients is steadily increasing, many of these individuals experience a variety of ongoing problems, such as physical limitations, psychological issues, and vocational concerns (Delisa, Miller, Melnick, Mikulic, & Gerber, 1985; Kurtzman et al., 1988; Lehmann et al., 1978). Quality-of-life issues have increasingly become an area of interest as a result of increasing life expectancy. Currently, many health-care providers recognize cancer as a chronic illness. Contributors to such recognition include the increase in the number of cancer survivors and documentation and research by cancer specialists regarding the extent of problems patients encounter as a result of the illness and its treatment. Rehabilitation of the cancer patient is now an important component of providing comprehensive care, because the number of individuals expected to survive cancer will continue to increase.

THE CONCEPT OF CANCER REHABILITATION

The origin of utilizing a rehabilitation approach to the treatment of cancer patients began with the National Cancer Act of 1971. This Act included cancer rehabilitation as one objective and directed funds toward the development of training, demonstration, and research projects. In 1972, the National Cancer Institute sponsored the National Cancer Rehabilitation Planning Conference. This conference identified four objectives related to the rehabilitation of cancer patients: (1) psychological support, (2) optimal physical functioning, (3) vocational counseling, and (4) optimal social functioning (Dudas & Carlson, 1988). With the increasing number of living cancer patients, these objectives are even more timely today.

A number of investigators have proposed definitions of cancer rehabilitation and delineated some related principles. Cromes (1978) defined *cancer rehabilitation* as assisting the person with cancer to obtain maximum physical, social, psychological, and vocational functioning within the limits created by the disease and resulting treatment. Baldonado and Stahl (1982) described *cancer rehabilitation* as the prevention, maintenance, restoration, and reeducation process that occurs over the course of the patient's disease. Mayer and O'Connor (1989) suggested that rehabilitation is a process assisting patients to achieve optimal functioning in their environments. In general, these definitions of rehabilitation contain the same basic components found in rehabilitation definitions used with other patient populations. Nonetheless, health-care professionals use and recognize rehabilitation principles less often with cancer than with other disorders, such as stroke, traumatic brain injury, spinal cord injury, neurological disorders, and heart disease (DeLisa, Martin, & Currie, 1988). However, due to beliefs, attitudes, and myths that surround cancer and its treatment, the language used to describe cancer rehabilitation has received considerable attention and resulted in refinements of the definition (Ganz, 1990; Watson, 1986, 1990). Dietz (1981), a pioneer in cancer rehabilitation, used the synonym *readaptation* instead of the term *rehabilitation,* emphasizing accommodation or adaptation to meet the ongoing needs of patients in the areas of psychological, physical, and vocational functioning. Dudas (1984) defined *cancer rehabilitation* as a dynamic, goal-directed process that enables patients to function at maximum levels in all aspects of their lives. The use of the word *dynamic* reflects a significant and fundamental difference in the concept of *rehabilitation* when applied to cancer as opposed to most other commonly recognized rehabilitation populations; namely, the nature and course of cancer is often a constantly changing experience for patients and results in fluctuating needs and challenges patients must face regarding daily functioning.

Rehabilitation efforts applied to stroke, spinal cord and brain injury patients typically begins after a discrete incident or accident results in medical problems and disabilities. Following the acute phase of medical treatment and stabilization, the health-care team initiates rehabilitation efforts and, barring additional medical complications, the patient enters the recovery phase. When applying the concept of rehabilitation to cancer patients the course can be substantially more complex due to the various forms of cancer, variety of treatments and their effects, and issues of recurrence and terminal illness. There is often no clear demarcation of the initiation of a recovery phase as found with other rehabilitation populations. Cancer rehabilitation specialists need to conduct the rehabilitation of their patients within the framework of regarding cancer as a long-term chronic illness, similar to the rehabilitation philosophy used with multiple sclerosis patients and others who may experience an unpredictable and variable medical course.

Dietz (1981) identified the following four phases or categories of cancer rehabilitation that address the scope and course of the illness and the variety of needs that can exist at different times: preventive, restorative, supportive, and palliative. Preventive interventions lessen the impact of expected disabilities through education and teaching. Preventive measures also include approaches to improve physical functioning and general health status prior to treatment. In addition, pretreatment psychological consultation can assist with early identification of adjustment issues and allow for prompt intervention. Restorative interventions are procedures that attempt to return the patient to previous levels of physical, psychological, social, and vocational functioning, such as range-of-motion exercises postoperatively for mastectomy patients and reconstructive surgery for head and neck cancer patients. Supportive rehabilitation efforts aim to teach patients to adapt to permanent disabilities and minimize changes from ongoing disease. Such efforts, include teaching the use of prosthetic devices after amputation and other devices and procedures that assist patients in preserving self-management, self-care abilities, and independent functioning. Other supportive efforts include the provision of emotional support regarding adjustment issues while learning to cope with physical and lifestyle changes. During the palliative phase, when there may be increasing disability and an advanced disease process, interventions and goals relate to minimizing or eliminating complications and providing comfort and support. Examples of palliative goals include pain control, prevention of contractures and bed sores, reduction of unnecessary deterioration due to inactivity, and psychological support for the patient and family.

Wells (1990) also addressed the issues associated with providing rehabilitation services for the entire range of cancer patients by classifying them into three major groups. The first group consists of individuals who have good life expectancy and no lasting disabilities or disfigurement. The primary needs for this group are counseling and education to help them change potentially detrimental lifestyle behaviors. Counseling also focuses on the transition from their identification primarily as a cancer patients in the sickness role, which they often adopt or others place on them to reidentification as a productive member of society. The second patient group also includes individuals who have good life expectancy, but have experienced significant psychological and/or physical changes as a result of treatment. These patients may require extensive physical and psychological therapies to assist in resumption of previous activities and lifestyle. The third group consists of those cancer patients who have experienced unsuccessful treatment attempts or have relapsed and, as a result, have a shortened life expectancy. Wells advocates that these patients also require rehabilitation services in order to allow them an optimum quality of life regardless of their remaining life span.

The rehabilitation needs of cancer patients have become prominent because of the increased attention given to the experience of being a "cancer survivor." Mullan (1985, 1990) supports the use of the term *survivor* over previously used terms, such as *cancer victim*. Cancer survivorship has become an experience shared by an increasing number of people and has resulted in a strong movement to address survivors needs. The National Coalition for Cancer Survivorship published a resource manual that covers a variety of topics from support services and communication with medical professionals to financial matters (Mullan & Hoffman, 1990). Their objective in this manual is to educate and instruct cancer survivors in managing the diverse challenges that confront them and their families.

Mullan (1990) outlined three stages of cancer survival: acute, extended, and permanent survival. Acute survival, the initial phase, typically involves diagnostic and treatment interventions aimed at arresting the disease process. Extended survival is the phase during which both the disease and treatment efforts may have produced a variety of physical and psychological complications, such as diminished strength and altered physical appearance. Although patients may have experienced some of these effects during the acute phase, these changes continue during the extended phase and interfere with patients' daily functioning as they resume previous activities at home and work. Emotional support regarding adjustment issues and ongoing therapies regarding physical functioning are crucial needs at this time. Permanent survival is the point at which the likelihood of recurrence is quite small and cancer specialists consider the disease under control or alleviated. During this phase, however, the patient may suffer from long-term effects of treatment or face major issues, such as attempting to obtain employment and insurance coverage.

It is apparent that a set program of therapies that health-care professionals initiate at a particular point in the course of treatment will not adequately address all potential concerns and needs of cancer patients and their families. Cancer rehabilitation is unique in that it potentially involves a vast number of patients with several different forms of cancer. Also, within a particular diagnostic group, patients have a wide range of rehabilitation needs based in part on the stage of cancer at diagnosis and the forms of treatment the patient has undergone. The different treatments may themselves result in a variety of secondary problems. The possibilities of recurrence and terminal illness present additional complicating factors. As a result, providing comprehensive rehabilitation services to cancer patients is vastly different from providing rehabilitation services to other patient populations. Rehabilitation needs for a particular cancer patient can vary greatly throughout all phases of the illness, from initial diagnosis and treatment through remission, possible recurrence, and a potentially terminal illness stage.

Lehmann and colleagues (1978) investigated the frequency of rehabilitation problems that cancer patients encounter. The investigators screened a sample of 805 cancer patients for psychological and physical medicine problems. Patients involved in the study represented a variety of different types of cancer, including leukemia, and head and neck, breast, respiratory, nervous system, bladder, and bone cancer.

Over 50% of the patients had physical medicine problems, a significant portion of whom experienced problems similar to those of other rehabilitation patients (e.g., individuals recovering from stroke and spinal cord injuries). A large percentage of the sample evidenced psychological problems. Psychological problems were more common among patients experiencing physical problems than those without physical involvement; whereas 52% of patients with physical involvement experienced psychological problems, about 29% of those without physical involvement evinced psychological difficulties. Also, patients with cancer of the nervous system had higher incidences of psychological problems than those with other cancer sites. The study concluded that physical medicine and psychological problems exist in a large number of cancer patients and that many of these patients could benefit from rehabilitation interventions because the nature of their problems are similar to those found in many other patient rehabilitation groups.

Fobair and colleagues (1986) surveyed over 400 cancer patients and found that about one third continued to experience problems for many years after diagnosis and treatment. Patients experienced decreased energy levels, problems at work, decreased sexual activity, and psychological symptoms. The mean number of years from time of diagnosis to survey time was 9 years. Wellisch (1987) reported that older cancer patients often experience more physical difficulties during the early phases of treatment and recovery. Early intervention with such patients could be beneficial in decreasing the time required to regain maximum energy levels, a factor that relates to psychological well-being (Fobair et al., 1986).

One group of investigators (Harvey, Jellinek, & Habeck, 1982) performed a survey of 36 cancer rehabilitation programs to investigate team member composition, organizational structure, and patient populations, among other factors. Results of the survey supported the use of an interdisciplinary-treatment team approach. The sample of referred patients included nearly equal numbers of individuals in groups classified as cure/control, possible control, and those with advanced or uncontrolled disease. This finding again illustrates the need for rehabilitation interventions at various points in the disease process. This study also found that many individuals accept the importance of cancer rehabilitation programs, particularly in community-hospital settings. Content of the surveyed programs included an emphasis on education, treatment protocols for specific cancer sites, and pain control.

COMMON BARRIERS TO CANCER REHABILITATION

Despite documentation substantiating the increasing number of cancer patients and the percentage of these patients with significant needs, there has not been universal acceptance of applying the rehabilitation approach to cancer patients. Investigators have identified several obstacles to the implementation of cancer rehabilitation programs.

One of the most difficult barriers to overcome is the negative perception of cancer by society at large and among health-care professionals (Brooks, 1979; Dent & Gouldton, 1982; Watson, 1986). Studies investigating the attitudes of medical professionals confirmed the existence of negative bias toward cancer, based partly on stereotypical views of the illness (Cooper, Bean, Alpert, & Baum, 1980). Ganz (1990) identified several myths commonly associated with cancer. One myth is that cancer is a contagious illness. Ganz reported that about 15 million Americans believe cancer is contagious, and an additional 20 million are unsure whether it is contagious. Second, many people view cancer survivors as incapable of resuming their previous lifestyles. Although some cancer patients do face long-term disabilities, most patients are not permanently affected by this type of physical and mental disability. The most common myth is that an individual with the diagnosis of cancer inevitably suffers from a terminal condition. As previously stated, current data suggest that quite the opposite is true (Wingo et al., 1995).

Haley, Huynh, Paiva, and Juan (1977) suggested that the attitudes of physicians can influence the quality of medical care. The pessimism that persists regarding cancer does influence frequency of referrals to rehabilitation specialists. Health-care practitioners often view cancer patients as poor rehabilitation candidates based on flawed perceptions of life expectancy and ability to participate in a therapy program (Lehmann et al., 1978; Clark, Moreton, Healey, & MacDonald, 1967). This negative view of cancer patients is ironic considering that 30% of coronary patients will not survive convalescence and approximately 50% of stroke patients will have died after one year, yet both these populations generally receive comprehensive rehabilitation services on a routine basis (Wells, 1990).

In addition to an overall pessimistic view toward cancer patients, those who are in the terminal phase of the disease process are even less likely to receive rehabilitation services, as are the elderly, whom some perceive as having reached the natural end of the life cycle (Wells, 1990). *Despite stage of disease or age of the patient, the issue of quality of life needs to be a prime consideration in providing comprehensive health care.* Although rehabilitation goals are typically less ambitious with the terminally ill or significantly debilitated patient than with other cancer patients, the maintenance of independent functioning and self-care is beneficial regarding effects of self-image and self-esteem. As stated earlier, palliative goals are valid objectives for rehabilitation. Such goals include providing comfort and emotional support and ameliorating complications (Dietz, 1981).

Still another obstacle to the timely use of rehabilitation services is the view of cancer as primarily an acute medical condition (Watson, 1986). Clearly, in the early phases of illness, diagnosis, and initial treatment interventions, the primary emphasis is on eliminating the disease process. However, clinicians who overemphasize the critical challenge of seeking curative objectives may inadvertently overlook the concurrent rehabilitation needs of patients. Once health-care professionals achieve the set curative goals, they may neglect the long-term consequences of the illness and treatment in light of the major victory they accomplished by preserving or prolonging a patient's life.

There are additional barriers to the expansion of rehabilitation efforts. Not all professionals have had the opportunity to train in settings in which there are rehabilitation departments offering services to cancer patients (Shedd & Aguilar-Markus, 1987). Also, there is a relative lack of research on the outcome of a coordinated rehabilitation approach toward treating specific types of cancer and associated problems (Mayer, 1991). Thus, health-care professionals must also deal with these issues.

OVERCOMING BARRIERS

The primary barriers that the health-care team must confront are negative and pessimistic attitudes toward cancer held by the public and by some health-care professionals. In order for the concept of cancer rehabilitation to attain the same degree of acceptance as rehabilitation with stroke, spinal cord injury, and other traditional rehabilitation populations, significant alterations in attitude are essential.

Watson (1986) contends that changing attitudes toward cancer is vital because attitudes often relate to one's behavior. For example, a negative attitude regarding a given topic may predispose an individual to have feelings of discomfort when confronted with that topic, whereas a positive attitude reflects a willingness to become involved (Watson, 1986). Behaviorally, a negative attitude may result in an avoidance of the topic. In essence, the consequences of negative attitudes toward cancer are often avoidance of the subject. From this perspective avoidant behavior may hamper rehabilitation efforts due to lack of awareness of patients' needs. A positive attitude indicates potential awareness of patients' needs and willingness to provide an increasing array of services as part of rehabilitation.

Watson (1986) proposed use of the rehabilitation philosophy as a method of changing attitudes toward cancer. The philosophy of rehabilitation is typically not a disease-focused treatment approach. Instead, it recognizes the limitations and impairments that result from an accident or illness and emphasizes interventions that enable patients to adapt to the imposed disabilities and resume optimal functioning. Within the framework of rehabilitation, the cancer patient is an individual with a cancer-related disability. Within this framework, the health-care team views cancer patients in the same manner as they view other patients facing limitations and thus as candidates to receive treatment aimed at circumventing those limitations. The rehabilitation philosophy confronts medical conditions and resultant limitations in a manner that engenders hope and suggests that obstacles are not necessarily insurmountable. Health-care providers who adopt the rehabilitation philosophy toward cancer patients are in a position to see opportunities for intervention versus barriers regarding the limitations resulting from the illness and its treatment.

Health-care professionals from a number of disciplines are likely to interact with cancer patients at some time during their careers. Professional training and education needs to directly address the many misconceptions regarding cancer in order to assist in changing the attitudes of health-care providers. Lebovits, Croen, and Goetzel (1984) found that participation in a clinical oncology program produced significant changes in medical students' attitudes toward cancer patients relative to students who did not enroll in the course. In general, the students were somewhat less pessimistic toward the illness. Interestingly, the course objectives were similar to the philosophy inherent in cancer rehabilitation: (1) recognition of cancer as a chronic disease, often managed on an outpatient basis; (2) identification of the roles of multiple disciplines in the treatment of cancer patients; and (3) an appreciation of the psychological and social aspects of treating cancer patients. The findings of this study are similar to those of previous studies on the importance of course work as a means to improve medical students' attitudes toward cancer (Blanchard et al., 1981; Cassileth & Egan, 1979). Greater exposure to rehabilitation programs that actively include cancer patients would illustrate that such patients are similar to other rehabilitation populations. Studies suggest that direct contact with cancer patients, particularly early in the medical education experience, can have a positive impact on changing stereotypical negative attitudes toward cancer and cancer patients (Cohen, Ruckdeschel, Blanchard, Rohrbaugh, & Horton, 1982; Haley et al., 1977). Including cancer rehabilitation as an integral component in the curricula of those specific disciplines that are likely to have contact with cancer patients would greatly assist in changing current attitudes and biases toward cancer. Practicum experiences with direct clinical contact would offer the best opportunity to alter negative attitudes. Continuing education courses regarding cancer rehabilitation could benefit those professionals currently working in health care.

Unfortunately, changing societal views toward cancer is a much more formidable task than altering the perspectives of health-care providers. Historically, views of dreaded illnesses change only after medical discoveries result in dramatic advances in diagnosis, treatment effectiveness, and prevention measures, such as immunizations. For example, attitudes toward tuberculosis and polio are quite different today than at the beginning of the century. However, at this time, the number of individuals diagnosed with cancer continues to increase each year, and this is not likely to allay concerns regarding the illness.

Changing public attitudes toward cancer, in light of the increasing numbers of newly diagnosed patients, will most likely rely on education regarding the survivability of the illness because the ideals of discovering the ultimate cure and/or complete prevention do not seem attainable within the foreseeable future. The efforts of the National Coalition for Cancer Survivors, in publishing a resource guide for cancer survivors (Mullan & Hoffman, 1990), is an excellent example of enlightening cancer patients and the public to the fact that cancer is no longer a death sentence. Continuing public education regarding the benefits of early diagnosis of cancer in addition to data regarding increasing survivability of the illness and services available to survivors will likely result in a gradual change in the general public's attitude about cancer.

Providing adequate reimbursement for treatment interventions related to cancer disabilities would assist in acknowledging that cancer treatment consists of more than initial diagnosis and treatment directed toward cure and remission. Support for cancer rehabilitation research is also essential in establishing cancer rehabilitation as a generally accepted component of comprehensive cancer treatment.

PRINCIPLES OF CANCER REHABILITATION

Rehabilitation specialists have proposed several general principles regarding rehabilitation interventions that are applicable to cancer patients (DeLisa et al., 1988; Dietz, 1981). Some important principles in the application of cancer rehabilitation follow.

Treatment requires an interdisciplinary-team approach. Due to the variety of potential problems that a cancer patient may face throughout the course of the illness, the availability of professionals from a broad range of disciplines is essential in order to offer comprehensive care. The needs of the patient will determine the number of team members involved on a particular case. Therefore, not all team members will necessarily work with each patient identified as a rehabilitation candidate.

The health-care team needs to develop rehabilitation goals within the limitations imposed by the illness, the patient's environment, and available social support. Goals must be objective, realistic, and attainable within a reasonable time frame. Setting unrealistic or unattainable goals can result in a disservice to the patient and family by providing false hope and expectations. Structuring goals such that they are attainable within a reasonable time frame often serves to motivate patients to maintain effort because patients are then able to appreciate therapy gains they obtain from active participation. This approach often requires breaking down a single goal into smaller components, each of which is in itself, a goal. For example, the clinician can conceptualize the goal of ambulation as a number of specific goals, such as balance and standing for increased lengths of time. Goals that appear unreachable and too difficult can overwhelm the patient. "Component goal setting" assists in altering patients' perceptions of the probability of attaining a goal. Setting short-term (1-week) and long-term (several weeks or months) goals is another common rehabilitation approach to goal setting. The health-care team needs to involve the patient in periodically assessing and amending goals, because a patient's status and limitations can change significantly.

The patient, family members, and significant others need to be active participants in the rehabilitation process. Patient and family involvement assists in goal setting. Treatment is the collaborative effort of professional members of the team with the patient and his or her support network. Active involvement assists in providing patients with some sense of control at a time when so much may appear beyond their control.

Most advocates of cancer rehabilitation agree that referral and intervention needs to occur at the time of diagnosis and continue throughout the course of the illness. Although need for specific patient interventions at the time of diagnosis may not be significant, contact with the rehabilitation team can serve the general purpose of educating the patient and family about services available if needs arise in the future. Also, pretreatment education and interventions can be of tremendous assistance with certain types of cancer. The rehabilitation team needs to provide services to cancer patients throughout the course of the illness and during different stages of the disease process even though the scope of the goals may vary. As stated previously, treatment providers must not base the initiation of rehabilitation efforts on life expectancy or age.

Treatment plans must be individualized to meet each patient's unique and specific needs. Rehabilitation team members consider all aspects of an individual's functioning when developing the treatment plan. Components of functioning that team members need to consider include physical, psychological, social, and vocational factors. Proper comprehensive evaluation and treatment needs to include consideration of all areas of the patient's life when developing the overall rehabilitation plan.

MEMBERS OF THE CANCER REHABILITATION TEAM

The wide range of difficulties cancer patients encounter necessitates the involvement of a large number of professionals from different disciplines. On cancer rehabilitation teams, each represented discipline provides a unique contribution to the rehabilitation process (DeLisa et al., 1985; Hirsch, Grabois, & Decker, 1988; Lehmann et al., 1978).

Physicians. Physicians from several different speciality areas serve on cancer rehabilitation teams. Primary-care physicians, surgeons, radiation oncologists, and medical oncologists actively contribute to rehabilitation efforts simultaneously to manage the disease process. The physiatrist, a specialist in physical medicine, diagnoses and treats neuromuscular disease, musculoskeletal disease, and functional deficits and performs electrodiagnostic procedures (i.e., nerve conduction studies, electromyography). The physiatrist also prescribes treatments that other disciplines perform, such as physical, occupational, and speech therapies. Another role of the physiatrist is that of liaison between team members. Such a liaison requires a considerable degree of coordination, especially when rehabilitation and clinical management of the disease are both ongoing at the same time.

Care Coordinator. The role of a clinical care coordinator is to assist in the organization and management of the team. An important aspect of this role is conducting initial evaluations of patients referred to the rehabilitation team for consultation. Care coordinators may come from nursing, social work, or other rehabilitation-related fields but must be familiar with functions of the other disciplines in order to effectively assess patient needs. Following initial screening, representatives from other disciplines conduct clinical assessments based on the needs the patient presents and/or those identified by the care coordinator.

Psychologist. Cancer patients and their families often experience a number of psychological and adjustment issues related to the illness, treatment, and resulting disabilities. The psychologist provides assessment and treatment to assist in management of cancer-related psychological distress. The psychologist's role may include work with patients, families, and others significantly involved with the patient's life. Another role of the psychologist on a rehabilitation team is to assist other team members when the psychological issues of patients and families are complicating their efforts to provide therapy in an effective manner. Psychological consultation with other team members has the goal of maximizing the benefit the patient receives in the rehabilitation process.

Physical Therapist. The role of the physical therapist includes evaluation of muscle strength, mobility, and joint range of motion (ROM). Treatment interventions range from providing exercises to maintain/increase ROM, endurance, and coordination, to training the patient in mobility and progressive gait activities. Physical therapists also administer treatment modalities, such as heat and cold, electrical stimulation, hydrotherapy, traction, and massage.

Occupational Therapist. Occupational therapists evaluate patients' self-care abilities involving activities of daily living (ADL) such as dressing, bathing, meal preparation and homemaking. These professionals also assist patients with increasing their independent ADL abilities, including the use of adaptive techniques and equipment. In addition, occupational therapists evaluate home environments for potential modification, provide instruction in driving with adaptive devices, and provide interventions to assist with upper extremity ROM, strength, endurance, and coordination.

Speech Pathologist. The speech pathologist evaluates and treats communication deficits, dysphagia, and cognitive dysfunction in addition to providing preoperative counseling for patients who may experience alterations in speech and swallowing as a result of the disease process and treatment. Speech pathologists are also responsible for training patients in the use of alternative means of speech and communication, including adaptive communication devices, alaryngeal speech (esophageal speech, use of a prosthetic larynx), and for treating patients who have intraoral defects or experience aphasia. Treatment of swallowing deficits, whether a result of illness or treatment, is another area of specialization for the speech pathologist.

Social Worker. The role of the social worker can vary significantly depending on the institution. Social workers often provide counseling services to patients and families regarding emotional support, community resources, finances, lifestyle changes, and treatment participation. In some settings, social workers often serve as leaders for support groups and may also actively aid in discharge planning activities, such as arranging home-care services and transfer to other health-care settings.

Oncology/Rehabilitation Nurse. The role of the nurse is pivotal in cancer rehabilitation. The nurse is typically an extension of other members of the team because they often assist with treatment interventions initiated by the physical, occupational, or speech therapists. Such interventions include assisting patients with exercises, mobility on the unit, self-care activities, and speech and swallowing techniques. Because nurses typically have extensive contact with patients and families, they are aware of the emotional stress and adjustment issues that are present and often function as counselors, providing significant emotional support for patients and families. In addition to their active involvement with most other disciplines regarding treatment interventions, nurses are responsible for skin care, bowel and bladder management, and patient–family education. Cancer nurses are crucial in promoting the rehabilitation goal of maintaining optimal independent functioning.

Dietician. Diet and nutrition are important factors in cancer rehabilitation. Proper diet and adequate nutritional status significantly influence a patient's ability to actively participate in an applied therapy program and are essential for patients undergoing radiation and chemotherapy treatment. The role of the dietician is to evaluate current nutritional status and provide recommendations regarding specific dietary needs. Cancer patients often require dietary supplements and alternative methods of receiving nutrition. Dieticians also assist in teaching patients and family members important dietary aspects of successful rehabilitation.

Vocational Counselor. Vocational counselors assist patients regarding the impact of cancer and treatment on a variety of employment issues. Functions of vocational counselors include evaluation, training, and liaison with employers. The vocational impact of cancer is an area that health-care providers often overlook in regard to potential for intervention (Conti, 1990; Taylor, 1984).

Although these professionals are most commonly cited as members of the cancer rehabilitation team, many other professionals provide important and valuable services. Other team members may include a chaplain, dentist, and prosthetist–orthotist. Additionally, rehabilitation programs benefit from consultation relationships with other care-providing organizations, such as home health-care agencies and community hospice centers.

EFFECTIVE FUNCTIONING OF THE CANCER REHABILITATION TEAM

Although it is beyond the scope of this chapter to provide an in-depth review of how to achieve productive team functioning, it is essential to address some of the most important factors in developing an effective cancer-rehabilitation team approach.

The premier difference between a team approach to treatment versus individual disciplines providing treatment in isolation is the degree of communication and interaction among professionals. Communication is a critical factor in team functioning (DeLisa et al., 1988). Each team member must develop excellent interpersonal communication skills if the team is to function in a productive manner. Important characteristics possessed by team members include assertiveness, willingness to listen and accept differing points of view, ability to tolerate review and challenge of one's ideas, ability to tolerate conflict, willingness to work toward resolution, and acceptance of the team approach to care. Although most team communication occurs during the team conference, informal contact occurs on an ongoing basis between members as patient issues arise and team members identify additional patient needs.

Rothberg (1981) cited a number of principles that assist in creating effective team participation. Two essential ingredients include teaching members how to work together and providing time for development. Education provides team members with an understanding of the roles and functions of other team members and enhances respect for the skills and knowledge of others. Development of definitive roles for team participants clarifies expectations regarding the responsibility of each member. The team leader must respect other members as exemplified via consultation, listening, and encouraging involvement. The rehabilitation team must develop a process for handling conflict, an accepted consequences of team interaction, in a productive fashion. The team leader must also promote and attend to activities that maintain the strength and cohesiveness of the team, and emphasize the establishment and maintenance of communication to remove obstacles to communication. A team leader should encourage the development of each members' full potential via support for continuing education and attendance at relevant professional meetings.

Effective team meetings are another essential component to successful team functioning. Team meetings must occur on a regular basis, and are typically scheduled once a week at a specific time and place. Team members must attempt to attend all regularly scheduled meetings. A good team meeting is productive, stimulating, and goal oriented, and it involves interaction, problem solving, and creativity (DeLisa et al., 1988). Common objectives of the meeting are to discuss patient status, review previous goals, set new goals, and discuss patient-related issues and concerns. The meetings work best when conducted in an organized manner, following a specified format for discussing each patient. A frequent approach in conducting a team meeting is for each discipline involved with a particular patient to provide a progress report. Following the report of each discipline, there is brief discussion regarding overall treatment goals.

The physiatrist usually serves as team leader. Other team members, however, can also function in the role of coordinator for the team meeting. Regardless of which member serves as leader of the meeting that individual has numerous responsibilities. There are a number of objectives that team members must achieve during team meetings, and the leader is responsible for conducting the meeting so that the team meets these objectives in a timely and efficient manner. The responsibility of the meeting leader is to keep the group focused on the objectives. The leader facilitates the discussion, clarifies issues and responsibilities, and ensures that members understand treatment goals.

Effective team functioning is an important variable in providing quality care. Melvin (1980) suggested that an interdisciplinary team working together toward common goals provides more to patient care than the total accomplished by each individual member treating the patient separately. An interdisciplinary team approach, a core component of cancer rehabilitation, has the potential to achieve results greater than the sum of the activities of individual disciplines.

MODELS OF CANCER REHABILITATION PROGRAMS

Several different models exist for handling referrals and initiating treatment interventions in cancer rehabilitation programs (Dietz, 1981; Lehmann et al., 1978; Watson, 1990). Health-care professionals have three primary means for initiating rehabilitation care for cancer patients (Harvey et al., 1982). First, individual team members are consulted regarding specific patient problems. Second, the rehabilitation physician or care coordinator receives a referral regarding a patient. Third, the entire team refers the patient for consultation. Differences of opinion also may exist in determining which cancer patients might benefit from cancer rehabilitation consultations. These differences relate to status of the program within the overall institutional structure and level of acceptance the program has achieved. For example, some programs may only receive referrals of patients with the particular diagnoses for which they have developed specific protocols; other programs may restrict their scope of services due to limited staff and resources. In addition, due to attitudes of some individual physicians, not all cancer patients who might potentially benefit from rehabilitation obtain referral to rehabilitation services. In order for a cancer rehabilitation team to be maximally effective, the institutional administration and medical staff must support the rehabilitation team by ensuring that all cancer patients have access to services of team members.

Lehmann and colleagues (1978) outlined a program model that utilized a physiatrist as liaison between the clinical oncology team and rehabilitation team. The clinical oncology team included a radiation oncologist, general surgeon, medical oncologist, plastic surgeon, gynecologist, otolaryngologist, and other medical specialists interested in cancer. The Patient Care Coordinator assisted with referrals from the clinical oncology team to the rehabilitation team. A Rehabilitation coordinator was responsible for screening all patients treated by the clinical oncology team. The physiatrist reviewed information regarding patients who exhibited potential rehabilitation problems and, in consultation with the attending physician, made recommendations regarding possible therapeutic interventions.

Watson (1990) proposed a cancer rehabilitation model that emphasizes the development of a comprehensive care program. Following the diagnosis of cancer, the patient enters an overall cancer health-care program in order to achieve the maximum level of functioning within the limits imposed by the disease process. The program consists of three simultaneous treatment approaches: (1) interventions to cure, control, or palliate the disease process; (2) interventions directed toward maintaining optimal physical functioning; and (3) educational information shared with the patient and family regarding shared prevention measures to avoid or reduce secondary problems. The final step in the comprehensive program is ongoing follow-up to monitor changing conditions and needs.

Most models have several common attributes. Ideally, all patients diagnosed with cancer would receive referral for an initial consultation to the cancer rehabilitation team. The care coordinator assists in efficient management of referrals and treatment initiation. Typically, the care coordinator makes the initial contact and conducts a preliminary needs assessment. Based on this assessment and communication with the referring physician and physiatrist, appropriate rehabilitation team members would receive referrals. This is a comprehensive and efficient means of referral similar to the referral process used with other rehabilitation populations, such a system is preferable to one that involves making referrals to individual team members or referrals requesting involvement of the entire team. Referrals to individual disciplines do not provide opportunity for utilization of a team approach in addressing patients' problems. Referrals to the entire team are not time efficient because they necessitate evaluations by each member, and often a patient may require services from only a portion of the team. An interdisciplinary team approach is preferable to other approaches because it provides more comprehensive treatment. Routine meetings are essential to update patient status, review goals, set new objectives, and solve difficult situations. Last, ongoing contact with cancer patients is vital because the disease process and treatment side effects can vary over time, resulting in need for different interventions throughout the course of illness.

REHABILITATION PROBLEMS ASSOCIATED WITH CANCER

Cancer is an illness that affects virtually all systems and regions of the body. Relative to other rehabilitation populations, cancer is a much more diverse illness in its presentation. Such diversity creates a tremendous range of potential rehabilitation problems. Also, as stated earlier, cancer is unlike stroke, spinal cord injury, traumatic brain injury, and other rehabilitation diagnoses in which the phase of recovery begins at a discrete point in time after an initial incident. Cancer can have a rather unpredictable course that involves an initial period of illness followed by remission but with possibility of recurrence. This fluctuating course results in rehabilitation problems arising anytime during the course of illness, and future needs are not always foreseeable at the time of diagnosis or initial treatment.

There are two broad, general categories of rehabilitation problems that relate to cancer and result in altered physical functioning: primary and secondary deficits. Primary deficits are a direct result of the location and action of disease process on a particular system, organ, or body part that produces changes in the patient's previous level of functioning. For example, a spinal cord tumor may result in paraplegia due to its location and direct effect on the spinal cord. The location of a brain tumor may cause gait and balance disturbances. Secondary deficits result from treatment measures that the health-care team has utilized to arrest the disease process but such treatments may also create changes in patient functioning. Examples of such treatments and deficits include: radical neck dissection surgery resulting in decrease of

ROM secondary to transection of the spinal accessory nerve (Herring, King, & Connelly, 1987) and chemotherapy induced peripheral neuropathies (Kaplan & Wiernik, 1982). Because emphasis of the rehabilitation team is on overall patient functioning, causal factors involved in development of deficits are not particularly important. Patients receive evaluation and treatment based on changes that have occurred in their functional abilities, not in relation to type of cancer or other variables. The following examples reveal potential cancer-rehabilitation problems.

Breast cancer accounts for the largest percentage of new cancer cases for adult women (Wingo et al., 1995). Following surgical intervention, patients may experience edema, pain, and restricted ROM (DeLisa et al., 1985; Hirsch et al., 1988; Scanlon & Feldman, 1988). Physical and occupational therapy exercises assist in reducing and eliminating these problems. Breast cancer patients also have significant psychosocial needs during the course of illness (Taylor et al., 1985). A variety of interventions, in addition to traditional psychotherapy, may assist patients to deal effectively with the psychological impact of breast cancer. Immediate breast reconstruction assists with psychological adjustment (DeLisa et al., 1985; Scanlon & Feldman, 1988). The Reach to Recovery Program, a program of volunteers who have undergone treatment for breast cancer, also significantly assists newly diagnosed patients regarding adjustment issues.

Primary bone tumors and metastatic bone cancer can produce several difficulties that a rehabilitation team can address (Hirsch et al., 1988). Amputation and limb-sparing procedures can significantly change the patient's functional status (DeLisa et al., 1985). Physical and occupational therapy actively aid in restoring function via prosthetic training and exercise programs. Psychological issues and vocational concerns may be present and require intervention.

About 25% of cancer patients will develop metastatic brain disease (Patchell & Posner, 1990). Patients with brain metastasis and primary tumors may experience a variety of rehabilitation problems similar to those of stroke and traumatic brain injury patients. Common deficits include sensory loss, impaired motor function, speech and swallowing difficulties, personality changes, and impaired cognition. Rehabilitation efforts for these patients require the same disciplines as those utilized by stroke and traumatic brain injury teams, physical and occupational therapy, speech pathology, psychology, nursing, and others. Despite an often poor or guarded prognosis, these patients can and do benefit from rehabilitation efforts (Hirsch et al., 1988).

Spinal cord tumors and metastases result in numerous rehabilitation problems. Spinal cord injury and neurological deficits often result from direct compression of the spinal cord by the tumor or extradural pressure from surrounding metastatic deposits (Hirsch et al., 1988). Primary sites for metastatic spinal disease are usually lung, breast, and prostate (Gilbert, Kim, & Posner, 1979). In one study, at least 50% of patients presenting with symptoms of spinal metastases were known to have malignant disease (Stark, Henson, & Evans, 1982). The majority of patients present with an initial complaint of pain often followed by onset of motor weakness, sensory loss, and bowel and bladder problems. Prognosis for functional recovery is better for patients with primary spinal cord tumors than for metastatic tumors. Although, survival in cases of spinal metastatic disease is typically 6 to 12 months, there is a wide range of variability, and studies indicate that treatment efforts are justifiable (Jameson, 1974; Murray, 1985). Rehabilitation procedures for cancer patients are much the same as techniques for traumatic spinal cord injury patients.

Cancer of the head and neck produces several significant functional and emotional difficulties that require a comprehensive rehabilitation approach. Compared to many other types of cancer, problems that result from head and neck cancer necessitate involvement of a large number of disciplines with specialized skills. The most common problem areas include nutrition and deglutition, impaired shoulder functioning, self-care issues, speech and communication deficits, and psychosocial issues (Shedd & Aguilar-Markulis, 1987). The dietician and speech pathologist are responsible for evaluation and treatment concerning issues of proper nutritional status and swallowing difficulties (DeLisa et al., 1985). Physical therapy and occupational therapy actively aid in treatment of shoulder dysfunction that results from damage to muscle and nerve tissue during surgical procedures (Herring et al., 1987). Head and neck cancers can potentially interfere with speech. For example, cancer of the larynx may require a total laryngectomy. Speech pathologists play an important role in assisting patients to utilize alternative means of voicing and communication (McKenna, Fornataro-Clerici, McMenamin, & Leonard, 1991; Schaefer & Johns, 1982). The rehabilitation nurse is instrumental in teaching self-care procedures to patients and in emphasizing the importance of patients' continuing such behavior at home. Cancer of the head and neck can have a profound impact regarding psychological status of patients (Argerakis, 1990). Patients face a potentially life-threatening illness and the possibility of significant functional changes involving speech, sight, taste, smell, and mobility along with alteration of their facial appearance. Due to the importance of facial features in social interaction and emotional expression, emotional investment to the head and neck area is greater than to any other body part (Breitbart & Holland, 1990). The patient may experience tremendous adjustment difficulties related to issues of self-image, identity, and self-esteem. Such difficulties often result in significant symptoms of anxiety and depression. Adequate psychological adjustment is often more difficult to obtain among head and neck cancer patients than among other cancer patients because many individuals who are at risk for developing head and neck cancer are alcohol abusers (Shedd, 1982). Continued alcohol abuse and related problems often result in poor compliance with treatment recommendations. Consultation for substance-abuse treatment is often an essential addition to efforts of the rehabilitation team. Due to complicated aspects of head and neck cancer, it is best if patients with these type of cancers contact the rehabilitation team soon after diagnosis and prior to surgery.

Virtually all cancer diagnoses and resulting treatment interventions have the potential to produce rehabilitation problems. In addition to specific deficits related primarily to cancer sites, cancer and treatment interventions produce other, more generalized problems, such as treatment-related neuropathy and encephalopathy and cerebrovascular complications (Grauss, Rodgers, & Posner, 1985; Hirsch et al., 1988). Cancer-related pain is common, occurring in about 40% of patients with intermediate disease and up to 80% of patients with advanced disease (Bond, 1985; Bonica, 1985). Inactivity due to illness results in deconditioning, can have serious consequences regarding the maintenance of independent functioning, and is also detrimental to psychological well-being (DeLisa et al., 1985). *Asthenia,* a syndrome involving fatigue and lethargy despite normal muscle strength, and *cachexia,* generalized weight loss with muscle weakness, are both symptoms often experienced by cancer patients (Hirsch et al., 1988). Sexual problems are a frequent concern of cancer patients. Sexual difficulties include a decline in sexual desire and loss of interest in sexual activity (Ganz, 1990). Cancer and its treatment can also lead to physical changes that result in difficulties with sexual functioning and reproduction (Auchincloss, 1990; Loescher et al., 1989).

Clinicians often overlook and neglect vocational problems related to cancer (Conti, 1990; Taylor, 1984). In 1985, for example, it was reported that only one half of one percent (0.50%) of all individuals who received vocational rehabilitation services were patients with the diagnosis of cancer. Thus, some investigators have proposed that vocational rehabilitation agencies make a concentrated effort to reach cancer patients who could benefit from services (Taylor & Crisler, 1988). Cancer patients who have utilized vocational rehabilitation services have reported positive experiences, and vocational rehabilitation costs for cancer cases are lower than for other populations (Conti, 1990).

Another vocational issue in relation to cancer is existence of discrimination toward hiring cancer patients. Approximately 25% of cancer survivors have experienced some form of employment discrimination (Hoffman, 1990). Discrimination often occurs due to belief in many incorrect myths about cancer (Ganz, 1990). Bordieri, Drehmer, and Taricone (1990) conducted a study with managers enrolled in MBA courses and found that cancer patients generally received lower hiring recommendations relative to applicants with pneumonia, regardless of qualifications. The diagnoses used included colon, pancreas, bone, thyroid, and liver cancer. Interestingly, the only cancer applicant given a rating similar to the rating given to the pneumonia patient was the applicant with liver cancer. This type of cancer has only a 3% five-year survival rate, further illustrating the public's incredible lack of knowledge about cancer. The findings of this study are consistent with results of previous studies (Bordieri & Drehmer, 1988; Schag & Heinrich, 1986). Hoffman (1990) suggested that increased efforts regarding education and provision of legal resources for survivors may decrease employment discrimination against cancer patients.

Related to the issues of employment are problems that patients often encounter regarding health-insurance coverage. Cancer patients are often the victims of health-insurance discrimination (Hoffman, 1990). Some cancer patients find their health insurance terminated after receiving a cancer diagnosis, and others have cancelled their insurance due to increased premiums. Some patients may feel "trapped" in their jobs due to the need to maintain health-insurance coverage (Mellette, 1985). The problems cancer patients encounter regarding employment, insurance, and discrimination warrant further attention because the number of cancer survivors continues to increase.

Investigators have extensively researched and documented psychological consequences related to cancer (Breitbart & Holland, 1990; Grzesiak, 1987; Holland & Rowland, 1990; Mahon, Cella, & Donovan, 1990; Welch-McCaffrey et al., 1989). The nature of psychological issues associated with cancer are numerous, diverse and complex. Psychological adjustment issues related to the experience of cancer can occur among many dimensions of the illness, including type and site of cancer, prognosis for survival, stage of cancer and age at time of diagnosis, degree of functional deficits in relation to the illness and treatment, and potential for recurrence. A review of the extent of these psychological issues is beyond the scope of this chapter; however, some important aspects require discussion. Psychological issues affect not only patients but also those individuals who feel closely connected to them, including immediate family members and close friends. Following the diagnosis of cancer, patients may experience disruption of previous social and emotional support systems due to their perceived feelings of alienation as they strive to adjust to the diagnosis. Family members and close friends of patients also experience significant adjustment issues at various stages of the illness, from diagnosis through treatment. Psychological interventions with significant others, apart from patients, may help to address their concerns and indirectly assist in maintenance of patients' support networks. Severity of psychological distress experienced by cancer patients varies widely and depends on several factors, including individual coping abilities and social support (Cooper & Watson, 1991; Rowland, 1990a, 1990b, 1990c). Investigators can ascertain predictors of patients' ability to adequately cope with cancer from knowledge of patients' previous personality styles and functioning. Among the most important predictors of poor adaptation to cancer are previous psychological problems, substance abuse, low socioeconomic status, negative philosophy toward life, social isolation, recent losses, and numerous obligations (Rowland, 1990a).

Approaches to assist cancer patients with the multitude of psychological problems that accompany diagnosis of cancer occur in many forms. Clinicians working with cancer patients have successfully utilized traditional individual psychotherapy, family and couple therapy, group psychotherapy, and support groups (Welch-McCaffrey et al., 1989). The psychological issues resulting from cancer are among the most complex problems that the patient may encounter because the illness requires constant adjustment and emotional strength throughout its often unpredictable course.

CONCLUSION

The goals of cancer treatment have always been the protection and prolongation of life. Survivorship through medical treatment plans that emphasize eradication of the cancer through a variety of means (i.e., surgery, radiation, chemotherapy) has always been the primary goal. The concept of *cancer rehabilitation* complements and extends these concepts of cancer care. The overall goal of this approach is to *improve quality of life for cancer patients and their families through a team-oriented, multidisciplinary approach that is set on restoring each patient's physical and emotional integrity and human dignity while living with the disease.*

As the number of surviving cancer patients continues to increase in the future, needs of these individuals will further demand attention. The use of a comprehensive rehabilitation approach addresses cancer patients' needs because it adequately and effectively meets the variety of challenges associated with this disease.

REFERENCES

American Cancer Society. (1983). *Cancer facts and figures.* New York: Author.
Argerakis, G. P. (1990). Psychosocial considerations of the post-treatment of head and neck cancer patients. *Dental Clinics of North America, 34*(2), 285–305.

Auchincloss, S. (1990). Sexual dysfunction in cancer patients: Issues in evaluation and treatment. In J. C. Holland & J. H. Rowland (Eds.), *Handbook of psychooncology* (pp. 383–412). New York: Oxford University Press.

Baldonado, A., & Stahl, D. (1982). *Cancer nursing.* New York: Medical Examination Publishing.

Blanchard, C. G., Ruckdeschel, J. C., Cohen, R. E., Shaw, E., McSharry, J., & Horton, J. (1981). Attitudes towards cancer: I. The impact of a comprehensive oncology course on second year medical students. *Cancer, 47,* 2756–2762.

Bond, M. R. (1985). Cancer pain: Psychological substrates and therapy. *Clinical Journal of Pain, 1,* 99–104.

Bonica, J. J. (1985). Treatment of cancer pain: Current status and future needs. *Advances in Pain Research and Therapy, 9,* 589–616.

Bordieri, J., & Drehmer, D. (1988). Causal attribution and the hiring recommendations for disabled job applicants. *Rehabilitation Psychology, 33,* 239–247.

Bordieri, J. E., Drehmer, D. E., & Taricone, P. F. (1990). Personnel selection bias for job applicants with cancer. *Journal of Applied Social Psychology, 20*(3), 244–253.

Breitbart, W., & Holland, J. C. (1990). Head and neck cancer. In J. C. Holland & J. H. Rowland (Eds.), *Handbook of Psychooncology* (pp. 232–239). New York: Oxford.

Brooks, A. (1979). Public and professional attitudes toward cancer: A view from Great Britain. *Cancer Nursing, 2,* 453–459.

Cassileth, B. R., & Egan, T. A. (1979). Modification of medical students perceptions of the cancer experience. *Journal of Medical Education, 54,* 797–802.

Clark, R. L., Moreton, R. D., Healey, J. E., & MacDonald, E. J. (1967). Rehabilitation of the cancer patient. *Cancer, 20,* 839–845.

Cohen, R. E., Ruckdeschel, J. C., Blanchard, C. G., Rohrbaugh, M., & Horton, J. (1982). Attitudes towards cancer: II. A comparative analysis of cancer patients, medical students, medical residents, physicians and cancer educators. *Cancer, 50,* 1218–1223.

Conti, J. V. (1990). Cancer rehabilitation: Why can't we get out of first gear? *Journal of Rehabilitation, 56*(4), 19–22.

Cooper, C. L., & Watson, M. (1991). *Cancer and stress: Psychological, biological and coping studies.* Chichester, UK: Wiley.

Cooper, S., Bean, G., Alpert, R., & Baum, J. (1980). Medical student attitudes toward cancer. *Journal of Medical Education, 55,* 434–439.

Cromes, G. F. (1978). Implementation of interdisciplinary cancer rehabilitation. *Rehabilitation Counseling Bulletin, 21,* 230–237.

DeLisa, J. A., Martin, G. M., & Currie, D. M. (1988). Rehabilitation medicine: Past, present and future. In J. A. DeLisa, D. M. Currie, B. M. Gans, P. F. Gatens, J. A. Leonard, & M. C. McPhee (Eds.), *Rehabilitation medicine: Principles and practice* (pp. 3–24). Philadelphia: Lippincott.

DeLisa, J. A., Miller, R. M., Melnick, R. R., Mikulic, M. A., & Gerber, L. H. (1985). Rehabilitation of the cancer patient. In V. T. DeVita, S. A. Rosenberg, & S. Hellman (Eds.), *Cancer: Principles and practice of oncology* (pp. 2155–2188). Philadelphia: Lippincott.

Dent, O., & Gouldton, K. (1982). Community attitudes to cancer. *Journal of Biosocial Science, 14,* 359–372.

Dietz, J. H. (1981). *Rehabilitation oncology.* New York: Wiley.

Dudas, S. (1984). Rehabilitation concepts of nursing. *Journal of Enterostomal Therapy, 11,* 6–15.

Dudas, S., & Carlson, C. E. (1988). Cancer rehabilitation. *Oncology Nursing Forum, 15*(2), 183–188.

Fobair, R., Hoppe, R. T., Bloom, J., Cox, R., Varghese, A., & Speigel, D. (1986). Psychosocial problems among survivors of Hodgkin's disease. *Journal of Clinical Oncology, 4,* 805–814.

Ganz, P. A. (1990). Abolishing the myths: The facts about cancer. In F. Mullan & B. Hoffman (Eds.), *An almanac of practical resources for cancer survivors* (pp. 7–30). Mt. Vernon, NY: Consumers Union.

Gilbert, R. W., Kim, J. H., & Posner, J. R. (1979). Epidural spinal cord compression from metastatic tumor: Diagnosis and treatment. *Annals of Neurology, 3,* 40–51.

Grauss, F., Rodgers, L. E., & Posner, J. B. (1985). Cerebrovascular complications in patients with cancer. *Medicine, 64,* 16–35.

Grzesiak, R. C. (1987). Psychological considerations in rehabilitation of the cancer patient. In M. G. Eisenberg & R. C. Grzesiak (Eds.), *Advances in clinical rehabilitation* (Vol. 1, pp. 268–288). New York: Springer.

Gunn, A. E. (1984). *Cancer rehabilitation.* New York: Raven.

Haley, H. B., Huynh, H., Paiva, R. E., & Juan, I. R. (1977). Students attitudes towards cancer: Changes in medical school. *Journal of Medical Education, 52,* 500–507.

Harvey, R. F., Jellinek, H. M., & Habeck, R. V. (1982). Cancer rehabilitation: An analysis of 36 program approaches. *Journal of the American Medical Association, 247*(15), 2127–2131.

Herring, D., King, A. I., & Connelly, M. (1987). New rehabilitation concepts in the management of radial neck dissection syndrome: A clinical report. *Physical Therapy, 67*(7), 1095–1099.

Hirch, D., Grabois, M., & Decker, N. (1988). Rehabilitation of the cancer patient. In J. A. DeLisa, D. M. Currie, B. M. Gans, P. F. Gatens, J. A. Leonard, & M. C. McPhee (Eds.), *Rehabilitation medicine: Principles and practice* (pp. 660–670). Philadelphia: Lippincott.

Hoffman, B. (1990). Taking care of business: Employment insurance and money matters. In F. Mullan & B. Hoffman (Eds.), *An almanac of practical resources for cancer survivors* (pp. 97–149). Mt. Vernon, NY: Consumers Union.

Holland, J., & Wellisch, D. (1988). Psychosocial issues and cancer. *CA-A Cancer Journal for Clinicians, 38*(3), 130–132.

Holland, J. C., & Rowland, J. H. (1990). *Handbook of psychooncology: Psychosocial care of the patient with cancer.* New York: Oxford University Press.

Jameson, R. M. (1974). Prolonged survival in paraplegia due to metastatic spinal tumor. *Lancet, 8,* 1209–1211.

Kaplan, R. S., & Wiernik, R. H. (1982). Neurotoxicity of antineoplastic drugs. *Seminars in Oncology, 9,* 103–128.

Kurtzman, S. H., Gardner, B., & Kellner, W. S. (1988, June). Rehabilitation of the cancer patient. *American Journal of Surgery, 155,* 791–803.

Lebovitz, A., Croen, M., & Goetzel, R. (1984). Attitudes towards cancer: Development of the cancer attitude questionnaire. *Cancer, 54,* 1124–1129.

Lehmann, J. F., DeLisa, J. A., Warren, C. G., deLateur, B. J., Bryant, P. L., & Nicholson, C. G. (1978). Cancer rehabilitation: Assessment of need, development, and evaluation of a model of care. *Archives of Physical Medicine and Rehabilitation, 59,* 410–419.

Loescher, L. J., Welsh-McCaffrey, D., Leigh, S. A., Hoffman, B., & Meyskens, F. L. (1989). Surviving adult cancers. Part 1: Physiological effects. *Annals of Internal Medicine, 111*(5), 411–432.

Mahon, S. M., Cella, D. F., & Donovan, M. I. (1990). Psychosocial adjustment to recurrent cancer. *Oncology Nursing Forum, 17*(3), 49–52.

Marcone, R. C. (1978). *En bloc* resections for osteogenic sarcoma. *Cancer Treatment Reports, 62,* 225–231.

Mayer, D. K. (1991). Rehabilitation of the person with cancer. *Recent Results in Cancer Research, 121,* 437–441.

Mayer, D., & O'Connor, L. (1989). Rehabilitation of persons with cancer: An ONS position statement. *Oncology Nursing Forum, 16*(3), 433.

McKenna, J. P., Fornataro-Clerici, L. M., McMenamin, P. G., & Leonard, R. J. (1991). Laryngeal cancer: Diagnosis, treatment and speech rehabilitation. *American Family Practice, 44,* 123–129.

Mellette, S. J. (1985). The cancer patient at work. *CA-A Cancer Journal for Clinicians, 35*(6), 360–372.

Melvin, J. L. (1980). Interdisciplinary and multidisciplinary activities and ACRM. *Archives of Physical Medicine and Rehabilitation, 61,* 379–380.

Mullan, F. (1985). Seasons of survival: Relections of a physician with cancer. *New England Journal of Medicine, 313,* 270–273.

Mullan, F. (1990). Survivorship: An idea for everyone. In F. Mullan & B. Hoffman (Eds.) *An almanac of practical resources for cancer survivors* (pp. 1–4). Mt. Vernon, NY: Consumers Union

Mullan, F., & Hoffman, B. (Eds). (1990). *An almanac of practical resources for cancer survivors.* Mt. Vernon, NY: Consumers Union.

Murray, P. K. (1985). Functional outcome and survival in spinal cord injury secondary to neoplasia. *Cancer, 55,* 197–201.

Patchell, R. A., & Posner, J. B. (1990). Cancer and the nervous system. In J. C. Holland and J. H. Rowland (Eds.), *Handbook of psychooncology* (pp. 327–341). New York: Oxford University Press.

Rothberg, J. S. (1981). The rehabilitation team: Future directions. *Archives of Physical Medicine and Rehabilitation, 62,* 407–410.

Rowland, J. H. (1990a). Intrapersonal resources: Coping. In J. C. Holland & J. H. Rowland (Eds.), *Handbook of psychooncology* (pp. 44–57). New York: Oxford University Press.

Rowland, J. H. (1990b). Interpersonal resources: Social support. In J. C. Holland & J. H. Rowland (Eds.), *Handbook of psychooncology* (pp. 58–71). New York: Oxford University Press.

Rowland, J. H. (1990c). Developmental stage and adaptation: Adult model. In J. C. Holland & J. H. Rowland (Eds.), *Handbook of psychooncology* (pp. 25–47). New York: Oxford University Press.

Scanlon, E. F., & Feldman, J. L. (1988). Rehabilitation of the breast cancer patient. *Seminars in Surgical Oncology, 4,* 268–273.

Schaefer, S. D., & Johns, D. F. (1982). Attaining functional esophageal speech. *Archives of Otolaryngology, 108,* 647–649.

Schag, C., & Heinrich, R. (1986). The impact of cancer on daily living: A comparison with cardiac patients and healthy controls. *Rehabilitation Psychology, 31,* 157–167.

Shedd, D. P. (1982). Cancer of the head and neck. In J. F. Holland & E. Frei (Eds.), *Cancer medicine* (2nd ed., pp. 167–185). Philadelphia: Lea & Febiger.

Shedd, D. P., & Aguilar-Markulis, N. V. (1987). Rehabilitation of the cancer patient. In S. Ariyan (Ed.), *Cancer of the head and neck* (pp. 785–789). St. Louis, MO: Mosby.

Silverberg, E., Boring, C. C., & Squires, T. S. (1990). Cancer statistics for 1990. *CA-A Cancer Journal for Clinicians, 40,* 9–26.

Stark, R. J., Henson, R. A., & Evans, S. J. (1982). Spinal metastases: A retrospective survey from a general hospital. *Brain, 105,* 189–213.

Taylor, C. M. (1984). The rehabilitation of persons with cancer: Is this the best we can do? *Journal of Rehabilitation, 50*(4), 60–71.

Taylor, C. M., & Crisler, J. R. (1988). Concerns of persons with cancer as perceived by cancer patients, physicians and rehabilitation counselors. *Journal of Rehabilitation, 54*(1), 23–27.

Taylor, S. E., Lichtman, R. P., Wood, J. V., Bluming, A. Z., Dosik, G. M., & Liebovitz, R. L. (1985). Illness-related and treatment-related factors in psychological adjustment to breast cancer. *Cancer, 55,* 2506–2513.

Watson, P. G. (1986). Rehabilitation philosophy: A means of fostering a positive attitude toward cancer. *Journal of Enterostomal Therapy, 13,* 153–156.

Watson, P. G. (1990). Cancer rehabilitation: The evolution of a concept. *Cancer Nursing, 13*(1), 2–12.

Welch-McCaffrey, D., Hoffman, B., Leigh, S. A., Loescher, L. J., & Meyskens, F. L. (1989). Surviving adult cancers. Part 2: Psychosocial implications. *Annals of Internal Medicine, 111*(6), 517–524.

Wellisch, D. K. (1987). Surviving and its effects of the family. In *Proceedings of the Fifth National Conference on Human Values and Cancer* (pp. 59–62). San Francisco: American Cancer Society.

Wells, R. J. (1990). Rehabilitation: Making the most of time. *Oncology Nursing Forum, 17*(4), 503–507.

Wingo, P. A., Tong, T., & Bolden, S. (1995). Cancer statistics, 1995. *CA-A Cancer Journal for Clinicians, 45*(1).

IV

PSYCHOLOGICAL ASPECTS OF VARIOUS DISEASE STATES

23

Recent Advances in Psychosocial and Behavioral Oncology

Denise M. Tope and Thomas G. Burish

Cancer is, in many ways, a behavioral problem. Since researchers estimate that we could prevent, or at least successfully treat, more than half of all cancers if people changed their behaviors so as to reduce risk of developing the disease and increase likelihood of early detection and treatment if it does develop (Tubiana, 1991). In addition to prevention and early detection, psychosocial and behavioral factors play a role in determining quality of life once individuals develop cancer, degree to which individuals can successfully manage some treatment-related symptoms and perhaps even outcome of treatment.

Over the last century, many authors have proposed theories regarding the role of personality and other psychological factors in the etiology and course of cancer. However, empirical support for the role of psychosocial and behavioral factors in the etiology, diagnosis, treatment, and rehabilitation of cancer patients is a relatively recent phenomenon. Similarly, psychosocial and behavioral oncology as a formal field of inquiry is relatively young, with targeted research funding, training opportunities, specialty journals, professional organizations, and other indications of the emergence of an independent field developing only within the last 20 years. Although a relatively young field, psychosocial and behavioral oncology has already produced a large number of important theoretical and clinical findings. Advances that have occurred within the last half-decade are manifest not only in new informa-

---

Denise M. Tope • Behavioral Medicine Institute, 5401 Kingston Pike, Suite 540, Knoxville, Tennessee 37919. **Thomas G. Burish** • Department of Psychology, Vanderbilt University, Nashville, Tennessee 37240.

Handbook of Health and Rehabilitation Psychology, edited by Anthony J. Goreczny. Plenum Press, New York, 1995.

tion and technologies, but also in fundamental, unifying strategies that researchers within the field have adopted. Recent progress is largely due to fieldwide efforts to (1) improve assessment strategies to better define target problems and refine treatment approaches; (2) conduct theory-based research; (3) explore interactions between physiological and psychosocial factors in disease development and progression on the one hand, and treatment-related symptoms on the other; and (4) establish interdisciplinary research programs.

The purpose of this chapter is to selectively review recent research in four relevant areas as examples of the breadth and clinical importance of the field and to suggest several of the most challenging areas for future inquiry. Accordingly, the chapter consists of five major sections. The first four sections cover the areas of prevention, symptom management, quality of life, and psychological factors predicting disease outcome. In each of these sections, we describe various research programs in some detail as examples of state-of-the-art research. In each section it would have been possible to describe many other excellent research findings. The focus on a small number of research programs is due to space limitations and desire to provide some detail about a limited number of programs rather than few details about a large number of programs. Moreover, the examples chosen represent coherent and thoughtful approaches to research that both address current needs and lay groundwork for further advancement within the discipline of psychosocial oncology. After describing research in these four areas, a final section provides concluding comments and suggestions for future inquiry.

PRIMARY PREVENTION

Most research in the area of primary prevention focuses on enabling individuals to refrain from adopting unhealthy behaviors, such as cigarette smoking, or, if they have developed them, to change from health-compromising to health-promoting behaviors (e.g., from sunbathing to not sunbathing, sedentary lifestyles to regular exercise programs, high-fat–low-fiber diets to low-fat–high-fiber diets). Because cigarette smoking appears to be the single most preventable cause of cancer in the United States (Office of the Surgeon General Report, 1988), and projections indicate smoking kills one of five individuals alive today in developed countries (Peto, Lopez, Boreham, Thun, & Heath, 1992), smoking prevention and cessation has received a great deal of research attention.

In spite of the considerable amount of research that clinicians have devoted to behavior change in general and smoking cessation in particular, most smoking-cessation programs have only limited success, with 80% or more of participants usually smoking again within one year or less (Glasgow & Lichtenstein, 1987). Current research by Prochaska and his colleagues suggests that researchers may have based past attempts to alter individuals' smoking habits on an oversimplistic notion of how people change behavior, and that a more sophisticated, theory-based approach can produce significantly better results. In fact, the National Cancer Institute recently acknowledged (see Shiffman et al., 1991) that recognition of the complexity and multifaceted nature of behavioral change has been a primary route through which successes in the area of primary prevention have occurred.

Prochaska and his colleagues base much of their work on the Transtheoretical

Stages of Change model (Prochaska, 1979). This model holds that rather than conceptualizing behavior changes as dichotomous events (e.g., either an individual does or does not smoke), it is better to view individuals as progressing through a series of five stages of change. The five stages are (1) *precontemplation,* in which individuals are not seriously considering change; (2) *contemplation,* in which people realize there is a problem, are thinking about overcoming it, and are intending to make a change within the next 6 months; (3) *preparation,* in which people are seriously planning to take some corrective action, usually within the next month; (4) *action,* in which people are actively working on changing their behavior; and (5) *maintenance,* during which people try to maintain the changes they have made. In general, people do not pass through these stages in a linear fashion but often move back and forth within them.

If the Transtheoretical Stages of Change model is correct, one would assume that extent to which individuals benefit from a traditional smoking-cessation program (i.e., an action-oriented program) is a direct function of their stage of change. Prochaska and DiClemente (1992) found that this is exactly what occurs. A study of 570 former smokers who stopped smoking after a home-based self-help program showed that amount of success in quitting directly related to the stage they were in prior to treatment. Specifically, individuals in the preparation stage were more likely to change than those in the contemplation stage, who, in turn, were more likely to change than those in precontemplation.

If likelihood for change relates to the stage one is in, then it is also quite likely that intervention packages that aim to move individuals through the stages, starting at whatever stage individuals are in, would be more effective than interventions that implicitly assume everyone is ready to take action, an assumption almost all current smoking-cessation programs make. Again, this is exactly what Prochaska and his colleagues (Prochaska, DiClemente, Velicer, & Rossi, 1993) found. The investigators randomly assigned 756 smokers, according to stage of development, to one of four conditions. Subjects in one condition received standard self-help smoking-cessation manuals (from the American Lung Society and the American Cancer Society); subjects in the other three conditions received manuals matched to the stage of change they were in (subjects in two of the conditions also received other intervention components not directly relevant to this discussion). Results indicated that over an 18-month follow-up period, groups that received stage-specific interventions stopped smoking at significantly greater rates than those who received a common (i.e., stage-irrelevant) intervention.[1] These results provide empirical support for the Transtheoretical Stages of Change model and suggest, for the first time, that self-help smoking cessation interventions can be effective with relatively large numbers of individuals if treatment providers identify the stage of change of each individual and match or tailor interventions for that particular stage. It is interesting and encouraging to note that these findings already appear to be having impact. For example, the American Lung Association has recently begun to organize "thinking-about-quitting" seminars as a preliminary step to its traditional, action-oriented smoking-cessation program.

---

[1] Prochaska et al. (1993) also conducted a second study that compared subjects assigned to a common intervention condition to those assigned to a stage-specific intervention. Surprisingly, in this study, stage-specific interventions generally were not superior to the common intervention. Prochaska and associates offer several plausible explanations for failure of this study to replicate the first study.

If the research of Prochaska and his colleagues ended here, the findings would be highly important, heuristically and clinically, but they go further. Prochaska and his colleagues (Prochaska et al., 1994) studied cognitive changes that accompany movement through the stages of change. As one might expect, when individuals are in the precontemplation stage, that is, when they do not recognize that their behavior is problematic and do not intend to change, their assessment notes that adisadvantages of changing their behavior outweigh advantages. As individuals move through the stages of change, this weighting of factors begins to reverse until, in the action and maintenance stages, they see perceived advantages of change outweighing disadvantages. This simple but important phenomenon characterizes at least 12 different health-related behaviors, including smoking, sun exposure, exercise, weight control, condom use, and mammography screening (Prochaska et al., 1994); that is, change does not occur until individuals regard "pros" of a behavior to outweigh "cons," and, in each case, this particular balance occurs in the action phase. Figure 23.1 displays the relationship between assessment of advantages and disadvantages of regular exercise and respective stages of change.

Prochaska (1992) further analyzed data for all 12 health behaviors in the prior set of studies and found a striking statistical consistency across behaviors in the amount of change in the decisional balance of advantages and disadvantages that was necessary in order for individuals to move from precontemplation to action. Two empirically derived equations summarize this consistency:

$$PC > A = 1 \ SD \ PROS_H$$

$$PC > A = 1 \ SD \ CONS_{unh}$$

The first equation indicates that moving individuals from the precontemplation (PC) to action (A) stage requires approximately a 1 SD increase in the value one places on pros of the healthy behavior $(PROS_H)$ in question. The second equation is simply a corollary of the first: It suggests that movement from precontemplation to action can also occur with a 1 SD increase in perceived cons of the unhealthy

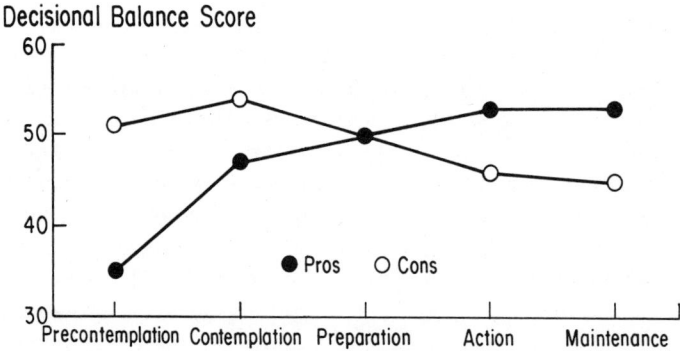

Figure 23.1. The decisional balance score (in T-scores) reflecting perceived advantages (Pros) and disadvantages (Cons) of regular exercise by individuals in various stages of change. (Adapted with permission from Prochaska et al., 1994.)

behavior ($CONS_{unb}$). A 1 *SD* change in perception of advantages and disadvantages of changing health-related behaviors requires, according to Prochaska (1992), an intervention strong enough to account for approximately 20% of the variance in treatment outcome.

If these projections hold up with further empirical testing by various research groups working on different problem behaviors, they would suggest that it may be possible to predict whether a particular treatment will be effective with a given group of individuals for a given problem. For instance, a meta-analysis of a given group of rigorous treatment-outcome studies might produce a fairly reliable indication of the likely effect size produced by a given treatment under certain circumstances. Knowing this effect size would, if Prochaska's preliminary work holds up, allow one to predict whether that treatment would move subjects from precontemplation to action. Further analyses might suggest that clinicians could combine certain treatments, interactively or additively, to produce desired treatment outcomes. For example, it may be that, by itself, a particular self-help smoking-cessation program is not likely to produce change, but that in combination with public policies restricting smoking or raising the tax on cigarettes, it will be effective. If one were able to develop clinically meaningful mathematical models of change and subsequently predict treatment outcome, psychosocial oncology and primary prevention of cancer would take a monumental step forward.

SYMPTOM MANAGEMENT

The behavioral sciences play a critical role, not only in the area of primary prevention, but also assisting in reduction of distress of individuals who have developed cancer and are receiving aggressive treatment for their disease. Initially, mental health clinicians trying to improve quality of life of cancer patients relied primarily on emotional and supportive counseling. In recent years, however, practitioners have developed techniques for behavioral management of treatment side effects and successfully applied these techniques with increasing frequency. In fact, recognition that physiological and psychosocial factors interact to create many symptoms and health outcomes experienced by cancer patients has become a mainstay of behavioral oncology. Specific disease and treatment-related problem areas targeted for behavioral intervention have included cancer-related pain, sexual dysfunctions, neuropsychological problems, negative affect, and chemotherapy-induced nausea and vomiting. Among these areas, chemotherapy-induced nausea and vomiting has received the most research attention.

As a systemic cytotoxic treatment, chemotherapy affects virtually every cell in the body, not only cancer cells. As a result, it can produce a wide variety of side effects, among the most debilitating being intense nausea, vomiting, and affective distress (Nerenz, Leventhal, & Love, 1982). Until the late 1970s, cancer specialists believed these side effects were due solely to pharmacological properties of chemotherapy drugs, and antiemetics were the treatment of choice for such effects. Researchers then discovered that as many as one third of cancer chemotherapy patients experienced conditioned side effects as well as pharmacologically induced effects. Conditioned symptoms are the result of an associative learning process in which stimuli associated with chemotherapy treatment settings (such as sight of nurses and smell of the drugs) begin to elicit nausea, vomiting, and negative affects, such as anxiety and depression. These conditioned symptoms can occur before (in which case we call them *anticipatory symptoms*), during, or after delivery of chemotherapy (Carey & Burish, 1988).

Several different research groups have demonstrated that various psychological interventions can successfully prevent or treat these conditioned side effects. For instance, in a recent study, Burish and his colleagues (Burish, Snyder, & Jenkins, 1991) randomly assigned 60 cancer chemotherapy patients to one of four treatments: (1) general coping preparation (PREP), (2) progressive muscle relaxation training with guided relaxation imagery (PMRT), (3) both PREP and PMRT, or (4) a standard treatment-control condition. The PREP intervention, administered at a separate 90-minute session prior to the first chemotherapy treatment, consisted of four major components: (1) guided tour of the clinic and treatment area; (2) videotape of patients receiving chemotherapy and discussing the treatment and how they coped with its side effects; (3) question-and-answer period with an oncology nurse; and (4) written materials about cancer, chemotherapy, and what to do for various symptoms and side effects. PMRT patients received the intervention immediately before and during the first three chemotherapy treatments, with patients asked to practice PMRT daily between treatments. Family members received invitations to accompany patients during all aspects of the study; most family members did attend. Results indicated that relative to standard treatment, the PREP intervention increased patients' knowledge of their disease and its treatment, reduced conditioned side effects, decreased negative affect, and improved general coping ability. PMRT patients showed some decrease in negative affect and vomiting relative to control patients. The combination of PREP and PMRT did not provide patients with significant advantages over one treatment alone. However, family members exposed to both the PREP and PMRT interventions reported coping significantly better with stress than those exposed to only one or to neither intervention. Overall, data suggest that a relatively simple coping-preparation procedure, and one that treatment teams can readily implement in a variety of clinical settings, can reduce many different types of distress associated with cancer chemotherapy. Other research on psychosocial treatment of the side effects of cancer chemotherapy also indicate substantial benefits (Carey & Burish, 1988; Morrow, Burish, & Bellg, 1992).

Although clinical researchers have developed effective interventions for prevention and treatment of conditioned side effects, two problems have plagued this research. First, the most common conditioned side effect of chemotherapy, nausea, is a subjective phenomenon that is difficult to measure and precludes objective comparison from one subject to another or from one study to another. Second, even though effective interventions for preventing development of conditioned side effects exist, it is not possible to predict, with clinically acceptable levels of accuracy, who will develop conditioned side effects and who will not (see Burish & Carey, 1986). As a result, most patients do not receive treatment until they have already developed conditioned symptoms, leading to needless suffering and more expensive intervention.

Recent research by Morrow may help to overcome both of these problems. Morrow has developed a portable physiological recording instrument that permits continuous recording of several autonomic nervous system indices, such as heart rate, pallor, blood volume pulse, and peripheral skin temperature, from a small sensor attached to the face. The device also allows patients to manually press a button to indicate certain events, such as when they feel nauseated and when they vomit. In preliminary research, Morrow and colleagues (1992) had cancer chemotherapy patients wear this device before, during, and after chemotherapy, and subsequently determined whether certain patterns of physiological activity reliably associated with nausea and vomiting. Preliminary results have been promising. On the basis of complex spectral analysis, Morrow has found that there appears to be a reliable linear relationship between total autonomic activity prior to chemotherapy and subsequent treatment-related nausea and vomiting. Moreover, peak activity in specific physiological indices appears to have predictable temporal relationships to subsequent vomiting. Although preliminary, these data have two important implications. First, they suggest that autonomic nervous system activity, measured before chemotherapy treatments, may be a reliable predictor of subsequent nausea and vomiting and, perhaps, of conditioned nausea and vomiting. Second, one or more autonomic nervous system indices may prove to be objective indices of nausea, at least for cancer patients undergoing cytotoxic chemotherapy treatment. If future research supports these findings, significant advances in measurement and control of chemotherapy side effects are likely to follow.

Redd, Bovbjerg, and colleagues have illustrated a third major advance in the area of conditioned side effects. These investigators hypothesized that if nausea and vomiting become conditioned to chemotherapy, then perhaps other responses also become conditioned, including immune system parameters. Researchers have known, for quite some time, that the immune system can become conditioned to cytotoxic drugs (Ader, 1981), at least in animals. Because chemotherapy is cytotoxic, Redd and Bovbjerg speculated that it may produce conditioned immunosuppression in humans. To test this notion, the investigators (Bovbjerg et al., 1990) assessed nausea and immune function in 20 ovarian cancer patients undergoing outpatient chemotherapy treatments. Experimenters measured patients' levels of nausea, anxiety, and immune function at home several days before chemotherapy treatment and again at the hospital as patients awaited treatment. Results indicated significantly greater immunosuppression, as indicated by proliferative responses to T-cell mitogens, when patients awaited chemotherapy relative to home measurements several days earlier. Results also indicated that these findings were not due to increased anxiety levels common immediately before chemotherapy. These findings confirm that a number of responses, including immune parameters, can become conditioned in the chemotherapy context. Because immune parameters can affect timing and dose of chemotherapy, understanding factors that affect drug levels is clinically important.

In summary, psychosocial oncology has made significant contributions reducing treatment-related distress in cancer patients. Research has led to the discovery that some side effects of cancer treatments, especially cytotoxic chemotherapy, are due to maladaptive learning and that several psychological interventions can prevent and treat these side effects. Moreover, preliminary data suggest that it may be possible to develop objective methods for measuring and predicting these side effects, which, in turn, might lead to efficient strategies for individualized treatment protocols. Finally, it appears that important immune functions might also become conditioned, possibly affecting decisions on chemotherapy administration and, in some cases, producing clinically significant alterations in the body's defense system. Many of these results are preliminary and require considerable additional research before we can fully appreciate their reliability and clinical usefulness. However, each of these results has potential to make a significant contribution to advancing psychological oncology and reducing distress of cancer patients.

ASSESSMENT OF QUALITY OF LIFE

In contrast to research described in the prior section, which focused on specific symptoms or side effects caused by cancer or its treatment, the next body of research we consider is more global, focusing on overall quality of life. As used in psychosocial oncology, the phrase *quality of life* incorporates information from multiple life domains, including disease- and treatment-related physical symptoms, perceptions of personal health, physical functional status, and psychological and social well-being (Aaronson, 1991).

Concern with cancer patients' quality of life has increased sharply during recent years. Initially, research attention and funding focused on understanding cancer and finding a cure or extending lives of cancer patients through aggressive treatment. Treatments did indeed become more effective, but often at a cost: They can be aversive and disfiguring, and require extended and demanding care. As a result of the success of cancer treatments in extending life, combined with their adverse side effects, both health-care professionals and patients became interested in improving quality as well as quantity of life. In fact, some individuals have raised concerns about whether the quantity of life resulting from some treatments is worth their effects on quality of life. Treatment-outcome research on large patient populations, often referred to as *clinical trials research,* now routinely assesses impact of treatments on quality of cancer patients' lives.

Perhaps one of the most exciting advances in assessing quality of life is incorporation of quality-of-life information into calculating survival rates of cancer patients. As noted earlier, length of survival and quality of life do not always positively correlate; in fact, in some situations they may well relate negatively. Gelber and his colleagues (Gelber & Goldhirsch, 1986; see Feldstein, 1991, for a brief review) have pioneered a mathematical strategy for adjusting patient-survival data through use of a weighting system that reflects value of time spent in various health states. The basic concept originated in economic theory, and other investigators have applied it in epidemiological research under the label of "quality-adjusted life years." Modification of this procedure, developed by Gelber and associates for use in psychosocial oncology, involves computation of an adjusted survival rate known as Time Without Symptoms and Toxicity, or TWiST. TWiST computation is essentially simple subtraction: amount of time that patients undergo cancer treatment, labeled *toxicity,* or experience unpleasant disease or treatment-related symptoms, labeled *symptoms,* minus patients' overall survival rates. For example, a woman with breast cancer who undergoes a 6-cycle regimen of adjuvant chemotherapy and is alive and disease-free 2 years following initiation of chemotherapy has a 24-month survival rate from the initiation of chemotherapy. To compute TWiST, health-care providers must assess and incorporate incidence and duration of symptoms. For example, if a patient experienced nausea for 2 months, TWiST score would be 2 months less than overall survival time. Table 23.1 contains a more detailed description of TWiST methodology.

The TWiST approach is very conservative in rating negative impact of symptoms and toxicity on patients' quality of life, adopting a worst-case perspective. It assumes that all negative events and symptoms are equally "bad," and, in fact, that they are so bad that individuals are not experiencing a quality of life worth living. In reality, of course, individuals tend to perceive varying degrees of "goodness" and "badness" for each symptom. In response to the need to incorporate value gradations for symptoms and toxicity experienced by cancer patients, Gelber and colleagues (1987) added a quality-adjusted component to TWiST analysis. *Q-TWiST* is an alternate measure of time benefit that allows for patient preferences or variable value ratings of time spent in certain health states, a mathematical procedure accomplished through assignment of weights or coefficients. In short, Q-TWiST calculation occurs by adding TWiST scores and a weighted sum of symptoms, toxicity, and recovery, as illustrated in the equation:

$$Q\text{-}TWiST = TWiST + (W_S \times \text{Symptoms}) + (W_T \times \text{Toxicity}) + (W_R \times \text{Recovery})$$

Coefficients can assume values from 0 to 1, inclusive. For instance, a coefficient of 1.00 for recovery indicates that quality of time in recovery from treatment, with its

Table 23.1. Construction of TWiST for Individual Breast Cancer Patients Undergoing Adjuvant Chemotherapy

	Event	Time removed from total survival
A.	Leukopenia, thrombocytopenia, and Grades 1 or 2 anemia (asymptomatic)	No penalty
B.	Any reversible subjective toxic effect[a] of any grade (excluding emenorrhea) reported during a cycle or month of treatment	Remove entire month
C.	Alopecia and weight gain	Remove an additional 3 months after last report to allow for recovery
D.	Isolated mastectomy scar or contralateral breast cancer alone	Remove 3 months to allow for recovery from local procedure
E.	Any appearance of relapse[b] (other than D) or second primary tumor (not breast)	Remove entire remaining survival

Note: From "Time Without Symptoms and Toxicity (TWiST): A Quality-of-Life Oriented Endpoint to Evaluate Adjuvant Therapy" by Gelber et al., 1987. Reprinted by permission.
[a]Subjective toxic effects include those noted and graded prospectively by the investigators: nausea, vomiting, anorexia, diarrhea, mucositis, infections, epigastric pain, neurotoxicity, headache, euphoria, depression, allergic skin disorders, alopecia, cystitis, muscle weakness, hypercalcemia, hot flashes, thrombosis, thromboembolism, edema, lymphedema, weight gain, eye disorders, joint pain, symptomatic anemia, hemorrhage, and nonmenstrual vaginal bleeding.
[b]Included skeletal recurrences when symptomatic or at initiation of systemic treatment.

associated symptoms and discomfort, was as good as time spent outside of treatment and recovery and, hence, would not negatively impact computed survival time. A coefficient of 0.50 suggests that the months spent in recovery were half as valuable to patients as time spent without recovery-related symptoms.

The TWiST and Q-TWiST procedures fit cleanly into clinical trial paradigms and provide information that is directly useful and interpretable to physicians. For example, Gelber, Goldhirsch, and Cavalli (1991) incorporated the Q-TWiST method into a large, international randomized clinical trial designed to compare effectiveness of three treatments for breast cancer: (1) single-cycle perioperative adjuvant chemotherapy in both pre- and postmenopausal women, (2) longer duration adjuvant chemotherapy for premenopausal women or chemoendocrine therapy for postmenopausal women, and (3) a combination treatment of peri- and postoperative chemo/chemoendocrine therapy. The sample consisted of 1,229 women, all of whom underwent evaluation 5 years after initiation of treatment. Results indicated that women who had undergone longer duration chemotherapy or chemoendocrine therapy had longer overall survival rates, improved probability of disease-free survival, and 22 more months of Q-TWiST relative to women who had undergone only the single cycle of chemotherapy. These data suggest that in spite of increased toxicity associated with prolonged treatment (which resulted in subtraction of at least 5 months from Q-TWiST), longer duration therapy was preferable in both medical and psychosocial outcome.

Although TWiST and Q-TWiST offer promising new ways to assess outcome of medical treatments, they are not without problems. Perhaps the major difficulty is the need to assign values to components in the equations. Relative unpleasantness of multiple symptoms and value of time are not easy for individuals to operationalize or measure. As a result, computation of TWiST and especially Q-TWiST involves a tremendous and uncomfortable degree of latitude regarding component values. For instance, amount of time required for "recovery" from a symptom, such as alopecia, is debatable. Also debatable is determining the threshold value of a symptom, such as depression, before it receives consideration in TWiST and Q-TWiST equations. Assignment of quality adjusted weights in Q-TWiST analysis can compound potential ambiguity. It remains an empirical question, for example, whether it would be best for information for these coefficients to come from patients' experiences alone or from health-care providers' and family members' perceptions as well. Appropriate timing of assessment of these value ratings during the course of treatment and illness is also uncertain but of considerable importance (Aaronson, 1991). Patients may rate value of time spent with severe nausea differently if asked for evaluations during episodes of postchemotherapy vomiting versus several weeks later.

In acknowledging the degree and potential bias afforded by assigning weights, Gelber and colleagues have offered two suggestions to improve reliability when comparing treatments in a Q-TWiST analysis. First, compute Q-TWiST equations multiple times using several feasible combinations of value ratings (Goldhirsch, Gelber, Simes, Glasziou, & Coates, 1989). Investigators could then compare findings from multiple calculations to determine degree of parallelism. Although considerably more complicated statistically, a second option is to conduct a threshold analysis and then present results of TWiST or Q-TWiST in terms of rough threshold, rather than specific assigned weights, along with confidence intervals to indicate certainty of conclusions (Glasziou, Simes, & Gelber, 1990).

If future investigations sufficiently address current methodological shortcomings in the TWiST and Q-TWiST methods, these procedures may become an increasingly valuable adjunct to clinical trials. Nevertheless, we have not yet witnessed their ultimate utility in clinical trials. In each of the published studies of which we are aware that incorporate TWiST and Q-TWiST methodology, treatment findings using traditional survival-time analyses and quality-of-life analyses have been similar; the situation has not yet arisen in which a TWiST or Q-TWiST analysis indicated that a treatment that seems to hold a clear medical advantage is so toxic and symptom-eliciting that quality-of-life issues have outweighed, at least statistically, time spent in survival. If researchers continue to refine and apply TWiST and Q-TWiST methodology, then such a controversial situation, in which medical findings and quality-of-life findings diverge, is likely to occur. In the end, usefulness of TWiST, Q-TWiST, and other quality-of-life findings depend in large part, on the degree to which we can reliably operationalize value preferences, and on whether studies determine these techniques validly represent patients' evaluations of the quality of their time alive, and whether health-care professionals give enough importance to quality-of-life assessment to change treatment decisions.

PSYCHOLOGICAL FACTORS AFFECTING THE COURSE OF CANCER

Although much, and perhaps most, of the research in the area of psychosocial oncology has been in the areas of primary prevention, symptom management, and quality of life, the topic that has received the most attention in the lay press has been whether psychological interventions can cure cancer. The issue of mind–body relationships has long intrigued scientists and the lay public, especially with regard to whether individuals can control physical phenomena through mental means. In recent years, several individuals have made claims about the power of mental phenomena on cancer, including claims regarding curative effects of specially designed behavior therapy (Grossarth-Maticek & Eysenck, 1991), mental imaging (Simonton, 1992), positive attitude (Siegel, 1986), and laughter (Cousins, 1979), to name just a few. Regrettably, there has not been acceptably rigorous scientific evidence for any of these claims. Moreover, correlational studies that have addressed relationships between psychological factors, such as mood, coping styles, and health beliefs, and cancer progression and mortality have produced largely negative findings (Cassileth, Lusk, D. Miller, Brown, & C. Miller, 1985; Jamison, Burish, & Wallston, 1987; Kaplan & Reynolds, 1988; Pettingale, Burgess, & Greer, 1988; Richardson Zarnegar, Bisno, & Levine, 1990; Silberfarb et al., 1991; Zonderman, Costa, & McCrae, 1989). As a result, most physicians and scientists have remained unconvinced. A recent study has begun to change that.

Spiegel (1985) and his colleagues (Spiegel, Bloom, & Yalom, 1981) undertook a study aimed at improving quality of life of metastatic breast cancer patients. Eighty-six randomly assigned patients received either group therapy and self-hypnosis, or standard clinic treatment only. Results of the study indicated that patients who received psychological intervention had significantly improved quality of life (e.g., they experienced significantly less depression, fatigue, confusion, and phobic responses, used more effective coping strategies, and reported suffering less due to pain) than patients in the control group. Years later, Spiegel, Bloom, Kraemer, and

Gottheil (1989) assessed whether the intervention also affected longevity. In a carefully conducted analysis of the data, they found that patients in the intervention condition lived an average of 18 months longer than control patients, as measured from date of study entry to death, approximately 15 months longer, as measured from date of first metastasis to death, and approximately 13 months longer, as measured from initial medical visit to death. The first two comparisons were statistically, as well as clinically, significant. These results provide important pilot data suggesting that psychological treatment may extend the lives of some cancer patients.

Although promising, we must cautiously view these results until researchers in the area address several issues. For example, it is critical to determine whether other researchers can replicate the results prospectively in other patient populations across multiple institutions. Future research must also determine whether treatment effects hold after controlling important biological and medical factors so as to ensure that the disease and medical treatments are similar (or statistically controlled) in all patients. Assessment of other individual-difference factors is also critical, so that one can determine whether treatments help only a small subset of patients, whether they might actually be detrimental to a small subset of patients, or whether they fairly generalize positive effects. Finally, if researchers are able to replicate the results, identification of specific causal mechanisms will become of utmost interest and importance. Research on each of these issues and others is currently underway at several different institutions in the United States and elsewhere.

SUMMARY AND FUTURE DIRECTIONS

The field of psychosocial oncology has burgeoned within the last decade and especially within the past 5 years. Because cancer is often preventable and prevention is dependent largely on changing individuals' behaviors, researchers and clinicians have devoted considerable attention to encouraging people to adopt healthy lifestyles. Although we have made steady progress in this area, new findings, perhaps best exemplified by Prochaska (1979, 1992) and colleagues' Transtheoretical Stages of Change model, may allow us to understand, predict, and control cancer-relevant behaviors much more effectively than was heretofore possible. Over the past decade, research has documented that psychological interventions can also play a unique role in improving quality of life of cancer patients, including reducing conditioned side effects that often result from aggressive cancer treatment. Recent empirical efforts promise to take these important early findings a step further by allowing us to objectively assess and anticipate occurrence of distressing symptoms, such as nausea, that many health-care professionals previously considered largely subjective phenomena not easily predicted or reliably measured. It also appears that aversive cancer treatments may also produce conditioning in other physiological systems, including conditioned immune suppression. This and other research aimed at reducing distress in cancer patients will significantly benefit from new measurement techniques assessing overall quality of life and from research determining how clinicians can best use this measurement in the overall assessment of cancer treatments. Finally, in one of the most exciting and heralded findings in recent years, it appears that legitimate psychological interventions may, under certain circumstances, help some types of cancer patients live longer. This finding is tentative and demands rigorous replication, but it promises to extend the field of psychosocial oncology to new frontiers that had primarily been the province of unscientific and untoward speculation and exaggeration.

Despite these advances, or more likely because of them and the groundwork they have laid, the field of psychosocial oncology faces significant challenges that remain unfulfilled and represent major targets for future work. Three of these challenges follow directly from research discussed in this chapter. First, many of the findings reported in this chapter relate, at least hypothetically to a general notion of social support. For example, from clinical experience we have found that behavioral techniques for managing conditioned side effects are more likely to be effective for patients who have spouses or family members who will provide encouragement and participate in the intervention program. Spiegel (1991) speculated that one of the mechanisms that may have contributed to increased longevity of their treatment patients involved social support provided by the group therapy experience. Past research on social support has included a curious blend of looseness and breadth (Kobasa et al., 1991); social support appears reliably related to longevity across several circumstances (House, Landis, & Umberson, 1988), but it is hard to measure, define, or apply in an individually useful manner. We need much more research to address these issues and uncover mechanisms through which social support exerts its impact. If the findings from this research are positive, they may constitute one of the most important advances in the next decade of research on psychosocial oncology.

Second, although researchers have given much attention to changing behaviors of cancer patients and those at risk of developing cancer, the notion of changing behaviors of health professionals has received relatively little attention. Many health professionals still model unhealthy behaviors to their patients, fail to recommend simple screening and preventative behaviors, and are unaware of advances in the psychosocial area and, hence, are unlikely to recommend these advances or incorporate them into their practices. Applying behavior-change principles to health-care providers presents as a major challenge for future research.

Finally, if psychosocial researchers are truly to have a major impact on changing behaviors in a variety of domains, their findings must lead to health-policy changes that extend research findings from laboratories and clinics to communities throughout the country. Public health policies, including subsidies for tobacco production, regressive health insurance that does not support prevention or early detection, and lack of support for making health education a priority in schools, must change if psychosocial oncology is to ever have a massive societal impact on diseases like cancer. Psychosocial researchers bear an important responsibility in the initial steps of changing policy. In contrast to the training and penchants characteristic of many, researchers must alert leaders in policy-making positions to psychosocial research findings, assist leaders in understanding practical implications of such findings, and coax them into considering such findings when making policy decisions. If our goal is large-scale application of basic and applied psychosocial research findings, this is an effort and a challenge that the field cannot afford to overlook.

REFERENCES

Aaronson, N. K. (1991). Methodological issues in assessing the quality of life of cancer patients. *Cancer, 67* (Suppl. 3), 844–850.

Ader, R. (Ed.). (1981). *Psychoneuroimmunology.* New York: Academic Press.

Bovbjerg, D. H., Redd, W. H., Maier, L. A., Holland, J. C., Lesko, L. M., Niedzwiecki, D., Rubin, S. C., & Hakes, T. B. (1990). Anticipatory immune suppression and nausea in women receiving cyclic chemotherapy for ovarian cancer. *Journal of Consulting and Clinical Psychology, 58,* 153–157.

Burish, T. G., & Carey, M. P. (1986). Conditioned aversive response in chemotherapy patients: Theoretical and developmental analysis. *Journal of Consulting and Clinical Psychology, 54,* 593–600.

Burish, T. G., Snyder, S. L., & Jenkins, R. A. (1991). Preparing patients for cancer chemotherapy: Effect of coping preparation and relaxation interventions. *Journal of Consulting and Clinical Psychology, 59,* 518–525.

Carey, M. P., & Burish, T. G. (1988). Etiology and treatment of the psychological side effects associated with cancer chemotherapy: A critical review and discussion. *Psychological Bulletin, 104,* 307–325.

Cassileth, B. R., Lusk, E. J., Miller, D. S., Brown, L. L., & Miller, C. (1985). Psychosocial correlates of survival in advanced malignant disease? *New England Journal of Medicine, 312,* 1551–1555.

Cousins, N. (1979). *Anatomy of an illness as perceived by the patient: Reflections on healing and regeneration.* New York: Norton.

Feldstein, M. L. (1991). Quality-of-life-adjusted survival for comparing cancer treatments: A commentary on TWiST and Q-TWiST. *Cancer, 67* (Suppl. 3), 851–854.

Gelber, R. D., & Goldhirsch, A. (1986). New endpoint for the assessment of adjuvant therapy in post-menopausal women with operable breast cancer. *Journal of Clinical Oncology, 4,* 1772–1779.

Gelber, R. D., Goldhirsch, A., Castiglione, M., Price, K., Isley, M., & Coates, A. (1987). Time without symptoms and toxicity (TWiST): A quality-of-life oriented endpoint to evaluate adjuvant therapy. In S. E. Salmon (Ed.), *Adjuvant therapy of cancer* (pp. 455–465). Philadelphia: Saunders.

Gelber, R. D., Goldhirsch, A., & Cavalli, F. (1991). Quality-of-life-adjusted evaluation of adjuvant therapies for operable breast cancer: The International Breast Cancer Study Group. *Annals of Internal Medicine, 114,* 621–628.

Glasgow, R. E., & Lichtenstein, E. (1987). Long-term effects of behavioral smoking cessation interventions: *Behavior Therapy, 18,* 297–324.

Glasziou, P. P., Simes, R. J., & Gelber, R. D. (1990). Quality adjusted survival analysis. *Statistics in Medicine, 9,* 1259–1276.

Goldhirsch, A., Gelber, R. D., Simes, R. J., Glasziou, P., Coates, A. S. (1989). Costs and benefits of adjuvant therapy in breast cancer: A quality-adjusted analysis. *Journal of Clinical Oncology, 7,* 36–44.

Grossarth-Maticek, R., & Eysenck, H. J. (1991). Creative novation behaviour therapy as a prophylactic treatment for cancer and coronary heart disease. *Behaviour Research and Therapy, 29,* 1–16.

House, J. S., Landis, K. R., & Umberson, D. (1988). Social relationships and health. *Science, 241,* 540–545.

Jamison, R. N., Burish, T. G., & Wallston, K. A. (1987). Psychogenic factors in predicting survival of breast cancer patients. *Journal of Clinical Oncology, 5,* 768–772.

Kaplan, G. A., & Reynolds, P. (1988). Depression and cancer mortality and morbidity: Prospective evidence from the Alameda County study. *Journal of Behavioral Medicine, 11,* 1–13.

Kobasa, S. C., Spinetta, J. J., Cohen, J., Crano, W. D., Hatchett, S., Kaplan, B. H., Lansky, S. B., Prout, M. N., Ruckdeschel, J. C., Siegel, R. & Wellisch, D. K. (1991). Social environment and social support. *Cancer, 67,* 788–793.

Morrow, G. R., Asbury, R., Hammon, S., Dobkin, P., Caruso, L., Pandya, K., & Rosenthal, S. (1992). Comparing the effectiveness of behavioral treatment for chemotherapy-induced nausea and vomiting when administered by oncologists, oncology nurses, and clinical psychologists. *Health Psychology, 11*(4), 250–256.

Morrow, G. R., Burish, T. G., & Bellg, A. (1992). Anticipatory nausea and vomiting. In M. Martin & D. Rubioe (Eds.), *Antiemetic therapy: Current status and future prospects* (pp. 181–199). Madrid, Spain: Glaxo.

Nerenz, D. R., Leventhal, H., & Love, R. R. (1982). Factors contributing to emotional distress during cancer chemotherapy. *Cancer, 50,* 1020–1027.

Office of the Surgeon General. (1988). The health consequences of smoking: Nicotine addiction (Report No. 223-672-0). Rockville, MD: U.S. Government Printing Office.

Peto, R., Lopez, A. D., Boreham, J., Thun, M., & Heath, C. (1992). Mortality from tobacco in developed countries: Indirect estimation from national vital statistics. *Lancet, 339,* 1268–1278.

Pettingale, K. W., Burgess, C. & Greer, S. (1988). Psychological response to cancer diagnosis—I. Correlations with prognostic variables. *Journal of Psychosomatic Research, 32,* 255–261.

Prochaska, J. O. (1979). *Symptoms of psychotherapy: A transtheoretical analysis.* Homewood, IL: Dorsey Press.

Prochaska, J. O. (1994). Strong and weak principles for progressing from precontemplation to action based on twelve problem behaviors. *Health Psychology, 13,* 47–51.

Prochaska, J. O., & DiClemente, C. C. (1992). Stages of change in the modification of problem behaviors. In M. Hersen, R. M. Eisler, & P. M. Miller (Eds.), *Progress in behavior modification* (pp. 184–218). Sycamore, IL: Sycamore Press.

Prochaska, J. O., DiClemente, C. C., Velicer, W. F., & Rossi, J. S. (1993). Standardized, individualized, interactive and personalized self-help programs for smoking cessation. *Health Psychology, 12,* 399–405.

Prochaska, J. O., Velicer, W. F., Rossi, J. S., Goldstein, M. G., Marcus, B. H., Rakowski, W., Fiore, C., Harlow, L. L., Redding, C. A., Rosenbloom, D., & Rossi, S. R. (1994). Stages of change and decisional balance for twelve problem behaviors. *Health Psychology, 13,* 39–46.

Richardson, J. L., Zarnegar, Z., Bisno, B., & Levine, A. (1990). Psychosocial status at initiation of cancer treatment and survival. *Journal of Psychosomatic Research, 34,* 189–201.

Shiffman, S., Cassileth, B. R., Black, B. L., Buxbaum, J., Celentano, D. D., Corcoran, R. D., Gritz, E. R., Laszlo, J., Lichtenstein, E., Pechacek, T. F., Prochaska, J., & Scholefield, P. G. (1991). Working group report: Needs and recommendations for behavior research in prevention and early detection of cancer. *Cancer, 67* (Suppl. 3), 800–804.

Siegel, B. S. (1986). *Love, medicine, and miracles.* New York: Harper & Row.

Silberfarb, P. M., Andersen, K. M., Rundle, A. M., Holland, J. C., Cooper, M. R., & McIntyre, O. R. (1991). Mood and clinical status in patients with multiple myeloma. *Journal of Clinical Oncology, 9,* 2219–2224.

Simonton, O. C. (1992). *The healing journey.* New York: Bantam.

Spiegel, D. (1991). A psychosocial intervention and survival time of patients with metastatic breast cancer. *Advances: The Journal of Mind–Body Health, 7,* 10–19.

Spiegel, D. (1985). The use of hypnosis in controlling cancer pain. *CA: Cancer, A Journal for Clinicians, 35,* 221–223.

Spiegel, D., Bloom, J. R., Kraemer, H. C., & Gottheil, E. (1989). Effect of psychosocial treatment on survival of patients with metastatic breast cancer. *Lancet, 2,* 888–891.

Spiegel, D., Bloom, J. R., & Yalom, I. (1981). Group support for patients with metastatic cancer. *Archives of General Psychiatry, 38,* 527–533.

Tubiana, M. (1991). Trends in primary and secondary prevention. *Cancer Detection and Prevention, 15,* 1–5.

Zonderman, A. B., Costa, P. T., & McCrae, R. R. (1989). Depression as a risk for cancer morbidity and mortality in a nationally representative sample. *Journal of the American Medical Association, 262,* 1191–1195.

24

Psychological Aspects of Chronic-Maintenance Hemodialysis Patients

Phillip J. Brantley and Polly B. Hitchcock

INTRODUCTION

End-stage renal disease (ESRD) is a condition involving irreversible failure of excretory and regulatory functions of the kidneys. As ESRD progresses, residual renal function can no longer sustain normal body functioning, and survival is impossible without some form of renal replacement therapy (Eknoyan, 1991). ESRD remained virtually untreatable and often resulted in death until the early 1960s, when hemodialysis treatment began prolonging life (Norton, 1982). Although suitable for only a few patients, renal transplantation and peritoneal dialysis can preclude the more prevalent ESRD treatment, chronic-maintenance hemodialysis (Wauters, Hunziker, & Brunner, 1983). Congress began funding hemodialysis treatment in 1972, thereby increasing its availability to ESRD patients, many of whom until then did not qualify for treatment based on their "social worth" (Kutner & Brogan, 1990). Medical advances continue to increase longevity, reduce infection risk, and improve hemodialysis procedures; however, the intrusive nature of this process can result in difficulty adjusting to maintenance hemodialysis. The lifestyle accompanying hemodialysis requires compliance with a complex and strict treatment regimen. For this reason, psychological problems associated with this regimented lifestyle have arisen,

---

Phillip J. Brantley • Department of Family Medicine, Louisiana State University Medical Center, Baton Rouge, Louisiana 70805.   **Polly B. Hitchcock** • Department of Psychology, Louisiana State University, Baton Rouge, Louisiana 70803.
Handbook of Health and Rehabilitation Psychology, edited by Anthony J. Goreczny. Plenum Press, New York, 1995.

including depression, anxiety, neuropsychological complications, noncompliance, and marital difficulties. Psychologists began addressing these issues and integrating into teams of treatment professionals in the early 1970s (Kirschenbaum, 1991). Health psychologists, in particular, have become involved in efforts to improve patient adherence to medical procedures and improve quality of life for hemodialysis patients. This chapter discusses ESRD, its prevalence, complications, and treatment, and psychological issues associated with chronic-maintenance hemodialysis.

Most human beings fail to appreciate the life-sustaining aspects of the kidneys and view their daily demands as nothing more than a nuisance. The three essential functions of the kidneys involve (1) regulation of volume and composition of body fluids, (2) excretion of metabolites, and (3) production or metabolism of hormones (Andreoli, 1988). Several diseases can compromise integrity of the kidneys. In the United States, the most common causes of ESRD include diabetes mellitus, hypertension, chronic glomerulonephritis, chronic pyelonephritis, and polycystic kidney disease (Kokko, 1988; Luke, 1988). Until recently, glomerulonephritis was the leading cause of chronic renal failure. Because of aggressive treatment of this heterogeneous group of glomerular disorders, however, diabetes and hypertension have become the primary agents of chronic renal failure (Brenner & Lazarus, 1991).

Due to their increased rates of diabetes and hypertension, African-Americans have a much higher incidence rate of ESRD than Native Americans, Asians, or whites. Several other demographic trends among chronic renal failure patients are striking (Department of Health and Human Services, 1991a). Incidence rates strongly relate to age. Whereas only 8 patients per 1 million under age 15 developed ESRD in 1988, 512 patients per 1 million in the 65- to 74-year age group developed the disorder in 1988. Males have a higher incidence rate than females (168 per 1 million vs. 133 per 1 million in 1988). Furthermore, between 1983 and 1985, total ESRD incidence has steadily increased at a 6.9% annual rate. In 1988, the year for which latest figures are available, 36,743 individuals experienced renal failure in the United States and the Medicare ESRD program had a total enrollment of 134,786 individuals (Department of Health and Human Services, 1991a).

MEDICAL ASPECTS OF END-STAGE RENAL DISEASE AND HEMODIALYSIS

When renal functioning decreases to 20–25% of normal capacity, the characteristic constellation of clinical symptoms marking the uremic syndrome appear (Cordova, Benabe, & Martinez-Maldonado, 1991). Renal insufficiency and failure lead to imbalances in the acid–base composition, electrolytes, and volume of extracellular fluid, along with accumulation of toxic metabolites and endocrine disturbances (Eknoyan, 1991). Clinical abnormalities of uremia are so pervasive that they affect functioning of the pulmonary, cardiovascular, neurological, dermatological, gastrointestinal, hematological, and immunological systems (Brenner & Lazarus, 1991). This combination of systemic biochemical derangement and multiple-organ dysfunction is lethal. When conservative ESRD management fails, more drastic medical interventions are necessary to preserve life and, optimally, patients begin receiving such interventions before irreversible stages of uremia develop (Luke, 1988).

Two major treatment options are available for ESRD patients: transplantation and dialysis. The preferred treatment is renal transplantation from either living or cadaverous donors (Evans, 1992). When this is not possible, as is often the case, physicians must resort to one of two forms of dialysis. In hemodialysis, patients' blood circulates extracorporeally through an artificial kidney that contains a semipermeable membrane and a dialysate similar in composition to normal plasma (Luke, 1988). The process of diffusion down a chemical concentration gradient removes extraneous fluid and toxic substances from the blood. Usually, arteriovenous fistula in the forearm provides permanent vascular access (Luke, 1988).

Hemodialysis helps to correct many, but not all, fluid, electrolyte, and acid–base ESRD imbalances (Hakim & Lazarus, 1986). Patients generally receive this procedure, which requires 3–6 hours to complete, three times weekly (Luke, 1988). Hemodialysis can take place during inpatient or outpatient sessions supervised by health-care professionals, or patients can attempt to manage treatment in their homes (Christensen, Smith, Turner, Holman, & Gregory, 1990). Outpatient hemodialysis is the most common ESRD treatment modality, providing therapy to 82.1% of all dialysis patients in 1989 (Department of Health and Human Services, 1991a).

In continuous ambulatory peritoneal dialysis (CAPD), peritoneal membranes serve as artificial kidneys and eliminate need for blood removal from patients' bodies. Instead, CAPD involves infusion and removal of dialysate solution from the abdominopelvic cavity several times daily in 30–60 minute cycles (Devins et al., 1990). Because this form of dialysis operates more continuously than hemodialysis, the accompanying treatment regimen is less restrictive than the hemodialysis regimen (Popovich et al., 1978). CAPD and self-directed home hemodialysis offer relatively more freedom to ESRD patients than traditional outpatient hemodialysis. Both procedures, however, tend to require supportive partners, adequate home environments, self-motivation by patients, and relatively stable medical status (Luke, 1988).

Kidney dialysis and transplantation costs are exorbitant. Before 1972, considerations of "social worth" (i.e., employment history and income), which tended to favor white males, influenced selection of dialysis and transplantation patients (Kutner & Brogan, 1990). Congress established a program in 1972 to ensure that ability of individuals to pay for treatment would not limit access to these treatments (Novello, 1991). The End-Stage Renal Disease Program of Medicare decrees that patients with chronic ESRD must receive either kidney transplants or regular dialysis treatments. Although this program entitles every kidney patient to receive some form of treatment, bias continues to operate in assignment of patients to treatment modality (Levenson & Glocheski, 1991).

Kidney transplantation relates to better health outcomes than other treatments (Evans, 1992), but few ESRD patients receive this treatment. For example, between 1985 and 1988, only 9% of ESRD patients were able to obtain a functioning graft within 1 year of renal failure (Department of Health and Human Services, 1991a). Patient selection for transplantation depends predominantly on age, renal diagnostic category, and availability of tissue-compatible grafts (Department of Health and Human Services, 1991a; Kutner & Brogan, 1990). For example, patients who are younger and those with renal failure attributed to glomerulonephritis and polycystic kidney disease have higher transplantation rates than older patients and those with hypertensive nephropathy (Department of Health and Human Services, 1991a). Higher rates of hypertension and diabetes among blacks, as well as their underrepresentation among kidney donors, make them less likely to receive transplants at this time (Kutner & Brogan, 1990).

Therefore, given medical and socioeconomic factors influencing treatment selection, it is not surprising that transplant, home hemodialysis, and CAPD patients are predominantly white, whereas blacks disproportionately represent outpatient hemodialysis groups (Novello, 1991). Furthermore, a recent study suggests women are less likely to receive transplants than men even though evidence exists suggesting women make better candidates for successful transplantation than men do (Kutner & Brogan, 1990). According to Kutner and Brogan, medical status alone cannot account for this gender discrepancy. These biases in treatment assignment, whether medically legitimate or resulting from discrimination, have profound implications because different outcomes are associated with different treatment forms (Levenson & Glocheski, 1991). Although measures are under way to investigate and correct such biases, the fact remains that patients maintained on outpatient hemodialysis tend to be older, sicker (Novello, 1991), and more economically disadvantaged than other ESRD patients. Sociodemographic composition of this patient population therefore provides an additional challenge to health-care professionals.

Although chronic-maintenance hemodialysis can slow ESRD progression, it is less than satisfactory for several reasons. Artificial kidneys cannot completely replace native kidneys' endocrine and regulatory functions (Luke, 1988), and dialysis patients vary in degree to which treatment successfully corrects their uremia. Several conditions that may persist despite treatment include anemia, renal osteodystrophy, pruritus, sodium and volume overload, hypertension, hyperkalemia, hypocalcemia, many metabolic derangements, accelerated cardiovascular disease, and pericarditis (Hakim & Lazarus, 1986).

Some of the most distressing complications for hemodialysis patients involve sexual dysfunction. Frequently reported problems include loss of libido, impotence, infertility, and amenorrhea (Cordova et al., 1991). Authors of much of the medical literature generally assume that sexual dysfunction relates to either physiological disturbances or pharmacological complications of ESRD, but psychological factors may also contribute to sexual problems (Levy, 1979). For example, patients may experience shame about altered body appearance and fear rejection by their partners. Physicians rarely address such concerns, and patients often feel too embarrassed to discuss the subject (Foulks & Cushner, 1986). Few, if any, empirical investigations appearing in the literature attempt to differentiate between relative contributions of physical and psychological factors in sexual dysfunction among hemodialysis patients. Therefore, incidence, nature, and most appropriate treatment of sexual problems in this population remain unclear.

Several complications also associate with the hemodialysis procedure itself. Besides being time-consuming and physically restrictive, treatments can be unpleasant. Technological improvements have virtually eliminated the more fatal complications of the dialysis procedure, such as air embolism (Luke, 1988), but several problems remain. For example, patients frequently experience severe muscle cramps and hypotensive episodes during dialysis. Excessive internal bleeding may result from use of anticoagulants, medications administered during dialysis to prevent blood from clotting when it travels outside the body through artificial kidneys. In addition, occlusion and aneurysm of vascular accesses are common. Vascular accesses also provide gateways for hepatitis and septicemia infections (Hakim & Lazarus, 1986).

Because of continued medical complications such as these, death rates for hemodialysis patients are extremely high. The latest figures from the national ESRD patient registry (Department of Health and Human Services, 1991a) indicate that survival rate 5-years post–renal failure is only 34.5%. Leading causes of death for patients maintained on hemodialysis are heart disease, stroke, and infections (Henderson, 1979). Death rates of ESRD patients are dependent on different causes of renal failure. Five-year survival rate, as reported by the Department of Health and Human Services is lowest for diabetics (21.3%) and highest for those patients with polycystic kidney disease (53.9%). These mortality patterns by diagnostic category, however, reflect underlying age distributions. Studies of survival rates of ESRD patients suggest mortality increases with advancing age irrespective of renal disease (e.g., Hellerstedt et al., 1986; Ruggiero, Brantley, Bruce, McKnight, & Cocke, 1992).

PSYCHOLOGICAL ASPECTS OF HEMODIALYSIS

In addition to numerous physical conditions associated with ESRD and its treatment, several psychological complications of maintenance hemodialysis exist. Central nervous system symptoms of uremia range from memory deficits and concentration problems to coma and seizures (Andreoli, 1988). Unusual behavior or organic psychoses may be present. Dialysis disequilibrium and dialysis dementia are two neurological disturbances unique to chronic dialysis patients.

Dialysis disequilibrium is an acute condition attributed to rapid reduction of blood urea nitrogen levels during initial dialysis treatments (Brenner & Lazarus, 1991). Symptoms include mental confusion and hallucinations. This disorder, although typically transient, may lead to convulsions and death if not controlled (McKee, Burnett, Raft, Batten, & Bain, 1982). Dialysis dementia is a progressively fatal disease of the central nervous system, characterized by speech and motor defects, dementia, and seizures. Initial accounts associated the disorder with long-term hemodialysis (Luke, 1988), prompting a spate of neuropsychological investigations in the early 1980s. Reports were inconclusive, however; some studies found little or no evidence of cognitive deterioration in chronic hemodialysis patients over time or compared to controls (e.g., McKee et al., 1982), but other investigators found impairments in memory or general cognitive functioning (e.g., Gilli & Bastiani, 1983; Ryan, Souheaver, & DeWolfe, 1981). Researchers in this area have yet to perform a systematic literature review to clarify incidence and nature of dialysis dementia or other neuropsychological dysfunction. Perhaps lack of interest in this area stems from a reported decline in incidence of dialysis dementia in recent years, which some researchers attribute to improvements in reduction of aluminum content of dialysate (Luke, 1988). Others have challenged aluminum's role in the pathogenesis of dialysis dementia, suggesting instead other mechanisms (e.g., slow virus infection) or even a multifactorial process (Gorelick et al., 1991).

Common psychological problems associated with surviving on maintenance hemodialysis include depression, suicide, anxiety, and phobic responses to treatment (Blodgett, 1981). Depression has been the most commonly reported (e.g., Czaczkes & De-Nour, 1978) and researched (Levenson & Glocheski, 1991) psychological symptom in the literature. Reported prevalence rates, however, have varied substantially (Levenson & Glocheski, 1991). Failures to control for length of time on dialysis may account for part of the discrepancy. Psychological adjustment appears to vary substantially over the course of treatment (N. Kutner, Fair, & M. Kutner, 1985). For example, at treatment onset, patients may experience a "honeymoon" phase accompanied by a euphoric sense of relief as physical symptoms of uremia decrease (Reichsman & Levy, 1972). Later, these patients may experience depression and resentment of their dependence on a machine for life (Novello, 1991).

Many depressive symptoms may represent incompletely treated uremia rather than psychopathology (Levenson & Glocheski, 1991). It has been difficult to differentiate psychological symptoms caused by uncleared uremic toxins from those caused by other concomitant diseases associated with ESRD or from those associated with psychopathology (Lundin, 1989). Pharmacological interventions associated with hemodialysis (e.g., steroids, antihypertensive medications) may also alter mood (Hong, Smith, Robson, & Wetzel, 1987). Unfortunately, most studies of psychological disturbance in ESRD have ignored or failed to control for such medical confounds (Levenson & Glocheski, 1991).

Anemia experienced almost universally by hemodialysis patients (Eschbach, Egrie, Downing, Browne, & Adamson, 1987), represents one example of a medical confound that investigators often fail to control. Anemia associated with chronic renal failure results, in part, from deficiency of erythropoietin, a hormone controlling red blood cell formation (Jelkman, 1986). The primary site for erythropoietin production in healthy adults is the kidneys (Eschbach & Adamson, 1988). Clinical features of anemia include weakness, fatigue, and poor exercise tolerance (Schwartz, Prior, Terzian, & Kahn, 1988). Uremic anemia may exacerbate preexisting medical conditions, such as coronary artery disease, gastrointestinal problems, and paresthesias (Keitt, 1988), but impact of ESRD anemia on psychological functioning and general quality of life has been unclear (Lundin, 1989). Purported psychological sequelae include decreased sense of well-being, impaired cognitive functioning, sleep disturbances, and sexual dysfunction (Schwartz et al., 1988).

Past treatments for anemia, such as iron supplements, androgen therapy, and red blood cell transfusions, have proven less than satisfactory (Eschbach et al., 1987). Recent development of recombinant human erythropoietin, however, has provided a significant advance in ESRD anemia management. The Food and Drug Administration approved Epoietin (Epo), a biologically engineered protein, in 1989 (Department of Health and Human Services, 1991b). Several clinical trials suggest Epo can correct anemia by increasing red cell production and improving hematocrit levels (Raine, 1988; Schwartz et al., 1988). Treatment with recombinant human erythropoietin may also provide a method for differentiating between psychological symptoms possibly caused by anemia and those caused by other factors (Lundin, 1989). Although several recent studies (e.g., Nissenson, 1989) have indicated that Epo increases exercise tolerance, central nervous system functioning, sexual potency, and general well-being, none of the studies were controlled double-blind comparisons with placebo. It will be interesting to see if reported rates of depression decrease as more patients take the drug.

In spite of several studies suggesting a large percentage of hemodialysis patients experience depression or general emotional distress (Levenson & Glocheski, 1991), systematic investigations examining efficacy of various psychological interventions are completely lacking in the literature. This paucity of treatment research may reflect actual clinical practice. Hong and associates (1987) found that 47% of hemodialysis patients with major depressive episodes received no psychological intervention. Such a finding may be due to attending physicians' assumptions that the disease process itself solely causes depressive symptoms. It therefore seems imperative that researchers compare outcomes of patients experiencing depressive symptomatology who receive combinations of medical and psychological interventions with those who receive medical treatment only.

Hemodialysis studies are now focusing on more global aspects of psychosocial adjustment. Despite uremia relief and the modest increase in longevity that dialysis provides, clinicians have questioned the quality of life of patients maintained on outpatient hemodialysis (e.g., Nehemkis & Gerber, 1986). The issue of quality of life is difficult to address because it is a multidimensional phenomenon encompassing such areas as social functioning, economic security, and psychological and physical adjustment (Greenwald, 1987; Gurin, Verhoff, & Feld, 1960). Hollandsworth (1988) delineated several quality-of-life factors particularly relevant for medical patients. These include survival, health status, medical complications, exercise tolerance, employment status, and general well-being. Given the significant morbidity and disability that occur with ESRD, it is not surprising that this disease is the second most represented disorder in quality-of-life literature (Hollandsworth, 1988).

Investigators generally agree that maintenance hemodialysis is the most intrusive of renal replacement therapies (Devins et al., 1983). ESRD and hemodialysis may disrupt virtually every facet of individuals' lives. Even if hemodialysis patients report favorable subjective adjustment, they do not work or function at the same level as the general population (Evans et al., 1985). For example, dialysis treatment schedules interfere with employment and leisure activities (Devins et al., 1990). Limited availability of dialysis centers may especially burden patients in rural areas, forcing them to travel considerable distances for treatment several times each week (Evans, 1992). Because of such problems, Devins and associates (1981) characterized ESRD as a "living stress laboratory" for studying chronic illness effects. The greatest stressor for these patients may be the mandate to comply with stringent dietary, fluid, and medication regimens accompanying hemodialysis.

COMPLIANCE ISSUES IN HEMODIALYSIS

As noted previously, hemodialysis only partially compensates for kidney failure. Dialysis patients must therefore modify their diets to reduce amount of waste, electrolytes, minerals, and fluids removed by the hemodialysis process. For example, dialysis patients must limit intake of protein, sodium, potassium, and phosphorus (Finn & Alcorn, 1986). Most patients must limit daily fluid intake to approximately 1000 cc, including beverages and foods that become liquid at room temperature (Blackburn, 1977). The treatment regimen also includes various supplemental medications to alleviate dietary deficiencies associated with ESRD and compensate for the hemodialysis process. These include vitamin and mineral supplements, phosphate binders, antihypertensives, and folic acid. Indeed, medication regimens of some patients may include instructions to ingest up to 50 pills per day (Finn & Alcorn, 1986; Nehemkis & Gerber, 1986).

Compliance with dietary regimen is probably the most difficult treatment consideration for hemodialysis patients because of the complexity and number of recommendations and the fact that it affects long-standing personal habits and alters lifestyles significantly (Hoover, 1989). Nonetheless, evidence suggests that deviations from prescribed dietary and fluid restrictions may result in several short- and long-term health problems. For example, excessive fluid intake may result in shortness of breath, hypotensive episodes during dialysis, pulmonary edema, and congestive heart failure (Robertson & Berl, 1986). Excessive serum concentrations of potassium ions can provoke cardiac arrthymias (Andreoli, 1988). In spite of dangers purportedly associated with noncompliance, literature reviews indicate 20% to 78% of dialysis patients fail to comply with treatment recommendations (e.g., Hartman & Becker, 1978; Wolcott, Maida, Diamond, & Nissenson, 1986).

Patient noncompliance also may take a toll on health-care professionals by straining already tenuous patient–staff relationships. The intimate nature of caring, almost daily, for patients with this chronic and ultimately fatal disease often leads to compromised therapeutic relationships (Wertzel, Vollerath, Ritz, & Ferner, 1977). Health-care workers may develop resentment and anger if they view patient noncompliance as passive–aggressive attempts to manipulate family members and staff, or if they believe patients are contributing less toward rehabilitation and survival than staff members are contributing. Even if health-care workers develop charitable attitudes toward ESRD patients, the frustration of patient noncompliance and high mortality rates may contribute to staff burnout and high employment turnover rates (Freyberger, 1973). Unfortunately, empirical data are scarce concerning effectiveness of psychological interventions with staff (e.g., stress management) and its effect on patients' moods or compliance.

Clinicians and researchers have speculated about and investigated various factors that contribute to noncompliance in hemodialysis patients. These include demographic factors (Procci, 1981), denial (De-Nour & Czaczkes, 1972), passive suicidal behavior (Abram, Moore, & Westervelt, 1971), ignorance of treatment regimen (Cummings, Becker, Kirscht, & Levin, 1982), and lack of social support (Hartman & Becker, 1978). Literature reviews have failed to find consistent and powerful support for any one of these factors (e.g., Hoover, 1989; Wolcott et al., 1986). More recently, cognitive factors, such as patients' preferences for involvement in treatment (Christensen et al., 1990) or perceived control of treatment (Schneider, Friend, Whitaker, & Wadhwa, 1991), have shown promise as important predictors of compliance.

The search for single determinants of compliance, however, may ultimately fail. No single factor may adequately explain compliance (German, 1988). It is best if we view compliance as a complex phenomenon subject to a variety of influences (Gerber & Nehemkis, 1986). Demographic, emotional, and cognitive variables, as well as other factors, no doubt interact in a multidimensional process. A composite of the more frequently reported findings in the literature suggests that "typical" abusers of diet and fluid restrictions are most likely unemployed, single, young males with little social support (e.g., Boyer, Friend, Chlouverakis, & Kaloyanides, 1990; Cummings et al., 1982; Oldenburg, MacDonald, & Perkins, 1988; Procci, 1981). Interestingly, Kutner and Brogan (1990) suggested that noncompliant males may actually receive rewards for their noncompliance; such patients may ultimately receive transplants to relieve dialysis staff from coping with disruptive behavior in the clinic.

Given the enormous amount of attention to the compliance issue, researchers have investigated surprisingly few interventions that deal specifically with dialysis patients. The traditional medical-model approach relies on patient-education programs grounded in the belief that compliance behaviors are directly proportional to patients' knowledge levels about prescribed regimens (Hoover, 1989). Knowledge obtained through such programs may be necessary, but not sufficient, to motivate this patient population to perform the enormous number of compliance behaviors required (Brantley, Mosley, Bruce, McKnight, & Jones, 1990). Some researchers (e.g., Boyer et al., 1990) have suggested applying findings from relapse prevention research to hemodialysis patients, but rarely have such interventions undergone evaluation in controlled trials.

For example, clinical researchers have successfully employed behavioral interventions in the form of token economies and behavioral contracting to assist in increasing compliance among dialysis patients (Finn & Alcorn, 1986). Finn and Alcorn's review of six behavioral studies suggests feedback to patients, staff praise, behavioral contracting, and token economies may increase patient compliance to dietary regimens. The majority of these early studies, however, involved single-case designs or uncontrolled treatments.

Recently Kirschenbaum (1991) described a program designed to improve treatment compliance by increasing self-directed care. Based on cognitive–behavioral principles, the program involves a 5-step approach that includes establishment of behavioral contracts and self-monitoring. Kirschenbaum presented case examples indicating that the program is beneficial in enhancing self-directed care, even among patients that nursing staff deemed hopeless. By the author's own admission, however, the individually administered program is somewhat labor intensive and may be impractical on a large scale.

Recent debate regarding reliability and validity of compliance measures, however, has waylaid implementation of controlled group evaluations of these different interventions. Some researchers have suggested that variations in measurement and definitions of compliance have contributed to inconsistent findings in the literature and impeded the search for effective treatments. For example, direct observations, staff ratings, and patients' self-reports of compliance behaviors show little consistency (Wolcott et al., 1986). Therefore, measurement of adherence to dietary and fluid restrictions in hemodialysis patients often involves objective indices. As such, biochemical indices of serum potassium (K+), blood urea nitrogen (BUN), and serum phosphorus may reflect adherence to dietary restrictions (Ferraro, Dixon, & Kinlaw, 1986). Intersession weight gain (IWG), which represents weight gained between dialysis treatments, is a measure of compliance to fluid restrictions. It is a function of fluid and dietary sodium intake (Wolcott et al., 1986).

Several investigators (e.g., Finn & Alcorn, 1986) have questioned the reliability and validity of casual use of these biochemical indices of compliance. Many of these measures appear sensitive to residual kidney function, individual differences in metabolism, and presence of concomitant diseases, leading some researchers to ask whether biochemical indices accurately reflect compliance behaviors. Several reviews (Ferraro et al., 1986; Wolcott et al., 1986) have provided useful guidelines for measuring compliance. For example, some authors recommend collecting multiple observations across different aspects of compliance (e.g., biochemical indices, patient self-report, and staff ratings). It is also important to remember that adherence to many aspects of treatment regimens may be relatively independent (Orme & Binik, 1989).

Kaplan (1990), however, criticized the recent trend of health psychology and behavioral medicine research to focus more on biochemical, rather than behavioral, outcomes. He argued forcefully that longevity and quality-of-life indicators are the most important consequences for patients. Although early hemodialysis research and commentary (e.g., Finn & Alcorn, 1986) emphasized the dire consequences associated with even minimal departures from treatment recommendations, the relationship between survival and noncompliance, as measured by biochemical indicators, is suspect.

Estimates of deaths directly attributable to noncompliance have ranged from 4–14% (De-Nour, 1982) to 60% (Abram et al., 1971), suggesting that our understanding of the association between moderate levels of noncompliance and mortality is less than complete. Ruggiero et al. (1992) investigated validity of dietary compliance parameters (BUN, K+, IWG) in relation to patient survival. Results suggested that biochemical indicators of compliance play a minimal role in predicting survival of ESRD patients on chronic hemodialysis. These patients are extremely ill, and mortality appears related more to age and diagnostic factors than to standard biochemical compliance indicators (Ruggiero et al., 1992).

Although total disregard of dietary and fluid restrictions will lead to certain death, stringent compliance may offer diminishing returns after patients achieve certain adherence levels. Continued admonishments for failing to strictly adhere to dietary restrictions may provide more frustration than benefit to these patients, especially if treatment team members do not address other psychological and socioeconomic stressors. Psychologists and other health-care professionals may better serve these patients by helping them enhance quality of life. Research indicates only a minority of hemodialysis patients receive any kind of rehabilitative services or assistance (Novello, 1991). Furthermore, studies suggest patients themselves rank dietary and fluid restrictions among the top stressors associated with their condition (e.g., Gurklis & Menke, 1988; Schneider et al., 1991).

Interestingly, Hitchcock, Brantley, Jones, and McKnight (1992) found evidence suggesting that minor stressful events themselves were predictive of variations in biochemical indices of dietary compliance. Minor stress (e.g., argument with spouse, inability to complete planned activities) may disrupt compliance with treatment recommendations in chronic-maintenance hemodialysis patients. It is somewhat intuitive to assume that minor stressful events, occurring on a daily or weekly basis, may interfere with performance of compliance behaviors in this population. An alternative explanation is that stress alters the association between dietary compliance behaviors and biochemical outcome by means of physiological effects on metabolism. Nonetheless, one implication of this study is that stress management training may enhance interventions seeking to improve compliance (Hitchcock et al., 1992).

Compliance research with dialysis patients tends to emphasize adherence to fluid and dietary recommendations, possibly at the expense of other equally important aspects of the treatment regimen. For example, an area virtually ignored involves behaviors to reduce infection risk, which ranks among the leading causes of death among hemodialysis patients (Bradley, Evans, & Calne, 1987). Dialysis patients receive instructions to cleanse their vascular access with an antibacterial agent for several minutes before dialysis initiation to decrease life-threatening septicemia infections (Luke, 1988). Behavioral observation of vascular access cleansing (VAC) procedures reveals that patients typically engage in only cursory washing (Mosley, Brantley, Jones, & McKnight, 1992).

One of the author and his colleagues (Brantley et al., 1990) examined effectiveness of four group interventions regarding ability to enhance VAC compliance in 56 hemodialysis patients. The four conditions were (1) patient education, (2) behavioral management with a monetary incentive, (3) a combination of patient education/behavioral management, and (4) attention control. The monetary incentive of the behavioral-management groups consisted of $25 given away at a raffle after the 2-week intervention. Patients obtained raffle tickets by properly cleansing their access before dialysis treatment. Whereas patients in the education, behavioral, and behavioral/education groups gave significantly more correct answers about VAC procedures at posttreatment than at pretreatment, only patients in the behavioral and behavioral/education groups completed significantly more VAC steps at posttreatment and 1-month follow-up than they did prior to treatment. However, neither group of patients maintained the gains after 1 year.

This finding is consistent with observations throughout the dialysis and general compliance literature (e.g., Boyer et al., 1990; Brownell & Jeffrey, 1987; Finn & Alcorn, 1986; Leventhal & Cameron, 1987) that patients with chronic illnesses tend to become lax in compliance over time and that they may need continuous treatment for long-term adherence. Periodic booster sessions of behavioral interventions may be all that are necessary to successfully maintain adherence (Brantley et al., 1990). Intermittent behavioral-group interventions may also serve to prevent noncompliance before it develops in new patients. Perhaps even more important is that behavioral interventions may motivate chronically ill patients to comply with treatment regimens without blaming them for compliance failures or adding pressure to their already-extensive burdens.

Treatment teams can easily administer to this patient population. Chronic maintenance hemodialysis is probably the only medical treatment administered *en masse*. Patients typically receive treatment in open units, with as many as 15–25 patients dialyzed at the same time on shifts (e.g., morning, afternoon, and evening) in some larger facilities. Although there has been much discussion regarding the aforementioned adversarial relationships that may develop between dialysis patients and staff, the comraderie that often arises among patients frequently goes unnoticed. For example, it is not uncommon for patients, waiting to be "hooked up," and their family members to socialize with others in waiting rooms.

During dialysis, patients typically receive their treatments at the same stations each session. Because stations are 10 feet apart, "neighbors" can talk during dialysis. Direct-care staff often utilize the support that patients can give to each other. A common practice is to assign new patients who may be especially apprehensive about dialysis to stations next to well-adjusted and compliant "old-timers." Besides being cost effective and logistically practical with this patient population, group interventions may exploit therapeutic effects of this ready-made support system.

In one of the few such reports in the literature, Tucker, Mulkerne, and Ziller (1982) outlined a group-treatment approach to facilitate global psychosocial adjustment among outpatient hemodialysis patients. The ongoing program, described as broad-based and cost-effective, addressed, in group sessions, issues such as marital and sexual adjustment, self-improvement, and coping with ESRD. The authors also utilized additional strategies, such as behavior management techniques, peer counseling, and deinstitutionalization of the center. Although the authors based their conclusions on a small sample, indices suggest the program contributed to positive psychosocial consequences for patients and direct-care staff. Interventions such as this, combined with behavioral approaches to enhance compliance, may provide the best strategy to assist ESRD patients in their general well-being. Incorporation of self-directed care may also benefit certain types of patients. Systematic outcome studies, however, are necessary to evaluate their effectiveness.

SUMMARY

Although hemodialysis attenuates ESRD progression and prolongs life, chronic-maintenance hemodialysis patients continue to face enormous psychological and socioeconomic pressures. Unfortunately, information regarding factors affecting psychosocial well-being of hemodialysis patients mainly comes from anecdotal reports and uncontrolled studies. For example, we need to obtain much more data concerning incidence of sexual dysfunction and depression among hemodialysis patients and information regarding to what extent such problems result from physical or psychological factors, or both. Future research must also develop and systematically study methods to enhance quality of life in hemodialysis patients.

In spite of these knowledge gaps, research in the field has increasingly concentrated on compliance issues. Psychologists, however, must avoid pitfalls of the medical-model approach to compliance, in which findings show medical professionals viewing patients as passive recipients of prescribed treatment mandates. In this framework, treatment providers expect obedience and strict adherence, and they believe that symptoms and functional deficits that persist result directly from noncompliance, which in turn result from various psychosocial aberrations. Research has indicated such a view is inappropriate and unrealistic for patients with a chronic degenerative disease, such as ESRD. Although compliance is an important goal, it must not be the only goal in rehabilitation of chronic-maintenance hemodialysis patients. Group interventions combining behavioral treatments to enhance compliance *and* strategies to facilitate global psychosocial adjustment may provide the best outcomes for this population.

REFERENCES

Abram, H. S., Moore, G. I., & Westervelt, F. G. (1971). Suicidal behavior in chronic dialysis patients. *American Journal of Psychiatry, 149,* 1624–1628.

Andreoli, T. E. (1988). Approach to the patient with renal disease. In J. B. Wyngaarden & L. H. Smith (Eds.), *Cecil textbook of medicine* (pp. 502–508). Philadelphia: Saunders.

Blackburn, S. L. (1977). Dietary compliance of chronic hemodialysis patients. *Journal of the American Dietetic Association, 70,* 31–37.

Blodgett, C. (1981). A selected review of the literature of adjustment to hemodialysis. *The International Journal of Psychiatry in Medicine, 11*(2), 97–117.

Boyer, C. B., Friend, R., Chlouverakis, G., & Kaloyanides, G. (1990). Social support and demographic factors influencing compliance of hemodialysis patients. *Journal of Applied Social Psychology, 20*(22), 1902–1918.

Bradley, J. R., Evans, D. B., & Calne, R. Y. (1987). Long-term survival in haemodialysis patients. *Lancet, 1,* 295–296.

Brantley, P. J., Mosley, Jr., T. H., Bruce, B. K., McKnight, G. T., & Jones, G. N. (1990). Efficacy of behavioral management and patient education on vascular access cleansing compliance in hemodialysis patients. *Health Psychology, 9*(1), 103–113.

Brenner, B. M., & Lazarus, J. M. (1991). Chronic renal failure. In J. D. Wilson, E. Braunwald, K. J. Issellacher, R. G. Petersdorf, J. B. Martin, A. S. Fauci, & R. K. Root (Eds.), *Harrison's principles of internal medicine* (12th ed., pp. 1150–1157). New York: McGraw-Hill.

Brownell, K. D., & Jeffrey, R. W. (1987). Improving long-term weight loss: Pushing the limits of treatment. *Behavior Therapy, 18,* 353–374.

Christensen, A. J., Smith, T. W., Turner, C. W., Holman, Jr., J. M., & Gregory, M. C. (1990). Type of hemodialysis and preference for behavioral involvement: Interactive effects on adherence in end-stage renal disease. *Health Psychology, 9*(2), 225–236.

Cordova, H. R., Benabe, J. E., & Martinez-Maldonado, M. (1991). In H. E. Jacobson, G. E. Striker, & S. Klahr, (Eds.), *The principles and practice of nephrology* (pp. 690–698). Philadelphia: Decker.

Cummings, K. M., Becker, M. H., Kirscht, J. P., & Levin, N. W. (1982). Psychosocial factors affecting adherence to medical regimens in a group of hemodialysis patients. *Medical Care, 20,* 567–580.

Czaczkes, J. W., & De-Nour, A. K. (1978). *Chronic hemodialysis as a way of life.* New York: Brunner/Mazel.

Department of Health and Human Services. (1991a). *Health care financing research report: End stage renal disease, 1989* (HCFA Publication No. 03319). Baltimore, MD: Health Care Financing Administration.

Department of Health and Human Services. (1991b). Medicare program: Coverage of Erythropoietin (EPO) used by competent home dialysis patients. *Federal Register, 56*(171), 43706–43710.

De-Nour, A. K. (1982). Psychosocial adjustment to illness scale (PAIS): A study of chronic hemodialysis patients. *Journal of Psychosomatic Research, 18,* 217–221.

De-Nour, A. K., & Czaczkes, J. W. (1972). Personality factors in chronic hemodialysis patients causing noncompliance with medical regimen. *Psychosomatic Medicine, 34,* 333–344.

Devins, G. M., Binik, Y. M., Hollomby, D. J., Barre, P. E., & Guttman, R. D. (1981). Helplessness and depression in end-stage renal disease. *Journal of Abnormal Psychology, 90,* 531–545.

Devins, G. M., Binik, Y. M., Hutchinson, T. A., Hollomby, D. J., Barre, P. E., & Guttmann, R. D. (1983). The emotional impact of end-stage renal disease. *Internal Journal of Psychiatry in Medicine, 13,* 327–343.

Devins, G. M., Mandin, H., Hons, R. B., Burgess, E. D., Klassen, J., Taub, K., Schorr, S., Letourneau, P. K., & Buckle, S. (1990). Illness intrusiveness and quality of life in end-stage renal disease: Comparison and stability across treatment modalities. *Health Psychology, 9*(2), 117–142.

Eknoyan, G. (1991). Treatment of the uremic syndrome and its complications. In H. R. Jacobson, G. E. Striker, & S. Klahr (Eds.), *The principles and practice of nephrology* (pp. 699–705). Philadelphia: Decker.

Engel, G. L. (1977). The need for a new medical model: A challenge for biomedicine. *Science, 196,* 129–136.

Eschbach, J. W., & Adamson, J. W. (1988). Recombinant human erythropoietin: Implications for nephrology. *American Journal of Kidney Diseases, 11*(3), 203–209.

Eschbach, J. W., Egrie, J. C., Downing, M. R., Browne, J. K., & Adamson, J. W. (1987). Correction of anemia of end-stage renal disease with recombinant human erythropoietin: Results of combined phase I and II clinical trials. *New England Journal of Medicine, 316,* 73–78.

Evans, R. W. (1992). Need, demand, and supply in kidney transplantation: A review of the data, an examination of issues, and projections through the year 2000. *Seminars in Nephrology, 12*(3), 234–255.

Evans, R. W., Manninen, D. L., Garrison, L. P., Hart, G., Blagg, C. R., Gutman, R. A., Hull, A. R., & Lowrie, E. G. (1985). The quality of life in patients with end-stage renal disease. *New England Journal of Medicine, 312*(9), 553–559.

Ferraro, K. F., Dixon, R. D., & Kinlaw, B. J. R. (1986). Measuring compliance among in-center hemodialysis patients. *Dialysis and Transplantation, 15*(5), 226–236, 266.

Finn, P. E., & Alcorn, J. D. (1986). Noncompliance to hemodialysis dietary regimens: Literature review and treatment recommendations. *Rehabilitation Psychology, 31,* 67–78.

Foulks, C. J., & Cushner, H. M. (1986). Sexual dysfunction in the male dialysis patient: Pathogenesis, evaluation, and therapy. *American Journal of Kidney Diseases, 8*(4), 211–222.

Freyberger, H. (1973). Six years as a psychosomaticist in a hemodialysis unit. *Psychotherapy and Psychosomatics, 22,* 226.

Gerber, K. E., & Nehemkis, A. M. (1986). Epilogue: The complex nature of compliance. In K. E. Gerber & A. M. Nehemkis, (Eds.), *Compliance: The dilemma of the chronically ill* (pp. 226–235). New York: Springer.

German, P. S. (1988). Compliance and chronic disease. *Hypertension, 11*(Suppl. 2), 56–60.

Gilli, P., & De Bastiani, P. (1983). Cognitive function and regular dialysis treatment. *Clinical Nephrology, 19*(4), 188–192.

Gorelick, P. B., Hier, D. B., Mangone, C., Robbins, S., Plioplys, A., & Kathpalia, S. (1991). Status of aluminum as a risk factor for dialysis encephalopy and Alzheimer's disease. *International Journal of Artificial Organs, 14*(2), 70–73.

Greenwald, H. P. (1987). The specificity of quality of life measures among the seriously ill. *Medical Care, 25,* 642–651.

Gurin, G., Verhoff, J., & Feld, S. (1960). *Americans view their health.* New York: Basic Books.

Gurklis, J. A., & Menke, E. M. (1988). Identification of stressors and use of coping methods in chronic hemodialysis patients. *Nursing Research, 37,* 236–239.

Hakim, R. M., & Lazarus, J. M. (1986). Management of the patient with renal failure. In B. M. Brenner & F. C. Rector (Eds.), *The kidney* (pp. 1791–1825). Philadelphia: Saunders.

Hartman, P. E., & Becker, M. H. (1978). Noncompliance with prescribed regimen among chronic hemodialysis patients: A method of prediction and educational diagnosis. *Dialysis and Transplantation, 7,* 978–989.

Hellerstedt, W. L., Johnson, W. J., Ascher, N., Kjellstrand, C. M., Knutson, R., Shapiro, F. L., & Sterioff, S. (1986). Survival rates of 2,728 patients with end-stage renal disease. *Mayo Clinic Proceedings, 59,* 776–783.

Henderson, L. W. (1979). Hemodialysis. In L. E. Earley & C. W. Gottschalk (Eds.), *Strauss & Welt: Diseases of the kidney* (3rd ed., pp. 442–448). Boston: Little, Brown.

Hitchcock, P. B., Brantley, P. J., Jones, G. N., & McKnight, G. T. (1992). Stress and social support as predictors of dietary compliance in hemodialysis patients. *Behavioral Medicine, 18,* 13–20.

Hollandsworth, J. G. (1988). Evaluating the impact of medical treatment on the quality of life: A 5-year update. *Social Science and Medicine, 26,* 425–434.

Hong, B. A., Smith, M. D., Robson, A. M., & Wetzel, R. D. (1987). Depressive symptomatology and treatment in patients with end-stage renal disease. *Psychological Medicine, 17,* 185–190.

Hoover, H. (1989). Compliance in hemodialysis patients: A review of the literature. *Journal of the American Dietetic Association, 89,* 957–959.

Jelkman, W. (1986). Erythropoietin research 80 years after the initial studies by Carnot and Deflandre. *Respiratory Physiology, 63,* 257–266.

Kaplan, R. M. (1990). Behavior as the central outcome in health care. *American Psychologist, 45*(11), 1211–1220.

Keitt, A. S. (1988). Introduction to the anemias. In J. B. Wyngaarden & L. H. Smith (Eds.), *Cecil textbook of medicine.* Philadelphia: Saunders.

Kirschenbaum, D. S. (1991). Integration of clinical psychology into hemodialysis programs. In J. J. Sweet, R. H. Rozensky, & S. M. Tovian (Eds.), *Handbook of clinical psychology in medical settings* (pp. 567–586). New York: Plenum Press.

Kokko, J. (1988). Chronic renal failure. In J. B. Wyngaarden & L. H. Smith (Eds.), *Cecil textbook of medicine* (pp. 563–573). Philadelphia: Saunders.

Kutner, N. G., & Brogan, D. (1990). Sex stereotypes and health care: The case of treatment for kidney failure. *Sex Roles, 24*(5/6), 279–290.

Kutner, N. G., Fair, P. L., & Kutner, M. H. (1985). Assessing depression and anxiety in chronic dialysis patients. *Journal of Psychosomatic Research, 29*(1), 23–31.

Levenson, J. L., & Glocheski, S. (1991). Psychological factors affecting end-stage renal disease: A review. *Psychosomatics, 32*(4), 382–389.

Leventhal, H., & Cameron, L. (1987). Behavioral theories and the problem of compliance. *Patient Education and Counseling, 10,* 117–138.

Leventhal, H., Zimmerman, R., & Gutmann, M. (1984). Compliance: A self-regulation perspective. In W. D. Gentry (Ed.), *Handbook of behavioral medicine* (pp. 369–436). New York: Guilford.

Levy, N. B. (1979). The sexual rehabilitation of the hemodialysis patient. *Sexuality and Disability, 2,* 60–65.

Luke, R. G. (1988). Dialysis. In J. B. Wyngaarden & L. H. Smith (Eds.), *Cecil textbook of medicine* (pp. 573–577). Philadelphia: Saunders.

Lundin, A. P. (1989). Quality of life: Subjective and objective improvements with recombinant human erythropoietin therapy. *Seminars in Nephrology, 9,* 22–29.

McKee, D. C., Burnett, G. B., Raft, D. D., Batten, P. G., & Bain, K. P. (1982). Longitudinal study of neuropsychological functioning in patients on chronic hemodialysis: A preliminary report. *Journal of Psychosomatic Research, 26*(5), 511–518.

Mosley, Jr., T. H., Brantley, P. J., Jones, G. N., McKnight, G. T. (1992). Predicting compliance of in-center patients to vascular access cleansing recommendations. *Dialysis and Transplantation, 21,* 216–225.

Nehemkis, A. M., & Gerber, K. E. (1986). Compliance and the quality of survival. In A. M. Nehemkis & K. E. Gerber (Eds.), *Compliance: The dilemma of the chronically ill* (pp. 73–97). New York: Springer.

Nissenson, A. R. (1989). Recombinant human erythropoietin: Impact on brain and cognitive function, exercise tolerance, sexual potency, and quality of life. *Seminars in Nephrology, 9*(1, Suppl. 2), 25–31.

Norton, J. C. (1982). *Introduction to medical psychology.* New York: Free Press.

Novello, A. C. (1991). Ethical, social, and financial aspects of ESRD. In B. M. Brenner & F. C. Rector (Eds.), *The kidney* (4th ed., pp. 2424–2443). Philadelphia: Saunders.

Oldenburg, B., MacDonald, G. J., & Perkins, R. J. (1988). Prediction of quality of life in a cohort of end-stage renal disease patients. *Journal of Clinical Epidemiology, 41*(6), 555–564.

Orme, C. M., & Binik, Y. M. (1989). Consistency of adherence across regimen demands. *Health Psychology, 8,* 27–43.

Pederson, J. A., Czerwinski, A. W., & Adams, R. L. (1983). Chronic renal failure, dialysis, and neuropsychological function. *Journal of Clinical Neuropsychology, 5*(4), 301–312.

Popovich, R. P., Moncrief, J. W., Nolph, K. D., Ghods, A. J., Twardowski, Z. J., & Pyle, W. K. (1978). Continuous ambulatory peritoneal dialysis. *Annals of Internal Medicine, 88,* 449–456.

Procci, W. R. (1981). Psychological factors associated with severe abuse of hemodialysis diet. *General Hospital Psychiatry, 3,* 111–118.

Raine, A. E. G. (1988). Hypertension, blood viscosity and cardiovascular morbidity in renal failure: Implications of erythropoietin therapy. *Lancet, 1,* 97–100.

Reichsman, R., & Levy, N. B. (1972). Problems in adaptation to maintenance hemodialysis: A four-year study of 25 patients. *Archives of Internal Medicine, 130,* 859–865.

Robertson, G. L., & Berl, T. (1986). Pathophysiology of water metabolism. In B. M. Brenner & F. C. Rector (Eds.), *The kidney* (pp. 385–432). Philadelphia: Saunders.

Ruggiero, L., Brantley, P. J., Bruce, B. K., McKnight, G. T., & Cocke, T. B. (1992). The role of dietary compliance in survival of hemodialysis patients. *Dialysis and Transplantation, 21*(1), 14–17.

Ryan, J. J., Souheaver, G. T., & DeWolfe, A. S. (1981). Halstead–Reitan test results in chronic hemodialysis. *Journal of Nervous and Mental Disease, 169*(5), 311–314.

Schneider, M. S., Friend, R., Whitaker, P. & Wadhwa, N. K. (1991). Fluid noncompliance and symptomatology in end-stage renal disease: Cognitive and emotional variables. *Health Psychology, 10*(3), 209–215.

Schwartz, A. B., Prior, J., Terizan, L., & Kahn, B. (1988). Erythropoietin for the anemia of chronic renal failure. *American Family Physician, 37,* 211–215.

Tucker, C. M., Mulkerne, D. J., & Ziller, R. C. (1982). An ecological and behavioral approach to outpatient dialysis treatment. *Journal of Chronic Diseases, 35,* 21–27.

Wauters, J. P., Hunziker, A., & Brunner, H. R. (1983). Regionalized self-care hemodialysis. *Journal of the American Medical Association, 250,* 59–62.

Wertzel, H., Vollerath, P., Ritz, E., & Ferner, H. (1977). Analysis of patient–nurse interaction in hemodialysis units. *Journal of Psychosomatic Research, 21,* 359–366.

Wolcott, D. L., Maida, C. A., Diamond, R., & Nissenson, A. R. (1986). Treatment compliance in end-stage renal disease patients on dialysis. *American Journal of Nephrology, 6,* 329–338.

25

Diabetes Mellitus
Considerations of the Influence of Stress

Virginia L. Goetsch and Deborah J. Wiebe

INTRODUCTION

Diabetes mellitus is a heterogeneous disorder of carbohydrate metabolism characterized by defects in insulin secretion or action. Insulin acts by allowing glucose to enter cells, where cellular actions metabolize glucose as an energy source. Insulin also promotes glucose storage and inhibits release of glucose from storage sites. Abnormally low insulin production or action thus contributes to chronic elevations of blood glucose (BG), the primary manifestation of diabetes. If prolonged, hyperglycemia leads to costly and life-threatening complications. Recent estimates indicate that 6.6% of the U.S. population currently has diabetes and prevalence of diabetes will increase as this population ages (Helms, 1992; Kovar, Harris, & Hadden, 1987).

There are two etiologically distinct types of diabetes. Insulin-dependent (Type I or juvenile-onset) diabetes mellitus (IDDM) manifests as an inability to produce adequate levels of insulin. Most experts now believe that a viral infection triggers an autoimmune response among genetically predisposed individuals; that response then destroys most or all insulin-producing beta cells in the pancreas (Craighead, 1978; Palmer & McCulloch, 1991). As a result, individuals with IDDM are unable to produce sufficient insulin and must take exogenous insulin on a daily basis to survive. Although onset can occur at any age, IDDM usually appears before age 30.

Non-insulin-dependent (Type II or adult-onset) diabetes mellitus (NIDDM) is

---

Virginia L. Goetsch • Department of Behavioral Medicine and Psychiatry, West Virginia University Health Sciences Center, Morgantown, West Virginia 26505.   **Deborah J. Wiebe** • Department of Psychology, University of Utah, Salt Lake City, Utah 84112.
Handbook of Health and Rehabilitation Psychology, edited by Anthony J. Goreczny. Plenum Press, New York, 1995.

more common, accounting for 80% of diabetes in the United States. Two defects—insulin resistance and insulin secretion—contribute to development of overt NIDDM (Banerji & Lebovitz, 1989; DeFronzo, Bonadonna, & Ferannini, 1992; Reaven, 1984). In many NIDDM patients, the primary defect involves impaired tissue sensitivity to insulin (i.e., insulin resistance). Although insulin resistance is initially offset by increased insulin secretion in these individuals, production of insulin eventually declines due to pancreatic exhaustion. In other NIDDM patients, the primary defect appears to be deficient insulin secretion; insulin resistance develops concomitantly with or subsequent to this defect (DeFronzo et al., 1992). Both defects appear genetically mediated, as evidenced by 90–100% concordance rates among monozygotic twins (Barnett, Eff, Leslie, & Pyke, 1981). However, environmental or behavioral factors also may be important; obesity increases risk for NIDDM, and weight reduction decreases insulin resistance in NIDDM patients (Wing, 1991). Onset of NIDDM is gradual and usually occurs after age 40.

Although IDDM and NIDDM are physiologically distinct, they share an inability to utilize glucose as a source of energy. This inability can have short- and long-term health consequences. In absence of insulin, the body catabolizes proteins and fats to provide an alternative energy source. Catabolism of body fat produces excessive amounts of ketoacids that, if untreated, can cause coma and death. Long-term diabetic complications are also severe. Diabetic individuals have heightened risk for development of macrovascular diseases, such as coronary heart disease and stroke. Diabetes is also a leading cause of blindness, kidney disease, and lower limb amputations in the United States (Keen & Jarrett, 1982; National Center for Health Statistics, 1980). It is not surprising that, as serious complications develop, patients with diabetes report decreasing quality of life and increasing anxiety and depression (Lloyd, Matthews, Wing, & Orchard, 1992; Wredling, Theorell, Roll, Lins, & Adamson, 1992).

Adequate control of BG can prevent or delay onset of diabetic complications (Knuiman, Welborn, McCann, Stanton, & Constable, 1986; Skyler, 1987). Thus, the treatment goal for both IDDM and NIDDM is to maintain BG levels within a relatively normal range. To this end, individuals with diabetes must engage in a complex self-management regimen, including various combinations of dietary restrictions, exercise, self-monitoring of blood or urine glucose, insulin, and/or oral medications.

Researchers have theorized that psychosocial factors influence progression and management of diabetes in many ways (see Cox, Gonder-Frederick, Pohl, and Pennebaker, 1986 and Cox, Gonder-Frederick, and Cox, Gonder-Frederick and Saunders, 1991, for reviews). The focus of the present chapter is the role of one such factor—psychological stress—in the etiology, progression, and management of both IDDM and NIDDM. In following sections, we initially describe interrelated physiological and psychological pathways theorized to link stressful events to parameters of diabetes control (e.g., BG levels). We then review the empirical literature to determine extent to which research has tested, and supported or refuted, one such pathway: direct effects of stressful events on BG and metabolism. Finally, we discuss theoretical, empirical, and clinical implications of this body of literature.

STRESS AND DIABETES

There are at least two mechanisms through which stressful events can affect blood glucose and other health-related parameters in individuals with diabetes.

Health status can be changed by deviations from the diabetic regimen, and stressful life events can exert a negative influence on adherence to the regimen. This is considered an *indirect* mechanism by which stress affects diabetes. All human beings are potentially susceptible to such stress-related deviations in health behaviors; it is likely that most people can recall at least one occasion when some stressful event or events led them to skip their daily exercise, go to bed without flossing their teeth, or indulge in chocolate rather than fruit for dessert. However, given the pathophysiology of diabetes, such deviations can have life-threatening implications. Nonadherence can trigger acute hyperglycemia and, if prolonged or repeated, can influence development of chronic health problems associated with diabetes. Diabetic individuals also may be particularly vulnerable to stress-related lapses in adherence simply because of complexity of their regimen (Marlatt & Gordon, 1985). Thus, stressful events may have important *indirect* effects on BG through influence on regimen adherence.

More germane to this chapter are the *direct* physiological effects of stressors on BG. Since early observations by Cannon (1941), there has been wide acceptance of the notion that stressful events provoke central nervous system (CNS) and peripheral physiological changes (i.e., increases in cortical activity, levels of peripheral hormones, heart rate, blood pressure, and perspiration, along with an altered distribution of blood flow). Another important component of this classic "fight or flight" response is an increase in BG. It makes inherent sense that increased availability of energy sources (i.e., glucose) would enhance likelihood of survival from threat. Increases in circulating glucose may not be adaptive for those with diabetes, however, especially if prolonged or if episodic hyperglycemia ensues.

Several pathways function to increase available energy in the face of threat. Figure 25.1 summarizes these pathways (Goetsch, 1989). The pancreas and liver receive alpha and beta innervation from the sympathetic nervous system (SNS; Young & Landsberg, 1979). Increased sympathetic activity inhibits insulin and stimulates glucagon release by the pancreas. Glucagon, in turn, stimulates gluconeogenesis, conversion of glycogen to glucose by the liver, and release of hepatic glucose stores into the bloodstream. Increased levels of circulating epinephrine and cortisol, released from the adrenals, affects the pancreas, liver, and peripheral tissues as well. For example, epinephrine increases peripheral insulin resistance, and inhibits insulin release by the pancreas and glucose storage by the liver. Cortisol increases peripheral insulin resistance and stimulates hepatic glucose production. Other hormones, in addition to classic "stress hormones," also influence glucoregulatory aspects of the stress response. For example, growth hormone and endogenous opiates also influence level of circulating glucose (McCubbin, Surwit, Kuhn, Cochrane, & Feinglos, 1987). Thus, researchers have identified multiple physiological mechanisms through which stressful events can affect BG, but in order to fully understand the complex interactions of various SNS and hormonal mediators, substantial work still remains to be done.

In addition to appreciation of physiological mechanisms through which stress affects BG, we must consider research investigating stress–BG relationships in a theoretical context. Although a thorough discussion of various conceptualizations of stress is not feasible, the interested reader can refer to Chapter 14 by Brantley and Thomason. In general, theorists adopt one of three broad conceptualizations of stress: stress as a response, stimulus, or "transaction" between individuals and the environment. Although many investigators do not explicitly state a theoretical mod-

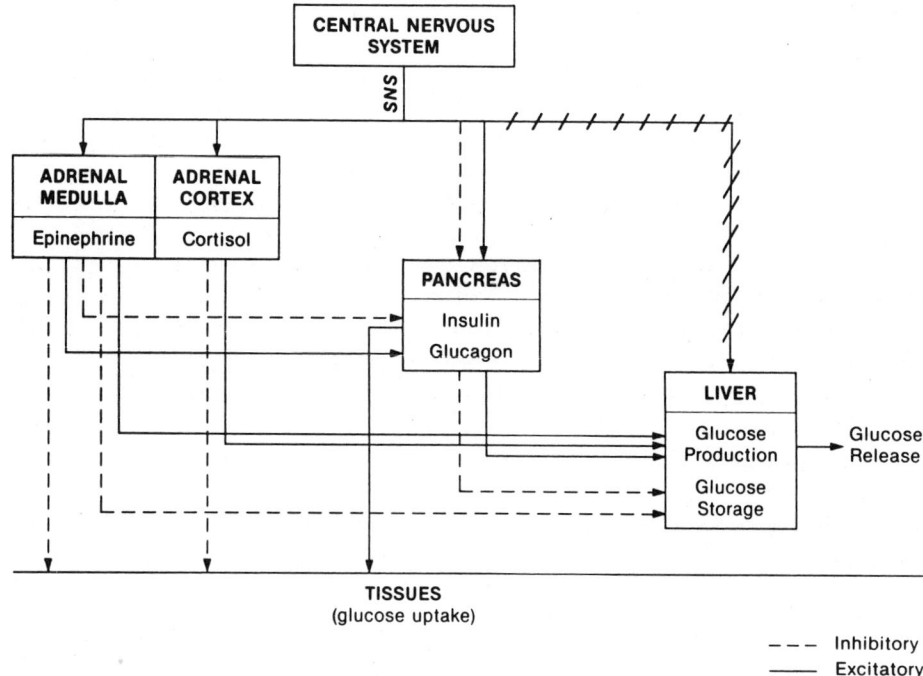

Figure 25.1. Schematic of some of the hormonal and sympathetic nervous system (SNS) influences on blood glucose (from Goetsch, 1989).

el, the experimental design or data interpretation they use usually indicates their orientation. As an example, physiologists interested in stress most often take an interest in responses, that is, the physiological consequences of various stress manipulations. Proponents of such response-based models have less concern regarding qualities of stimuli necessary to elicit a response and place more interest in physiological characteristics of responses. In contrast, other professionals have focused on characteristics of events classified as stressors. Work in this area has focused on definition and characterization of naturally occurring events (e.g., major and minor life experiences) that people find stressful.

Many stress researchers have taken a "transactional" stance (Lazarus & Folkman, 1984), recognizing that we must consider characteristics of individuals (i.e., physiological, psychological, and/or behavioral responses), situations (i.e., antecedent stressors or life experiences), and the interaction of these two domains; that is, consequences of any event are a function of both quality and intensity of the event and various characteristics of individuals' responses (e.g., perceived threat, avoidant coping response) to the event. Such a model acknowledges that individuals do not all respond in the same manner to an identical stressor, and each individual may respond differently to different stressors. Thus, research that incorporates measures of individuals, stimulus conditions, and complex interactions of these two domains seems likely to provide the most comprehensive, meaningful information.

REVIEW OF THE EMPIRICAL LITERATURE

Studies of effects of stressful events on BG regulation have employed several paradigms, each with its own inherent strengths and drawbacks. Most paradigms either explicitly or implicitly adopt a stimulus or response-based approach to stress. For example, studies employing laboratory animal models of diabetes, and chemical infusion and laboratory stress-induction procedures with diabetic individuals focus on BG and other physiological responses to a wide variety of stressors. Retrospective and prospective studies regarding the influence of daily stress and major life events primarily focus on stimulus conditions in which dysregulation occurs. Few studies of individual differences or interactions of individuals and environments exist. The following sections give readers an appreciation of the current status of research investigating effects of stressful events on BG in individuals with diabetes.

Animal Models

Researchers have used several laboratory animal models of diabetes to examine effects of acute stressors on development of overt diabetes and on physiological responses of animals with established diabetes. For example, animal models of IDDM have included surgical (i.e., pancreatectomy) and chemical (B-cell cytotoxin) manipulations, and at least two animal models of IDDM spontaneously develop diabetes. Restraint (Capponi, Kawada, Varela, & Vargas, 1980) and a combination of stressors (crowding, random home-cage reassignment, and rotational stress; Carter, Hermann, Stokes, & Cox, 1987) hasten development of overt diabetes in these animals. In contrast, Huang, Plaut, Taylor, and Wareheim (1981) found that shock inhibited development of diabetes in a chemical model of IDDM, and Ader, Johnson, Huang, and Riley (1991) found evidence that high emotionality associated with delayed onset of IDDM in an animal model that spontaneously develops diabetes.

Only two studies have evaluated the influence of stressors on BG in animals with established IDDM. Ader, Kreutner, and Jacobs (1963) found significantly higher BG and mortality rates in a chemically induced animal model of IDDM when animals lived in groups rather than being housed individually, but individually housed animals showed more emotionality. It is hard to explain the seemingly opposing effects of stressful group-housing conditions versus emotionality produced by individual caging (Ader et al., 1963; Ader et al., 1991). The former appears to hasten onset of IDDM and exacerbate glycemic responses in IDDM animals, and the latter appears to provide a protective effect. Nor is it clear why shock had a protective effect regarding development of diabetes (Huang et al., 1981). However, a second investigation with a standard stressor (foot shock) demonstrated hyperglycemic responses in rats with established chemically induced diabetes as well as in nondiabetic comparison animals (Lee, Konorska, & McCarty, 1989). Thus, there is some support for diabetogenic and hyperglycemic effects of stressful conditions in animal models of IDDM as well as data to suggest that stressors can produce hyperglycemic responses in nondiabetic animals. Our current state of knowledge does not permit us to adequately explain inconsistencies in the findings, particularly the distinction between emotionality and stressor effects and contradictory effects of shock. There are, however, inherent differences in the pathophysiology of various animal models of IDDM represented in the empirical literature that may someday help explain the different effects. In spite of the contradictory effects of shock and emotionality, stressful housing conditions, restraint, and combined stressors do have consistently deleterious effects on BG in animal models of IDDM.

Probably most well known is work by Surwit, Feinglos, and colleagues, who investigated effects of standard stressors and various chemicals on BG and mechanisms of such effects in an animal model of NIDDM, the obese ob/ob mouse (Kuhn, Cochrane, Feinglos, & Surwit, 1987; Surwit & Feinglos, 1983; Surwit, Feinglos, Livingston, Kuhn, & McCubbin, 1984; Surwit, McCubbin, Kuhn, McGee, Gerstenfeld, & Feinglos, 1986). The ob/ob strain is obese and suffers from hyperglycemia and peripheral insulin resistance and, thus, is a valuable animal model of NIDDM. Not all mice in a given litter develop obesity and other characteristics of NIDDM, and these animals carry the ob/? label. They serve as an excellent comparison group in studies of influence of stressors on BG. Surwit and colleagues found that a standard stressor, restraint and shaking, produced increases in BG and decreases in insulin in ob/ob mice; the stressor also produced increases in BG, although to a lesser extent, in their lean ob/? littermates. Another group of researchers demonstrated hyperglycemic effects due to intubation with an earlier, chemically induced animal model of NIDDM using sand rats (Mikat, Hackel, Cruz, & Lebovitz, 1972).

Kuhn, Cochrane, Feinglos, and Surwit (1987) found effects similar to these studies when they infused epinephrine in lean (ob/?) and obese (ob/ob) mice. In addition, phentolamine, an alpha antagonist, resulted in insulin increases that were greater in obese than lean mice. This last finding suggested that effects of stressors on BG and insulin in ob/ob mice result from alpha-adrenergic mediation and replicated earlier work with a chemically induced animal model of NIDDM, KK mice (Fujimoto, Sakaguchi, & Ui, 1981).

These studies are remarkable in their relatively consistent demonstration of hyperglycemic and, in some cases, hypoinsulinemic effects of standard stressors in various animal models. The advantage of such work is the great degree of experimental control that is possible. The obvious problem is the difficulty generalizing such data to humans with diabetes.

Chemical Infusion

Some researchers have conducted response-based hormone infusion studies, similar to those with animal models, with diabetic and nondiabetic humans. This work often attempts to simulate "normal" hormone responses to stressful events in a controlled manner to examine subsequent effects on BG and insulin. A large number of studies have shown a relatively consistent pattern of hyperglycemic responses secondary to infusion of epinephrine, cortisol, and glucagon, or combinations of these hormones, in nondiabetic and diabetic adults and children (Baker, Kaye, & Haque, 1967; Fernqvist, Gunnarsson, & Linde, 1988; Gerich, Lorenzi, Tsalikian, & Karem, 1976; Hamberg, Hendler, & Sherwin, 1980; Ortiz-Alonzo et al., 1991; Shamoon, Hendler, & Sherwin, 1980; Soman, Shamoon, & Sherwin, 1980). IDDM and NIDDM subjects tend to show exaggerated hyperglycemic responses compared to modest hyperglycemic effects found in nondiabetics (Gerich et al., 1976; Ortiz-Alonzo et al., 1991). Epinephrine also decreases pancreatic beta cell sensitivity to glucose (i.e., epinephrine results in a blunted insulin response to increased BG) in nondiabetic subjects and decreases maximal beta cell secretory capacity in NIDDM subjects (Ortiz-Alonzo et al., 1991).

Thus, as a whole, these studies consistently support the notion that stressful events have hyperglycemic and hypoinsulinemic effects. However, endogenous physiological responses to stress involve a myriad of interacting neural and hormonal influences that are impossible to completely mimic with exogenous hormone infusions. These data also are much more consistent than those with psychological stressors, so generalization to physiological effects of naturally occurring stressors seems unwarranted at this point.

Laboratory Stress Induction

Numerous studies regarding influence of psychological stress on BG in individuals with diabetes have employed brief laboratory stressors to elicit neural and hormonal "fight or flight" responses. This research is notable for its inconsistent findings, particularly in contrast to the relatively clear-cut results with animal models and chemical infusion. Various laboratory stressors have produced hyperglycemic, hypoglycemic, or nonsignificant effects on BG in IDDM, NIDDM, and nondiabetic subjects. Rather than rejecting this paradigm, a closer examination of discrepancies in methodology and design may help reconcile the current data and provide a framework for more successful and consistent investigations.

Brief laboratory stressors, such as mental arithmetic and threat of shock, have produced increases in BG in NIDDM subjects (Goetsch, VanDorsten, Pbert, Ullrich, & Yeater, 1987; Goetsch, Wiebe, Veltum, & VanDorsten, 1990); some investigators, however, have found that stressful imagery, mental arithmetic, and a physical stressor (repeated grip-strength testing) resulted in no effects on BG in NIDDM subjects (Goetsch et al., 1987; Naliboff, Cohen, & Sowers, 1985). Still other researchers have found nonsignificant group effects on BG in IDDM adults and children after mental arithmetic (Carter, Gonder-Frederick, Cox, Clarke, & Scott, 1985; Gonder-Frederick, Carter, Cox, & Clarke, 1990; Kemmer et al., 1984), noise (Carter et al., 1985), digit symbol subtest of the Wechsler Adult Intelligence Scale-Revised (Edwards & Yates, 1985), public speaking (Gilbert, Johnson, Silverstein, & Malone, 1989; Kemmer et al., 1984), video games (Cox, Gonder-Frederick, Clarke, & Carter, 1988), and viewing a gory film (Gonder-Frederick et al., 1990).

Numerous methodological differences characterize these studies. Probably the most readily obvious difference is number and diverse types of stressors chosen. The duration of stressors and intervals between stressor administrations and blood samplings have also varied, as have prestressor baseline BGs (i.e., some studies employed an overnight fast prior to the laboratory session, whereas in others, subjects ate a standard meal immediately prior to the session). This last point may be particularly critical; Cox et al. (1988) demonstrated that a video game stressor had differential effects on the same subjects depending on whether their BG at prestressor baseline was relatively high and rising or low and falling. The stressor had a significant effect relative to a no-stress condition only in the second condition.

Also, not all studies have documented that stressors were indeed stressful; some studies failed to measure subjective and physiological changes, such as epinephrine, cortisol, electrodermal activity, heart rate, and/or blood pressure. Although we usually presume manipulations such as arithmetic and stressful imagery are stressful, such presumptions may not always be valid. The findings of McLesky, Lewis, and Woodruff (1978) highlight this point. These researchers found that surgical stress produced increases in glucagon that were significantly greater in a mixed group of NIDDM and IDDM subjects relative to nondiabetics. Although they did not report BG data, given the nature of physiological effects of glucagon, one might expect that surgical stress also produced increases in BG that were greater in diabetic subjects than nondiabetics. Although this study must undergo replication with separate groups of IDDM and NIDDM subjects, contrast between probable intensity of surgical stress compared with relatively mild laboratory stressors described earlier emphasizes the necessity of validating "stressfulness" of stressors.

Furthermore, individual differences in response to various stressors and differences across individuals in response to the same stressor may result in difficulty detecting a stress effect that is consistent across all subjects. For example, one group of investigators in two studies has demonstrated that BG response to stressors in IDDM subjects is idiosyncratic, but a delayed retest with the same stressor revealed that subjects were highly consistent regarding direction and magnitude of BG response (Carter et al., 1985; Gonder-Frederick et al., 1990). This group also demonstrated that absolute BG response was greater with an active stressor (mental arithmetic) than with a passive one (viewing a gory film; Gonder-Frederick et al., 1990). Thus, both individual differences in physiological response and differences across various types of stressors are important considerations. This point is reminiscent of the earlier theoretical discussion advocating a transactional model of stress. Specific (and ideally, causal) characteristics of individuals who are more or less responsive to stressors, or who respond with hyperglycemia versus hypoglycemia, remain unknown. Such characteristics, discussed in a later section of this chapter, may be dispositional/psychological (e.g., emotional lability, anxiety), behavioral (e.g., avoidant coping style), physiological (e.g., autonomic neuropathy or hyperresponsive adrenals), and/or constitutional (e.g., aerobic fitness). Further investigations regarding influences of various types of stressors (e.g., active vs. passive), as well as demonstration of external validity of laboratory data, will likely help reconcile current discrepancies.

Stressful Life Events

Some researchers have investigated relationships between naturally occurring life stressors and various diabetes parameters. Robinson and associates found that individuals with IDDM report having experienced more severe life stressors in the time prior to diagnosis than do nondiabetic siblings or neighborhood controls (Robinson & Fuller, 1985; Robinson, Lloyd, Fuller, & Yateman, 1988). It is possible that onset of diabetes creates stress in people's lives and that presence of a life-threatening illness biases recall of previously experienced events. Nevertheless, such findings are consistent with the hypothesis that psychological stress contributes to development of IDDM.

Numerous studies have also investigated the relationship between life stress and glycosylated hemoglobin (HbA1c), an index of BG control over the preceding 6 to 8 weeks (Nathan, Singer, Hurxthal, & Goodson, 1984). Because higher HbA1c levels reflect poorer metabolic control, a positive relationship suggests that stress disrupts BG control. Resulting data have been highly inconsistent regardless of type of diabetes studied. Several authors have reported significant positive correlations between life stress and HbA1c independent of regimen adherence (Chase & Jackson, 1981; Cox, Taylor, Nowacek, Holley-Wilcox, Pohl, & Guthrow, 1984; Demmers, Neale, Winsloff, Gronsman, & Jaber, 1989; Hanson, Henggeler, & Burghen, 1987a, 1987b), but others have found nonsignificant relationships (Delamater, Kurtz, Bubb, White, & Santiago, 1987; Griffith, Field, & Lustman, 1990; Halford, Cuddihy, & Mortimer, 1990; Neimcryk, Speers, Travis, & Gary, 1990; Rhodewalt & Marcroft, 1988; Wilson et al., 1986).

Numerous problems with this methodological approach preclude clear interpretations of the data. First, measurement of stress varies dramatically across studies. Some investigators have measured life stress by scoring items that participants subjectively evaluated as undesirable and, at other times, by scoring experienced events regardless of subjective impact. Consistent with the transactional model of stress discussed earlier, such measurement differences alter the pattern of stress–HbA1c relationships in the same subject samples; negatively evaluated events consistently have greater impact (Brand, J. Johnson, & S. Johnson, 1986; Frenzel, McCaul, Glasgow, & Schafer, 1988; Jacobson, Rand, & Hauser, 1985). Second, we cannot draw causal inferences due to the correlational nature of the data. It is quite possible that poorly controlled diabetes increases level of stress in one's life rather than vice versa. Third, long-term measures of both life stress and BG control may represent insensitive tests of potentially acute effects of stress on BG levels. Indeed, some authors have argued that daily stress is more predictive of general health status than are major life events (DeLongis, Coyne, Dakof, Folkman, & Lazarus, 1982). For example, Halford et al. (1990) found no relationship between life stress and HbA1c measures among subjects with IDDM; however, when the investigators measured association between daily stress and daily BG levels, half of the subjects were stress responsive. These data are consistent with the notion that life stress methodologies provide relatively weak tests of the stress–BG hypothesis.

Home-Monitoring Studies

Home-monitoring studies represent a relatively new approach toward studying relationships between stress and BG levels in individuals with diabetes. With this approach, subjects monitor naturally occurring stressors as they transpire on a daily basis. Researchers can then assess associations between these acute measures of life stress and BG both within and across subjects. This approach has several distinct advantages. First, it allows one to assess relationships between daily-life stress and acute BG fluctuations. Individuals with diabetes generally believe such relationships exist (Cox et al., 1984), but tests of accuracy of these beliefs have been rare. Second, if we obtain multiple measures of daily stress and BG within the same individuals, it is possible to determine whether some individuals are stress responders whereas others are not. Finally, this methodology provides an opportunity to determine whether acute BG responses observed in the laboratory generalize to patients' ongoing lives.

Hanson and Pichert (1986) studied adolescents with IDDM for 3 days during a diabetes camp. Each day, subjects recorded both occurrence and positive or negative impact of any stressors they had experienced. Measurement of diet and exercise also occurred on a daily basis. Between-subjects analyses revealed that negatively evaluated stress significantly and positively correlated with average daily BG levels. Although negative stress also associated with some diet and exercise measures, the stress–BG relationship remained significant after statistically controlling for effects of self-care behaviors.

Halford et al. (1990) asked 15 adults with IDDM to measure their BG three times daily for 8 weeks. Each evening, subjects also completed one-item measures of stress, aerobic exercise, and diet. The investigators then used daily stress measures to predict average daily BG levels for each subject. Seven subjects displayed a significant positive stress–BG relationship (i.e., stress responders) that remained significant after statistically controlling for influence of diet and exercise. Eight subjects displayed no significant stress–BG relationships. The only identifiable difference between stress responders and nonresponders was that responders had more variability on daily stress scores.

In a third home-monitoring study, IDDM subjects completed daily stress and adherence measures on six discrete occasions over a 6-week time period (Aikens, Wallander, Bell, & Cole, 1992). Average daily stress did not relate to HbA1c levels, an index of BG control over the 6-week interval. However, higher daily stress variability did associate with poorer glycemic control, and this relationship occurred independent of adherence. Although daily stress variability is not a standard stress measure, these data are consistent with the Halford et al. (1990) findings that stress responders had more variability on stress scores than did nonresponders. The possibility that fluctuations in stress levels are more harmful than chronically elevated stress levels deserves additional empirical attention.

Only one home-monitoring study has utilized NIDDM subjects (Goetsch et al., 1990). In this study, the investigators behaviorally, rather than statistically, controlled effects of diet and exercise. After monitoring all food intake and activity levels for 3 days, subjects repeated this 3-day diet and activity regimen four times across a 12-day period. Assessment of BG levels occurred four times daily. The investigators measured stress prior to each BG assessment (acute stress) as well as at the end of each day (daily stress). Average BG ranges were larger on high versus low daily stress days. In addition, 4 of 6 subjects displayed significant positive correlations between acute stress and BG levels. Interestingly, among subjects with positive stress–BG relationships, strength of stress–BG correlations were perfectly consistent with the relative magnitude of BG reactions to a laboratory stressor (mental arithmetic).

In summary, a variety of home-monitoring procedures with both IDDM and NIDDM subjects have consistently found positive stress–BG relationships. Although none of the studies measured neuroendocrine processes presumed to mediate stress effects, all of the home-monitoring studies found that stress–BG relationships occur independent of adherence. Thus, stress-related increases in BG did not appear to occur via indirect behavioral mechanisms. As discussed in more detail later, further research is necessary to explain why some individuals reliably display increased BG levels in response to stress while others do not. We believe the home-monitoring paradigm offers a particularly well-suited methodology for identifying such individual vulnerabilities to stress. In this process, however, it may prove necessary to refine methodological and statistical procedures in order to capture accurate pictures of stress–BG relationships in everyday life (see Stone, Kessler, and Haythornwaite, 1991, Tennen, Suls, and Affleck, 1991, and Wheeler and Reis, 1991, for reviews of such issues).

Stress-Management Interventions

In this section, we review investigations regarding glycemic effects of stress-management interventions among individuals with diabetes. This review serves two major purposes. First, such investigations provide additional information about relationships between stress and BG levels. If pharmacological or behavioral reduction of stress improves glycemic control, this offers additional evidence that stress has a deleterious effect on BG levels. Second, this literature provides important information for health psychologists who work with diabetic populations and have interests in utilizing psychological/behavioral interventions to enhance clinical management of this disease.

Pharmacological Interventions

Researchers have not systematically investigated pharmacological interventions to alter effects of stress on glycemic control. Baker and colleagues, however, reported suggestive evidence that beta-blocking medication (propranolol) improves diabetes control in IDDM children responsive to psychological and physiological stressors (Baker, Barcai, Kaye, & Hague, 1969; Baker, Kaye, & Hague, 1967). Alprazolam, a benzodiazepine, also lowered BG responsivity to stress in an animal model of NIDDM (Surwit et al., 1986). Such data suggest that pharmacological interventions may be useful to modify stress-induced hyperglycemia in some diabetic patients. It is important to note, however, that this possibility needs further empirical support and that long-term use of some medications, notably beta-blockers, can deleteriously affect diabetes control (Surwit, Ross, & Feinglos, 1991).

Stress-Management and Relaxation Interventions

Studies employing relaxation training have shown that relaxation decreases both adrenocortical activity and circulating catecholamines. Given that such neuroendocrine processes theoretically mediate stress effects on BG, it is not surprising that researchers have attempted to improve diabetes control through relaxation interventions. Case studies and single-subject designs provide suggestive evidence that biofeedback and relaxation training improve parameters of glycemic control, such as insulin requirements, daily BG levels, and BG excursions (e.g., Fowler, Budzynski, & Vandenbergh, 1976; Lammers, Naliboff, & Straatmeyer, 1984; Landis et al., 1985; Rosenbaum, 1983; Seeburg & DeBoer, 1980). Unfortunately, these data are difficult to interpret due to small and imprecisely defined subject samples, lack of control groups, simultaneous applications of multiple treatments, and lack of evidence that the relaxation intervention was effective.

Recently, investigators have conducted several well-controlled studies. Feinglos, Hastedt, and Surwit (1987) investigated 20 patients with IDDM who had histories of poor glycemic control. Subjects randomly assigned to a treatment condition received progressive muscle-relaxation training and EMG biofeedback during a 1-week hospitalization, and they engaged in daily practice at home subsequent to discharge. Subjects in the control group were hospitalized under identical conditions but received no relaxation intervention. EMG changes revealed that treatment subjects learned more how to relax than control subjects. However, treatment and control subjects did not differ on any measure of diabetes control (i.e., glucose tolerance, insulin dose, and hbA1c levels).

Surwit and Feinglos (1983) utilized a very similar design with a sample of poorly controlled adults with NIDDM. Relaxation subjects displayed improved glucose tolerance and postprandial BG levels relative to control subjects. Subjects in the relaxation condition also displayed decreases in plasma cortisol from pre- to posttreatment assessments, whereas those in the control group displayed cortisol increases (Surwit & Feinglos, 1984). Such data suggest that relaxation-induced improvements in BG control occurred via altered adrenal cortical activity. In a more recent study of patients with NIDDM, Surwit, Lane, McCaskill, Ross, and Feinglos (1992) assessed benefits of adding relaxation training to intensive conventional therapy. Although relaxation training did not improve long-term glycemic control or glucose tolerance for all subjects, individuals with high trait-anxiety scores appeared to benefit from relaxation interventions more than did individuals with low anxiety.

To summarize, the most well-controlled studies indicate that relaxation training improves glycemic control among patients with NIDDM but not among patients with IDDM. Furthermore, recent data suggest that NIDDM patients who are dispositionally anxious are most likely to benefit from such psychological interventions. As a result of these data, Surwit and colleagues have argued that stress effects on glycemic control are generally more profound among persons with NIDDM and that clinicians need to direct interventions to manage stress primarily at this population (Feinglos et al., 1987; Surwit & Feinglos, 1988; Surwit et al., 1991). However, it may be premature to disregard potential benefits of relaxation training in IDDM subjects given the paucity of well-controlled research in this area.

Exercise Interventions

Multiple studies with other populations have demonstrated that aerobic fitness can attenuate physiological reactivity to stressful events (Crews & Landers, 1987). Training appears to have its effect by buffering catecholamine release (Blumenthal et al., 1990). Thus, one would predict that exercise interventions and comparisons of subjects who are aerobically fit with those who are sedentary will reveal similar palliative effects that extend to BG. Only one unpublished study has examined this possibility with NIDDM subjects. Goetsch, Pbert, VanDorsten, Yeater, and Ullrich (1988) found that BG response to laboratory stress (threat of shock) attenuated after 3 months of thrice weekly aerobic training. It is unclear whether attenuation of catecholamine response or some other mechanism mediated effects of training, but these preliminary findings encourage further research in the area.

FACTORS MODERATING THE STRESS–BLOOD GLUCOSE RELATIONSHIP

A recurring theme in the literature reviewed previously is that although stress does not uniformly disrupt glycemic control, it does have an adverse impact among some diabetic individuals. Carter et al. (1985) and Gonder-Frederick et al. (1990) reported that a subgroup of individuals with IDDM displayed BG increases in response to a laboratory stressor; those responses were reliable over time. Halford et al. (1990) found that approximately half of their IDDM subjects displayed positive daily stress–BG relationships whereas the remaining subjects did not. Similarly, Goetsch et al. (1990) found that 4 of 6 NIDDM subjects demonstrated positive acute stress–BG associations. In this section, we review literature regarding various factors that may distinguish stress responders from nonresponders.

Physiological Factors

Numerous physiological factors, such as beta-blocking medications, oral hypoglycemic agents (Gerich, 1989; Peters & Davidson, 1992), and physical fitness (American Diabetes Association, 1991) may alter SNS processes and/or insulin secretion and action. Studies of stress and diabetes often fail to measure or control for these variables, which may be contributing to the inconsistent picture regarding stress–BG relationships.

Because diabetic autonomic neuropathy compromises SNS functions, neuropathic subjects may be less likely to display sympathetically mediated BG fluctuations than nonneuropaths. Locatelli et al. (1989) found that IDDM patients with autonomic neuropathy displayed smaller heart rate increases to mental arithmetic than did nonneuropathic patients and nondiabetic controls; patients without neuropathy displayed heart rate responses that were not different from nondiabetic controls. Although no group displayed increased BG levels in response to the stressor, such data suggest that autonomic neuropathy may make some diabetic individuals physically incapable of displaying significant BG reactions to stress.

As mentioned earlier, Surwit et al. (1991; Surwit & Feinglos, 1988) argued that stress influences BG in NIDDM but not IDDM individuals. They based this hypothesis on differential responses to relaxation training among the two populations as well as on differences in alpha-adrenergic sensitivity and lability of glycemic control. Although this notion must undergo direct tests, the possibility that type of diabetes moderates stress–BG relationships could also explain some inconsistencies in the literature.

Individual Differences

There have been several attempts to identify personality variables that distinguish stress responders from nonresponders. Stabler, Lane, Ross, Morris, Litton, and Surwit (1988) asked IDDM children who were Type A or Type B to play a challenging video game while receiving negative performance feedback. Subjects with the Type A pattern displayed larger hyperglycemic responses than did those with the Type B pattern. Although Rhodewalt and Marcroft (1988) found that Type A behavior also associated with poorer long-term glycemic control in adults with IDDM, two other studies have failed to find this relationship (Cox et al., 1984; Stabler et al., 1988). Trait anger, a characteristic that appears related to the Type A pattern, also has related to poorer glycemic control (Lane, Stabler, Ross, Morris, Litton, & Surwit, 1988; Peyrot & McMurry, 1985).

Numerous studies have attempted to determine effects of trait anxiety on diabetic control. Although some authors have found trait anxiety associated with poorer long-term BG control (Neimcryk et al., 1990; Turkat, 1982), the bulk of this literature indicates that trait anxiety does not relate to objective indices of glycemic control (Delamater et al., 1987; Lane et al., 1988; Simonds, Goldstein, Walker, & Rawlings, 1981; Wilson et al., 1986). Nonetheless, the finding that trait-anxious NIDDM patients receive more benefit from relaxation training than low-anxious patients (Surwit et al., 1992) suggests this variable deserves additional empirical attention.

Dispositional variables theorized to "buffer" stress effects have also undergone investigation. Lane et al. (1988) found that high trait curiosity and sociability associated with better long-term BG control and lower mean BG levels during home-monitoring. The authors hypothesized that curiosity and sociability had this positive impact because they buffered against adverse effects of stress by enhancing coping flexibility. Although this hypothesis is interesting, potential mediational processes that went unmeasured limit conclusions we can draw. Aikens and colleagues (1992) studied influence of learned resourcefulness, a variable theorized to improve one's ability to self-regulate behavioral and psychophysiological responses to stress (Rosenbaum, 1983). In contrast to expectations, learned resourcefulness negatively related to BG control.

In summary, despite numerous attempts to document dispositional differences in BG–stress responsivity, it is difficult to draw firm conclusions from existing literature. The data are highly inconsistent and, with only a few exceptions, have utilized IDDM populations. This is significant in light of the suggestion that stress has stronger effects among NIDDM than IDDM subjects. In addition, instruments used to measure specific personality variables have varied widely across studies and, in some cases, may not represent the most reliable or valid choices. In the case of Type A behavior, for example, no study has utilized the Structured Interview, despite the fact that this is the only Type A measure that relates to objective long-term health outcomes (Matthews, 1988). Finally, theoretical processes underlying relationships among personality, stress, and glycemic control have only rarely undergone investigation and study. Clinicians and researchers have often theorized that individual differences affect health by exacerbating or attenuating adverse effects of stress (Wiebe & Smith, in press). Such models imply that personality and stress interact to affect health outcomes, such as glycemic control. Although there are some exceptions, interactive effects of personality and stress have received inadequate evaluation in the diabetes literature.

Social Support

A large body of literature has evolved around the notion that social support protects one's health by moderating or buffering adverse effects of stress (Cohen & Wills, 1985). In the diabetes literature, measures of social support and/or social competence have been found uncorrelated with long-term BG control when analyzed independently of stress (Cox et al., 1984; Griffith et al., 1990; Hanson et al., 1987a, 1987b; Wilson et al., 1986). However, when evaluating interactions between stress and social support, significant stress-buffering effects have evolved in some (Griffith et al., 1990; Hanson et al., 1987b), but not all cases (Cox et al., 1984). Reported interactions reveal that stress disrupts glycemic control primarily among diabetic individuals with low levels of social support or social competence. Additional research is clearly necessary to establish reliability of such findings. If social support does moderate stress, interventions that improve social support could be beneficial for diabetic patients who are stress responders.

Taken together, the literature reviewed in this section suggests that research studies have identified no factors that consistently mediate or moderate effects of stressful events on glucose metabolism. Part of the reason for this is certainly the relatively recent application of the idea that physiological and/or psychological factors may moderate individuals' responses to stressors. Further systematic characterization of individuals who are more or less vulnerable to effects of stressful events is a worthy endeavor.

SUMMARY AND FUTURE DIRECTIONS

The one question around which this chapter revolves is "Do psychological stressors have a direct effect on BG in individuals with diabetes?" The answer is "Probably, in some cases," but more research must take place before making any firm conclusions. Prior research has largely identified physiological mechanisms through which stressful events might influence BG, and some research paradigms have produced data suggesting that psychological stressors can activate these mechanisms. Results from studies employing laboratory animal models are fairly consistent, such animals are susceptible to stressors (e.g., restraint, crowding, and rotation). These stressor stimuli hasten development of overt diabetes in IDDM models and produce hyperglycemic effects in animals with established IDDM and NIDDM. Studies employing chemical infusion in individuals with IDDM and NIDDM have consistently produced results consistent with those obtained using laboratory animal models. "Stress hormone" infusions that attempt to mimic endogenous stress responses produce hyperglycemic responses in diabetic subjects, and to a lesser extent, in nondiabetic subjects. In addition, three prospective home-monitoring studies with IDDM subjects and one with NIDDM subjects demonstrated a direct relationship between stressful events and BG. One controlled study of relaxation training with NIDDM subjects supports the stress–BG relationship in that this stress management procedure produced improvements in glucose tolerance and BG. A second study with NIDDM subjects did not entirely replicate the first, but suggested that relaxation training was more beneficial to subjects with high trait anxiety.

In contrast, laboratory stress-induction paradigms and retrospective studies of major life events in subjects with established diabetes have produced mixed or negative results. The data regarding brief laboratory stressors are inconsistent; some studies demonstrate increased BG, but a larger number of studies find no change or decreased BG. Retrospective studies suggest that major life events may associate with onset of diabetes, although effects of life events on metabolic control (i.e., glycosylated hemoglobin) in established diabetes are equivocal.

What remains is to determine if we can reconcile these findings and, if so, to then consider a meaningful direction or directions for future research. We must also evaluate clinical importance of stress–BG data. The literature review and methodological/theoretical discussion presented here highlights strengths and difficulties in some areas. For example, although laboratory animal models and chemical infusion studies produce relatively consistent data, research to date has not demonstrated, and may not warrant, generalization to effects of naturally occurring stress.

Retrospective studies of life stress and onset of diabetes are mostly consistent with the stress–BG hypothesis, but are likely to contain a bias related to distress of recent diagnosis of an ongoing, chronic disease. Thus, this paradigm will probably not provide additional, "clean" data that will clearly advance the hypothesis.

Although laboratory stress-induction studies have produced the most inconsistent data, this paradigm still has some experimental appeal. Its strengths are the degree of control allowed by a laboratory setting and closer approximation of naturally occurring stressors relative to chemical infusions. Furthermore, laboratory stress-induction procedures allow one to evaluate the "person" part of the person–environment transactional model. Possible reasons for discrepant and negative data are many (and discussed in some detail earlier), but they are apparent enough throughout this literature to argue against dismissing this paradigm. Careful designs incorporating recent findings and more theoretically valid stressors may lead to more consistent data. For example, the search for a universal stressor that produces hyperglycemic responses in all subjects is no longer tenable. Recent data highlight two important ideas that must help direct future research. First, not all stressors have the same impact on all people, and second, different stressors have different effects on the same individual. Nonetheless, individuals' responses to the same stressor are likely reliable. These ideas are not new to stress research in other areas (e.g., cardiovascular reactivity; see additional chapters in this text) but have not received adequate attention in examinations of stress effects with diabetic subjects. Thus, designs that identify and distinguish "responders" from "nonresponders," characterize types of stressors (e.g., passive vs. active) that produce varying degrees of responses in "reactors," and identify characteristics that mediate or moderate effects of stressors (e.g., coping responses, social support) will likely advance the hypothesis. This approach adopts the transactional view of stress advanced by Lazarus and Folkman (1984).

Possibly most compelling are findings from the handful of prospective home-monitoring studies. Every study has demonstrated direct hyperglycemic effects of stressful events. However, it is a difficult paradigm to employ because it requires a great deal of effort on the part of subjects, and experimenters must contend with many factors that can influence BG in the natural environment; it is, nonetheless, an appealing approach. Such monitoring studies are intrusive but are probably the best available studies for capturing what truly happens to individuals during daily experiences. This paradigm readily lends itself to examination of influences of individual differences and different types of stressors, an important extension of this work.

Examination of data from various paradigms also points out several other patterns in the way this research has progressed. The vast majority of studies, particularly laboratory stress-induction and home-monitoring studies, utilized IDDM subjects, and no single study compared groups of IDDM and NIDDM subjects. Surwit and Feinglos (1988) discussed several lines of research that suggest individuals with NIDDM may be more vulnerable than those with IDDM and nondiabetic subjects to effects of stress. Hyperresponsivity to catecholamines may be inherent in the pathophysiology of NIDDM. If this is the case, then the stress–BG hypothesis clearly needs additional testing.

Even if future research adequately identifies individuals vulnerable to stressful events and conditions most debilitating for these individuals, we must question the clinical significance of stress-related hyperglycemic responses. Although it is true that poor metabolic control is a predictor of morbidity and mortality, it is unclear whether stressful events contribute to metabolism to such a large extent as to increase risk. Answering this question probably requires longitudinal studies of "responsive" individuals. Such studies do not yet exist.

If clinical significance of stress-related BG increases in vulnerable individuals is uncertain, one also must consider clinical importance of stress management strategies. At present, there is not unequivocal evidence that relaxation training or other stress management strategies produce clinically meaningful and cost-effective improvements in diabetic metabolism. However, only three controlled group studies exist, and none provide longitudinal follow-up; thus, they do not permit us to even begin to address clinical significance of such interventions. It is likely that stress management would not be useful for everyone with diabetes; the second study with NIDDM subjects by Surwit et al. (1992) is an important start to understanding who might best benefit. As this research continues, it will be important to consider the multiple ways in which stress management interventions might be beneficial. In addition to buffering direct impact of stressors on BG, stress management might also attenuate stress-related deteriorations in adherence to the diabetic regimen and enhance quality of life by enhancing psychological adjustment. Likewise, although intervention studies are far from conclusive regarding clinical significance, they do partially support the stress–BG hypothesis; that is, the fact that stress management improves diabetic metabolism in some subjects suggests that stress has an impact on metabolism in those subjects.

Taken as a whole, this literature review and discussion have identified strengths of current research and attempted to make suggestions for future research. There is enough evidence from data presently published to encourage further examination regarding direct effects of stressful events on blood glucose in individuals with diabetes, but there is not enough evidence to state unequivocally that psychological stressors cause hyperglycemia. Further work will characterize vulnerable individuals and conditions, with the ultimate goal of not only understanding influences of stressful events on diabetes but of enhancing health and quality of life of individuals with this lifelong disease.

REFERENCES

Ader, D., Johnson, S., Huang, S., & Riley, W. (1991). Group size, cage shelf level, and emotionality in nonobese diabetic mice: Impact on onset and incidence of IDDM. *Psychosomatic Medicine, 53,* 313–321.

Ader, R., Kruetner, A., & Jacobs, H. (1963). Social environment, emotionality, and alloxan diabetes in the rat. *Psychosomatic Medicine, 25,* 60–68.

Aikens, J. E., Wallander, J. L., Bell, D. S. H., & Cole, J. A. (1992). Daily stress variability, learned resourcefulness, regimen adherence, and metabolic control in Type I diabetes mellitus: Evaluation of a path model. *Journal of Consulting and Clinical Psychology, 60,* 113–118.

American Diabetes Association (1991). Diabetes mellitus and exercise. Position statement of the American Diabetes Association. *Diabetes Care, 14,* 36.

Baker, L., Barcai, A., Kaye, R., & Hague, N. (1969). Beta adrenergic blockage and juvenile diabetes. *Journal of Pediatrics, 75,* 19–29.

Baker, L., Kaye, R., & Hague, N. (1967). Studies on metabolic homeostasis in juvenile diabetes mellitus II: Role of catecholamines. *Diabetes, 16,* 504–505.

Banerji, M. A., & Lebovitz, H. E. (1989). Insulin-sensitive and insulin-resistant variants of NIDDM. *Diabetes, 38,* 784–792.

Barnett, A. H., Eff, C., Leslie, R. D. G., & Pyke, D. A. (1981). Diabetes in identical twins. *Diabetologia, 20,* 87–93.

Blumenthal, J., Fredrikson, M., Kuhn, C., et al. (1990). Aerobic exercise reduces levels of sympathoadrenal responses to mental stress in subjects without prior evidence of myocardial ischemia. *American Journal of Cardiology, 65,* 93.

Brand, A. H., Johnson, J. H., & Johnson, S. B. (1986). Life stress and diabetic control in children and adolescents with insulin-dependent diabetes. *Journal of Pediatric Psychology, 11,* 481–495.

Cannon, W. (1941). *Bodily changes in pain, hunger, fear, and rage.* New York: Macmillan.

Capponi, R., Kawada, M., Varela, C., & Vargas, L. (1980). Diabetes mellitus by repeated stress in rats bearing chemical diabetes. *Hormone and Metabolic Research, 12,* 411–412.

Carter, W., Gonder-Frederick, L., Cox, D., Clarke, W., & Scott, D. (1985). Effects of stress on blood glucose in IDDM. *Diabetes Care, 8,* 411–412.

Carter, W., Herman, J., Stokes, K., & Cox, D. (1987). Promotion of diabetes onset by stress in the BB rat. *Diabetologia, 30,* 674–675.

Chase, H. P., & Jackson, G. G. (1981). Stress and sugar control in children with insulin-dependent diabetes mellitus. *Journal of Pediatrics, 98,* 1011–1013.

Cohen, S., & Wills, T. A. (1985). Stress, social support, and the buffering hypothesis. *Psychological Bulletin, 98,* 310–357.

Cox, D., Gonder-Frederick, L., Clarke, W., & Carter, W. (1988). Effects of acute experimental stressors on insulin-dependent diabetes mellitus. *Diabetes, 37* (Suppl.), 51A.

Cox, D. J., Gonder-Frederick, L., Pohl, S., & Pennebaker, J. W. (1986). Diabetes. In K. A. Holroyd & T. L. Creer (Eds.), *Self-management of chronic diseases: Handbook of clinical interventions and research* (pp. 305–346). New York: Academic Press.

Cox, D. J., Gonder-Frederick, L., & Saunders, J. T. (1991). Diabetes: Clinical issues and management. In J. J. Sweet, R. H. Rozensky, & S. M. Tovian (Eds.), *Handbook of clinical psychology in medical settings* (pp. 473–495). New York: Plenum Press.

Cox, D. J., Taylor, A. G., Nowacek, G., Holley-Wilcox, P., Pohl, S. P., & Guthrow, E. (1984). The relationship between psychological stress and insulin-dependent diabetic blood glucose control: Preliminary investigations. *Health Psychology, 3,* 63–75.

Craighead, J. E. (1978). Current views on the etiology of insulin-dependent diabetes mellitus. *New England Journal of Medicine, 299,* 1439–1445.

Crews, D., & Landers, D. (1987). A meta-analytic review of aerobic fitness and reactivity to psychosocial stressors. *Medical Science in Sports and Exercise, 19* (Suppl.), S114.

DeFronzo, R. A., Bonadonna, R. C., & Ferannini, E. (1992). Pathogenesis of NIDDM: A balanced overview. *Diabetes Care, 15,* 318–368.

Delamater, A. M., Kurtz, S. M., Bubb, J., White, N. H., & Santiago, J. V. (1987). Stress and coping in relation to metabolic control of adolescents with Type I diabetes. *Developmental and Behavioral Pediatrics, 8,* 136–140.

DeLongis, A., Coyne, J. C., Dakof, G., Folkman, S., & Lazarus, R. (1982). Relationship of daily hassles, uplifts, and major life events to health status. *Health Psychology, 1,* 119–136.

Demmers, R. Y., Neale, A. V., Wensloff, N. J., Gronsman, K. J., & Jaber, L. A. (1989). Glycosylated hemoglobin levels and self-reported stress in adults with diabetes. *Behavioral Medicine, 15,* 167–172.

Edwards, C., & Yates, A. (1985). The effects of cognitive task demand on subjective stress and blood glucose levels in diabetics and nondiabetics. *Journal of Psychosomatic Research, 29,* 59–69.

Feinglos, M. N., Hastedt, P., & Surwit, R. S. (1987). Effects of relaxation therapy on patients with Type I diabetes mellitus. *Diabetes Care, 10,* 72–75.

Fernqvist, E., Gunnarsson, R., & Linde, B. (1988). Influence of circulating epinephrine on absorption of subcutaneously injected insulin. *Diabetes, 37,* 694–701.

Fowler, J. E., Budzynski, T. H., & VandenBergh, R. L. (1976). Effects of an EMG biofeedback relaxation program on the control of diabetes. *Biofeedback and Self-Regulation, 1,* 105–112.

Frenzel, M. P., McCaul, K. D., Glasgow, R. L., & Schafer, L. C. (1988). The relationship of stress and coping to regimen adherence and glycemic control of diabetes. *Journal of Social and Clinical Psychology, 6,* 77–87.

Fujimoto, K., Sakaguchi, T., & Ui, M. (1981). Adrenergic mechanisms in the hyperglycaemia and hyperinsulinaemia of diabetic KK mice. *Diabetologia, 20,* 568–572.

Gerich, J. E. (1989). Oral hypoglycemic agents. *New England Journal of Medicine, 321,* 123–145.

Gerich, J., Lorenzi, M., Tsalikian, E., & Karem, J. (1976). Studies of the mechanism of epinephrine-induced hyperglycemia in men. *Diabetes, 25,* 65.

Gilbert, B., Johnson, S., Silverstein, J., & Malone, J. (1989). Psychological and physiological responses to acute laboratory stressors in insulin-dependent diabetes mellitus adolescents and nondiabetic controls. *Journal of Pediatric Psychology, 14,* 577–591.

Goetsch, V. (1989). Stress and blood glucose in diabetes mellitus: A review and methodological commentary. *Annals of Behavioral Medicine, 11,* 102–112.

Goetsch, V., Pbert, L., Van Dorsten, B., Yeater, R., & Ullrich, I. (1988, March). *The effect of aerobic training on blood glucose reactivity in type II Diabetics.* Paper presented at the Meetings of the Society of Behavioral Medicine, Boston, MA.

Goetsch, V. L., Van Dorsten, B., Pbert, L. A., Ullrich, I. H., & Yeater, R. A. (1993). Acute effects of laboratory stress on blood glucose in noninsulin-dependent diabetes. *Psychosomatic Medicine, 55,* 492–496.

Goetsch, V., Wiebe, D., Veltum, L., & Van Dorsten, B. (1990). Stress and blood glucose in Type II diabetes mellitus. *Behaviour Research and Therapy, 28,* 531–537.

Gonder-Frederick, L., Carter, W., Cox, D., & Clarke, W. (1990). Environmental stress and blood glucose change in insulin-dependent diabetes mellitus. *Health Psychology, 9,* 503–515.

Griffith, L. S., Field, B. J., & Lustman, P. J. (1990). Life stress and social support in diabetes: Association with glycemic control. *International Journal of Psychiatry in Medicine, 20,* 365–372.

Halford, W. K., Cuddihy, S., & Mortimer, R. H. (1990). Psychological stress and blood glucose regulation in Type I diabetic patients. *Health Psychology, 9,* 516–528.

Hamberg, D., Hendler, R., & Sherwin, R. (1980). Influence of small increments of epinephrine on glucose tolerance in normal humans. *Annals of Internal Medicine, 13,* 160–183.

Hanson, C. L., Henggeler, S. W., & Burghen, G. A. (1987a). Model of associations between psychosocial variables and health-outcome measures of adolescents with IDDM. *Diabetes Care, 10,* 752–758.

Hanson, C. L., Henggeler, S. W., & Burghen, G. A. (1987b). Social competence and parental support as mediators of the link between stress and metabolic control in adolescents with insulin-dependent diabetes mellitus. *Journal of Consulting and Clinical Psychology, 55,* 529–533.

Hanson, S. L., & Pichert, J. W. (1986). Perceived stress and diabetes control in adolescents. *Health Psychology, 5,* 439–452.

Helms, R. B. (1992). Implications of population growth on prevalence of diabetes: A look at the future. *Diabetes Care, 15,* 6–9.

Huang, S., Plaut, S., Taylor, G., & Wareheim, B. (1981). Effect of stressful stimulation on the incidence of streptozotocin induced diabetes in mice. *Psychosomatic Medicine, 43,* 431–437.

Jacobson, A. M., Rand, L. I., & Hauser, S. T. (1985). Psychologic stress and glycemic control: A comparison of patients with and without proliferative diabetic retinopathy. *Psychosomatic Medicine, 47,* 372–380.

Keen, H., & Jarrett, J. (1982). *Complications of diabetes* (2nd ed.). London: Arnold.

Kemmer, F., Bisping, R., Steingruber, H., Baar, H., Hardtmann, R., Schlaghecke, R., & Berger, M. (1984). Psychological stress and metabolic control in patients with type I diabetes mellitus. *New England Journal of Medicine, 314,* 1078–1084.

Knuiman, M. W., Welborn, I. A., McCann, V. J., Stanton, V. J., & Constable, I. J. (1986). Prevalence of diabetic complications in relation to risk factors. *Diabetes, 35,* 1332–1339.

Kovar, M. G., Harris, M. I., & Hadden, W. (1987). The scope of diabetes in the United States population. *American Journal of Public Health, 77,* 1549–1550.

Kuhn, C., Cochrane, C., Feinglos, M., & Surwit, R. (1987). Exaggerated peripheral responsivity to catecholamines contributes to stress-induced hyperglycemia in the ob/ob mouse. *Physiology, Biochemistry, and Behavior, 25,* 491–495.

Lammers, C. A., Naliboff, B. D., & Straatmeyer, A. J. (1984). The effects of progressive relaxation on stress and diabetic control. *Behavioral Research and Therapy, 22,* 641–650.

Landis, B., Jovanovic, L., Landis, E., Peterson, C. M., Groshen, S., Johnson, K., & Miller, N. E. (1985). Effect of stress reduction on daily glucose range in previously stabilized insulin-dependent diabetic patients. *Diabetes Care, 8,* 624–626.

Lane, J. D., Stabler, B., Ross, S. L., Morris, M. A., Litton, J. C., & Surwit, R. S. (1988). Psychological predictors of glucose control in patients with IDDM. *Diabetes Care, 11,* 798–800.

Lazarus, R., & Folkman, S. (1984). *Stress, appraisal, and coping.* New York: Springer.

Lee, J., Konorska, M., & McCarty, R. (1989). Physiological responses to acute stress in alloxan and streptozotocin diabetic rats. *Physiology and Behavior, 45,* 483–489.

Lloyd, C. E., Matthews, K. A., Wing, R. R., & Orchard, T. J. (1992). Psychosocial factors and complications of IDDM: The Pittsburgh epidemiology of diabetes complications study. *Diabetes Care, 15,* 166–172.

Locatelli, A., Franzetti, I., Lepore, G., Maglio, M. L., Gaudio, E., Caviezel, F., & Pozza, G. (1989). Mental arithmetic stress as a test for evaluation of diabetic sympathetic autonomic neuropathy. *Diabetic Medicine, 6,* 490–495.

Marlatt, G. A., & Gordon, J. R. (1985). *Relapse prevention: Maintenance strategies and addictive behavior change.* New York: Guilford.

Matthews, K. A. (1988). Coronary heart disease and Type A behaviors: Update on and alternative to the Booth-Kewley and Friedman (1987) quantitative review. *Psychological Bulletin, 104,* 373–380.

McCubbin, J., Surwit, R., Kuhn, C., Cochrane, C., & Feinglos, M. (1987). Effect of opiate antagonism on stress-induced hyperglycemia in obese mice. *Diabetes, 36* (Suppl.), 18A.

McLesky, C., Lewis, S., & Woodruff, R. (1978). Glucagon levels during anesthesia and surgery in normal and diabetic patients. *Diabetes, 27,* 492.

Mikat, E., Hackel, D., Cruz, P., Lebovitz, H. (1972). Lowered glucose tolerance in the sand rat (psammonys obesus) resulting from esophageal intubation. *Proceedings of the Society for Experimental Biology and Medicine, 139,* 1390–1391.

Naliboff, B., Cohen, M., & Sowers, J. (1985). Physiological and metabolic responses to brief stress in non-insulin dependent diabetic and control subjects. *Journal of Psychosomatic Research, 29,* 367–374.

Nathan, D. M., Singer, D. E., Hurxthal, K., & Goodson, J. D. (1984). The clinical information value of the glycosylated hemoglobin assay. *New England Journal of Medicine, 310,* 341–346.

National Center for Health Statistics (1980). *National Health and Nutrition Examination Survey (1976–1980).* Washington, DC: Department of Health and Human Services.

Niemcryk, S. J., Speers, M. A., Travis, L. B., & Gary, H. E. (1990). Psychosocial correlates of hemoglobin A1c in young adults with Type I diabetes. *Journal of Psychosomatic Research, 34,* 617–627.

Ortiz-Alonzo, F., Herman, W., Zobel, D., Perry, R., Smith, M., & Halter, J. (1991). Effect of epinephrine on pancreatic B-cell and A-cell function in patients with NIDDM. *Diabetes, 40,* 1194–1202.

Palmer, J. L., & McCulloch, D. K. (1991). Prediction and preventions of IDDM—1991. *Diabetes, 40,* 943–947.

Peters, A. L., & Davidson, M. B. (1992). Does insulin + sulfonylureas = effective treatment of NIDDM? *Clinical Diabetes, 10,* 19–21.

Peyrot, M., & McMurry, J. F. (1985). Psychosocial factors in diabetes control: Adjustment of insulin-treated adults. *Psychosomatic Medicine, 47,* 542–557.

Reaven, G. M. (1984). Insulin secretion and insulin action in non-insulin-dependent diabetes mellitus: Which defect is primary? *Diabetes Care, 7,* 17–24.

Rhodewalt, F., & Marcroft, M. (1988). Type A behavior and diabetic control: Implications of psychological reactance for health outcomes. *Journal of Applied Social Psychology, 18,* 139–159.

Robinson, N., & Fuller, J. H. (1985). Role of life events and difficulties in the onset of diabetes mellitus. *Journal of Psychosomatic Research, 29,* 583–591.

Robinson, N., Lloyd, C. E., Fuller, J. H., & Yateman, N. A. (1988). Psychosocial factors and the onset of Type I diabetes. *Diabetic Medicine, 6,* 53–58.

Rosenbaum, L. (1983). Biofeedback-assisted stress management for insulin-treated diabetes mellitus. *Biofeedback and Self-Regulation, 8,* 519–532.

Rosenbaum, M. (1990). The role of learned resourcefulness in the self-control of health behavior. In M. Rosenbaum (Ed.), *Learned resourcefulness: On coping skills, self-control, and adaptive behavior* (pp. 3–30). New York: Springer.

Seeburg, K. N., & DeBoer, K. F. (1980). Effects of EMG biofeedback on diabetes. *Biofeedback and Self-Regulation, 5,* 289–293.

Shamoon, H., Hendler, R., & Sherwin, R. (1980). Synergistic interactions among anti-insulin hormones in the pathogenesis of stress hyperglycemia in humans. *Journal of Clinical Endocrinology, 52,* 1235–1241.

Simonds, J., Goldstein, D., Walker, B., & Rawlings, S. (1981). The relationship between psychological factors and blood glucose regulation in insulin-dependent diabetic adolescents. *Diabetes Care, 4,* 610–615.

Skyler, J. S. (1987). Why control diabetes: Influence on chronic complications of diabetes. *Pediatric Annals, 16,* 713–724.

Soman, V., Shamoon, H., & Sherwin, R. (1980). Effects of physiological infusion of epinephrine in normal humans: Relationship between the metabolic response and B-adrenergic binding. *Journal of Clinical Endocrinology and Metabolism, 50,* 294–297.

Stabler, B., Lane, J. D., Ross, S. L., Morris, M. A., Litton, J., & Surwit, R. S. (1988). Type A behavior pattern and chronic glycemic control in individuals with IDDM. *Diabetes Care, 11,* 361–362.

Stabler, B., Surwit, R. S., Lane, J. D., Morris, M. A., Litton, J., & Feinglos, M. N. (1987). Type A behavior pattern and blood glucose control in diabetic children. *Psychosomatic Medicine, 49,* 313–316.

Stone, A. A., Kessler, R. C., & Haythornthwaite, J. A. (1991). Measuring daily events and experiences: Decisions for the researcher. *Journal of Personality, 59,* 575–607.

Surwit, R. S., & Feinglos, M. N. (1983). The effects of relaxation on glucose tolerance in non-insulin-dependent diabetes. *Diabetes Care, 6,* 176–179.

Surwit, R. S., & Feinglos, M. N. (1984). Relaxation-induced improvement in glucose tolerance is associated with decreased plasma cortisol. *Diabetes Care, 7,* 203–204.

Surwit, R., & Feinglos, M. (1988). Stress and autonomic nervous system in Type II diabetes: A hypothesis. *Diabetes Care, 11,* 83–85.

Surwit, R., Feinglos, M., Livingston, E., Kuhn, C., McCubbin, J. (1984). Behavioral manipulation of the diabetic phenotype in ob/ob mice. *Diabetes, 33,* 616–618.

Surwit, R. S., Lane, J. D., McCaskill, C. C., Ross, S. L., & Feinglos, M. N. (1992, March 25–28). Relaxation training for Type II diabetes: Predicting who will benefit. Paper presented at the Society of Behavioral Medicine, New York.

Surwit, R. S., McCubbin, J. A., Kuhn, C. M., McGee, D., Gerstenfeld, D. A., & Feinglos, M. N. (1986). Alprazolam reduces stress hyperglycemia in ob/ob mice. *Psychosomatic Medicine, 48,* 278–282.

Surwit, R. S., Ross, S. L., & Feinglos, M. N. (1991). Stress, behavior, and glucose control in diabetes mellitus. In P. M. McCabe, N. Schneiderman, T. M. Field, & Skyler, J. S. (Eds.), *Stress, coping, and disease* (pp. 97–117). Hillsdale, NJ: Erlbaum.

Tennen, H., Suls, J., & Affleck, G. (1991). Personality and daily experience: The promise and the challenge. *Journal of Personality, 59,* 313–337.

Turkat, I. D. (1982). Glycosylated hemoglobin levels in anxious and nonanxious diabetic patients. *Psychosomatics, 23,* 1056–1058.

Wheeler, L., & Reis, H. T. (1991). Self-recording of everyday life events: Origins, types, and uses. *Journal of Personality, 59,* 339–354.

Wiebe, D. J., & Smith, T. W. (in press). Personality and health: Progress and problems in psychosomatics. In S. R. Briggs, R. Hogan, & W. Jones (Eds.), *Handbook of personality psychology.* New York: Academic Press.

Wilson, W., Ary, D. V., Biglan, A., Glasgow, R. E., Toobert, D. J., & Campbell, D. R. (1986). Psychosocial predictors of self-care behaviors (compliance) and glycemic control in non-insulin-dependent diabetes mellitus. *Diabetes Care, 9,* 614–622.

Wing, R. R. (1991). Behavioral weight control for obese patients with Type II diabetes. In P. M. McCabe, N. Schneiderman, T. M. Field, & Skyler, J. S. (Eds.), *Stress, coping, and disease* (pp. 147–167). Hillsdale, NJ: Erlbaum.

Wredling, R. A. M., Theorell, P. G., Roll, H. M., Lins, P. E. S., & Adamson, U. K. C. (1992). Psychosocial state of patients with IDDM prone to recurrent episodes of severe hypoglycemia. *Diabetes Care, 15,* 518–521.

Young, J., & Landsberg, L. (1979). Sympathoadrenal system: The regulation of metabolism. In S. Ingbar (Ed.), *Contemporary endocrinology.* New York: Plenum Press.

26

Systemic Lupus Erythematosus

Linda R. Kostyak

Medical professionals have often called systemic lupus erythematosus (SLE) a "mysterious" illness because its confusing symptomatology has baffled the medical community for centuries. It is the product of an immune system gone awry, and, for this reason, it is capable of producing a variety of curious symptoms in virtually any organ or system of the body. A formal definition of SLE is "a chronic, inflammatory disease in which the body's immune system, instead of serving its normal protective function, forms antibodies that attack healthy tissues and organs" (Lupus Foundation of America, Inc., 1990, p. 2). SLE is sometimes fatal, often debilitating, and, once diagnosed, always present; to date, research has found no definite cause, course, or cure. Current classifications list three types of lupus: (1) discoid lupus, which affects only skin by causing rashes and lesions; (2) drug-induced lupus, caused by a reaction to medications; and (3) systemic lupus erythematosus, which is most serious and systemwide. Although all three types of lupus receive mention in this chapter, the primary focus is on the most severe form, SLE, tracing the history, diagnosis, treatment, and implications for the field of psychology.

HISTORY OF SLE

A 13th-century physician, Rogerius, first coined the term *lupus* (Latin for wolf) to describe inflamed, destructive facial lesions that resemble a "wolf's bite" (Blotzer, 1983). Although reports of similar skin ulcerations dotted medical literature for the next five centuries, a systematic description and formal name for the disease, *lupus*

Linda R. Kostyak • Western Psychiatric Institute and Clinic, University of Pittsburgh Medical Center, Pittsburgh, Pennsylvania 15213.
Handbook of Health and Rehabilitation Psychology, edited by Anthony J. Goreczny. Plenum Press, New York, 1995.

erythematosus, awaited von Hebra in 1845 (cited in Graninger, Smolen, & Zielinski, 1987) and Cazanave in 1851 (Cazanave & Chausit, 1851). The disease remained merely a skin disorder until 1872, when Kaposi recognized that patients occasionally presented with a concurrent set of symptoms that included fever, arthritis, lymphadenopathy, and anemia (cited in Graninger et al., 1987). His report prompted formation of a distinction between *disseminated lupus erythematosus* and forms limited to skin. In 1904, Osler from Baltimore, Maryland, and Jadassohn from Vienna simultaneously identified additional symptoms, such as renal failure, endocarditis, delirium, aphasia, and hemiplegia (Dubois & Wallace, 1987), shifting emphasis from the skin to the diffuse or systemic nature of the disease. Through work of pathologists during the 1920s and 1930s (e.g., Baehr, Klemperer, & Schifrin, 1935; Friedberg, Gross, & Wallach, 1936; Libman & Sacks, 1924), they more fully and adequately described clinical characteristics of the disease, and SLE became a distinct clinical entity within the medical community (Lahita, 1987).

A search for laboratory tests that could identify SLE in the blood ensued. Researchers initially believed that a particular cell, named the LE cell, described by Hargraves, Richmond, and Morton in 1948, could serve as a unique marker of SLE, but later research linked LE cells to rheumatoid arthritis and other illnesses (Ropes, 1976). Moore and Lutz (1955), among others, found that a false-positive syphillis or Wasserman test frequently occurred in patients with SLE and often predated diagnosis. In 1953, Elliott and Mathieson associated lowered blood complement levels with SLE. However, it was not until Witebsky, Rose, Terplan, Paine, and Egan (1957) proposed the concept of autoimmunization that attention turned toward presence of *autoantibodies* in the blood of SLE patients, and hence, the notion that SLE was an autoimmune disease.

WHAT IS SLE?

Clinical research and animal models have indeed determined SLE is an autoimmune disease whereby "the immune system in all of its complexity 'turns against itself' and attacks the body's own tissues" (Lahita, 1987, p. 1). Although a thorough discussion of the immune response is beyond the scope of this chapter, some basic knowledge of the process is necessary.

Essentially, the immune system defends the body against foreign, potentially harmful invaders, such as viruses and bacteria, by first recognizing such substances or *antigens* and subsequently responding in ways to remove them from the body. One mechanism for ridding the body of foreign antigens is through production of *antibodies*. Antibodies are "molecules made by the immune system that bind to foreign antigens with great specificity . . . (and) direct their removal from the body" (Seaman, 1990, p. 7). Two divisions of the immune system regulate this production. The first, or *humoral* division, consists of B cells produced in bone marrow that circulate through plasma or white blood cells searching for infection. The second, or *cellular* division, consists of two types of T cells, T helpers and T suppressors, also produced in bone marrow but recycled through the thymus before circulating through the body (Roitt, Brostoff, & Male, 1989). In a normal immune response, B cells detect foreign antigens and begin production of antibodies. T-helper cells signal further production of antibodies to eliminate the antigens. T-suppressor cells tell B cells to discontinue production when antibodies have surrounded or destroyed the antigen. However, the system can run amok at any stage in the process. For example, a congenital deficiency of B cells does not allow production of antibodies and thus leaves the body susceptible to all foreign invaders. A virus, such as human immunodeficiency virus (HIV), depresses T-helper cell response so that the body is unable to produce enough antibodies to fight invading substances. Autoimmunity occurs when B cells mistake the body's own cells for foreign invaders and create *autoantibodies* that attack a variety of healthy cells. In addition, T-suppressor cells fail to stop B-cell production of antibodies. When the autoantibody and mistaken antigen meet, they pull *complements,* or circulating protein, out of the body and form a large molecule called the *immune complex.* This large complex clogs different vessels or joints within the body. The result is inflammation of virtually any organ or system of the body, including joints, skin, bones, serous membranes (those surrounding the lungs, heart, and abdomen), kidneys, gastrointestinal tract, cardiovascular system, and brain (Lahita, 1987).

Inflammation produces an array of symptoms. Table 26.1 lists frequencies of common SLE symptoms (Schur, 1985; Wallace, 1993).

In addition to the common complaints, a review of the literature from 1956 through 1982 cites 66 clinical and laboratory manifestations of SLE, including a range of psychological and neurological (often referred to as neuropsychiatric) symptoms addressed later (Dubois & Wallace, 1987). Profound fatigue, believed to be the result of general weakness or part of the immune response (Schwartz, 1989), often accompanies disease activity. Rothfield (1989) reported moderate to severe fatigue in nearly all cases. However, a classic pattern of symptoms does not exist, and SLE can affect any system or organ in any combination. Likewise, the course of SLE is unpredictable and chronic in nature; in other words, symptom exacerbations intersperse with remissions. Overall, tendency of the disease is toward remission (Ropes, 1976); however, factors controlling the course and symptoms remain unclear.

Genetic predisposition appears to play an important role in development and expression of SLE. Studies have shown that 10–12% of patients with SLE have a relative with the disease (Dubois & Wallace, 1987). For male patients, familial SLE may be even higher, as reported by Buckman, Moore, Ebbin, Cox, and Dubois

Table 26.1. Common Symptoms of SLE[a]

Symptom	Frequency (%)
Arthralgia (achy joints)	95
Fever over 100° F (38° C)	90
Arthritis (swollen joints)	90
Skin rashes	74
Anemia	71
Kidney involvement	50
Pleurisy	45
Butterfly (malar) rash	42
Photosensitivity	30
Hair loss (alopecia)	27
Raynaud's phenomenon	17
Seizures	15
Mouth ulcers	12

[a]Adapted from Schur (1985) and Wallace (1993).

(1978), who studied 340 patients and found that 30% of the males had additional family members afflicted with the disease. Heredity, however, does not fully explain presence of SLE. Studies of monozygotic (identical) twins, reared together and apart, reveal less than 100% concordance (Arnett, Bias, & Schulman, 1972; Brunner, Horwitz, Shann, Sturgill, & Davis, 1973). In other words, although genetic factors may predispose individuals to develop SLE, environmental factors may also be necessary to signal onset of symptoms.

A variety of environmental factors may contribute to either disease onset or exacerbations. For example, certain medications, such as hydralazine, procainamide, D-penicillamine, tetracycline, isoniazid, and many oral contraceptives, produce lupus-like symptoms that remit upon discontinuation of the drug (Fernandez-Herlihy, 1989; Yung & Richardson, 1994). Occupational exposure to industrial agents, such as polyvinylchloride (Cordasco et al., 1980), hydrazines, tartrazines (Reidenberg et al., 1983), and silicone (Suratt, Winn, Brody, Bolton, & Giles, 1977; Ziskind, Jones, & Weill, 1976) may also play a role in autoimmunity. Moreover, the Food and Drug Administration (FDA) recently halted use of silicone in cosmetic surgery, particularly for breast augments, because of its suspected link to autoimmune disorders (Fock, Feng, & Tey, 1984; Kumagai, Shiokawa, Medsger, & Rodnan, 1984). Other suspected environmental factors are viruses. Studies of the virus responsible for Acquired Immunodeficiency Syndrome (AIDS), human immunodeficiency virus (HIV), have led to speculation that SLE may also result from a virus. However, attempts to isolate a lupus-causing virus have failed (Talal, 1983). Dietary factors, such as alfalfa seeds, have also received attention as possibly linked to SLE (Bardana et al., 1982), but findings remain inconclusive. Ultraviolet radiation appears to produce disease exacerbations (commonly called *flares*), especially when the skin is involved (Lahita, 1987). Studies of the role of sex hormones in development of SLE seem promising, because these hormones appear to regulate immune responses (Dubois & Wallace, 1987).

Physical and emotional trauma are other environmental factors that may cause the immune system to go awry. Dubois and Wallace (1987, p. 31) state that "there is little doubt that physical or emotional trauma can exacerbate a preexisting inflammatory arthritis, but . . . no study has convincingly demonstrated that this occurrence is more than coincidence." Nevertheless, patients' reports continue to associate symptoms with physical or emotional stress.

In summary, the causes and relative contributions of heredity and environment in the emergence of SLE remain unclear. Some researchers have proposed a "lupus diathesis (model)—a genetic or environmental set of factors which place a normal person at risk of acquiring or developing SLE" (Dubois & Wallace, 1987, p. 453). Just how these factors interact to produce SLE is unclear, but examination of the epidemiology of SLE may offer some insights.

Epidemiology is "the study of the distribution of a disease within a population with particular reference to demographic characteristics" (Hopkinson, 1991, p. 291). In other words, epidemiologists seek to describe diseases by the numbers and types of people afflicted. Investigators in the field of epidemiology trace, and often compare, incidence, prevalence, age, race, sex, and mortality to provide a profile of the phenomenon of interest. *Incidence* refers to the number of new cases of a disease that occur in a specific group of people over a specific period of time. Incidence of SLE in the United States is about 5 per 100,000 per year (Dubois &

Wallace, 1987) and has increased over the years. *Prevalence,* on the other hand, denotes the total number of cases, old and new, at a particular point in time. Like incidence, prevalence of SLE in the United States has increased, and current estimates place prevalence rates at 30–50 per 100,000 (Hopkinson, 1991); Thus, approximately 84,000 to 140,000 people have SLE. Unfortunately, as Tuffanelli (1991) indicated, these numbers, for the most part, reflect only patients who have been hospitalized and do not include those with discoid (skin) lupus or those with marginal diagnoses. When adjusted for these omissions, prevalence of SLE rises to 500,000 to 750,000 individuals within the United States. Approximately 90% of SLE patients are women, usually between the ages of 16 and 55 (Lahita, 1987). The disease appears to be four times more common in blacks than whites (Hopkinson, 1991) and possibly more often fatal in blacks (Petri, Perez-Gutthann, Longenecker, & Hockberg, 1991). These data appear to support genetic and/or hormonal factors as causes of SLE. However, researchers have not thoroughly studied socioeconomic status and psychological factors, and thus it is possible that the disparity between males and females and between blacks and whites is the result of underreporting symptoms, less access to medical facilities or insurance, noncompliance with medical regimens, or poor health practices. Although etiology of the disease remains unknown, diagnostic and treatment methods have improved overall survival rates in the past three decades. Among others, Swaak, Nossent, and Bronsveld (1989) suggested a survival rate of 94% five years after diagnosis. Of course, *survival* means only that patients are alive; it does not describe conditions or quality of life with which afflicted individuals must contend.

PSYCHOLOGICAL ASPECTS OF SLE

Chronic illness in general can lead to a host of difficulties for both patients and their families. Pitzelle (1985) described chronic illness as: (1) permanent; (2) the cause of frequent and costly medical intervention; and (3) the cause of substantial modification of lifestyle, life goals, vocational choices and opportunities, recreational activities, interpersonal relationships, and family role or position. Chronic illness means that life will never be the same as it was prior to disease development. The strength and vitality that are necessary to cope with life changes and stressors may no longer consistently be available. Pain and discomfort may make even the most minor tasks difficult. Moreover, the unpredictable, often debilitating, nature of chronic diseases may impose great limitations on future goals and aspirations. In this respect, SLE is no exception. SLE demands continual philosophical, physical, occupational, educational, social, financial, and family adjustments. The stress of these adjustments can trigger many physiological and psychological responses that further aggravate the immune system and increase the level of stress (Stein & Schleifer, 1985). As this cycle of stress continues, risk of psychological symptoms increases.

Psychological distress may occur at any time during the course of the disease; but, for several reasons, distress often begins long before diagnosis and treatment. Initial symptoms are often vague and transitory; consequently, patients often become labeled "neurotic" or otherwise go misdiagnosed by well-meaning or uninformed physicians. Moreover, laboratory tests to detect SLE do not always correlate with subjective reports of symptoms, and thus, the disease remains undiagnosed (and untreated) for long periods (McCarty, 1985). Patients in rural areas may not have access to major medical centers and the latest diagnostic techniques. Above all, patients with SLE do not usually look sick, and others may dismiss them as malingerers. According to Dubois and Wallace (1987, p. 496), "Because the time from onset of symptoms to diagnosis averages 3 years, many patients are already frustrated by the time they are told they have lupus." Having a concrete diagnosis may initially have a calming or even euphoric effect on patients, until they discover that there are no easy remedies. Subsequent responses range from denial to anger, but the endless nature of the disease often gives way to feelings of hopelessness and helplessness. As the unpredictable symptoms wax and wane, patients' senses of control may diminish and self-images may become distorted (Steptoe, 1989). Fear of death may be prominent, as reported by nearly one fourth of the SLE patients studied by Liang et al. (1984). Additionally, we could conceptualize and describe the seemingly interminable losses of physical function and independence as a series of grief processes repeatedly encountered but never quite resolved.

Medical treatments notwithstanding, it is essential that patients adapt their lifestyles to ensure health and longevity. The profound fatigue that accompanies SLE demands frequent rest periods, which may limit employment, educational, or social pursuits (McCarty, 1985). Decreased mobility due to joint pain, pleurisy, or heart involvement may dramatically reduce activity levels. Exposure to sunlight exacerbates symptoms (Epstein, Tuffanelli, & Dubois, 1965; Freeman, Knox, & Owen, 1969); thus patients need to curtail outdoor activities and sometimes require sunscreened windows for automobiles. Devices such as splints, canes, and wheelchairs may be necessary for functioning.

In addition to these lifestyle adjustments, social support systems may dwindle as patients become less able to participate in social activities. Family relationships may become strained in several different ways. For example, other family members may need to undertake duties once performed by patients. Changes in roles, power, and communication patterns, essentially the whole family structure, can lead to further stress on patients. Because SLE affects more women than men, traditional families, in which women assume the majority of child-care responsibilities, may no longer be in balance, creating role and identity confusion. Children may receive less than adequate direction or may become parentified as they assume roles of parent and caregiver. On the other hand, men with SLE who once fulfilled the role of primary wage earner may no longer be able to do so. In addition to role changes, extended family relationships may also become strained as members of extended families begin to receive requests for help with finances, child care, or patient caregiving. The need for expensive medications and procedures can financially burden families. Frequent hospital admissions, physician visits, and laboratory tests compound financial problems. Moreover, individuals with SLE are a "special-risk" population; thus, medical or life insurance may be difficult to obtain (Moynihan, 1990).

Individual development may become sidetracked, particularly because SLE primarily affects young and middle-age adults. As described by Ireys and Burr (1984), there are a variety of developmental tasks for young adults, including leaving their families of origin, developing a capacity for intimacy, choosing vocations, creating lives with their partners, and establishing a niche in society. Young adults with SLE may remain dependent on their families of origin, fearful of sexuality because of pain or disfigurement, too fatigued or physically debilitated to sustain a career, and without income, status, or civic responsibilities that ensure a role in society. Similarly, middle-age adults must negotiate a range of developmental tasks, such as assisting teenage children to become adults, developing leisure activities, accepting physiological changes, and adjusting to aging parents (Rustad, 1984). For middle-age adults with SLE, these tasks may be virtually impossible to complete, hindered again by dependency, limited social relationships, and weakness and pain.

Clearly, psychosocial stressors associated with chronic illness in general, and SLE in particular, can disrupt many facets of patients' lives. Psychological responses to such stress vary, and often patients experience symptoms of depression or anxiety (Cassileth et al., 1984). Previous maladaptive patterns of responding may also become exaggerated, and patients may exhibit characterological traits associated with dependent, narcissistic, avoidant, and passive–aggressive personality disorders. In a few cases, psychosis may evolve. Chronicity, as well as secondary gains, can maintain or worsen psychological symptoms. Unlike many other chronic illnesses, SLE itself may produce psychological problems. When SLE affects the central nervous system, a wide range of neurological, psychological, and cognitive problems can emerge, as discussed in the following section.

CENTRAL NERVOUS SYSTEM SLE

Central nervous system SLE may result from any of a number of disease effects on the central nervous system, such as cerebral vasculitis (inflammation of blood vessels), a cross-reaction of specific antibodies with brain tissue, and blocking of neurotransmitters by particular antibodies (Bresnihan et al., 1979; Denburg & Temesvari, 1983). Whatever the cause, identification of central nervous system SLE is difficult. Effects of central nervous system SLE can manifest in neurological, psychological, and cognitive impairments, alone or in combination. Most telltale is presence of neurological problems. Hughes (1980) reported that neurological signs appear in 50–70% of patients with SLE. Seizures occur in 10–15% of SLE patients. Most commonly, seizures in SLE patients are grand mal type, but petit mal, temporal lobe, focal, and Jacksonian seizures may also occur (Bluestein, 1987). Cranial neuropathies, which occur in about 12% of SLE patients (Bluestein, 1987), may affect the optic nerve and diminish the field of vision. Cerebrovascular accidents (strokes or intracranial hemorrhage) may also develop (Asherson, Denburg, Denburg, Carbotte, & Futrell, 1993), as may movement disorders. Occasionally, SLE also affects the peripheral nervous system.

Accurate diagnosis of central nervous system SLE is most likely when only neurological signs are evident. However, neurological signs often coexist with psychological symptoms that are similar to those suggested as responses to psychosocial stressors. For example, mood disorders, such as depression, commonly exist in patients with central nervous system SLE (Dubois & Wallace, 1987). Personality problems, characterized by dramatic changes in behavior, may also develop. General psychosis, marked by hallucinations and/or delusions, may be present in up to 55% of patients (O'Connor & Musher, 1966), but recent figures suggest a much lower incidence. In a few cases, clinicians have linked schizophrenia to SLE activity (Dubois & Wallace, 1987).

In addition to neurological and psychiatric difficulties, cognitive functions, such as general intellectual abilities, attention, perception, memory, language, reasoning, and spatial abilities, may become impaired. Standardized neuropsychological tests sample these abilities, and clinicians can use such tests to describe deficits in cognitive functioning as well as detect possible neural injury or central nervous system dysfunction (Koffler, 1987). Although evaluation of SLE patients with neuropsychological test batteries is a relatively new assessment approach, several studies have revealed interesting results. For example, Koffler (1987) tested 45 patients and found consistent abnormalities in visual, arithmetic, and writing skills as well as general intelligence relative to rheumatoid arthritis patients and normal controls. Likewise, Kutner, Busch, Mahmood, Racis, and Krey (1988) compared 22 SLE patients with rheumatoid arthritis patients and normal controls and found that SLE patients were significantly lower in visuomotor skills. In addition, those with SLE had lower scores on tests of vocabulary and long-term verbal and visual memory. Carbotte, S. Denburg, and J. Denburg (1986) found that 80% of SLE patients considered to have central nervous system involvement, versus 14% of rheumatoid arthritis patients, demonstrated cognitive dysfunction. On the other hand, a study of 20 SLE patients by Wekking, Nossent, van Dam, and Swaak (1991) disputed these findings and suggested only difficulties with concentration.

Overall, incidence of psychological symptoms associated with SLE ranges from 12–71%. However, lack of consistent diagnostic criteria, variable research methods, and researcher bias represent methodological confounds extant in most studies (Dubois & Wallace, 1987). Nevertheless, there is general consensus that SLE disease activity, as well as psychosocial stressors, can produce psychological symptoms in many patients. Increased susceptibility of SLE patients to any number of other diseases, such as cancer, uremia, or hypertension, that also have psychological ramifications further compounds risk for developing psychological difficulties. Furthermore, medications used to treat SLE can produce *iatrogenic* effects, that is, inadvertent effects caused by the medication that are sometimes psychological in nature.

Treatment of mental health difficulties often demands that clinicians distinguish symptoms caused by disease or medication (i.e., *organic* disorders) from symptoms imposed by reactions to psychosocial stressors (i.e., *functional* disorders). Unfortunately, similarity in features of organic and functional disorders often complicates differential diagnosis. For example, features of clinical depression (e.g., sleep disorders, appetite disturbance, depressed mood, and suicidality) can accompany chronic stress, central nervous system involvement, or medication. These symptoms may represent any two, or all three etiological sources, and sifting through this quagmire can be tedious and frustrating for health-care providers and patients alike. Several methods exist to aid in this determination. One method, detailed patient history, can reveal premorbid psychological problems, gradual versus acute onset of psychological symptoms, previous sensitivity to medications, and general patterns of psychological disturbance. If a patient's history suggests, for example, recurrent depressions with or without disease activity, clinicians might assume that a current depression is reactive (i.e., functional). If, on the other hand, depressions appear to coincide with increases in medication or disease activity, a diagnosis of organic depressive disorder might be more accurate. However, this historical method of assessment is not completely satisfactory, because it is possible that patients can experience both functional and organic disorders throughout the course of their disease.

As an alternative to the patient-history method, Jacobs, Bernhard, Delgado, and Strain (1977) proposed the use of a brief mental status questionnaire to assess current cognitive functioning. This questionnaire, previously used to screen for organic mental disorders in the medically ill, is effective in determining if patients are suffering from delirium or dementia (often assumed to result from organic processes). Other various questionnaires that assess a broad array of psychological symptoms and processes may provide assistance for diagnostic purposes, but a lack of specificity limits their usefulness. Thus, many methods for securing differential diagnoses have focused on physiological correlates. Early attempts tested cerebrospinal fluid for autoantibodies that might point to central nervous system involvement. Recent research has attempted to specify autoantibodies that may react with brain tissue associated with central nervous system functions. S. Denburg, Carbotte, Long, and J. Denburg (1988) tested a particular antibody called *serum lymphocytotoxic antibody* in 98 female SLE patients and observed an association between antibodies and cognitive impairment. With limited success, other studies have used brain scanning techniques and EEGs to identify anomalies that occur in the presence of psychological symptoms (Denburg & Temesvari, 1983). Most encouraging is a recent study by Schneebaum et al. (1991) that sought to link elevated levels of anti-P antibodies (an antibody that reacts with neuronal tissue) with psychological symptoms. The authors concluded that this particular autoantibody, easily detected in blood, appears to be a specific marker for SLE and relates to presence of depression and psychosis. Further research is still necessary to develop definite procedures for this test.

As mentioned previously, when only neurological signs are apparent, such as seizures or neuropathies, clinicians can generally limit diagnoses to organic processes. Similarly, effects of medications used to treat SLE have undergone significant research, and adequately trained professionals can fairly easily identify presence of *steroid psychosis,* especially when patients have used 40 mg or more of steroids per day (Hall, Popkin, Stickney, & Gardner, 1979). Probable symptoms of steroid psychosis (emotional lability, anxiety, distractibility, pressured speech, sensory flooding, insomnia, depression, perplexity, agitation, auditory and visual hallucinations, intermittent memory impairment, mutism, disturbance of body image, apathy, and hypomania) will generally remit when patients reduce dosage or discontinue use of steroids. In short, psychological problems related to SLE can be organic or functional in origin, or a combination of both. Accurate differential diagnosis continues to be elusive except in a few cases in which clinicians can isolate definite neurological impairment or medication effects; therefore, management of psychological symptoms is sometimes a matter of trial and error.

TREATMENT AND MANAGEMENT OF SLE

Effective treatment of SLE begins with a thorough and comprehensive assessment that yields an accurate diagnosis. Therefore, it seems appropriate to first present a brief overview of the general diagnostic process and criteria. According to Reeves and Lahita (1987), "a careful history and physical examination form the basis upon which SLE is diagnosed" (p. 358). History includes presence of SLE or other autoimmune disorders in family members, a drug and medication history to rule out drug-induced SLE, previous allergies to antibiotics, and onset of various types of symptoms. The general physical examination also includes laboratory tests known to correlate with SLE activity. Table 26.2 lists the accepted criteria for diagnosis of SLE (in abbreviated form) as determined by an appointed subcommittee of the American Rheumatism Association (Dubois & Wallace, 1987).

Individuals receive a diagnosis of SLE when they have met either simultaneously or in sequence, at least 4 of these 11 criteria. Clinicians must then determine severity of the disease. Mild SLE can include fatigue, arthritis, arthralgia, and occasional rash. Moderate SLE activity involves occurrence of additional symptoms, such as pleuritis, pericarditis, mouth ulcers, Raynaud's phenomenon (cold fingers and toes due to vascular problems), headaches, or abdominal pain. The most severe form of the disease includes these symptoms as well as major organ involvement (Ropes, 1976). Although there is no cure for SLE at the present time, a variety of medical, physical, and psychological treatments help manage the disease.

Of the medical treatments, immunosuppressive therapy and anti-inflammatory drugs represent the primary mode of treatment (Currey & Hull, 1987). Corticosteroids, such as prednisone, have amazing success reducing inflammation, but they are not without side effects. The most common side effects include: Cushing's syndrome; muscle atrophy, osteoporosis, atrophy of adrenal glands, susceptibility to infections, aseptic bone necrosis, cataracts, and steroid psychosis (Drug Facts and Comparisons, 1993; Miescher & Beris, 1984; U.S. Pharmacopeia, 1993). Efforts to control side effects of corticosteroids, such as using the lowest possible dosage or

Table 26.2. 1982 Revised Criteria for Classification of SLE[a]

Criterion	Definition
Malar	Fixed erythema about the cheeks
Discoid rash	Erythematous raised patches, which may produce scarring
Photosensitivity	Skin rash as a reaction to sunlight
Oral ulcers	Usually painless in mouth or nose
Arthritis	Nondeforming arthritis of two or more joints with tenderness and swelling
Serositis	Pleuritis (inflammation of the membrane surrounding the lung) or pericarditis (inflammation of the membrane surrounding the heart)
Renal disorder	Effects on the kidney determined by laboratory tests
Neurologic disorder	Seiures or psychosis in absence of known causative factors
Hematologic disorder	Hemolytic anemia, leukopenia, lymphopenia, or thrombocytopenia
Immunologic disorder	Positive LE cell, particular autoantibodies, or a false-positive syphilis test
Antinuclear antibody	Abnormal titer of this particular antibody

[a]Adapted from Dubois and Wallace (1987) and Tan et al. (1982).

alternating days when dosages are taken, have proven somewhat effective (Wallace, 1993). However, the toxic effects of corticosteroids often limit their use to moderate and severe cases of SLE.

Antimalarial drugs of the quinine family (e.g., Plaquenil, quinacrine) also assist in treatment of SLE, particularly mild to moderate SLE. For reasons still unclear, these medications appear to reduce fatigue and arthritis pain and improve skin lesions (McCarty, 1985). Side effects, although usually minimal, can include yellow skin pigmentation, loss of hair, skin dryness, gastrointestinal upset, muscle weakness, headaches, and damage to the retina. However, occasional serious side effects, such as mental confusion and convulsions, may also occur (Gluck, 1990). Nonsteroidal anti-inflammatory drugs (NSAIDs), such as motrin, indomethacin, and aspirin, have limited effectiveness controlling serious complications but may provide relief for arthritis and arthalgia pain. When disease activity is severe and uncontrolled, cytotoxic drugs often used in organ transplantations, can suppress immune system activity and lower the necessary dosage of steroids (Dubois & Wallace, 1987). This serious treatment, however, also produces unwanted effects, particularly nausea and vomiting, hormonal deficiencies, susceptibility to infection, and possible development of cancers (Klippel, 1987). Anticonvulsants and psychotropic medications help control neurological and psychiatric symptoms. Steroid creams, readily prescribed for discoid SLE, appear to heal and reduce lesions. Medical researchers continue to experiment with other pharmacological agents, such as sex hormones (Huston, 1989), and with other treatments, such as plasmapheresis, which involves exchange of blood plasma (Miescher & Beris, 1984), and antibody therapy (Huston, 1987), but studies remain inconclusive.

Physicians often prescribe exercise and physical therapy for patients with SLE. Dubois and Wallace (1987) suggested SLE patients engage in exercises that sustain isometric contractions to increase muscle strength, but cautioned against exercises that place stress on the body's supporting structures. Thus, swimming may enhance overall tone and strength, but it is probably best if SLE patients avoid jogging. Formal physical therapy can help develop an individual program of exercise as well as train gait control. Occupational therapy can assist patients in modifying household structures or obtaining proper supportive devices, such as canes and splints, for efficient movement and functioning. With reference to diet, only a well-balanced regimen significantly affects SLE; however, fish oil derivatives may also diminish arthritis symptoms often experienced by patients with SLE (Lee et al., 1985). Proper rest is imperative for SLE patients and is even more important for periods following corticosteroid reduction. Patients with discoid lupus (and many others with SLE) must also avoid ultraviolet light. Sunscreens and sunscreened automobile windows are usually effective in diminishing flares.

In addition to medical and physiologically oriented treatments, there are many psychological treatments that can help SLE patients and family members to understand the disease, reduce both physical and psychological symptoms, cope with chronic stress, reduce marital and family discord, and generally adapt to modified lifestyles. Treatment approaches include individual, family, and group modalities and span a broad range of theoretical viewpoints and therapeutic techniques.

Individual psychological treatments primarily aim at providing patients with self-awareness and self-efficacy. Depending upon patients' presenting complaints, therapists can accomplish this goal through biological, behavioral, cognitive, or emotional interventions. Behavioral medicine techniques help "modify the impact of biological and autonomic systems on the experience of being ill" (Tunks & Bellissimo, 1991, p. 55). Techniques utilized by behavioral medicine practitioners can provide relief from some of the most prominent and often most distressing symptoms and thus enable patients to attain a measure of personal competence. In general, basic stress management skills can help patients understand their physiological and psychological responses to stress and provide methods to minimize or eliminate these responses. Similarly, principles of progressive muscle relaxation or autohypnosis can reduce anxiety rooted in the out-of-control feelings that often accompany chronic illness (Mineka & Kelly, 1989). In particular, common symptoms, such as headaches and Raynaud's phenomenon (see Table 26.1), respond well to biofeedback and thermal feedback measures, as shown by Sappington and Fiorito (1985), who followed a single SLE patient with Raynaud's phenomenon and found that benefits from an intensive 5-week thermal feedback protocol extended over an 8-year period. Pain management and stress management programs might also include detailed analyses of patients' maladaptive behaviors and provide suggestions for precise behavioral changes. For example, an individualized weight-loss program could lead to reduced strain on arthritic joints, or a psychoeducational program offering advice to family members could reduce secondary gains.

Other psychological treatments include cognitive interventions that teach patients to monitor their irrational thoughts or beliefs, substitute more realistic perceptions, or engage in more appropriate problem solving (Keefe, Dunsmore, & Burnett, 1992). Such cognitive techniques are also useful in effectively treating depression (Beck, 1976).

Alternatively, traditional, or psychodynamic psychotherapeutic approaches, can facilitate working through the many losses associated with SLE, treat characterological disturbances that exacerbate symptoms or situations, and remediate interpersonal difficulties. Vocational counseling is often necessary, and treatment teams can include such counseling with any of the various types of interventions.

SLE patients do not exist in a vacuum; their disease affects entire families. Marital and family interventions aim at improving communication, adjusting roles, shifting power structures, and helping members negotiate developmental tasks. Education about the disease may be a helpful addition, especially in the context of family therapy, where each member can openly voice particular fears, and therapists can then dispel any preexisting myths.

Use of group therapy for SLE patients has been minimal; however, SLE patients with primarily psychological complaints may find group treatments helpful. Most group treatments focus on stress management or forms of relaxation. One interesting study by Rider and Kibler (1990) used progressive muscle relaxation with background music to enhance health-directed imagery and improve physical functioning. Although small sample size limited the study, their report of positive results warrants further exploration of group treatment.

Support groups have probably received the most attention as group treatments for SLE. In 1986, the Western Pennsylvania Chapter of the Lupus Foundation of America designed a psychoeducational support group program, currently distributed to over 200 cities in the United States and Canada. The task force assigned to program development identified two distinct groups of SLE patients: (1) newly diagnosed patients who were "fact hungry" and in need of medical information, and (2) patients with established diseases who were "support hungry" and in need of coping assistance. The complete program offers advice from and contact with professional facilitators, such as physicians, psychologists, and allied health-care providers, who educate patients and their families about medical and psychological aspects of SLE. In addition, participants receive encouragement to discuss their personal experiences. Efficacy of the program remains untested; however, in the first year of operation, 315 individuals in the western Pennsylvania area attended groups, and participation has continued to increase. Moreover, funding from the Pennsylvania Department of Health has enabled establishment of similar support groups in 21 Pennsylvania counties. Research is now under way to assess the program; preliminary results suggest that this type of support-group intervention may indeed prove fruitful in helping SLE patients manage the disease.

Of course, treatment teams cannot ignore the problem of organic versus functional disorders when selecting patients' treatments. Patients' failures to respond to ongoing treatments of any type may signal presence of organic processes. In this case, appropriate referrals for medical services are necessary. On the other hand, organic disorders do not preclude additional psychological problems; in this case, psychological interventions may supplement medical treatments.

Clearly, management of this complex disease requires a multidisciplinary approach as well as cooperation and motivation of patients. As mentioned, a wide range of treatment choices include medication; exercise and physical therapy; individual psychotherapy based on behavioral, cognitive, or behavioral medicine approaches; vocational counseling; family therapy; and group therapy, including support groups. At present, psychological approaches have a well-established role in the treatment of SLE. However, there is great need in this area for further research efforts aimed at designing additional methods of management and evaluating relative efficacy of various treatments and treatment combinations.

FUTURE DIRECTIONS

Growing prevalence of HIV, responsible for AIDS, has stimulated great interest in the immune system and its dysregulation. Although AIDS may represent a disease process that is opposite of SLE—AIDS causes the immune system to underreact, whereas SLE causes the immune system to overreact—research into intricacies of the immune response will no doubt advance understanding of both SLE and AIDS and their underlying processes. Similarly, medical, pharmacological, and technological research directed at discovering causes and cures for SLE and AIDS has abounded in recent years, and as these diagnoses become more common, such research will continue well into the future.

The role of psychologists in exploration, management, and even prevention of SLE is virtually limitless. First, SLE provides an excellent model of mind–body interaction. It is a widely accepted premise in the field of psychoneuroimmunology that immune responses influence neural and endocrine function and, hence, behavior (Ader & Cohen, 1985). However, SLE clearly suggests that behavior also affects immune responses and, thus, flares of the disease. Psychological research into SLE may shed further light on this delicate process and possibly describe behavioral methods of balancing immune system functioning. Second, despite much research into genetic and hormonal origins of SLE, it appears likely that environmental triggers and personal behaviors are also necessary ingredients for disease development. Research into environmental and behavioral risk factors may point the way to prevention and amelioration of SLE.

Third, there is a dearth of carefully conducted research into the perceptions, attitudes, and beliefs of SLE patients regarding their disease. Armed with a thorough understanding of the patients' experiences, psychologists would be better able to design more appropriate educational materials and programs as well as community campaigns aimed at early detection. Fourth, the sometimes toxic and usually uncomfortable results of many medical treatments for SLE may encourage patients to seek alternative behavioral approaches. Enhancement of existing, or development of additional, behavioral methods for pain management and symptom relief could diminish need for toxic medications or invasive medical techniques. Single-case design studies utilizing innovative techniques (e.g., biofeedback for psychological conditions, visual imagery to reduce migrating arthralgias) may prove invaluable in this search.

Fifth, although psychologists are already instrumental in providing clinical assistance to SLE patients and their families, further investigations of therapeutic outcomes are necessary to expand the scope of psychological intervention and encourage patients to seek psychological help. Again, single-case design studies can afford clinicians opportunities to lend evidence to the efficacy of their services and provide a base of knowledge upon which more programmatic research efforts can develop. Sixth, SLE is unique in that it affects both women and blacks disproportionately. Research into gender and racial differences may serve to delineate additional risk factors and possibly point to alternative treatment methods. Seventh, medical research alone may not resolve the problem of organic versus functional psychological disorders. Development of psychological and neuropsychological screening tools to detect organic processes could assist in this dilemma and eliminate long periods of patient frustration and overmedication. And finally, research regarding SLE, called "the Great Imitator" because its presentation mimics a myriad of diseases and psychological conditions, may provide valuable information about other disease processes. By understanding SLE and its many implications, psychologists and other health-care professionals are apt to gain a better understanding of conditions that surround and contribute to disease and health.

Acknowledgments

Special thanks to Ruth Ann Seilhamer for her helpful comments, to Jean Mientus and Deborah Nigro for their assistance through the Lupus Foundation of America, and to Paul Kostyak for his patience and assistance with the preparation of this chapter.

REFERENCES

Ader, R., & Cohen, N. (1985). CNS–immune system interactions: Conditioning phenomena. *The Behavioral and Brain Sciences, 8,* 379–394.

Aladjem, H. (1985). *Understanding lupus: What it is, how to treat it, how to cope with it.* New York: Scribner's.

Aladjem, H., & Schur, P. H. (1988). *In search of the sun: A woman's courageous victory over lupus.* New York: Macmillan.

American Psychiatric Association. (1987). *Diagnostic and statistical manual of mental disorders* (3rd ed. rev.). Washington, DC: Author.

Arnett, F. C., Bias, W. B., & Shulman, L. E. (1972). Studies in familial systemic lupus erythematosus. *Arthritis and Rheumatism, 15,* 102.

Asherson, R. A., Denburg, S. D., Denburg, J. A., Carbotte, R. M., & Futrell, N. (1993). Current concepts of neuropsychiatric systemic lupus erythematosus (NP-SLE). *Postgraduate Medical Journal. 69(1),* 602–608.

Baehr, G., Klemperer, P., & Schifrin, A. (1935). A diffuse disease of the peripheral circulation usually associated with lupus erythematosus and endocarditis. *Transactions of the Association of American Physicians, 50,* 139.

Bardana, E. J., Jr., Malinow, M. R., Houghton, D. C., McNulty, W. P., Wuepper, K. D., Parker, F., & Pirofsky, B. (1982). Diet-induced systemic lupus erythematosus (SLE) in primates. *American Journal of Kidney Disease, 1(6),* 345–352.

Beck, A. T. (1976). *Cognitive therapy and the emotional disorders.* New York: International Universities Press.

Blotzer, J. W. (1983). Systemic lupus erythematosus I: Historical aspects. *Maryland State Medical Journal, 32,* 439–441.

Bluestein, H. G. (1987). Neuropsychiatric disorders in systemic lupus erythematosus. In R. G. Lahita (Ed.), *Systemic lupus erythematosus* (pp. 593–614). New York: Churchill Livingstone.

Bluestein, H. G. (1987). Neuropsychiatric manifestations of systemic lupus erythematosus. *The New England Journal of Medicine, 317(5),* 309–311.

Bresnihan, B., Hohmeister, R., Cutting, J., Travers, R. L., Waldburger, M., Black, C., Jones, T., & Hughes, G. R. V. (1979). The neuropsychiatric disorder in systemic lupus erythematosus: Evidence for both vascular and immune mechanisms. *Annals of the Rheumatic Diseases, 38,* 301–306.

Brunner, C. M., Horwitz, D. A., Shann, M. K., Sturgill, B. A., & Davis, J. S. (1973). IV: Clinical and immunologic studies in identical twins discordant for systemic lupus erythematosus. *American Journal of Medicine, 55,* 249–254.

Buckman, K. J., Moore, S. K., Ebbin, A. J., Cox, M. B., & Dubois, E. L. (1978). Familial systemic lupus erythematosus. *Archives of Internal Medicine, 138,* 1674–1676.

Carbotte, R. M., Denburg, S. D., & Denburg, J. A. (1986). Prevalence of cognitive impairment in systemic lupus erythematosus. *The Journal of Nervous and Mental Disease, 174(6),* 357–364.

Cassileth, B. R., Lusk, E. J., Strouse, T. B., Miller, D. S., Brown, L. L., Corss, P. A., & Tenaglia, A. N. (1984). Psychosocial status in chronic illness: A comparative analysis of six diagnostic groups. *The New England Journal of Medicine, 311(8),* 506–511.

Cazanave, P. L., & Chausit, M. (1851). Annales des maladies de la peau et de la syphilis. *Conference du 4 Juin 1851 Paris, 3,* 297–299.

Cope, N. R., & Hall, H. R. (1985). The health status of black women in the U.S.: Implications for health psychology and behavioral medicine. *SAGE, II(2),* 20–24.

Cordasco, E. M., Demeter, S. L., Kerkay, J., van Ordstrand, H. S., Lucas, E. V., Chen, T., & Golish, J. A. (1980). Pulmonary manifestations of vinyl and polyvinylchloride interstitial lung disease. *Chest, 78,* 828–834.

Currey, H. L. F., & Hull, S. (1987). *Rheumatology for general practitioners.* Oxford: Oxford University Press.

Darby, P. L., & Schmidt, P. J. (1988). Psychiatric consultations in rheumatology: A review of 100 cases. *Canadian Journal of Psychiatry, 33,* 290–292.

Denburg, J. A., Carbotte, R. M., & Denburg, S. D. (1987). Neuronal antibodies and cognitive function in systemic lupus erythematosus. *Neurology, 37,* 464–467.

Denburg, S. D., Carbotte, R. M., Long, A. A., & Denburg, J. A. (1988). Neuropsychological correlates of serum lymphocytotoxic antibodies in systemic lupus erythematosus. *Brain, Behavior and Immunity, 2,* 222–234.

Denburg, J. A., & Temesvari, P. (1983). Current review: The pathogenesis of neuropsychiatric lupus. *Canadian Medical Association Journal, 128,* 257–260.

Drug facts and comparisons. (1993). St. Louis, MO: Facts and Comparisons, Kluwer.

Dubois, E., & Wallace, D. J. (1987). *Lupus erythematosus* (3rd ed.). Philadelphia: Lea & Febiger.

Dvoredsky, A. E., & Cooley, H. W. (1986). Comparative severity of illness in patients with combined medical and psychiatric diagnoses. *Psychosomatics, 27(9),* 625–630.

Elliott, J. A., Jr., & Mathieson, D. R. (1953). Complement in disseminated (systemic) lupus erythematosus. *Archives of Dermatology and Syphilology, 68,* 119–128.

Epstein, J. H., Tuffanelli, D. L., & Dubois, E. L. (1965). Light sensitivity and lupus erythematosus. *Archives of Dermatology, 91,* 483–485.

Fernandez-Herlihy, L. (1989). Drug-induced lupus may hold the key. *Local Lupus, XVI,* 10.

Fock, K. M., Feng, P. H., & Tey, B. H. (1984). Autoimmune disease developing after augmentation mammoplasty: Report of three cases. *Journal of Rheumatology, 11(1),* 98–100.

Freeman, R. G., Knox, J. M., & Owen, D. W. (1969). Cutaneous lesions of lupus erythematosus induced by monochromatic light. *Archives of Dermatology, 100,* 677–682.

Friedberg, C. K., Gross, L., & Wallach, K. (1936). Nonbacterial thrombotic endocarditis associated with prolonged fever, arthritis, inflammation of serous membranes and widespread vascular lesions. *Archives of Internal Medicine, 58,* 662–684.

Fukase, M. (Ed.). (1980). *Systemic lupus erythematosus.* Tokyo: University of Tokyo Press.

Ginzler, E., Diamond, H., Kaplan, D., Weiner, M., Schlesinger, M., & Seleznick, M. (1978). Computer analysis of factors influencing frequency of infection in systemic lupus erythematosus. *Arthritis and Rheumatism, 21(1),* 37–44.

Gluck, O. (1990). Antimalarials and lupus. *Facts about lupus, 14.* Rockville, MD: Lupus Foundation of America, Inc.

Graninger, W., Smolen, J. S., & Zielinski, C. C. (1987). Description of systemic lupus erythematosus: A historical perspective. In J. S. Smolen & C. C. Zielinski (Eds.), *Systemic lupus erythematosus: Clinical and experimental aspects* (pp. 2–5). Berlin/Heidelberg, Germany: Springer-Verlag.

Gupta, S., & Talal, N. (1985). *Immunology of rheumatic diseases.* New York: Plenum Press.

Hall, R. C. W., Popkin, M. K., Stickney, S. K., & Gardner, E. R. (1979). Presentation of steroid psychoses. *Journal of Nervous and Mental Disease, 167(4),* 229–235.

Hargraves, M. M., Richmond, H., & Morton, R. (1948). Presentation of two bone marrow elements: The tart cell and LE cell. *Proceedings of the Staff Meeting of the Mayo Clinic, 23,* 25.

Honer, W. G., & Prohovnik, I. (1989). Organic affective disorder and vascular dysregulation in systemic lupus erythematosus. *Canadian Journal of Psychiatry, 34,* 134–136.

Hopkinson, N. (1991). Systemic lupus erythematosus: Epidemiological clues to aetiology. *British Journal of Hospital Medicine, 45(5),* 291–293.

Hughes, G. R. V. (1980). Central nervous system lupus—diagnosis and treatment. *The Journal of Rheumatology, 7(3),* 405–411.

Huston, D. P. (1987). Experimental therapy in systemic lupus erythematosus. In R. G. Lahita (Ed.), *Systemic lupus erythematosus* (pp. 947–972). New York: Churchill Livingstone.

Ireys, H. T., & Burr, C. K. (1984). Apart and a part: Family issues for young adults with chronic illness and disability. In M. G. Eisenberg, L. C. Sutkin, & M. A. Jansen (Eds.), *Chronic illness and disability through the life span: Effects on self and family* (pp. 184–206). New York: Springer.

Jacobs, J. W., Bernhard, M. R., Delgado, A., & Strain, J. J. (1977). Screening for organic mental syndromes in the medically ill. *Annals of Internal Medicine, 86,* 40–46.

Kaell, A. T., Shetty, M., Lee, B. C. P., & Lockshin, M. D. (1986). The diversity of neurologic events in systemic lupus erythematosus. *Archives of Neurology, 43,* 273–276.

Keefe, F. J., Dunsmore, J., & Burnett, R. (1992). Behavioral and cognitive–behavioral approaches to chronic pain: Recent advances and future directions. *Journal of Consulting and Clinical Psychology, 60(4),* 528–536.

Kimmel, D. C. (1980). *Adulthood and aging: An interdisciplinary, developmental view* (2nd ed.). New York: Wiley.

Klippel, J. H. (1987). Immunosuppressive therapy. In R. G. Lahita (Ed.), *Systemic lupus erythematosus* (pp. 923–945). New York: Churchill Livingstone.

Knippen, M. A. (1988). The relationship among selected variables associated with fatigue in women with systemic lupus erythematosus (Doctoral dissertation, The Catholic University of America). *Dissertation Abstracts International, 50,* 2338.

Koffler, S. (1987). The role of neuropsychological testing in systemic lupus erythematosus. In R. G. Lahita (Ed.), *Systemic lupus erythematosus* (pp. 847–853). New York: Churchill Livingstone.

Kumagai, Y., Shiokawa, Y., Medsger, T. A., Jr., & Rodnan, G. P. (1984). Clinical spectrum of connective tissue disease after cosmetic surgery. *Arthritis and Rheumatism, 27(1),* 1–12.

Kutner, K. C., Busch, H. M., Mahmood, T., Racis, S. P., & Krey, P. R. (1988). Neuropsychological functioning in systemic lupus erythematosus. *Neuropsychology, 2,* 119–126.

Labrie, V. Y. (1987). Lupus: Managing a complex chronic disability (Doctoral dissertation, University of California, San Francisco). *Dissertation Abstracts International, 48(2)*, DA8708450.

Lahita, R. G. (Ed.). (1987). *Systemic lupus erythematosus*. New York: Churchill Livingstone.

Lee, T. H., Hoover, R. L., Williams, J. D., Sperling, R. J., Ravalese, J., III, Spur, B. W., Robinson, D. R., Corey, E. J., Lewis, R. A., & Austin, K. F. (1985). Effect of dietary enrichment with eicosapentanaenoic docosahexaenoic acids on in vitro neutrophil and monocyte leukotrine generation and neutrophil function. *New England Journal of Medicine, 312(19)*, 1217–1224.

Liang, M. H., Rogers, M., Larson, M., Eaton, H. M., Murawski, B. J., Taylor, J. E., Swafford, J., & Schur, P. H. (1984). The psychosocial impact of systemic lupus erythematosus and rheumatoid arthritis. *Arthritis and Rheumatism, 27(1)*, 13–19.

Libmann, E., & Sacks, B. (1924). A hitherto undescribed form of valvular and mural endocarditis. *Archives of Internal Medicine, 33*, 701–737.

Lupus Foundation of America, Inc. (1990). *Facts about lupus* (A series of pamphlets available from 4 Research Place, Suite 180, Rockville, MD 20850-3226).

Makarova, O. V. (1978). Effect of systemic lupus erythematosus antibodies against DNA on RNA synthesis. *Arthritis and Rheumatism, 21(1)*, 45–50.

McCarty, D. J. (1985). *Arthritis and allied conditions: A textbook of rheumatology*. Philadelphia: Lea & Febiger.

Miescher, P. A., & Beris, P. (1984). Treatment of SLE. In P. H. Lambert, L. Perrin, & S. Izui (Eds.), *Recent advances in systemic lupus erythematosus* (pp. 349–359). London: Academic Press (Harcourt Brace).

Mineka, S., & Kelly, K. A. (1989). The relationship between anxiety, lack of control and loss of control. In A. Steptoe & A. Appels (Eds.), *Stress, personal control, and health* (pp. 163–191). Chichester: Wiley.

Mitchell, W. D., & Thompson, T. L. (1990). Psychiatric distress in systemic lupus erythematosus outpatients. *Psychosomatics, 31(3)*, 293–300.

Moore, J. E., & Lutz, W. V. (1955). The natural history of systemic lupus erythematosus: An approach to its study through chronic biologic false positive reaction. *Journal of Chronic Diseases, 1*, 297–316.

Moynihan, T. C. (1990). Lupus: Underwriting an enigma. *Broker World, 10(2)*, 144–150.

National Institute of Arthritis and Musculoskeletal and Skin Diseases (1986, December). *Update: Lupus erythematosus research* (DHHS No. NIH 87-460). Washington, DC: U.S. Government Printing Office.

O'Connor, J. F., & Musher, D. M. (1966). Central nervous system involvement in systemic lupus erythematosus: A study of 150 cases. *Archives of Neurology, 14*, 157–164.

Perry, S. W. (1987). Psychiatric aspects of systemic lupus erythematosus. In R. G. Lahita (Ed.), *Systemic lupus erythematosus* (pp. 821–846). New York: Churchill Livingstone.

Petri, M., Perez-Gutthann, S., Longenecker, J. C., & Hockberg, M. (1991). Morbidity of systemic lupus erythematosus: Role of race and socioeconomic status. *American Journal of Medicine, 91*, 345–353.

Pitzelle, S. K. (1985). *We are not alone: Learning to live with chronic illness*. Minneapolis, MN: Thompson.

Reeves, W. H., & Lahita, R. G. (1987). Clinical presentation of systemic lupus erythematosus in the adult. In R. G. Lahita (Ed.), *Systemic lupus erythematosus* (pp. 355–382). New York: Churchill Livingstone.

Reidenberg, M. M., Durant, P. J., Harris, R. A., de Boccardo, G., Lahita, R., & Stenzel, K. H. (1983). Lupus erythematosus-like disease due to hydrazine. *American Journal of Medicine, 75*, 365–370.

Rider, M. S., & Kibler, V. E. (1990). Treating arthritis and lupus patients with music-mediated imagery and group psychotherapy. *The Arts in Psychotherapy, 17*, 29–33.

Roitt, I., Brostoff, D., & Male, D. (1989). *Immunology* (2nd ed.). St. Louis, MO: Mosby.

Ropes, M. W. (1976). *Systemic lupus erythematosus*. Cambridge, MA: Harvard University Press.

Rothfield, N. F. (1989). Systemic lupus erythematosus: Clinical aspects and treatment. In D. J. McCarty (Ed.), *Arthritis and allied conditions—A textbook of rheumatology, 11th ed.* (pp. 1022–1048). Philadelphia: Lea & Febiger.

Rustad, L. C. (1984). Family adjustment to chronic illness and disability in midlife. In M. G. Eisenberg, L. C. Sutkin, & M. A. Jansen (Eds.), *Chronic illness and disability through the life span: Effects on self and family* (pp. 222–242). New York: Springer.

Sappington, J. T., & Fiorito, E. M. (1985). Thermal feedback in Raynaud's phenomenon secondary to systemic lupus erythematosus: Long-term remission of target symptoms. *Biofeedback and Self-Regulation, 10(4)*, 335–341.

Schneebaum, A. B., Singleton, J. D., West, S. G., Blodgett, J. K., Allen, L. G., Cheronis, J. C., & Kotzin, B. L.

(1991). Association of psychiatric manifestations with antibodies to ribosomal P Proteins in systemic lupus erythematosus. *American Journal of Medicine, 90,* 54–62.

Schur, P. H. (1985). Introduction: An overview of lupus. In H. Aladjem, (Ed.), *Understanding lupus: What it is, how to treat it, how to cope with it* (pp. XV–XXXI). New York: Scribner's.

Schwartz, R. S. (1989). Fatigue and the vexed, tired lupus patient. *Lupus News, 9(2),* 1–2. Rockville, MD: Lupus Foundation of America, Inc.

Seaman, W. P. (1990). The cellular requirements for immunity and autoimmunity. *Lupus News, 10(1),* 7–9.

Siekert, R. G., & Clark, E. C. (1955). Neurologic signs and symptoms as early manifestations of systemic lupus erythematosus. *Neurology, 5,* 84–88.

Stein, M., & Scheifler, S. J. (1985). Frontiers of stress research: Stress and immunity. In M. R. Zales (Ed.), *Stress in health and disease* (pp. 97–114). New York: Brunner/Mazel.

Steptoe, A. (1989). The significance of personal control in health and disease. In A. Steptoe & A. Appels (Eds.), *Stress, personal control, and health* (pp. 309–318). Chichester, UK: Wiley.

Suratt, P. M., Winn, W. C., Brody, A. R., Bolton, W. K., & Giles, R. D. (1977). Acute silicosis in tombstone sandblasters. *American Review of Respiratory Diseases, 115,* 521–529.

Swaak, A. J. G., Nossent, J. C., & Bronsveld, W. (1989). Systemic lupus erythematosus. I. Outcome and survival: Dutch experiences with 110 patients studied prospectively. *Annals of Rheumatic Diseases, 48,* 447–454.

Talal, N. (1983). A clinician and a scientist look at acquired immune-deficiency syndrome (AIDS). A validation of immunology's theoretical foundation. *Immunology Today, 4,* 180.

Tan, E. M., Cohen, A. S., Iries, J. F., Masi, A. T., McShane, D. J., Rothfield, N. F., Schaller, J. G., Talal, N., & Winchester, R. J. (1982). The 1982 revised criteria for the classification of systemic lupus erythematosus. *Arthritis and Rheumatism, 25(2),* 1271–1277.

Tuffanelli, D. L. (1991). What is the magnitude of the problem of lupus erythematosus? *Lupus News: The Official Newsletter of the Lupus Foundation of America, Inc., 11(2),* 1–2.

Tunks, E., & Bellissimo, A. (1991). *Behavioral medicine: Concepts and procedures.* New York: Pergamon.

United States pharmacopeia dispensing information: Drug information for the health care professional (13th ed.). (1993). Massachusetts: Rand McNally.

Urowitz, M. B., & Gladman, D. D. (1980). Late mortality in SLE—"The price we pay for control." *Journal of Rheumatology, 7(3),* 412–416.

van Dam, A. P., Wekking, E. M., & Oomen, H. A. P. C. (1991). Psychiatric symptoms as features of systemic lupus erythematosus. *Psychotherapy and Psychosomatics, 55,* 132–140.

Voss, E. W., Jr. (Ed.). (1988). *Anti-DNA antibodies in SLE.* Boca Raton, FL: CRC Press.

Wallace, D. J. (1993). The clinical presentation of SLE. In D. J. Wallace & B. H. Hahn (Eds.), *Dubois' lupus erythematosus, 4th ed.* (pp. 317–321). Philadelphia: Lea & Febiger.

Wallace, D. J. (1993). Steroid sparing drugs in lupus. *Lupus News: The Official Newsletter of the Lupus Foundation of America, Inc., 9(2),* 2.

Wallace, D. J., Podell, T., Weiner, J., Klinenberg, J. R., Forouzesh, S., & Dubois, E. L. (1981). Systemic lupus erythematosus—survival patterns: Experience with 609 patients. *Journal of the American Medical Association, 245(9),* 934–938.

Wekking, E. M., Nossent, J. C., van Dam, A. P., & Swaak, A. J. J. G. (1991). Cognitive and emotional disturbances in systemic lupus erythematosus. *Psychotherapy and Psychosomatics, 55,* 126–131.

Western Pennsylvania Chapter, Inc., Lupus Foundation of America, Inc. (1986). *In-hospital lupus support group program manual.* Pittsburgh, PA: Author.

Willner, P. (1984). Cognitive functioning in depression: A review of theory and research. *Psychological Medicine, 14,* 807–823.

Witebsky, E., Rose, N. R., Terplan, K., Paine, J. R., & Egan, R. W. (1957). Chronic thyroiditis and autoimmunization. *Journal of the American Medical Association, 164,* 1439–1447.

Yung, R. L., & Richardson, B. C. (1994). Drug-induced lupus. *Rheumatic Disease Clinics of North America, 20(1),* 61–86.

Ziskind, M., Jones, R. N., & Weill, H. (1976). Silicosis. *American Review of Respiratory Diseases, 113,* 643–665.

V
EMERGING TOPICS

27

Theoretical Models Applied to AIDS Prevention

Janet S. St. Lawrence, Ted L. Brasfield, Kennis Jefferson, and Edna Alleyne

Human immunodeficiency virus (HIV) infection and acquired immunodeficiency syndrome (AIDS) offer an unprecedented challenge to psychologists. When researchers first identified the underlying cause of the epidemic as a retrovirus, it was apparent that behavior change would be the only means of curtailing HIV infection for literally years into the future while biomedical research searched for a vaccine or cure. AIDS is now well into its second decade, and behavioral methods remain the cornerstone of prevention efforts. Because of the retrovirus's complex properties, biomedical solutions are slow to emerge and behavioral prevention remains at the forefront of efforts to interrupt the escalating spread of HIV infection and AIDS. For the first time in recorded history, psychologists, rather than biomedical professionals, are the key response to an epidemic. Psychologists can respond through behavior-change interventions on an individual, group, or community level; by altering the social stigma attached to these diseases through attitude-change programs; and by consultation with health educators, health-care providers, public health specialists, and policy-making bodies to aid in translating the scientific database into sound programs and policies.

The HIV/AIDS epidemic is not a monolithic event (Hinman, 1991) and no single method of response will surmount this epidemic. The AIDS health crisis incorporates several epidemics, each with different means of transmission, differences in illness progression, regional and geographic variations, and different effects upon

---

Janet S. St. Lawrence, Ted L. Brasfield, Kennis Jefferson, and Edna Alleyne • Community Health Program, Jackson State University, Jackson, Mississippi 39217.
Handbook of Health and Rehabilitation Psychology, edited by Anthony J. Goreczny. Plenum Press, New York, 1995.

various population segments. Many AIDS prevention efforts are atheoretical becausecommunity-based groups reacted quickly to a perceived health threat, developed and implemented programs based on their face validity, and gave little attention to either theory or program evaluation. However, after-the-fact implicit theoretical assumptions are often detectable. As AIDS prevention has matured, scientists have begun to advance theoretical models but sometimes still use these models *post hoc* to supply conceptual foundations. Empiricism has been slower to evolve, and evaluation research remains sparse. There is wide latitude found in this literature base. In some cases, heuristic programs remain virtually untested. In others, developers have based their programs on theoretical health models, with stringent attention to evaluation. Most available efforts fall somewhere between these two extremes.

Five theoretical models appear in the AIDS education and prevention literature. These conceptual "families" are (1) psychoeducational theories, which stress information provision; (2) cognitive theories, which emphasize internal decision-making processes; (3) models based on learning theory; (4) applications based on theories of motivation and emotional arousal; and (5) social marketing and social influence theories, adapted to AIDS prevention. These five theoretical models have heterogenous origins. Some have evolved specifically to explain health behavior. Nonetheless, some researchers have extracted other models from social and clinical psychology and extended them to health behavior or adopted models from other disciplines because they seemed relevant. In addition to their conceptual diversity, their applications vary. Some theories are more applicable at individual or small-group levels, whereas others are more applicable with larger populations or on a community level. In the sections that follow, we discuss these theoretical models and review their applications to AIDS prevention.

PSYCHOEDUCATIONAL THEORIES STRESSING INFORMATION PROVISION

AIDS education programs are the most prominent response to this health threat. Reliance on education alone is fraught with difficulties, and evidence suggests that educational campaigns are a necessary, although insufficient, component to slow the spread of HIV infection. AIDS educational programs share the goals of (1) imparting information so that recipients develop an understanding of HIV transmission; (2) influencing attitudes and behaviors so target audiences will translate newly acquired knowledge into practice; and (3) as the end result, lowering HIV infection. Despite these common elements, AIDS educational materials and programs vary widely with respect to content, coverage, depth, educational level, emotional maturity, social sensitivity, explicitness, and target audience.

A national study of educational campaigns found that widespread media campaigns alert the general public to the issues, but that more specific programs usually are necessary to generate behavior change among individuals who are most at risk (Ross & Carson, 1988). This is consistent with several studies that have found little correlation between knowledge and behavior among individuals at potential risk for HIV infection (St. Lawrence & Betts, 1989; St. Lawrence, Kelly, Hood, & Brasfield, 1987). Despite these apparently grim findings, mathematical modeling strategies show that, over the long term, AIDS educational programs do reduce HIV transmission (Kaplan & Abramson, 1989). These mathematical projections indicate that it is shortsighted to limit AIDS prevention efforts only to interventions that demonstrate an immediate, measurable impact, such as the behavior skills model. Although education may, by comparison, be "ineffectual" in the short term, evidence that reasonable long-term benefits accrue justifies channeling continued resources into education programs.

COGNITIVE THEORIES APPLIED TO AIDS PREVENTION

Cognitive models emphasize relationships between decision making and behavior and view cognitive factors as causal determinants of behavior. Although these approaches are highly popular as explanatory models in the AIDS prevention literature, there is less empirical, evaluative data on cognitive models than on behavioral models, based on learning theory, or social marketing/social influence models. Cognitive models, generally encountered in survey research however, do provide frameworks to help explain correlative relationships, identified in surveys, between cognitive beliefs and specific behaviors. Each cognitive model of AIDS prevention shares the assumption that cognitive variables are causal, predisposing factors that result in risky behavior.

The Health Belief Model

Derived from cognitive expectancy theory, the Health Belief Model (HBM) (Becker, 1974; Rosenstock & Kirscht, 1979) serves as a theoretical framework to explain and predict a large variety of health-related behaviors in the public health literature (Brown, DiClemente, & Reynolds, 1991). Given the popularity of the HBM in general health research, it is not surprising that investigators extended it to AIDS prevention. The HBM proposes that cognitive mediators, such as (1) perceived vulnerability to a health threat, (2) perceived severity of the threat, (3) belief in effectiveness of precautionary action, (4) perceived costs of implementing action, and (5) presence of environmental cues, interact with one another to produce behavior change. When applied to AIDS prevention, the Health Belief Model presumes that safer sexual intentions develop from personal beliefs regarding susceptibility to HIV infection, perceived consequences of becoming infected, and extent to which one believes safer sexual practices are effective in reducing susceptibility. Additionally, the model hypothesizes that perceived efficacy of safer sexual behaviors subsequently balance against perceived social, physical, and psychological barriers to change. Finally, the model assumes that specific identifiable stimuli are necessary to trigger the decision-making process. These cues to action might be, for example, educational or mass media campaigns designed to raise public awareness of the health threat. When applying the Health Belief Model to condom-promotion campaigns, for example, one would predict condom use will increase as individuals (1) perceive themselves susceptible to HIV infection, (2) regard consequences of infection as severe, (3) believe condoms effectively prevent transmission, (4) perceive minimal barriers to condom use, (5) have visible reminders in the environment, and (6) are able to acquire and use condoms to protect themselves.

The HBM, originally proposed in the 1950s, was an effort to understand the general public's low compliance with preventive health recommendations. Later, it became widely adopted as an explanatory framework for factors that determine responses to any health threat (Janz & Becker, 1984). In 1974 and 1984, review articles examined research evaluating the Health Belief Model (Becker, 1974; Janz & Becker, 1984). In the 1974 review, 10 of 11 studies found that perceived susceptibility predicted preventive behavior, whereas the remaining components were significant in 70% to 80% of the studies reviewed. A decade later, a very different pattern emerged from the literature review. This later review found that perceived impediments to adopting safer practices were the most significant predictors of behavior change (all 10 of the studies reviewed), whereas severity of perceived health threat was least important, and perceptions of vulnerability and beliefs regarding efficacy of health recommendations were of intermediate importance. However, none of the reviewed studies addressed behaviors similar to those implicated in the AIDS epidemic. They addressed health issues, such as attending health-screening programs, compliance with immunizations, or keeping follow-up clinic appointments. Only one study among the articles included in the review dealt with a potentially threatening health issue, but it did not require any difficult behavior changes (Becker, Kaback, Rosenstock, & Ruth, 1975).

Nonetheless, a considerable body of literature supports the worth of the Health Belief Model as a framework for understanding health promotion (Becker, 1974; Janz & Becker, 1984; Kegeles, 1980; Nathanson & Becker, 1983). Nathanson and Becker used the model in a pilot study that improved beliefs about contraception, sexual knowledge, and contraceptive use by adolescents following participation in a 15-hour program, but the authors did not analyze the model's individual components or their unique contribution to the outcome. When Petosa and Jackson (1991) dissected the Health Belief Model and computed a regression equation to assess each component's contribution to safer sexual intentions, explained variance was moderate among 7th graders ($R^2 = .435$) but demonstrated an inverse relationship with educational level, decreasing to $R^2 = .169$ by 11th grade. The model received empirical support from only 1 of 3 samples that participated in the Petosa and Jackson study. Their study generated some doubt about replicability of isolated studies that reported the Health Belief Model's usefulness in predicting health-relevant attitudes.

Several other studies have investigated relationships between individual components of the Health Belief Model and behavior change. Most of the authors of these studies did not design the studies specifically to test the Health Belief Model. In most cases, these projects investigated variables selected for pragmatic, rather than theoretical, reasons. However, we can still interpret the findings in context of the HBM. For example, Klein et al. (1987) found that individuals who believed they were in a high-risk category and felt vulnerable to AIDS were more likely to reduce their risky behavior. Although Klein had not designed the study to test the HBM, the concluding discussion tied the finding into the HBM *post hoc*. Several other studies have also reported correlations between perceptions of threat and subsequent risk reduction (Coates et al., 1987; Keeter & Bradford, 1988; Valdiserri et al., 1988), but much less information is available to indicate whether other components of the HBM are relevant for AIDS prevention. The number of research studies that have found perceptions of susceptibility, severity, and benefits to be significant predictors of subsequent risky behavior is about the same as the number of studies that have no significant relationship at all (Coates et al., 1987; Emmons et al., 1986; Joseph et al., 1987; McCusker, Zapka, Stoddard, & Mayer, 1989; McKusick, Horstman, & Coates,

1985a; McKusick et al., 1985b; Validserri et al., 1988). Findings from AIDS prevention research using the Health Belief Model are, at best, equivocal. McCusker et al. (1989) concluded that, given the model's proven usefulness for explaining other health threats and its limited predictive value in AIDS prevention research, the "dynamics of an individual's adoption of preventive behaviors related to AIDS may be largely independent of other health protective behaviors" (p. 27).

There are several weaknesses in the Health Belief Model that may account for the inconsistent findings when extending it to AIDS prevention. First, many studies that provided correlational support for a predictive relationship between the HBM and health behavior actually account for only a modest amount of the behavioral variance. Second, although the model predicts perceived risk leads to behavior change, it does not explain the origin of interpretations of risk (Cleary et al., 1986). Third, the model does not describe how health beliefs develop or persist over time (Prochaska, Albrecht, Levy, Sugrue, & Kim, 1990). In addition, we can also challenge the assumption that beliefs precede behavior. Because this claim relies on correlational data, it is equally valid to claim that beliefs are a consequence, rather than a precursor, of behavior. The Health Belief Model has contributed very little to program development or intervention research at present but remains a popular framework to explain relationships between variables in survey research.

The Theory of Reasoned Action

The Theory of Reasoned Action (TRA; Ajzen & Fishbein, 1980; Fishbein & Ajzen, 1975) is conceptually similar to the Health Belief Model. Both offer cognitive variables as causal explanations for behavior change but significant differences between the two models do exist. The TRA assumes that people are rational organisms who systematically process and utilize available information before selecting a course of action. Behavior change occurs, as in other cognitive models, by altering underlying cognitions rather than by intervening with behavior (Fishbein & Middlestadt, 1989). The theory attempts to yoke attitudes and behavior by incorporating attitudes, subjective norms, cognitive intentions, and behavior into a predictive model. According to the theory, behavior results from cognitive intentions. Intentions, in turn, are the culmination of a quasi-mathematical equation combining attitudes (perceived costs and benefits of a behavior × perceived likelihood of occurrence) and subjective norms (perceived norms of significant others × motivation to comply with these norms) (Gallois, Kashima, Hill, & McCamish, 1990).

What distinguishes the TRA from the HBM is its emphasis on intentions as immediate precursors and determinants of behavior. According to the TRA, four factors interact to determine an intention: (1) an individual's attitudes toward a specific behavior, (2) beliefs about the behavior, (3) perceptions regarding peers' attitudes toward the behavior, and (4) extent to which the individual values the peer group's approval. Although this theory is similar to other cognitive theories in viewing behavior as an outcome of beliefs, inclusion of referent groups' norms as contributing factors and emphasis on cognitive intentions distinguish the TRA from other cognitive theories. In attending to peer norms, the TRA bears some similarity to social influence models. An intuitively appealing feature of the TRA lies in its attempt to quantify relationships between knowledge, beliefs, attitudes, and behavior. In the AIDS prevention literature, investigators have usually employed the TRA in survey research to explain observed correlations between attitudes and precautionary behavior, or intentions to engage in safer behavior in the future (cf. L. Jemmot & J. Jemmot, 1991). Support for one component of the TRA came from a study that found the only reliable predictor of gay men's shifts to safer sex was perceived peer support for precautionary behavior change (Joseph et al., 1987), but researchers also cite this same study as support for the social influence theory.

Like the HBM, the TRA assumes that information alters beliefs and attitudes thereby changing behavior, but researchers have found little evidence to support whether beliefs and attitudes are predecessors of behavior. This has been particularly true in health education campaigns, which generally produce large increases in knowledge, minimal change in attitudes, and almost no behavioral change (cf. Bartlett, 1981). Information alone is often insufficient to produce health-related behavioral change (Bartlett, 1981; Winett, 1986).

A second problem lies in this theory's logic. While the TRA attributes a causal role to intentions as determinants of subsequent behavior, supporters of the theory base this conclusion on correlational, rather than experimental, research. It is equally possible that it is behavior (i.e., use of condoms in the past) that generates future intentions (i.e., intention to use condoms in the future) rather than the reverse. Or there may be another causative factor that produces *both* intentions and behavior. It is also possible that even when intentions shift, behavior may remain stable or recalcitrant to change. To date, supporters of the TRA have not ruled out these alternative explanations.

Gallois et al. (1990) specifically tested the model with a large Australian sample; the study offered limited support for the model. Findings of the study showed that (1) denial was the prevailing strategy used to assess personal risk, (2) influencing participants' behaviors the most were preferences of their sexual partners followed by attitudes of their friends, and (3) perceived norms of the general public were inconsequential. Thus, their results offered greater support for the diffusion of innovation and social marketing models (discussed later) than for the Theory of Reasoned Action.

Decision-Making Theory

Decision-making theory also offers a cognitive framework for AIDS prevention, but it is less popular than the Health Belief Model and Theory of Reasoned Action. Decision-making theory relies on the assumption that people make rational choices that they believe will increase positive outcomes and enable them to avoid negative experiences (Abelson & Levi, 1985; Fishhoff, 1989). Historically, researchers have used decision theory to describe a wide array of situations, ranging from decisions to go to war (Lebow & Stein, 1987) to surgical decisions made on the basis of X-rays (Eddy, 1982).

Applied to AIDS prevention, decision theory acknowledges the myriad decisions that confront individuals at HIV risk, such as whether to undergo testing for HIV, change behaviors for self-protection, change behaviors out of consideration for others, or guard confidentiality. The model offers an explanatory framework for how decisions *should* be made and then examines differences between decisions that lead to risk taking and those that maximize safety. Given the complexity of these decisions, it is not surprising that the model is intricate.

Leviton (1989) identified four problems that arise when extending this model to AIDS prevention. First, individuals engaging in high-risk sex or drug use anticipate immediate gratification and have to juggle both immediate positive (i.e., sexual gratification, income, effects of substance use) and long-term negative consequences of their behavior (i.e., possible infection, illness in the future). Second, individuals often make decisions under conditions of uncertainty (i.e., wanting to have sex with a partner who may or may not have HIV). Third, individuals often fail to use probabilistic reasoning. Fourth, when individuals encounter the certainty of immediate gratification and uncertain long-term ramifications, they fix their attention on the immediate pleasure, and delay of gratification is a less appealing alternative (Mischel & Ebbeson, 1970).

At present, very little experimental work has substantiated the relevance or practicality of decision-making theory for AIDS prevention. As presented by Fishoff (1989), the model is highly quantifiable and lends itself to empirical evaluation, but whether the model will prove useful when extended to AIDS prevention remains unclear.

THEORIES BASED ON THE PRINCIPLES OF LEARNING

Learning theories emphasize environmental conditions implicated in the acquisition and maintenance of behaviors. Two general models based on learning theories are present in the AIDS prevention literature: operant theory, which make no assumptions about cognitive processes, and social learning theory, which incorporates cognitive mediating variables.

Operant Learning Theory

Operant learning theory does not rely on inaccessible mentalistic events to explain behavior. Instead, it relies on observable environmental events (reinforcers and discriminitive stimuli) implicated in the acquisition, performance, and maintenance of behavior (Ferster & Skinner, 1957; Skinner, 1969). Clinicians use operant approaches extensively in behavioral interventions for smoking cessation, medication, adherence, and weight loss (Brownell, 1982; Chesney, 1984; Pechacek, 1979). In the context of AIDS prevention, operant strategies can assist people who engage in high-risk behavior to regain control over their behavior by identifying and rearranging environmental influences and reinforcers. Operant approaches involve analysis of three components: (1) the behavior, (2) current reinforcers strengthening or maintaining the behavior, and (3) discriminative stimuli that serve as cues and "trigger" behavior.

Behaviors targeted for intervention using operant approaches could be, for example, condom use or entering settings associated with risky behavior in the past. *Discriminative stimuli* are any antecedent events that set in motion the behavioral sequence. Thus, we can interrupt the chain of behavior by modifying setting stimuli in an individual's environment (i.e., changing the route traveled between work and home so as to avoid temptation to stop at a location associated with risky behavior in the past, or taking enough money for only two drinks if overindulgence and undercontrol led to previous risky behavior). *Reinforcers* are any consequences that make it more likely individuals will repeat an act in the future. Types of reinforcement include positive reinforcement (e.g., sexual pleasure, drug high, appreciation from a partner for using a condom) and negative reinforcement (e.g., staying safe to avoid unwanted infection and subsequent illness). Patients and therapists can modify risky behaviors through selective manipulation of reinforcers or punishers contingent on those behaviors, and by rearranging antecedent conditions that preceded those behavior in the past.

Social Learning Theory

Social learning theory (Bandura, 1986) recognizes that individuals also learn in a social context by observing others and then imitating observed actions. Models may be media figures, peers, family, or others in the social environment. Modeled behavior and observed consequences mold observers' expectations, thereby influencing whether observers adopt similar behaviors. Individuals do not need to experience reinforcement directly; they also learn from observing others receiving reinforcement. This cognitive acquisition is what distinguishes social learning theory from operant learning theory. AIDS prevention based on social learning theory incorporates three intervention components: (1) reconceptualizing cognitive and emotional meanings attached to past risky behavior patterns, (2) modeling needed behavioral competencies to produce needed behavior changes, and (3) reinforcement for using these newly acquired skills (Des Jarlais & Friedman, 1988; Kelly & St. Lawrence, 1988a, 1988b).

Self-Efficacy Theory

Derived from social learning theory, self-efficacy theory may also be applicable to AIDS prevention. Social learning theory predicts that individuals who sense they have control and power over their lives are more likely to lower their risky behaviors than those who do not have that control. Self-efficacy refers to individuals' perceptions about whether they are capable of performing actions (Bandura, 1977a, 1977b, 1986, 1989). The concept of self-efficacy has proven useful in other areas of health promotion, such as smoking cessation (Pechacek & Danaher, 1979). When applied to AIDS prevention, self-efficacy assumes that individuals who continue engaging in risky behavior doubt their own ability to implement changes that will protect them from further risk. Those who made some effort to lower risk in the past, but failed or relapsed, may also have little self-efficacy. According to Bandura (1989), even when individuals know what to do and possess the necessary skills, they may be unable to self-manage if they lack a sense of self-efficacy. Thus, self-efficacy theory implicates individuals' beliefs about their capabilities, how those beliefs affect what they do, how much effort they can mobilize, how long they persevere, whether they engage in self-defeating thought patterns, and their stress in situations requiring change (Bandura, 1989).

Montgomery and her colleagues (1989) cited self-efficacy theory to explain a relationship between educational attainment and greater precautionary change among gay men, except for men at the very highest risk levels. They interpreted educational attainment as a proxy for self-efficacy and also extended this line of reasoning to explain the absence of any relationship between education (or any other demographic factor) and sustained risk for men at highest risk when their study began. Although seemingly a paradox, they speculated that both observations are consistent with self-efficacy; men at highest risk may have held negative expectations regarding their own futures that are not independent of self-efficacy beliefs.

Behavior skills training may both train needed competencies and simultaneously improve one's sense of self-efficacy, thereby increasing one's persistence in implementing behavior change. For example, condom use by gay men increased substantially following skills training that taught men how to discuss safer sex with partners and involved practice rehearsals (Kelly, St. Lawrence, Hood, & Brasfield, 1989a; Valdiserri et al., 1989). In acquiring the new behavioral competencies, self-efficacy may have undergone a parallel increase as participants practiced and gained confidence in their newly acquired skills. Then, as participants shared their successes with the group in subsequent sessions, they became role models giving evidence that individuals can successfully implement precautionary changes, thereby overcoming self-doubt in participants who had not yet begun using the newly acquired skills. At this stage, social learning theory predicts change due to peer modeling, whereas self-efficacy theory predicts modeling would empower others to believe they too can succeed, which may simply be a substitute phrase for self-efficacy. Among Hispanic intravenous drugs users, for example, role models were critical to the success of prevention campaigns (Jiminez, 1987). Street outreach health educators who were former prostitutes were highly effective in educating street prostitutes in Seattle (Cohen et al., 1988). Self-efficacy theory assumes these successful campaigns resulted from both information provision and the elevated sense of self-efficacy that participants gained from seeing peer models attest that they successfully made changes.

Several studies have found self-efficacy theory useful as a predictor of behavior change. Charles (cited in Stall, Coates, and Huff, 1988) examined differences between gay men at high, medium or low risk using a predictive model that included personal efficacy beliefs, response efficacy beliefs, perceptions of vulnerability, social skills, perceived peer support, and self-esteem measures. Personal efficacy was the only significant predictor of precautionary behavior. In other words, men who were at lowest risk had the highest self-efficacy scores, a relationship replicated by Joseph et al. (1987).

No intervention has isolated a strategy to test change resulting from interventions mediating self-efficacy changes alone, because the same studies that address self-efficacy also involve information provision, skills training, peer modeling, and other components of learning theory. Thus, it remains unclear whether self-efficacy is pivotal to change or, perhaps, an end stage after individuals have already made successful changes.

Applications of Learning Theory to AIDS Prevention

To date, no intervention has relied exclusively on operant or social learning theory. Instead, behavioral interventions tend to be multicomponent in nature, integrating both operant and social learning theory models into interventions. Our research team in Mississippi conducted a prototypical behavioral AIDS prevention program to assist homosexual men at imminent risk for HIV infection in reducing behavior that placed them at risk (Kelly, St. Lawrence, Hood, & Brasfield, 1989a).

This project illustrates both strengths and disadvantages of behavioral models when applied to AIDS prevention.

The program took place in a small southern city at a time when AIDS incidence was modest but increasing. The program's developers met with staff in community settings frequented by gay men, gay organizations, and health department personnel prior to announcing the program. Based on these community inputs, a recruitment strategy evolved. We introduced the intervention, termed Project ARIES (an acronym for **A**IDS **R**isk **I**ntervention and **E**ducation **S**eries), through brochures and posters placed in bars, adult bookstores, churches, health department test sites, and college campuses, and we mailed the brochures and posters to health-care providers within a 25-mile radius. At the suggestion of staff in one of the gay clubs, we prepared a video and projected it several times each evening in the gay bars. Project staff were highly visible in the clubs and bars, wearing shirts with the project logo and circulating among patrons discussing the program, offering to answer questions, and indicating their willingness to get together to talk about the program outside the bar setting. Members of the project team personally responded to invitations to meet with small groups in potential participants' homes to describe the program and answer questions. Individuals who expressed interest received encouragement to contact a restricted telephone line to schedule an assessment.

Recruitment developed slowly as project staff established their credibility and became trusted within social networks. Recruitment continued for approximately 9 months before 104 men entered the study cohort. Some individuals within the sample were at exceedingly high risk; some were low risk but seeking support to maintain their precautionary behavior; and some episodically engaged in high-risk practices. For example, the average number of different sexual partners reported for the preceding year was 16.2. The *SD* of 30.4 reflects a skewed distribution wherein many participants reported low frequencies, while some reported exceedingly high frequencies. This pattern was consistent across all sexual-practice variables, and because sexual-practice patterns were highly idiosyncratic, the same individuals were not in the high-frequency tail of the distribution across all variables.

Prior to intervention, each participant completed an assessment battery, which included an AIDS Knowledge Test (Kelly, St. Lawrence, Hood, & Brasfield, 1989b); the Beck Depression Inventory (Beck, Ward, Mendelson, Mock, & Erbaugh, 1961); the state version of the State–Trait Anxiety Inventory (Spielberger, Gorsuch, & Lushema, 1970); the Health Locus of Control Inventory (K. Wallston, B. Wallston, & Devillis, 1978); self-reported sexual and substance-use behavior for the preceeding year, 2 months, and biweekly period on a Risk History Record; and role-played simulated situations involving coercions to engage in risky behavior. Subjects also completed biweekly measures throughout the intervention to monitor the intervention's immediate impact and provide a more finely grained record than the 2-month data would allow.

When recruitment ended, participants received random assignment to either an immediate intervention group ($N = 51$) or a delayed intervention group ($N = 53$). The immediate intervention group met in small groups for 12 weekly sessions. After their intervention, all participants repeated the assessment before the delayed intervention group began the same intervention. Given the length of the intervention and long delays for some participants between recruitment and intervention, we expected some attrition. By the postintervention assessment, 42 individuals remained in the immediate intervention group and 43 in the delayed intervention group.

The intervention illustrates a multicomponent application of behavioral principles to AIDS risk reduction. The multicomponent program included the following:

1. *Education about AIDS and risk-reduction strategies.* In 3 of the 12 sessions, staff presented basic information about HIV infection and transmission, corrected misconceptions, and identified sexual practices of varying risk levels, along with the rationale for its classification as high, moderate, or low risk.

2. *Self-management training.* During another 3 sessions, staff helped participants identify and change antecedents of their personal risk patterns. In one exercise, for example, each participant wrote a description of three recent episodes of high-risk behavior, including information about the setting, substance use, mood, cognitive intentions, and characteristics of the other person (without identifying information). Based upon their vignettes, each participant identified antecedents associated with unsafe episodes in the past and examined common denominators across situations. Once having identified personally relevant antecedents, each individual developed self-management strategies and rehearsed, within the group, how to implement the plan. After in-session practice, participants received encouragement to try the practiced strategies *in vivo* during the coming week. During the following session, participants then discussed successes and problems that arose. The types of solutions participants generated included environmental rearrangements (e.g., having condoms available where sexual activity might take place, avoiding settings associated with risk in the past), cognitive modification strategies (e.g., self-reinforcement for staying safe or thought stopping to control temptations), and operant strategies (e.g., expressing appreciation to a partner who complied with safety).

3. *Sexual assertion training.* Three sessions followed standard assertion-training procedures, but staff adapted the procedures to contexts relevant for AIDS prevention with gay men. Group leaders first described and then modeled characteristics of effective assertion, and participants followed with in-session practice. The larger group subdivided into dyads or triads for rehearsal, and group leaders moved between small groups reinforcing, shaping, and providing feedback as participants rehearsed how to initiate precautionary discussions with potential partners and refuse coercive pressures to engage in unsafe activities.

4. *Generating social supports for safety and health beliefs.* Affirmative supports among peer social networks facilitate risky behavior change and maintenance (Coates et al., 1987; Joseph et al., 1987; Kelly & St. Lawrence, 1988a, 1988b). Therefore, in the final 3 sessions, staff initiated discussion, peer feedback, and problem-solving training as participants evaluated personal lifestyle issues, goals, constructive versus maladaptive behavior patterns, relationship patterns, and involvement in community activities that generated a sense of pride and community support. During the last session, each participant disclosed specific steps he had taken to reduce his risk and how he had made these changes. In this way, each participant became a coping model reinforcing and normalizing risk reduction from within the social network.

In order to evaluate effectiveness of the intervention we compared the immediate intervention group with the delayed intervention group. Results indicated that individuals in the experimental group became more knowledgeable about AIDS and more skilled initiating discussions about safety with potential partners and refusing high-risk coercions, displayed significantly lower rates of unprotected anal intercourse, and increased condom use during sexual activity to a greater degree than individuals in the delayed intervention group. The paper-and-pencil inventories, with scores in the normative ranges even at preintervention, did not show significant change.

Taken together, the results documented that risk reduction based on operant and social learning principles produced robust behavioral change among individuals who displayed high frequencies of risky behavior immediately prior to intervention. A later study evaluated an abbreviated version of the same intervention condensed into a 6-session format (Kelly, St. Lawrence, Betts, Brasfield, & Hood, 1990). The change produced by the abbreviated intervention paralleled results from the 12-week intervention, suggesting the program could be made less time-intensive without sacrificing its impact.

The advantage of basing interventions on learning theory is that they are not dependent upon difficult-to-measure internal dispositions to explain the behavior or evaluate outcome. Instead, the focus is on environmental variables that are both observable and measurable. Although behavioral principles may seem manipulative to some (Leviton, 1989), they place control squarely on individuals by helping them recognize and rearrange "triggers" and consequences associated with past behavior patterns. The behavioral approach's greatest strength—attention to environmental contingencies—may also be its greatest weakness (Leventhal, Meyer, & Gutman, 1980). The program described here is typical of the "weaknesses" in multicomponent behavioral programs in that it is impossible to know which elements were responsible for producing outcome changes. The intervention included education, behavioral self-monitoring, behavior contracting, thought stopping, assertion training, problem solving, modeling, goal setting, rehearsal, shaping, and reinforcement. It may be that we can delete some of these elements from the intervention without compromising its effectiveness and the prevention program as it presently stands may include nonessential components that are neither cost- nor time-effective.

However, the behaviors that place individuals at risk for HIV infection are multifaceted and individuals at risk for infection need to maintain behavior change for an indefinite period of time; thus, interventions that include a variety of components may serve individuals at risk better than single-component programs. Multicomponent approaches send participants forth with varied armamentaria to deal with the myriad situations that will inevitably arise in the natural environment. Especially for AIDS prevention, it may be premature to test individual components before we have a better idea of the comparative effectiveness of different intervention models and their relative efficacy with different population subgroups. It is therefore best if we reserve "fine-tuning" until we find an optimal intervention package of proven superiority.

THEORIES OF MOTIVATION AND EMOTIONAL AROUSAL

Researchers have also proposed use of programs based on classical theories of emotional arousal and drive reduction for AIDS education and prevention efforts.

Among the theories in this "family" contained in the AIDS prevention literature are: (1) the Fear–Drive Model (Leventhal, Safer, & Panagis, 1983), (2) the Dual Process Model (Leventhal et al., 1983), and (3) Protection–Motivation Theory (Maddux & Rogers, 1983; Rogers, 1983).

The Fear–Drive and Dual Process Models

The Fear–Drive Model asserts that fear generates subjective discomfort that, in turn, motivates action to reduce the unpleasant emotional state (Leventhal et al., 1983). The Dual Process Model (Leventhal et al., 1983) extends the Fear–Drive Model to regard fear as an effective motivator when associated with a health threat. In addition, the Dual Process Model recognizes that fear-generated behaviors may be irrational and fail to alleviate the health threat but may instead reduce the unpleasant emotional state while leaving actual behavioral risk levels intact. Denial is an example of emotional coping that is behaviorally maladaptive because it minimizes the likelihood that individuals will act to reduce their risk. The Dual Process Model also implicates helplessness in its explanation for failure to react to perceived threats by recognizing that when intense fear generates feelings of helplessness, individuals are less likely to embark on any course of action.

Protection–Motivation Theory

Protection–motivation theory (Maddux & Rogers, 1983; Rogers, 1983) is conceptually similar to the previous model. This theory asserts that fear induced by a health threat initiates a generalized coping appraisal that, in turn, generates coping responses that may be adaptive or maladaptive. The particular coping responses that individuals ultimately choose are dependent on individuals' perceptions and beliefs regarding available options and their ability to implement those options. Several studies have used this framework to study other areas of health behavior, such as cardiovascular risk, and concluded that high-threat appeals that incorporate high-response efficacy information produce the strongest behavior change or intentions to change (Rippetoe & Rogers, 1987; Wurtel & Maddux, 1987).

What these three models (i.e., Fear–Drive Model, Dual Process Model, and protection–motivation theory) share is an emphasis on health messages that arouse fear in an effort to motivate action without exceeding some critical level of fear that will generate despair instead of mobilizing action. Like the cognitive theories, emotional models of preventive health behavior recognize that perception of risk is a prerequisite for behavior change. Emotional models differ from cognitive models by their emphasis on anxiety or fear as the motivating force that must precede action (Cummings, Becker, & Mailes, 1980). Although recognizing that the risk of inducing psychological distress is high, practitioners who rely on such models believe anxiety induction is necessary and that interventions must (1) maintain a level of anxiety that motivates precautionary behavior, (2) assist individuals to maintain psychological equilibrium in the face of this anxiety, and (3) contain the anxiety below a debilitating threshold level (Bauman & Siegel, 1987). These theories are less specific in delineating how to accomplish this delicate balance.

Rhodes and Wolitski (1990) evaluated messages with varying levels of threat and found the most fear inducing were, in fact, the most memorable. However, their study did not evaluate the behavioral impact of these communications, and their conclusion that fear-oriented appeals are an effective route for behavior change has not received wide support. In this respect, it is typical of the literature based on motivation/emotion theories in that it failed to validate the relationship of anxiety induction to subsequent behavioral performance.

There is, in fact, relatively little evidence to support the contention that anxiety induction is a constructive motivating force and considerable evidence suggesting that individuals frequently use denial to manage the resulting anxiety. Under some circumstances, denial can be adaptive, such as when it maintains homeostasis long enough for an individual to marshal coping resources (Lazarus, 1981; Taylor, 1983). However, in the context of AIDS, denial is not functional, not even in the short term. Even infrequent risky activity confers exceedingly high risk. Thus, emotional-arousal theories present a conundrum when applied to AIDS risk reduction. On the one hand, individuals at risk need to embark on safer behavior-change efforts if they are to preserve their health. Yet, if they elect not to use denial as a coping strategy, they leave themselves vulnerable to high levels of anxiety. The alternative is to react to their anxiety with denial, undermining the likelihood they will adopt precautionary behavior.

Confrontational health messages may well promote denial rather than safety in response to the anxiety they generate. Considerable evidence attests to the fact that many individuals whose behavior places them at high risk greatly underestimate their personal-risk levels, adapt recommendations in ways that allow them to perpetuate unsafe behavior, or generate idiosyncratic beliefs that confer a false sense of security (e.g., individuals who learn they did not test positive for HIV despite having engaged in risky behavior and mistakenly conclude that they must be impervious to HIV infection; Bauman & Siegel, 1987). Thus, fear-generating approaches may be counterproductive if they generate avoidance rather than promote adoption of protective behavior (Job, 1988).

The classic example of a failed anxiety-induction approach was a costly mass media effort in Australia called the "Grim Reaper" campaign. The advertising campaign was a national effort aired on Australian television. Announcements featured a shrouded figure, the grim reaper, with a bowling ball in his hand, which he released to strike down human figures arranged as bowling pins. Evaluation of the campaign showed that people recalled its dramatic presentation, but that it did not influence behavior or leave any constructive residual message about AIDS. This is consistent with information attesting to the fact that low-threat communications are superior to high-fear or high-threat appeals in promoting constructive responses (Rhodes & Wolitski, 1990).

Although fear-induction techniques are some of the methods commonly proposed for AIDS education/prevention, there are several cautions regarding their use (Leventhal, Meyer, & Gutman, 1980). First, we do not have a very good understanding of the effectiveness of high-fear versus low-fear inducing messages in influencing behavior change, nor do fear-inducing messages always operate in consistent directions. Second, fear induction can alienate intended audiences and create disregard of intended health messages. Shilts (1987) described how the gay community disregarded early AIDS warnings by suspecting political motives were the underlying impetus for the messages. Linking the sources who are providing prevention messages to authorities who have negatively interacted with the target group in the past compromises effectiveness of the message. This is probably why outreach workers and community-based programs offered from within existing social networks are often effective, whereas individuals in the target groups often disregard "official" channels. Many of the population subgroups devastated by AIDS have traditionally had a distrustful regard of many official agencies and authority figures.

Another hazard is that when fear induction is the vehicle for communication, individuals may become fatalistic and feel helpless to protect themselves. These feelings of impotence may, in turn, perpetuate continued risk levels. Finally, as discussed earlier, these campaigns generate denial, which may be adaptive in the sense that they minimize emotional distress but maladaptive when it precludes needed behavior changes. Obviously, fear-based messages can generate a myriad of responses; some are adaptive, whereas others are more likely to preserve risky behavior. Thus, fear-generating messages have the potential to impede constructive change and may compromise prevention efforts.

SOCIAL INFLUENCE THEORIES

Community-wide programs can reach a critical mass of individuals with information, motivation, and skills to foster changes in the social norms regulating behavior (Miller, Turner, & Moses, 1990). Social marketing theories and diffusion of innovation theory generally form the basis of such programs.

Social Marketing

Social marketing strategies use commercial marketing techniques for health promotion. Such strategies reflect implicit belief that the knowledge, beliefs, attitudes, and needs of the target groups—the "consumers" of information—are the most important determinants of effective prevention. Embedded in the social context of the targeted "consumer," social marketing approaches attempt to offer individuals personal benefits they value in language that is familiar, and at a "price" (not necessarily monetary) they are willing to pay in order to achieve a meaningful goal (MacDonald & Schneider, 1991). Public health programs have promoted social marketing concepts for decades and are now adapting these concepts to respond to AIDS. Silvestre et al. (1986) defined *social marketing* as "the design, implementation, and control of programs seeking to increase the acceptability of a social idea or practice in a target group" (p. 223).

Diffusion of Innovation Theory

Diffusion of innovation theory (Rogers, 1983) involves the process by which influential members within social networks disseminate trends through their social networks into the general population. Public health researchers have widely advocated and implemented AIDS prevention strategies that seek to influence entire communities, but they have rarely evaluated such interventions.

Applications to AIDS Prevention

STOP AIDS (Puckett & Bye, 1987) was the first major AIDS prevention intervention using social marketing/diffusion of innovation methods. The STOP AIDS campaign, begun in San Francisco, capitalized on community mobilization by using members of the local gay community to provide risk-reduction information and skills to other gay men. The developers modeled the program on home-marketing methods used to sell housewares and personal-care products. Epidemiological evidence suggests there were dramatic behavior changes in individuals in San Francisco and other urban AIDS epicenters, but there is no data that can extricate the contribution of STOP AIDS to these changes.

Researchers and others across the country have widely adopted the STOP AIDS model (Beeker & Rose, 1989; Miller, Booraem, Flowers, & Iverson, 1989). While its beginnings were atheoretical and there was no direct program evaluation, Miller, Booraem, Flowers, and Iverson (1990) replicated and evaluated the STOP AIDS program in southern California. Pre- and postdiscussion assessments of participants' knowledge, attitudes, and intentions to change their behaviors found significant postdiscussion changes on all measures. However, there was no longitudinal measurement to assess extent to which the program impacted on actual behavior or to assess whether the results were durable. Until researchers conduct more rigorous outcome evaluation studies, we cannot generate any conclusions regarding effectiveness of this strategy.

As discussed earlier, although AIDS educational campaigns are common, the knowledge they disseminate does not always translate into behavioral change. Studies indicating that individuals who successfully implement risk-reduction changes perceive precautionary behavior is the expected norm within their peer group suggest that community-level interventions promoting shifts in peer norms are a viable risk-reduction strategy (Kelly et al., 1991a; McKusick, Coates, Wiley, Morin, & Stall, 1987). Diffusion theory suggests that engaging key individuals to serve as disseminators of information and expectations through a population can facilitate populationwide behavior changes (Rogers, 1983). Applied to AIDS prevention, this implies that trends, such as safer sex, are more likely to diffuse through a population if popular individuals within the social group serve as behavior-change innovators within their own peer group.

Our research team evaluated this theoretical model in an experimentally tested community-level intervention in three small cities (Kelly et al., 1991b, 1992). The cities each had one or two gay clubs patronized by relatively stable populations, constituting compact and isolated environments in which to test an intervention designed to promote population-wide behavioral shifts. Before intervention began, we conducted anonymous surveys in gay clubs in each city to assess HIV risk levels among gay men who patronized the clubs. Over 85% of the patrons completed surveys, thereby yielding cross-sections of risk behavior among these men. We repeated the population-wide surveys twice, establishing baseline behavior rates in all three cities. The experimental design for the project was a multiple baseline across cities, with each city receiving the intervention at 6-month lagged intervals.

Bartenders in the gay clubs identified socially influential gay men. We then recruited nominees to participate in four weekly training sessions. The sessions provided detailed educational information on HIV transmission and risk reduction along with social skills training to teach participants how to convey risk-reduction information to others in their social networks (Kelly et al., 1991b, 1992). Each opinion leader contracted to initiate conversations with at least 14 friends in the weeks that followed. Each participant wore a button with a logo matching the same logo on posters placed in each club, which helped stimulate conversational opportunities.

Three months after the intervention and at 6-month intervals thereafter, we repeated population-wide surveys to detect whether the intervention produced changes in the risky behavior levels of gay men in each city. These population-wide surveys revealed consistent and substantial reductions in the proportion of gay men who engaged in risky behavior following intervention in each city. The proportion of men who engaged in unprotected anal intercourse was reduced between 15% and 22% from baseline levels. Because changes followed the stepwise introduction of the program in each city, it was clear that the intervention was responsible for these reductions.

The results of this study were substantial, and the changes went well beyond what one could expect from any of the standard, ongoing AIDS educational activities that occured over the course of the project. This study indicated that health-care providers can enlist key-opinion leaders into risk-reduction interventions and train them to serve as peer health educators and that disseminated information can produce populationwide decreases in risky behavior. This suggests that interventions harnessing marketing strategies similar to the one employed in the project described here may be a cost-effective means of quickly disseminating information not only among gay men, but also for other groups, such as adolescents, women, inner-city dwellers, or substance users.

A conceptually similar project in San Francisco evaluated a peer-led community level intervention in three West Coast cities to assist young homosexual men in reducing AIDS risk behaviors (Hays, Kegeles, & Coates, 1990). This program centered around three key elements: (1) peer outreach efforts in formal and informal settings, (2) peer-led risk-reduction workshops, and (3) an ongoing publicity campaign about the program to establish legitimacy for the intervention and provide ongoing cues for safer sex.

FUTURE DIRECTIONS

The goal for AIDS prevention is exceedingly clear and straightforward—to persuade people not to engage in practices that transmit HIV infection. However, the means of achieving this goal remain unclear, even after a decade of effort. A variety of approaches will likely be necessary to change the prevalence of high-risk behaviors that transmit HIV infection. Both sexual behavior and drug use are complex behavioral topographies, provide immediate and powerful gratification, and are usually private acts. Acts that occur outside public settings and among groups that often feel alienated from mainstream society, acts that provide powerful reinforcement and have negative consequences that are temporally distant, and acts about which we know relatively little other than that they are difficult behaviors to change even under ideal circumstances, present difficult challenges for both primary and secondary prevention efforts. Further complications arise from the fact that many of the population segments that could benefit from prevention programs also have unique social and psychological qualities, value systems, information channels, and patterns of behavior that investigators must incorporate into program development, intervention content, and service delivery.

Education has been foremost among AIDS prevention efforts. Educational programs may attempt to reach a broad cross-section of society, focus on smaller targeted subgroups, or operate at an individual level. On a community level, such programs usually attempt to provide the general public with factual information. Public health programs have invested substantial resources in educational campaigns in the United States. For example, every household in the country received a copy of the Surgeon General's pamphlet, *Understanding AIDS,* and mass media advertisements, such as the "America Responds to AIDS" campaign repeatedly are broadcast over public airwaves, displayed in communities across the country, and featured in print media. Even though informational campaigns successfully convey factual information about how the virus transmits from one individual to another, such campaigns do not necessarily dispel misconceptions about transmission. Unfortunately, misconceptions seem impervious to informational campaigns, and programs must specifically address such misconceptions before they can be dispelled. Upwards of 95% of Americans are aware of AIDS and know that sexual intercourse and sharing drug apparatus can spread HIV infection (Hardy, 1990). However, upwards of 25% of the American public continues to believe insects can transmit AIDS or that they can be infected by eating in a restaurant where the cook has HIV infection. It appears that educational efforts must both transmit correct information and attempt to change misconceptions.

Community-level primary prevention could include educational programs within the schools. School-based programs were effective deterrents to smoking and alcohol use in past prevention campaigns, and there is no apparent reason why programs similar to those used to deter smoking and alcohol use could not delay onset of sexual activity, discourage drug use, or promote condom use among youth who are sexually active. To be maximally effective, school-based primary prevention programs will need to incorporate skills training as well as information provision (Stover & Eichler, 1991). In a national survey of high school students, approximately half had received HIV instruction in their schools. Information was associated with greater knowledge about HIV and its means of transmission (Holtzman et al., 1991). However, proposals to provide educational programs within the schools have been controversial, precluding widespread prevention via this route. As an aside, in a smaller study, Hingson and his colleagues (1991) found that foreign-born high school students did not possess the same amount of information as nonimmigrant students within the same classrooms, thereby underscoring the importance of tailoring educational messages to specific audiences.

The benefits of education may not be immediately apparent, but research and mathematical modeling studies suggest education may impact on future behavior to a greater degree than it influences present actions.

Studies have repeatedly shown that peer social norms influence behavior. Because official government and health agencies often are not credible or do not have established ties with populations at risk for HIV infection, the presence of community-based organizations and outreach workers are crucial in reaching individuals at highest HIV-infection risk. Peer-initiated programs are also more likely to incorporate needed sensitivity and be more linguistically appropriate than programs generated from outside the social network.

Many programs employ outreach workers drawn from the population targeted for intervention. The Centers for Disease Control and Prevention (1990) currently supports more than 600 community-based organizations involved in such outreach service delivery (Hinman, 1991). For example, recovering addicts contact injecting drug users who are not in drug-treatment programs. These outreach workers convey the need for precautionary behavior changes and information on how to eliminate or reduce infection risk, endorse the benefits of making these changes, and serve as credible and visible role models promoting precautionary norms. A demonstration project in San Francisco documented significant change in both needle sharing and disinfection following such an outreach program (Centers for Disease Control, 1990; Siegel, Weinstein, & Fineberg, 1991). A Seattle project using peer influence to establish condom use as the social norm showed significant reductions in high-risk sexual activity by men who engaged in sex with men (O'Reilley et al., 1989). Prostitutes trained to become peer educators were effective in promoting condom use among street prostitutes (Cohen et al., 1988). In each of these successful programs, members of the targeted population received training to provide health outreach to their peers, and these efforts gave impetus to communitywide shifts in behavior.

Counseling before and after HIV testing provides another prime opportunity to discuss strategies for reducing or eliminating infection risk and has been the cornerstone of efforts to educate the public on an individual level. Although HIV testing remains controversial as an AIDS prevention strategy, measurable behavior changes have resulted among individuals who undergo counseling and testing; however, it is difficult, if not impossible, to disentangle the effects of counseling from those due to knowledge of serostatus and other programs that are simultaneously available. Pre- and posttest counseling are usually brief single sessions, with no opportunity to extend the counseling for longer duration. A single session is unlikely to have a strong impact on behavior changes that individuals need to sustain indefinitely, and repetitive sessions may permit reinforcement of precautionary behavior shifts. However, multisession programs are rare. Nonetheless, successful coping strategies are more likely to result from sustained counseling than from a single contact.

The public health intent of counseling and testing is to help uninfected individuals initiate and sustain precautionary changes that reduce their infection risk and deter individuals who are already seropositive from engaging in behavior that will infect others. Ideally, testing and counseling could also be a vehicle into other needed services, such as drug-treatment programs, although this is rarely the case. Most often, practitioners use testing and counseling sessions as a starting point for partner tracing and notification efforts in which they identify sexual and needle-sharing partners and subsequently contact these partners for HIV counseling and testing.

HIV-antibody testing and pretest–posttest counseling services are available in more than 5,000 publicly funded test sites in the United States. As of December 1990, those sites had performed more than 4 million tests, and approximately 5% of the tests identified individuals who were HIV seropositive (Hinman, 1991). An unknown, but probably large, number of people prefer to undergo testing in the private sector. At the present time, demographic characteristics of individuals who seek testing are shifting to parallel the changing demographics of HIV infection. Women, heterosexual men, and racial and ethnic minorities have become increasingly represented among test seekers and among those found HIV seropositive. HIV counseling is also necessary in a broader array of service delivery settings, such as sexually transmitted diseases (STD) and prenatal clinics. Chirgwin, De Hovitz, Dillon, and McCormack (1991) found that nearly 20% of STD clinic clients who consented to an HIV test were seropositive.

Many individuals have advocated partner-contact tracing and notification as an opportunity for one-to-one education with sexual or needle-sharing partners of individuals infected with HIV. Marks, Richardson, and Maldonado (1991) found that 52% of individuals who were sexually active and HIV seropositive had not disclosed their HIV status to sexual partners. Several studies have found that from 12% to 30% of contacted partners were also HIV infected, but most were unaware of their HIV status before becoming sensitized to the need for testing as a result of partner-contact tracing. Partner-notification programs are present in all 50 states, but the emphasis and resources allocated to these programs vary considerably, and the integrity of confidentiality protections is critical to their effectiveness.

The only assured way of preventing HIV transmission is to avoid sex and needle-sharing with HIV infected individuals. However, sexual abstinence is not an achievable goal, and only a fraction of injecting drug users become permanently drug free (Hinman, 1991). Consequently, it is also important to provide information about harm reduction (e.g., condom use, avoiding anal intercourse, not sharing needles, and cleaning used needles with bleach).

In addition to educational efforts, other clinical services, such as protection of the national blood supply, are also necessary. Availability of clinical services for treatment of genital ulcer disease (repeatedly associated with seropositivity) or drug use and contraceptive provision can become an entry into AIDS prevention programs. Another important problem not yet addressed is development of effective programs to increase adherence to universal precautions among health-care workers, thereby reducing nosocomial transmission.

In all likelihood, no single prevention methodology is sufficient unto itself, and multiple channels are necessary to converge upon this now-entrenched health crisis. In addition, many existing prevention models have received inadequate evaluation. As a result, they risk becoming self-perpetuating in absence of data affirming their effectiveness. Challenges for program evaluation are myriad because we must somehow extract the effects of a specific intervention from ongoing behavioral, social, and scientific influences that confound program-evaluation efforts. Evaluation will ultimately require longitudinal studies to establish which approaches best promote sustained behavior change and characteristics of those individuals who are most receptive to particular approaches.

The urgent and compelling need for service delivery has made it imperative to develop short-term and immediate prevention efforts. We desperately need to conduct outcome evaluations, but process evaluation is often the compromise between immediate clinical demands and empiricism. The acute need to design and implement careful evaluation methodologies is one of the chief immediate challenges facing AIDS prevention efforts.

Agencies also need to sustain prevention efforts in a manner that is relevant for the target population addressed. All too often, program reports describe isolated "one-shot" interventions the developers then dismantle after collection of the data.

In addition, many prevention programs regard complex social groups as homogenous, overlooking the complexity among their members. For example, men who gay-identify may require different strategies than men who self-identify as bisexual or heterosexual, even though all three may engage in sex with other men. The same strategies that are effective with floral designers in New York City may not be effective, for example, with offshore oil workers in Louisiana. Program developers also need to appropriately tailor interventions and education programs for different ages, genders, races, ethnicities, socioeconomic levels, and geographic regions. Several surveys have found that younger gay men continue to report significantly higher frequencies of unprotected anal intercourse, stressing the importance of additional prevention efforts for young men who have sex with men (Hays et al., 1990; Kelly et al., 1990). Gay men in rural areas and small cities also engage in higher rates of unsafe behavior and do not possess as much information as men in urban areas (St. Lawrence, Hood, Brasfield, & Kelly, 1989), confirming the need for greater penetration of prevention efforts outside urban centers. Men who intermittently or continuously have unsafe contacts, or who only recently became sexually active, may require very different intervention approaches than those who implemented risk-reduction efforts and are now beginning to lapse. Because 24% of homosexual and 42% of bisexual men with AIDS are black or Hispanic, prevention programs clearly need to consider the social and cultural background of racial and ethnic minorities (Chu, Peterman, Doll, Buehler, & Curran, 1992).

It is also important to focus prevention efforts on heterosexuals. Even in AIDS-endemic areas, heterosexuals continue to minimize their risk of contracting HIV infection. One recent population-based study in San Francisco, the most AIDS-sensitized city in the world, found that only 9% of heterosexual males reported always using condoms, and the percentage was even lower for those reporting multiple sexual partners (Catania et al., 1992). Preventing infection and transmission among bisexual men is also important in preventing transmission to their female partners and subsequent vertical transmission to their offspring. Nor can we regard any of these populations as homogeneous because each incorporates diversity.

Relapse prevention is another area requiring attention. Many individuals have successfully made major reductions in risk behavior since the beginning of the AIDS health crisis. Particularly among gay-identified men, these reductions have been substantial and positive (Centers for Disease Control, 1987; Martin, 1987). However, as with other health-related patterns such as smoking, overeating, or exercise adherence, relapse is not uncommon. Relapse-prevention programs are necessary to sustain and reinforce risk-reduction changes subsequent to implementation of the changes (Adib, Joseph, Ostrow, Tal, & Schwartz, 1991; Kelly et al., 1991a; Stall, Ekstrand, Pollack, McKusick, & Coates, 1990).

Each prevention model probably has some impact on slowing the escalating HIV-infection rate. No single theoretical model has emerged to explain, predict, or intervene with the variety of behaviors implicated in HIV transmission, nor can we regard any single model as clearly superior at the present time. Given complexity of the practices that transmit HIV, limited information regarding effective programs, difficulties inherent in changing practices that are immediately reinforcing but confer distant health risks, and the social sensitivity needed to intervene with sexual or substance-use behaviors, no single theory is likely to prove adequate unto itself.

Prevention efforts based on any one heuristic model may result in less than optimal success. The complexity of the problem may well require different theoretical "tools" to address different facets of the threat. For maximum immediate impact, the best current recommendation is to use the full range of approaches while continuing to develop and evaluate better intervention and evaluation methodologies.

Condom promotion is essential if prevention efforts are to succeed. Social marketing and diffusion of innovation theories, in particular, appear well suited to condom promotion. In the past two decades, campaigns based on these models dramatically increased condom use in Sweden and Japan (Ajax, 1974; Matsumoto, Koizumi, & Nohara, 1972). There is little reason to believe that campaigns similar to those used in Sweden and Japan would not achieve similar results in the United States if we can resolve the social barriers to their implementation. Health-care practitioners have even implemented social marketing campaigns promoting condom use in countries with deeply entrenched religious and social sanctions again population control, even under restraints limiting advertising of specific products (Arnold & Lubic-Finkel, 1974; El-Ansary & Kramer, 1973). Under these circumstances, successful campaigns have emphasized family planning and STD prevention, often keyed around logos that gain public recognition as the campaign theme and serve as visible prompts in the community.

Successful campaigns share several elements. They reflect understanding of target audiences' needs, wants, and desires rather than institutional decisions about what the target audience "should" want (Solomon & DeJong, 1986). Staff of such campaigns deliver information with clear, specific, coordinated, and consistent messages through communication channels that access the target audience. They incorporate incentives to promote safety and generate supports—both material and social—for change. Finally, successful efforts rely on intermediaries embedded in the target audience who lend credibility to the prevention message and are effective in redefining social norms.

Social marketing/diffusion of innovation models have relevance for HIV-prevention efforts on a community level because these models change the social norms that influence risk taking. This approach is also likely to enhance maintenance subsequent to conclusion of the intervention because the supports remain in the social network, even after the active intervention ends. However, for some individuals, more time-intensive interventions will be necessary. Behavioral skills approaches will continue to be necessary for individuals who either do not possess or have little experience in the behavioral competencies needed to implement change. Durability of these changes is also critical because even occasional relapses place individuals at life-threatening risk. Community-level social marketing and diffusion of innovation models appear to be time- and cost-effective strategies for quickly disseminating change through existing groups. In the final analysis, social endorsements within groups may be the critical ingredient in establishing a climate in which individuals feel that others expect, sanction, and approve of precautionary behavior (Solomon & DeJong, 1986; Potterat, 1985).

Over the past decade, extensive efforts defined how to deliver risk-reduction messages, how to tailor interventions to different audiences, and what expected benefits would likely follow. In the next decade, we face the challenge of developing and delivering a coordinated, concerted effort at the local, regional, national, and international levels.

Acknowledgment

Support for the preparation of this chapter was provided by National Institutes of Mental Health and Health & Human Services Grant 1R01 MH48848 (HD).

REFERENCES

Abelson, R. P., & Levi, A. (1985). Decision making and decision theory. In G. Lindzay & E. Aronson (Eds.), *Handbook of social psychology* (3rd ed. pp. 167–183). New York: Random House.

Adib, S. M., Joseph, J. G., Ostrow, D. G., Tal, M., & Schwartz, S. A. (1991). Relapse in sexual behavior among homosexual men: A 2-year follow-up from the Chicago MACS/CCS. *AIDS, 5,* 757–760.

Ajax, L. (1974). How to market a nonmedical contraceptive: A case study from Sweden. In M. H. Redford, G. W. Duncan, & D. J. Prager (Eds.), *The condom: Increasing utilization in the United States* (pp. 88–94). San Francisco: San Francisco Press.

Ajzen, I., & Fishbein, M. (1980). *Understanding attitudes and predicting social behavior.* Englewood Cliffs, NJ: Prentice-Hall.

Altman, D. L., & Piotrow, P. T. (1984). Social marketing: Does it work? *Population Reports, 21,* 41–56. Baltimore, MD: Johns Hopkins University.

Arnold, C. B., & Lubic-Finkel, M. (1974). Free condom distribution projects for adolescent males. In M. H. Redford, G. W. Duncan, & D. J. Prager (Eds.), *The Condom: Increasing utilization in the United States* (pp. 425–434). San Francisco: San Francisco Press.

Bandura, A. A. (1977a). *Social learning theory.* Englewood Cliffs, NJ: Prentice-Hall.

Bandura, A. A. (1977b). Self-efficacy: Toward a unifying theory of behavioral change. *Psychological Review, 84,* 191–215.

Bandura, A. A. (1986). Self-efficacy mechanism in human agency. *American Psychologist, 40,* 359–373.

Bandura, A. A. (1989). Perceived self-efficacy in the exercise of control over AIDS infection. In V. M. Mays, G. W. Albee, & S. F. Schneider (Eds.), *Primary prevention of AIDS: Psychological approaches* (pp. 128–141). Newbury Park, NY: Sage.

Bartlett, E. E. (1981). The contribution of school health education to community health promotion: What can we realistically expect? *American Journal of Public Health, 71,* 1384–1391.

Bauman, L. J., & Siegel, K. (1987). Misperception among gay men of the risk for AIDS associated with their sexual behavior. *Journal of Applied Social Psychology, 17,* 329–350.

Beck, A. T., Ward, C. H., Mendelson, M., Mock, J., & Erbaugh, J. (1961). An inventory for measuring depression. *Archives of General Psychiatry, 4,* 561–571.

Becker, H. M. (1974). The Health Belief Model and personal health behavior. *Health Education Monographs, 2,* 236–473.

Becker, M. (1979). Psychosocial aspects of health-related behavior. In H. Freeman, S. Levine, & I. Reeder (Eds.), *Handbook of medical sociology* (pp. 253–274). Englewood Cliffs, NJ: Prentice-Hall.

Becker, M. H., Kaback, M. M., Rosenstock, I. M., & Ruth, M. V. (1975). Some influences on public participation in a genetic screening program. *Journal of Community Health, 1,* 3–14.

Beeker, C., & Rose, T. (1989, June). *The Stop AIDS model for community change: Acceptability in a low-incidence areas for AIDS.* Paper presented to the 5th International Conference on AIDS, Montreal, Canada.

Brown, L. K., DiClemente, R. K., & Reynolds, L. A. (1991). HIV prevention for adolescents: Utility of the health belief model. *AIDS Education and Prevention, 3,* 50–59.

Brownell, K. D. (1982). Obesity: Understanding and treating a serious, prevalent, and refractory disorder. *Journal of Consulting and Clinical Psychology, 50,* 820–840.

Catania, J. A., Coates, T. J., Kegeles, S., Fullilove, M. T., Peterson, J., Marin, B., Siegel, D., & Hulley, S. (1992). Condom use in multi-ethnic neighborhoods of San Francisco: The population based AMEN (AIDS in multi-ethnic neighborhoods) study. *American Journal of Public Health, 82,* 284–287.

Centers for Disease Control. (1987). Self-reported changes in sexual behaviors among homosexual and bisexual men from the San Francisco City Clinic Cohort. *Morbidity and Mortality Weekly Report, 36,* 187–189.

Centers for Disease Control. (1990). Update: Reducing HIV transmission in intravenous drug users not in drug treatment—United States. *Morbidity & Mortality Weekly Report, 39,* 535–538.

Chesney, M. (1984). Behavior modification and health enhancement. In J. D. Matarrazo, S. M. Weiss, J. A. Herd, N. E. Miller, & S. M. Weiss (Eds.), *Behavioral health: A handbook of health enhancement and disease prevention* (pp. 658–663). New York: Wiley.

Chirgwin, K., DeHovitz, J. A., Dillon, S., & McCormack, W. M. (1991). HIV infection, genital ulcer disease and crack cocaine use among patients attending a clinic for sexually transmitted diseases. *American Journal of Public Health, 81,* 1576–1579.

Chu, S. Y., Peterman, T. A., Doll, L. S., Buehler, P. W., & Curran, J. W. (1992). AIDS in bisexual men in the United States: Epidemiology of disease and transmission to women. *American Journal of Public Health, 82,* 220–224.

Cleary, P. D., Rogers, T. F., Singer, E., Avorn, J., Van Devanter, N., Perry, S., & Pindyck, J. (1986). Health education about AIDS among seropositive blood donors. *Health Education Quarterly, 13,* 317–329.

Coates, T. J., Stall, R., Mandel, J. S., Boccelleri, A., Sorenson, J. L., Morales, E. F., Morin, S. F., Wiley, J. A., & McKusick, L. (1987). AIDS: A psychosocial research agenda. *Annals of Behavioral Medicine, 9,* 21–28.

Cohen, J. B., Poole, L. E., Lyons, C. A., Lockett, G. J., Alexander, P., & Wofsy, C. B. (1988, June). *Sexual behavior and HIV infection risk among 354 sex industry women in a participant based research and prevention program.* Paper presented to the 4th International Conference on AIDS, Stockholm, Sweden.

Cummings, K. M., Becker, M. H., & Mailes, M. C. (1980). Bringing the models together: An empirical approach to combining variables used to explain health actions. *Journal of Behavioral Medicine, 3,* 123–145.

Des Jarlais, D. C., & Friedman, S. R. (1988). The psychology of preventing AIDS among intravenous drug users. *American Psychologist, 43,* 865–870.

Eddy, D. M. (1980). Probabilistic reasoning in clinical medicine: Problems and opportunities. In D. Kahneman, P. Slovic, & A. Tversky (Eds.), *Judgment under uncertainty: Heuristics and biases* (pp. 46–53). New York: Cambridge University Press.

El-Ansary, A. L., & Kramer, O. E. (1973). Social marketing: The family planning experience. *Journal of Marketing, 37,* 1–7.

Emmons, C. A., Joseph, J. G., Kessler, R. C., Wortman, C. B., Montgomery, S. B., & Ostrow, D. G. (1986). Psychosocial predictors of reported behavior change in homosexual men at risk for AIDS. *Health Education Quarterly, 13,* 331–345.

Ferster, C. B., & Skinner, B. F. (1957). *Schedules of reinforcement.* New York: Appleton-Century-Crofts.

Fischhoff, B. (1989). Making decisions about AIDS. In V. M. Mays, G. W. Albee, and S. P. Schneider (Eds.), *Primary prevention of AIDS: Psychological approaches* (pp. 168–206). Newbury Park, CA: Sage.

Fishbein, M., & Ajzen, I. (1975). *Belief, attitude, intention, and behavior.* Reading, MA: Addison-Wesley.

Fishbein, M., & Middlestadt, S. E. (1989). Using the Theory of Reasoned Action as a framework for understanding and changing AIDS-related behaviors. In V. M. Mays, G. W. Albee, & S. F. Schneider (Eds.). *Primary prevention of AIDS: Psychological approaches* (pp. 93–110). Newbury Park, NY: Sage.

Franzini, L. R., Sideman, L. M., Dexter, K., & Elder, J. P. (1990). Promoting AIDS risk reduction via behavioral training. *AIDS Education and Prevention, 2,* 313–321.

Gallois, C., Kashima, Y., Halls, R., & McCamish, M. (1990, June). *Preferred strategies for safe sex: Relation to past and actual behaviour among sexually active men and women.* Paper presented to the 6th International Conference on AIDS, San Francisco, CA.

Hardy, A. M. (1990, June 25). AIDS knowledge and attitudes for October to December 1989. *Vital and Health Statistics,* No. 186. Washington, DC: National Center for Health Statistics.

Hays, R. B., Kegeles, S. M., & Coates, T. J. (1990). High HIV risk-taking among young gay men. *AIDS, 4,* 901–907.

Hingson, R. W., Strunin, L., Grady, M., Strunk, N., Carr, R., Berlin, B., & Craven, D. E. (1991). Knowledge about HIV and behavioral risks of foreign-born Boston public school students. *American Journal of Public Health, 81,* 1638–1641.

Hinman, A. R. (1991). Strategies to prevent HIV infection in the United States. *American Journal of Public Health, 81,* 1557–1559.

Holtzman, D., Anderson, J. E., Kann, L., Arday, S. L., Truman, B. I., & Kolbe, L. J. (1991). HIV instruction, HIV knowledge, and drug infection among high school students in the United States. *American Journal of Public Health, 81,* 1596–1601.

Janz, N., & Becker, M. (1984). The health belief model: A decade later. *Health Education Quarterly, 11,* 1–47.
Jemmot, L. S., & Jemmot, J. B. (1991). Applying the Theory of Reasoned Action to AIDS risk behavior: Condom use among black women. *Nursing Research, 30,* 228–234.
Jiminez, R. (1987). *AIDS: Primary and secondary prevention strategies targeting Hispanics.* Houston: AIDS Foundation of Houston.
Job, R. F. S. (1988). Effective and ineffective use of fear in health promotion campaigns. *American Journal of Public Health, 78,* 163–167.
Joseph, J. G., Montgomery, S. B., Emmons, C. A., Kessler, R. C., Ostrow, D. G., Wortman, C. B., O'Brien, K., Eller, M., & Eshleman, S. (1987). Magnitude and determinants of behavioral risk reduction: Longitudinal analysis of a cohort at risk for AIDS. *Psychology and Health, 1,* 73–96.
Joseph, J. G., Montgomery, S., Kirscht, J., Kessler, R. C., Ostrow, D. G., Emons, C. A., & Phair, J. P. (1987, June). *Behavioral risk reduction in a cohort of homosexual men: Two year follow-up.* Paper presented to the 3rd International Conference on AIDS, Washington, DC.
Kaplan, E. H., & Abramson, P. (1989). A mathematical model of AIDS education: So what if the program ain't perfect? *Evaluation Review, 13,* 107–122.
Keeter, S., & Bradford, J. B. (1988). Knowledge of AIDS and related behavior change among unmarried adults in a low-prevalence city. *American Journal of Preventive Medicine, 4,* 146–152.
Kegeles, S. (1980). The health belief model and personal health behavior. *Social Science and Medicine, 146,* 227–229.
Kelly, J. A., Kalichman, S. C., Kauth, M. R., Kilgore, H. G., Hood, H. V., Campos, P. E., Rao, S. M., Brasfield, T. L., & St. Lawrence, J. S. (1991c). Situational factors associated with AIDS risk behavior lapses and coping strategies used by gay men who successfully avoid lapses. *American Journal of Public Health, 81,* 1335–1338.
Kelly, J. A., & St. Lawrence, J. S. (1988a). AIDS prevention and treatment: Psychology's role in the health crisis. *Clinical Psychology Review, 8,* 255–284.
Kelly, J. A., & St. Lawrence, J. S. (1988b). *The AIDS health crisis: Psychological and social interventions.* New York: Plenum Press.
Kelly, J. A., St. Lawrence, J. S., Betts, R., Brasfield, T. L., & Hood, H. L. (1990). A skills training group intervention model to assist persons in reducing risk behaviors for HIV infection. *AIDS Education and Prevention, 2,* 24–35.
Kelly, J. A., St. Lawrence, J. S., & Brasfield, T. L. (1991a). Predictors of vulnerability to AIDS risk behavior relapse. *Journal of Consulting and Clinical Psychology, 59,* 163–167.
Kelly, J. A., St. Lawrence, J. S., Diaz, Y. E., Stevenson, L. Y., Hauth, A. C., Brasfield, T. L., Kalichman, S. C., Smith, J. E., & Andrew, M. E. (1991b). HIV risk behavior reduction following intervention with key opinion leaders of population: An experimental analysis. *American Journal of Public Health, 81,* 168–171.
Kelly, J. A., St. Lawrence, J. S., Hood, H. V., & Brasfield, T. L. (1989a). Behavioral intervention to reduce AIDS risk activities. *Journal of Consulting and Clinical Psychology, 57,* 60–67.
Kelly, J. A., St. Lawrence, J. S., Hood, H. V., & Brasfield, T. L. (1989b). An objective test of AIDS risk behavior knowledge: Scale development, validation, and norms. *Journal of Behavior Therapy and Experimental Psychiatry, 20,* 227–234.
Kelly, J. A., St. Lawrence, J. S., Stevenson, L. Y., Hauth, A. C., Kalichman, S. C., Diaz, Y. E., Brasfield, T. L., Koob, J. J., & Morgan, M. G. (1992). Producing population-wide reductions in HIV risk behavior among small city gay men: Results of an experimental field trial in three cities. *American Journal of Public Health, 52,* 1483–1490.
Klein, D., Sullivan, G., Wolcott, D., Ladsverk, J., Namir, S., & Fawzy, F. (1987). Changes in AIDS risk behaviors among homosexual male physicians and university students. *American Journal of Psychiatry, 144,* 742–747.
Lazarus, R. S. (1981). The costs and benefits of denial. In B. S. Dohrenwend & B. P. Dohrenwend (Eds.), *Stressful life events and their contexts* (pp. 131–156). New York: Prodist.
Lebow, R. N., & Stein, J. (1987). Beyond deterrence. *Journal of Social Issues, 43,* 5–72.
Leventhal, H., Meyer, D., & Gutman, M. (1980). The role of theory in the study of compliance to high blood pressure regimens. In R. B. Haynes, M. E. Mattson, & O. E. Tillner (Eds.), *Patient compliance to prescribed antihypertensive medication regimens: A report to the National Heart, Lung, and Blood Institutes.* Washington, DC: U.S. Department of Health and Human Services.

Leventhal, H., Safer, M. A., & Panagis, D. M. (1983). The impact of communications on self-regulation of health beliefs, decisions, and behavior. *Health Education Quarterly, 10,* 3–31.

Leviton, L. (1989). Theoretical foundations of AIDS prevention. In R. O. Valdiserri (Ed.), *Preventing AIDS: The design of effective programs.* New Brunswick, NJ: Rutgers University Press.

MacDonald, G., & Schneider, A. (1991, June). *The importance of social marketing techniques in creating effective media campaigns.* Paper presented to the 7th International Conference on AIDS, Florence, Italy.

Maddux, J. E., & Rogers, R. W. (1983). Protection motivation and self-efficacy: A revised theory of fear appeals and attitude change. *Journal of Experimental Social Psychology, 19,* 469–479.

Marks, G., Richardson, J. L., & Maldonado, N. (1991). Self-disclosure of HIV infection to sexual partners. *American Journal of Public Health, 81,* 1321–1323.

Martin, J. L. (1987). The impact of AIDS on gay male sexual behavior patterns in New York City. *American Journal of Public Health, 77,* 578–581.

Matsumoto, Y. S., Koizumi, A., & Nohara, T. (1972). Condom use in Japan. *Studies in Family Planning, 3,* 251–255.

McCusker, J., Zapka, J. G., Stoddard, A. M., & Mayer, K. H. (1989). Responses to the AIDS epidemic among homosexually active men: Factors associated with preventive behavior. *Patient Education and Counseling, 13,* 15–30.

McCusick, L., Coates, T. J., Wiley, J. A., Morin, S. F., & Stall, R. (1987, June). *Prevention of HIV infection among gay and bisexual men: Two longitudinal studies.* Paper presented to the 3rd International Conference on AIDS, Washington, DC.

McKusick, L., Hurstman, W., & Coates, T. J. (1985a). AIDS and sexual behavior reported by gay men in San Francisco. *American Journal of Public Health, 75,* 493–496.

McKusick, L., Wiley, J., Coates, T. J., Stall, R., Saika, G., Morin, S., Charles, K., Horstman, W., & Conant, M. A. (1985b). Reported changes in the sexual behavior of gay men at risk for AIDS, San Francisco 1982–1984: The AIDS Behavioral Research Project. *Public Health Reports, 100,* 622–629.

Miller, H. G., Turner, C. F., & Moses, L. E. (1990). *AIDS: The second decade.* Washington, DC: National Academy Press.

Miller, T., Booraem, C., Flowers, J., & Iverson, A. (1989, June). *Short- and long-term results of an AIDS prevention program.* Paper presented to the 5th International Conference on AIDS, Montreal, Canada.

Miller, T., Booraem, C., Flowers, J., & Iverson, A. (1990). Changes in knowledge, attitudes, and behavior as a result of a community-based AIDS prevention program. *AIDS Education and Prevention, 2,* 12–23.

Mischel, W., & Ebbeson, E. B. (1970). Attention in delay of gratification. *Journal of Personality and Social Psychology, 16,* 329–337.

Montgomery, S. B., Joseph, J. G., Becker, M. H., Ostrow, D. G., Kessler, R. C., & Kirscht, J. P. (1989). The health belief model in understanding compliance with preventive recommendations for AIDS: How useful? *AIDS Education and Prevention, 1,* 303–323.

Nathanson, C., & Becker, M. (1983). Contraceptive behavior among unmarried young women: A theoretical framework for research. *Population and the Environment, 6,* 39–59.

O'Reilly, K. R., Higgins, D. L., Galavoti, C., Sheridan, J., Wood, R., & Cohn, D. (1989, June). *Perceived community norms and risk reduction: Behavior change in a cohort of gay men.* Poster presented to the 5th International Conference on AIDS, Montreal, Canada.

Pechacek, T. F. (1979). Modification of smoking behavior. In N. Krasnegor (Ed.), *The behavioral aspects of smoking.* National Institute on Drug Abuse Research Monograph 26. Rockville, MD: U.S. Department of Health, Education, and Welfare.

Pechacek, T. F., & Danaher, B. G. (1979). How and why people quit smoking. In P. C. Kendall & S. M. Hollon (Eds.), *Cognitive behavioral interventions: Theory, research, and procedures.* New York: Academic Press.

Petosa, R., & Jackson, K. (1991). Using the Health Belief Model to predict safer sex intentions among adolescents. *Health Education Quarterly, 18,* 475–476.

Potterat, J. J. (1985). Gonorrhea as a social disease. *Sexually Transmitted Diseases, 12,* 25–52.

Prochaska, T. R., Albrecht, G., Levy, J. A., Sugrue, N., & Kim, J.-H. (1990). Determinants of self-perceived risk for AIDS. *Journal of Health and Social Behavior, 31,* 384–394.

Puckett, S. B., & Bye, L. L. (1987). *The STOP AIDS Project: An interpersonal AIDS prevention program.* San Francisco: The STOP AIDS Project, Inc.

Rhodes, F., & Wolitski, R. J. (1990). Perceived effectiveness of fear appeals in AIDS education: Relationship to ethnicity, gender, age, and group membership. *AIDS Education and Prevention, 2,* 1–11.

Rippetoe, P. W., & Rogers, R. W. (1987). Effects of components of protection-motivation theory on adaptive and maladaptive coping with a health threat. *Journal of Personality and Social Psychology, 52,* 596–604.

Rogers, E. M. (1983). *Diffusion of innovations.* New York: Free Press.

Rogers, R. W. (1983). Cognitive and physiological processes in fear appeals and attitude change: A revised theory of protection motivation. In J. T. Cacioppo & R. E. Petty (Eds.), *Social psychophysiology: A sourcebook* (pp. 153–217). New York: Guilford.

Rosenstock, I. M. (1974). The Health Belief Model and preventive health behavior. *Health Education Monographs, 2,* 354–386.

Rosenstock, I. M., & Kirscht, J. P. (1979). Why people seek health care. In G. C. Stone, F. Cohen, & N. E. Adler (Eds.), *Health psychology* (pp. 173–187). San Francisco: Jossey-Bass.

Ross, M. W., & Carson, J. A. (1988). Effectiveness of distribution of information on AIDS: A national study of six media in Australia. *New York State Journal of Medicine, 88,* 239–241.

St. Lawrence, J. S., & Kelly, J. A. (1989). AIDS prevention: Community and behavioral interventions. In A. S. Bellack & M. Hersen (Eds.), *Progress in behavior modification* (Vol. 24, pp. 11–59). New York: Sage.

St. Lawrence, J. S., & Betts, R. (1989, June). *Comparison of the knowledge, attitudes, and AIDS-risk behaviors of college students in the southeastern United States.* Paper presented to the 5th International Conference on AIDS, Montreal, Canada.

St. Lawrence, J. S., Hood, H. V., Brasfield, T. L., & Kelly, J. A. (1989). Differences in gay men's AIDS risk knowledge and behavior patterns in high and low AIDS prevalence cities. *Public Health Reports,* 391–395.

St. Lawrence, J. S., Hood, H. V., Brasfield, T. L., & Kelly, J. A. (1988, November). *AIDS risk knowledge and sexual risk behavior among homosexual men in high versus low AIDS prevalence areas.* Symposium presented to the Association for the Advancement of Behavior Therapy, New York.

St. Lawrence, J. S., Kelly, J. A., Hood, H. V., & Brasfield, T. L. (1987, June). *The relationship of AIDS risk knowledge to actual risk behavior among homosexually active men.* Paper presented to the 3rd International Conference on AIDS, Washington, DC.

Shilts, R. (1987). *And the band played on: Politics, people, and the AIDS epidemic.* New York: St. Martin's Press.

Siegel, J. E., Weinstein, M. C., & Fineberg, H. V. (1991). Bleach programs for preventing AIDS among IV drug users: Modeling the impact of HIV prevalence. *American Journal of Public Health, 81,* 1273–1279.

Silvestre, A., Lyter, D. W., Rinaldo, C. R., Kingsley, L. A., Forrester, R., & Huggins, J. (1986). Marketing strategies for recruiting gay men into AIDS research and education projects. *Journal of Community Health, 11,* 222–231.

Skinner, B. F. (1969). *Contingencies of reinforcement: A theoretical analysis.* New York: Appleton-Century-Crofts.

Solomon, M. Z., & DeJong, W. (1986). Recent sexually transmitted disease prevention efforts and their implications for AIDS health education. *Health Education Quarterly, 13,* 301–316.

Spielberger, C. D., Gorsuch, R. L., & Lushema, R. E. (1970). *Manual for the State-Trait Anxiety Inventory.* Palo Alto, CA: Consulting Psychologists.

Stall, R. D., Coates, T. J., & Huff, C. (1988). Behavioral risk reduction for HIV infection among gay and bisexual men. *American Psychologist, 43,* 878–885.

Stall, R., Ekstrand, M., Pollock, L., McKusick, L., & Coates, T. L. (1990). Relapse from safer sex: The next challenge for AIDS prevention efforts. *AIDS, 3,* 1181–1187.

Stover, E., & Eichler, A. (1991, June). *Preventing AIDS infection among adolescents: Coordinating ongoing research efforts.* Paper presented to the 7th International Conference on AIDS, Florence, Italy.

Taylor, S. E. (1983). Adjustment to threatening events: A theory of cognitive adaption. *American Psychologist, 11,* 161–173.

Valdiserri, R. O., Lyter, D. W., Leviton, L. C., Callahan, C. M., Kingley, L. A., & Rinaldo, C. R. (1988). Variables influencing condom use in a cohort of gay and bisexual men. *American Journal of Public Health, 78,* 801–805.

Valdiserri, R. O., Lyter, D. W., Leviton, L. C., Callahan, C. M., Kingley, L. A., & Rinaldo, C. R. (1989). AIDS prevention in homosexual and bisexual men: Results of a randomized trial evaluating two risk reduction interventions. *AIDS, 3,* 21–26.

Wallston, K. A., Wallston, B. S., & Devillis, R. (1978). Development of the Multi-Dimensional Health Locus of Control (MHLOC) scales. *Health Education Monographs, 6,* 160–170.

Winett, R. A. (1986). *Information and behavior: Systems of influence.* Hillsdale, NJ: Erlbaum.

Wurtel, S. K., & Maddux, J. E. (1987). Relative contributions of protection motivation theory components in predicting exercise intentions and behavior. *Health Psychology, 6,* 453–466.

28

Aging
Issues in Health and Neuropsychological Functioning

Paul D. Nussbaum

The purpose of this chapter is to review some of the relevant issues of aging for health psychology. The initial section is a review of the demographics of the *elderly* (defined as age 65 and older) in the United States. The next section consists of a brief overview of some of the theories of aging from gerontological, psychological, and biological sciences. The third section comprises a review of some common psychiatric and other medical disorders from which older adults suffer. A focus of the present chapter involves the impact of illness upon the elderly individual's neuropsychological functioning. The final section includes suggestions for future research and a recommendation for interdisciplinary collaboration.

DEMOGRAPHICS

Older adults in the United States represent one of the fastest growing segments of the population. Rowe and Katzman (1992) reported that the number of individuals older than 65 increased from 3 million in 1900 to 25 million in 1980, and estimates indicate the number of older individuals will be approximately 31 million by the year 2000. Older adults comprised 4% of the entire population in 1900. Today, they represent approximately 11% of the population, and projections indicate this percentage will increase to 17% by the early part of the next century (U.S. Bureau of the Census, 1981). Albert (1988) reviewed the gerontological literature

---

This chapter is written in loving memory of Gail I.

Paul D. Nussbaum • Aging Research and Education Center, Lutheran Affiliated Services, 500 Wittenberg Way, Mars, Pennsylvania 16046.
Handbook of Health and Rehabilitation Psychology, edited by Anthony J. Goreczny. Plenum Press, New York, 1995.

and reported that whereas the average life span of human beings remained constant during the early 1800s, ranging from 30 to 40 years, a change in the human life span began in the late 1800s. Today, on average, an American can expect to live to age 75. The increase in the number of older adults is even higher for individuals over the age of 75. Indeed, scientists have created the term *old-old* to categorize this segment of the elderly population (i.e., age 75 and older) as separate from *old* persons, age 65–74. There were approximately 900 thousand individuals over the age of 75 in the United States in 1900. This number increased to nearly 10 million by 1980 and will likely reach 15 million by the middle of the next century (Rowe & Katzman, 1992).

Several factors are responsible for the increased life span of human beings. These include improvements in sanitation, nutrition, medical and mental health service, and adherence to exercise. Both infant and childhood mortality has markedly declined because of these improvements as well as the development of new antibiotics. In addition, improved diagnostic and treatment procedures have produced a decline of serious medical conditions, such as cardiac and cerebrovascular disease in the elderly (Albert, 1988).

The increase in the number of older adults, particularly those considered old-old, underscores the need for an increase of health-care professionals with specialization in geriatrics (Horton & Puente, 1990; Peterson, 1986; Satin, 1986; Storandt, 1977). Indeed, Rowe and Katzman (1992) described the increased interest in the neurology of aging as a recent development. Clinical psychology needs to implement doctoral, internship, and postdoctoral programs that provide specialized course work, clinical practicums, and scientific methodology in the study and treatment of older adults. At present, patients receive mental health services from a variety of professional disciplines, including psychology, nursing, medicine, rehabilitation, and psychiatry. Research on the provision of mental health services for the elderly has demonstrated that the number of older patients treated is small (Smyer, Zarit, & Qualls, 1990). The reasons elderly individuals do not utilize mental health services include negative attitudes of mental health professionals and social services toward older adults and negative expectations by both patients and professionals concerning treatment effectiveness (Butler, 1975; Lutsky, 1980; Nussbaum, Thompson, & Robinson, 1989; Wetle & Levkoff, 1984). Likewise, professionals are reluctant to treat older adults because of poor reimbursement for services and lack of referrals from health-care providers (Smyer et al., 1990). Other research involving the mental-health professions suggests that age-related bias is less evident than are negative beliefs about treatment efficacy (Gatz & Pearson, 1988).

The development of interdisciplinary programs that train professionals in the study and treatment of older adults might represent a first step in improving attitudes of professionals. The interaction between scientists and clinicians with expertise in the area of geropsychiatry is necessary to improve the mental health care of the older adult (Schacter, Kaszniak, & Kihlstrom, 1991; Smyer et al., 1990). It is also important to continue educating society about the benefits of mental health because this might assist in reduction of older adults' reluctance to seek effective treatment.

MODELS OF AGING

It is impossible to review all of the different models of aging in the present chapter. This section, therefore, will first present a discussion of the definition of aging. Then, a brief overview of theories of aging derived from the social and biological sciences will follow.

Despite the enormous literature on aging, a universally accepted definition of aging has been slow to develop (J. Birren & B. Birren, 1990; Katzman, 1983). Birren (1988) defined *aging* as "an orderly or regular transmission with time of representative organisms living under representative environments" (p. 160). Aiken (1982) asserted that identification of old age depends both on the characteristics of the elderly and on the needs of society. In addition, Aiken reminded the reader of the fact that an individual's stage of development also contributes to the perception of what *old* is. One reason researchers have not produced a consistent definition of aging is because there exist too few interdisciplinary efforts. In an attempt to produce an accepted theory of aging, J. Birren and B. Birren (1990) proposed the need for an integrative theory of aging that would include contributions from different scientific disciplines. The authors cautioned, however, that such an integrative theory would require both methodological sophistication and, more important, cooperative and motivated collaborators across different disciplines.

J. Birren and B. Birren (1990) defined the *psychology of aging* as the study of changes in behavior that typically occur after early adulthood. Nussbaum and colleagues (1989) reviewed four of the major theories of successful aging from the social sciences. The first was *disengagement theory* (Cumming, Dean, Newell, & McCaffrey, 1960), which posits that an aging individual gradually withdraws from society and that society, in turn, slowly withdraws from the individual. Hypothetically, the process of withdrawal is mutual and beneficial to society. Cumming and associates asserted that individuals accomplish successful aging by the process of withdrawal and that maladaptive aging occurs when one does not disengage from society. The second theory, outlined by Nussbaum et al. (1989) was *activity theory* (Lebo, 1953; Tobin & Neugarten, 1961) which hypothesizes individuals can successfully age by maintaining an active lifestyle. The third theory of aging, *continuity theory* (Atchley, 1989; Neugarten, Havighurst, & Tobin, 1968) proposes successful aging is a function of individual personality. An aging individual must continue to interact with the environment in a manner that maximizes personal needs and maintains adaptation. The fourth theory included *social-environmental theory* (J. Hendricks & C. Hendricks, 1986), which posits successful aging occurs when an individual's social environment, including people and physical structures, is functional and reinforcing. Birren (1988) recently presented a theory of aging that relates to development, but is not identical to it. This theory of aging rests on the premise that, with age, an organism experiences a decline in structure and function that results in deterioration of social, biological, and behavioral capacities. Even more recently, life-span developmental psychology has presented a multidetermined model of aging that involves interacting influences (e.g., individual, age-related, historical–social, biological, and environmental; see Horton and Puente, 1990).

Scientists within the biological sciences have also studied aging and the effects of aging on the central nervous system (see Katzman & Terry, 1992). Nussbaum et al. (1989) noted that the aging process is as common to human beings as it is to single cell organisms. The aging human body experiences changes of the internal and external organs and systems (Aiken, 1982). Indeed, Katzman (1983) pointed out that death is age-related. Although biological theories have existed since Hippocrates, who believed aging was secondary to a loss of body heat (see Aiken, 1982), several biological theorists have developed more modern theories of aging. Biological theories of aging divide into *breakdown theories* that posit aging results from wear and tear, stress, or fatigue of organs and cells (Shock, 1977) and *substance theories* that postulate aging is a result of the production of substances unfamiliar to the body. Examples of breakdown theories include the homeostatic imbalance theory, autoimmune theory, and reservoir theory (see Aiken, 1982; Curtis, 1966; Makinodan, 1977). The autoimmune theory, although considered a breakdown theory, is also a substance theory. Other examples of biological theories include the cross-linkage theory, free radical theory, and hormonal theory (see Aiken, 1982; Shock, 1977). Another biological theory (Hayflick, 1974) postulates that certain animals have innate built-in time clocks that count down years of life. The presumption of this theory is that the organism has an *a priori* specified amount of life based on the cells' ability to reproduce and remain functional. Several environmental factors relate to biological variables and influence the aging process. For example, proper diet, no use of nicotine, and regular exercise reduce cardiovascular and other potentially fatal diseases (Rowe & Kahn, 1987).

AGING AND THE CENTRAL NERVOUS SYSTEM

Perhaps no other organ or cluster of organs is so vulnerable to the aging process as the brain. Normal aging of the central nervous system (CNS) involves "aging changes that occur in individuals free of overt diseases of the nervous system" (Katzman & Terry, 1992, p. 18). The aging of the CNS hypothetically encompasses a slow and perhaps continuous change in specific functional abilities. Katzman and Terry present a review of the effects of the aging process on neurological status, neurotransmitters, cerebral blood flow, electrophysiology, cell integrity, and brain morphology. The present review concentrates on the effects of aging on cognitive functioning.

The most studied area of normal aging, as it relates to the CNS, involves issues related to changes in cognitive functioning. The literature has demonstrated that different domains of cognitive functioning appear relatively more vulnerable to the effects of aging than other domains (Albert, 1988; Bayles & Kaszniak, 1987; Goldstein, 1983; Katzman & Terry, 1992; Rinn, 1988; Villardita, Cultrera, Cupone, & Mejia, 1985). Speed of cognitive processing and motor speed, for example, begin to slow relatively early (Katzman & Terry, 1992), and this slowing is evident even in very healthy older adults (Mitrushina & Satz, 1991). Cerella (1990) theorized that the increased latency of information processing in older adults is attributable to defects distributed across an aging neural network and not to a dysfunction at a discrete stage of information processing.

The pattern of findings derived from studies assessing age-related cognitive decline suggests that the cognitive functions most vulnerable to aging are those that require rapid information processing, necessitate processing of novel information, or demand the most effortful processing (Bayles & Kaszniak, 1987; Craik & McDowd, 1987; Hasher & Zacks, 1979; Villardita et al., 1985). The elderly appear to have some difficulty spontaneously engaging in deeper levels of information processing (see Craik & Lockhart, 1972). In contrast, older adults' performance is similar to that of younger adults on tasks of automatic processing (Craik & McDowd, 1987). One compensatory mechanism that appears to assist the older adult with engaging in deeper levels of cognitive process is provision of external cues and organization of material (Bayles & Kaszniak, 1987). The effortful processing deficit in older age manifests across different cognitive domains and appears to represent a unifying theory for explaining age-related cognitive changes.

Rinn (1988) argued that although a decline in mental abilities occurs with aging, the deterioration is not natural. He asserted that normal age-related mental deterioration may represent a subclinical dementia. Furthermore, Rinn reported that age-related cognitive decline relates to brain atrophy and reduced cerebral blood flow. For example, he noted that a small amount of cortical atrophy accompanies normal aging, beginning in the second decade and continuing until the sixth decade, with a dramatic increase in cortical atrophy occurring after age 60. In addition, normal aging relates to reduced cerebral blood flow beginning around age 25 and declining at increasing rates thereafter, with the most noticeable decline occurring after age 69. Others have also suggested that age-related decrements in cognitive functioning might be secondary to general age-related brain changes (Albert & Stafford, 1988; Doraiswamy et al., 1991; Williamson et al., 1990).

Based on a review of the changes in cognitive functioning that accompany normal aging, it seems reasonable to speculate (as some have) that anterior areas of the brain are perhaps most vulnerable to the effects of aging (Craik, L. Morris, R. Morris, & Loewen, 1990; Kobari, Stirling, & Ichijo, 1990; Mittenberg, Seindenber, O'Leary, & DiGiulio, 1989; Schacter, Kaszniak, Kihlstrom, & Valdiserri, 1991; Squire, 1987). Squire noted that, relative to other brain regions, the prefrontal cortex suffers approximately 15–20% neuronal loss with old age and represents an area vulnerable to the aging process. Schacter and colleagues (1991) cautioned, however, that *frontal lobe dysfunction* remains a broad term encompassing multiple functional and cognitive systems. The relationship of frontal lobe dysfunction to specific memory and other cognitive processes is somewhat equivocal and demands increased investigation. Indeed, Boone, Miller, Lesser, Hill, and D'Elia (1990) found minimal evidence for age-related differences in frontal lobe capacity compared to healthy middle-aged adults. Similarly, Valdois, Joanette, Poissant, Ska, and Dehaut (1990) demonstrated that cognitive profiles of normal elderly are heterogeneous, and investigators might have difficulty relating the different profiles to a specific region of cortical dysfunction.

Recent studies have employed magnetic resonance imaging (MRI) technology with normal elderly (I. Awad, Spetzler, Hodak, Catherine, C. Awad, & Carey, 1986; Coffey, Figiel, Djang, & Weiner, 1990; Gerard & Weisberg, 1986; Lechner et al., 1987; Steingart et al., 1987; Sullivan, Pary, Telang, Rifai, & Zubenko, 1990; Zubenko et al., 1990). Results from MRI studies indicate that approximately 25% to 30% of older adults without dementia demonstrate leukoaraiosis or decreased density of the white matter (Hachinski, Potter, & Merskey, 1987). From review of these articles, it is interesting to note that investigators frequently cite anterior cortical and subcortical regions, areas intimately connected with the frontal cortex, as vulnerable to leukoaraiosis. Increased age and the presence of hypertension, diabetes, or stroke predict the presence of leukoaraiosis in the elderly. The effect of leukoaraiosis on cognitive functioning in older adults remains unclear. In addition to the frontal cortex, advanced age affects other brain regions as well (Hoyer, 1990; Squire, 1987). For example, the hippocampus, a neuroanatomic structure important for the learning of new information, suffers age-related neurobiological changes (Hoyer, 1990; Lim, Zipursky, Murphy, & Pfefferbaum, 1990; Squire, 1987).

Finally, comorbid physical (Hoyer, 1990) or mental disease might also contribute to the decline in cognitive functioning. However, Albert (1988) asserted that age-related declines in intellectual processing are evident even among the most healthy elderly. Scientists need to take great care when reviewing the normal aging literature because interpretation of the results can differ based on whether the studies consisted of cross-sectional or longitudinal designs (see Albert & Moss, 1988; Rinn, 1988). In addition, most of the literature on cognitive functioning in older adults consists of samples of healthy, well-educated individuals and thus may present external validity problems.

PSYCHIATRIC DISORDERS OF THE ELDERLY

Aging individuals can experience emotional crises similar to those of younger adults. Older adults, however, have likely accumulated more losses and experienced a higher number of stressors than younger persons simply because of living longer. In addition, the capacity to cope with the accumulation of losses in older age may decrease because of individuals' potential decline in adaptive capacity. In contrast, older adults have acquired a lifetime of experience successfully coping with emotional crises that might render them more able to handle difficult situations in later life. Perhaps against general stereotyping, *most older adults are in good cognitive, behavioral, and emotional health* (Birren & Renner, 1980). Unfortunately, there exist elderly persons who suffer some forms of psychopathology. The following section reviews some common psychiatric illnesses experienced by the elderly.

Mood Disorders

Mood disorders, defined by the *Diagnostic and Statistical Manual of Mental Disorders* (DSM-III-R; American Psychiatric Association, 1987), include depressive disorders and bipolar disorders. This chapter focuses on depression, which represents the most common emotional or affective disorder of advanced age (Breslau & Haug, 1983). Prevalence estimates of major depression in the elderly vary according to diagnostic criteria employed and whether the patient is residing in an institution. For example, using DSM-III-R criteria, prevalence estimates of major depression in community-dwelling elderly range from 1% for men to 3.64% for elderly women (Hendrie & Crossett, 1990). In addition, 26.8% of community-dwelling elderly complain of dysphoric symptoms (Blazer, Hughes, & George, 1987). Blazer and colleagues argued that DSM criteria for major depression do not adequately capture most older adults in community populations who display depressive symptoms. Other studies have reported that major depression is present in approximately 4% of the elderly population while dysthymia is present in a somewhat larger number, 5% to 8% (Ruegg, Zisook, & Swerdlow, 1988). Prevalence estimate of major depression for institutionalized elderly range from 12% to over 40% (Parmelee, Katz, & Lawton, 1989). An NIH study (1991) estimated the rate of new cases of depression in nursing home residents to be about 12.6%, with an additional 18% developing new depressive symptoms over a 1-year period. Another study found major depression in 11.5% of elderly hospitalized medical patients with 23% of the patients reporting depressive symptomatology (Koenig, Meador, Cohen, & Blazer, 1988).

Suicide Risk in the Elderly

A primary concern for the clinician treating the older depressed patient is the risk of suicide. Indeed, although the elderly comprise 11% of the population, they account for nearly 25% of all suicides, with older white males representing the highest risk group (Aiken, 1982). By the mid-1970s, the ratio of men to women who committed suicide had risen to seven to one. As Jenike (1988) pointed out, risk factors for suicide in older adults include alcohol abuse, a sudden calm in a previously depressed patient, a psychiatric history or previous suicide attempt, rigid personality style, previous or present physical illness, numerous losses, and patients' perceptions of being alone without friends or emotional support. In a recent retrospective study (Younger, Clark, Lindroth, & Stein, 1989) employing psychological autopsy methodology of older suicide victims, however, a high percentage of victims were married and not living alone. Nonetheless, a large number (46%) of the victims did evidence despondency over a potential terminal illness, such as cancer. Conwell, Caine, and Olsen (1990) reviewed the literature and found physical illness to be a common risk factor for suicide in late life. Of the physical diseases, cancer was the most frequently occurring disease related to suicide in older adults. Because adults older than 65 account for nearly 65% of all deaths attributable to cancer, clinicians dealing with such individuals must recognize the risk for suicide. Indeed, most older adults who commit suicide visit their physicians shortly prior to death. In contrast, although premorbid psychopathology occurs in a significant percentage of suicide victims, very few of these patients visit mental health settings. Nonetheless, some investigators (Pearlman & Uhlmann, 1988; Younger et al., 1990) have argued that a patient's concern about a terminal illness is a multidimensional construct, does not predict suicide, and is one of a variety of risk factors that contributes to a patient's decision to end his or her life. In an attempt to understand contributors to suicide, one study demonstrated that several factors affect the acceptability of suicide (Deluty, 1989). Evaluations of suicide were more acceptable when evaluators were male, victims wee male, victims were elderly, and the patient was suffering a terminal cancer.

The issue of suicide in the elderly population remains an extremely important area for clinical and scientific concern. Investigators need to continue conducting research aimed at clarifying risk factors for suicide. For example, whether physical illness represents a risk factor for suicide in older adults needs continued investigation. An additional area of investigation might include the ability of physicians to recognize suicide risk in older adults, because the physician is usually the professional with whom older patients visit prior to ending their lives.

Cognitive Impairment in Elderly Depressed

From 10% to 20% of elderly depressed persons suffer significant cognitive impairment (Reynolds et al., 1988). The labels *pseudodementia* (Kiloh, 1961), *dementia syndrome of depression* (Folstein & McHugh, 1978), *depression-induced organic mental disorder* (McAllister, 1983), and *depression-related cognitive dysfunction* (Stoudemire, Hill, Gulley, & Morris, 1989) describe the severe, but reversible, cognitive impairment that mimics a progressive dementia in older depressed patients. Over 30 years ago, Kiloh (1961) stated that pseudodementia frequently occurred in older depressed patients. Since that time, authors have written numerous articles describing the clinical features of pseudodementia and its differential from progressive dementia (Bulbena & Berrios, 1986; Cummings, 1989; Folstein & Rabins, 1991; Jeste, Gierz, & Harris, 1990; Kaszniak, 1987; Stoudemire et al., 1989; Wells, 1979).

Several investigators have conducted critical analyses of the label *pseudodementia* (Arie, 1983; Nussbaum, 1994; Reifler, 1982; Shaberg, 1978, 1980). Although these authors have agreed that the label *pseudodementia* alerts clinicians to the existence of potentially treatable forms of cognitive impairment, they have argued for the abandonment of the term for the following reasons:

1. It implies that the patient has either an organic or a functional illness, when many patients present with both.
2. Clinicians often mistakenly use the term as a diagnosis rather than its intended use as a descriptive label only.
3. It confuses the complicated interaction of depression and the aging brain.
4. It oversimplifies the division between cognitive and affective illness.
5. It does not clarify the relationship between degenerative neurophysiological changes in aging and depression.
6. It does not answer questions regarding the clinical response of depression in patients with dementia to antidepressant medication.
7. It does not elucidate the association between dementia and depression.
8. The term itself does not specify the etiology of the illness.

In an effort to address the need for investigation of the neurobiology of cognitive impairment in elderly depressed, Folstein and Rabins (1991) argued that "persons who suffer from both cognitive impairment and depression have abnormalities of common neural structures" (p. 37). For example, they argued that patients with major depression, Parkinson's, Huntington's, or Alzheimer's disease suffer a dysfunction of the cortical pathways that bridge aminergic fibers from the brain stem to the cortex. Folstein and Rabins proposed the *syndrome of the aminergic nuclei* (SOTAN) to replace pseudodementia and describe the coexistence of changes in mood, cognition, and movement often present in older patients. The authors asserted that this concept might alleviate confusion within the literature and assist in understanding the pathological mechanisms and etiology of cognitive impairment in elderly depressed persons. The model that Folstein and Rabins proposed is consistent with one characterization of depression in the elderly as a *subcortical dementia* (see King and Caine, 1990).

MRI in Assessment of Elderly Depressed Persons

Similar to research on normal aging, investigators have recently utilized MRI technology in the assessment of older depressed patients. Studies involving MRI have consistently indicated that older depressed patients have a significantly high incidence of leukoaraiosis and subcortical pathology relative to normal controls (Coffey, Figiel, Djang, Saunders, & Weiner, 1989; Coffey et al., 1990; Krishnan et al., 1988; Nasrallah, Coffman, & Olson, 1989; Zubenko et al., 1990). These studies have found that severity of subcortical pathology relates to later age of depression onset, vascular disease, presence of hypertension, smoking history, and perhaps hypercholesterolemia. Indeed, one study (Figiel et al., 1991) found that basal ganglia hyperintensities occur more frequently (60% vs. 11%) in late-onset depressed patients (after age 60) than in early-onset depressed patients (before age 60). For each late-onset patient, MRI indicated the location of the lesion was the dorsal aspect of the head of the caudate nucleus. The two groups did not differ in the number of subjects with deep white matter hyperintensities nor in the average number of white matter hyperintensities. The late-onset depressed group, however, evinced larger deep white matter lesions (>1 cm) than the early-onset group. Figiel and colleagues noted that depressed patients' frontal lobes were most vulnerable to the presence of deep white matter hyperintensities whereas parietal and occipital lobes were minimally susceptible, and the temporal lobe was free of hyperintensities. These authors speculated that the white matter hyperintensities of the frontal lobe and caudate might induce depression via disconnection of the cerebral cortex from the limbic system. This hypothesis supports the Folstein and Rabins (1991) model and provides additional evidence for a subcortical–frontal neuropathology of depression in older patients.

The clinical significance of the leukoaraiosis and subcortical pathology in elderly depressed remains unknown. Coffey and colleagues (1989) found an association between severity of white matter lesions and memory impairment using a standard scale of verbal and figural recall. In addition, another group of investigators (Nussbaum, Kaszniak, Allender, & Rapcsak, 1995) found that subcortical lesions in a sample of cognitively intact elderly depressed predicted later cognitive decline. Finally, Wolfe, Linn, Babikian, Knoefel, and Albert (1990) found that the presence of multiple lacunar infarcts, as measured by computed axial tomography, correlated with neuropsychological signs of frontal lobe dysfunction in older patients. These three studies represent preliminary attempts to relate the presence of deep white matter lesions and subcortical pathology to cognitive impairment and depressed mood.

Additional evidence for a subcortical–frontal neuropathology underlying late-onset depression comes from the literature on cerebrovascular disease and depression (Robinson, 1987; Robinson, Morris, & Federoff, 1990; Starkstein et al., 1991). The authors conducting research in this area have demonstrated that depressive disorder is a common sequela of stroke. Patients with left dorsal–lateral–frontal cortical lesions and left basal ganglia lesions have a significantly higher frequency of major depression than patients with lesions in other locations. In addition, a study employing positron emission tomography, a measure of glucose metabolism, demonstrated an association between major depression and left anterolateral–prefrontal cortical abnormality (Baxter et al., 1989). Likewise, a study employing single photon emission tomography, a measure of cerebral blood flow, demonstrated an association between major depression and decreased blood flow in all cortical areas, with notable decreases in frontal and subcortical areas (O'Connell et al., 1989).

Neuropsychological Findings

A review of the cognitive and neuropsychological literature regarding elderly depressed persons suggests deficits of effortful processing (Weingartner, 1986), a conservative response bias (Niederehe, 1986), psychomotor slowing (Hart & Kwentus, 1987), reduced verbal fluency (Cassens, Wolfe, & Zola, 1990; Hart, Kwentus, Wade, & Hamer, 1987), poor concept formation (Cassens et al., 1990; Hart, Kwentus, Wade, & Taylor, 1988), impaired abstract thinking, and poor sustained concentration

(Raskin, Friedman, & DiMascio, 1982). Caine (1981) found depressed patients impaired on tasks that demand attention, mental processing speed, and spontaneous elaboration, whereas cortically mediated functions, such as reading, naming, repetition, mathematics, and motor praxis were intact. Caine asserted that depressed patients maintain cortically based cognitive capacity but suffer impairment of the arousal–attention–concentration system. This conclusion supports Weingartner (1986), who attributed impaired cognitive functioning in depressed patients to a deficit in effortful processing. King and Caine (1990) reviewed the literature on late-life depression and concluded that the basal ganglia appear to be a primary region of neuropathology in elderly depressed patients with cognitive impairment. They also noted that the neuroanatomical basis of depression in older adults remains speculative and in need of continued research.

In summary, this review suggests a neuroanatomical basis for depression in some elderly. Specifically, depression appears to result from lesions of the left frontal cortex and basal ganglia. The existence of deep white matter lesions in elderly depressed patients might also contribute to onset of depressed mood and cognitive impairment through disruption of cortical–subcortical neurochemical pathways. The Folstein and Rabins (1991) model appears to have the support of the present review. Depression in some older adults appears related to a dysfunction of the subcortical–frontal neural system.

Other Psychiatric Disorders of Later Life

Depression is certainly not the only psychiatric disorder of late life. Mania occurs in 5–8% of patients admitted to psychogeriatric hospitals (Jenike, 1988; Molinari, 1991). An additional 13% of older patients diagnosed with affective disorders complain primarily of manic symptoms. It is relatively uncommon, however, for mania to occur for the first time after age 65 (Jefferson, 1983), but older manic patients have a high rate of recidivism (Molinari, 1991). Approximately 2% to 10% of geriatric psychiatric admissions carry the diagnosis of schizophrenia or other psychotic disorder not secondary to a dementia or mood disorder (Rabins, Pauker, & Thomas, 1984; Rosse, Ciolino, & Gurel, 1985). One study (Molinari, 1991) using a sample of geriatric male veterans found a relatively high incidence (23%) of schizophrenia as a discharge diagnosis, but the investigator did not exclude dementia and mood disorders. In another study assessing psychiatric disturbance among older adults, Christenson and Blazer (1984) estimated the prevalence of persecutory ideation to be about 4% in a geriatric community population.

Alcohol Abuse in the Elderly

The abuse of alcohol and drugs in the elderly population is common, especially after retirement or other life stressors (Christison & Blazer, 1988; Rinn, 1988). Elderly individuals also tend to abuse prescribed medications. Indeed, older adults use more medications than younger adults (Graveley & Oseasohn, 1991). Research has found that the elderly receive nearly 25% of all prescribed medications and represent the largest consumers of sedative-hypnotics and tranquilizers (Christison & Blazer, 1988; Simon, 1980). Christison and Blazer reported that drug-related problems in the elderly include abuse, intoxication, dependence–withdrawal, overmedication, drug reactions, interactions, and side effects. Alcohol represents the most frequently used drug of the older population. Approximately 10% of adults over the age of 60 suffer from alcohol abuse or dependence (Christison & Blazer, 1988), and this rate increases substantially when sampling inpatient settings (Parette, Hourcade, & P. Parette, 1990). Molinari (1991) found that about 3% of geriatric male veterans carried a discharge diagnosis of alcohol dependence. Atkinson, Tolson, and Turner (1990) found nearly 15% of an outpatient sample of older men (over age 59) suffered their first onset of alcohol-related problems after age 60, and 29% had their first experience of alcohol-related difficulties after age 65. Compared to early-onset cases, older onset alcohol problems tended to be more mild and circumscribed, and individuals with older onset alcohol difficulties evidenced less family alcoholism and greater psychological stability than their early-onset counterparts. Late-onset patients were also more compliant with outpatient treatment regimens (Atkinson et al., 1990).

Rinn (1988) reviewed the negative consequences of alcoholism for older adults and reported that the damaging effects of alcohol on the aging brain tend to be more significant than with younger adults. Indeed, older alcoholics can develop cognitive deterioration related to an alcohol dementia (Reisberg & Berglund, 1987), Korsakoff's syndrome (Brandt & Butters, 1986), or a toxic-metabolic confusional state. Recovery from alcohol-induced brain damage is also slower in older than younger adults (Rinn, 1988). Other negative consequences of alcohol abuse in the elderly include increased risk of stroke, decreased cerebral blood flow (Shaw, 1987), severe sleep disturbance that manifests as a decrease in the rapid-eye-movement stage of sleep, fragmentation of sleep, and increased daytime fatigue (see Rinn, 1988).

Dementia

Dementia refers to a disturbance of intellect, personality, and communication functioning (Bayles & Kaszniak, 1987). There are many different causes of dementia, and some forms of dementia are reversible whereas others are progressive (Hasse, 1977). The prevalence of dementia in the elder is estimated at 15% of the population older than 65 (Katzman, 1976). The most frequent cause of dementia in the elderly is Alzheimer's disease (AD). Based on autopsy data (Tomlinson, Blessed, & Roth, 1970), AD alone, or with another disorder, accounts for 50% to 70% of dementia in persons older than 65. A recent clinical study (Evans et al., 1989) suggested that the number of individuals with AD is nearly 4 million, suggesting that the Katzman (1976) estimate of dementia prevalence is low. Evans and colleagues demonstrated that the risk of developing AD increases with age. Koff (1986) reported that the number of AD patients will likely increase to beyond 8 million by the year 2050. This finding raises serious concerns for the health-care system in the United States. Because the progressive nature of the disease results in complete debilitation of the patient, the responsibility of caring for these unfortunate individuals rests on family members, health-care providers, and society in general. Questions remain regarding the readiness of the current health-care system to provide the necessary care (Berg et al., 1991; Jarvik, 1991; Koff, 1986; Rutledge, 1990). Some authors have proposed the development of progressive special-care units and alternative day-care treatment programs to assist in the care of AD patients in order to remove total responsibility for the care of the patient from the family. The study of AD must remain a major focus of research during the next century. Khachaturian

(1985) addressed the need for AD research and underscored the opportunities for behavioral scientists in this regard.

PHYSICAL DISORDERS OF THE ELDERLY

This section highlights some of the major medical disorders that afflict the elderly and the impact of these disorders on neuropsychological functioning. Whereas a complete review is impossible for the present chapter, the following sections focus on hypertension, cancer, diabetes, and head injury.

Hypertension

Heart disease represents the primary cause of death among individuals over the age of 65 (Crawford & Cohen, 1984). A disturbance of heart function can result in a variety of neurological impairments. These include generalized hypoxia or acute anoxic episode, cerebral infarction, and cerebral embolization (Rosenberg, 1981). Neuropsychological impairments might also result from cardiac disease (Rinn, 1988). Areas of cognitive deficit might include memory, language, visuospatial skills, finger motor speed, executive functions, and emotional reactions (Kuhn et al., 1988; Nussbaum & Goldstein, 1992; Roose, Dalack, & Woodring, 1991; Savageau, Stanton, Jenkins, & Klein, 1982).

The relationship of hypertension to cognitive functioning is less clear. Rinn (1988) argued that hypertension often relates to abnormal changes in the brain and cerebrovascular system and therefore likely contributes to neuropsychological deficits. Indeed, information presented earlier in this chapter indicated that hypertension in older adults predicts the presence of MRI-assessed leukoaraiosis. In a recent study (Schmidt et al., 1991), asymptomatic hypertensive individuals performed significantly worse than normal controls on neuropsychological tests measuring verbal memory, total learning, and memory capacity. Additionally, hypertensive subjects demonstrated twice as many punctate high-signal intensities of the white matter (leukoaraiosis) as controls. However, against the prediction of Rinn (1988), Schmidt et al. found no relationship between presence of leukoaraiosis and cognitive impairment. Goldstein (1992) reviewed the literature on hypertension and cognitive functioning in the elderly and concluded that although deficits in cognitive functioning occur in older hypertensive individuals, they tend to be mild. Areas of particular cognitive deficit include memory functions that require sustained attention and psychomotor abilities. Goldstein reached the same conclusions regarding the effects of antihypertension medication. Finally, several investigators have demonstrated that certain nonpharmacological treatments for hypertension are effective with the elderly (Abrahamson, 1987; Black, 1989; Buby, Elfner, & May, 1990; Irvine, Johnston, Jenner, & Marie, 1986; Pearce, Engel, & Burton, 1989). These treatments include nutrition, exercise, behavior modification techniques, relaxation training, and biofeedback.

Cancer

Cancer risk increases with age and represents the second leading cause of death among individuals over the age of 65 (Crawford & Cohen, 1984). Although individuals 65 years of age and older comprise 11% of the population, they account for nearly 60% of all cancer deaths (D'Agostino, Gray, & Scanlon, 1990). In addition, cancer is the primary medical illness of suicide victims in the elderly population (Conwell et al., 1990). The incidence of cerebral tumors also increases with age. A commonly used classification scheme divides tumors into primary tumors of the CNS (e.g., gliomas and meningiomas) and secondary tumors that represent metastases from regions outside the CNS. The most frequent origins for metastatic CNS tumors include the lungs, breast, gastrointestinal tract, kidney, and prostate (Wedding & Cody, 1990). The most frequently occurring 82% of all tumors) cerebral tumors in the elderly (over age 60) include glioblastoma, meningioma, acoustic neuroma, and metastatic cancer (Wolfson & Katzman, 1992). According to Wedding and Cody (1990), the effect of a cerebral tumor in the elderly is similar to the effect on younger adults and depends on the type, location, and rate of growth of the tumor. However, Wolfson and Katzman (1992) reported that adults older than 60 have poorer prognoses than younger patients. Tumors generally result in increased intracranial pressure that can cause acute confusional behavior and cognitive impairment (D'Agostino et al., 1990; Wedding & Cody, 1990). Psychiatric symptomatology might occur early in the growth of a frontal tumor. Likewise, headache is a common symptom of cerebral tumor growth. Thus, when elderly individuals complain about headaches, clinicians need to be alert regarding the possible presence of a tumor (Wedding & Cody, 1990). Treatment of cerebral tumors is similar for older and younger adults. However, physicians rarely use chemotherapy with the elderly, and older patients are more vulnerable than younger adults to complications from long-term steroid treatment (Wolfson & Katzman, 1992). One preventive measure of cancer for the elderly includes enforced dietary restriction (Horwath, 1991).

Diabetes

The occurrence of diabetes increases with age. Common sequelae of diabetes mellitus include mild neuropsychological impairments (Rinn, 1988) and severe atherosclerotic complications, including stroke (Horwath, 1991). One study found the risk for cerebral infarction was 2.6 times greater in diabetic men and 3.1 times greater in diabetic women compared to nondiabetic controls (Wolf, Kannel, & Verter, 1984). Atherosclerosis accompanies diabetes mellitus and may lead to diabetic encephalopathy, a condition that involves focal and diffuse cerebral neuronal damage (Lavis, 1981). There exists some controversy regarding diabetes as a predictor of MRI-measured leukoaraiosis. One study (Lechner et al., 1987) found diabetes to be a risk factor for the presence of leukoaraiosis, whereas another study did not (Sullivan et al., 1990). According to Rinn (1988), only one study on the cognitive effects of diabetes in the elderly has emerged. The identified deficits include problems with list learning and mental manipulation of information.

Head Injury in the Elderly

A relatively new area of research with clinical importance is the prevalence and effects of heady injuries on older adults. An early review (Holden, 1988) of the head injury literature found increased mortality with increased age, particularly due to complications (e.g., surgical risks, severity and length of coma, and length of posttraumatic amnesia). The mortality rate for the group aged 15–24, however, was higher than for those 65 years and older. Holden noted that head injuries in younger adults were due primarily to road–traffic accidents, whereas older adults suffered head injuries secondary to falls. Indeed, Jennett (1982) conducted a survey of Scottish citizens and reported that older adults involved in traffic accidents were more likely than younger adults to be pedestrians or passengers. Also, falls in the elderly appear related to alcohol consumption. Men experienced more head injuries across all age groups with one exception: Women over age 75 suffered more head injuries than men, perhaps due to the fact that women outlive men. Data collected from a U.S. population revealed many similarities to the Jennett study, but some differences were apparent. For example, Kraus et al. (1984) reported that the rate of head injuries in the elderly due to pedestrian traffic accidents were lower in the United States than in Scotland. In addition, head injury related to traffic accidents occurred primarily in the 15- to 25-year-old group and not in the elderly population as the data in Scotland indicated. Kraus and associates attributed the differences to the possibility that pedestrians are more common in Great Britain, where fewer elderly have access to a car. A final difference was that brain injury due to firearms was higher in U.S. men over the age of 65 than in elderly British males.

More recently, Fields (1991) reviewed this scant literature and found that older adults who suffer traumatic brain injury (TBI) are more susceptible than younger victims to increased mortality, increased length of hospitalization, and decreased potential to return home. Consistent with previous literature, Fields reported that older adults suffer more falls, but fewer motor vehicle accidents than younger adults. Fields discussed three problems in comparing older versus younger TBI patients. First, there is the issue of cause and effect: Was the older adult's head injury the cause or the result of degenerative changes? Second, researchers need to control statistically for the severity of TBI and total body injury when making comparisons between different age groups. Third, researchers need to statistically control for the nature of the accident. Controlling for the aforementioned points, Fields conducted a prospective study of the negative effects of TBI in newly admitted head injured patients ($N = 2326$). The investigator stratified patients across seven age spans from ages 25–34 to age 85 and above. Consistent with previous literature, results of this study demonstrated a substantial increase in negative outcomes when TBI occurred in an older adult. Fields concluded that such results have both practical (prognosis) and conceptual (risk factors) importance for the study of TBI in the elderly. Interestingly, head injury may be a risk factor for development of AD (Heyman et al., 1986; Mortimer, French, Hutton, & Schuman, 1985).

Finally, Holden (1984) argued that despite the negative outcome typically related to brain injury in the older adult population, clinicians must attempt aggressive treatment and rehabilitation of patients, and cautioned against unnecessary ageism, encouraging research investigation into the efficacy of rehabilitation with older patients who suffer head injuries.

FUTURE DIRECTIONS

This chapter has reviewed some of the common psychiatric and other medical disorders the elderly experience, highlighting each disorder's effect on cognitive functioning. The issue of cognitive functioning and cognitive decline in normal aging represents an exciting area of investigation. Continued research employing neuroimaging technology might provide support for the theory of age-related frontal lobe dysfunction. Rinn's notion of a subclinical dementia as a function of aging might also find support with continued longitudinal study of "healthy" elderly. Depression in the older adult has already become a major area of investigation. Consistent findings across different disciplines suggest that depression in the older adult results from a subcortical–frontal dysfunction, although this theory needs additional evidence to support it. The clinical significance of MRI-measured leukoaraiosis in elderly depressed patients is not yet known and deserves investigation. The impact of physical illness on aging central nervous systems also deserves continued investigation, particularly because older adults represent a large percentage of the population. Researchers need to aggressively study suicide, alcoholism, and head injury in the elderly in order to reduce the prevalence of these problems. The recognition of risk factors for suicide in the elderly must remain a critically important issue for clinicians and physicians working with older adults. Finally, models of successful aging become even more important because a growing number of individuals are living longer. In summary, the older adult population will soon demand the primary attention of the health-care system. The health-care community must make efforts to address the needs of this growing population segment. Professionals working with the elderly must attempt to integrate clinical and scientific interests to produce a multidisciplinary approach to the understanding, treatment, and care of the elderly. Educators need to develop programs to train specialists in the sociology, psychology, and biology of the aging human being. Society must also begin to understand the aging process in order to minimize fears and unfounded ageism. The next century will likely witness an increased understanding of the aging process and perhaps a more acceptable attitude toward the elderly.

REFERENCES

Abrahamson, C. F. (1987). Response to the challenge: Effective treatment of the elderly through thermal biofeedback combined with progressive relaxation. *Biofeedback and Self-Regulation, 12,* 121–125.

Aiken, L. R. (1982). *Later life* (2nd ed.). New York: Holt, Rinehart & Winston.

Albert, M. S. (1988). General issues in geriatric neuropsychology. In M. S. Albert & M. B. Moss (Eds.), *Geriatric neuropsychology* (pp. 3–12). New York: Guilford.

Albert, M. S., & Moss, M. B. (1988). *Geriatric neuropsychology.* New York: Guilford.

Albert, M. S., & Stafford, J. L. (1988). Computed tomographic studies. In M. S. Albert & M. B. Moss (Eds.), *Geriatric neuropsychology* (pp. 211–227). New York: Guilford.

American Psychiatric Association. (1987). *Diagnostic and statistical manual of mental disorders* (3rd ed. rev.). Washington, DC: Author.

Arie, T. (1983). Pseudodementia. *British Medical Journal, 286,* 1301–1302.

Atchley, R. C. (1989). A continuity theory of normal aging. *Gerontological Society of America, 29,* 183–190.

Atkinson, R. M., Tolson, R. L., & Turner, J. A. (1990). Late versus early onset problem drinking in older men. *Alcoholism: Clinical and Experimental Research, 14,* 574–579.

Awad, I. A., Spetzler, R. F., Hodak, J. A., Awad, C. A., & Carey, R. (1986). Incidental subcortical lesions identified on magnetic resonance imaging in the elderly: I. Correlation with age and cerebrovascular risk factors. *Stroke, 17,* 1084–1089.

Baxter, L. R., Schwartz, J., Phelps, M. E., Mazziota, J. C., Guze, B. H., Selin, C. E., Gerner, R. H., & Sumida, R.

M. (1989). Reduction of prefrontal cortex glucose metabolism common to three types of depression. *Archives of General Psychiatry, 46,* 243–249.

Bayles, K. A., & Kaszniak, A. W. (1987). *Communication and cognition in normal aging and dementia.* Boston: College-Hill Press.

Berg, L., Buckwalter, K. C., Chafetz, P. K., Gwyther, L. P., Holmes, D., Koepke, K. M., Lawton, M. P., Lindeman, D. A., Magasiner, J., Maslow, K., Sloane, P. D., & Teresi, J. (1991). Special care units for persons with dementia. *Journal of the American Geriatrics Society, 39,* 1229–1236.

Birren, J. E. (1988). A contribution to the theory of aging: As a counterpart of development. In J. E. Birren & V. L. Bengtson, (Eds.), *Emergent theories of aging* (pp. 153–176). New York: Springer.

Birren, J. E., & Birren, B. A. (1990). The concepts, models, and history of the psychology of aging. In J. E. Birren & K. W. Schaie (Eds.), *Handbook of the psychology of aging* (pp. 3–20). San Diego: Academic Press.

Birren, J. E., & Renner, J. (1980). Concepts and issues of mental health and aging. In J. E. Birren & R. B. Sloane (Eds.), *Handbook of mental health and aging* (pp. 3–33). Englewood Cliffs, NJ: Prentice-Hall.

Black, H. R. (1989). Nonpharmacologic therapy for hypertension in the elderly. *Geriatrics, 44,* 20–29.

Blazer, D., Hughes, D. C., & George, L. K. (1987). The epidemiology of depression in an elderly community population. *Gerontologist, 27,* 281–287.

Boone, K. B., Miller, B. L., Lesser, I. M., Hill, E., & D'Elia, L. D. (1990). Performance on frontal lobe tests in healthy, older individuals. *Developmental Neuropsychology, 6,* 216–223.

Brandt, J., & Butters, N. (1986). The alcoholic Wernicke–Korsakoff syndrome and its relationship to long-term alcohol abuse. In I. Grant & K. M. Adams (Eds.), *Neuropsychological assessment of neuropsychiatric disorders* (pp. 441–477). New York: Oxford University Press.

Breslau, L., & Haug, M. R. (1983). *Depression and aging.* New York: Springer.

Buby, C., Elfner, L. F., & May, J. G. (1990). Relaxation pretraining, pulse wave velocity, and thermal biofeedback in the treatment of essential hypertension. *International Journal of Psychophysiology, 9,* 225–230.

Bulbena, A., & Berrios, G. E. (1986). Pseudodementia: Facts and figures. *British Journal of Psychiatry, 148,* 87–94.

Butler, R. N. (1975). *Why survive? Being old in America.* New York: Harper & Row.

Caine, E. D. (1981). Pseudodementia: Current concepts and future directions. *Archives of General Psychiatry, 38,* 1359–1364.

Cassens, G., Wolfe, L., & Zola, M. (1990). The neuropsychology of depressions. *Journal of Neuropsychiatry and Clinical Neurosciences, 2,* 202–213.

Cerella, J. (1990). Aging and the information processing rate. In J. E. Birren & K. W. Schaie (Eds.), *The psychology of adult development and aging* (pp. 201–219). Washington, DC: American Psychological Association.

Christenson, R., & Blazer, D. (1984). Epidemiology of persecutory ideation in an elderly population in the community. *American Journal of Psychiatry, 141,* 1088–1091.

Christison, C., & Blazer, D. (1988). Clinical assessment of psychiatric symptoms. In M. S. Albert & M. B. Moss (Eds.), *Geriatric neuropsychology* (pp. 82–99). New York: Guilford.

Coffey, E. C., Figiel, G. S., Djang, W. T., Saunders, W. B., & Weiner, R. D. (1989). White matter hyperintensity on magnetic resonance imaging: Clinical and neuroanatomic correlates in depressed elderly. *Journal of Neuropsychiatry and Clinical Neurosciences, 6,* 135–144.

Coffey, E. C., Figiel, G. S., Djang, W. T., & Weiner, R. D. (1990). Subcortical hyperintensity on magnetic resonance imaging: A comparison of normal and depressed elderly subjects. *American Journal of Psychiatry, 147,* 187–189.

Comfort, A. (1974). *The biology of senescence* (2nd ed.). New York: Elsevier.

Conwell, Y., Caine, E. D., & Olsen, K. (1990). Suicide and cancer in late life. *Hospital and Community Psychiatry, 41,* 1334–1338.

Craik, F.I.M., & Lockhart, R. S. (1972). Levels of processing: A framework for memory research. *Journal of Verbal Learning and Verbal Behavior, 11,* 671–684.

Craik, F.I.M., & McDowd, J. M. (1987). Age difference in recall and recognition. *Journal of Experimental Psychology: Learning, Memory, and Cognition, 13,* 474–479.

Craik, F.I.M., Morris, L. W., Morris, R. G., & Loewen, E. R. (1990). Relations between source amnesia and frontal lobe functioning in older adults. *Psychology and Aging, 5,* 148–151.

Crawford, J., & Cohen, H. J. (1984). Aging and neoplasia. *Annual Review of Gerontology and Geriatrics, 4,* 3–32.

Cumming, E., Dean, L., Newell, D., & McCaffrey, I. (1960). Disengagement tentative theory of aging. *Sociometry, 23,* 23–35.

Cummings, J. (1989). Dementia and depression: An evolving enigma. *Journal of Neuropsychiatry and Clinical Neurosciences, 1,* 236–242.

Curtis, H. (1966). *Biological mechanisms of aging.* Springfield, IL: Thomas.

D'Agostino, N. S., Gray, G., & Scanlon, C. (1990). Cancer in the older adult: Understanding age-related changes. *Journal of Gerontological Nursing, 16,* 12–15.

Deluty, R. H. (1989). Factors affecting the acceptability of suicide. *Omega, 19,* 315–326.

Doraiswamy, P. M., Figiel, G. S., Husain, M. M., McDonald, W. M., Shah, S. A., Boyko, O. B., Ellinwood, E. H., & Krishnan, K.R.R. (1991). Aging of the human corpus collosum: Magnetic resonance imaging in normal volunteers. *Journal of Neuropsychiatry and Clinical Neurosciences, 3,* 392–297.

Evans, D. A., Funkenstein, H. H., Albert, M. S., Scherr, P. A., Cook, N. R., Chown, M. J., Hebert, L. E., Hennekens, C. H., & Taylor, J. O. (1989). Prevalence of Alzheimer's disease in a community population of older adults. *Journal of the American Medical Association, 262,* 2551–2556.

Fields, R. B. (August, 1991). *The effects of head injuries on older adults.* Paper presented at the 99th Annual Meeting of the American Psychological Association, San Francisco. CA.

Figiel, G. S., Krishnan, R. R., Doraiswamy, P. M., Rao, V. P., Nemeroff, C. B., & Boyko, O. B. (1991). Subcortical hyperintensities on brain resonance imaging: A comparison between late age onset and early onset elderly depressed subjects. *Neurobiology of Aging, 26,* 245–247.

Folstein, M. F., & McHugh, P. R. (1978). Dementia syndrome of depression. In Katzman, R., Terry, R. D., & Bick, K. L. (Eds.), *Alzheimer's disease: Senile dementia and related disorders* (pp. 281–289). New York: Raven.

Folstein, M. F., & Rabins, P. V. (1991). Replacing pseudodementia. *Neuropsychiatry, Neuropsychology, and Behavioral Neurology, 4,* 36–40.

Gatz, M., & Pearson, C. G. (1988). Ageism revised and the provision of psychological services. *American Psychologist, 43,* 184–188.

Gerard, G., & Weisberg, L. A. (1986). MRI periventricular lesions in adults. *Neurology, 36,* 998–1001.

Goldstein, G. (1983). Normal aging and the concept of dementia. In C. J. Golden & P. J. Vincente (Eds.), *Foundations of clinical neuropsychology* (pp. 249–271). New York: Plenum Press.

Goldstein, G. (1992). Hypertension and cognitive function in the elderly. *Medical Progress, 2,* 127–132.

Graveley, E. A., & Oseasohn, C. S. (1991). Multiple drug regimens: Medication compliance among veterans 65 years and older. *Research in Nursing and Health, 14,* 51–58.

Hachinski, V. C., Potter, P., & Merskey, H. (1987). Leuko-araiosis. *Archives of Neurology, 44,* 21–23.

Hart, R. P., & Kwentus, J. A. (1987). Psychomotor slowing and subcortical-type dysfunction in depression. *Journal of Neurology, Neurosurgery, and Psychiatry, 50,* 1263–1266.

Hart, R. P., Kwentus, J. A., Wade, J. B., & Hamer, R. M. (1987). Digit symbol performance in mild dementia and depression. *Journal of Consulting and Clinical Psychology, 55,* 236–238.

Hart, R. P., Kwentus, J. A., Wade, J. B., & Taylor, J. R. (1988). Modified Wisconsin Card Sorting Test in elderly normal, depressed, and older neuropsychiatric patients. *Clinical Neuropsychologist, 2,* 49–56.

Hasher, L., & Zacks, R. T. (1979). Automatic and effortful processes in memory. *Journal of Experimental Psychology, 108,* 356–388.

Hasse, E. R. (1977). Diseases presenting as dementia. In C. E. Wells (Ed.), *Dementia* (pp. 27–68). Philadelphia: Davis.

Hayflick, L. (1974). The strategy of senescence. *Journal of Gerontology, 14,* 37–45.

Hendricks, J., & Hendricks, C. D. (1986). *Aging in mass society: Myths and realities* (3rd ed.). Boston: Little, Brown.

Hendrie, H. C., & Crossett, J.H.W. (1990). An overview of depression in the elderly. *Psychiatric Annals, 20,* 64–70.

Heyman, A., Wilkinson, W. E., Stafford, J. A., Helms, M. J., Sigmon, A. G., & Weinberg, T. (1986). Alzheimer's disease: A study of epidemiologic aspects. *Annals of Neurology, 15,* 335–341.

Holden, U. (1984). Head injury and older people. In U. Holden (Ed.), *Neuropsychology and aging* (pp. 154–176). New York: New York University Press.

Horton, A. M., & Puente, A. E. (1990). Life-span neuropsychology: An overview. In A.M.H. Horton (Ed.), *Neuropsychology across the lifespan* (pp. 1–15). New York: Springer.

Horwath, C. C. (1991). Nutrition goals for older adults: A review. *Gerontologist, 31,* 811–821.

Hoyer, S. (1990). Brain glucose and energy metabolism during normal aging. *Aging, 2,* 245–258.

Irvine, M. J., Johnston, D. W., Jenner, D. A., & Marie, G. V. (1986). Relaxation and stress management in the treatment of essential hypertension. *Journal of Psychosomatic Research, 30,* 437–450.

Jarvik, L. F. (1991, February). VA and the Alzheimer patient: Projections and partnerships. *VA Practitioner,* pp. 57–62.

Jefferson, J. W. (1983). Lithium and affective disorder in the elderly. *Comprehensive Psychiatry, 24,* 166–178.

Jenike, M. (1988). Depression and other psychiatric disorders. In M. S. Albert & M. B. Moss (Eds.), *Geriatric neuropsychology* (pp. 115–144). New York: Guilford.

Jennett, B. (1982). Head injury in the elderly. In F. I. Caird (Ed.), *Neurosurgical disorders in the elderly.* Bristol, UK: Wright.

Jeste, D. V., Gierz, M., & Harris, M. J. (1990). Pseudodementia: Myths and realities. *Psychiatric Annals, 20,* 71–79.

Kaszniak, A. W. (1987). Neuropsychologiacal consultation to geriatricians: Issues in assessment of memory complaints. *Clinical Neuropsychologist, 1,* 35–46.

Katzman, R. (1976). The prevalence and malignancy of Alzheimer's disease. *Archives of Neurology, 33,* 217–218.

Katzman, R. (1983). Demography, definitions, and problems. In R. Katzman & R. Terry (Eds.), *The neurology of aging* (pp. 1–15). Philadelphia: Davis.

Katzman, R., & Terry R. (1992). Normal aging of the central nervous system. In R. Katzman & J. W. Rowe (Eds.), *Principles of geriatric neurology* (pp. 18–58). Philadelphia: Davis.

Khachaturian, Z. S. (1985). Progress of research on Alzheimer's disease. *American Psychologist, 40,* 1251–1255.

Kiloh, L. G. (1961). Pseudo-dementia. *Acta Psychiatrica Scandinavica, 37,* 336–351.

King, D. A., & Caine, E. P. (1990). Depression. In J. L. Cummings (Ed.), *Subcortical dementia* (pp. 218–230). New York: Oxford University Press.

Kobari, M., Stirling, M., & Ichijo, M. (1990). Leuko-araiosis, cerebral atrophy, and cerebral perfusion in normal aging. *Archives of Neurology, 47,* 161–165.

Koenig, H. G., Meador, K. G., Cohen, H. J., & Blazer, D. G. (1988). Depression in elderly hospitalized patients with medical illness. *Archives of Internal Medicine, 148,* 1929–1936.

Koff, T. (1986, Summer). Nursing home management of Alzheimer's disease. *American Journal of Alzheimer's Care and Related Disorders,* pp. 12–15.

Kraus, J. P., Black, M. A., Hessol, N., Lcy, F., Rokaw, W., Sullivan, C., Bowyers, S., Knowlton, S., & Marshall, L. (1984). The incidence of acute brain injury and serious impairment in a defined population. *American Journal of Epidemiology, 119,* 186–201.

Krishnan, K. R., Goli, V., Ellinwood, E., France, R. D., Blazer, D. G., & Nemeroff, C. B. (1988). Leukoencephalopathy in patients diagnosed as major depressive. *Biological Psychiatry, 23,* 519–522.

Kuhn, W. F., Myers, B., Brennan, A. F., Davis, M. H., Lippmann, S. B., Gray, L. A., & Pool, G. E. (1988). Psychopathology in heart transplant candidates. *Journal of Heart Transplantation, 7,* 223–226.

Lavis, V. R. (1981). Psychiatric manifestations of endocrine disease in the elderly. In A. J. Levenson & R.C.W. Hall (Eds.), *Neuropsychiatric manifestations of physical disease in the elderly* (pp. 59–82). New York: Raven.

Lebo, D. (1953). Some factors said to make for happiness in old age. *Journal of Clinical Psychology, 9,* 384–390.

Lechner, H., Schmidt, R., Bertha, G., Justich, E., Offenbacher, H., & Schneider, G. (1987). Nuclear magnetic resonance image white matter lesions and risk factors for stroke in normal individuals. *Stroke, 19,* 263–265.

Lim, K. O., Zipursky, R. B., Murphy, G. M., & Pfefferbaum, A. (1990). *In vivo* quantification of the limbic system using MRI: Effects of normal aging. *Psychiatry Research, 35,* 15–26.

Lutsky, N. (1980). Attitudes toward old age and elderly persons. *Annual Review of Geriatrics,* 287–336.

Makinodan, T. (1977). Immunity and aging. In C. Finch & L. Hayflick (Eds.), *Handbook of the biology of aging.* New York: Van Nostrand Reinhold.

McAllister, T. W. (1983). Overview: Pseudodementia. *American Journal of Psychiatry, 140,* 528–533.

Mitrushina, M., & Satz, P. (1991). Changes in cognitive functioning associated with normal aging. *Archives of Clinical Neuropsychology, 6,* 49–60.

Mittenberg, W., Seidenberg, M., O'Leary, D. S., & Digiulio, D. V. (1989). Changes in cerebral functioning associated with normal aging. *Journal of Clinical and Experimental Neuropsychology, 11,* 918–932.

Molinari, V. A. (1991). Demographic and psychiatric characteristics of 390 consecutive discharges from a geropsychiatric inpatient ward. *Clinical Gerontologist, 10,* 35–45.

Mortimer, J. A., French, L. R., Hutton, L. R., & Schuman, L. M. (1985). Head injury as a risk factor for Alzheimer's disease. *Neurology, 35,* 264–267.

Nasrallah, H. A., Coffman, J. A., & Olson, C. A. (1989). Structural brain imaging findings in affective disorders: An overview. *Journal of Neuropsychiatry and Clinical Neurosciences, 1,* 21–26.

National Institute of Health (1991, November). *Diagnosis and treatment of depression in late life.* Consensus Development Conference Statement, Washington, DC.

Neugarten, B. L., Havighurst, R. J., & Tobin, S. S. (1968). Personality and patterns of aging. In B. L. Neugarten (Ed.), *Middle age and aging* (pp. 173–177). Chicago: University of Chicago Press.

Niederehe, G. (1986). Depression and memory impairment in the aged. In L. W. Poon (Ed.), *Clinical memory assessment of older adults* (pp. 226–237). Washington, DC: American Psychological Association.

Nussbaum, J. F., Thompson, T., & Robinson, J. D. (1989). *Communication and aging.* New York: Harper & Row.

Nussbaum, P. D. (1994). Pseudodementia: A slow death. *Neuropsychology Review, 4,* 71–90.

Nussbaum, P. D., & Goldstein, G. (1992). Neuropsychological sequelae of cardiac transplantation: A preliminary review. *Clinical Psychology Review, 12,* 475–484.

Nussbaum, P. D., Kaszniak, A. W., Allender, J., & Rapcsak, S. (1995). Depression and cognitive decline in the elderly: A follow-up study. *The Clinical Neuropsychologist, 9,* 101–111.

O'Connell, R. A., Van Heertum, R. I., Billick, S. B., Holt, A. R., Gonzalez, A., Notardonato, H., Luck, D., & King, L. N. (1989). Single photon emission computed tomography with IMP in the differential diagnosis of psychiatric disorders. *Journal of Neuropsychiatry and Clinical Neurosciences, 1,* 145–153.

Parette, H. P., Hourcade, J. J., & Parette, P. C. (1990). Nursing attitudes toward geriatric alcoholism. *Journal of Gerontological Nursing, 16,* 26–30.

Parmelee, P. A., Katz, I. R., & Lawton, M. P. (1989). Depression among institutionalized aged: Assessment and prevalence estimation. *Journal of Gerontology, 44,* 22–29.

Pearce, K. L., Engel, B. T., & Burton, J. R. (1989). Behavioral treatment of isolated systolic hypertension in the elderly. *Biofeedback and Self-Regulation, 14,* 207–217.

Pearlman, R. A., & Uhlmann, R. F. (1988). Quality of life in chronic diseases: Perceptions of elderly patients. *Journal of Gerontology, 43,* M25–M30.

Peterson, D. A. (1986). Extent of gerontology instructions in American institutions of higher education. *Educational Gerontology, 12,* 519–530.

Rabins, P., Pauker, S., & Thomas, J. (1984). Can schizophrenia begin after age 44? *Comprehensive Psychiatry, 25,* 290–293.

Raskin, A., Friedman, A. S., & DiMascio, A. (1982). Cognitive and performance deficits in depression. *Psychopharmacology Bulletin, 18,* 196–202.

Reifler, B. V. (1982). Arguments for abandoning the term pseudodementia. *Journal of American Geriatrics Society, 30,* 665–668.

Reynolds, C. F., Hoch, C. C., Kupfer, D. J., Buysse, D. J., Houck, P. R., Stack, J. A., & Campbell, D. W. (1988). Bedside differentiation of depressive pseudodementia from dementia. *American Journal of Psychiatry, 145,* 1099–1103.

Rinn, W. E. (1988). Mental decline in normal aging: A review. *Journal of Geriatric Psychiatry and Neurology, 1,* 144–158.

Reisberg, J., & Berglund, M. (1987). Cerebral blood flow and metabolism in alcoholics. In O. A. Parsons, N. Butters, & P. E. Nathan (Eds.), *Neuropsychology of alcoholism: Implications for diagnosis and treatment* (pp. 64–75). New York: Guilford.

Robinson, R. G. (1987). Depression and stroke. *Psychiatric Annals, 17,* 731–740.

Robinson, R. G., Morris, P.L.P., & Fedoroff, J. P. (1990). Depression and cerebrovascular disease. *Journal of Clinical Psychiatry, 51,* 26–33.

Roose, S. P., Dalack, G. W., & Woodring, S. (1991). Death, depression, and heart disease. *Journal of Clinical Psychiatry, 52,* 34–39.

Rosenberg, G. M. (1981). Neuropsychiatric manifestations of cardiovascular disease in the elderly. In A. J. Levinson & R.C.W. Hall (Eds.), *Neuropsychiatric manifestations of physical disease in the elderly* (pp. 29–40). New York: Raven.

Rosse, R. B., Ciolino, C. P., & Gurel, L. (1986). Utilization of psychiatric consultation with an elderly medically ill inpatient population in a VA hospital. *Military Medicine, 151,* 583–586.

Rowe, J. W., & Kahn, R. L. (1987). Human aging: Usual and unusual. *Science, 237,* 143–149.

Rowe, J. W., & Katzman, R. (1992). Principles of geriatrics as applied to neurology. In R. Katzman & J. W. Rowe (Eds.), *Principles of geriatric neurology* (pp. 3–17). Philadelphia: Davis.

Ruegg, R. G., Zisook, S., & Swerdlow, N. R. (1988). Depression in the aged: an overview. *Psychiatric Clinics of North America, 11,* 83–99.

Rutledge, M. E. (1990, September). Adult day health care: An up-and-coming necessity. *VA Practitioner,* pp. 69–74.

Satin, D. G. (1986). The future of geriatric and interdisciplinary education. *Educational Gerontology, 12,* 549–561.

Savageau, J. A., Stanton, B., Jenkins, & Klein, M. D. (1982). Neuropsychological dysfunction following elective cardiac operation: I. Early assessment. *Journal of Thoracic Cardiovascular Surgery, 84,* 585–594.

Schacter, D. L., Kasniak, A. W., & Kihlstrom, J. F. (1991). Models of memory and the understanding of memory disorders. In T. Yanagihara & R. C. Petersen (Eds.), *Memory disorders: Research and clinical practice* (pp. 111–134). New York: Marcel Dekker.

Schacter, D. L., Kaszniak, A. W., Kihlstrom, J. F., & Valdiserri, M. (1991). The relation between source memory and aging. *Psychology and Aging, 6,* 559–568.

Schmidt, R., Fazekas, F., Offenbacher, H., Lytwyn, H., Blematl, B., Niederkorn, K., Horner, S., Payer, F., & Friedl, W. (1991). Magnetic resonance imaging white matter lesions and cognitive impairment in hypertensive individuals. *Archives of Neurology, 48,* 417–420.

Shaw, T. G. (1987). Alcohol and brain function: An appraisal of cerebral blood flow. In O. A. Parsons, N. Butters, & P. E. Nathan (Eds.), *Neuropsychology of alcoholism: Implications for diagnosis and treatment* (pp. 129–154). New York: Guilford.

Shock, N. (1977). Biological theories of aging. In J. Birren & K. W. Schaie (Eds.), *Handbook of the psychology of aging.* New York: Van Nostrand Reinhold.

Shraberg, D. (1978). The myth of pseudodementia: Depression and the aging brain. *American Journal of Psychiatry, 135,* 601–603.

Shraberg, D. (1980). Questioning the concept of pseudodementia. *American Journal of Psychiatry, 137,* 260.

Simon, A. (1980). The neuroses, personality disorders, alcoholism, drug use and misuse, and crime in the aged. In J. E. Birren & R. B. Sloane (Eds.), *Handbook of mental health and aging* (pp. 653–670). Englewood Cliffs, NJ: Prentice-Hall.

Smyer, M. A., Zarit, S. H., & Qualls, S. H. (1990). Psychological intervention with the aging individual. In J. E. Birren & K. W. Schaie (Eds.), *Handbook of the psychology of aging* (pp. 375–404). New York: Van Nostrand Reinhold.

Squire, L. R. (1987). *Memory and brain.* New York: Oxford University Press.

Starkstein, S. E., Bryer, J. B., Berthier, M. L., Cohen, B., Price, T., & Robinson, R. G. (1991). Depression after stroke: The importance of cerebral hemisphere asymmetries. *Journal of Neuropsychiatry and Clinical Neurosciences, 3,* 276–285.

Steingart, A., Hachinski, V. C., Lau, C., Fox, A. J., Diaz, F., Cape, R., Lee, D., Inzitari, D., & Merskey, H. (1987). Cognitive and neurologic findings in subjects with diffuse white matter lucencies on computed tomographic scan. *Archives of Neurology, 44,* 32–35.

Storandt, M. (1977). Graduate education in gerontological psychology: Results of a survey. *Educational Gerontology, 2,* 141–146.

Stoudemire, A., Hill, C., Gulley, L. R., & Morris, R. (1989). Neuropsychological and biomedical assessment of depression–dementia syndromes. *Journal of Neuropsychiatry and Clinical Neurosciences, 1,* 347–361.

Sullivan, P., Pary, R., Telang, F., Rifai, A. H., & Zubenko, G. S. (1990). Risk factors for white matter changes detected by magnetic resonance imaging in the elderly. *Stroke, 21,* 1424–1428.

Tobin, S. S., & Neugarten, B. L. (1961). Life satisfaction and social interaction in aging. *Journal of Gerontology, 16,* 344–346.

Tomlinson, B. E., Blessed, G., & Roth, M. (1970). Observations on the brains of demented old people. *Journal of Neurological Science, 11,* 205–242.

United States Bureau of the Census. (1981). *Facts about older Americans.* DHHS Publication No. 81-200006. Washington, DC: U.S. Government Printing Office.

Valdois, S., Yves, J., Poissant, A., Ska, B., & Dehaut, F. (1990). Heterogeneity in the cognitive profiles of the elderly. *Journal of Clinical and Experimental Neuropsychology, 12,* 587–598.

Villardita, C., Cultrera, S., Cupone, V., & Mejia, R. (1985). Neuropsychological test performance and normal aging. *Archives of Gerontology and Geriatrics, 4,* 311–319.

Wedding, D., & Cody, S. (1990). Neurological disorders in the elderly. In A. M. Horton (Ed.), *Neuropsychology across the life span* (pp. 65–80). New York: Springer.

Weingartner, H. (1986). Automatic and effortful demanding cognitive processes in depression. In L. W. Poon (Ed.), *Clinical memory assessment of older adults* (pp. 218–225). Washington, DC: American Psychological Association.

Wells, C. (1979). Pseudodementia. *American Journal of Psychiatry, 136,* 895–900.

Wetle, T., & Levkoff, S. E. (1984). Attitudes and behaviors of service providers toward elder patients in the VA system. In T. Wetle & J. W. Rowe (Eds.), *Older veterans: Linking VA and community resources* (pp. 205–230). Cambridge: Harvard University Press.

Williamson, P. C., Mersky, H., Morrison, S., Rabheru, K., Fox, H., Wands, K., Wong, C., & Hachinski, V. (1990). Quantitative electroencephalographic correlates of cognitive decline in normal elderly subjects. *Archives of Neurology, 47,* 1185–1188.

Wolf, P. A., Kannel, W. B., & Verter, J. (1984). Cerebrovascular diseases in the elderly: Epidemiology. In M. L. Albert (Ed.), *Clinical neurology of aging* (pp. 458–477). New York: Oxford University Press.

Wolfe, N., Linn, R., Babikian, V. L., Knoefel, J. E., & Albert, M. L. (1990). Frontal systems impairment following multiple lacunar infarcts. *Archives of Neurology, 47,* 129–132.

Wolfson, L., & Katzman, R. (1992). The neurological consultation at age 80. II: Some specific disorders observed in the elderly. In R. Katzman & J. W. Rowe (Eds), *Principles of geriatric neurology* (pp. 339–351). Philadelphia: Davis.

Younger, S. C., Clark, D. C., Lindroth, R. O., & Stein, R. J. (1990). Availability of knowledge informants for a psychological autopsy study of suicides committed by elderly people. *Journal of the American Geriatrics Society, 38,* 1169–1175.

Zubenko, G. S., Sullivan, P., Nelson, J. P., Belle, S. H., Huff, J., & Wolf, G. L. (1990). Brain imaging abnormalities in mental disorders of late life. *Archives of Neurology, 47,* 1107–1111.

29

Computer Applications in Behavioral Medicine

Gerhard Werner

INTRODUCTION

Conceived in the 1970s, behavioral medicine has since outgrown its original conceptual foundations of learning and conditioning; it has assimilated aspects of cognitive therapy, behavioral family therapy, and social skills training and also blended these approaches, to some extent, with pharmacotherapy. It has also extended its scope from assessment and therapy to prevention and rehabilitation (Kaptein & Rooijen, 1990). Despite this increase in scope and diversity, behavioral medicine has adhered to essential principles of behavior therapy, insisting on quantitative measures of observables, emphasis on performance and action, and the priority of manifest current functioning over inferred psychological processes (Bellack & Hersen, 1990; Wixted, Bellack, & Hersen, 1990). Operational, objective, and quantitative characteristics of these principles seem to be promising candidates for computer-based procedures of one kind or another. A few innovative and forward looking clinician–investigators had already recognized this during the formative stages of behavioral medicine. Yet, despite fairly consistent reports of satisfactory results, current health-care practitioners have not applied computer-based approaches in behavioral medicine as widely as seems warranted by the apparent match between the tasks and the computer's potential as assistive tool. Agras (1987) addressed this issue in his Presidential Address to the 20th Annual Meeting of the Association for Advancement of Behavior Therapy; in his discussion—"Where Do We Go from

---

Gerhard Werner • Highland Drive Veterans Affairs Medical Center and University of Pittsburgh School of Medicine, Pittsburgh, Pennsylvania 15206.
Handbook of Health and Rehabilitation Psychology, edited by Anthony J. Goreczny. Plenum Press, New York, 1995.

Here?"—he drew attention to the desirability of building on already existing, successful computer applications, and stressed the potential of developing promising new applications. However, Greist (1989), one of the pioneers of computer-administered behavior therapy since the early 1970s, recently contrasted this vision with some realistic constraints; referring to limited penetration of such applications into clinical practice, he concluded his assessment with a quote from Darwin's *The Origin of Species:* "I look with confidence to the future—to young and rising naturalists, who will be able to view both sides of the question with impartiality."

My intent in this chapter is to review development of computer applications that are most germane to behavioral medicine's conceptual framework. Accordingly, automated psychological testing (e.g., Minnesota Multiphasic Personality Inventory [MMPI]), database management, and office logistics are outside the scope of this chapter. Several anthologies and monographs address these subjects in detail: A book by Ager and Bendall (1991) reviews use of computer in clinical psychology; Romanczyk (1986) discusses clinically relevant aspects of microcomputer technology; a monograph edited by Sidowski, Johnson, and Williams (1980) provides a valuable summary of the state of computer applications in mental health care in the 1980s; and mental health information systems have been reviewed by McCoullough, Farrell, and Longabaugh (1986) and Mezzich (1986). Computer applications in clinical practice of mental health professionals (Schwartz, 1984) and agencies (Slavin, 1982) have undergone review in comprehensive multiauthored texts, and *Computers in Psychology* (Mulder, Maarse, Sjouw, & Akkerman, 1991) covers a wide spectrum of topics. Eiduson, Brooks, Motto, Platz, and Carmichael (1968) conceived an imaginative approach to organizing and storing patient information for research and clinical service; and Greist and Klein (1980) appropriately advocated advantages for storage, access, and retrieval of information collected by computers from patients along with possibilities computers offer regarding formatting patient data for convenient review by clinicians. Interested readers can refer to these sources.

The expectation is that clarification of apparent impediments will pave the way for recognition that such impediments are more apparent than real and indicate the potential for overcoming them. One important consideration is that many pioneering efforts began at a time when computer technology was in its infancy (seen from the current vantage point), but the present state of computer science offers vastly superior conceptual and technological tools. In light of these advances, early pioneering successes may appear pale in comparison to the effectiveness, efficiency, economy, and conceptual opportunities now available for imaginative clinical applications. The current chapter reviews computer applications in general areas of practice that have relevance for behavioral medicine.

ASSESSMENT PROCEDURES

Computer Support for Patient Interviews and Interview Evaluation

A notable event in the history of computing offered the opportunity to put a novel idea to the test; that event was development of the first small, general-purpose, free-standing LINC computer (Clark & Molnar, 1964). Molnar and Clark (1990) recently discussed the exciting history regarding development of this computer. The idea behind its development was to apply computers to taking medical histories directly from patients, and the innovators who seized this opportunity were a group of physicians at the University of Wisconsin. These investigators sought to determine whether computer interviewing has advantages over self-administered patient questionnaires, because interactive communication with patients would permit exploring particularities of abnormal findings on an individual basis. The computer-mediated dialogue emulated, at least to some extent, the experienced physician as diagnostic interviewer. Slow and small as the LINC computer was by today's standards, an impressive success story unfolded in rapid succession with subsequent development of computer programs for a variety of medical topics. Slack (1982), one of the principal architects of that work and an associate of the Wisconsin group at that time, reviewed details of the story of that progression. Careful design of the interview programs ensured their adequacy from the professional point of view; what the developers did not fully anticipate, yet served as a gratifying surprise, was the enthusiastic reaction of patients to the computer-based interviewing process (Slack & Van Cura, 1968).

Successes with computer-based patient interviewing in medical problem areas also led to exploratory applications in psychiatry. Maultsby and Slack (1971) set out to answer two questions: (1) Will psychotherapists find computer-generated patient interviews useful for psychiatric evaluation? and (2) Will psychiatric patients accept undergoing interviews conducted by computers? Their approach and emphasis was decisively different from two other computer developments occurring at about the same time: (1) Colby's attempt with computers to simulate psychotherapy (Colby, Watt, & Gilbert, 1966) and model human belief systems and psychopathological syndromes (Colby, 1973), and (2) the much-debated and misunderstood program ELIZA, which the developers really designed as an object lesson in computer science, albeit creating the illusion of a genuine conversational dialog with psychotherapeutic jargon (Weizenbaum, 1976). Nonetheless, the program's originator himself forcefully repudiated its application in psychotherapeutic settings (Weizenbaum, 1977). In contrast to these more esoteric considerations, Maultsby and Slack designed their program for an immediate practical application; namely, computer-based, self-administered interviews of medical–surgical patients referred for psychiatric evaluation interviews and some patients in a mental health clinic. Initial results were encouraging; when clinicians read computer-generated evaluation reports prior to seeing patients, those reports facilitated and expedited diagnostic decisions in about two thirds of the test cases, but clinicians did occasionally note omission of some important information. Patients found computer interviews generally interesting and enjoyable. The patient sample in this study apparently did not present significant psychopathology; they often experienced relief and reassurance from computer interviews themselves and did not require further psychiatric intervention.

These results encouraged the Wisconsin Group to proceed in the following years to extend the conceptual basis of psychiatric interviewing programs and determine patient reactions in more detail and for a larger diversity of psychopathology. Computer interviews were effective for eliciting target-symptom identification (Greist, Klein, & Cura, 1973) and suitable for administration of standard psychiatric evaluation instruments. For suicide-risk prediction, the computer interview was superior to clinical judgment (Greist, Gustafson, Laughren, & Chiles, 1973). Other applications for specific purposes evolved in quick succession. These applications encompassed a computer-generated advisor for psychotropic medication (Sletten, Altman, Evenson, & Cho, 1973); a program to forecast elopement risk (Altman, Brown, & Sletten, 1972); a dietary interview program for use by nutritionists (Slack et al., 1976); a computer-based headache interview (Bana, Leviton, Swindler, Slack, & Graham, 1980); and a computer-generated lithium advisor (Greist, Jefferson, Combs, Schou, & Thomas, 1977) that subsequently expanded to a computer-generated Lithium Information Center (Greist et al., 1985). An extensive computer-assessment interview for phobic patients that included categorization of phobia type, screening for concurrent depression, and definition of behavioral targets suitable for desensitization therapy was the preferred mode of assessment, relative to personal interviews, for a substantial majority of patients (Carr & Ghosh, 1983). Concurrent and subsequent studies in other centers corroborated and supported viability of computer-based self-reports of psychiatric patients (Carr, Ghosh, & Ancill, 1983; Johnson, Gianetti, & Williams, 1979; Klinger, Miller, Johnson, & Williams, 1977; Williams, Johnson, & Bliss, 1975) and corroborated usefulness of such programs for diagnostic assessment in terms of *Diagnostic and Statistical Manual of Mental Disorders* (DSM) categories (Zetin, Warren, Lanssens, & Tominaga, 1987). A program for psychiatric diagnosis performed its task with an accuracy comparable, or superior, to clinicians (Glueck & Stroebel, 1969). Numerous more recent studies have pursued use of computers for diagnostic applications in psychiatry, but because this work falls outside the specific scope of behavioral medicine, I will not review it in this chapter but, instead, will list a few notable recent references to which interested readers can refer (Maurer, Biel, Kuhner, & Loffler, 1989; Mauer, Hillig, Freyberger, & Velthausen, 1991; Murphy, Neff, Sobol, Rice, & Olivier, 1985; Overby, 1987; Werner & Smith, 1989).

Contrary to researchers' expectations, acutely disturbed psychiatric patients were able to interact reliably with computers (Klein, Greist, & Cura, 1975). Patients generally felt more comfortable revealing personal and sensitive information (e.g., drug use, bizarre thoughts) to computers than to clinicians. This comfort level increased still further upon repeating computer interviews, to the point that patients often expressed their preference of computer over clinician interviewers (Greist & Klein, 1980). Patients' favorable comments included appreciation of privacy of the interview, absence of time pressure, open-endedness and directness of questions, and effects of the program for gaining insight into their own problems; however, a minority of patients reported having some initial difficulty answering the computer's questions and did experience the computer interaction as impersonal. The rapidly increasing popularity of self-administration of psychological tests and inventories (Angle, L. Hay, W. Hay, & Ellinwood, 1977; Johnson et al., 1979; Stout, 1981) motivated Canoune and Leye (1985) to undertake a carefully designed comparison of results obtained with human- and computer-conducted interviews. Their findings identified distinct differences in interview results, primarily with test items involving social values. For example, subjects seemed to feel more pressure to respond in accord with expected social values if interviewed by a human rather than by a computer. The point is that we must not necessarily consider interview data equivalent in the two interview situations, but computer interviews seem to offer the possibility of obtaining sensitive and private information that patients may not readily share in human interviews. Subjects in the Canoune and Leye (1985) study were volunteers enrolled in a psychology course, and test items concerned questions of interpersonal values. Findings with volunteers are in accord with results obtained among clinical populations. Patients report more clinical symptoms, tell fewer lies, and more freely admit having performed socially undesirable acts when participating in computer interviews as opposed to paper-and-pencil questionnaires (Evans & Miller, 1969). One group of investigators reported that computer-administered psychiatric histories contained, on the average, five items per patient that were not included in clinicians' records; missing items included having a criminal record, repeated firings from jobs, and suicide attempts (Carr et al., 1983).

The observations reported previously also bear on interpretations of test results with patients undergoing evaluation for alcohol and drug-related problems. Careful selection of test questions with high information value and discriminatory power to diagnose alcoholism showed that a mere five questions, administered on the basis of a decision tree, sufficed as a reliable screening test for alcoholism (Reich et al., 1975). This study focused exclusively on efficiency of computer-administered screening tests for clinical purposes and did not examine patient reactions to test procedures. On the other hand, Lucas, Mullin, Luna, and McInroy (1977) paid particular attention to comparisons between clinicians and computers as interrogators; when rated on a semantic differential scale, patients found computer interviews highly acceptable. These results are in agreement with the less formally validated observations of prior investigators. Most significant, however, was that in computer interviews, patients reported appreciably more alcohol consumptions than they disclosed to their human interlocutors. Other, more recent studies found the same tendency for underreporting of alcohol intake in personal interviews relative to computer-elicited histories (Duffy & Waterton, 1984; Malcolm, Sturgis, Anton, & Williams, 1989). However, one set of investigators using a group of patients in an addiction-treatment center found no differences between face-to-face interviews, paper-and-pencil questionnaires, or computer interrogations (Skinner & Allen, 1983). Because patients in this study referred themselves for treatment, it is conceivable that their motivation for treatment overshadowed the preference patients frequently have for apparent anonymity of computer interviews. Hence, underreporting in face-to-face interviews may vary from situation to situation and depend upon patients' motivations to seek professional assistance. A further obstacle to generalizing findings across studies, and even within one study, is that agreement between computer and face-to-face elicited data depends on the format of the questions. Agreement is generally better with questions requiring a dichotomous "yes" or "no" answer than for interval data (such as volume of alcohol consumed); moreover, discrepancies between direct computer and clinician interviews increase sharply with higher levels of alcohol consumption (Bernadt, Daniels, Blizard, & Murray, 1989). Another variable is patients' prior experiences with computers (Skinner, Allen, McIntosh, & Palmer, 1985). Actually undergoing computer interviews generally raises patients' preferences for automated interviews relative to preinterview expectations. Surprisingly, the increase of preference for computer interviewing in the posttest is highest with computer novices. A significant variable noted in the primary-care setting relates to the process of data entry; data entry by clinicians while interviewing patients was much less acceptable than direct data entry by patients (Brownbridge, Fitter, & Sime, 1984). Considerably more work is necessary to determine individual and sociocultural differences. For example, elderly patients experience some discomfort with computer interviewing (Carr, Wilson, Ghosh, Ancil, & Woods, 1982), but prior training seems to readily alleviate this impediment (Johnson & White, 1980). Future research needs to focus on identification of such differences.

Behavioral Interviews

Because functional relationships between behavior and environment are among the principal distinguishing characteristics of behavioral medicine, practitioners in the field place premium value on behavioral assessment. Although the importance of assessment is not in question, there is debate about extensiveness of assessment. Some authors prefer a broad-spectrum assessment, but others prefer a more targeted approach. Angle and coworkers (1977) advocated computer implementation of assessment, primarily to ensure that certain clinically essential questions consistently get asked. When conducted by experienced and sensitive clinicians, unstructured clinical interviews are, of course, valuable, but in terms of reliably asking certain questions, human interviewers cannot match the computer's predictability. One early study, for example, demonstrated that clinicians, even when using structured interviews, accidentally omit up to 5% of required questions (Fairbairn, Woods, & Fletcher, 1959).

Angle (1981) introduced a new version of the previously released behavioral interview program. This program presents over 3,500 multiple-choice questions covering developmental, psychosocial, and medical information. Patients receive questions in a linear sequence, but the program skips clearly redundant or superfluous questions based on information already reported. A summary report highlighted excess and deficiency conditions and produced a form of problem-oriented record. Efficacy of computer-administered assessments exceeded that of unstructured interviews by a considerable margin, at least with regard to documentation of critical findings (Angle, Johnson, Grebenkemper, & Ellinwood, 1979). The assessment program was also applicable for gathering follow-up data, treatment progress, and outcome research.

A more limited objective of computer-mediated interviewing is to obtain a summary of target complaints (Farrell, Camplair, & McCullough, 1987). In their study comparing computer interviews and assessment protocols consisting of unstructured intake interviews, the Symptoms Checklist-90, and the MMPI, Farrell et al. found low agreements between target complaints identified during computer interviews and those noted by therapists. Nevertheless, the authors of this study seemed satisfied that overall agreement of interview results warrants application of their program for standardizing target-complaint assessment. A computer-based method to measure employment handicap is one of the more unique computerized applications available (Floyd & Kettle, 1991). This program showed striking differences between individuals' self-ratings of aptitudes and level of education. This area is in its infancy and needs additional refinement before being put into widespread clinical use.

In the spirit of behavioral medicine's striving for objectivity, Lang (1969), over 20 years ago, designed a very imaginative approach. To bypass semantic vagaries of statements about patients' feeling states, Lang displayed a sketch of a person on the computer screen (the Self-Assessment Mannequin, SAM); using joy sticks, patients could vary aspects of facial expression and body image along the continua of happy–unhappy, excited–calm, and submissive–dominant. Although there has been no comprehensive evaluation of this technique, there are suggestive indications that children, as well as adults, readily identify with the display of SAM and appreciate relationships between graphic displays under their control and relevant semantic dimensions. Moreover, subjects appear to prefer this mode of reporting feeling states over pencil-and-paper questionnaires (Lang, 1980).

Despite generally positive experiences with computer-based assessment in the hands of the originators of various methods referred to previously, impact on general practice remains marginal, except for a few research settings. Nonetheless, some programmers developed several notable special-purpose assessment programs during the 1980s, but with a shift in emphasis; instead of following the approach of self-reporting, computer programs scored tape-recorded interviews. Howland and Siegman (1982) designed a program to automate the task of rating voice and speech samples for parameters characteristic of Type A behavior (Rosenman, 1978). Intent of the program was to achieve uniformity of rating and eliminate costly and time-consuming efforts of training raters. The promising results, with regard to accuracy, also revealed a significant correlation between interviewers' and interviewees' speech styles. This observation indicates the need for standardization of interviewers' styles. Recorded verbal samples were also the starting point for automated scoring with content analysis scales (Gottschalk & Bechtel, 1982).

Although computers offer reliability, consistency, and capacity for storing large quantities of data for preparation of reports, there do remain some issues for further investigation before we decisively proclaim computer superiority and general applicability for individual patient assessments. Consider, for instance, that experienced clinicians' carefully and sensitively conducted interviews are important factors in building therapeutic relationships and interpersonal rapport between patients and clinicians (Lockshin & Harrison, 1991). Does replacement of this phase by computers affect treatment outcome? The answer to this question remains unknown. There are also justified concerns regarding reliability and quality of computer software for interpreting test results, both in regard to quality of the software itself and uncritical acceptance by clinicians of generated reports. However, software discussed in this regard largely applies to psychometric tests and is thus outside the realm of this chapter. Interested readers can refer to the debate of this topic in an article by Lockshin and Harrison (1991).

Assessment in behavioral medicine requires considerably more than elicitation of symptoms and complaints. It includes a functional analysis of factors that contribute and maintain problem behaviors. Such assessments also require awareness of life circumstances and appreciation of expectations placed on patients by themselves and significant others (Kanfer & Goldstein, 1991). When considering range of data needed for effective intervention planning, it is surprising that behavioral medicine practitioners have not used computer assistance more widely than the literature reflects. Knowledge-based expert systems of the type used for "intelligent" data acquisition and consultation in many medical specialties are strikingly absent from current behavioral medicine practices.

Behavior Monitoring

The single most important contribution of behavioral psychology to behavioral medicine is emphasis on measurement of individualized, operationally defined, overt behaviors (Kazdin, 1981). Methodological considerations, measures taken (e.g., frequency, duration, antecedents, and consequents of target behaviors), and questions regarding whether recording of behaviors influences occurrence have received significant attention by Nelson (1977) and in a handbook of behavioral assessment (Hersen & Bellack, 1981). Readers can refer to these citations for detailed information. What follows is a cursory review of information important to the current chapter.

Practical considerations assume an important role in selecting what, when, and how to monitor behavior, including self-monitoring (Mahoney, 1977). The objective of self-monitoring is to improve reliability of reports and avoid faulty recollections and distortions caused by omissions or intruding influences in the anamnesis. Ambulatory monitoring of abnormal behavior under naturalistic conditions is an ideal goal that traditional methods can rarely achieve. Taylor and colleagues (1986) designed an original approach to achieve this objective for ambulatory monitoring of anxiety attacks. They used a microcomputer interfaced with motion sensors and ECG electrodes to identify panic attacks as episodes of high heart rates during low activity. The microcomputer was useful for storage and subsequent cross-validation with subjective reports. Apart from gathering data, either in initial evaluations or during determinations of treatment progress, self-monitoring can be effective in impressing on patients the relationships between target behaviors and context in which they occur. Self-monitoring can thus contribute to appreciation of conceptual foundations of employed treatment approaches (Tunks & Bellissimo, 1991).

The rapidly advancing miniaturization of computing devices offers attractive possibilities to replace conventional approaches of tape recorders and diaries, the latter often associated with the drawback of *post facto* entries. Programmable handheld computers with adequate memory for storing data in a format suitable for later retrieval as printouts or graphs are becoming valuable enrichments of self-monitoring techniques (Paggeot, Kvale, Mace, & Sharkey, 1988; Taylor, Fried, & Kenardy, 1990). Computer-assisted self-observation has evolved as a valuable clinical tool for assessing effectiveness of situation-specific coping strategies (Perrez, 1988).

Computers and Family Therapy

Computer applications in family therapy cut across the lines of assessment, data analysis, and interventions to such a degree that it makes separation of those modalities artificial, even though assessment is a substantial segment of the entire spectrum of activities in behavioral marital therapy. I have, therefore, decided to include this topic as an assessment procedure, despite some blurring of distinctions. A book edited by Figley reflects the state of the field as of 1985; notwithstanding some remarkable and ingenious applications, the distance between the vision of what suitably designed computer applications could contribute and what, in fact, is operational in many centers and private offices is considerable. Aradi (1985) and Constantine (1985a) presented exciting visions of potential applications that could support work of family therapists and for which current technology is available, but careful planning and software design are still lacking. A paper by Erdman and Foster (1986) is a virtual treasure box filled with ideas to underscore potential computer applications within the framework of theories of marital and family therapy. Nonetheless, wide application of most of these ideas has not occurred.

A notable exception to this underuse of computers involves the work of Friedman (1985), who applies the close interdigitation of computer applications for various purposes in full-time clinical practice. The author uses a commercially available computer program[1] to obtain comprehensive intake information that clients supply in a multiple-choice format on computer. The program records progress notes and test scores on spreadsheets for computer-generated graphic displays; computer games are available to the individuals in the waiting room while the therapist spends time with another member of the family. Of course, billing and client correspondence are also part of this integrated computer environment.

Although database management systems are outside the scope of this review, I do mention the following one because the developers specifically designed it to assist with clinical decision making in a family therapy clinic (Mead, Cain, & Steele, 1985). The database of the program accommodates problem/goal lists, intervention lists, progress notes, severity ratings, and expected goal outcomes, all in both English prose and coded form. Uniformity of the database is of value for insuring continuity of treatment, for instance, when supervisors change, and for deriving hypotheses for clinicians to test in treatment. The system is still undergoing evaluation, but it appears that this approach holds much promise. The program, titled "The Family Recorder," serves to gather and organize information on a family in treatment, track information, display genograms, and can also serve as a training tool (Gerson, 1985).

Particularly intriguing is the diversity of approaches for applying computers directly to the study of family dynamics. The first significant effort in this area associated with the Reiss (1971) theory of family problem solving. The author programmed a computer to present cognitive problems to individual family members, score each member's responses, and monitor ensuing exchanges between family members. A computer orchestrated the task for the purpose of characterizing the family interaction in its entirety. Note that this sophisticated computer application originated over 20 years ago! ENRICH is a self-assessment program of more recent vintage that provides detailed summaries of couples' relationships and listings of the areas requiring specific work (Olson, 1985). In addition to expediting identification of problem areas for therapists, the computer interview increases marriage partners' own appreciation of the nature of their difficulties and promotes their investment in the treatment process. Lehtinen and Smith (1985) designed two versions of a program (MATESIM) that applies data gathered in computer interviews of the marriage partners to assist therapists with identifying incompatibilities, and this program can indicate targets of self-directed change to the marriage partners. The authors based both versions of the program on procedures for rational decision making and thus, therapists can also apply this program to premarital counseling interventions. The programs PARA (Paradigm and Regime Assessment) and Micro-Kvebaek, although not yet fully developed at time of publication in 1985, illustrate new conceptual possibilities (Constantine, 1985b). Clinicians receive computer display frames that represent a state-space in two dimensions (e.g., dependence–independence and stability–change). Clinicians then position a cursor in the frame at a point that represents their clinical judgment regarding the families with whom they work. The computer can then either superimpose frames of different paradigmatic dimensions for visual inspection or summarize information of the different frames in verbal reports. MicroKvebaek, based on the family sculpture technique

---

[1] Rainwater, G. & Coe, D. S. (1982). *Psychological/Social/History Report.* Indiatlantic, FL: Psychologist Inc., P. O. Box 3896.

(Cromwell, Fournier, & Kvebaek, 1980), proceeds in the format of a video game. Family members use a joy stick to position themselves as tokens on the computer screen along various dimensions, such as enmeshment–disengagement and isolation. When family members have placed all tokens, the computer records the "sculpture" of the family; the computer can then retrieve the "sculpture" on the video screen in tabular form or as narrative reports. A. Baldwin, C. Baldwin, and Cole (1982) designed a natural language-coding system for representing families' free play interactions; the computer then analyzes encoded narratives for type and frequency of interactional events as indicators of family dynamics.

The Multiple Vantage Profile (MVP) is a computer program that evolved over several years to measure how family systems perceive their relationship structures. The program asks each family member to rank the dyadic relationship between all family members, both as currently perceived and as beliefs regarding desired relationships. Computer users can enter estimated values in numerical form (using a Likert-type scale) or graphically by positioning two stick figures on the computer screen. Graphic displays of closeness scores facilitate therapists' abilities to form hypotheses about coalitions and alliances within family systems. Investigators from the same institution (Texas Technological University) also deserve credit for another contribution: the computer-implemented "Personalized Spouse Observation Checklist" (Atkinson & McKenzie, 1984). This system allows marital partners to define for themselves reinforcing and aversive events and to record occurrence during the day.

COMPUTERS IN BEHAVIORAL TREATMENT

The decade of the 1970s marked the same flurry of activity regarding exploration of computer applications for behavioral treatments as it did with assessment. Design of new machines that reached the market at that time were particularly appropriate for behavioral treatment protocols, notably automated biofeedback training. Lang (1980) told the story of his pioneering experimental work with feedback training to control human heart rate (Lang, 1969, 1974). Other investigators quickly enlisted principles of the new methodology for a number of applications, generating new insights and facilitating new clinical approaches. This methodology enabled elucidation of relationships between heart rate feedback and anxiety (Gatchel, 1974) and permitted evolution of efficacy of an automated system for response-contingent training strategies in EMG biofeedback-assisted relaxation training (Pope & Gerstein, 1977). Beatty (1971) used a computer to study differential effects of response-contingent versus noncontinent feedback in operant conditioning of alpha and beta wave activity. Lang, Melamed, and Hart (1970) were the first group to develop a fully automated procedure for systematic desensitization of phobic patients. There is even one case of successful automated desensitization (Wolpe & Migler, 1967) as well as documentation of successful automated group desensitization for test anxiety (Donner & Guerney, 1969). Placing subject and computer in a closed loop for selecting episodes of cortical quiescence to study evoked cortical potentials (Mulholland, 1977) and closed-loop setups to train eye-fixation for removal of artifacts from electroencephalograph records are samples that illustrate the versatility of the automated method. But this new methodology also raised new questions, particularly regarding individual differences in the control of visceral functions by feedback (Lang, 1980) and differences between normal and clinically impaired subjects (e.g., patients with ischemic heart disease; Lang, Troyer, Twentyman, & Gatchel, 1975).

These initial experiences set the stage for numerous applications of automated interventions in treatment according to the principles of behavioral medicine. Range of applications could, of course, be as large as the number of appropriate treatment approaches *per se,* and the computer could serve merely as an assisting tool in conduct of treatment protocols, collection and analysis of data, and detection of complex response patterns. There are, however, aspects of automation that go beyond the mere assistance aspect. The considerable variance in the clinical literature regarding effectiveness of biofeedback training is, at least in part, attributable to variability in feedback modalities, accuracy of instrumentation, and precision of data acquisition and analysis. Roemer (1975) suggested that many errors of this kind remain undetected until introduction of computer controls. Automation can contribute to standardization of procedures and protocols and, thus, eliminate a significant source of variance (Kolotkin, 1981). Furthermore, parameters of the training procedure (e.g., criterion levels for feedback signals) are under program control and, therefore, are readily adjustable to individual-patient characteristics (Price & Gatchel, 1979).

In light of the initial upsurge of computer-assisted biofeedback, potential applicability of an automated approach, and its previously listed advantages, it is surprising that the number of recent clinical reports is relatively small. One comparison of computer-administered therapy consisting of cognitive elements and systematic desensitization versus group therapy for alleviating test anxiety showed both approaches were equally effective (Buglione, De Vito, & Mulloy, 1990). Biglan, Villwock, and Wick (1979) also achieved a significant reduction of debilitating test anxiety with use of computer assisted therapy. The desensitization program allowed the therapist to spend less than 2 hours of therapy contact time over a 3-week period. Another study involving computer-instructed treatment of phobias by means of self-administered *in vivo* exposure found no reduction in time spent with therapists relative to therapist-instructed treatment; all instruction methods were equally effective, but book instruction, relative to computer instruction and therapist instruction, required the least amount of therapist time (Ghosh, Marks, & Carr, 1984). Nonetheless, some anxiety disorder patients do seem to prefer computers over therapists. In one treatment study of phobic individuals, patients chose to continue with computer-supervised treatment even when offered the alternative of personal consultation with a psychiatrist (Carr, Ghosh, & Marks, 1988). Chandler, Burck, and Sampson (1988) effectively developed a generic program for systematic desensitization that clinicians can use with a variety of patients.

Straddling the line between treatment and education is a program called SAFEDRINK for heavy drinkers. It offers conversational interaction with users and displays audiotape dramatizations of patients' problems. The program offers encouragement and reassurance and explains strategies for treatment (Carr, 1991).

Although reduction of blood pressure (Agras, Taylor, Kraemer, Allen, & Schneider, 1980; Wadden, Luborsky, Greer, & Crits-Christoph, 1984), headache (van der Helm-Hylkema, 1990), chronic pain (Groenman, Vlaeyen, Eck, & Schuerman, 1990), gastrointestinal disorders (van der Ploeg, 1990), cardiac rehabilitation (Erdman, 1990), and insomnia (Zwart, 1990) are conditions with established records of being amenable to behavioral intervention in a sizable proportion of patients, there is a surprising dearth of attempts to design and evaluate computer-assisted approaches. Greist (1989) underscored this gap between the evidence of promise and lack of significant propagation and listed numerous fundamental issues that await systematic study and clarification. Many untapped opportunities for effective and economic treatment, in addition to those already mentioned, remain unexplored, such as possible computer-assisted interventions with chronic cancer patients (Couzijn, Ros, & Winnubst, 1990), post-traumatic stress syndrome sufferers (Foy, Resnick, Carroll, & Osato, 1990), and clients receiving consultation–liaison psychiatry services (Hammer, Hammond, Strain, & Lyons, 1985).

Nonetheless, there are encouraging new trends. Behavioral medicine practitioners have successfully treated patients with orthopedic difficulties via computer-enhanced electromyograph biofeedback (F. Crofts & J. Crofts, 1988) as well as patients with scoliosis, who received automated posture feedback (B. Dworkin & S. Dworkin, 1988). Although computer-based dietary counseling has been available since the mid-1970s (Witschi et al., 1976), automated behavioral interventions for treatment of obesity and for weight control became the recent target of concerted efforts by a few active groups of clinician–investigators. Pursuing what appropriately received the label of "a new frontier for behavior therapy," some behavioral medicine practitioners programmed portable microcomputers for response cuing, immediate feedback of goal attainment for target behaviors, and response-contingent positive reinforcement and instruction. Such innovations afford the opportunity of applying well-established principles of these behavior change interventions (Bandura, 1969) "on-line" throughout subjects' daily routines. In an initial pilot study, subjects equipped with the microcomputer lost 2.5 times as much weight as subjects in the control group who used the paper-and-pencil method for record keeping (Burnett, Taylor, & Agras, 1985). A later study subsequently confirmed and expanded the initial findings: resultant analyses revealed that computer treatment was the most cost-effective treatment employed and additional group support may enhance long-term maintenance of weight loss (Agras, Taylor, Feldman, Losch, & Burnett, 1990; Taylor, Agras, Losch, & Plante, 1991). Another group of investigators also found that computer-assisted weight-loss treatment was superior to therapist-conducted treatment (Foree-Gavert & Gavert, 1980). A unique method of treating a patient with obsessive–compulsive behavior consisted of equipping the patient with a portable (handheld) computer for recording incidence of obsessional-checking urges; the computer then issued instructions to resist the urge for a few minutes, generated some reassuring statements, and counted down time. The computer also stored a frequency of urges and level of coping success. Improvement was good but required continued computer use to persist (Baer, Minichiello, Jenike, & Holland, 1988).

Although on the fringes of behavioral medicine in a narrow sense, a potentially very significant application concerning compliance with medication regimens warrants attention. Sorrell, Greist, Klein, Johnson, and Harris (1982) designed computer programs that not only monitor on-line adherence to treatment with tricyclic antidepressants but also record side effects or negative attitudes about the medication, thus providing clinicians with indications that patients may require increased attention.

COUNSELING AND PSYCHOTHERAPY

To the extent to which affective engagement in patient–therapist interaction is of significant therapeutic efficacy, some authors believe computers fulfill, at best, an ancillary role in therapy (Selmi, Klein, Greist, Johnson, & Harris, 1982), such as tracking progress in therapy (Block, 1986; McCullough et al., 1984). However, others have also advocated computer-assisted instruction as an adjunct to psychotherapy (Sampson, 1984, 1986). Some of the existing learning models for computer counseling seem to help users develop and improve understanding of their abilities and, to some extent, assist with acquiring decision-making skills (Davidson, 1984). In some instances, such programs provide career knowledge, professional guidance counseling, and instruction in study skills (Sampson, 1983). Requests for vocational or academic information may, at times, indirectly relate to emotional problems (Sampson & Pyle, 1983), but the programs, in this regard, generally provide very limited, if any, usefulness (Cairo, 1983). However, McLemore and Fantuzzo (1982) designed a program to clarify feelings, reframe problems, and suggest helpful solutions, and they obtained beneficial results with a group of college students. Programs for pastoral counseling (Cassel, 1977) and drug counseling for parolees (Cassel, 1971) have appeared in the literature, but insufficient details of design and evaluation limit one's ability to judge their usefulness. Advertising companies sometimes promote self-help computerized programs with exaggerated claims (Caruso, 1984), and these programs require careful review and circumspection prior to being recommended to clients.

The program ELIZA (Weizenbaum, 1976), briefly referred to in an earlier section, aroused considerable surprise, discussion, and controversy. Contrary to the designer's intention, some individuals perceived the program as a model or parody, of Rogerian psychotherapy. The most surprising finding was the high degree of emotional involvement users of the program developed. Factors contributing to such attachment included psychological effects of interactive conversation, wishes (or urges) to trust machines, the prevailing climate of machine-dispensed knowledge, and propensity to view machines in an anthropomorphic illusion (Shore, 1986), aspects possibly reinforced by the program's predictability (Turkle, 1980) and its nonjudgmental, seemingly empathic responses (Holden, 1977). However, Weizenbaum wished to dissociate himself from what he considered the false pretense of the program that led to experiences of interpersonal respect, understanding, and love; Weizenbaum (1976) noted, "When the computer says 'I understand,' it is a lie and deception." Perhaps the real issue is to sort out which areas and forms of psychotherapy are, and which ones are not, suitable for computer applications. However, despite many reservations and objections, anyone involved in advanced computer programming finds the vision of computers as psychotherapists intriguing and fascinating (Plutchik & Karasu, 1991), if for no other reasons than it would be a formidable challenge to capture therapists' flexible strategies of interventions in terms of program instructions. But realistic appraisals regarding magnitude of the task must temper one's enthusiasm, in part because of the appreciable complexity of computer-assisted analysis of free conversation (Gervasio, 1984), which still remains largely limited to relatively simple forms of text analysis and falls short of capturing the richness of language in psychotherapeutic dialogues.

Psychotherapy based on cognitive (Turk & Salovey, 1985) and problem-solving interventions (D'Zurilla, 1986) appears to offer less controversial opportunities for applying problem-solving computer programs of the type developed in artificial intelligence. In a series of careful studies of computer counseling, Wagman and coworkers (Wagman, 1988; Wagman & Kerber, 1980, 1984) arrived at circumspect conclusions with their counseling program, PLATO; underscoring constraints imposed by concepts of artificial intelligence on the one hand and concepts of psychotherapy on the other, they introduced a valuable distinction between the conceptual level of counseling theory and counseling technique. The largely technique-guided and didactic orientation of cognitive therapy can account for the reported effectiveness of these authors' computer-based Dilemma Counseling System (PLATO-DCS). Lawrence (1986) also listed reasons in support of computer implementations of cognitive therapy: (1) interventions and expectations are sufficiently explicit, and (2) cognitive therapy involves instruction and exercises amenable to precise specification. Initial efforts in this direction with limited application seemed to launch computer-assisted psychotherapy on a promising path (Colby, Faught, & Parkinson, 1979; Colby et al., 1966). Selmi et al. (1982) described an interactive computer program for treatment of mild to moderate depressive disorders based on principles of cognitive-behavior therapy; we are still awaiting more complete assessment of its efficacy. Although some progress has been achieved, some caution is still in order before we accept without reservation the optimism that motivated Colby and colleagues to proclaim that "computer-assisted psychotherapy has arrived" (Colby, Gould, & Aronson, 1989). They based this view on some success with a therapeutic learning program that reflects Gould's theory of adult development (Gould, 1988). Patients attending Gould's program met in groups to interact with a therapist and the computer for short-term psychotherapy.

Wisely choosing a well-defined problem area amenable to a blending of cognitive–behavioral psychotherapy and counseling, two groups of investigators approached sex therapy as their target. The Reitman (1984) program puts premium value on cognitive restructuring in interactive dialogue with the computer program; Binik, Servan-Schreiber, Freiwald, and Hall (1988) and Servan-Schreiber and Binik (1989) adopted a rule-based program design modeled after a principle known as Expert Systems (Beaumont, 1991) to design an intelligent tutorial program (SEXPERT) that also contains a diagnostic module for sexual dysfunction. This program supports a flexible dialogue and emulates, in a fairly convincing manner, natural discourse with a clinician. The programs are sufficiently self-contained for use in a self-help mode. Clinical evaluation in extensive field tests is still under way.

The pros and cons of computer use in psychotherapy have aroused much debate. Typically, there are two principal arguments against such use. The first of these is that no program can take into account the virtually endless variety of problems psychotherapy patients may present. It is easy to dispel this argument because it misses the point; general-purpose psychotherapy programs are not under discussion. As suggested earlier, selection of circumscript problem areas and adoption of a cognitive–behavioral stance is definitely in the realm of achievement. The second argument against use of computers in psychotherapy is that dehumanizing effects of computers are an insult to human dignity. This argument has, at best, limited force. First, these are the words of therapists and not the words of persons who are allegedly the victims of dehumanization. Patients (the victims) have overwhelmingly demonstrated a readiness to accept computers as partners for dialogue. Second, this argument misses the point that computers have become companions in virtually everybody's lives already, either through use at the workplace or in the home.

The need for meticulous care in designing programs prior to routine clinical application and for carefully designed and executed evaluation is not controversial. Those who have worked with programs of this kind know better than anyone how much thought and deliberate care programmers must invest in development. Bluhm (1988) offered a thoughtful review of these and related considerations that are valuable guidelines for anyone wishing to undertake work in this field. Lawrence (1986) presented a commendable perspective on this debate:

> The most important question is not whether a machine can do psychotherapy, or even whether a machine can do psychotherapy as well as a human . . . (or) whether a computer should do therapy . . . What we need to know is whether the computer can do anything useful for people who need help with the sorts of problems that bring them to human therapists and counselors, whatever the machine process may be called.

Two telling arguments in support of computer-administered psychotherapy are that (1) it would make psychotherapy accessible to a larger segment of patients than is currently feasible (McLemore & Fantuzzo, 1982; Zarr, 1984), and (2) therapy would be uniform and thus more amenable to rigorous outcome evaluation of different treatment approaches (Ghosh & Greist, 1988).

Like all of psychotherapy, some screening of patients is advisable to determine in advance their suitability for computer-mediated therapy to (1) safeguard ethical considerations; (2) eliminate those who either lack, or are unwilling to acquire, the minimal skills for interacting with a computer; and (3) eliminate those who have substantial emotional problems that might interfere with computer-administered therapy (Sampson & Pyle, 1983; Zarr, 1984).

GERONTOLOGY AND GERIATRICS

Normal and pathological aging associates with several conditions that could offer singular opportunities for helpful interventions that computer and information technology can provide. Few programs of this type are in existence or under development, but many unexplored possibilities suggest extraordinary potential for improving quality of life, risk prevention, and clinical management of geriatric patients (Frydenberg, 1988; Stinson, 1989). Safety monitoring is one application that is essential for preserving autonomous living arrangements for elderly individuals who require minor forms of assistance and safeguards of a kind that current microprocessor technology can assure. Englehardt and Edwards (1986) have been eloquent spokespersons for applications of service robotics to improve home safety and have contributed substantially to development of prototypes. Specific target applications include assistance with ambulation, safety devices for housekeeping tasks ("smart kitchen"), surveillance monitoring, vital signs monitoring, and cognitive aids. Many more applications are on the drawing boards of forward-looking investigators and developers. There is substantial fermentation in this field, with many devices displayed and discussed at conferences, but nothing yet formally reported or evaluated in the published literature. Feedback training for regaining bladder and bowel continence and muscle control after strokes has been successful (Cardozo, Krishnan, & Polkey, 1984; Solomon, 1984). Following a visit to the American Association of Retired Persons Technology Center, acceptance of these and related innovations by potential users varied for different applications between 60% and 80% (Edwards & Engelhardt, 1989). However, despite extraordinary potential, consumer interest, and presentations at Congressional hearings on the savings of health-care expenditures by postponing nursing home care, available technological potential and realistic applications remain lightyears apart.

According to Hollander and Plummer (1986), computers are also capable of making contributions to therapeutic and educational enrichment of elderly individuals. An interesting observation of these investigators was that thought-provoking games receive the highest level of attention and interest of a group of clients ranging from 61 to 96 years of age. About half of the participants in this study expressed an interest in learning new and more challenging software. Therapists can also use computer games to provide nonthreatening assessments of cognitive or psychological difficulties (Weisman, 1983).

It is especially important that developers make computer systems user-friendly for elderly individuals, given the high degree of computer phobia among elderly individuals. One multimodal user-interface with voice, mouse, and keyboard input specifically designed for elderly individuals requires virtually no training (Christensen, Chaudhary, Gottshall, Hartman, & Yatcilla, 1989). Contrary to common expectations, experiences with elderly individuals who become enthusiastic computer users abound and thus dispel the deleterious prejudice that "you can't teach an old dog new tricks." The most dramatic example is the Senior Net, operating in several states on the West Coast; it is a system for computer mail (E-mail) for access from the homes of elderly individuals whose social intercourse has become restricted for various reasons. Existing reports indicate that communication through E-mail alleviates the sense of loneliness that many elderly individuals feel and marks a turning point in their regaining a sense of social integration and well-being. Moreover, the computer net provides its elderly users, through "bulletin boards," current information on health-care issues, Medicare, and other issues of relevance.

The extensive literature on health behavior across the life cycle, with emphasis on elderly individuals (George & Siegler, 1985; Leventhal, Prohaska, & Hirschman, 1985), offers innumerable suggestions for interventions and strategies. Many of the elderly would be amenable to educational and informational computer-assisted implementations, but none are as yet in existence. Poon and Siegler's (1991) observation that behavioral medicine pays only lip service to health-promoting behavior among elderly individuals is thus supported by the lack of application tools that could augment effectiveness of such measures. In 1990, the U.S. Department of Health and Human Services published its voluminous list of objectives for "Healthy People 2000," which included targets for older adults, but means to achieve the goals are not part of the report. Future computer developments could assist in meeting these goals.

Complicating careful clinical assessment in geriatrics is the multidisciplinary nature of the task. Requirement for accuracy of diagnosis and the disastrous consequences of misdiagnosis of disorders causing dementia are notorious (Katzman, Lasker, & Bernstein, 1986). Therefore, one would expect computer-assisted clinical decision-making tools to be more useful in geriatrics than in any other field of medicine. Some computer programs have indeed provided significant clinical assistance. Schnelle and Traughber (1983) found that the Geriatric Assessment Inventory (GAI) for monitoring behavior of nursing home patients was useful for identifying those patients who did not require nursing home care and could likely live independently. Independent control assessments validated discriminative ability of the GAI (Schnelle & Traughber, 1983). Zemcov, Barclay, Brush, and Blass (1984) designed an extensive computer-compatible assessment and documentation system with particular emphasis on the differential diagnosis of dementia. The National Resident Assessment Instrument for Nursing Homes (Morris et al., 1990) is a remarkable assessment instrument, but it is not yet available in computerized form. A computer-assisted diagnostic program for consultation in geriatric psychiatry, originally designed for use by primary-care physicians (Werner & Smith, 1989) suffered the fate of virtually all diagnostic expert systems in medicine by being too time-consuming for practical use in clinical settings (Werner, 1991), despite its satisfactory clinical performance. The program, subsequently redesigned, operates in interactive mode and asks important questions at appropriate junctures during interviews (Werner & Smith, 1992). The program then prepares a succinct summary of clinical and psychosocial findings for review by clinicians and issues alerting messages of potentially adverse drug interactions and abnormal laboratory findings.

COGNITIVE REHABILITATION

A decisive assessment of computer-assisted cognitive treatment interventions is premature because research studies have been forthcoming in significant numbers only during the past half-dozen years, and available studies have generally involved only small numbers of patients. Also, comparison between investigations is difficult because of the varieties and degree of cognitive deficits and differences in treatment procedures (Robertson, 1990; Skilbeck, 1991). Discussion of this topic must also observe distinctions between restitution of function; compensation for impaired functions, possibly based on the brain's plasticity for compensatory reorganization; and compensation for deficits by external aids. Although most of the work in this field involves patients with traumatic brain injury, some of the considerations also apply to elderly patients with degenerative dementia or strokes. This work rests largely on Luria's theory of brain function (Luria, Naydin, Tsvetkova, & Vinarsky, 1969) and the ideas of Ben-Yishay et al. (1983). Both groups of investigators emphasize analysis of cognitive impairment into modular components, massive training, and overlearning (Butler & Namerow, 1988).

One study utilizing computers for cognitive rehabilitation reported impressive results with visual–perceptual retraining in three patients with one-sided visual neglect (Robertson, Gray, & McKenzie, 1988). Other studies have reported successes similar to those of Robertson and colleagues with a visual search and left-right orientation (Bradley, Welch, & Skilbeck, 1991) and with individually designed training tasks to treat attentional deficits (Gray & Robertson, 1989). This sample of case reports conveys the possibilities of automating retraining procedures that presumably often require individualized design to meet the specific nature of deficit. Unfortunately, discussion of remedial instrumentation for specific sensory and speech impairments (M. Grossfeld & C. Grossfeld, 1986) is outside the scope of this chapter, as is discussion of the numerous applications of information and computer technology in the service of physical rehabilitation (Soede, 1989). In addition, although guidelines for acquisition of cognitive-retraining equipment are available (Lynch, 1990b), space limitations preclude review of those guidelines.

Rehabilitation of global cognitive deficits generally requires continued compensatory assistance, but lasting functional improvement is also possible. Several studies involving cognitively impaired individuals illustrate the potential of computer-assisted cognitive retraining. Lynch (1990a) described a computer system, intended to be prosthetic, that enabled a subject to be self-sufficient with regard to writing documents and managing finances after just a few training sessions. In another study, investigators using a computer-based program successfully trained two patients with traumatic brain injury to organize informational material, and the patients ultimately gained some restitution of work efficiency (Kreutzer, Conder, Wehman, & Morrison, 1989). Computer-assisted home-care therapy, individually tailored to the requirements of three patients in another study, enabled the patients to develop skills that generalized to applications outside the therapeutic environment (Purdy & Nerri, 1989). Johnson (1990) showed that memory training resulted in some generalization of coping skills in a young patient with neuropsychological deficits. However, in a group of closed-head-injury patients with severe to extremely severe impairment, computer-assisted cognitive training did not improve memory, attention, and higher cognitive functioning relative to conventional remedial measures (Batchelor, Shores, Marosszeky, & Sandaman, 1988). Thus, more information is necessary before declaring such programs effective.

An exciting new area is the use of computers to assist in development of prosthetic devices. One group of investigators described a cognitive prosthesis that enabled stepwise development of a speech prosthesis for the one patient in their study. This case illustrates the emergent concept of microcomputer-assisted ProsthesisWare as aids for daily living (Chute, Conn, DiPasquale, & Hoag, 1988). Expert systems may potentially offer assistance in the future design of this type of instrumentation (Napper, Robey, & McAfee, 1989).

The impressive casuistry sketched in the foregoing paragraphs faces the criticisms of lack of controls and absence of large-group studies (McGuire, 1990). Against this, I submit that this is in the very nature of the problems undergoing treatment. Such problems do not readily allow placement of patients with different deficits and degrees of traumatic brain damage into homogeneous groups. As Meehl (1978) brilliantly discussed, patients with localized brain damage cannot be subject to experimental design and data analysis modeled after agricultural plots. Thus, there is still room for casuistry and the design of individual treatments. This is, in fact, the very advantage of the programmable computer in this application. However, this is not to discount the possibility of more or less general-purpose programs, presumably best suited for cognitive–communicative impairments due to diffuse, degenerative cortical deficits (Story & Sbordorne, 1988). Moreover, computer-assisted cognitive rehabilitation is only one component in the total treatment plan of impaired patients, and pretreatment evaluations for predictors of training success will ultimately help select the most suitable patients for cognitive rehabilitation programs (Malec, Goldstein, & McCue, 1991).

PATIENT EDUCATION

Behavioral epidemiology has identified a considerable number of conditions that place patients at risk for developing diseases at a later time (Epstein & Porte, 1978). Patient education is an important factor for monitoring such risks (secondary prevention) or avoiding them when possible (primary prevention; Luiselli, 1989). Computer-assisted educational approaches have assisted with a variety of conditions and situations. Their range of topics is considerable and varies widely. The first example of computer-based patient education in the literature illustrates an eminently practical application for patients suffering from chronic urinary tract infection. In addition to observing their medication regimen, patients must participate in treatment by collecting clean urine specimens to prevent contamination. Developers of the educational program designed an interactive computer program to assist with the ordinarily cumbersome and time-consuming instructions for collecting clean voided urine specimens. The program assisted users by offering explanations and suggestions and answering questions at a self-paced rate and in privacy. A patient group receiving computer instruction had significantly fewer urine contaminations than a group receiving written instructions (Fisher, Johnson, Porter, Bleich, & Slack, 1977). This study demonstrated a principle that is applicable to numerous situations: Patients can learn, via instruction, how to take part in their own treatment.

As another example of patient education, computer games serve as microcomputer-based lessons in preventive-health maintenance topics in several hospital waiting rooms (Beck, Ellis, Scott, Raines, & Hakanson, 1982; Ellis & Raines, 1981). Weight control, a risk factor for coronary heart disease, and smoking are the primary targets of such games. Computers collect patients' answers and inform health-care personnel of patients' knowledge deficiencies. Effectiveness of the programs is difficult to assess, but patients generally accept the approach (Ellis, 1987). One study found that degree of acceptance of a program on risk factors for heart disease related to patients' educational level, and the majority of patients responded favorably (Chen, Houston, & Burson, 1983).

Adolescents can receive nonjudgmental and confidential information on alcohol, drugs, diet, sexuality, and smoking from the Body Awareness Resource Network (BARN) at the University of Wisconsin (Bosworth, Gustafson, Hawkins, Chewing, & Day, 1983). Behavioral health scientists have also developed and applied nutrition (Witschi et al., 1976) and dietary counseling programs (L. Wheeler, M. Wheeler, Ours, & Swider, 1983). Another group of investigators approached general health habits in teenagers with an elaborate protocol: Subjects completed daily paper-and-pencil questionnaires on exercise, smoking, and eating habits. A computer then processed this information to generate reports. In addition, subjects had a handheld microcomputer that reminded them to report their data, discussed dietary goals, and offered praise when warranted (Burnett, Magel, Harrington, & Taylor, 1989).

Drug addiction and dependence hold much promise for effective prevention efforts with computers due to the frequent preference of addicts for self-help approaches over formal therapy (Barber, 1990). On this premise, thee have been recommendations for development of programs for preventing heroin and alcohol relapse, but no formal programs are available yet. On the other hand, a computer-delivered smoking-cessation program is available and is somewhat effective in reducing smoking, but the results were far from dramatic (Burling, Marotta, Gonzales, & Moltzen, 1989). A program developed by Schneider, Walter, and O'Donnell (1990) offered a computer network to over 1,100 subscribers, allowed for individual consideration of smoking history, and followed each participant's progress during treatment; in addition, one group of subjects had access to a computer forum on smoking cessation. Combined participation in the complete program and the forum achieved the highest success rates.

New patient educational applications include the interactive videodisc method, which predictably enriches the didactic effect. Olevitch and Hagan (1991) reported considerable gains on a wellness-maintenance questionnaire with chronically mentally ill patients using an interactive videodisc simulation. They designed the program to teach stress management, medication compliance, and community-living skills. Prevention of acquired immune deficiency syndrome (AIDS) is the educational subject of one microcomputer (Schinke, Orlandi, Gordon, & Weston, 1989) and one interactive videodisc program (McGrane, Allely, & Toth, 1990).

Staff education has also received the benefit of computer education, and such an approach has definite advantages (Hannah et al., 1989). The findings of Devine, O'Connor, Cook, Wenk, and Curtin (1988) underscore the far-reaching implications of staff education: A 3-hour workshop for staff nurses on psychoeducational patient care significantly reduced amount of sedatives and hypnotics dispensed to patients after surgery and enabled somewhat earlier hospital discharge. This was not computer-assisted education, but I cite the observation to stress the importance of staff education as a strategic place for introducing behavioral medicine principles at all levels of health care, an area receiving increased attention (Johnston, Weinman, & Marteau, 1990).

Few investigators have compared effectiveness of computerized health education with that of traditional methods. Using textbook material on sexually transmitted diseases, Deardorff (1986) ascertained that recall of information was about the same for written instructions and computer presentations and lowest for a face-to-face presentation. Prior familiarity with computers did not make any difference in outcome. The investigator rightly discussed a shortcoming of this study that may seriously impair generalization of results: The investigators did not prepare the computer-presented material specifically for computer presentation and thus did not capitalize on the essential interactive relationship between study material and user.

Computer-assisted instruction has thus far found fewer applications than video material, for which there are better evaluation data available (Gagliano, 1988). Of course, this is not surprising in view of the difference in time during which these media have been available. Consider also that theory and practice of computer-aided instruction in other fields has made quantum jumps in recent years (Blomeyer & Dianne, 1991; Nix & Spiro, 1990), as has availability of authoring tools from software producers. I submit that initial efforts to apply computers to health education, pioneering as they were, had limited applicability because of the (in retrospect) rudimentary methods at the disposal of investigators. Final determinations of the usefulness of computers in health education is therefore premature. The same applies with even stronger force to interactive videodisc applications.

DRAWING THE BALANCE

Computer applications in behavioral medicine have clearly advanced during the past 20 years from novel and innovative pilot developments to increasingly sophisticated tools. On the other hand, computers have not become the "Fourth Quantum Advance" that Rome (1967) predicted they would be for psychiatry, nor have they influenced physicians' styles of practice to the extent envisioned by the enthusiastic innovators of artificial intelligence in medicine. The lag in clinical applications is in stark contrast to the computer's pervasive role for administrative and actuarial tasks in clinicians' offices and clinics (Hedlund, Evenson, Sletten, & Cho, 1980). Why are clinician–patient transactions of assessment, diagnosis, and treatment seemingly more refractory, despite claims of increased efficiency, improved quality of clinical care, and increased access to treatment for those who do not have it now? These same concerns motivated Ager and Bendall (1991) to declare the exploration of clinical computer applications in behavioral medicine an "ethical imperative."

Pervasive concerns during the early years of clinical computer applications included patients' acceptance and the fear of introducing a "dehumanizing" element into patient–clinician relationships. These concerns are largely dispelled by the cumulative evidence now available in the literature. Moreover, computers have literally become daily companions to large segments of the new "information society," both at work and in the home. In fact, the "home computer phenomenon" and its impact on families (Wakefield, 1985) is liable to become a new clinical problem for behavioral medicine interventions, as it can be for professional or amateur computer addicts (Turkle, 1984). If, on the other hand, the problem is computer anxiety, then behavioral medicine offers its own effective methods for breaking the vicious cycle of negative anticipations and stress (Bloom, 1985).

In several contexts of the preceding review, I referred to the discrepancy between hardware and software available for earlier applications and the incredibly rapid advances of computer methodology in recent years. Hence, we cannot base a realistic appraisal of the future contribution of information technology and computers to behavioral medicine merely on extrapolations from the past, notwithstanding the notable achievements. Diffusion of new methods in clinical practice can be slow and depends on many factors beyond conceptual validity and practical merit, economy being one. However, it is possible to state categorically that there are certain things computers can do for behavioral medicine that no other method can accomplish equally effectively. One such example is self-monitoring in patients' naturalistic environments, including some notable examples cited earlier. Another example is automated feedback and desensitization training. Once again, satisfactory baseline experiences exist, and new methodology can most certainly make such methods more efficient and versatile and less expensive.

Regarding direct patient assessment with computers, ample experience from feasibility and demonstration projects warrants taking the next step of studying implications of the process for clinical practice and research (Erdman, Klein, & Greist, 1985). Nonetheless, diagnosis and assessment are much more complex issues, as are applications in psychotherapy, areas in which clinicians' value judgments and idiosyncratic modes of relating to patients play a significant role. I submit that lessons learned in the three decades of artificial intelligence in medicine are applicable. Recall that these efforts started with the rallying cry that what physicians needed was assistance with making medical diagnoses. Expert systems would supposedly capture the cumulative knowledge of experts and represent them as computer algorithms, mostly rule-based. But, as it turned out, this is not what physicians by and large wanted. It was like building a car without caring for the customer's preferences. Gradually, program development shifted to computer-based consultation and systems that would critique clinicians' decisions. This improved use by clinicians to some extent. But one major hurdle remained: No matter how elegant and "clever" the program was, and how fast the computer responded, in many clinical settings, it was next to impossible to spend the time it takes to consult the computer expert and to fit this consultation in established work routines.

What is the lesson? The most important factor for ensuring success of new programs is close and direct involvement of prospective users and program designers ("knowledge engineer") in the joint enterprise of determining, in meticulous detail, conditions of use, programs' objectives, and degree to which new methods increase clinical efficiency within the limits of established practice patterns. Developers and users must jointly participate in an iterative process, prototype development alternating with application and field testing. This is a very laborious and costly undertaking (Erdman, Greist, Klein, Jefferson, & Getto, 1981), but the price of shortcuts is generally wasteful failure. Finding the right program "off the shelf" is tricky, unless careful review is possible prior to acquisition for routine use. Even after passing initial user criteria, there must exist the possibility for modifying the software to particular requirements (Johnson, Williams, Klingler, & Gianetti, 1977). Unfortunately, programs designed for a particular clinic or investigator frequently remain at the site of their development and do not readily become available for sharing. Lack of standardization and generally acceptable conventions contribute, of course, to this state of affairs and cause much duplication of effort. One survey (Levitan & Willis, 1985) identified finding the right software and cost and time of new software development as two principal obstacles to utilization of current information technology. The same survey also raised ethical considerations, primarily as concerns for thoughtful deliberation rather than as barriers. Miller, Schaffner, and Meisel (1985) discussed issues related to confidentiality, liability, and who "should" use a program under what conditions, issues that will continue to require considerable debate until we can reach consensus. However, despite the most careful evaluation of computer programs, their place is, and must remain, assistive, consultative, and advisory, with no claim to infringe on clinicians' ultimate authority and responsibilities (Dombal, 1987).

REFERENCES

Ager, A., & Bendall, S. (Eds.). (1991). *Microcomputers and clinical psychology.* New York: Wiley.

Agras, W. S. (1987). So where do we go from here? (Presidential Address). *Behavior Therapy, 18,* 203–217.

Agras, W. S., Taylor, C. B., Feldman, D. E., Losch, M., & Burnett, K. F. (1990). Developing computer-assisted therapy for the treatment of obesity. *Behavior Therapy, 21,* 99–109.

Agras, W. S., Taylor, B., Kraemer, H. C., Allen, R. A., & Schneider, J. A. (1980). Relaxation training. *Archives of General Psychiatry, 37,* 859–863.

Altman, H., Brown, M. L., & Sletten, I. W. (1972). And silently steal away: A study of elopers. *Diseases of the Nervous System, 33,* 52–58.

Angle, H. V. (1981). The interviewing computer: A technology for gathering comprehensive treatment information. *Behavior Research Methods and Instrumentation, 13,* 607–612.

Angle, H. V., Hay, L. R., Hay, W. M., & Ellinwood, E. H. (1977). Computer assisted behavior assessment. In J. D. Cone & R. P. Hawkins (Eds.), *Behavioral assessment* (pp. 369–380). New York: Brunner/Mazel.

Angle, H. V., Johnson T. J., Grebenkemper, N. S., & Ellinwood, C. H. (1979). Computer interview support for clinicians. *Professional Psychology, 10,* 49–51.

Aradi, N. S. (1985). The application of computer technology to behavioral marital therapy. *Journal of Psychotherapy and the Family, 1*(1/2), 167–177.

Atkinson, B. J., & McKenzie, P. N. (1984). The Personalized Spouse Observation Checklist: A computer-generated assessment of marital interaction. *Journal of Marital and Family Therapy, 10*(4), 427–429.

Baer, L., Minichiello, W. E., Jenike, M., & Holland, A. (1988). Use of a portable computer program to assist behavioral treatment in a case of obsessive–compulsive behavior. *Journal of Behavior Therapy and Experimental Psychiatry, 19,* 237–240.

Baldwin, A. L., Baldwin, C. P., & Cole, R. E. (1982). Family free-play interaction: Setting and methods. *Monographs of the Society for Research in Child Development, 47*(Ser. No. 197, No. 5), 36–44.

Bana, D. S., Leviton, A., Swindler, C., Slack, W., & Graham, J. R. (1980). A computer-based headache interview: Acceptance by patients and physicians. *Headache, 20,* 85–89.

Bandura, A. (1969). *Principles of behavior modification.* New York: Holt, Rinehart & Winston.

Barber, J. (1990). Computer-assisted drug prevention. *Journal of Substance Abuse Treatment, 7*(2), 125–131.

Batchelor, J., Shores, E. A., Marosszeky, J. E., & Sandaman, J. (1988). Cognitive rehabilitation of severely closed-head-injured patients using computer-assisted and noncomputerized treatment techniques. *Journal of Head Trauma Rehabilitation, 3*(3), 78–84.

Beatty, J. (1971). Effects of initial alpha wave abundance and operant training procedures on occipital alpha and beta wave activity. *Psychonomic Science, 23,* 197–199.

Beaumont, J. G. (1991). Expert systems and the clinical psychologist. In A. Ager (Ed.), *Microcomputers and clinical psychology* (pp. 175–193). New York: Wiley.

Beck, R. J., Ellis, L.B.M., Scott, D., Raines, J. R., & Hakanson, N. (1982). Microcomputer as patient educator. *American Journal of Hospital Pharmacy, 39,* 2105–2108.

Bellack, A. S., & Hersen, M. (1990). *Handbook of comparative treatments for adult disorders.* New York: Wiley.

Ben-Yishay, Y., Diller, L., Rattock, J., Ross, B., Schaier, A., & Scherger, P. (1983). *Working approaches to remediation of cognitive deficits in brain damage.* In 7th Annual Workshop for Rehabilitation Professionals, New York.

Berndt, M. W., Daniels, O. J., Blizard, R. A., & Murray, R. M. (1989). Can a computer reliably elicit an alcohol history? *British Journal of Addiction, 84*(4), 405–411.

Biglan, A., Villwock, C., & Wick, S. (1979). The feasibility of a computer controlled program for the treatment of test anxiety. *Journal of Behavior Therapy and Experimental Psychiatry, 10,* 47–49.

Binik, Y. M., Servan-Schreiber, D., Freiwald, S., & Hall, K. (1988). Intelligent computer-based assessment and psychotherapy: An expert system for sexual dysfunction. *Journal of Nervous and Mental Disease, 176*(7), 387–400.

Block, B. (1986). Computer-assisted psychotherapy. *Journal of Contemporary Psychotherapy, 16*(1), 72–75.

Blomeyer, R. L., & Dianne, M. C. (1991). *Case studies of computer aided learning.* London: Falmer.

Bloom, A. J. (1985). An anxiety management approach to computerphobia. *Training and Development Journal, 39*(1), 90–92.

Bluhm, H. P. (1988). *Computers in guidance, counseling and psychotherapy.* Springfield, IL: Thomas.

Bosworth, K., Gustafson, D. H., Hawkins, R. P., Chewing, B., & Day, T. (1983). Adolescents, health education, and computers. *Health Education, 14*(6), 58–60.

Bradley, V., Welch, J. L., & Skilbeck, C. E. (1991). *Cognitive retraining using microcomputers.* London: Taylor & Francis.

Brownbridge, G., Fitter, M., & Sime, M. (1984). The doctor's use of a computer in the consulting room: An analysis. *International Journal of Man–Machine Studies, 21,* 65–90.

Buglione, S. A., DeVito, A. J., & Mulloy, J. M. (1990). Traditional group therapy and computer-administered treatment for test anxiety. *Anxiety Research, 3*(1), 33–39.

Burling, T. A., Marotta, J., Gonzales, R., & Moltzen, J. O. (1989). Computerized smoking cessation program for the worksite: Treatment outcome and feasibility. *Journal of Consulting and Clinical Psychology, 57*(5), 619–622.

Burnett, K. F., Magel, P. M., Harrington, S., & Taylor, C. B. (1989). Computer-assisted behavioral health counseling for high school students. *Journal of Counseling Psychology, 36,* 63–67.

Burnett, K. F., Taylor, C. B., & Agras, W. S. (1985). Ambulatory computer-assisted therapy for obesity: A new frontier for behavior therapy. *Journal of Consulting and Clinical Psychology, 53*(5), 698–703.

Butler, R. W., & Namerow, N. S. (1988). Cognitive retraining in brain-injury rehabilitation: A critical review. *Journal of Neurologic Rehabilitation, 2*(3), 93–101.

Cairo, P. C. (1983). Evaluating the effects of computer-assisted counseling systems: A selective review. *The Counseling Psychologist, 11,* 55–59.

Canoune, H. L., & Leyhe, E. W. (1985). Human versus computer interviewing. *Journal of Personality Assessment, 49*(1), 103–106.

Cardozo, L., Krishnan, K. R., & Polkey, C. E. (1984). Urodynamic observations in patients with sacral anterior root stimulation. *Paraplegia, 22,* 201–209.

Carr, A. C., & Ghosh, A. (1983). Response of phobic patients to direct computer assessment. *British Journal of Psychiatry, 142,* 60–65.

Carr, A. C., Ghosh, A., & Ancill, R. J. (1983). Can a computer take a psychiatric history? *Psychological Medicine, 13,* 151–158.

Carr, A. C., Ghosh, A., & Marks, I. M. (1988). Computer-supervised exposure treatment for phobias. *Canadian Journal of Psychiatry, 33,* 112–117.

Carr, A. C., Wilson, S. L., Ghosh, A., Ancil, R. J., & Woods, R. T. (1982). Automated testing of geriatric patients using a microcomputer-based system. *International Journal of Man–Machine Studies, 28,* 297–300.

Carr, T. C. (1991). Microcomputers and psychological treatment. In A. Ager (Ed.), *Microcomputers and clinical psychology* (pp. 65–78). New York: Wiley.

Caruso, D. (1984, September). Software probes the minds. *InfoWorld, 6,* pp. 34–39.

Cassel, R. N. (1971). Systems analysis approach to computer-based counseling for addiction treatment. *The International Journal of Addictions, 6,* 493–495.

Cassel, R. N. (1977). A computerized pastoral counseling system. *Psychology, 14,* 20–23.

Chandler, G. M., Burck, H., & Sampson, J. P. (1988). The effectiveness of a generic program for systematic desensitization. *Computers in Human Behavior, 4,* 339–346.

Chen, M., Houston, T., & Burson, J. (1983). Microcomputer-based health education in the waiting room. *Journal of Computer-Based Instruction, 9,* 90.

Christensen, M., Chaudhary, S. S., Gottshall, R., Hartman, J., & Yatcilla, D. (1989). EASE: A user interface for the elderly. In G. Salvendy & M. J. Smith (Eds.), *Designing and using human-computer interfaces and knowledge based systems* (pp. 428–435). Amsterdam: Elsevier.

Chute, D. L., Conn, G., DiPasquale, M. C., & Hoag, M. (1988). ProsthesisWare: A new class of software supporting the activities of daily living. *Neuropsychology, 2*(1), 41–57.

Clark, W. A., & Molnar, C. E. (1964). The LINC: Description of a laboratory instrument computer. *Annals of the New York Academy of Sciences, 274,* 194–198.

Colby, K. M. (1973). Simulations of belief systems. In R. C. Schank & K. M. Colby (Eds.), *Computer models of thought and language* (pp. 251–286). San Francisco: Freeman.

Colby, K. M., Faught, W. S., & Parkinson, R. C. (1979). Cognitive therapy of paranoid conditions: Heuristic suggestions based on a computer simulation model. *Cognitive Therapy and Research, 3*(1), 55–60.

Colby, K. M., Gould, R. L., & Aronson, G. (1989). Some pros and cons of computer-assisted psychotherapy. *The Journal of Nervous and Mental Disease, 177*(2), 105–108.

Colby, K. M., Watt, J. B., & Gilbert, J. P. (1966). A computer method of psychotherapy: Preliminary communication. *The Journal of Nervous and Mental Diseases, 142*(2), 148–152.

Constantine, J. A. (1985a). Computers and family therapy: An epilogue. In C. R. Figley (Ed.), *Computers and family therapy.* New York: Haworth Press.

Constantine, L. L. (1985b). Computer-aided assessment: Design considerations. In C. R. Figley (Ed.), *Computers and family therapy* (pp. 89–103). New York: Haworth Press.

Couzijn, A. L., Ros, W.J.G., & Winnubst, J.A.M. (1990). Cancer. In A. A. Kaptein, H. M. van der Ploog, B. Garssen, P.J.G. Schreurs, & R. Beunderman (Eds.), *Behavioral medicine: Psychological treatment of somatic disorders* (pp. 231–246). Chichester, UK/New York: Wiley.

Crofts, F., & Crofts, J. (1988). Biofeedback and the computer. *British Journal of Occupational Therapy, 51*(2), 57–59.

Cromwell, R., Fournier, D., & Kvebaek, D. (1980). *The Kvebaek family sculpture technique.* Jonesboro, TN: Pilgrimage.

D'Zurilla, T. J. (1986). Problem solving training. In T. J. D'Zurilla (Ed.), *Problem solving therapy* (pp. 93–142). New York: Springer.

Davidson, R. S. (1984). Applications of computer technology to learning therapy. *Journal of Organizational Behavior Management, 6,* 155–168.

Deardorff, W. W. (1986). Computerized health education: A comparison with traditional forms. *Health Education Quarterly, 13*(1), 61–72.

Devine, E. C., O'Connor, F. W., Cook, T. D., Wenk, V. A., & Curtin, T. R. (1988). Clinical and financial effects of psychoeducational care provided by staff nurses to adult surgical patients in the post-DRG environment. *American Journal of Public Health, 78*(10), 1293–1297.

Dombal, F. T. (1987). Ethical considerations concerning computers in medicine in the 1980s. *Journal of Medical Ethics, 13,* 179–184.

Donner, L., & Guerney, B. G. (1969). Automated group desensitization for test anxiety. *Behavior Research and Therapy, 7,* 1–13.

Duffy, J. C., & Waterton, J. J. (1984). Under-reporting of alcohol consumption in sample surveys: The effect of computer interviewing in fieldwork. *British Journal of Addiction, 79*(3), 303–308.

Dworkin, B., & Dworkin, S. (1988). The treatment of scoliosis by continuous automated postural feedback. In R. Ader, H. Weiner, & A. Baum (Eds.), *Experimental foundations of behavioral medicine: Conditioning approaches* (pp. 67–86). Hillsdale, NJ: Erlbaum.

Edwards, R., & Engelhardt, K. G. (1989). Microprocessor-based innovations and older individuals: AARP survey results and their implications for service robotics. *International Journal of Technology and Aging, 2*(1), 42–55.

Eiduson, B. T., Brooks, S. H., Motto, R. L., Platz, A., & Carmichael, R. (1968). New strategy for psychiatric research, utilizing the Psychiatric Case History Event System. In N. S. Kline & L. E. (Eds.), *Computers and electronic devices in psychiatry.* New York: Grune & Stratton.

Ellis, L.B.M. (1987). Computer-based patient education. *Computers in Human Services, 2*(3/4), 117–130.

Ellis, L.B.M., & Raines, J. R. (1981). Health education using microcomputers: Initial acceptability. *Preventive Medicine, 10,* 77–84.

Engelhardt, K. G., & Edwards, R. (1986). Increasing independence for the aging. *Byte, 11*(3), 191–198.

Epstein, L. H., & Porte, R. L. (1978). Behavioral epidemiology. *AABT Newsletter, 1,* 3–5.

Erdman, H. P., & Foster, S. W. (1986). Computer-assisted assessment with couples and families. *Family Therapy, 13*(1), 23–40.

Erdman, H. P., Greist, J. H., Klein, M. H., Jefferson, J. W., & Getto, C. (1981). The computer psychiatrist: How far have we come? Where are we heading? How far do we dare to go? *Behavior Research Methods and Instruments, 13*(4), 393–398.

Erdman, H. P., Klein, M. H., & Greist, J. H. (1985). Direct patient computer interviewing. *Journal of Consulting and Clinical Psychology, 53*(6), 760–773.

Erdman, R.A.M. (1990). Myocardial infarction and cardiac rehabilitation. In A. A. Kaptein, M. H. van der Ploog, B. Garssen, P.J.G. Schreurs, & R. Beunderman (Eds.), *Behavioral Medicine: Psychological treatment of somatic disorders* (pp. 127–145). New York: Wiley.

Evans, W. M., & Miller, J. R. (1969). Differential effects on response bias of computer vs. conventional administration of social science questionnaire. *Behavioral Science, 14,* 216–227.

Fairbairn, A. S., Woods, C. H., & Fletcher, C. M. (1959). Variability in answers to a questionnaire on respiratory symptoms. *British Journal of Preventive and Social Medicine, 13,* 175–192.

Farrell, A. D., Camplair, P. S., & McCullough, L. (1987). Identification of target complaints by computer interview: Evaluation of the computerized assessment system for psychotherapy evaluation and research. Special Issue: Eating disorders. *Journal of Consulting and Clinical Psychology, 55*(5), 691–700.

Figley, C. R. (Ed.). (1985). *Computers and family therapy: An introduction.* New York: Haworth Press.

Fisher, L. A., Johnson, S., Porter, D., Bleich, H. L., & Slack, W. V. (1977). Collection of a clean voided urine specimen: A comparison among spoken, written and computer-based instructions. *American Journal of Public Health, 67*(7), 640–644.

Floyd, M., & Kettle, M. (1991). A computer-based approach to measurement of employment handicap. *International Journal of Rehabilitation Research, 14,* 37–47.

Foree-Gavert, S., & Gavert, L. (1980). Obesity: Behavior therapy with computer-feedback versus traditional starvation treatment. *Scandinavian Journal of Behavior Therapy, 9,* 1–14.

Foy, D. W., Resnick, H. S., Carroll, E. M., & Osato, S. S. (1990). Behavior therapy. In A. S. Bellak & M. Hersen (Eds.), *Handbook of comparative treatments for adult disorders* (pp. 302–315). New York: Wiley.

Friedman, P. H. (1985). The use of computers in marital and family therapy. *Journal of Psychotherapy and the Family,* 1(1-2), 37-48.

Frydenberg, H. (1988). Computers: Specialized applications for the older person. *American Behavioral Scientist,* 31(5), 595-600.

Gagliano, M. E. (1988). A literature review on the efficacy of video in patient education. *Journal of Medical Education,* 63, 785-792.

Gatchel, R. J. (1974). Frequency of feedback and learned heart rate control. *Journal of Experimental Psychology,* 103, 274-283.

George, L. K., & Siegler, I. C. (1985). Stress and coping in later life. In E. Palmore, E. W. Busse, & G. L. Maddox (Eds.), *Normal Aging III.* Durham, NC: Duke University Press.

Gerson, R. (1985). Systems psychotherapy, the micro-computer, and the American family. *Marriage and Family Review,* 8(1-2). 155-165.

Gervasio, A. H. (1984). Computer-assisted analysis of conversation. *Behavior Research Methods and Instrumentation,* 16(2), 158-161.

Ghosh, A., & Greist, J. H. (1988). Computer treatment in psychiatry. *Psychiatric Annals,* 18(4), 246-250.

Ghosh, A., Marks, I. M., & Carr, A. C. (1984). Controlled study of self-exposure treatment for phobics: Preliminary communication. *Journal of the Royal Society of Medicine,* 77, 483-487.

Glueck, B. C., Jr., & Stroebel, C. F. (1969). The computer and the clinical decision process II. *American Journal of Psychiatry,* 125 (Suppl.), 2-7.

Gottschalk, L. A., & Bechtel, R. J. (1982). The measurement of anxiety. *Psychiatry,* 23(4), 364-369.

Gould, R. (1988). Adulthood. In H. I. Kaplan & B. J. Sadock (Eds.), *Comprehensive textbook of psychiatry.* Baltimore, MD: Williams & Wilkins.

Gray, J. M., & Robertson, I. (1989). Remediation of attentional difficulties following brain injury: Three experimental single case studies. *Brain Injury,* 3, 163-170.

Greist, J. H. (1989). Computer-administered behavior therapies. Special Issue: Behavioural psychotherapy into the 1990's. *International Review of Psychiatry,* 1(3), 267-274.

Greist, J. H., Gustafson, D. H., Laughren, T. P., & Chiles, J. A. (1973). A computer interview for suicide-risk prediction. *American Journal of Psychiatry,* 130(12), 1327-1332.

Greist, J. H., Jefferson, J. W., Combs, A. M., Schou, M., & Thomas, A. (1977). The lithium librarian. *Archives of General Psychiatry,* 34, 456.

Greist, J. H., Jefferson, J. W., Ackerman, D. L., Baudhuin, M. G., Erdman, H. P., & Carroll, J. A. (1985). Lithium information center: The lithium library revisited. *Journal of Clinical Psychiatry,* 46(8), 327-331.

Greist, J. H., & Klein, M. H. (1980). Computer programs, for patients, clinicians and researchers in psychiatry. In J. B. Sidowski, J. H. Johnson, & T. A. Williams (Eds.), *The use of computers in the delivery of mental health care: The necessary background conditions* (pp. 161-181). Norwood, NJ: Ablex.

Greist, J. H., Klein, M. H., & Cura, L.J.V. (1973). A computer interview for psychiatric patient target symptoms. *Archives of General Psychiatry,* 29, 247-253.

Groenman, N. H., Vlaeyen, J.W.S., Eck, H., & Schuerman, J. A. (1990). Chronic pain. In A. A. Kaptein, H. M. van der Ploog, B. Garssen, P.J.G. Schreurs, & R. Beunderman (Eds.), *Behavioral medicine: Psychological treatment of somatic disorders* (pp. 51-66). New York: Wiley.

Grossfeld, M. L., & Grossfeld, C. A. (1986). *Microcomputer applications in rehabilitation of communicative disorders.* Rockville, MD: Aspen.

Hammer, J. S., Hammond, D., Strain, J. J., & Lyons, J. S. (1985). Microcomputers and consultation psychiatry. *General Hospital Psychiatry,* 7, 119-124.

Hannah, K. J., Conlay-Rice, P., Fenty, D., McKiel, E., Soltes, D., Hogan, T., & Wiens, D. (1989). Computer applications for staff development and patient education. *Method. Inform. Med.,* 28, 261-266.

Hedlund, J. L., Evenson, R. C., Sletten, I. W., & Cho, D. W. (1980). The computer and clinical prediction. In J. B. Sidowski, J. H. Johnson, & T. A. Williams (Eds.), *The use of computers in the delivery of mental health care: The necessary background conditions* (pp. 201-235). Norwood, NJ: Ablex.

Hersen, M., & Bellack, A. S. (Ed.). (1981). *Behavioral assessment: A practical handbook.* New York: Pergamon.

Holden, C. (1977). The empathic computer. *Science,* 198, 32.

Hollander, E. K., & Plummer, H. R. (1986). An innovative therapy and enrichment program for senior adults utilizing the personal computer. *Activities, Adaptation and Aging,* 8(1), 59-68.

Howland, E. W., & Siegman, A. W. (1982). Toward the automated measurement of the type-A behavior pattern. *Journal of Behavioral Medicine, 5*(1), 37–53.

Johnson, D. F., & White, C. B. (1980). Effects of training on computer test performance in the elderly. *Journal of Applied Psychology, 65,* 357–358.

Johnson, J. J., Gianetti, R. A., & Williams, T. A. (1979).Psychological Systems Questionnaire: An objective personality test designed for on-line computer presentation, scoring and interpretation. *Behavior Research Methods and Instrumentation, 11*(2), 257–260.

Johnson, J. J., Williams, T. A., Klingle, D. E., & Gianetti, R. A. (1977). Interventional relevance and retrofit programming: Concepts for the improvement of clinician-acceptance of computer-generated assessment reports. *Behavior Research Methods and Instrumentation, 9*(2), 123–132.

Johnson, R. (1990). Modifying memory function: Use of a computer to train mnemonic skills. *British Journal of Clinical Psychology, 29*(4), 437–438.

Johnston, M., Weinman, J., & Marteau, T. M. (1990). Health psychology in hospital settings. In A. A. Kaptein, H. M. van der Ploog, B. Garssen, P.J.G. Schreurs, & R. Beunderman (Eds.), *Behavioral medicine: Psychological treatment of somatic disorders* (pp. 15–31). New York: Wiley.

Kanfer, F. H., & Goldstein, A. P. (1991). *Helping people change* (4th ed.). New York: Pergamon.

Kaptein, A. A., & Rookjen, E. (1990). Behavioral medicine—some introductory remarks. In A. A. Kaptein, H. M. van der Ploog, B. Garssen, P.J.G. Schreurs, & R. Beunderman (Eds.), *Behavioral medicine: Psychological treatment of somatic disorders* (pp. 3–13). New York: Wiley.

Katzman, R., Lasker, B., & Bernstein, N. (1986). Accuracy of diagnosis and consequences of misdiagnosis of disorders causing dementia. In *Office of technology assessment* (pp. 1–110). Washington, DC: U.S. Government Printing Office.

Kazdin, A. E. (1981). Behavioral observation. In M. Hersen & A. S. Bellack (Eds.), *Behavioral assessment: A practical handbook* (pp. 101–124). New York: Pergamon.

Klein, M. H., Greist, J. H., & Cura, L.J.V. (1975). Computers and psychiatry: Promises to keep. *Archives of General Psychiatry, 32,* 837–843.

Klingler, D. E., Miller, D. A., Johnson, J. J., & Williams, T. A. (1977). Process evaluation of an on-line computer-assisted unit for intake assessment of mental health patients. *Behavior Research Methods and Instrumentation, 9*(2), 110–116.

Kolotkin, R. L. (1981). Computers in biofeedback research and therapy. *Behavior Research Methods and Instrumentation, 13*(4), 532–542.

Kreutzer, J. S., Conder, R., Wehman, P., & Morrison, C. (1989). Compensatory strategies for enhancing independent living and vocational outcome following traumatic brain injury. *Cognitive Rehabilitation, 7*(1), 30–35.

Lang, P. (1980). Behavioral treatment and bio-behavioral assessment. In J. B. Sidowski, J. H. Johnson, & T. A. Williams (Eds.), *The use of computers in the delivery of mental health care: The necessary background conditions* (pp. 119–137). Norwood, NJ: Ablex.

Lang, P. J. (1969). The "on-line" computer in behavior therapy research. *American Psychologist, 24,* 236–239.

Lang, P. J. (1974). Learned control of human heart rate in a computer directed environment. In P. A. Obrist, A. H. Black, J. Brener, & L. V. DiCara (Eds.), *Cardiovascular physiology* (pp. 392–405). Chicago: Aldine.

Lang, P. J., Melamed, B. J., & Hart, J. (1970). A psychophysiological analysis of fear modification using an automated desensitization procedure. *Journal of Abnormal Psychology, 76,* 220.

Lang, P. J., Troyer, G. W. Twentyman, C. T., & Gatchel, P. J. (1975). Differential effects of heart rate modification training on college students, older males and patients with ischemic heart disease. *Psychosomatic Medicine, 37,* 429–446.

Lawrence, G. H. (1986). Using computers for the treatment of psychological problems. *Computers in Human Behavior, 2,* 43–62.

Lehtinen, M. W., & Smith, G. W. (1985). MATESIM: Computer assisted marriage analysis for family therapists. In C. R. Figley (Ed.), *Computers and family therapy* (pp. 117–131). New York: Haworth Press.

Leventhal, H., Prohaska, T. R., & Hirschman, R. S. (1985). Preventive health behavior across the life-span. In J. Rosen & L. J. Solomon (Eds.), *Preventing health risk behaviors and promoting coping with illness.* Hanover, NH: University Press of New England.

Levitan, K. B., & Willis, E. A. (1985). Barriers to practitioners' use of information technology utilization: A discussion and results of a study. In C. R. Figley (Ed.), *Computers and family practice* (pp. 21–35). New York: Haworth Press.

Lockshin, S., & Harrison, K. (1991). Computer-assisted assessment of psychological problems. In A. Ager (Ed.), *Microcomputers and clinical psychology* (pp. 47–63). New York: Wiley.

Lucas, R. W., Mullin, P. J., Luna, C.B.X., & McInroy, D. C. (1977). Psychiatrist and a computer as interrogators of patients with alcohol-related illnesses: A comparison. *British Journal of Psychiatry, 131,* 160–167.

Luiselli, J. K. (1989). Health-threatening behaviors. In J. K. Luiselli (Ed.), *Behavioral medicine and developmental disabilities* (pp. 114–151). New York: Springer.

Luria, A. R., Naydin, F. L., Tsvetkova, L. S., & Vinarksy, E. N. (1969). Restoration of higher cortical function following local brain injury. In P. J. Vinken & G. W. Bruyn (Eds.), *Handbook of clinical neurology* (Vol. 3). Amsterdam: North Holland.

Lynch, W. J. (1990a). Cognitive prostheses for the brain impaired. *Journal of Head Trauma Rehabilitation, 5*(3), 78–80.

Lynch, W. J. (1990b). Selecting a computer for rehabilitation. *Journal of Head Trauma Rehabilitation, 5*(4), 101–103.

Mahoney, M. J. (1977). Some applied issues in self-monitoring. In J. D. Cone & R. P. Hawkins (Eds.), *Behavioral assessment* (pp. 241–254). New York: Brunner/Mazel.

Malcolm, R., Sturgis, E. T., Anton, R. F., & Williams, L. (1989). Computer-assisted diagnosis of alcoholism. *Computers in Human Services, 5*(3–4), 163–170.

Malec, E. A., Goldstein, G., & McCue, M. (1991). Predictors of memory training success in patients with closed heady injury. *Neuropsychology, 5*(1), 29–34.

Maultsby, M. C., & Slack, W. V. (1971). A computer-based psychiatric history system. *Archives of General Psychiatry, 25,* 570–572.

Maurer, K., Biel, H., Kuhner, C., & Loffler, W. (1989). On the way to expert systems: Comparing DSM-III computer diagnoses with CATEGO (ICD) diagnoses in depressive and schizophrenic patients. *European Archives of Psychiatry and Neurological Sciences, 239*(1), 127–132.

Mauer, K., Hillig, A., Freyberger, H. J., & Velthausen, S. (1991). Erfahrungen mit den "Schedules for Clinical Assessment in Neuropsychiatry" im Rahmen einer multizentrischen Feldstudie. *Schweizer Archiv fuer Neurologie und Psychiatrie, 142*(3), 235–245.

McCullough, L., Farrell, A. D., & Longabough, R. (1984). The making of a computerized assessment system: Problems, pitfalls and pleasures. In M. D. Schwartz (Ed.), *Using computers in clinical practice.* New York: Haworth Press.

McCullough, L., Farrell, A. D., & Longabaugh, R. (1986). The development of a microcomputer-based mental health information system. *American Psychologist, 41*(2), 207–214.

McGrane, W. L., Alley, E. B., & Toth, F. J. (1990). The use of interactive media for HIV/AIDS prevention in the military community. *Military Medicine, 155*(6), 235–240.

McGuire, B. E. (1990). Computer-assisted cognitive rehabilitation. *Irish Journal of Psychology, 11*(4), 299–308.

McLemore, C. W., & Fantuzzo, J. W. (1982). CARE: Bridging the gap between clinicians and computers. *Professional Psychology, 13,* 501–510.

Mead, D. E., Cain, M. W., & Steele, K. (1985). A computer data based management system for a family therapy clinic. In C. R. Figley (Ed.), *Computers and family therapy* (pp. 49–88). New York: Haworth Press.

Meehl, P. (1978). Theoretical risks and tabular asterisks: Sir Karl, Sir Ronald, and the slow progress of soft psychology. *Journal of Consulting and Clinical Psychology, 46*(4), 806–834.

Mezzich, J. E. (Ed.). (1986). *Clinical care and information systems in psychiatry.* Washington, DC: American Psychiatric Press.

Miller, R. A., Schaffner, K. F., & Meisel, A. (1985). Ethical and legal issues related to the use of computers in clinical medicine. *Annals of Internal Medicine, 102*(4), 529–536.

Molnar, C. E., & Clark, W. A. (1990). Development of the LINC. In B. I. Blum & K. Duncan (Eds.), *A history of medical informatics* (pp. 119–130). New York: ACM Press.

Morris, J. N., Hawes, C., Fries, B. E., Phillips, C. D., Mor, V., Katz, S., Murphy, K., Drugovich, M. L., & Friedlob, A. S. (1990). Designing the National Resident Assessment Instrument for nursing homes. *Gerontologist, 30*(3), 293–302.

Mulder, L.J.M., Maarse, F. J., Sjouw, W.P.B., & Akkerman, A. E. (Ed.). (1991). *Computers in psychology.* Amsterdam: Swets & Zeitlinger.

Mulholland, T. (1977). *Testing hypotheses with feedback methods.* In International Conference on Biofeedback and Self-regulation, Tuebingen, Germany.

Murphy, J. M., Neff, R. K., Sobol, A. M., Rice, J. X., & Olivier, D. C. (1985). Computer diagnosis of depression and anxiety: The Stirling County study. *Psychological Medicine, 15,* 99–112.

Napper, S. A., Robey, B. L., & McAfee, P. H. (1989). An expert system for use in the prescription of electronic augmentative and alternative communication devices. *AAC Augmentative and Alternative Communication, 5*(2), 128–136.

Nelson, R. O. (1977). Methodological issues in assessment via self-monitoring. In J. D. Cone & R. P. Hawkins (Eds.), *Behavioral assessment* (pp. 217–240). New York: Brunner/Mazel.

Nix, D., & Spiro, R. J. (1990). *Cognition, education and multimedia.* Hillsdale, NJ: Erlbaum.

Olevitch, B. A., & Hagan, B. J. (1991). An interactive videodisc as a tool in the rehabilitation of the chronically mentally ill: A preliminary investigation. *Computers in Human Behavior, 7*(1), 57–73.

Olson, D. H. (1985). Microcomputers for couple and family assessment: ENRICH and other inventories. In C. R. Figley (Ed.), *Computers and family therapy* (pp. 105–115). New York: Haworth Press.

Overby, M. A. (1987). PSYEXPERT: An expert system prototype for aiding psychiatrists in the diagnosis of psychotic disorders. *Compu Biol Med, 17* (6), 383–393.

Paggeot, B., Kvale, S., Mace, F. C., & Sharkey, R. W. (1988). Some merits and limitation of hand-held computers for data collection. *Journal of Applied Behavior Analysis, 21,* 429.

Perrez, M. (1988). Bewaltigung von Alltagsbelastungen und seelische Gesundheit: Zusammenhange auf der Grundlage computer-unterstutzter Selbstbeobachtungs- und Fragebogendaten. *Zeitschrift fur Klinische Psychologie Forschung und Praxis, 17*(4), 292–306.

Plutchik, R., & Karasu, T. (1991). Computers in psychotherapy: An overview. *Computers in Human Behavior, 7*(1–2), 33–44.

Poon, L. W., & Siegler, I. C. (1991). Psychological aspects of normal aging. In J. Sadavoy, L. W. Lazarus, & L. F. Jarvick (Eds.), *Comprehensive review of geriatric psychiatry* (pp. 117–145). Washington, DC: American Psychiatric Press.

Pope, A. T., & Gerstein, C. D. (1977). Computer automation of feedback training. *Behavior Research Methods and Instrumentation, 9*(2), 164–168.

Price, K. P., & Gatchel, R. J. (1979). A perspective on clinical feedback. In R. J. Gatchel & K. P. Proce (Eds.), *Clinical applications of biofeedback: Appraisal and status* New York: Pergamon.

Purdy, M., & Nerri, L. (1989). Computer-assisted cognitive rehabilitation in the home. *Cognitive Rehabilitation, 7*(6), 34–38.

Reich, T., Robins, L. N., Woodruff, R. A., Taibleson, M., Rich, C., & Cunningham, L. (1975). Computer-assisted derivation of a screening interview for alcoholism. *Archives of General Psychiatry, 32,* 847–852.

Reiss, D. (1971). Intimacy of problem solving. *Archives of General Psychiatry, 25,* 442–455.

Reitman, R. (1984). The use of small computers in self-help sex therapy. In M. D. Schwartz (Ed.), *Using computers in clinical practice: Psychotherapy and mental health applications* (pp. 363–380). New York: Haworth Press.

Robertson, I. (1990). Does computerized cognitive rehabilitation work? *Aphasiology, 4,* 381–405.

Robertson, I., Gray, J., & McKenzie, S. (1988). Microcomputer-based cognitive rehabilitation of visual neglect: Three multiple-baseline single case studies. *Brain Injury, 2,* 151–163.

Roemer, R. A. (1975). Some interactive computer applications in a physiological psychology laboratory. *American Psychologist, 30,* 295–298.

Romanczyk, R. G. (1986). *Clinical utilization of microcomputer technology.* New York: Pergamon.

Rome, H. P. (1967). Prospects for a Psi-Net: The fourth quantum advance in psychiatry. *Comprehensive Psychiatry, 8*(6), 450–454.

Rosenman, R. H. (1978). The interview method of assessment of the coronary-prone behavior pattern. In T. Dembroski, S. Weiss, J. Shields, S. Haynes, & M. Feinleib (Eds.), *Coronary-prone behavior.* New York: Springer.

Sampson, J. P. (1983). An integrated approach to computer applications in counseling psychology. *Counseling Psychologist, 11*(8), 65–74.

Sampson, J. P. (1984). Maximizing the effectiveness of computer applications in counseling and human development: The role of research and implementation strategies. *Journal of Counseling and Development,63,* 187–191.

Sampson, J. P., Jr. (1986). The use of computer-assisted instruction in support of psychotherapeutic processes. *Computers in Human Behavior, 2,* 1–19.

Sampson, J. P., & Pyle, K. R. (1983). Ethical issues involved with the use of computer-assisted counseling, testing and guidance systems. *Personnel and Guidance Journal, 61*(5), 283–286.

Schinke, S. P., Orlandi, M. A., Gordon, A. N., & Weston, R. E. (1989). AIDS prevention via computer-based intervention. *Computers in Human Services, 5*(3–4), 147–156.

Schneider, S. J., Walter, R., & O'Donnell, R. (1990). Computerized communication as a medium for behavioral smoking cessation treatment: Controlled evaluation. *Computers in Human Behavior, 6*(2), 141–151.

Schnelle, J. F., & Traughber, B. (1983). A behavioral assessment system applicable to geriatric nursing facility residents. *Behavioral Assessment, 5*(3), 231–243.

Schwartz, M. D. (Ed.). (1984). *Using computers in clinical practice.* New York: Haworth Press.

Selmi, P. M., Klein, M. H., Greist, J. H., Johnson, J. H., & Harris, W. G. (1982). An investigation of computer-assisted cognitive-behavior therapy in the treatment of depression. *Behavior Research Methods and Instrumentation, 14*(2), 181–185.

Servan, Schreiber, D., & Binik, Y. M. (1989). Extending the intelligent tutoring system paradigm: Sex therapy as intelligent tutoring. *Computers in Human Behavior, 5*(4), 241–259.

Shore, J. (1986). Conversation with a computer. *Computer and People, 35*(7/8), 7–11.

Sidowski, J. B., Johnson, J. H., & Williams, T. A. (1980). *The use of computers in the delivery of mental health care: The necessary background conditions.* Norwood, NJ: Ablex.

Skilbeck, C. (1991). Microcomputer-based cognitive rehabilitation. In A. Ager (Ed.), *Microcomputers and clinical psychology* (pp. 95–118). New York: Wiley.

Skinner, H. A., & Allen, B. A. (1983). Does the computer make a difference? Computerized versus face-to-face versus self-report assessment of alcohol, drug, and tobacco use. *Journal of Consulting and Clinical Psychology, 51*(2), 267–275.

Skinner, H. A., Allen, B. A., Mcintosh, M. D., & Palmer, W. H. (1985). Lifestyle assessment: Applying microcomputers in family practice. *British Medical Journal, 290,* 212–214.

Slack, W., Porter, D., Witschi, J., Sullivan, M., Buxbaum, R., & Stare, F. J. (1976). Dietary interviewing by computer. *Journal of the American Dietetic Association, 69,* 514–516.

Slack, W. V. (1982). A history of computerized medical interviews. *MD Computing,* 52–59.

Slack, W. V., & Van Cura, L. J. (1968). Patient reaction to computer-based medical interviewing. *Computers and Biomedical Research, 1,* 527–531.

Slavin, S. (Ed.). (1982). *Applying computers in social service and mental health agencies.* New York: Haworth Press.

Sletten, I. W., Altman, H., Evenson, R. C., & Cho, D. W. (1973). Computer assignment of psychotropic drugs. *American Journal of Psychiatry, 130,* 595–598.

Soede, M. (1989). The use of information technology in rehabilitation: An overview of possibilities and new directions for applications. *Journal of Medical Engineering and Technology, 13*(1/2), 5–9.

Solomon, M. (1984). Neuromuscular stimulation: Applications in orthopedic medicine. *Orthopedics* (**Special Issue**), *7,* 1111–1200.

Sorrell, S. P., Greist, J. H., Klein, M. H., Johnson, J. H., & Harris, W. G. (1982). Enhancement of adherence to tricyclic antidepressants by computerized supervision. *Behavior Research Methods and Instrumentation, 14*(2), 176–180.

Stinson, C. H. (1989). Roles for computers in geriatric health care. *International Journal of Technology and Aging, 2*(1), 77–93.

Story, T. B., & Sbordorne, R. J. (1988). The use of microcomputers in the treatment of cognitive-communicative impairments. *Journal of Head Trauma Rehabilitation, 3*(2), 45–54.

Stout, R. L. (1981). New approaches to the design of computerized interviewing and testing systems. *Behavior Research Methods and Instrumentation, 13*(4), 436–442.

Taylor, C. B., Agras, W. S., Losch, M., & Plante, T. G. (1991). Improving the effectiveness of computer-assisted weight loss. *Behavior Therapy, 22,* 229–236.

Taylor, C. B., Fried, L., & Kenardy, J. (1990). The use of a real-time computer diary for data acquisition and processing. *Behavior Research and Therapy, 28*(1), 93–97.

Taylor, C. B., Sheik, J., Agras, W. S., Roth, W. T., Margraf, J., Maddock, R. J., & Gossard, D. (1986). Ambulatory heart rate changes in patients with panic attacks. *American Journal of Psychiatry, 143,* 478–482.

Tunks, E., & Bellissimo, A. (1991). *Behavioral medicine: Concepts and procedures.* New York: Pergamon.

Turk, D. C., & Salovey, P. (1985). Cognitive structures, cognitive processes, and cognitive behavior modification: I. Client Issues. *Cognitive Therapy and Research, 9*(1), 1–17.

Turkle, S. (1980). Computers as Rorschach. *Society, 17*(2), 15–24.

Turkle, S. (1984). *The second self.* New York: Simon & Schuster.
van der Helm-Hylkema, H. (1990). Headache. In A. A. Kaptein, H. M. van der Ploog, B. Garssen, P.J.G. Schreurs, & R. Beunderman (Eds.), *Behavioral medicine: Psychological treatment of somatic disorders* (pp. 67–81). New York: Wiley.
van der Ploeg, H. M. (1990). Gastrointestinal disorders. In A. A. Kaptein, H. M. van der Ploog, B. Garssen, P.J.G. Schreurs, & R. Beunderman (Eds.), *Behavioral medicine: Psychological treatment of somatic disorders* (pp. 205–216). New York: Wiley.
Wadden, T. A., Luborsky, L., Greer, S., & Crits-Christoph, P. (1984). The behavioral treatment of essential hypertension: An update and comparison with pharmacological treatment. *Clinical Psychology Review, 4,* 403–429.
Wagman, M. (1988). *Computer psychotherapy systems.* New York: Gordon & Breach.
Wagman, M., & Kerber, K. W. (1980). PLATO DCS, an interactive computer system for personal counseling: Further development and evaluation. *Journal of Counseling Psychology, 27*(1), 31–39.
Wagman, M., & Kerber, K. W. (1984). Computer-assisted counseling: Problems and prospects. *Counselor Education and Supervision, 24,* 142–154.
Wakefield, R. A. (1985). Computers, family empowerment, and the psychotherapist: Conceptual overview and outlook. In C. R. Figley (Ed.), *Computers and family therapy* (pp. 9–20). New York: Haworth Press.
Weisman, S. (1983). Computer games for the frail elderly. *Gerontologist, 23*(4), 361–363.
Weizenbaum, J. (1976). *Computer power and human reason.* San Francisco: Freeman.
Weizenbaum, J. (1977). Computers as "therapists" [Letter to the Editor]. *Science, 198,* 354.
Werner, G. (1991). Evolving paradigms of decision support systems for health professions. *Heuristics, 4*(1), 66–76.
Werner, G., & Smith, E. T. (1989). Conferring with an expert diagnostic consultant in geriatric psychiatry. *Annual International Conference of the IEEE Engineering in Biology and Medicine Society, 11,* 1215–1218.
Werner, G., & Smith, E. T. (1992). Computer-assisted geriatric patient evaluation by physician extenders. In *MEDINFO-92.* Geneva, Switzerland.
Wheeler, L. A., Wheeler, M. L., Ours, P., & Swider, C. (1983). Use of CAI/VIDEO in diabetes patient nutritional education. In R. E. Dayhoff (Ed.), *Seventh Annual Symposium on Computer Applications in Medical Care* (pp. 961-964). New York: Institute of Electrical and Electronic Engineers.
Williams, T. A., Johnson, J. H., & Bliss, E. L. (1975). A computer-assisted psychiatric assessment unit. *American Journal of Psychiatry, 132*(1), 1074–1076.
Witschi, J., Porter, D., Vogel, S., Buxbaum, R., Stare, F. J., & Slack, W. (1976). A computer-based dietary counseling system. *Journal of the American Dietetic Society, 69,* 385–390.
Wixted, J. T., Bellack, A. S., & Hersen, M. (1990). Behavior therapy. In A. S. Bellack & M. Hersen (Eds.), *Handbook of comparative treatments for adult disorders* (pp. 17–33). New York: Wiley.
Wolpe, J., & Migler, B. (1967). Automated desensitization: A case report. *Behavior Research and Therapy, 5,* 133.
Zarr, M. L. (1984). Computer-mediated psychotherapy: Toward patient-selection guidelines. *American Journal of Psychotherapy, 38*(1), 47–62.
Zemcov, A., Barclay, L. L., Brush, D., & Blass, J. P. (1984). Computerized data base for evaluation and follow-up of demented outpatients. *Journal of the American Geriatrics Society, 32,* 801–842.
Zetin, M., Warren, S., Lanssens, E., & Tominaga, D. (1987). Computerized psychiatric diagnostic interview. In *SCAMC* (pp. 292–298). Washington, DC.
Zwart, F. M. (1990). Insomnia. In A. A. Kaptein, H. M. van der Ploog, B. Garssen, P.J.G. Schreurs, & R. Beunderman (Eds.), *Behavioral medicine: Psychological treatment of somatic disorders* (pp. 83–94). New York: Wiley.

30

The Marketing of Professional Health-Care Services

Wade Lancaster

INTRODUCTION

Revolution is changing the American health-care system. Changes taking place are unquestionably some of the most dramatic in the history of American health care. Impact of the trends now affecting the health-care system undoubtedly will influence structure and functioning of the system well into the 21st century.

The decade of the 1980s witnessed the procompetition environment, which supported deregulation and encouraged intensive competition as a way to correct some of the health-care system's problems. With shifts in federal policies came pressure for cost containment. Disgusted with years of rising health-care costs, big purchasers (e.g., governments, businesses, and unions) began forcing changes regarding use and payment of physicians, hospitals, and other providers. As a result, Medicare adopted the prospective payment system whereby reimbursement and length of hospital stay became predetermined by diagnosis. Similarly, many other third-party payers adopted prospective payment systems, often through managed care programs. These fixed reimbursements affected health-care providers by reducing revenues which, in turn, led to an increase in competition among traditional providers, ushering in a new wave of profit and nonprofit organizations.

As these newer health-care organizations, many which emphasized wellness, became more acceptable to consumers and competition increased, primary purchasers of health care began hoping that informed consumers would help contain

---

Wade Lancaster • Health Sciences Center, University of Virginia, Charlottesville, Virginia 22903.
Handbook of Health and Rehabilitation Psychology, edited by Anthony J. Goreczny. Plenum Press, New York, 1995.

rapidly escalating costs by choosing the best providers at the lowest prices and therefore the inefficient would not survive (Duda, 1990). Something did not work, however, because health-care costs continued to increase.

A growing concern focused on how to best (1) maintain or improve current service levels in the face of increasing demand for health-care products and services by consumers with decreasing ability and/or willingness to pay for those services, and, at the same time, (2) effectively deal with changes in federal policies, reductions in funding, pressures for cost containment, and dramatic increases in competition. These are some of the environmental factors that forced many health-care providers to turn in desperation to marketing to solve the problem of declining revenues.

With the market playing an increasingly more important role, health-care services marketing emerged as an area of paramount importance to provider organizations. Hospitals were among the earliest adopters of marketing, seeking improvements in their utilization and competitive positions. Unfortunately, the concept and practice of marketing, with many of its own unique terms, was foreign and misunderstood by many of these providers, most of whom had limited views regarding its nature and scope as well as unrealistic expectations as to what it could accomplish. Consequently, early reactions to marketing were mixed.

Some organizations viewed marketing as an unprofessional, inappropriate application of crass commercialism, often associated with hucksterism. Given these negative images held by people outside the marketing field, one might ask why health-care professionals should become immersed in such a tawdry area? The truth is that modern marketing suffers from an identity crisis.

Much of this misunderstanding comes from the tendency to narrowly associate marketing with only one or two of the major components involved in the total marketing process. For example, to the uninformed, marketing may raise images of attractively packaged goods of marginal quality, offensive and misleading advertising, or deceptive selling tactics. Consequently some individuals view marketing as the task of influencing and persuading others to buy goods and services. Many individuals resent these persuasive attempts and develop negative images of marketing. Unfortunately, these individuals often overlook, forget, or simply do not understand the remaining components of the marketing process.

Although descriptions of the appropriate use of marketing techniques frequently appear in forums, workshops, professional journals, and a few specialized books, for some health professionals, marketing represents no more than a set of buzzwords, with little or no understanding of concepts. One study, for example, reported that 66% of the physicians surveyed believe that marketing is merely a synonym for advertising (Folland, 1987). In short, there appears to be a considerable gap between what many health professionals understand about marketing and what marketers do and say. In light of this confusion regarding some of the fundamentals of marketing, this chapter focuses on marketing concepts that are particularly useful for health-care professionals.

In this chapter, I describe the nature and scope of modern marketing, explain the contemporary philosophy of marketing known as *consumer orientation,* and outline a planning framework that centers on key strategic issues facing health-care marketers.

WHAT IS MARKETING?

The process of marketing is as old as humankind, having been in existence since barter, trade, or exchange began among primitive peoples. In contrast, formal study of marketing as a discipline is relatively new. Since its inception, the marketing discipline has been in a constant state of transition; the concept of marketing has undergone several conceptual as well as perceptual changes.

Although vigorous debate concerning the basic notion of marketing had alternately waxed and waned since the early 1900s, most individuals have traditionally associated marketing with the sale of physical products and consumer services. Initial investigations involved in formal study of marketing dealt primarily with creation, stimulation, facilitation, and valuation of transactions between profit-seeking business firms and want-gratifying consumers. For the most part, marketing scholars focused their attention on managerial problems of large consumer goods producers who catered to the needs of the mass market. In contrast, these scholars devoted relatively little attention to the marketing of services in the private sector and even less attention to the marketing of public sector services. During the late 1960s and 1970s, not only did scholars challenge the traditional view of marketing, they also vigorously debated the possibility of expanding the scope of marketing.

Broadened Concepts of Marketing

In 1969, Kotler and Levy's landmark article criticized the then-prevailing view of marketing as "a function peculiar to business firms." They suggested that marketing is a more pervasive societal activity performed by different organizations in a wide variety of contexts. They observed that nonbusiness organizations have products and services, as well as customers, and use marketing tools; however, it was business organizations that developed and used the science of effective marketing. Therefore, Kotler and Levy argued that because all organizations perform marketing, or at least marketing-like activities the choice facing managers is not whether to market but whether to market well or poorly.

The movement to expand the concept of marketing achieved a major milestone in 1971, when the *Journal of Marketing* devoted an entire issue to marketing's changing social and environmental role. In this issue, Kotler and Zaltman (1971, p. 5) coined the term social marketing, which they defined as

> the design, implementation, and control of programs calculated to influence the acceptability of social ideas and involving considerations in product planning, pricing, communication, distribution, and marketing research.

Also published in this issue was one of the earliest health-care marketing articles, written by Zaltman and Vertinsky (1971) and considered one of the cornerstones of the discipline's literature. In their article, they discussed social marketing in a health context and development of a psychosocial model of health-related behavior. The model has helped to sensitize health-care organizations to certain key health factors and has permitted an evaluation of the consequences of a chosen marketing strategy.

Shortly thereafter, Kotler (1972) reevaluated his earlier positions about broadening the concept of marketing and articulated a *generic* concept of marketing. He proposed that marketing involves "how transactions are created, stimulated, facilitated, and valued" (p. 49). The focus is on transaction, which is "the exchange of values between two parties." Thus, marketing takes place whenever (1) there are two social units, (2) one is seeking a specific response from another, (3) the response probability is not constant, and (4) one attempts to produce the desired response by creating and offering values to the market. When one adopts a functional view of marketing, the generic concept does not limit marketing to specific institutions.

In summary, the thrust of these articles was to emphasize the fundamental character of marketing in business and other contexts, identifying its root character in the nature of exchange. All human interactions are then potentially susceptible to marketing analyses so that, in addition to transactions included in traditional business marketing, there is the possibility of other types of marketing, such as social marketing, and the marketing of organizations, individuals, and places. From mass marketing phenomena to intimate marketing in private dyadic relationships, elements basic to giving and receiving are at work.

In its broadest sense, *marketing* is simply a conscious, systematic approach to the planning, implementation, and evaluation of exchange relationships. Applied to health care, marketing is the process of providing want-satisfying goods and services in exchange for value. The value may be profit, as in the traditional business definition, or it may also be money used to staff a hospital and buy the latest equipment or the psychic value of "doing something for someone else," as perceived by volunteers. There are two parties to the exchange, and both buyers (users or consumers) and sellers (or providers) must receive benefits.

Marketing-Practice Philosophies

The role of marketing and its relative importance to an organization depends upon the philosophy of that organization's management. Four different managerial orientations under which organizations practice marketing are prevalent: production, product, selling, and marketing.

A *production orientation* is one of the oldest philosophies guiding organizations. The basis of this philosophy is the supposition that consumers will demand products and services that are available and affordable, and, therefore, the organization must focus on pursuing efficiency in production and distribution (Kotler & Clarke, 1987). This philosophy is appropriate under two sets of circumstances. First, when demand exceeds supply, organizations must attempt to increase output. In the second case, when production costs are high, improvements in productivity are necessary to reduce such costs.

Some health-care organizations focus on running a smooth production process, even if it means compromising human needs to meet the requirements of that process. Many medical and dental practices use assembly-line principles. Large numbers of patients may wait long periods in waiting rooms so that practitioners can maximize their efficiency in seeing patients. Although this way of operating results in handling many cases per hour, many individuals view it as unfriendly and impersonal.

A *product orientation* entails a managerial viewpoint that the major task of organizations is to deliver products or services they think would be good for the market. Under this orientation, management subscribes to the notion that by "building a better mousetrap, the world will beat a path to your door." This orientation assumes consumers will recognize that products or services offering the most quality, performance, and features are superior and therefore demand those products or services.

Organizations that never grow beyond a product orientation have marketing myopia, which eventually leads to their demise. A classic example is the railroad industry; its management thought consumers wanted trains rather than transportation, and ignored competitive offerings by the trucking industry, such as door-to-door pickup and delivery (Cooper, 1985).

A product orientation is a paternalistic approach to marketing that assumes organizations know best what is good for consumers. This orientation is especially prevalent in the health-care field. If new equipment or technology means better patient care, organizations then acquire that equipment or technology. Health-care providers often become so enamored with the quality, sophistication, and technology of medical care they deliver that they do not recognize the consumer dissatisfaction and discomfort it causes. Their focus is with the number of patients seen or with the number of procedures or tests administered. Emphasis is on service-delivery quality, as perceived by the professional. Patients' needs receive little consideration. After all, how effectively could patients evaluate health care?

A *selling orientation* holds that consumers will not buy enough unless organizations stimulate consumer interest in existing products and services by undertaking large selling and promotion efforts. There are three basic tenets underlying this concept. First, consumers do not buy products and services; organizations sell them. The second tenet is that consumers are plentiful: some may buy again; others will not. In either case, there is no great concern about repeat business. The third basic tenet underlying this concept is that a variety of sales-stimulating devices, such as advertisements, personal selling, and promotional giveaways can effectively convince consumers to buy (Cooper, 1985).

Although the selling orientation may not be prevalent in health care, some organizations believe they can substantially increase the size of their market by becoming more selling oriented. Rather than modify their products or restructure their services to make them more attractive, these organizations increase their budgets for advertising, outreach, personal selling, and other forms of sales promotion. For example, some home health-care agencies react to declining patient volumes by increasing the frequency of visits made by liaison nurses to referring hospitals, increasing their public relations budgets, and developing new agency brochures. Many hospitals must confront the problem of empty beds, and some try "selling" their community on using the local hospital. Physicians in major cities find extreme competition for patients, and some of them attempt to "sell" to patients by advertising. The focus in each of these examples is on short-term results: increasing patient volume.

A *marketing orientation* recognizes that achieving organizational goals depends on determining needs, wants, and values of target markets and satisfying them through design, communication, pricing, and delivery of appropriate and competitively viable products and services. It begins with a well-defined market, focuses on consumer needs, integrates all consumer-affecting marketing activities, and generates profits by creating consumer satisfaction.

This orientation consists of three tenets. The first is that an active plan of marketing research is essential to determine consumer wants, needs, and values. Organizations must systematically study customers' needs, wants, perceptions, preferences, and satisfaction using surveys, focus groups, and other means. Organizations must then constantly act on this information to improve their offerings to better meet consumer needs. The second tenet is that organizations must integrate all target market or consumer-related activities. The third tenet is that successfully satisfying consumers will result in repeat business, consumer loyalty, and organizational support, all of which contributes to the satisfaction of organizations' primary goals (Cooper, 1985).

It may be instructive, at this juncture, to briefly compare the selling and marketing orientations because many individuals confuse these orientations. Whereas the selling orientation focuses on needs of organizations, the marketing orientation focuses on needs of consumers. The selling orientation takes an inside-out perspective. It starts within organizations, focuses on what they have to offer, and uses various sales-stimulating devices, such as heavy selling and promoting, as a means to achieve profitable sales. In contrast, the marketing orientation takes an outside-in perspective. It begins with existing or potential consumer needs, plans a coordinated set of programs and services to serve those wants, needs, and values, and, in return, satisfies its goals through creating satisfaction. In short, the marketing orientation is really the antithesis of the selling orientation. As Peter Drucker (1973) stated,

> The aim of marketing is to make selling superfluous. The aim of marketing is to know and understand the consumer so well that the product or service fits him and sells itself. (p. 64)

Historically, the production and product orientations have dominated the health-care field. More recently, there has been a shifting trend toward the selling and, even more important, the marketing orientations. One impediment to a more rapid transition involves the difference between needs and perception of needs.

More specifically, the responsibility of identifying and responding to consumer health needs has traditionally fallen on health professionals who have defined these needs from the health profession's perspective rather than consideration of the actual utilities sought by consumers, or the motivations that influence human behavior. It is the focus on consumers to determine needs that makes marketing different relative to the predominant mode of patient service planning (Cooper, 1985).

The marketing orientation focuses on the concept that health-care organizations must meet consumer wants and needs, as determined by consumers, in order to survive. Marketing is, in part, a "state of mind." It is a willingness always to think of clients or patients first, recognizing that when patients feel satisfied, organizations can achieve their other goals as well.

The starting point for marketing is putting consumers first. It makes little sense to spend money developing a marketing strategy to increase the patient load of a private health-care provider's practice while ignoring basic "antimarketing" behavior among employees. For example, the same practitioners who are often willing to pay for marketing studies fail to see that they are losing patients every day because of the way the receptionist, nurse, or other caregiver is interacting with patients. In contrast, practitioners who realize that marketing means more than filling appointments or beds, and who provide services that consumers want, have been more successful than their less enlightened competitors.

There remains, however, a certain degree of skepticism with regard to applying the marketing concept to health care. Few companies object to the patient or consumer orientation but do object to the hard-sell and similar tactics sometimes used in aggressive marketing.

Few organizations, health-care or otherwise, have managed to truly adopt the philosophy of a consumer orientation. Many organizations only pay lip service to the philosophy and then wonder why marketing does not work as well as they expected. A major factor underlying a marketing orientation is that organizations must invest resources to determine what consumers truly want. This can be time-consuming and expensive. However, if marketing takes its rightful place at the center of provider decision making and focuses on consumers, it can have a significant impact on many of the important factors affecting cost (Duda, 1990).

What Marketing Is Not

Confusion and misunderstanding of marketing extends beyond the philosophies mentioned earlier, to the tools and tactics used in their practice. One must be careful not to equate marketing with either advertising or selling. As Peter Drucker (1973) noted, "Selling and marketing are antithetical rather than synonymous or even complementary" (p. 64). Advertising and personal selling are only two of the promotional tools available to the marketer. Ideally, companies select appropriate promotion tools after they have determined the appropriate consumer group (target market), designed services to satisfy those consumers, priced services at levels acceptable to both consumers and the organization, and developed a plan to make services available where consumers can obtain them.

Advertising through mass media (newspapers, magazines, radio, television, outdoor boards, and direct mail) and personal selling (direct one-to-one contact) are two of the ways a marketer can communicate with the target market. Advertising is a small but visible part of the marketing plan. Marketers sometimes select advertising as the most efficient way to communicate with consumers about an organization's offering. Marketers often use personal selling to communicate with small, narrowly defined target markets of decision makers who influence many other consumers. Because it is time consuming and extremely expensive, marketers direct personal selling primarily to employers who choose various health-care options for their companies; caregivers whose recommendations influence many potential consumers; and purchasers of goods that facilitate delivery of health care, such as medical equipment and supplies.

The Uniqueness of Marketing Services

There are some differences between services and physical products, as well as between services and service that health care organizations, as services providers, need to understand if they are to effectively practice marketing. A physical product is an object, device, or thing, whereas a service is a deed, performance, or effort (Berry, 1980). Consumers can touch, inspect, and store products until they are needed. Services, in contrast, are intangible. Consumers cannot feel, inspect, store, or return services if the purchase is unsatisfactory.

Organizations first manufacture and sell products before purchasers consume them. In contrast, services get sold prior to being produced and consumed. With services, provision and consumption often occur simultaneously. For example, patients first make appointments (are sold), and then psychologists are physically present (the product) to ask questions and develop diagnostic impressions of patients who participate in the process (consumption). Providers directly deliver services to consumers. Generally, with services, there are few intermediaries (channels of distribution) between providers of services and users of services. Some managed-care plans or hospital-based home health-care programs, nursing homes, or urgent-care centers could be considered intermediaries.

Because services are inseparable, one cannot inventory them. Even when a clinic has no appointments scheduled during certain hours, the facility and staff are still available. There is the capacity to produce services but no patients to consume them. If demand exceeds the number of appointment slots available, clinics must turn patients away because there is no inventory. In short, an important task of health-care providers is to match services' availability with services' demand.

Finally, services are, in many regards, more heterogeneous than physical products. Manufacturing companies can regulate quality of products within rather strict standards. Quality of health-care services, however, can vary from one provider to another in the same practice or hospital. Moreover, quality of care by the same caregiver will vary from day to day. People-based services (as opposed to machine-based services) are very difficult to standardize. Therefore, it is important to recognize that although patients may receive the same services, the services may be different (Zeithaml, Parasuraman, & Berry, 1990).

HEALTH-CARE CONSUMERS

The health-care market consists of a wide diversity of consumers, which includes patients, physicians, and other caregivers, third-party payers including managed care programs, and a variety of other consumers. One of the problems facing health-care marketers is to identify all of the diverse consumer groups in the market that health-care providers must satisfy and then focus on a specific target group. When an organization identifies its consumers in global, generic terms, such as "the market" or "everyone," it is clear that the managers do not understand marketing. Eventually, every organization realizes that trying to be everything to everybody is impractical.

Health-care organizations by nature have some inherent specializations (e.g., ambulatory care, long-term care, emergency medicine, psychological services) that determine who the consumers are. Yet, within these specialty areas, there are consumers with varying needs, wants, and desires. In order to focus on more meaningful, manageable groups of consumers, marketers engage in market segmentation and target marketing. This consists of identifying recognizable groups that make up the market and then selecting a group as the target market. Although organizations can target several groups, each group requires different marketing activities in order to achieve customer satisfaction.

Segmentation for a general psychology practice is more challenging than for a specialized addiction-treatment center. Even in addiction treatment, segments could include people addicted to alcohol, food, tobacco, or gambling. Also, the market in general psychology could be segmented by age (i.e., children or adults). Specialization of a hospital, nursing home, or physician's or psychologist's practice would be a first step in the segmentation process, but company planners must also consider other demographic, psychographic, geographic, and benefits factors as well.

Patients are consumers. However, the buyer–seller relationship of traditional exchange processes is different from the buyer–seller relationship in much of health care because patients depend on professional providers. Most people have no knowledge of medical terminology or the complexity of a medical diagnosis or care, and cannot accurately evaluate the health care provided. Hence, patients are dependent on professionals.

At one time, patients would never have questioned their providers' choices and decisions. Today, however, patients are more prone to shop for physicians who have privileges at the health-care institutions the patients prefer. In addition, third-party payers and the popular press have encouraged consumers to get second opinions for medical diagnoses and to express their preference for a particular hospital. Thus, choice of both physician and hospital has become part of the decision-making process. Moreover, providers who make the original diagnoses may not be the ones who continue the patients' care.

Largely because of changes in the health-care climate, health-care providers have directed a variety of marketing efforts toward patients. For example, health-care providers have used advertising to communicate with patients concerning the benefits (satisfaction) that they, the providers, have available. However, these providers must carefully develop the services offered in order to satisfy consumers *before* advertising will be effective. Public relations activities, such as heart-transplant recipient reunions, health fairs, baby fairs, and others, are additional ways that health-care providers can make information available to the public.

Physicians are another important target market because they often refer their patients to other health-care providers. Physicians are important consumers for hospitals because almost all patients admitted to a particular hospital are there because their physicians have staff privileges at, and recommended admission to that facility. If physicians choose not to admit patients to a given hospital, that hospital will have no patients. Thus, hospitals often devote significant efforts toward marketing to physicians.

Physicians use a referral system when patients need care that is outside their expertise. With the abundance of specialists, physicians are learning that marketing to other physicians is also important. Because physicians often recommend treatment in long-term care facilities, nursing homes, rehabilitation centers, home health-care organizations, and others have targeted physicians with their marketing efforts. Typically, patients or responsible caregivers choose facilities from the groups recommended by their physicians. If particular health-care providers are not in the suggested groups, there is little chance patients will consider the providers.

Third-party payers, which include insurance companies, managed care groups, governments, and employers, are another important consumer group that health-care providers must satisfy. Their fundamental concern is that health-care providers are efficiently treating patients while keeping costs under control. For example, AT&T entered into an agreement with three insurance companies in an attempt to contain health-care costs. By using designated health-care providers, employees pay a $150 deductible and receive 90% reimbursement for nonhospital procedures. If employees choose not to use designated providers, the deductible is $200 and reimbursement is set at 80% (Winslow, 1990).

As payers, insurance companies are important target markets for nursing homes, hospitals, and health-care institutions. If insurance companies do not feel satisfied with the quality of care or charges for procedures, they use their considerable financial influence to make changes. In addition, if the consumers of insurance companies (the patients) do not feel satisfied with the health care provided, those companies will feel compelled to react in order to satisfy their customers.

Other important target markets include state health departments, contributors, volunteers, and employees. State health departments actively compete with other agencies for public funding. It is important that the community (the health department's customer) and the legislators (the elected representatives for the general public) are aware of and understand the service provided by the health department. If the general public is not aware of the benefits that the health department is providing, government funding will be difficult to obtain. Similarly, hospitals and other health-care providers have community, state, and federal regulatory groups and funding agencies to satisfy.

Contributors and volunteers are especially important to nonprofit health-care organizations. Both groups have needs that these organizations must satisfy. Contributors want to think that their donations go to worthwhile organizations and that they can make a difference.

Volunteerism is an important part of the nonprofit health-care organization's ability to appear less institutional and more caring and friendly. Patients appreciate the pink ladies and candy stripers who are common in many nonprofit hospitals and extended-care facilities. Because of the increased number of women in the workforce, the ranks of volunteers have thinned, and there are many organizations that compete for their time. Therefore, organizations that depend on volunteers must satisfy volunteers' needs if such organizations expect volunteers to continue to contribute their time and energies to those organizations.

It is also important to consider needs of current and potential employees. Because of shortages of health-care professionals (current and projected), recruiting becomes a marketing activity aimed at satisfying needs of potential employees, not just at the time of hiring, but over their careers as well. Retention of the best and brightest employees has the potential to ease marketing efforts, especially in people-based services.

Organizations must remember to assess the impact of changes in marketing strategies toward one group in terms of potential impact on other groups. As an example, one hospital recognized that patients would favorably perceive the institution of a patient-advocacy program but that physicians might perceive such a program as inconvenient or even threatening. By positioning the advocacy program as a time-saving aid for physicians' hospital practices, both patients and physicians felt more satisfied (Koger & Perry, 1983).

Because there are many diverse consumer groups to serve, health-care institutions must direct a coordinated effort toward their various target markets. Each target market requires different marketing efforts and activities to successfully satisfy it. Because health-care organizations have several different target markets to satisfy, strategic marketing assumes an important role.

THE NEED FOR STRATEGIC MARKETING

Strategic marketing emphasizes long-term implications, corporate inputs (purpose, vision, mission, objectives, culture, resources, and publics), varying roles for service and market matching, and relationships between the marketing function and the rest of the organization. The need for strategic marketing has heightened in the current environment of increased competition, deregulation, acquisition of nonmarketing-type companies by marketing-driven companies, and demographic changes.

Too many hospital beds, the surging number of medical school graduates, and deregulation have collectively increased competition. Typically, when marketing-oriented firms enter an industry that has not focused on marketing, changes occur, and the health-care industry has been no exception. Many of the new marketing and profit-oriented organizations are sophisticated competitors. They are driving less effective competitors from the market by capturing profitable customers and leaving low-paying and charity cases. These are some of the complex issues that current health-care reform is attempting to address; it eventually may require renewed regulation or, at a minimum, changes in the way customers consume health care.

Increasing numbers of older individuals and patients with AIDS along with other demographic changes, will also affect the need for strategic marketing thought. For example, many women have now entered the workforce and are most often responsible for making household health-care choices. Employed women have less time than women who do not have gainful employment, so convenience is an increasingly important factor to them.

All of these factors have served to increase health-care managers' awareness of the strategic importance of marketing. The objective of strategic marketing is to create unique ways of satisfying consumers so that they will become loyal users of the health-care providers' services. In marketing terms, the objective is to attain a sustainable competitive advantage. There are numerous differentiation strategies available to health-care organizations. The myriad possibilities mean that there are no "cookbook" formulas or sweeping generalizations that organizations can readily apply. Determining the competitive advantage and the strategies for sustaining it are the result of the strategic-marketing process (Duncan, Ginter, & Swayne, 1992).

The Strategic-Marketing Process

The strategic-marketing process includes developing a market definition; conducting a thorough situational analysis; understanding the organization's purpose, vision, mission, and objectives; developing marketing objectives that will accomplish corporate objectives; and determining marketing strategies that will accomplish marketing objectives.

Market Definition

Developing a market definition is an important first step; managers can usually deduce a market definition from the mission statement, and such a definition is central to identifying the market served, competition, and key environmental factors that will determine the best strategic-marketing alternatives.

Marketers use a variety of methods to arrive at market definitions. Identifying the market has important implications for strategic planning, and thus marketers expend a great deal of effort to accurately define the market served.

Using multiple methods to identify the market is important because this helps to avoid overlooking some aspect of the organization's offerings, thereby minimizing an opportunity for others. Some health-care providers, by their very nature, predefine their market. Community hospitals, regional hospitals, and county public health departments, for example, serve specific markets.

One facet of defining the market is describing the *scope* or *segment* providers choose to serve. More specifically, providers identify consumer groups in terms of geography, demographics, or by benefits desired. Providers may limit services offered to specific procedures such as open-heart surgery, or to diseases such as AIDS. Providers might define their geographic or service area in terms of number-of-miles radius around a clinic that represents the distance patients would travel to see a provider. Obviously, willingness to travel will vary from one patient to another, depending on providers' reputations, referrals, access, parking, and proximity to patients' homes or workplaces. The scope could be a city, county, or regional area. Some health-care providers (particularly for-profit hospitals and nursing home chains) have determined that they want to be national in scope, whereas others have set goals to be international in scope. Providers may define their demographic scope by age (children's hospitals, elderly care), gender (birthing centers, mammography clinics), religion (Catholic, Presbyterian, or other denominational hospitals), and other specific, identifiable, and quantitative characteristics of the population.

Health-care managers must define scope in terms of benefits that consumers want, not those that health-care professionals consider desirable. Some patients want to use the same physicians that celebrities use. The benefit sought is prestige. Some patients want admission to a specific hospital because it has the reputation of having performed a necessary procedure most frequently. The perceived benefit is risk reduction through experience. Patients will consider the hospital that has performed the most heart–lung transplants as the most experienced. Some patients want admission to the hospital that has the latest technology or most up-to-date equipment. The benefit sought is risk reduction through advances in technology.

Health-care providers, like other service providers, often must narrow their market scope when there are limited resources, whether financial, natural, or human. Nursing shortages in some areas have caused hospitals to close units until the hospital could recruit the necessary number of nurses. It is easy (and often preferable) to narrow market scope when there exists a large enough set of consumers who feel satisfied by a specific benefit. Generally, health-care providers broaden the scope with successes over time as additional resources become available and they can achieve economies of scale.

Another aspect of market definition is identifying distinctive competencies and assets. Johns Hopkins Hospital has become known for its research and experimentation in bone marrow transplants for leukemia patients. This is a distinctive competency, something it does better than many others. To maintain distinctive competence is a never-ending pursuit as competitors identify, improve, and adopt new ideas, services, and benefits to better satisfy consumers.

An asset is something the health-care provider has that is more valuable than what other providers possess. For example, a clinic located in a densely populated, built-up area may prevent other clinics from being able to build in that location. For either a distinctive competence or an asset to be of true value, consumers must perceive that competence or asset as beneficial. Consumers form this perception in connection with competitive offerings.

Definition of markets can also be in terms of growth opportunities, such as service or market development, market penetration, and diversification. When organizations introduce new services, they are pursuing *service development*. Adding an AIDS clinic or a hospital wing dedicated to adolescent-addiction treatment, which introduces new services for a hospital, is an example of service development.

Entering new markets with the same services previously offered is *market development*. A psychologist, for instance, who opens a satellite office in a nearby community is attempting to grow by market development.

Market penetration is attempting to increase the number of the type of consumers who need the same type of existing services. An example would be a group practice attempting to increase market share by directing marketing efforts toward increased usage by consumers in the area who currently are served by the practice.

Diversification is seeking new opportunities in new markets with new services. It is the riskiest endeavor, and it is not without frustration. Health-care organizations, as well as many others industries, have discovered that diversification can be very expensive and fraught with pitfalls. Unfamiliarity with products or services and the market has led to many business failures.

Situational Analysis

Health-care providers must understand their current market situation to develop the most effective marketing strategy. A situational analysis is one phase in the process of marketing-strategy development. The key to developing a situational analysis that will assist in providing organizations with strategic direction lies in determining market definition. Questions that organizations must focus on include what business they are in, what consumers needs and wants are, and how well they are satisfying consumers (Duncan et al., 1992).

Consumer Analysis

Research provides the means of conducting consumer analyses. Data sources will be both internal and external; providers must collect data from infrequent users and nonusers as well as current clients. Marketing research firms or consultants can serve to gather information about a market.

Health-care organizations can use secondary data already collected by someone else. Although this type of data has the advantage of being quickly available at low or no cost, the information may not answer specific questions that health-care organizations want answered. For example, census data by ZIP code may be available and sufficient for some purposes, but for other, more complex marketing decisions concerning new service offerings, office location, and other decisions, primary research may be necessary. Patient records, a form of secondary data, can provide a great deal of information about such things as percentages of patients covered by third-party payers, addresses, repeat business (If a mother comes to the hospital for her second delivery, which facility did she use for the first?), and other important patient data.

Primary data are data that organizations collect for their own use, and it likely answers specific questions. Disadvantages of primary data collection are high cost and length of time it takes to generate information. To delve into individuals' attitudes toward health care at a particular practice, clinic, or hospital, it may be necessary to conduct primary research, such as surveying previous patients, potential patients, and nonpatients (those who use competitors). Focus groups (usually a group of 10 to 15 individuals who come together for an hour or two to discuss issues presented by an impartial moderator) can provide useful information about how consumers perceive services, hospitals, clinics, or practices.

Competitor Analysis

In times of provider and facility shortage there is less concern about competition. With the current oversupply, however, most health-care providers are competing for patients. In order to develop effective marketing strategies, it is important to identify which health-care institutions are direct competitors and which are indirect competitors.

Competition occurs at various levels in the environment. The most general level of competition is *generic competition*. Consumers have a need for health care, which a variety of health-care providers can satisfy. At the generic level, those providers might include hospitals, clinics, urgent-care centers, physicians' or psychologists' offices, or home health care.

Specific competition would include "like kind" providers of health care. Examples include hospitals that compete directly for both patients and physicians, nursing homes that compete, or physicians who compete in the same specialty.

Services competition occurs at the product level. Emergency rooms, delivery rooms, or surgery are examples of services offered by hospitals. The most specific level of competition would be at the brand level. Although most hospitals and other health-care providers have not branded the services they offer, a few have. "New Life," a psychiatric service for Christians, is a brand of product offered by Western Medical Center in Anaheim, California. Other wings of the medical center offer different products. "Free Home Care" is a product of Olsten Health Care Services, Inc., a home health-care agency. When patients use Olsten's services as a result of hospital referrals, the hospitals build up credits for days of care that it can use to provide home health care for other patients who cannot afford it and do not have insurance or other benefits to pay for it. "CareBank" is a similar product offered by CareTeam Management Services, Inc.

Health-care providers must identify competition in terms of quantity and quality. There may be many providers of health care in a given region, but they will not all be of the same quality. It is important that strategic marketing managers accurately identify competition in order to develop a sustainable competitive advantage.

Primary competitors offer the same or very similar services and are direct competition. Secondary competitors provide some of the same services, but they may be worse (or better) at it, or they may be farther from the service area. This type of competition is more indirect. Tertiary competitors offer an alternative or substitute product; they are indirect competitors. For example, if a nursing home is full, patients might choose to use home health care as a substitute until space becomes available in a nursing home.

Because marketing professionals identify competition in customers' terms, it is often necessary to conduct marketing research to identify competition from customers' points of view rather than providers' points of view. A few questions to recent maternity patients could determine competition for the obstetrics service of a hospital: Which hospitals did your physician recommend? If the hospital you selected had been full, where would you have gone for delivery? Which hospitals did you consider? Which hospitals did you visit? Why did you choose this hospital for your baby's delivery? How satisfied were you with the experience? Would you choose the same hospital for the birth of your next child?

Marketing Objectives

Setting marketing objectives follows a hierarchical structure. Thus, after any situational analysis, a review of organizational missions and objectives is the starting point for determining marketing objectives. If organizations achieve their marketing objectives, those objectives will likely help them accomplish their overall objectives. Marketing objectives typically include revenues, market share, growth, innovation, and public responsibility (Duncan et al., 1992).

It is important to set *revenue* objectives and tie them to other objectives. Merely setting an objective for some dollar amount expected to come into a healthcare organization is shortsighted because outflow of money is also crucial. An example of a marketing revenue objective would be to generate revenues of $12.5 million by year's end while holding expenses to budgeted amounts.

Market share objectives are tricky because percentages depend on quantity and quality of competitors in the selected markets. For example, a local community hospital could say that is has a 100% share of the market (town) that it serves because it is the only hospital located in that town or community. But the important question is: How many people leave town for their medical care? Consequently, hospitals use a variation of market share based on occupancy rates or bed census data.

Growth is usually set as a percentage over the previous year in terms of revenue, market share, or census rates. Growth for growth's sake is not always desirable, which is sometimes a difficult lesson to learn. Almost any organization can reach growth objectives, but at what cost? Often, remaining the same size and increasing profitability is a more important objective.

Innovation objectives could include new services that providers will offer, speeding up service delivery, or being the leader in developing or offering new technology.

Most nonprofit hospitals, nursing homes, and hospices have publicly mandated *public responsibility* objectives. Many for-profit providers have also included public or social responsibility in their objectives. For example, some hospitals aim to serve a certain percent of indigent patients or to return a certain amount of money to their communities in the form of health benefits.

MARKETING IMPLEMENTATION STRATEGIES

No position of leadership lasts forever. The dynamic health-care market and ever-changing technology mean that no provider can sustain competitive advantage in the long run without a great deal of thought and effort. To further complicate the strategic process, the long run itself is becoming shorter as the rate of change becomes increasingly rapid. Managed care has changed many of the business relationships and patterns in health care. However, the need for marketing strategies remains keen.

There is no single, established way in which health-care organizations can ensure success; rather, several possibilities exist. To achieve a sustainable competitive advantage, there are four basic marketing implementation strategies: differentiation, low cost, focus, and horizontal integration (Duncan, Ginter, & Swayne, 1992). Health-care organizations can accomplish these marketing strategies in a variety of ways.

Differentiation Strategies

Differentiation strategies center around services offered but go beyond the fundamental core service. They include quality of service, faster service delivery, technological innovation, services innovation, and reliability.

Most health-care providers like to think they can differentiate their institution on the basis of the service they offer to consumers. Health-care providers often mention *quality*, but they only partially determine quality. It is consumers' perceptions of what constitutes quality that consumers will use to judge quality of service. To consumers, providers achieve quality service only when the service meets or exceeds expectations.

Realistically, consumers can only perceive quality from other environmental cues because few people have the expertise to actually judge competent medical care. Thus, consumers use cues they observe, such as friendly nurses, clean and pleasant surroundings, prompt responses to patient call buzzers/lights and questions, and convenient hours of operation to judge quality for many hospitals, long-term care providers, and private practices.

Individual consumers are not the only health-care customers to judge quality, however. Physicians and other health-care professionals are more likely to judge quality of an institution by assessing equipment, physicians who are currently on staff (or who have staff privileges), competence of nursing staff, and organization and leadership provided by nonmedical staff.

Health-care organizations can formulate strategies to improve or maintain quality over time. When these organizations allow quality to deteriorate, whether planned or unplanned, public use of their facilities will eventually decline as well. Hospitals' emergency rooms are generally resource consumers, but they can increase admissions by 25% or more. If a community hospital's emergency room is using cash and does not lead to at least some increase in admissions, hospital administrators might neglect it and allow it to deteriorate over time, and it is likely that this perception of deterioration would also carry over to the rest of the institution. To avoid this unplanned side effect, it might be better to face the issue squarely. Especially in the case of community hospitals, those hospitals could hold public meetings to demonstrate to citizens that the hospitals cannot afford to provide quality emergency care and, with group consensus, decide to close the units.

Consumers are increasingly impatient. They value their time and will not wait for service. Consumers share horror stories about such things as long waits in emergency rooms and sick patients being left in wheelchairs outside X-ray rooms with family and friends. To avoid negative word-of-mouth communication, caregivers need to think about *faster service delivery*. To "speed service delivery" does not mean to do things faster but to rethink why delays occur and correct underlying reasons. Faster responsiveness can develop into a sustainable competitive advantage.

Waiting time in providers' offices represents another opportunity. One busy professional calls the physician's office on the morning of his appointment and politely informs the receptionist that it is his policy to wait no longer than 15 minutes. He then inquires as to the physician's current schedule. If the doctor is behind, for whatever reason, and the caller would have to wait longer than 15 minute, he reschedules the appointment. If it happens more than once, he changes doctors. Most people understand emergencies, but when a doctor's staff consistently overschedules so that patients have long waiting times, many patients will find new physicians.

Another way a health-care organization may improve patients' or potential patients' perception that it provides quality care is to inform them about some of the special diagnostic capabilities and treatment expertise that the hospital or clinic offers. When organizations select differentiation through *technological innovation,* large sums of money must be available, because breakthroughs in medical equipment are costly. The price for new technology generally decreases over time, but in order to maintain technological innovation as a competitive strategy, there must be money to purchase new equipment as soon as it becomes available. Communicating information about new technology to patients is another necessary and expensive part of maintaining technological innovation as a competitive advantage.

Being a *services innovator* can provide differentiation opportunities. The first hospitals to offer physician referral services met needs of two of their consumers— patients and physicians. The hospital that developed the referral service first could use it as a differentiating strategy. When others copy the new service with a similar offering, there is less opportunity to differentiate.

Reliability, or standardization to achieve consistent quality, is another differentiating strategy. Service reliability is a goal for most health-care organizations. Services are difficult to standardize because consumers participate in the simultaneous production and consumption of services and, as previously indicated, human beings involved in health-care delivery (patients, physicians, nurses, therapists) are not capable of performing in the same way every time they might encounter the same situation. However, prescribed routines known to all can achieve some level of consistency in admitting procedures, new-patient procedures, preoperative preparation, and discharge planning.

Many freestanding urgent-care facilities have attempted to standardize procedures and thereby provide the additional benefit of "avoiding long emergency-room waiting time." However, patients who need procedures that are more complex and do not fit the standards of the urgent-care facility are generally sent to a hospital emergency room.

Using Differentiation Strategies

Corporations must exercise some caution when selecting any of the differentiation strategies. Differentiation will not work when the superior attribute highlighted is meaningless or unimportant to consumers. Additionally, if health-care providers have differentiating attributes that provide benefits but consumers do not know about it, there is no advantage. One possible example would be a new technology that helps better to diagnose patients' problems but for which the patients are unconscious when the equipment is in use. Patients will not perceive the benefit unless told that the hospital cares enough to purchase the wonderful, new equipment that works so much faster (or is less intrusive, or whatever the benefit may be).

It is important for health-care managers to realize that there is a cost in not providing quality in the delivery of health care. As previously mentioned, lawsuits abound. In addition, there are costs associated with doing things incorrectly. Consider hospital or nursing homes' billing statements that contain errors. Not only is there the cost of finding the errors and redoing the statements, there is also the cost of losing positive consumer attitudes and perhaps patients.

Cost-Leadership Strategies

Although cost-leadership strategies generally produce low costs that organizations can then translate into low prices, a high-priced strategy can effectively position organizations as quality health-care providers. However, consumers must perceive that the benefits (aesthetically pleasant surroundings, attentive care, or latest technology) are worth the higher price.

In manufacturing, being the low-cost producer in an industry can be a significant competitive advantage. It allows firms to make many more choices about price, quality, and profitability of their products. Cost-leadership strategies include reduction of overhead, control of raw materials, reduction of labor costs, redesign of the offering, automation, location, increase of government subsidy, absence of frills, and combination of low cost and high quality (Duncan et al., 1992). Many of these cost strategies seem manufacturing-oriented, but they have important marketing implications. However, health-care providers must carefully select and evaluate low-cost strategies before implementing them. Few people want to think that they are receiving "cheap" health are.

Organizations usually select *reduced overhead* strategy when they are mature. Overhead generally consists of rent, utilities, and other expenses that would occur even if there were no patients. It can also include administrative salaries, insurance, and other ongoing costs.

It might be that certain health-care providers invest too much money in overhead during times of growth. Many organizations are quick to add employees and facilities when times are good, but they rarely cut back when times are difficult. The result is excessive overhead. One way for hospitals to reduce overhead is to close wings or eliminate infrequently-used departments. Sometimes spending more money can reduce overhead, as when a physician moves to a newer building with more energy-efficient heating and cooling.

Control of raw materials or factors of production can provide a competitive advantage in terms of price as well as availability. When the University of Virginia was having difficulty recruiting nurses, the administration decided to provide financial assistance to those nursing students who agreed to practice nursing at the medical center after graduation. This gave the administration much more control over the hospital's major factor in service production—its nurses.

Reducing labor costs is a difficult strategy to implement for today's health-care organizations. As with other service industries, health care is labor intensive. In addition, the industry requires skilled labor. With the shortage of trained personnel, wages and salaries are going up rather rapidly. Moreover, qualified personnel must meet certification standards. Thus, certification standards, skilled-labor shortages, and wage inflation make it difficult to reduce labor costs. Rather than focus on reducing costs of labor, health-care organizations must place greater emphasis on proper scheduling, job redesign, and other forms of efficiency. By better matching consumer demand and labor availability, organizations can reduce costs.

Another cost-leadership strategy is to *redesign the offering,* changing the product offered so that it becomes less costly but no less desirable. Extended-care facilities that enjoy excellent reputations in their communities for cleanliness, good food, and competent and sympathetic caregivers could probably reduce square footage in patients' rooms—and thereby reduce cost of construction, heating and cooling, and maintenance—without harming their image.

Labor-intensive services are difficult, but not impossible, to *automate.* Blood pressure checks have become automated. Additionally, it may be possible to automate finger sticks for routine blood work by using a machine, but would the public accept a machine instead of a nurse? In another service industry, many bankers held on to their belief that consumers would want to talk to real people when cashing checks or depositing money. Those banks that were the first to automate with teller machines have been very profitable. Can health-care organizations achieve results similar to those in the banking industry?

A *location* that is attractive because of its proximity to patients' homes and work is a valuable asset, especially if other health-care providers cannot duplicate its convenience. Because people do not want to travel great distances for most health care, demographic studies of population are an important part of choosing a location for a facility. Satellite offices and hospital branches have become increasingly important in order to be available where patients want to receive care. Although satellite offices/hospitals do not typically cut costs for organizations, they do cut costs for patients, which can lead to increased market share and improved efficiency for health-care providers.

Some hospitals are finding it worthwhile to establish education centers in shopping malls. These centers can enhance hospitals' reputations by demonstrating their commitment to provide easily accessible outpatient health care and increase the hospitals' visibilities, which in turn can lead to increased bed census rates and economies of scale.

Mobile units are another method of achieving the optimum in health-care delivery. Long practiced by the Red Cross to gain more blood donations, other institutions are using movable diagnostic equipment in order to be closer to patients.

Increased Government Subsidy

Many nonprofit hospitals, extended-care facilities, and hospices have *government subsidies.* Organizations that have done a good job of keeping the public and lawmakers informed of the benefits they provide often find it easier to obtain increased subsidies.

A *no-frills* strategy eliminates all "extras" from services, a rather direct approach that tells consumers from the beginning that there will be no frills and in return they will receive a lower price. Home health care offered by hospitals seems to fit this strategy. On the other hand, many individuals admitted to large hospital wards perceive few "frills." Health-care providers must exercise caution in positioning "no frills" so that patients perceive the providers have only eliminated extras. Otherwise, the perception may be of poor care.

The *combination low cost and high quality* offers higher cost services only to consumers who prefer it. Organizations can then actually reduce overall costs by moving along the experience curve and achieving economies of scale (brought about by increased market share). Accurate assessment of demand, careful planning, and increased expertise (actual movement along the experience curve) are crucial to successful implementation of this strategy.

Focus Strategies

Organizations that have limited resources often implement focus strategies. Such organizations do not compete across the board, but only in selected areas. These organizations narrow market definition to identify select groups to serve. Thus, those companies can then devote enough resources to targeted consumer groups to achieve some degree of prominence or even dominance. In addition, increased specialization may lead to development of greater understanding and satisfaction on the part of the particular groups targeted, which may in turn increase usage and loyalty.

A sharply focused strategy has the benefit of being difficult for competition to attack. At the same time, such a strategy often restricts organizations' abilities to grow. Focus strategies include service, segment, geographic area, and low-share markets (Duncan et al., 1992).

A focused *service* is one part of a service line. Rather than attempting to offer a complete line of services, which usually includes low revenue producers and some services that yield high revenue, organizations offer only a part of a service line. Usually, organizations will focus on services in which they have greater expertise and when they believe that they can achieve some economies of scale with smaller service lines.

A teen counseling center has selected a focus strategy based on the *segment* served. A nursing home that focuses on Alzheimer's patients has also selected a focus strategy. Most community hospital use the *geographic area* strategy. They serve a specific geographic market and are the only hospital in the area. Private practices of individual psychologists generally use geographic-area focus strategies as well. As the practices develop and flourish, those psychologists may open second offices that extend their geographic areas.

Low-share markets are markets that are not of sufficient size to interest larger health-care providers. Hospital or physicians' practices that specialize in less common diseases can satisfy smaller markets extremely well and thereby service virtually all of the patients with those diseases. This strategy can be more profitable than trying to capture very small parts of larger markets that include many large and knowledgeable competitors. This strategy emphasizes profitability rather than size or growth.

Horizontal Integration

Horizontal integration occurs when one competitor buys out another. The competitors are essentially on the "same level," thus the term *horizontal integration*. In essence, organizations that are buying competitors are buying market shares. From a marketing perspective, the concern is which competitor will best enhance those organizations' strategies.

Many nonprofit organizations do not have choices, but receive orders from their governing or regulating bodies that they will take over operations of another facility (usually one that is performing poorly). For-profit organizations buy out others for a variety of reasons: to increase market share, to achieve economies of scale, to gain the other organizations' experiences in the market, or to eliminate aggressive competitors.

With horizontal integration, companies must consider organizational issues as well as matches between purchasing organizations' marketing strategies and purchased organizations' strategies. If the organizations are similar, integration can occur smoothly. But if the strategies are different, organizational executives must decide whether to change strategies to be more like purchasing organizations' strategies (or vice versa), or to broaden the services offered by maintaining strategies of both the purchased and purchasing organizations. Executives of purchasing organizations must discuss these considerations before the acquisition to determine if there is good strategic fit.

IMPLEMENTING THE STRATEGY

Once organizational executives have selected general implementation strategies, marketing management's task is to translate generalities of the strategies into meaningful distinctions for consumers. Selected strategies become marketing strategies when managers select target markets and develop marketing mixes to meet target markets' needs. Marketers must design and coordinate elements of a marketing mix—product, price, distribution (location of delivery), and promotion—to present the competitive advantage to targeted consumers. Answers to each of the questions posed in the exhibit are different depending on which marketing implementation strategy company executives select—differentiation, cost leadership, or focus strategies.

Once company personnel have identified target markets and determined marketing mixes, marketing strategies will provide sustainable comparative advantages and serve as cornerstones for making decisions. In addition, it is important for company executives to review their marketing strategies on a periodic basis to make sure their organization's competitive advantage still exists and remains desirable to consumers. When competitive pressure is increasing, revenue is decreasing or static during expected periods of growth, or excess of revenues over expenses is declining, health-care managers must reassess whether the competitive advantage is still meaningful to consumers.

The market naturally works to cut competitive advantages of leaders by technological and environmental changes that erode protective barriers. Additionally, competitors learn how to imitate leaders and negate or equalize competitive advantages. Organizations themselves might not take action to protect their positions. This passive reaction may occur either because companies do not perceive a threat from competitors or because those companies dismiss the threat as unimportant. Sometimes organizations do not respond because they consider any action detrimental to their overall strategy.

Organizations can engage in defensive moves to thwart prospective challengers. One defensive move is to signal intentions to defend a position. If smaller hospitals announce their intention to build specialized labor/delivery rooms, larger competitors in the region might increase their advertising budgets to promote their already-in-place specialized maternity care. The larger competitors have then signaled that they will defend their positions.

Another move to thwart prospective challengers is to attempt to foreclose avenues for attack, such as when large group practices add previously uncovered specialties in order to provide comprehensive care. "Raising the stakes" is another way to combat competition. Hospitals that purchase high-tech diagnostic equipment that no other hospital in the area can afford are raising the stakes.

Finally, competitors attempting to thwart prospective challengers might attempt to reduce attractiveness of challengers' markets by using mass media, which has covered health care extensively. For example, several individuals have written articles about financial and personnel difficulties that home health-care organizations face. Potential entrants to the industry may find it less attractive if they have exposure to such articles or similar commentaries in mass media.

The final step in implementing any strategy is assessment or control. Marketing audits look at all marketing activities to determine if there are areas where marketing could improve, if marketing efforts are supporting organizational missions, goals, and strategic objectives, and if results of marketing efforts were as planned.

SUMMARY AND CONCLUSIONS

Marketing is relatively new to most health-care organizations. This chapter has traced evolution of acceptance that most organizations follow from a production orientation through a selling orientation to a marketing orientation. The basics of marketing-oriented health-care providers include customer satisfaction, integrated marketing efforts, and provision of value for both parties (i.e., customers and providers) in the exchange process.

This chapter has discussed the variety of health-care customers—including physicians, patients, third-party payers, volunteers, and employees—and has illustrated their interdependence. Physicians admit patients to hospitals; third-party payers influence physicians' choices, patients' lengths of stay in the hospital, and other factors; volunteers and employees may also be patients; and government entities interpret need for additional health-care subsidies for the public.

Because of competition and complexity in the market, health-care providers must implement strategic marketing in order to survive. The strategic-marketing process involves determining markets served, analyzing situations (i.e., customers, competitors, and environmental factors), reviewing organizational missions and objectives, setting marketing objectives, and determining marketing strategies.

This chapter has illustrated how companies realize divisional positioning strategies—differentiation, cost leadership, focus, and horizontal integration—through marketing-implementation strategies. Finally, company executives develop marketing strategies through decisions regarding target market, product, promotion, price, and distribution. Successful health-care organizations use marketing strategies to drive their efforts.

REFERENCES

Berry, L. L. (1980). Services marketing is different. *Business, 30,* 24–30.
Cooper, P. D. (1985). *Health care marketing: Issues and trends.* Germantown, MD: Aspen Systems Corporation.
Drucker, P. F. (1973). *Management, tasks, responsibilities, practices.* New York: Harper & Row.
Duda, D. F. (1990, April 16). Marketing must turn savage. *Modern Healthcare,* p. 50.
Duncan, W. J., Ginter, P. M., & Swayne, L. E. (1992). *Strategic management of health care organizations.* Boston: PWS-Kent.
Folland, S. T. (1987). Advertising by physicians: Behavior and attitudes. *Medical Care, 25,* 311–326.
Koger, D. A., & Perry, F. L. (1983, May–June). Physician-centered marketing: A practical step to hospital survival. *Hospital and Health Services Administration,* pp. 43–53.
Kotler, P. (1972). A generic concept of marketing. *Journal of Marketing, 36,* 46–54.
Kotler, P., & Clarke, R. N. (1987). *Marketing for health care organizations.* Englewood Cliffs, NJ: Prentice-Hall.
Kotler, P., & Levy, S. J. (1969). Broadening the concept of marketing. *Journal of Marketing, 33,* 10–15.
Kotler, P., & Zaltman, G. (1971). Social marketing: An approach to planned social change. *Journal of Marketing, 35,* 3–12.
Winslow, R. (1990, July 19). AT&T's plan on health costs may set pattern. *The Wall Street Journal,* pp. B-1, B-3.
Zaltman, G., & Vertinsky, I. (1971). Health services marketing: A suggested model. *Journal of Marketing, 35,* 19–27.
Zeithaml, V. A., Parasuraman, A., & Berry, L. L. (1990). *Delivering quality service.* New York: The Free Press.

VI
EPILOGUE

31

The Future of Psychology in Health Care

Anthony J. Goreczny and Colleen M. O'Halloran

INTRODUCTION

The areas of health and rehabilitation psychology have grown tremendously. They are two of the fastest growing areas within the American Psychological Association. However, these areas, as well as all of the areas within the health professions, face enormous changes as health-care reform takes shape. There will be an increase in pressure on health-care professionals to provide evidence that their programs are effective and cost efficient. Health-care professionals also face challenges posed by changing demographics within the United States. Psychology as a discipline faces renewed challenges, and practitioners within the field must ensure that those outside our discipline recognize the contributions we have to offer. In this chapter, we review the changing health-care environment and psychology's role in it, discuss the importance of continuing to develop cooperative ventures with other disciplines and promoting recognition of psychology's achievements, highlight the need for advances in assessment, emphasize the importance of health psychologists becoming more involved in consulting on policy-making decisions without ignoring economic and political realities, and present one possible proposal for decreasing rates of one of the most significant risk factors contributing to premature death—smoking. Following these segments is a section in which we emphasize the need to step away from a provincial view of health care toward an international perspective. The chapter concludes with a summary section.

Anthony J. Goreczny • Highland Drive Veterans Affairs Medical Center and University of Pittsburgh School of Medicine, Pittsburgh, Pennsylvania 15206. **Colleen M. O'Halloran** • Highland Drive Veterans Affairs Medical Center, Pittsburgh, Pennsylvania 15206.
Handbook of Health and Rehabilitation Psychology, edited by Anthony J. Goreczny. Plenum Press, New York, 1995.

HEALTH-CARE COVERAGE

This section examines problems that have occurred in the age of managed mental health care, suggests the need for a different delivery system in the new reform packages, discusses advantages of including adequate mental health benefits, and outlines the important future directions for health psychologists' treatment and research in light of political influences and economic constraints.

Managed mental health care (MMHC) presents numerous difficulties for mental health professionals and can, in fact, contribute to rising health-care costs. One significant problem is the inherent financial incentives in MMHC to provide inpatient versus outpatient care and to deny outpatient care beyond an arbitrary number of visits without regard for various presenting problems. For example, consumers often feel financially coerced into choosing a 20% inpatient copayment versus a 50% outpatient copayment.

The systems for approving inpatient versus outpatient care also differ in important ways. Individuals conducting precertification for inpatient care often have affiliations with admitting hospitals and thus have an interest in filling beds rather than in reducing inpatient utilization (Welch, 1993c). Utilization review boards for outpatient care, on the other hand, usually have affiliations with managed-care organizations and thus feel financially driven to deny care. One survey found that utilization review boards denied outpatient psychotherapy extensions to 60% of patients not using "preferred provider" psychologists (Adler, 1991). Also, authorities on utilization boards do not have requirements mandating that they possess the same educational qualifications as individuals in the professional service they are reviewing, thereby making their judgments questionable and possibly negligent to consumers. The utilization board process has a particularly negative effect on psychological services because confidentiality and cohesive, continuous treatment may be impossible to maintain.

Inpatient incentives and limited initial assessments that often occur in MMHC systems (Welch, 1992b) lead to an inefficient and ineffective distribution of health-care resources. The largest drain on inpatient mental health care is an almost exclusive use of inpatient stays for acting-out adolescents and substance abusers. Researchers have found that as many as half of these individuals could receive treatment in outpatient settings with similar or improved results, most likely because patients and therapists are better able to evaluate environmental effects on the problem behaviors. Inpatient incentives also encourage consumers to rely on the most expensive treatments and providers (i.e., physicians).

Some reformers of health care believe mental health benefits themselves are simply too expensive for inclusion in reform plans. However, it is important to note that mental health problems often lead to increased medical utilization and thus to a rise in overall health-care costs. For example, patients may unnecessarily receive very expensive diagnostic tests for psychosomatic complaints. Evidence found in 21 of 22 studies revealed a 46% decrease in medical utilization after substance-abuse treatment and a 26% decrease in utilization after general mental health treatment (Youngstrom, 1991). Mental health problems can also lead to difficulties in the workplace, including a decrease in productivity and a rise in absenteeism. As a benefit in their policies, 140 Canadian and Australian life insurance companies have offered 12 visits to a psychologist per year. Independent evaluators have conducted assessments of this benefit for some of the companies and already have found a subsequent drop in disability benefits, use of psychotropic medication, and absenteeism in the work place (DeAngelis, 1991).

Policy makers who have suggested health-care reform plans have continued to skew plans in favor of the more expensive treatment options. For example, consultants to the National Institutes of Mental Health suggested a plan in which consumers pay a 20% copayment for psychotropic medicines and a 50% copayment for psychotherapy (Barron, 1992). The Russo Bill allows for 20 outpatient psychotherapy visits and 45 inpatient visits per year. In that plan, however, partial hospitalization can substitute for inpatient days (Youngstrom, 1992). President Clinton's Health Security Act provides 30 visits of outpatient psychotherapy at a 50% copayment and 60 days of inpatient treatment at a 20% copayment. If the particular plan allows, patients can substitute four outpatient psychotherapy visits for one inpatient day. However, the plan does not mandate that option at this time (Sleek, 1993).

One problem with the suggested health-care plans is the lack of provision for preventive and specialty psychological services. Health psychologists, for instance, can provide services that teach consumers how to have healthy lifestyles. Such treatment would include smoking cessation, weight control through proper nutrition and exercise, stress management, and relaxation training. These preventive services are extremely important in decreasing overall health-care costs, because 7 out of the 10 major medical illnesses are "lifestyle diseases" (DeAngelis, 1992). Also, health psychologists can offer specialty services, such as pain management, biofeedback, communication skills training, and chronic illness management, including compliance with treatment regimens and preprocedures or presurgery anxiety reduction. Clinicians can provide most of these preventive and specialty services in group settings, which further decreases the overall cost to the health-care system. Also, evaluation of interventions can occur in the context of interdisciplinary teams so that services can build on one another and health-care teams can avoid duplication of treatment. These preventive and specialty provisions rely on good front-end assessment, however. As stated earlier, the current MMHC system does not consist of well-trained individuals conducting initial assessments. Preventive/specialty services have the potential to increase the speed at which consumers' problems are effectively solved and decrease their need for more extensive services. However, in order to do this, patients must receive referrals to those services correctly and efficiently.

The American Psychological Association's Integrated Care Plan (Welch, 1992a) offers some improvements on the current system. One aspect is a focus on initial assessment through psychological assessment procedures, including psychological testing. This plan necessitates that highly educated personnel conduct initial evaluations because of the importance of sending patients to the most appropriate services the first time. Thus, the emphasis is not only on cost-effective treatment but also on quality treatment.

Another important part of the plan is elimination of a managed-care entity (Newman, 1993). Providers of psychological services deal directly with third-party payers, which may be the patient's employers, for example. Thus, the utilization review process is different. Individuals conducting reviews act more as case managers than as outside reviewers (Welch, 1993a). This type of arrangement allows for more equitable treatment-limit decisions because reviewers will be integrated team members and have educational backgrounds similar to those of providers.

The utilization review process in this plan also places the most restrictions on the most expensive benefits (i.e., inpatient treatment; Welch, 1992a). In fact, utilization review would not even take place on outpatient mental health services unless patients used more than 52 sessions per year (Michaelson, 1993). These is some evidence to support use of the Integrated Care Plan in that Bell South in New Orleans successfully implemented it, which subsequently resulted in a decrease in mental health benefit costs to that corporation (Moses-Zirkes, 1993).

Although a plan such as Integrated Care offers improvements on the current method of MMHC, psychologists must also make changes in order to realistically survive in the marketplace. Fox (1994) suggested that psychologists move away from an emphasis on diagnosing and treating mental illness and instead move toward broader behavioral health problems. According to Fox, the direction for psychology is to provide a wide range of services to enhance human effectiveness. This focus not only allows psychologists to become integral members of the health-care process, but also places health psychologists in the prime position to provide these services. Nonetheless, in this age of cost effectiveness, psychologists must demonstrate that they have clear treatment goals that are continent on presenting problems and supporting assessment materials, and also provide evidence that their treatments are effective with the problem behaviors in the least amount of time, relative to other potential treatments.

Use of treatment contracts with time limits on psychological services is one way to demonstrate well-devised, front-end assessments and clearer goals. Also, health and rehabilitation psychologists could assist in development of practice guidelines for specified problem areas, such as those developed for management of cancer-related pain and poststroke rehabilitation (Clinton, McCormick, & Besteman, 1994). Psychologists could develop practice guidelines for other specific services rendered, such as treatment for bereavement and trauma of a psychosocial nature. Such guidelines would demonstrate psychologists' willingness to hold themselves accountable for their treatments. Of course, in order to provide effective treatment, patients must be agreeable to suggested treatment plans and adhere appropriately. Thus, psychologist–patient communication must be a priority as well.

It is important to note that adequate outcome research and outcome measures are necessary if psychologists are to effectively market their services to reform politicians and to corporations that may potentially fund plans mandated by Clinton's Health Security Act. In order to reach the goals established by President Clinton's health plan, it appears that we must conduct research on the "dose-effect" relationship (Howard, Kopta, Krause, & Orlinsky, 1986) as it applies to particular treatments for specific problem areas. Psychologists must show how many sessions are necessary to assist a certain percentage of patients' return to adequate functioning. We also need to conduct studies on effectiveness of interdisciplinary treatment plans that include psychotherapy and psychotropic medications.

COMPETITIVE COOPERATION

The diseases of lifestyle, which are currently the primary killers in the United States, require multidisciplinary treatment—team cooperation to effectively and efficiently assess, diagnose, treat, and rehabilitate affected patients. Most hospitals have some type of multidisciplinary team available. However, in this highly competitive marketplace, we must not be so blind as to believe that cooperation will always take place. In our capitalistic society, an emphasis on profits drives companies and individuals to compete. In this increasingly competitive health-care arena, different disciplines will jockey for competitive advantage. Miller (1992) recognized this concern but also noted that it has the positive potential to force practitioners to demonstrate cost efficacy of their procedures. Although this has some advantages for the population at large, we must monitor the situation in order to ensure that no one field attempts to achieve a monopoly by excluding other fields.

Disciplines can attempt to achieve a monopoly on services in any one of several ways. For instance, McKegney and Schwartz (1986) used the guise of improving treatment quality and access to behavioral medicine practitioners as a means of recommending that behavioral medicine practitioners serve under departments of psychiatry, with physicians as gatekeepers to behavioral medicine services. Such an organizational structure places behavioral medicine practitioners in a secondary role, with limited power or access to independent resources. This serves to create a monopoly on mental health services, limiting competition to produce better services and stifling creative endeavors. In the end, all diseases have their end points as biological factors. However, this does not mean that emotional, social, and behavioral factors have only ancillary roles. We must continue to strike a balance between the amount of attention (and research funding) given to each field. Each has its place in health care, and we must ensure that policies reflect this. Psychologists and other behavioral medicine practitioners must remain able to provide services independent of other fields.

Human immunodeficiency virus (HIV) serves as one example of a lifestyle disease that requires multidisciplinary intervention. The virus is clearly a matter for physicians, physiologists, and pharmaceutical researchers. We need their expertise to develop a cure and vaccine. However, with no cure or vaccine foreseeable in the immediate future, the social and behavioral sciences must play an important role in attempting to minimize the spread of HIV. Once we have developed a cure and vaccine for HIV, such cure or vaccine would clearly be the indicated treatment. Until then, additional funding is necessary to assist social and behavioral scientists in continuing to identify those individuals at highest risk of contracting HIV and in finding ways to prevent them from engaging in high-risk behaviors. Treatments developed by behavioral and social scientists will not likely eliminate the problem posed by HIV. Eradicating the HIV problem will probably require some type of physical (e.g., pharmacological) intervention. When we find that, however, we must not disparage efforts made by social and behavioral scientists as inadequate because we can never know what the effect would have been without such interventions. Current efforts in this field will likely assist in minimizing spread of the virus, but we can only make projections about what would have resulted without implementation of current programs. Thus, although marketplace forces may promote competition between disciplines, we, as health care providers, must recognize that cooperation between disciplines is essential if we are to strive toward better health outcomes.

ASSESSMENT ISSUES

As indicated earlier in this chapter, we can most efficiently treat problems if we first conduct a thorough assessment of target complaints. A behavioral psychology orientation promotes thorough and efficient assessments. The hallmark of behavioral psychology has been an emphasis on direct assessment of behavior and minimization of constructs, such as depression and anxiety. Out of necessity, however, clinicians must sparingly use terms that represent constructs in order to effectively communicate with other health-care professionals. Nonetheless, such representation obscures assessment and creates significant measurement difficulties.

Assessment of depression among medical populations (those most likely to present to health and rehabilitation psychologists) is one area that is particularly noteworthy. Not only is depression relatively common among individuals with medical conditions (National Institutes of Health, 1993), many depression symptoms overlap with symptoms of coexisting physical problems, making detection of depression and subsequent treatment difficult. Further complicating assessment of depression among medical patients is that there are many depression assessment methods and instruments. Although there is bound to be some discrepancy between different methods (i.e., self-report instruments vs. structured interviews vs. biochemical assays) and even between different instruments using the same method, recent research suggests that clinical evaluations may produce vastly different clinical impressions depending upon assessment method and instrument used. Goreczny and Nussbaum (1994) addressed the importance of obtaining clinical concordance among different assessment instruments. *Clinical concordance* refers to agreement of diagnosis and clinical impressions. This is an important concept that has gone largely untested by psychometricians and assessment instrument developers. Most psychometricians assess reliability and validity of newly developed instruments using correlational methods only. Clinical concordance, on the other hand, requires that assessment instruments not only correlate highly with each other but that they also produce similar clinical impressions. For example, it is important that depression scales have high agreement regarding presence or absence of depression.

Goreczny and Nussbaum (1994) recently challenged the clinical concordance of two frequently used assessment instruments—the Minnesota Multiphasic Personality Inventory (MMPI) and Symptom Checklist 90-Revised (SCL-90-R). (The authors also used the Derogatis Stress Profile [1984], but we do not focus on those results here.) The results from this study found that the two instruments did highly correlate with each other ($r = .78, p < .0001$) but that there was substantial disagreement on presence of clinical depression. Using a cutoff of T-scores greater than 69 ($2\ SD$ above the mean) for each scale, the MMPI classified 95 of 134 subjects in the clinically depressed range, but the SCL-90-R classified only 3 of the 134 subjects in this range! Thus, depending on the scale that one uses for assessing depression, different impressions result.

Interestingly, the means of the two scales (79.05 and 49.30 for the MMPI and SCL-90-R, respectively) were significantly different, $F(2, 133) = 468.69, p < .0001$. This is important because clinicians often use these two instruments for screening purposes, often using one without the other, and given increased pressures on clinicians to improve efficiency (i.e., cost efficacy), it is likely that increased use of screening instruments will permit clinicians to assess more individuals. Use of the SCL-90-R only may result in underassessment of depression and subsequently fail to provide needed treatment services. Other recent studies have argued against use of the SCL-90-R as a clinical assessment instrument (Brackstone, Delehanty, Mann, & Pain, 1995). However, it is important to note that Goreczny and Nussbaum (1994) found that the SCL-90-R standard deviation for the sample (9.88) approached the theoretical *SD* of 10, whereas the *SD* of the MMPI (18.40) was almost twice the theoretical standard deviation. Implications of this are not clear. What appears clear is that psychometricians may need to begin reporting sensitivity and specificity statistics along with reliability and validity data of new assessment instruments. However, psychologists and other health-care practitioners must first develop an agreed-on benchmark for what constitutes depression and other measurable constructs.

UNDERSTANDING THE SIMPLE COMPLEXITY OF HUMAN BEHAVIOR

Health psychologists and rehabilitation psychologists, incorporating a behavioral medicine perspective, must approach each lifestyle disorder by recognizing the complex interplay of behavioral, emotional, genetic, physiological, social, and cultural determinants. Only after we take these factors into account can we begin to combat the medical problems currently afflicting human beings. We must approach these medical problems by recognizing not only different disciplines, but also factors at different levels of interaction. These include intrapersonal (e.g., genetic and constitutional factors, learning history, current skills and beliefs), interpersonal (e.g., social support, family interactions, occupational and peer relations), and environmental (e.g., legal issues, physical environment, and current policies) factors (Weiss, 1992).

Failure to appreciate the complex arena in which health behavior occurs will likely result in poor development and maintenance of change. For example, assisting injured individuals to become independent following a period of dependency on hospital staff and family members requires addressing issues regarding their beliefs about being able to return to premorbid functioning (i.e., intrapersonal issues) and conflicts among family members that might sabotage rehabilitation efforts (i.e., interpersonal issues). Although many treatment facilities currently attempt to address such issues, they may fail to address, or lack adequate resources to address concerns about whether the physical arrangement of the home environment will promote continued development of independent living skills. Similarly, if we are to promote healthy behavior, we must work toward changing the environment into one that encourages positive, healthy lifestyle behaviors (Brownell, Marlatt, Lichtenstein, & Wilson, 1986).

Furthermore, we must clearly delineate factors involved in development, change, and maintenance of healthy behaviors and lifestyles (Weiss, 1992). The factors involving each process (i.e., development, change, maintenance) may be different, and these factors may interact with the components described earlier, thereby further complicating our mission. For example, developing nutritious eating habits will likely differ if we focus on young children, adolescents, young adults, or older adults. As well, individuals' changing to or maintaining certain nutritious eating habits will certainly differ depending upon their age.

One of the most difficult issues for behavioral medicine specialists is helping individuals maintain behavior change once they have achieved it. Although behavior-change technologies have proven fairly successful in assisting individuals to achieve behavior change, we have been largely unsuccessful in assisting them to maintain it

(Marlatt & Gordon, 1985). Nonetheless, individuals can repeat previously successful treatment strategies or even attempt new ones if relapse occurs. However, we do not know the full ramifications and effects of repeated attempts at making certain specific changes. For instance, there is some evidence that weight cycling (repeated cycles that involve loss of weight secondary to dieting followed by subsequent weight regain) presents with its own health-damaging consequences (Lissner et al., 1991; Rodin, Radke-Sharpe, Rebuffe-Scrive, & Greenwood, 1990). HIV presents a unique problem with respect to maintenance of healthy behaviors. Individuals who relapse to a point that they begin engaging in behaviors that place them at high risk for contracting HIV place themselves in circumstances that may have serious consequences.

Another area of concern is the area of women's health status. Although women receive 70% of all prescriptions for psychoactive drugs (Ogur, 1986) and undergo about two thirds of all surgical procedures in this country (Travis, 1988), most of the research on health-related issues and prescription drugs has excluded women (Rodin & Ickovics, 1990). Researchers have excluded women from serving as subjects in studies because of methodological concerns, including problems related to hormonal variability (Bullock, 1984). However, the differing physiologies of men and women raise serious concerns about external validity of studies that utilize only men. Subsequently, results of studies on men have, at best, questionable generalizability to women. In addition, there are several health-related issues that predominantly or exclusively affect women (e.g., obstetrical and gynecological concerns, issues related to childbirth, osteoporosis, and breast cancer).

The need for clinical research into women's health problems is essential. Indeed, comparative studies may help answer questions about why women live longer than men and why women, relative to men, have lower age-adjusted mortality rates for all 12 of the leading causes of death in the United States (Wingard, 1984). Comparative studies may also help explain why the mortality advantage for women over men has evidenced declines over the past decade (U.S. Bureau of the Census, 1990). Such studies would undoubtedly provide answers that would help both men and women.

The issue of demographic differences is somewhat of a problem for scientists, however. Clinically, it is important to identify how demographic factors (e.g., age, gender, race) influence our therapies, such as pharmaceutical interventions. However, we cannot randomize demographic variables, thereby making true experimental designs unattainable. We must rely on quasi-experimental and correlational designs, but these designs do not permit us to adequately rule out competing alternative hypotheses. Although we must continue to be sensitive to issues related to specific groups, such as women and ethnic minorities, our primary overriding goal must be to identify general rules of health behavior as they relate to all people. When we begin adding influences of demographic variables, we begin adding variables that make identifying general rules of behavior more difficult. We can continue to add variables until the model becomes so complicated that it has no value to scientists. Therefore, as clinical scientists, we face a unique challenge: We must continue to guide our studies via theoretical propositions in an effort to identify general rules of behavior, but we must also identify how demographic variables relate to clinical interventions and outcomes.

Because of the complexity of health behaviors, in order for health-care professionals to have their greatest impact on healthy behaviors of others, health psychologists and others must intervene at all levels within the health-care system. First, these professionals must continue to treat patients individually and in groups. Through such interventions, health-care professionals help promote healthy behaviors (e.g., exercise, positive stress-management techniques, eating healthy nutritional meals) and eliminate unhealthy behaviors (e.g., smoking). Modification of one's lifestyle thereby helps eliminate risk factors associated with disease. Clinical and research work needs to continue to identify parameters of effective treatment (i.e., Which techniques work with which individuals? How can we develop techniques to move individuals to the contemplation and maintenance stages of change from earlier stages?).

In addition, we must continue to implement educational programs on large-scale, community-based levels in order to effect change in a cost-efficient manner. We must continue to expand large-scale health promotion programs, similar to those described by St. Lawrence in this volume, to areas not yet addressed.

Nonetheless, although health-promotion advocates can promote health of the nation's individuals by working directly with patients in individual, group, and community-based programs, those with expertise in such matters must also focus on extending leadership onto larger areas of influence, such as policy issues, both national and international. However, when using empirical data to suggest policy changes, those individuals involved cannot ignore economic and political issues either.

SMOKING: A PUBLIC HEALTH CONCERN

One of the most publicized health-policy concerns of recent years, other than health-care reform, involves taxing tobacco products. Tobacco use is clearly one of the main risk factors associated with a large proportion of premature deaths in the United States (see DeBon & Klesges, this volume), and basic economics explains that as cost of products increases demand decreases. Therefore, it seems reasonable to suggest that placing a tax on tobacco products is a policy that will raise badly needed revenue and increase health of the nation's individuals by decreasing one of the major risk factors (i.e., tobacco use) for premature death. Smoking-cessation programs at the interpersonal and intrapersonal levels have thus far been largely ineffective. The vast majority (95%) of people who stop smoking quit on their own, using information they obtained or techniques they learned from books or magazine articles rather than through use of a specified treatment program (Koop, 1983).

Raising taxes represents an intervention at the environmental level. However, in our democratic society that relies on market-based economics, such a policy decision is not likely to become law without first developing strong support from the multitude of individuals likely affected by any changes. Therefore, policy makers must first identify those groups of individuals most directly affected by any change in tobacco tax rates and include proper incentives to satisfy large numbers of those individuals.

The number of individuals affected by a tobacco tax is much broader than one might expect. First, and most obvious, are the users of tobacco products. A second group that policy makers must consider are the tobacco companies, who stand to lose enormous amounts of money as current smokers quit due to rising costs and fewer nonsmokers begin to smoke. A third group of individuals who would suffer significantly from increased taxes on tobacco products are the workers at factories, whose job it is to produce tobacco products. Fourth are the farm owners who currently receive significant subsidies from the government for production of tobacco products.

Although it may appear that this list delineates all of those groups of individuals affected by changes in taxes on tobacco products, there are several other groups that policy makers cannot ignore if they wish to successfully garner support for increased tobacco taxes. Two of these groups are spouses and children of workers involved in the tobacco industry, and advertising companies, which make large profits from developing advertising campaigns and promoting use of tobacco products. Spouses and children of tobacco-industry workers will not support policies that appear to threaten their livelihood, nor will advertising companies support policies that will decrease their profits. Thus, advertising companies, unions of tobacco workers, farm owners, and tobacco companies will all use their considerable clout to lobby against such policies unless they see benefits they can derive from proposed changes. Ultimately, these lobbying efforts would likely result in defeat of an important and beneficial health-promoting policy.

Another important consideration in raising taxes on tobacco products is the economic impact. A large and immediate increase in tobacco taxes and decrease in tobacco subsidies would likely have significant adverse effects on the U.S. economy. Executives of tobacco and advertising companies may find that they must substantially reduce their workforces. This would result in decreased income taxes for the U.S. Treasury, a decrease large enough that it might not offset the increased tax revenues from tobacco products. Given current concern about the U.S. budget deficit and debt and increasing uneasiness regarding the current world economy, policy makers must consider the significant economic and political implications of a large and immediate tax increase.

Thus, some well-minded individuals who want to immediately raise tobacco taxes may not be considering the overall implications of such a policy. Health advocates and the researchers who serve as consultants to policy makers cannot attempt to forge new policies based upon empirical considerations alone. They can assist lawmakers, but they must also consider influences of the market, political concerns, and the welfare of those groups of individuals affected by changes in tax rates. They must also consider prices of products in other countries (especially bordering countries) so that tax increases do not inadvertently produce a black market for the product. Finally, rather than approaching the tobacco problem from an adversarial stance, policy makers must include individuals from affected groups to formulate a program that addresses the issue as a cooperative venture offering incentives to all involved. Any committee designed for this purpose must include medical specialists; those with expertise in behavioral management; economists; experts on political implications of policies; and representation for farm owners, unions representing tobacco workers and their families, smokers' rights advocates, and the tobacco and advertising industries.

A Working Proposal

We offer the following proposal as one attempt to delineate a policy that both serves the health of Americans and takes into account the considerations discussed in the previous section. We recognize our limited appreciation of the complexity of such matters and lack of expertise in some vital areas. However, we intend this model only as a working model, one that will hopefully inspire others with expertise in the area to build upon this and other existing proposals in order to cultivate initiatives that enhance the health of Americans while also promoting sound economic and political policies.

In an effort to promote health, provide incentives for current smokers to quit smoking, and establish reasons for nonsmokers to remain abstinent from tobacco products, the U.S. government could slowly increase taxes and decrease subsidies on tobacco. A panel of experts on tobacco use and economics, appointed by the President and approved by Congress, would set the yearly rate of increase such that the number of smokers would not drop so drastically as to have adverse economic consequences. The increased tax revenues would go to six categories of expenditure: (1) 20% to tobacco companies to help them switch to a different product, (2) 20% to farm owners to compensate them for their losses and enable them to prepare for growing a different product, (3) 20% to workers and their families to retrain tobacco workers and their family members to begin different vocations or to enter (or reenter) the workforce, (4) 20% to advertising companies and magazines to pursue contracts from companies that produce health-promoting products, (5) 15% to research on treatment of cancer and development of increasingly effective smoking-cessation programs, and (6) 5% to the general U.S. Treasury to aid in deficit reduction. The panel of experts would have the authority to adjust these figures yearly such that all categories of affected individuals would receive sufficient monies to help compensate for losses.

INTERNATIONAL CONSIDERATIONS: A WORLDVIEW

As we become more able to traverse the world than we were just 30 or 40 years ago, and as economic and political barriers continue to decline, nations having highly advanced medical technology must consider assisting nations with underserved populations. Assisting countries to make changes to reduce or eliminate certain infectious diseases, increase potable water, and build better sanitation facilities, however, will undoubtedly lead to an increase in chronic diseases, similar to what has happened in the United States and many European countries. As countries grow in their abilities to overcome some of the unhealthy circumstances they face (e.g., inadequate sanitation), they may begin to emulate some of the behaviors and lifestyles found in our culture. We must incorporate what we have learned about our own unhealthy lifestyles to prevent other countries from making mistakes similar to our culture's mistakes (e.g., high stress, low exercise, high dietary fat, substance abuse/dependence). However, making changes in ways that other societies and cultures find acceptable is a difficult feat requiring international and interdisciplinary cooperation and diplomacy (Weiss, 1992).

As representatives from the country that is the leader in medical technology advances, health-care professionals in the United States have the privilege and opportunity (some might also say that we have the obligation) to assist other countries—assistance that they would likely welcome. As Koop (1983), who served as Surgeon General and represented the United States at the World Health Organization, noted,

"The world looks to [the United States] to set the standard by which humanity will make progress in health and medical care" (p. 309). We must recognize that not only is it humanitarian to help others, it is also in our best interests. As Mann (1991) cautioned, the rapid spread of HIV around the world highlights our call to action because

> conditions of the modern world are uniquely favorable to rapid global spread of infectious disease. AIDS demonstrated how swiftly remote or seemingly obscure health events elsewhere can become tomorrow's health care crisis here. (p. 247)

He later stated, "A global approach is needed now to detect, as rapidly as possible, the pandemics yet to come" (p. 247).

In addition to addressing concerns regarding infectious diseases, we must help prevent the spread of lifestyle diseases to other countries. As some countries, such as the United States, continue to place more restrictions on smoking, tobacco companies will seek to make their profits elsewhere. There have already been large increases in rates of cigarette smoking in Asian and African countries (Kaplan, Carriker, & Wakdeon, 1990; Shelton, 1988). In an effort to promote the health of all peoples, it is essential we offer our guidance and disseminate the lessons we have learned.

We have already begun establishing international societies to address issues of global concern. We must also begin disseminating information through international journals. We can no longer take a provincial view of the world, focusing only on problems of the United States and Western Europe. Western researchers must take a genuine interest in helping develop international networks aimed at assisting those in underserved communities and those who do not have access to current technological advances.

SUMMARY

The fields of health and rehabilitation psychology have evidenced tremendous growth over the past three decades. With emphasis of health-care reform on prevention of health-related problems and cost containment, psychologists, whose focus is on helping change unhealthy risk factors for disease into behaviors associated with good health, may benefit from health-care reform. Psychologists who insist on continuing to treat patients over long periods of time without assessing outcome of their treatments will likely find it difficult to survive in the new, more competitive health-care arena. Nonetheless, the health-care reform packages continue to emphasize expensive treatments over less expensive alternatives. In addition, mental health benefits under the different plans vary widely. Therefore, the future role psychologists will have after health-care reform remains uncertain.

Health and rehabilitation psychologists, however, have great reason for optimism. The health-care problems currently confronting our nation are those that behavioral management specialists (i.e., psychologists) can significantly influence. Lifestyle factors, such as eating habits, smoking, exercise, stress management practices, practicing safe sex, and adherence to prescribed medical regimens, are among the primary contributors to the major causes of premature death (i.e., heart disease, cancer, stroke). Changes in these lifestyle factors may provide more direct benefit in health outcome than any medication currently available. However, there is insufficient data to indicate that we can effectively alter behavioral risk factors for disease, and where convincing data do exist, there is little to confirm that making such changes actually results in better health outcomes. Technological advances have also enabled many individuals who previously would have died from health-related problems (i.e., stroke, motor vehicle accidents) live longer lives. One result of this, however, is an increased need for rehabilitation efforts.

Despite a need for more outcome-oriented studies of behavioral risk-factor change, there is also a need for empirical investigations into etiological mechanisms behind such change. Without adequate theories to guide scientific exploration of health and mind–body (or behavior–body) interactions, our understanding of these areas will be inadequate to address future health problems as they arise. In order to investigate these complicated and interesting issues, we will need to rely even more heavily on multidisciplinary and interdisciplinary communication than in the past.

Finally, we live in a dynamic world, and the rate of change in our world currently appears staggering. Our changing world carries with it the need for health and rehabilitation psychologists to adjust to changing conditions. Future demands require that we (1) prepare for an aging population and the challenges that brings, (2) perform more research into how demographic variables interact with our assessment and treatment procedures while keeping in mind the overall scientific goal of finding general rules of behavior as they relate to health outcomes, (3) incorporate modern technological advances (e.g., computers) into our health care more broadly than we have in the past, (4) utilize our expertise to help shape policy decisions, and (5) continue to strengthen our assessment procedures. Last, the need to take an international perspective when addressing health care is now essential. We must view the health-care crisis as a global crisis, not as one limited to the United States.

REFERENCES

Adler, T. (1991). Utilization review standards sought. *American Psychological Association Monitor, 22,* 18–19.

Barron, S. (1992). Mental health benefits plan draws fire. *American Psychological Association Monitor, 23,* 34.

Brackstone, M. J., Delehanty, R., Mann, B., & Pain, K. (1995). The nature and severity of distress among rehabilitation hospital patients. *International Journal of Rehabilitation and Health, 1,* 37–48.

Brownell, K. D., Marlatt, G. A., Lichtenstein, E., & Wilson, G. T. (1986). Understanding and preventing relapse. *American Psychologist, 41,* 765–782.

Bullock, T. H. (1984). Comparative neuroscience holds promise for quiet revolutions. *Science, 225,* 473–478.

Clinton, J. J., McCormick, K., & Besteman, J. (1994). Enhancing clinical practice: The role of practice guidelines. *American Psychologist, 49,* 30–33.

DeAngelis, T. (1991). Therapy part of Canadian package. *American Psychological Association Monitor, 22,* 19.

DeAngelis, T. (1992). Healthy psychology grows both in stature, influence. *American Psychological Association Monitor, 23,* 10–11.

Derogatis, L. R. (1984). *The Derogatis Stress Profile: A Summary Report.* Baltimore, MD: Author.

Fox, R. E. (1994). Training professional psychologists for the twenty-first century. *American Psychologist, 49,* 200–206.

Goreczny, A. J., & Nussbaum, P. D. (1994). Measuring depressive symptomatology of patients referred to a behavioral medicine clinic: Concordance of self-report measures. *Journal of Clinical Psychology in Medical Settings, 1,* 255–259.

Howard, K. I., Kopta, S. M., Krause, M. S., & Orlinsky, D. E. (1986). The dose–effect relationship in psychotherapy. *American Psychologist, 41,* 159–164.

Kaplan, M., Carriker, L., & Wakdeon, J. (1990). Gender differences in tobacco use in Kenya. *Social Science and Medicine, 30,* 305–310.

Koop, C. E. (1983). Perspectives on future health care. *Health Psychology, 2,* 303–312.

Lissner, L., Odell, P. M., D'Agostino, R. B., Stokes, J., Kreger, B. E., Belanger, A. J., & Brownell, K. D. (1991). Variability of body weight and health outcomes in the Framingham population. *New England Journal of Medicine, 324,* 1839–1844.

Mann, J. M. (1991). Global AIDS: Critical issues for prevention in the 1990's. *International Journal of Health Sciences, 21,* 553–559.

Marlatt, A. G., & Gordon, J. R. (1985). Relapse prevention: Maintenance strategies in the treatment of addictive behaviors. New York: Guilford.

McKegney, F. P., & Schwartz, C. E. (1986). Behavioral medicine: Treatment and organizational issues. *General Hospital Psychiatry, 8,* 330–339.

Michaelson, R. (1993). Utilization review inhibits quest to provide therapy. *American Psychological Association Monitor, 24,* 23.

Miller, N. E. (1992). Some trends from the history to the future of behavioral medicine. *Annals of Behavioral Medicine, 14,* 307–309.

Moses-Zirkes, S. (1993). Practice briefs senate, stresses outpatient care. *American Psychological Association Monitor, 24,* 18.

National Institutes of Health. (1993). Diagnosis and treatment of depression in late life: The NIH Consensus Development Conference Statement. *Psychopharmacology Bulletin, 29,* 87–95.

Newman, R. (1993). With integrated care, quality is not spared. *American Psychological Association Monitor, 24,* 38.

Ogur, B. (1986). Long day's journey into night: Women and prescription drug abuse. *Women and Health, 11,* 99–115.

Rodin, J., & Ickovics, J. R. (1990). Women's health: Review and research agenda as we approach the 21st century. *American Psychologist, 45,* 1018–1034.

Rodin, J., Radke-Sharpe, N., Rebuffe-Scrive, M., & Greenwood, M.R.C. (1990). Weight cycling and fat distribution. *International Journal of Obesity, 14,* 303–310.

Shelton, A. (1988). Spotlight on China: 1,397 billion still not enough. *Tobacco Reporter, 115,* 24–28.

Sleek, S. (1993). Mental health picture better in Clinton's health reform bill. *American Psychological Association Monitor, 24,* 1, 22.

Travis, C. B. (1988). *Women and health psychology: Biomedical issues.* Hillsdale, NJ: Erlbaum.

U.S. Bureau of the Census. (1990). Statistical abstracts of the United States: 1990 (110th ed.). Washington, DC: Author.

Weiss, S. M. (1992). Behavioral medicine on the world scene: Toward the year 2000. *Annals of Behavioral Medicine, 14,* 302–306.

Welch, B. L. (1992a, May). Managed care focus of marketing initiative. *American Psychological Association Monitor, 23,* 21.

Welch, B. L. (1992b). The best care: Integrated, not managed. *American Psychological Association Monitor, 23,* 30.

Welch, B. L. (1993a). Case-not-cost-management important in integrated care. *American Psychological Association Monitor, 24,* 19.

Welch, B. L. (1993b, March). Health care reformers: Bite the political bullet. *American Psychological Association Monitor, 24,* 24.

Welch, B. L. (1993c). Spend mental health dollars wisely, Welch says. *American Psychological Association Monitor, 24,* 18–19.

Wingard, D. L. (1984). The sex difference in morbidity, mortality, and lifestyle. *Annual Review of Public Health, 5,* 433–458.

Youngstrom, N. (1991). Mandated insurance benefits debated. *American Psychological Association Monitor, 22,* 24–25.

Youngstrom, N. (1992). National health system could boost psychology. *American Psychological Association Monitor, 23,* 1, 41.

Index

Abdominal obesity, 158, 168
Ability Testing Anxiety Scale Questionnaire, 417
Abstinence violation effect, 142, 314-315
Acceptable Maximal Effort, 371
Achalasia, 90, 92
Action limit, 377
Action stage, 142, 483
Activity level evaluation, 164-165
Activity theory, 585
Adaptation, 7, 9
   models of, 345-347
Adjustment
   headache, 12
   spinal cord injury, 350-351
Adrenal excretion, 101
Adrenal function, 41
Adrenal medula, 119
Adrenocorticotrophic hormone, 84
Aging, 583-597, 675
   activity theory, 585
   alcohol abuse, 592-593
   breakdown theories, 586
   cancer, 594-595
   central nervous system and, 586-588
   cognitive impairment in elderly depressed, 589-590
   continuity theory, 585
   dementia, 593-594
   demographics of, 583-584
   diabetes, 595
   disengagement theory, 585
   head injury, 595-596
   hypertension, 594
   models of, 584-586
   mood disorders, 588-592
   MRI in assessment of elderly depressed persons, 590-591
   neuropsychological findings, 591-592

Aging (*cont.*)
   physical disorders, 594-596
   psychiatric disorders, 588-594
   social-environmental theory, 585
   substance theories, 586
   suicide risk, 589
AIDS, 555-576, 674
   cognitive theories, 557-561
   decision-making theory, 560-561
   diffusion of innovation theory, 569
   dual process models, 567
   emotional arousal theories, 566-569
   fear-drive models, 567
   health belief model, 557-560
   learning-based theories, 561-566
      applications of, 563-566
   motivation theories, 566-569
   operant learning theory, 561-562
   protection-motivation theory, 567-569
   psychoeducational theories, 556-557
   self-efficacy theory, 562-563
   social influence theories, 569-571
   social learning theory, 562
   social marketing, 569
   theory of reasoned action, 559-560
AIDS Knowledge Test, 564
Alaryngeal speech, 467
Alcohol
   abuse in the elderly, 592-593
   and hypertension, 223-224
   and sleep, 107-108
Alcoholics Anonymous, 310
Alexithymia, 226
Allergens, 33, 38
Allergy Foundation of America, 32
Alopecia, 489
Ambulatory monitoring, 124, 128, 224, 226, 229-230, 251

677

American Asthma Report, 42
Americans with Disabilities Act, 377, 382, 450
Amitriptyline, 12, 22, 23, 190, 365, 446
Anger management, 148, 208, 313
Angina pectoris, 91, 240, 250
Anorexia; *See* Eating disorders
Anterior brain, susceptibility of, to traumatic damage, 433-434
Antibodies, 536
Antigens, 536
Antihistamines, 159
Antinuclear tests, Raynaud's disease, 122
Anxiety, 665, 668
   Crohn's disease, 84-86
   eating disorders, 176-180, 184, 188, 192
   esophageal motility disorders, 91
   headache and, 7
   hypertension, 226
   insomnia, 101-105, 107-112
   irritable bowel syndrome, 81-83
   obesity, 163
   pain, 332-333
   peptic ulcer disease, 88-89
   relapse prevention, 312
   spinal cord injury, 346, 349
   stress, 285
   surgery preparation, 292, 297-298, 303
   temporomandibular disorders, 60, 62-64, 66-67, 71
Arteriovenous anastomoses; *See* Shunts
Arthralgic model of temporomandibular disorders, 58-59
Arthritis, 8, 157
Articular disk, 56
Articular fossa, 56
Assertiveness training, 313
Assessment
   asthma, 35-36
   cognitive disabilities, 407-411
   coronary-prone behavior, 211-212
   eating disorders, 183-186
   multiple sclerosis, 403-411
   physical activity and exercise, 257-262
   quality of life, 488-491
   sexual dysfunction, 404-405
   temporomandibular disorders, 67
   traumatic brain injury, 441-445
Assessment issues, 667-669
Associative biases, 192
Asthenia, 472
Asthma, 31-50
   allergens, 33, 38
   antecedent stimuli, 48
   aspirin, 33
   assessment, 35-36
   characteristics of, 32-33
   consequences of, 41-45, 49
   context and, 46-47

Asthma (*cont.*)
   contextual variables and, 47
   corticosteroids, 42
   definition of, 31-32
   emotional reactions, 33, 39, 40-41
   environmental factors, 39
   establishing operations, 47
   establishing stimuli, 47
   exercise, 33, 38-40
   information collection, 48
   information processing and evaluation, 48-49
   intermittency of attacks, 32
   linkage of stimuli to responses, 34-35
   medication compliance, 36-38
   pathophysiology, 33-35
   perennial, 32
   psychological implications, 35
   psychological side effects of asthma medications, 41-43
   quality of life, 43-45
   relapse prevention, 49-50
   reversibility of attacks, 33
   risk-factor analysis, 38-40, 48
   seasonal, 38
   self-management, 45-50
   setting events, 47
   stimuli, 33, 36-41
   stimulus control, 48
   theophylline, 41-42
   triggers, avoidance or escape from, 38
   variability of attacks, 33
Asthma Quality of Life Questionnaire, 44
Asthma Self-Efficacy Scale, 35
Asthma Symptom Checklist, 44
Attitudes to Asthma Scale, 44
Aura, 4-7
Autoantibodies, 536-537
Autogenic training, 124-127, 129
Autonomic nervous system, 146, 374-375, 390
Aversive strategies, smoking cessation, 141
Avoidant coping, 9
Azathioprine, 84, 413

Back school, 381
Balanced-deficit diet, 166
Beck Depression Inventory
   AIDS, 564
   exercise, 162
   headache, 20
   multiple sclerosis, 398, 404, 406, 414, 417, 419
   obesity, 163
   spinal cord injury, 355
   temporomandibular disorders, 63
Behavior Change Inventory, 444
Binge eating, 159-160
Binge Eating Disorder, 159

Biofeedback, 665
  cardiovascular disorders, 248-250
  esophageal motility disorders, 91-92
  headache, 3, 9-13, 15-24
  insomnia, 102, 110-111
  irritable bowel syndrome, 82
  multiple sclerosis, 420-421
  peptic ulcer disease, 89-90
  Raynaud's disease, 123-129
  stress, 282-283
  surgery preparation, 303
  temporomandibular disorders, 61, 68-72
Biological models
  eating disorders, 180-182
  smoking, 136-137
Biomechanical model, temporomandibular disorders, 59
Blanching, 117
Body Dysmorphic Disorder, 180
Body fat, 157-158, 160
Body Image Assessment, 183, 186
Body image assessment, 185-186
Body Image Automatic Thoughts Questionnaire, 183, 185-186
Body image theories, 179-180
Body mass index, 158, 161, 191
Body mechanics coaching, 381
Body Perception Index, 185
Body Self-Relations Questionnaire, 183, 185-186
Body Shape Questionnaire, 183, 185
Brachial artery, 119-121, 126
Brain anatomy, 434-435
Brain stem pain-modulating systems, 6
Breakdown theories, 586
Brocha's aphasia, 439
Bronchial hyperreactivity, 34-35
Bronchiolitis, 32
Bronchitis, 32
Bruxism, 55, 57, 59-60, 62, 67, 69, 72
Bulimia, 160; see also Eating disorders
Bulimia test (BULIT), 183-185
Buproprion, 188, 191
Buss-Durkee Hostility Inventory, 211

Cachexia, 472
Caffeine, 106-108, 139, 146, 229
California Psychological Inventory, 35
Caloric intervention, 166
Cancer, 135, 143-144, 157, 162, 594-595, 674; see also Cancer rehabilitation; Oncology
Cancer rehabilitation, 457-474
  barriers to, 461-462
    overcoming, 462-464
  cancer rehabilitation team
    effective functioning of, 468-469
    members of, 465-467

Cancer rehabilitation (cont.)
  care coordinator, role of, 466
  concept of, 458-461
  dietician, role of, 467
  models of, 469-470
  occupational therapist, role of, 466
  oncology/rehabilitation nurse, role of, 467
  physical therapist, role of, 466
  physicians, role of, 465-466
  principles of, 464-465
  psychologist, role of, 466
  rehabilitation problems, 470-474
  social worker, role of, 467
  speech pathologist, role of, 466-467
  vocational counselor, role of, 467
Cardiovascular disorders, 239-252
  etiological considerations, 239-246
  health promotion efforts, 246-251
  neuroendocrine response to stress, 244
  prevailing state hypothesis, 244
  prevention programs, 246
  psychosocial risk factors, pathophysiological mechanisms for, 242-246
  recurrent activation hypothesis, 245-246
  risk-factor interactions, 240-242
  risk-factor reduction
    cardiovascular reactivity to stress, 247-250
    psychosocial risk, 247
  risk factors, 240
  stress and lipid function, 243-244
Central nervous system SLE, 541-543
Change Assessment Questionnaire, 444
Child Anxiety Scale, 35
Children's Depression Inventory, 35
Chlormezanone, 23
Cholecystokinin, 181
Chronic obstructive pulmonary disease, 135, 144
Chronic pain, 57, 63-65, 81, 325-336
  affective domain, 332-333
  behavioral domain, 333
  central models, 327-329
  cognitive domain, 331-332
  cognitive-behavioral model, 329
  family/social domain, 333-334
  gate control theory, 327
  integrative diathesis-stress model, 329-331
  neurotransmitter models, 327-328
  operant/behavioral model, 328-329
  peripheral neural mechanisms, 326-327
  personality models, 328
  theories of, 326-334
Cimetidine, 88
Circadian rhythm phase shift, 101
Clinical concordance, 668
Clinical Eating Disorder Rating Instrument (CE-DRI), 183-184
Clonidine, 118-121, 138

Index

Cognitive activation, in insomnia, 101–103
Cognitive-Behavior Rating Scale, 443
Cognitive-behavior therapy
    headache, 11–15, 20
    multiple sclerosis, 417
    temporomandibular disorders, 68, 70
Cognitive Capacity Screening Examination, 408–411
Cognitive screening
    brief, 408–409
    intermediate-length, 409–411
Cognitive rehabilitation
    cancer rehabilitation, 446–447
    computers and, 621–623
Cognitive restructuring, 111–112
Cognitive theories
    AIDS prevention, 557–561
    chronic pain, 329
    eating disorders, 178–179
Collagen vascular disease, 117
Colon hyperreactivity, 82
Colon motility, 80, 82
Committee for Accreditation of Rehabilitation Facilities, 380
Community reintegration
    spinal cord injury, 341–343
    traumatic brain injury, 450–451
Competitor analysis, 650–651
Compliance issues, 665
    asthma, 32, 36–39, 49
    chronic illness, 36
    diary cards, 36–37
    headache, 23–24
    hemodialysis, 503–508
    pill counts, 36–37
    smoking cessation, 140
Comprehensive care model, multiple sclerosis treatment, 411–412
Computer applications in behavioral medicine, 605–626, 675
    assessment procedures, 606–614
    behavior monitoring, 611–612
    behavioral interviews, 610–611
    behavioral treatment, 614–617
    cognitive rehabilitation, 621–623
    counseling and psychotherapy, 617–619
    family therapy, 612–614
    gerontology, 619–621
    headache, 4–5
    interview evaluation, 606–609
    patient education, 623–624
    patient interviews, 606–609
Computerized axial tomography, 61–62, 65, 392, 398, 441–442
Condylar displacement, 59
Condyle, 56, 59
Consumer analysis, 649–650
Consumer orientation, 638

Contemplation stage, 142, 483, 671
Contingency contracting, 141
Continuity theory, 585
Continuous ambulatory peritoneal dialysis, 499–450
Continuous headache pattern, 18
Contrecoup damage, 432
Controlled Oral Word Association Test, 410, 443–444
Controlled smoking, 142
Coping
    asthma, 50
    Crohn's disease, 87
    headache and, 8–9, 11–12, 16
    irritable bowel syndrome, 83
    relapse prevention and, 312–313
    smoking, 147–148
    surgery preparation, 295–296, 347–350
    temporomandibular disorder, 59–60, 63
Cornell Medical Index, 84
Coronary heart disease, 162, 198–203, 206, 208, 210, 213
Coronary-prone behavior, 197–213
    assessment, 211–212
    health outcomes, association with, 198–200
    hostility, 199–200
    intervention, 212–213
        efficacy of, 207–208
    modification of, 208
    psychological mechanisms, 205–207
    psychophysiological reactivity, 200–202
    psychosocial vulnerability, 202–203
    recurrent coronary prevention project, 207–208
    transactional model, 203–205
    Type A pattern, broadly defined, 198–199
Corticosteroids, asthma and, 42–43
Corticotropin releasing hormone, 181
Cost containment, 637–638
Cost-leadership strategies, 654–656
Craniomandibular malalignment, 59
Critical Incident Technique, 347
Crohn's disease, 83–87
Cultural issues in relapse prevention, 317–319
Cushing's syndrome, 159
Cyanosis, 117
Cyproheptadine, 190

Daily Drinking Diary, 311
Daily life stressors, 9
Daily Stress Inventory, 280
Decision-making theory, 560–561
Defense-defeat model, 221–223
Delayed sleep phase, 107
Delusional disorder, 180
Demand-control model, 223–224
Dementia, 593–594
Dementia Rating Scale, 409

Demyelinization, 391
Depression, 668-669
  asthma, 41
  coronary heart disease, 210
  Crohn's disease, 84-86
  eating disorders, 176, 178, 180, 184, 188, 192
  esophageal motility disorders, 91
  headache, 7-8, 12, 15, 20
  insomnia, 104, 107
  irritable bowel syndrome, 81, 83
  multiple sclerosis, 413-414
  obesity, 163
  pain, 326, 328, 330, 332, 334, 336
  peptic ulcer disease, 88-89
  relapse prevention, 312
  smoking, 145
  spinal cord injury, 344-349, 351, 355
  temporomandibular disorder, 62-63, 66-70
Depression screening instruments, 406-407
Desipramine, 188, 191
Dexamethasone Suppression Test, 20
Dexfenfluramine, 138, 168
Diabetes mellitus, 8, 149, 157-158, 161-162, 221, 241, 513-529, 595
  animal models, 517-518
  chemical infusion, 518-519
  exercise interventions, 524
  home-monitoring studies, 521-522
  individual differences, 525-526
  laboratory stress induction, 519-520
  pharmacological interventions, 523
  physiological factors, 525
  relaxation interventions, 523-524
  social support, 526-527
  stress and, 514-516
  stress management interventions, 523-524
  stress-blood glucose relationship, 524-527
  stressful life events, 520-521
Diagnosis
  asthma, 31-32
  headache, 4-6
  multiple sclerosis, 391-393
  temporomandibular disorders, 57-58
Diagnostic and Statistical Manual of Mental Disorders, 82, 91, 159, 175-177, 180, 185, 191-192, 276, 365, 588, 608
Diathesis-stress model of chronic pain, 329-331
Diazepam, 23
Differentiation strategies, 652-654
Diffuse esophageal spasm, 90-91
Diffusion of innovation theory, 569
Digital blood flow, 117-119, 126
Digital vasoconstriction, 118-119
Digital vasospasms, 117
Discriminative stimuli, 47, 561
Disengagement theory, 585
Disseminated lupus erythematosus, 536
Diuretics, 160
Divergent reasoning, 439
Diversification, 649
Dual process models, 567
Dual Process Preparation Hypothesis, 294
Duodenal ulcers, 87-90
Duodenum, 87
Dysfunctional families, 42
Dyspepsia, 80
Dysphagia, 90, 92
Dyspnea, 32

Eating Attitudes Test (EAT), 183, 185
Eating Disorder Examination, 183-184
Eating Disorder Inventory (EDI), 183, 185
Eating Disorder Not Otherwise Specified, 176, 192
Eating disorders, 175-193; *see also* Obesity
  assessment of, 183-186
  biological theories, 180-182
  cognitive-behavioral theories, 178-179
  comorbidity, 175-177
  diagnosis, 175-177
  endorphin theories, 181-182
  etiology of, 177-182
  family studies, 182
  family theories, 178
  genetic theories, 182
  information-processing paradigm, 192-193
  metabolic theories, 182
  neuroendocrine theories, 181
  neurotransmitter theories, 181
  pharmacological therapy, 190-191
  prevalence of, 177
  psychodynamic theories, 177-178
  psychological therapy, 186-190
  self-report symptom inventories, 184-185
  structured interviews, 184
  treatment-outcome research, 186-191
  twin studies, 182
Eating habits, 162-163
Echolalia, 440
ELIZA, 617
Emotional factors
  asthma, 33, 39, 40-41
  insomnia, 101, 104-105, 107
  Raynaud's disease, 121
  temporomandibular disorders, 60, 62-63, 67
Emphysema, 33
End stage renal disease, 497-504, 508
Endorphin theories, 181-182
Energy expenditure, 158, 160
Energy intake, 158, 160-161
Environmental programming, 48
Environmental prompts, 265
Environmental Status Scale, 404

Epidemiological studies
   headache, 3, 7, 17
   systemic lupus erythematosus, 538-539
   temporomandibular disorders, 56-57
   traumatic brain injury, 431-432
Epinephrine, 119, 127, 129
Ergonomic job analysis, 367, 376-377, 381
Ergotamine, 18-19, 23
Esophageal manometric recordings, 90-91
Esophageal motility disorders, 90-92
Estrogen, 147, 159
Ethnic minorities, 137, 143, 149, 268-269, 670
Etiology, 675
   cardiovascular disorders, 239-246
   eating disorders, 177-182
   headache, 6
   multiple sclerosis, 396-397
   temporomandibular disorders, 58-62
Excessive medication use, 13, 15, 18-20, 24, 328
Executive functions and regulation of behavior, 439, 443-445
Exercise, 255-271, 665, 671, 673-674
   assessment of, 257-262
   asthma, 33, 38-40
   behavioral observation methods, 258
   cognitive distraction, 267
   contracting, 265, 267
   decision balance sheet, 265
   diabetes, 595
   elderly, 270
   environmental prompts, 265
   ethnic minorities, 268-269
   exercise testing, 266
   goal setting, 266, 267
   health, 255-257
   insomnia, 108
   interventions, 264-268
   lifestyle exercise, 266
   lottery, 265
   phone call prompts, 266
   physiological assessment methods, 258-259
   programmed exercise, 266
   psychological models of, 262-264
   relapse prevention in, 262-263, 267
   self-monitoring, 266
   self-report methods, 259-262
   special populations, 268-270
   staff feedback, 266
   stages of change, 263-264, 267
   stimulus control, 265
   transtheoretical model, 263-264
   women, 269-270
Expanded Disability Status Scale, 403-404
Eysenck Personality Inventory, 81, 84

Family Environment Scale, 445
Family, role of in traumatic brain injury, 441, 444-445, 448-450
Family studies, eating disorders, 182
Family theories, eating disorders, 178
Fargo Activity Times/Sampling Survey, 258
Fat distribution, 158
Fear-drive models, 567
Fenfluramine, 168
Finger Tapping Test, 443
Fluoxetine, 138, 168, 365
Focus strategies, 656-657
Follicular phase, 147
Free fatty acids, 244
Frontal lobes, 434-437
Frontalis EMG, 102, 124-125, 128
Functional capacity, 370-372, 381
Functional Systems Scale, 403-404

Gastric bypass, 166
Gastric ulcers, 87, 89
Gastrointestinal disorders, 8, 79-93
   Crohn's disease, 83-87
      definition and description, 83-84
      psychological factors, 84-86
      treatment, 86-87
   esophageal motility disorders, 90-92
      definition and description, 90-91
      psychological factors, 91
      treatment, 91-92
   irritable bowel syndrome, 80-83
      definition and description, 80
      psychological factors, 80-82
      treatment, 82-83
   peptic ulcer disease, 87-90
      definition and description, 87-88
      psychological factors, 88-89
      treatment, 89-90
Gate control theory of pain, 327
General Adaptation Syndrome, 276
Gerontology
   computers and, 619-621
   headaches, 17
Glasgow Coma Scale, 442
Gluteal-femoral obesity, 158
Gold Standard Patients, 49
Gold Standard Physicians, 49
Growth hormone deficiency, 159

Halstead Category Test, 444
Halstead-Reitan Neuropsychological Battery, 408-409, 443
Halstead-Reitan Neuropsychological Test Battery for Children, 36
Hamilton Depression Inventory, 162
Hamilton Depression Rating Scale, 414, 417
Hassles scale, 12, 280, 419
Head injury in the elderly, 595-596
Headache Classification Committee of the International Headache Society, 4, 18

Index

Headache, 3-25, 55, 61, 82, 106, 372
 aura, 4-7
 behavioral factors, 3-4
 biofeedback therapies, 3, 9-13, 15-24
  cephalic vasomotor, 10-11
  electromyograph, 10-13, 17, 23
  thermal, 10-12, 15-16
 central mechanisms, 6-7
 cerebral blood flow, 6-7
 cerebral neural function, 6
 classification, 4-6
 cognitive-behavior therapy, 11-12
 concurrent psychiatric disorder, 20-21
 continuous headaches, 19-20
 coping, 9
 diagnostic/classification, 4-6
 disability, 8, 12
 excessive medication use, 18-19
 expectancies, 8
 geriatric population, 17
 integrating drug and nondrug therapies, 21-24
 limited-contact treatment, 14-16
 maintenance of treatment gains, 13-14
 medication adherence, 23-24
 migraine, 12, 16-17, 21-23
 nonpharmacological treatment, 10-21
 pathophysiology, 6-7
 pediatric migraine, 16-17, 22-23
  limited contact treatment, 16
 postconcussion syndrome, 438
 psychological assessment, 7-9
 quality of life, 8
 relaxation, 10-24
 small-group treatment, 15
 special populations, 15-17
 stress, 9
 tension-type headache, 12, 17, 23
 treatment nonresponders, 17-21, 24
Headache index, 23
Health belief model, 557-559
Health promotion, 133-319
Health-care consumers, 644-647
Health-care coverage, 664-666
Health-care reform, 663, 674
Health Locus of Control Inventory, 564
Heart Smart Cardiovascular Health Promotion Program, 246
Hemodialysis, 497-508
 compliance issues, 503-508
  medical aspects, 498-501
  psychological aspects, 497-498, 501-503
Home-monitoring studies, 521-522
Horizontal integration, 657
Hormonal fluctuations, 8
Hostility, 199-200, 226, 229, 343, 346
 irritable bowel syndrome and, 81
 modification of, 208

Human immunodeficiency virus, 555-557, 560-561, 563, 565-566, 568, 570-576, 667, 670, 674
Hypercholesteremia, 149, 168, 241, 243,
Hyperinsulinism, 159
Hyperreactivity of the airways, 32, 34
Hypertension, 8, 82, 140, 157, 161, 219-233, 241
 defense-defeat model, 221-223
 demand-control model, 223-224
 effort-distress models, 223-224
 personality variables, 225-226
 psychological factors, individual differences in susceptibility to, 226-231
 psychological stress, environmental sources of, 220-225
 reactivity
  physiological and demographic factors affecting, 228-229
  prognostic significance of, 230-231
  psychological factors influencing differences in, 229
 reactivity hypothesis, 227-228
 socioecological stress, models of, 224-225
 stress, individual psychological factors and the perception of, 225-226
Hypertensive lower esophageal sphincter, 90
Hyperventilation, 41
Hypocapnea, 41
Hypochondriasis, 81, 88
Hypoganodism, 159
Hypothalamic syndromes, 159
Hypothyroidism, 159
Hypoxia, 60
Hysteria, 81-82

Idiopathic insomnia, 99
Illness behaviors, 82, 89
Imipramine, 188, 191
Immune complex, 537
Incapacity Status Scale, 403-404
Individual differences
 diabetes, 525-526
 headache treatment maintenance, 14
 hypertension, 226-231
 surgery preparation, 296-298
Inflammatory bowel disease, 81, 87
Information-processing paradigm, 192-193
Insomnia, 99-112, 160
 biofeedback, 110-111
 clinical management of, 106-112
 cognitive activation, 102-103
 cognitive restructuring, 111-112
 definition, 99-101
 emotional dysfunction, 104
 epidemiology, 99-101
 evaluation, 106-108

Insomnia (cont.)
  medical examination, 106–107
  personality dysfunction, 104
  physiological hyperarousal, 101–102
  relaxation training, 110–111
  sleep history, 107–108
  sleep logs, 108
  sleep restriction, 110
  stimulus control, 109–110
  theoretical formulations, 101–106
  treatment, 108–112
Insomnoids, 105
Integrated Care Plan, 665–666
Intelligence, 443
  asthma and, 35–36
Internal derangement, 55, 60, 66
Internal-External Control Scale, 417
Internal-External Locus-of-Control Scale, 419–420
Interocclusal appliances, 68–69
Interview for Diagnosis of Eating Disorders (IDED), 183–184
Inventory of Drinking Situations, 311
Irritable bowel syndrome, 80–83, 87, 91
Ischemia, 60
Isoproterenol, 118–119

Jenkins Activity Survey, 199, 202, 209
Job-task analysis, 376-377
John Henryism 224–225
Johns Hopkins Precursors Study, 231
Joy, relapse prevention, 316–317

Kaufman Assessment Battery for Children, 35–36
Ketanserin, 122

Laboratory stress induction, 519–520
Lactose malabsorption, 81
Language, 439–440, 444
Left ventricular hypertrophy, 227
Leukopenia, 489, 544
Lidocaine, 120
Life change units, 279–280
Life Events Inventory, 14
Life Experiences Survey, 280
Lifestyle exercise, 266
Lifestyle modification and balance, 315–317
Limited-contact treatment, 14–16, 24
Linkowski Acceptance of Disability Scale, 355
Lithium, 159, 446
Living with Asthma Questionnaire, 44
Locus of control, 8–9, 69
Low-share markets, 657
Lower body obesity, 158
Luria-Nebraska Neuropsychological Battery, 36
Luteal phase, 147

Magnetic resonance imaging
  assessment of elderly depressed persons, 590–591
  multiple sclerosis, 392, 394, 397, 401–402
  traumatic brain injury, 441–442
Maintenance, 483, 669–671
  headache, 13–14
  obesity, 168–169
Managed mental health care, 664–666
Mandible, 56–57
Mania, 413
Manifest Anxiety Scale, 84
Market definition, 648–649
Market development, 649
Market orientation, 641–642
Market penetration, 649
Marketing, 637–659
  broadened concepts of marketing, 639–640
  competitor analysis, 650–651
  consumer analysis, 649–650
  consumer orientation, 638
  cost-leadership strategies, 654–656
  differentiation strategies, 652–654
  focus strategies, 656–657
  government subsidy, 656
  health-care consumers, 644–647
  horizontal integration, 657
  implementation strategies, 652–657
  implementing the strategy, 657–658
  low-share markets, 657
  market definition, 648–649
  market development, 649
  market penetration, 649
  objectives, 651–652
  philosophies, 640–643
  product orientation, 640–642
  selling orientation, 641–642
  service development, 649
  situational analysis, 649–651
  social marketing, 639–640
  strategic marketing
    need for, 647–652
    process of, 647–649
Masseter muscle, 60–61
Masticatory muscles, 55, 57, 59–60, 67
Maximal permissible limit, 377
McGill–Melzack Pain Questionnaire, 376
McMaster Family Assessment Device, 445
Mecamylamine, 138
Media, and smoking, 136–138
Medical evaluation
  insomnia, 106–107
  obesity, 164
  traumatic brain injury, 441–442
Medical Outcomes Study, 8
Meditation, relapse prevention and, 313–314
Memory, 438–439
Menstrual cycle, 4, 147–149

Menstrual phase, 147
Mental status examination, 442-443
Metabolic rate, 158-159, 168
Metabolic theories, eating disorders, 182
Metastatic brain disease, 471
Metropolitan Life Insurance Company Height-Weight Tables, 157-158
Middlesex Elderly Assessment of Mental State, 409
Millon Behavioral Health Inventory, 91
Millon Health Locus of Control Scale, 349
Minimal Record of Disability, 404
Mini-Mental State Examination, 408-411
Minnesota Multiphasic Personality Inventory (MMPI), 668-669
   asthma, 35
   back pain, 366
   headache, 20
   hostility scale, 199, 201-202, 211
   insomnia, 104
   irritable bowel syndrome, 81
   multiple sclerosis, 404-406, 417, 421
   obesity, 159
   temporomandibular disorders, 63, 66
Modeling, 49
Mood disorders
   aging and, 588-592
   multiple sclerosis, 413-414
Motor functions, 438, 443
Multiaxial Assessment of Pain, 64-65
Multidimensional Personality Questionnaire, 343
Multifactorial model, 7
Multiple Risk Factor Intervention Trial (MRFIT), 199
Multiple sclerosis, 389-422
   acute-rapid progressive, 394
   assessment, 403-411
   benign relapsing-remitting, 393
   benign sensory, 393
   biofeedback, 420-421
   chemotherapeutic treatments, 412-414
   chronic-progressive disease course, 394
   chronic relapsing-progressive, 394
   cognitive-behavioral group therapy, 417
   cognitive disabilities, assessment of, 407-411
   cognitive screening
     brief, 408-409
     intermediate-length, 409-411
   comprehensive care model of treatment, 411-412
   depression, 413-414
   depression screening instruments, 406-407
   diagnosis, 391-393
   disease course, 393-394
   etiology, 396-397
   general symptoms, 412-413
   group psychotherapy, 416-418

Multiple sclerosis (cont.)
   incidence, 397-399
   individual psychotherapy, 418-420
   insight-oriented group therapy, 417-418
   mania, 413
   Minnesota Multiphasic Personality Inventory (MMPI), 405-406
   mood disorders, 413-414
   neurological processes, 390-391
   neuropsychological deficits, 399-403
   physical disabilities, 403-404
   physical symptoms, 396
   psychological disorders, 396-399, 405-407
   psychotherapy, 416-421
   relapsing-remitting disease course, 393-394
   sexual dysfunction, 396
     assessment of, 404-405
     treatment of, 414-416
   stress management group therapy, 418
   symptomatology, 394-403
   treatment, 411-421
Multiple Sleep Latency Test, 102
Muscle contraction model of tension headache, 4, 6
Muscle hyperarousal, 55, 59, 60, 67, 69-70
Muscle metabolism, 101
Myocardial infarction, 8, 207-208
Myofascial pain-dysfunction, 55, 66
Myofascial pain-dysfunction model, temporomandibular disorders, 59-62
   research on, 60-62
Myogenic models of temporomandibular disorders, 58-59

Nebulizer chronolog, 37
Negative emotional states
   obesity, 159
   relapse prevention, 311-312
   smoking, 147-149
Neurobehavioral Cognitive Status Examination, 409
Neurobehavioral Rating Scale, 443
Neuroendocrine response to stress, 244
Neuroendocrine theories, eating disorders, 181
Neurogenic vasoconstriction, 126
Neurological processes underlying MS, 390-391
Neuropsychological assessment, traumatic brain injury, 443-444
Neuropsychological deficits, multiple sclerosis, 399-403
Neuropsychological findings, aging, 591-592
Neuropsychological functioning, asthma, 36
Neuroticism, 81, 84
Neurotransmitter models
   chronic pain, 327-328
   eating disorders, 181

Index

Nicotine, 107, 146, 159
　gum, 139-140
　patches, 139-140
　replacement therapy, 138-141
　tolerance, 136
　withdrawal, 142
Nifedipine, 122, 128
Night eating syndrome, 160
Norepinephrine, 118-119, 126-127, 129
Normal sleep pattern, defined, 100
Nutcracker esophagus, 90-91
Nutritional evaluation, 165
Nutritional goals, 161-162

Obesity, 149, 157-169
　activity level evaluation, 164-165
　balanced-deficit diet, 166
　behavioral goals, 162-163
　behavioral programs, 165-166
　body image, 163
　caloric intervention, 166
　causes, 158-161
　　medical, 159
　comprehensive assessment, 163-165
　definition, 157-158
　eating habits, 162-163
　energy intake, 160-161
　genetic factors, 158
　goals of treatment, 161-162
　maintenance, 168-169
　medical evaluation, 164
　medical goals, 161
　nutritional evaluation, 165
　nutritional goals, 161-162
　patient-treatment matching, 165
　pharmacotherapy, 168
　physical activity, 160, 162
　physiological factors, 158-159
　psychological evaluation, 164
　psychological factors, 159-160
　psychological goals, 162-163
　psychological status, 163
　surgical interventions, 166
　treatment, 161-169
　treatment modalities, 165-168
　very-low-calorie diets, 166
　weight cycling, 168
Obsessive-compulsiveness, 63
Occlusal model; See Structural disharmony model
Occupational disability, determinants of, 363-367
Occupational musculoskeletal disability, 361-383
　autonomic data, 374-375
　back school, 381
　behavioral self-regulation training, 380-382
　biomechanical risk factors, 366-367

Occupational musculoskeletal disability (cont.)
　body mechanics coaching, 381
　controversies in occupational rehabilitation, 382-383
　demographics, 364-365
　determinants of, 363-367
　electromyographic data, 372-374
　evaluation components, 367-377
　functional capacity, 370-372
　job-task analysis, 376-377
　pain self-report, 376
　pain-related deconditioning, 363-364
　physical reconditioning, 378-379
　psychological distress, 365-366
　psychophysiological data, 372-376
　self-efficacy enhancement technologies, 381-382
　treatment components, 377-382
　work environment perceptions, 366
　work reconditioning, 379-380
Olfaction, in traumatic brain injury, 440
Oncology, psychosocial and behavioral, 481-403
　primary prevention, 482-485
　psychological factors affecting course of cancer, 491-492
　quality of life, 488-491
　symptom management, 485-488
Operant theory
　AIDS prevention, 561-562
　chronic pain, 328-329
Oral dysfunction, 58
Osteoarthritis, 57, 327
Ovaco Working Posture Analysis System, 377
Overeaters Anonymous, 165
Ovulation, 147

Paced Auditory Serial Addition Test, 410
Paffenbarger Activity Questionnaire, 268
Pain Disability Index, 376
Pain-related deconditioning, 363-364
Passive smoking, 135
Pathophysiology
　asthma, 33-35
　headache, 6-7
　psychosocial risk factors, 242-246
　Raynaud's disease and phenomenon, 119-122
　traumatic brain injury, 432-434
Patient education
　computers in, 623-624
　irritable bowel syndrome, 82
　temporomandibular disorders, 71
Patient-treatment matching, obesity, 165
Paykel Life Events Questionnaire, 86
Peak expiratory flow rates, 39-40
Peak flow meters, 37-38

Peak flow values; *See* Peak expiratory flow rates
Pediatric headache, 16-17, 22-23
 migraine, 22-23
Peptic ulcer disease, 87-90
Peptic ulcers, 82
Perceived Stress Scale, 281
Pericranial muscle activity, 6-7
Periodic limb movement disorder, 107
Peripheral neural mechanisms, chronic pain, 326-327
Personality
 asthma and, 35
 chronic pain and, 328
 hypertension and, 225-226, 229
 insomnia and, 101, 104-105
 obesity, 159
 temporomandibular disorders and, 63, 67
Personality Inventory for Children, 35
Pharmacological interventions
 diabetes, 523
 eating disorders, 190-191
 obesity, 168
 Raynaud's disease, 122-123
 smoking, 138-141
 traumatic brain injury, 445-446
Phenothiazines, 159
Phenylephrine, 118-119, 121
Phenylpropanolamine, 138
Physical activity, 160; *see also* Exercise
 health and, 255-257
 level of, 162
 in the United States today, 256-257
Physical Capacities Scale, 381
Physical reconditioning, 378-379
Physiological assessment methods, 258-259
Physiological control, finger blood flow, 117-119
Physiological factors
 diabetes, 525
 obesity, 158-159
Physiological hyperarousal, insomnia, 101-102
Piers-Harris Children's Self-Concept Scale, 35
Plethysmography, 120
Polycystic ovary syndrome, 159
Porteus Mazes, 36
Posttraumatic amnesia, 443
Posttraumatic epilepsy, 437-438, 446
Posttraumatic hydrocephalus, 438
Practice effects, smoking and, 136
Practice guidelines, 666
Preauricular area, 55
Precertification, 664
Precontemplation stage, 142, 483
Prednisone, 42
Pregnancy, 139-140, 144
Premack principle, 49

Premenstrual phase, 147-148
Preparation, 483
Prevailing state hypothesis, 227, 244
Prevalence
 alcohol and other drug use, spinal cord injury, 352-354
 anorexia and bulimia nervosa, 177
 binge eating, 168
 insomnia, 100
Primary appraisal, 284
Primary insomnia, 100, 102
Problem avoidance, 9
Problem solving, 313
Product orientation, 640-642
Profile of Mood States, 418
Progesterone, 147, 159
Programmed exercise, 266
Propanolol, 21-22, 119, 126, 446
Prostaglandin, 128
Protection-motivation theory, 567-569
Pseudodementia, 589-590
Pseudohypoparathyroidism, 159
Pseudotherapy, 10
Psychiatric disorders of the elderly, 588-594
Psychoeducational theories, AIDS prevention, 556-557
Psychological aspects
 headache, 9
 hemodialysis, 497-498, 501-503
 systemic lupus erythematosus, 539-541
 various disease states, 481-548
Psychological disorders, multiple sclerosis, 396-399, 405-407
Psychological factors
 cancer course, 491-492
 Crohn's disease, 84-86
 esophageal motility disorders, 91
 headache, 3-4
 irritable bowel syndrome, 80-82
 obesity, 159-160
 peptic ulcer disease, 88-89
 reactivity differences, 229
 temporomandibular disorders, 62-67, 71
Psychological models, physical activity and exercise participation, 262-264
Psychophysiological biases, 193
Psychophysiological data, occupational musculoskeletal disability, 372-376
Psychophysiological disorders, 3-131
Psychophysiological insomnia, 99
Psychophysiological model, temporomandibular disorders, 59-62, 66, 68
Psychophysiological reactivity, coronary-prone behavior, 200-202
Psychosocial risk factors, cardiovascular disease, 242
Psychosocial vulnerability, coronary-prone behavior, 202-203

Psychotherapy, 665-666
  Crohn's disease, 86
  headache, 21
  insomnia, 107-108
  irritable bowel syndrome, 84
  multiple sclerosis, 416-421
  temporomandibular disorders, 70
Pulmonary physiology, 39

Q-TWiST, 489-491
Quality of life
  asthma, 43-45
  end stage renal disease, 503
  gastrointestinal disorders, 93
  headache, 7-9
  oncology, 488-491
  spinal cord injury, 341-343
Quebec Task Force on Spinal Disorders, 367-369, 382

Ranitidine, 88
Rating of Perceived Exertion Scale, 377
Raven Progressive Matrices, 444
Raynaud's disease and phenomenon, 117-129, 537
  behavioral treatment, 125-128
  familial aggregation, 122, 128
  medical treatments, 122-123
  pathophysiology, 119-122
  physiological control of finger blood flow, 117-119
  secondary Raynaud's phenomenon, 128
Reactions to Impairment and Disability Inventory, 346
Reactivity hypothesis, hypertension, 227-228
Recovery of function, 445
Recurrent activation hypothesis, 227, 245-246
Recurrent Coronary Prevention Project, 207-208, 247
Recurrent Illness Impairment Profile, 8
Rehabilitation, 325-474, 675
  cancer, 470-474
  traumatic brain injury, 445-450
Reitan-Indiana Aphasia Screening Test, 444
Relapse assessment, 311-312
Relapse fantasies, 312
Relapse prevention, 307-319
  anger management, 313
  applications in behavioral medicine, 317
  approach, 307-308
  assertiveness training, 313
  asthma, 46, 49-50
  communication skills, 314
  conditioning factors, 308-309
  coping skills training, 312-313
  cultural issues, 317-319
  disability risk reduction, 382
  high-risk situations, 311

Relapse prevention (cont.)
  joy, 316-317
  lapses, 314-315
  lifestyle modification and balance, 315-317
  meditation, 313-314
  models of helping and coping, 309-310
  negative emotional states, 311-312
  problem solving, 313
  relapse assessment, 311-312
  relapse fantasies, 312
  relaxation, 313-314
  self-efficacy, 318-319
  self-monitoring, 311
  smoking, 141-142, 148-149
  social marginalization, 318-319
  social pressure, 312
  social skills, 314
  strategies, 312-315
  urges and cravings, 314
  use of, 310-311
Relaxation, 665
  asthma, 49
  cardiovascular disorders, 246
  diabetes, 523-524
  eating disorders, 189-190
  esophageal motility disorders, 91
  headache, 10-24
  insomnia, 102-103, 109-111
  irritable bowel syndrome, 82
  peptic ulcer disease, 89
  Raynaud's disease, 124-125, 129
  relapse prevention, 313-314, 316
  smoking, 141
  stress, 282-283
  surgery preparation, 293, 303
  temporomandibular disorders, 68-69, 71-72
  Type A behavior, 207-208, 213
Respiratory disorders, 32-33
Response theories, stress, 277-278
Resting metabolic rate, 158
Restless Legs Syndrome, 107
Revised Asthma Problem Checklist, 35
Riboflavin, 37
Risk-factor analysis, asthma, 38-40, 48
Risk-factor interactions, cardiovascular disorders, 240-242
Role Repertory Technique, 347
Rosenberg Self-Esteem Scale, 417

Schedule for Affective Disorders and Schizophrenia, 414
Schedule of Recent Events, 279
Scleroderma, 117, 120, 128
Second International Workshop on Drug-Related Headache, 18
Secondary appraisal, 284
Secondary brain damage, 433
Secondary gain, 62, 67

Secondary psychopathology, 440
Secondary Raynaud's phenomenon, 128
Selective Reminding Test, 410
Self-efficacy,
  asthma, 35, 46, 49
  enhancement technologies, 381-382
  relapse prevention, and 318-319
  theory, AIDS and, 562-563
Self-hypnosis, 22
Self-management
  AIDS, 565
  asthma, 9, 24
  headache, 38, 40, 45-50
  smoking, 148
Self-monitoring
  exercise, 266
  relapse prevention, 311
  smoking cessation, 141
  traumatic brain injury, 444
Self-report inventories
  eating disorders, 184-185
  traumatic brain injury, 444
Self-report methods, exercise, 259-262
Selling orientation, 641-642
Sensate focus, 415
Sequelae of traumatic brain injury, 437-441
Serotonin, 7, 168, 328, 332, 365
Serum lymphocytotoxic antibody, 543
Service development, 649
Sexual behavior, traumatic brain injury, 440
Sexual Disorder Not Otherwise Specified, 180
Sexual dysfunction, multiple sclerosis, 396
Shearing forces, 432-433
Short sleeper, 100
Shunts, 117-119
Situational analysis, marketing, 649-651
Situational Competency Test, 311
Situational Confidence Questionnaire, 311
Situational variables, surgery preparation, 298-299
Sleep apnea, 100, 106, 157, 161
Sleep efficiency, 110
Sleep history, 107-108
Sleep hygiene, 107
Sleep logs, 108
Sleep restriction therapy, 110
Sleep state misperception, 100
Smoking and smoking cessation, 135-150, 241, 243, 665, 671-674
  behavioral models, 136
  behavioral strategies, 141-143
  biological models, 136-137
  pharmacological approaches, 138-141
  practice effects, 136
  relapse, 136-137, 141-142, 145-148
  smoking cessation strategies, 138-150
  social models, 137-138
  theoretical models, 136

Smoking and smoking cessation (*cont.*)
  weight, 136, 139-140, 142, 145-146, 149
  women and, 143-150
Social-environmental theory, 585
Social influence theories, 569-571
Social learning theory, 9, 79, 562
Social marginalization, relapse prevention, 318-319
Social marketing, 569, 639-640
Social models, continued smoking, 137-138
Social pressure, relapse prevention, 312
Social support
  AIDS, 565
  diabetes, 526-527
  smoking, 141-142, 145, 147-149
  spinal cord injury, 350-351
Social Position Index, 355
Social Readjustment Rating Scale, 279
Social worth, 497
Socioecological stress, models of, 224-225
Somatognathic system, 59
Somatization, 63, 66, 81
Spatial Recall Test, 410
Spinal cord injury, 341-357, 463, 470
  adaptation, models of, 345-347
  adjustment, 350-351
  community reintegration, 341-343
  coping models, 347-350
  quality of life, 341-343
  social support, 350-351
  stress models, 347-350
  substance abuse, 351-355
    effects on rehabilitation process, 354-355
    prevalence of, 352-354
    treatment for, 354
  theoretical concepts, 343-345
Speading depression, 6
Splint therapy, 68, 70-71
Stage of Change model, 142
State-Trait Anxiety Inventory, 63, 406, 419-420
Steroid psychosis, 543
Steroids, 159
Stimulus control
  asthma, 46, 48
  eating disorders, 186
  exercise, 265
  headache, 109-110
  insomnia, 109-110
  smoking, 141-142
Stimulus theories, stress, 277
Strategic marketing process, 647-649
Stress and stress management, 275-286, 665, 671, 673-674
  behavior, 283-284
  biology, 282-283
  cardiovascular disorders, 243-248, 250-251

Stress and stress management (*cont.*)
  cognition, 284-285
  Crohn's disease, 84-87
  definition, 276-279
  diabetes, 514-516, 523-524
  eating disorders, 181
  esophageal motility disorders, 91
  exercise, 256
  headache, 8-9, 11-12, 14, 23
  history of, 275
  hypertension, 219-221, 223-230, 232
  insomnia, 101, 105, 110, 112
  interaction theories, 278-279
  irritable bowel syndrome, 80-82
  lipid function, 243-244
  measurement of, 279-281
  multiple sclerosis group therapy, 418
  pain, 325, 330-331, 333-336
  peptic ulcer disease, 88-90
  Raynaud's disease, 117, 122, 128
  relapse prevention, 308, 313, 316-317
  response theories, 277-278
  smoking, 141, 147-148
  spinal cord injury, 347-350, 353, 356
  stimulus theories, 277
  surgery preparation, 292-293, 295-296, 299-303, 347-350
  temporomandibular disorders, 59-62, 66-72
  Type A behavior, 200-204, 207, 209-210, 212
Stress Inoculation Training, 285, 419-420
Stress management, 281-285; see also Biofeedback; Relaxation
Stressful life events, diabetes, 520-521
Stroke, 135, 144, 162, 241, 463, 470-471, 674-675
Stroop Word Color Test, 444
Structural disharmony model, temporomandibular disorders, 59, 68, 70
Structured interviews, eating disorders, 184
Subcortical dementia, 590
Substance abuse and spinal cord injury, 351-355
Substance theories, 586
Suicide risk in the elderly, 589
Sunk cost effect, 47
Surgery, preparation for, 291-304
  individual differences, 296-298
  models of
    current, 292-296
    historical, 292
  situational variables, 298-299
  theoretical considerations, 292-296
  time, 299-300
  timing, 299-300
Surgical interventions, obesity, 166
Surgical sympathectomy, 122, 128

Sympathetic nervous system
  hypertension, 225
  Raynaud's disease, 118-119, 126-127, 129
  smoking, 136
  temporomandibular disorders, 60
Symptom Checklist 90 Revised, 63, 349, 668-669
Systemic lupus erythematosus, 535-548
  central nervous system SLE, 541-543
  history, 535-536
  psychological aspects, 539-541
  treatment and management, 543-547

Temperature biofeedback; *See* Thermal biofeedback
Temporomandibular disorders, 55-73, 139-140
  anatomy, 56
  assessment, 67
  biofeedback, 61, 68-72
  biomechanical model, 59
  diagnostic problems, 57-58
  emotional distress, 60, 62-63, 67
  epidemiology, 56-57
  etiological models, 58-62
  interocclusal appliances, 68-69
  mechanisms of change, 70-71
  myofascial pain-dysfunction model, 59-62
  nature of, 55-58
  physiology, 56
  predictors of outcome, 69
  psychological distress, association with subcategories of TMD, 66-67
  psychological factors, 62-67, 71
  psychometric problems, 58
  psychophysiological model, 59-62
  relaxation training, 68-69, 71-72
  structural disharmony model, 59
  subgroups, based on psychological factors, 63-65
  treatment, 71-72
  treatment efficacy, 68-71
  treatment nonresponders, 70, 72
Thermal biofeedback, 123-129
Thermal imagery, 123
Thermic effect of food, 158
Thermic effect of physical activity, 158
Theophylline, asthma, 41-43
Theoretical considerations
  chronic pain, 326-334
  learning theories, AIDS prevention, 561-566
  motivation and emotional arousal, AIDS prevention, 566-569
  primary insomnia, 101-106
  reasoned action, AIDS prevention, 559-560
  smoking, 136
  spinal cord injury adjustment, 343-345

Theoretical considerations (*cont.*)
  surgery preparation, 292–296
Third party payers, 637, 645–646, 665
Thrombocytopenia, 489, 544
Time Without Symptoms and Toxicity (TWiST), 488–491
Transactional model
  coronary-prone behavior, 203–205
  exercise, 263–264
  stress, 278
Transcortical motor aphasia, 440
Transient ischemic attacks, 240
Transtheoretical Stages of Change Model, 482–485
Traumatic brain injury, 431–451
  anatomy, 434–435
  anterior brain, susceptibility of, to traumatic damage, 433–434
  assessment, 441–445
  behavioral approaches, 447–448
  behavioral sequelae, 438–440
  cognitive rehabilitation, 446–447
  community reintegration, 450–451
  demographic characteristics, 431–432
  divergent reasoning, 439
  epidemiologic characteristics, 431–432
  executive functions and regulation of behavior, 439, 443–444
  expression of deficits, 437
  family and, 441, 444–445, 448–450
  frontal lobes, 434–437
  headaches, 438
  intelligence, 443
  interdisciplinary team approach, 445
  language, 439–440, 444
  medical sequelae, 437–438
  medical/neurological evaluation, 441–442
  memory, 438–439
  mental status examination, 442–443
  motor functions, 438, 443
  neuropsychological assessment, 443–444
  nonneurological sequelae, 438
  olfaction, 440
  pathophysiology, 432–434
  pharmacological interventions, 445–446
  postconcussion syndrome, 438
  posttraumatic epilepsy, 437–438
  posttraumatic hydrocephalus, 438
  recovery of function, 445
  rehabilitation, 445–450
  secondary brain damage, 433
  secondary psychopathology, 440
  self-monitoring, 444
  self-report inventories, 444
  sequelae of, 437–441
  sexual behavior, 440
  treatment, 445–451
  types of, 432–433

Treatment
  Crohn's disease, 86–87
  eating disorders, 165–168
  esophageal motility disorders, 91–92
  headache, 10–24
    integrating drug and nondrug therapies, 21–24
  irritable bowel syndrome, 82–83
  multiple sclerosis, 411–421
  obesity, 161–169
  occupational musculoskeletal disability, 377–382
  peptic ulcer disease, 89–90
  primary insomnia, 108–112
  sexual dysfunction, 414–416
  substance use problems, 354, 664
  systemic lupus erythematosus, 543–547
  temporomandibular disorders, 68–71
  traumatic brain injury, 445–451
Treatment nonresponders
  headache, 17–21, 24
  temporomandibular disorders, 70
Trigeminal neuralgia, 66
Type A pattern, broadly defined, 198–199
  cardiovascular disease, 242, 245, 247
  hypertension, 226, 229
  peptic ulcer disease, 88
Tyramine, 118–119

Ulcerative colitis, 87
Uplifts scale, 280
Upper body obesity, 158
Upper extremity cumulative trauma disorder, 361
Utilization review, 664–666

Vagal bronchoconstriction, 41
Vagal stimulation, 90
Vascular access cleaning, 507
Vascular model of migraine, 4, 6
Vasospastic attacks, 120–123, 127–129
Venous occlusion plethysmography, 121, 126
Vertical banded gastroplasty, 166
Very-low-calorie diets, 166

Ways of Coping Checklist, 348–349, 419–420
Wechsler Adult Intelligence Scale-Revised, 400, 443
Wechsler Intelligence Scale for Children-Revised, 36
Wechsler Memory Scale, 400
Weight cycling, 168, 670
West Haven Yale Multidimensional Pain Inventory (MPI), 64, 73
Western Collaborative Group Study, 199–200, 226
Wide Range Achievement Test-Revised, 36

Wisconsin Card Sorting Test, 443-444
Women, 670
    exercise, 269-270
    headache, 13
    insomnia, 101
    smoking, 137, 143-150
    temporomandibular disorders, 57

Woodcock-Johnson Psycho-Educational Battery, 36
Work environment perceptions, 366
Work reconditioning, 379-380
Workers' Compensation, 362, 365, 382

Zung Self-Rating Depression Scale, 398

ISBN 0-306-44970-6